THE
ADULT SPINE

PRINCIPLES and PRACTICE

Volume 2

THE
ADULT SPINE
PRINCIPLES and PRACTICE

Volume 2

EDITOR-IN-CHIEF

John W. Frymoyer, M.D.
Professor of Orthopaedics
Director, McClure Musculoskeletal Research Center
Department of Orthopaedics and Rehabilitation
University of Vermont
Burlington, Vermont

ASSOCIATE EDITORS

Thomas B. Ducker, M.D.
Clinical Professor, Division of Neurosurgery
University of Maryland
Associate Professor, Department of Neurosurgery
The Johns Hopkins University
School of Medicine
Baltimore, Maryland

Nortin M. Hadler, M.D.
Professor of Medicine and
Microbiology/Immunology
School of Medicine
University of North Carolina
at Chapel Hill
Chapel Hill, North Carolina

John P. Kostuik, M.D.
Professor of Orthopaedic Surgery
University of Toronto
Director, Spinal Surgery
Director, Biomechanics Laboratory
The Toronto Hospital
Toronto, Ontario

James N. Weinstein, D.O.
Associate Professor
Department of Orthopaedic Surgery
Director
Spine Diagnostic and Treatment Center
University of Iowa Hospital
Iowa City, Iowa

Thomas S. Whitecloud III, M.D.
Professor and Acting Chairman
Department of Orthopaedic Surgery
Tulane University School of Medicine
New Orleans, Louisiana

Raven Press **New York**

Raven Press, 1185 Avenue of the Americas, New York, New York 10036

Made in the United States of America

Library of Congress Cataloging-in-Publication Data

The Adult spine: principles and practice/editor-in-chief, John W. Frymoyer; associate editors, Thomas B. Ducker . . . [et al.].
    p. cm.
  Includes bibliographical references.
  Includes indexes.
  ISBN 0-88167-689-6 (set)
  1. Spine—Abnormalities. 2. Spine—Wounds and injuries. 3. Spine—Diseases—Treatment. 4. Spine—Surgery. I. Frymoyer, John W. II. Ducker, Thomas B., 1937–
  [DNLM: 1. Spinal Diseases. 2. Spine. WE 725 A244]
RD768.A32 1991
617.5′6—dc20
DNLM/DLC
for Library of Congress   90-9101
                                            CIP

9 8 7 6 5 4 3 2 1

The major chapters in the history of spinal disorders are brief. In fact, most of the major insights have come within the past sixty years. All of the editors can identify within two generations our links with the historical personages in spinal disorders. Each of us has been influenced by the next generation of "pioneers," those who took the early principles established by such innovators as Mixter and Barr and combined them with new clinical and scientific insights, which have been so influential on the approach to spinal disorders taken today.

These individuals have served as our teachers and to them we dedicate this book: *F. P. Dewar, Harry Farfan, John Hall, Ian Macnab, Edgar Kahn, Ludwig Kempe, William Kirkaldy-Willis, Stephen Krane, Henry Metzger, Alf Nachemson, Richard Schneider, Edward Simmons, Henk Verbiest, Patrick Wall,* and *Leon L. Wiltse.*

The Editor-in-Chief also dedicates this volume to *William Luginbuhl, M.D.,* who, as Dean of the University of Vermont College of Medicine for twenty years, has provided consistent commitment to an environment of scholarly excellence and unstinting support to the Department of Orthopaedics and Rehabilitation and to spinal research.

Contents

VOLUME 1

Part III: Generalized Disorders of the Spine

Subject index follows page 904

Volume 2

Part IV: Cervical Spine

Traumatic Disorders of the Cervical Spine

Degenerative Conditions of the Spine

Subject index follows page 2178

Contributors

David B. Allan, M.B., Ch.B., F.R.C.S.
Senior Orthopaedic Registrar
The West of Scotland Back Pain Research
  Unit
Orthopaedic Department
Western Infirmary
Glasgow, G11 6NT Scotland

Gunnar B. J. Andersson, M.D., Ph.D.
Professor and Associate Chairman
Department of Orthopedic Surgery
Rush-Presbyterian-St. Luke's Medical
  Center
1653 West Congress Parkway, 1471 Jelke
Chicago, Illinois 60612

Charles Neuville Aprill, III, M.D.
Spine Radiologist
Diagnostic Conservative Management, Inc.
3715 Prytania Street, Suite 101
New Orleans, Louisiana 70115

M. C. Battié, Ph.D.
Research Associate
Department of Orthopaedics
University of Washington School of Medicine
Seattle, Washington 98195

Ulrich Batzdorf, M.D.
Professor of Surgery/Neurosurgery
University of California, Los Angeles
School of Medicine
10833 Le Conte Avenue
Los Angeles, California 90024

Jean C. Beckham, Ph.D.
Duke University Medical Center
Pain Management Program
Box 3159
Durham, North Carolina 27710

Daniel R. Benson, M.D.
Professor of Orthopaedic Surgery
Chief of Spine Service
Department of Surgery
University of California, Davis
2230 Stockton Boulevard
Sacramento, California 95817

Thomas N. Bernard, Jr., M.D.
Clinical Assistant Professor
Department of Orthopaedics
Tulane University School of Medicine
New Orleans, Louisiana
Hughston Orthopaedic Clinic
P.O. Box 9517
Columbus, Georgia 31995

S. J. Bigos, M.D.
Associate Professor
Department of Orthopaedics
Director, Spine Resource Clinic
University of Washington School of Medicine
Seattle, Washington 98195

Henry H. Bohlman, M.D., F.A.C.S.
Professor
Department of Orthopaedics
Case Western Reserve University
School of Medicine
Cleveland, Ohio
Chief, Acute Spinal Cord Injury Service
Veterans Administration Medical Center
Cleveland, Ohio
Chief, Reconstructive and Traumatic Spine
  Surgery Center
University Hospitals of Cleveland
2074 Abington Road
Cleveland, Ohio 44106

Michael J. Bolesta, M.D.
Assistant Professor
Department of Orthopaedics
Case Western Reserve University
School of Medicine
Cleveland, Ohio 44106

D. J. Botsford, M.D.
Faculty of Medicine
University of Toronto
One King's College Circle
Toronto, Ontario
Canada M5S 1A8

Richard H. Brown, Ph.D.
Director, Surgical Research Division
Research Director, Spine Center
11311 Shaker Boulevard
Saint Luke's Hospital
Cleveland, Ohio 44104

J. David Cassidy, D.C., M.Sc. (Orth.),
  F.C.C.S.(C)
Research Associate
Department of Pathology and Orthopaedics
University Hospital Saskatoon
Saskatoon, Saskatchewan
Canada S7N 0W0

John R. Cassidy, M.D.
Neurological Associates
1888 Hillview Street
Sarasota, Florida 34239

William L. Cats-Baril, Ph.D.
Associate Professor of Information and
  Decision
School of Business and
Rehabilitation Engineering Center
University of Vermont
Burlington, Vermont 05405

Charles R. Clark, M.D.
Professor of Orthopaedic Surgery
Director, Orthopaedic Spine Fellowship
University of Iowa College of Medicine
Iowa City, Iowa 52242

Andrew H. Cragg, M.D.
Assistant Professor
Department of Radiology
University of Iowa Hospital
Iowa City, Iowa 52242

Gregory R. Criscuolo, M.D.
Assistant Professor of Neurosurgery,
  Pediatrics, and Oncology
Division of Neurological Surgery
Yale University School of Medicine
333 Cedar Street
New Haven, Connecticut 06510; and
Instructor in Neurosurgery
Department of Neurological Surgery
The Johns Hopkins University
School of Medicine and
The Johns Hopkins Hospital
600 North Wolfe Street
Baltimore, Maryland 21205

Henry V. Crock, A.O., M.D., M.S.,
  F.R.C.S., F.R.A.C.S
Consultant Spinal Surgeon
Senior Lecturer/Honorary Consultant
Royal Postgraduate Medical School
Cromwell Hospital
Cromwell Office Road
London, SW5 0TU England

Rick B. Delamarter, M.D.
Assistant Professor
Division of Orthopaedic Surgery
UCLA School of Medicine
Chief, Orthopaedic Surgery
West Los Angeles Veterans Administration
  Medical Center
1000 Veteran Avenue, Room 22-70
Los Angeles, California 90024

Richard A. Deyo, M.D., M.P.H.
Associate Professor
Departments of Medicine and Health
  Services
University of Washington; and
Director, Northwest Health Services
  Research and Development Field Program
Seattle Veterans Administration Medical
  Center
1660 South Columbian Way
Seattle, Washington 98108

Ronald G. Donelson, M.D.
Assistant Professor
Department of Orthopedic Surgery
State University of New York
Health Science Center
Syracuse, New York 13202
Medical Director,
Acute Spinal Pain Program
St. Camillus Hospital and Rehabilitation
* Center*
Syracuse, New York
Orthopaedic Consultant
The McKenzie Institute
550 Harrison Street
Syracuse, New York 13202

Thomas B. Ducker, M.D.
Clinical Professor
Division of Neurosurgery
University of Maryland
Baltimore, Maryland
Associate Professor
Department of Neurosurgery
The Johns Hopkins University
School of Medicine
600 North Wolfe Street
Baltimore, Maryland 21205

Anne-Christine Duhaime, M.D.
Associate Neurosurgeon
Children's Hospital of Philadelphia
Assistant Professor
Department of Neurosurgery
University of Pennsylvania School of
* Medicine*
34th and Civic Center Boulevard
Philadelphia, Pennsylvania 19104

Stephen I. Esses, M.D., M.Sc., F.R.C.S.
Assistant Professor
Department of Surgery
University of Toronto
Consultant, Dewar Spine Unit
The Toronto Hospital
200 Elizabeth Street
Toronto, Ontario
Canada M5G 2C4

Roger B. Fillingim, Ph.D.
Duke University Medical Center
Pain Management Program
Box 3159
Durham, North Carolina 27710

Ernest M. Found, Jr., M.D.
Assistant Professor
Department of Orthopaedics
Assistant Director
Spine Diagnostic and Treatment Center
University of Iowa Hospitals and Clinics
Iowa City, Iowa 52242

Bruce Fredricksen, M.D.
Associate Professor
Department of Orthopaedic Surgery
State University of New York
Health Sciences Center at Syracuse
Syracuse, New York 13202

Gary E. Friedlaender, M.D.
Professor and Chairman
Department of Orthopaedics and
* Rehabilitation*
Yale University School of Medicine
333 Cedar Street
New Haven, Connecticut 06510

John W. Frymoyer, M.D.
Professor of Orthopaedics
Director, McClure Musculoskeletal Research
* Center*
Department of Orthopaedics and
* Rehabilitation*
University of Vermont
Burlington, Vermont 05405

Francis W. Gamache, Jr., M.D.
Associate Professor of Neurosurgery
Department of Surgery
The New York Hospital-Cornell Medical
* Center*
525 East 68 Street
New York, New York 10021

Kevin Gill, M.D.
Clinical Associate Professor of Orthopaedic
* Surgery*
University of Texas Southwestern Medical
* Center*
5920 Forest Park Road, Suite 400
Dallas, Texas 75235

Russell H. Glantz, M.D.
Associate Professor of Neurology
Department of Neurological Sciences
Rush Medical College
Rush-Presbyterian-St. Luke's Medical
*   Center*
1725 West Harrison Street
Professional Building, Suite 1140
Chicago, Illinois 60612

Vijay K. Goel, Ph.D.
Professor
Department of Biomedical Engineering
University of Iowa
Iowa City, Iowa 52242

Leon J. Grobler, M.D.
Assistant Professor
Department of Orthopaedics
University of Vermont
Staff Orthopaedic Surgeon
Orthopaedics and Spinal Service
Medical Center Hospital of Vermont
Burlington, Vermont 05405;
Director of Surgical Services
Spine Institute of New England
2 Hurricane Lane
Williston, Vermont 05495

Nortin M. Hadler, M.D., F.A.C.P.
Professor of Medicine and Microbiology/
*   Immunology*
University of North Carolina at Chapel Hill
School of Medicine
932 Faculty Laboratory Office Building
*   231H*
Chapel Hill, North Carolina 27599

Scott Haldeman, D.C., M.D., Ph.D.
Assistant Clinical Professor
Department of Neurology
University of California, Irvine
Irvine, California;
1125 East 17 Street, W-127
Santa Ana, California 92701

Nachman Halpern, M.A.
Hospital for Joint Diseases
Orthopaedic Institute
Bernard Aronson Plaza
301 East 17 Street
New York, New York 10003

Edward N. Hanley, Jr., M.D.
Chairman
Department of Orthopaedic Surgery
Carolinas Medical Center
1000 Blythe Boulevard
Charlotte, North Carolina 28232

Rowland G. Hazard, M.D.
Assistant Professor of Medicine and of
*   Orthopaedics and Rehabilitation*
University of Vermont; and
New England Back Center
2 Hurricane Lane
Williston, Vermont 05495

Kenneth B. Heithoff, M.D.
Medical Director
Center for Diagnostic Imaging
5775 Wayzata Boulevard, Suite 190
St. Louis Park, Minnesota, 55416

John G. Heller, M.D.
Assistant Professor
Department of Orthopaedic Surgery
Emory University School of Medicine
1365 Clifton Road, N.E.
Atlanta, Georgia 30322

Robert J. Henderson, M.D.
Dallas Spine Group
6161 Harry Hines Boulevard
Dallas, Texas 74235

Richard J. Herzog, M.D.
Medical Director
San Francisco Neuro Skeletal Imaging
1850 Sullivan Avenue, Suite 100
Daly City, California 94015; and
San Francisco Spine Institute
1850 Sullivan Avenue, Suite 140
Daly City, California 94015

Serena S. Hu, M.D.
Assistant Professor
Department of Orthopaedic Surgery
University of Minnesota Hospital
420 Delaware Street S.E.
Minneapolis, Minnesota 55455

Robert J. Huler, M.D.
Toronto General Hospital
200 Elizabeth Street
Toronto, Ontario
Canada M5G 2C4

Michael Huo, M.D.
Assistant Professor
Department of Orthopaedic Surgery
Georgetown University
Washington, D.C. 20007

Roger P. Jackson, M.D.
Clinical Assistant Professor
University of Kansas School of Medicine; and
Co-Director
Kansas University Medical Center
Rae R. Jacobs' Memorial Spine Fellowship
  Program at Kansas City
2750 Hospital Drive, 600
North Kansas City, Missouri 64116

William J. Kane, M.D., Ph.D.
Professor
Department of Orthopedic Surgery
Northwestern University Medical School
Hennepin County Medical Center
701 Park Avenue South
Minneapolis, Minnesota 55415

Constantine P. Karakousis, M.D.
Associate Chief, Surgical Oncology
Chief, Soft Tissue Melanoma Service
Roswell Park Memorial Institute
Clinical Professor
State University of New York at Buffalo
666 Elm Street
Buffalo, New York 14263

Jeffrey N. Katz, M.D., M.S.
Instructor in Medicine
Harvard Medical School
Department of Rheumatology/Immunology
Brigham and Women's Hospital
75 Francis Street, Tower 16B
Boston, Massachusetts 02115

Francis J. Keefe, Ph.D.
Associate Professor
Department of Psychology
Duke University Medical Center
Pain Management Program
Box 3159
Durham, North Carolina 27710

Lee A. Kelley, M.D.
Department of Orthopaedic Surgery
Tulane University School of Medicine
1430 Tulane Avenue
New Orleans, Louisiana 70112

John P. Kostuik, M.D., F.R.C.S.(C)
Professor of Orthopaedics
University of Toronto
Toronto, Ontario; and
  Director, Spinal Surgery; and
Director, Biomechanics Laboratory
The Toronto Hospital
200 Elizabeth Street
Toronto, Ontario
Canada M5G 2C4

Martin H. Krag, M.D.
Associate Professor
McClure Center for Musculoskeletal
  Research
Vermont Rehabilitation Engineering Center
Department of Orthopaedics and
  Rehabilitation
University of Vermont
Burlington, Vermont 05405

Thomas K. Kristiansen, M.D.
Associate Professor
Department of Orthopaedics and
  Rehabilitation
Director, Residency Program
McClure Musculoskeletal Research Center
University of Vermont
College of Medicine
Burlington, Vermont 05405

Noshia A. Langrana, Ph.D.
Professor
Mechanical Engineering
Rutgers University
Piscataway, New Jersey 08903

Henry La Rocca, M.D.
Clinical Professor of Orthopaedic Surgery
Tulane University School of Medicine
1201 South Clearview Parkway, Suite 140
New Orleans, Louisiana 70121

Casey K. Lee, M.D.
Professor
Orthopaedic Surgery
UMD-New Jersey Medical School
Newark, New Jersey 07103

Matthew H. Liang, M.D., M.P.H.
Associate Professor of Medicine
Harvard Medical School
Department of Rheumatology/Immunology;
* and Director*
Robert B. Brigham Multipurpose Arthritis
* Center*
Brigham and Women's Hospital
75 Francis Street, Tower 16B
Boston, Massachusetts 02115

John D. Loeser, M.D.
Director, Multidisciplinary Pain Center
University of Washington
Chief, Division of Neurosurgery
Children's Hospital and Medical Center
Seattle, Washington 98195

Donlin M. Long, M.D., Ph.D.
Director and Chairman
Neurosurgeon in Chief
Department of Neurological Surgery
The Johns Hopkins Hospital
600 North Wolfe Street
Baltimore, Maryland 21205

Paul C. McAfee, M.D.
Associate Professor
Departments of Orthopaedic Surgery and
* Neurosurgery*
The Johns Hopkins Hospital
Baltimore, Maryland 21205
Chief of Spinal Surgery
St. Josephs Hospital Spinal Center
Towson, Maryland
Orthopaedic Associates, P.A.
1217 St. Paul Street
Baltimore, Maryland 21202

John A. McCulloch, M.D.
Professor of Orthopaedics
Northeastern Ohio Universities
College of Medicine
Rootstown, Ohio 44304; and
75 Arch Street
Suite 501
Akron, Ohio 44304

Robin McKenzie, F.N.Z.S.P., Dip. M.T.
McKenzie Institute International
P.O. Box 93
Waikanae, New Zealand

Arnold H. Menezes, M.D.
Professor
Division of Neurosurgery
University of Iowa Hospitals
Iowa City, Iowa 52242

Eugene R. Mindell, M.D.
Professor
Department of Orthopaedic Surgery
Director, Orthopaedic Oncology Division
State University of New York at Buffalo
School of Medicine and Biomedical Sciences
100 High Street
Buffalo, New York 14203

Vert Mooney, M.D.
Professor of Orthopaedic Surgery
University of California, Irvine
Medical Director, Physical Assessment and
* Reactivation Center*
Irvine, California 92714
Irvine Medical Center
101 City Drive South
Orange, California 92668

Roland W. Moskowitz, M.D.
Professor of Medicine
Case Western Reserve University
School of Medicine
Director
Division of Rheumatic Diseases
University Hospitals
Cleveland, Ohio 44106

Alf Nachemson, M.D., Ph.D.
Professor and Chairman
Department of Orthopaedics
Gothenburg University
Gothenburg, Sweden

Clyde L. Nash, Jr., M.D.
Clinical Professor of Orthopaedics
Case Western Reserve
School of Medicine; and
Director, Department of Orthopaedics
Medical Director, Spine Center
Saint Luke's Hospital
11311 Shaker Boulevard
Cleveland, Ohio 44104

Mary Newton, B.A., M.Ed., M.C.S.P.
Research Physiotherapist
The West of Scotland Back Pain Research
* Unit*
Orthopaedic Department
Western Infirmary
Glasgow, G11 6NT Scotland

Eugene J. Nordby, M.D.
Associate Clinical Professor
Department of Orthopaedics
University of Wisconsin Medical School
6234 South Highlands Avenue
Madison, Wisconsin 53705

Margareta Nordin, R.P.T., Dr.Sci.
Director, Occupational and Industrial
  Orthopaedic Center
Hospital for Joint Diseases
Orthopaedic Institute
Bernard Aronson Plaza
301 East 17 Street
New York, New York 10003

J. Desmond O'Duffy, M.B.
Staff Consultant
Division of Rheumatology
Mayo Clinic
Professor of Medicine
Mayo Medical School
220 First Street, S.W.
Rochester, Minnesota 55905

T. Okuma, M.D.
Orthopaedic Surgeon
184 4-12-3 Kajino-Cho
Koganel-Shi
Tokyo, Japan

David Johnston Openshaw, M.D., B.S.,
  F.C.A., F.R.C.P.(C.)
Assistant Professor
Department of Anaesthesia
University of Toronto
The Toronto Hospital
200 Elizabeth Street
Toronto, Ontario
Canada M5G 2C4

John R. Parsons, Ph.D.
Associate Professor
Orthopaedic Surgery
UMD-New Jersey Medical School
Newark, New Jersey 07103

Eric D. Phillips, M.D.
Medical Director
Kansas City Spine Center
Baptist Medical Center
6601 Rockhill Road
Kansas City, Missouri 64131

Reed B. Phillipps, D.C., D.A.C.B.R.,
  M.C.S.M., Ph.D.
Research Director
Los Angeles College of Chiropractic
16200 East Amber Valley Drive
Whittier, California 90609

Malcolm H. Pope, Dr.Med.Sc., Ph.D.
Professor
McClure Center for Musculoskeletal
  Research
Vermont Rehabilitation Engineering Center
Department of Orthopaedics and
  Rehabilitation
University of Vermont
Given Building
Burlington, Vermont 05405

Wolfgang Rauschning, M.D., Ph.D.
Department of Orthopaedic Surgery
Uppsala University Academic Hospital
Uppsala, Sweden S-75185; and
Swedish Medical Research Council

Marilyn G. Rothwell, R.N.C.
Clinical Instructor in Medicine
Given Health Care Center;
University of Vermont
Burlington, Vermont 05405

John Schlegel, M.D.
Assistant Professor
Department of Orthopaedics
University of Texas Southwestern Medical
  Center
Dallas, Texas 74235

Luis Schut, M.D.
Professor
Departments of Neurosurgery and Pediatrics
University of Pennsylvania School of
  Medicine
Chief, Neurosurgery
Children's Hospital of Philadelphia
34th and Civic Center Boulevard
Philadelphia, Pennsylvania 19104

David K. Selby, M.D.
Clinical Professor
Department of Orthopaedic Surgery
University of Texas Southwestern Medical
  Center
Dallas Spine Group
6161 Harry Hines Boulevard
Dallas, Texas 74235

Henry H. Sherk, M.D.
Professor and Chief
Department of Orthopaedics and
*   Rehabilitation*
Medical College of Pennsylvania
3300 Henry Avenue
Philadelphia, Pennsylvania 19129

James W. Simmons, M.D.
Alamo Bone and Joint Clinic
4330 Medical Drive, Suite 200
San Antonio, Texas 78229

John W. Skubic, M.D.
Assistant Professor
Department of Orthopaedics
Loma Linda University Medical Center
Loma Linda, California 92350

Tony P. Smith, M.D.
Assistant Professor of Radiology
Department of Radiology
University of Iowa Hospital
Iowa City, Iowa 52242

Dan M. Spengler, M.D.
Professor and Chairman
Department of Orthopaedics and
*   Rehabilitation*
Vanderbilt University Medical Center
5400 Stanford Drive
Nashville, Tennessee 37232

E. Shannon Stauffer, M.D., F.R.C.S.
Professor and Chairman
Division of Orthopaedics and Rehabilitation
Southern Illinois University
School of Medicine
P.O. Box 19230
Springfield, Illinois 62708

Leslie N. Sutton, M.D.
Associate Neurosurgeon
Children's Hospital of Philadelphia
Associate Professor
Departments of Neurosurgery and Pediatrics
University of Pennsylvania School of
*   Medicine*
34th and Civic Center Boulevard
Philadelphia, Pennsylvania 19104

Henry M. Tufo, M.D.
President
Given Health Care Center;
Professor of Medicine
University of Vermont
Burlington, Vermont 05405

Gurvinder S. Uppal, M.D.
Department of Orthopaedic Surgery
Medical College of Pennsylvania
3300 Henry Avenue
Philadelphia, Pennsylvania 19129

Kent A. Vincent, M.D.
Assistant Professor
Division of Orthopedics and Rehabilitation
Oregon Health Sciences University and
*   Shriners Hospital for Crippled Children*
3181 S.W. Sam Jackson Park Road
Portland, Oregon 97201

Gordon Waddell, B.Sc., M.D., F.R.C.S.
Consultant Orthopaedic Surgeon
Director, The West of Scotland Back Pain
*   Research Unit*
Western Infirmary
Glasgow, G11 6NT Scotland

Robert L. Waters, M.D.
Clinical Professor
Department of Orthopaedic Surgery
University of Southern California
Los Angeles, California
Medical Director
Rancho Los Amigos Medical Center
7601 Imperial Highway
Harriman Building, Room 117
Downey, California 90241

James N. Weinstein, D.O.
Associate Professor
Department of Orthopaedics
Director, Spine Diagnostic and Treatment
*   Center*
University of Iowa Hospitals and Clinics
Iowa City, Iowa 52242

Sherri Weiser, Ph.D.
Hospital for Joint Diseases
Orthopaedic Institute
Bernard Aronson Plaza
301 East 17 Street
New York, New York 10003

Thomas S. Whitecloud III, M.D.
Professor and Acting Chairman
Department of Orthopaedic Surgery
Tulane University School of Medicine
New Orleans, Louisiana 70112

David G. Wilder, Ph.D., P.E.
Research Assistant Professor
McClure Center for Musculoskeletal
*   Research*
Vermont Rehabilitation Engineering Center
Department of Orthopaedics and
*   Rehabilitation*
University of Vermont
Burlington, Vermont 05405

Harold A. Wilkinson, M.D., Ph.D.
Professor and Chairman
Division of Neurosurgery
University of Massachusetts Medical School
55 Lake Avenue North
Worcester, Massachusetts 01655

Leon L. Wiltse, M.D.
Clinical Professor
Department of Orthopaedic Surgery
University of California, Irvine
Irvine, California
Long Beach Memorial Hospital
Long Beach, California
Wiltse Spine Institute
2888 Long Beach Boulevard
Suite 400
Long Beach, California 90806

Philip L. Witt, Ph.D., P.T.
Division of Physical Therapy
University of North Carolina at Chapel Hill
Medical School Wing E 222H
Chapel Hill, North Carolina 27599-7135

Hansen A. Yuan, M.D.
Professor and Chairman
Department of Orthopaedic Surgery
State University of New York
Health Sciences Center at Syracuse
Syracuse, New York 13202

Thomas A. Zdeblick, M.D.
Assistant Professor
Division of Orthopaedic Surgery
University of Wisconsin Hospital
600 Highland Avenue
Madison, Wisconsin 53792

Mark C. Zimmerman, M.D.
Assistant Professor
Orthopaedic Surgery
UMD-New Jersey Medical School
Newark, New Jersey 07103

Preface

Two decades ago a small handful of books and no journals were available to physicians and surgeons who daily encountered spinal disorders. Today, multiple journals and texts are devoted to this topic; yet a comprehensive text has been unavailable to bring together the epidemiology and socioeconomic consequences of spinal disease, its causation and diagnosis, its prevention, and the myriad of non-operative and operative approaches that are used with varying degrees of success.

The editors and publisher of *The Adult Spine* identified this important need two years ago. Our overall goal was simple: create a book that would serve as *the* reference text for every physician treating adult spine disorders. Our approach was somewhat more complex: Identify all of the important topics in spinal disorders from the foramen magnum to the coccyx, and get the recognized authorities to produce chapters that give the reader the most up-to-date information on those topics. Write chapters that can stand alone so that the reader can find the needed information, illustrated with original drawings and radiographs, and supported by a complete bibliography. At the same time, our editorial group was charged with the important task of making the individual chapters form a comprehensive whole.

The task has been complex. The effort has been monumental to produce a two-volume text comprising 104 chapters, over 400 original illustrations and 2,000 images, and a bibliography of nearly 9,000 references. To complete such a project in two years and thus keep the text at the "cutting edge" has required remarkable devotion from the editors, publisher, illustrators, and librarians.

All of us associated with this project are proud of the final product. We hope you, who read this text, will find it contains all of the important, timely information you need to understand and treat your patients with spinal disorders. If you and they benefit, then our efforts will have been well worth it.

John W. Frymoyer
Thomas B. Ducker
Nortin M. Hadler
John P. Kostuik
James N. Weinstein
Thomas S. Whitecloud III

Acknowledgments

The editors and publisher of *The Adult Spine* committed themselves early in the development of this project to a publication that was to be comprehensive and to contain the latest information in the rapidly evolving field of spinal disorders. From the time the editorial group was assembled to final production took two years. To accomplish a task of this magnitude in this time required unusual commitment and dedication from many people: the authors, who withstood our constant exhortations to timeliness and completeness; Kathey Alexander and her assistant Sandra Casperson; Cynthia Fairbanks, Linda Lotz, and Elinor Lindheimer of the Faye Zucker Editorial Group; the production staff at Raven Press, who remained stalwart in their commitment to complete the many publishing tasks; Donna Cavi who completed numerous illustrations and yet maintained a high standard of quality; and the staff of the Dana Medical Library at the University of Vermont, who rigorously checked the many references that will make this book particularly valuable to its readers.

Undoubtedly, each author has unsung heroes who deserve individual recognition but can here be thanked only collectively. The editorial group has the luxury of acknowledging the assistance of those who worked many hours in reading, editing, typing, and retyping manuscripts, including Barbara Burns, Beverly McGuire, Elizabeth Montgomery, Jill Hallam, Margie Loomer, Peggy Stover, Judy Clay, Anna Marie Hamori, and Jackie Durfee. A particularly important and key role was played by Ruth Jewett, who functioned with incredible diligence, commitment, and good humor. Without her multiple talents, the task would not have been completed.

The other unsung heroes are, of course, the wives of the editors, who withstood and survived their husbands' involvement in this project.

We hope you will find the efforts of all of us have resulted in a source of important, timely information, which will provide a basis for the rational diagnosis and treatment of your patients. If this occurs and your patients benefit, then our efforts will indeed have been worthwhile.

John W. Frymoyer
Thomas B. Ducker
Nortin M. Hadler
John P. Kostuik
James N. Weinstein
Thomas S. Whitecloud III

THE
ADULT SPINE
PRINCIPLES and PRACTICE

Volume 2

PART IV

Cervical Spine

The Adult Spine: Principles and Practice,
J. W. Frymoyer, Editor-in-Chief.
Raven Press, Ltd., New York © 1991.

CHAPTER 44

Anatomy and Pathology of the Cervical Spine

Wolfgang Rauschning

Increasingly detailed studies of the anatomy of the spine have been necessitated both by the development of new surgical techniques and improved instrumentations, as well as by the advent of the computerized imaging techniques, especially computed tomography (CT) and magnetic resonance (MR) tomography (2,3,4,11,13,14,15, 16,17,18).

The classical descriptive gross anatomy, systematized into categories such as osteology, myology, syndesmology, angiology, and so forth is necessary for the elementary understanding of structures, their function, and of basic designative terms. For the clinician, diagnostician, and surgeon alike, topographic relational and clinical anatomy are of greater value. Topographic relationships in two dimensions, such as displayed in computerized tomograms, are extremely difficult to interpret and comprehend in their three-dimensional context.

These recent developments have prompted surgeons and radiologists (and a few anatomists) to study various aspects of clinical and imaging anatomy (2,7,11,13, 14,15,16,17,18). New techniques, such as plastination, casting, cryodissection, and injection moulding, have been developed. The images in the current chapter have

been created with the Uppsala Cryoplaning Technique, which allows detailed assessment of bone and soft tissue relationships in frozen and undecalcified specimens (14).

In this chapter the running text briefly alludes to some clinically significant anatomical features of the cervical spine. The normal and imaging correlation anatomy has been described elsewhere and in greater detail (15). Anatomy can neither be taught ex cathedra nor be verbalized in writing; it can only be seen and explored hands-on. This chapter contains only a small selection from a database of more than 30,000 images from more than 100 cervical spinal cadaveric studies. Along with illustrations of some normal anatomical relationships, examples of clinically relevant pathological anatomy are presented.

Figures 1–3 are from the upper cervical spine and craniocervical junction. The unique atlanto-axial motion segment was formed by the assimilation of the bodies of C1 and C2. In these two segments roughly half of the rotatory movement of the entire cervical spine occurs (8). The atlanto-axial articulation (similar to the shoulder joint) lacks bony congruity and stability. Only ligaments and joint capsules resist excessive motion. A true synovial joint is located between the lateral masses of the atlas and axis and between the anterior arch of the atlas and the odontoid process (6). Another synovial joint is found between the transverse ligament (strictly

W. Rauschning, M.D., Ph.D.: Department of Orthopaedic Surgery, Uppsala University Academic Hospital, Uppsala, Sweden; Swedish Medical Research Council.

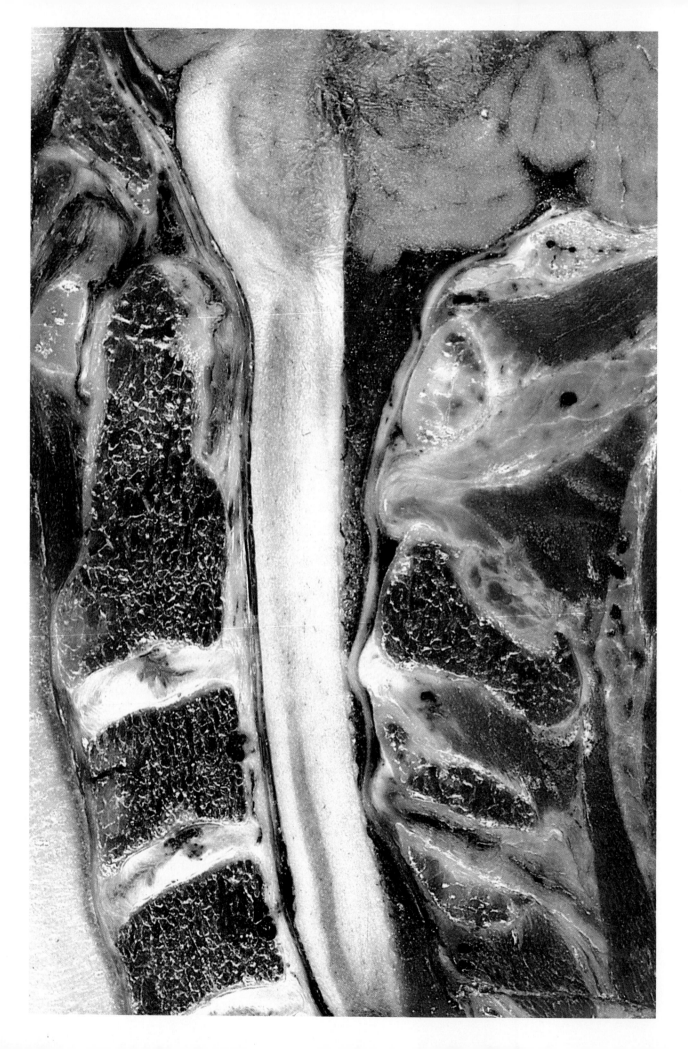

speaking: the transverse portion of the cruciate ligament) and the dens (Figs. 1 and 3). Far thicker than the transverse ligament and probably more important are the alar ligaments (Fig. 2). In addition, the tectorial membrane anchors the odontoid process directly to the skull base (foramen magnum).

The tip of the odontoid process abuts the lower pons and the medulla oblongata (Fig. 1). Posteriorly, the wide cisterna magna provides spatial reserve for a translatory posterior movement of the dens. The posterior soft tissue elements of the cervical spine are comparatively thin and resilient. These include the interlaminar ligamentum flavum, sparse strands of interspinous process ligament, and the flaccid joint capsules.

The spinous processes of the cervical spine are short and carry bifid tips. Contrary to textbook descriptions there is no supraspinous ligament. A complex suspensory system comprises a mid-sagittal septum of fibrous strands extending posteriorly in the midline and attaching to the strong elastic yellow ligamentum nuchae which is continuous with the superficial layers of the thoracic aponeurosis and stretches from the spinous process of C7 to the occipital tubercle. In the neutral position, the ligamentum flavum bulges slightly anteriorly. This bulge is more pronounced in extension and disappears in flexion.

The anterior wall of the cervical vertebral canal is perfectly straight in normal specimens (Fig. 1). In extension, this wall displays no bulge from the discs but a segmental "shingling," which is caused by the retrolisthesis of the upper vertebra in relation to the lower vertebra. This retrolisthesis is caused by the obliquity of the facet joints (Figs. 4 and 5) which induces this translatory movement through coupled motion.

The cervical intervertebral discs allow this sagittal translation whereas the uncinate processes effectively resist lateral movement which could have deleterious effect on the vertebral artery (2,6,7,9). The artery is tightly held in the costotransverse foramina of C3 to C6 and then runs through a knee-shaped, bony tunnel in the lateral mass of the axis and finally curves around the lateral aspect of the atlanto-axial joint (10). Instability at this level and/or osteoarthrotic lipping of the joint surfaces may erode the vertebral artery or cause arterial thrombosis (Figs. 6 and 7).

Figure 5 also displays meniscoid synovial folds in the facet joints of the mid-cervical spine. Little is known about their function and their potential role in post-traumatic, degenerative, and inflammatory neck pain (6,12,15). The author has observed significant post-traumatic changes, such as fresh ruptures, entrapment, and late fibrosis in these meniscoids (16,18).

In the cervical spine below C2, the segmental nerves have to transgress a distance of about 2 cm from the piercing of the thecal sac to the tubercles of the transverse process. Whereas the lumbar nerves invariably curve around the inner, inferior border of the pedicle of the upper vertebra of the motion segment, the cervical nerves run over the upper border of the pedicles and slope laterally and antero-inferiorly along the upper surface of the composite transverse process which is formed by the transverse process proper posteriorly and the anterior assimilated rib equivalent (*Anlage* in German). Both bony processes are connected by the distally convex intertransverse bar which forms the lateral border of the costotransverse foramen. The cervical spinal nerves exit their root canals through a musculotendinous slit between the scalenus muscles/tendons which insert into the tubercles of the transverse process and the rib anlage process (4,9,12,15).

Figure 4 also shows the topographic relationships in a C5-C6 motion segment of a spine which had been frozen in situ in moderate flexion. The epidural veins of the cervical spine are not a rete or convolute of veins but a system of wide communicating sinusoids which can fill and empty rapidly. This hydraulic system facilitates the swift and considerable volume variations of the osseoligamentous conduits which occur during the movements of the highly mobile cervical spine (15).

Extension decreases the sagittal diameter of the cervical vertebral canal. Retrolisthesis of the upper vertebra of the motion segment pushes its lower endplate towards the spinal cord which is bound anterolaterally by the roots which in turn are attached to the walls of the root canals. This does not occur in the more rigid thoracic spine (Fig. 8).

Extension allows the ligamentum flavum to retract and thicken by volume redistribution and relaxation of its pretension. This thickening occurs underneath the lamina. This dynamic effect of extension is even more accentuated in the root canals because the posterior movement of the lower endplate of the suprajacent vertebra compresses the neural bundle against the anterior surface of the superior articular process.

The "root" is a complex structure composed of structurally and neurophysiologically high dissimilar elements: the root sleeve, housing intrathecal motor and sensory roots, the highly vascularized and pressure-sensitive dorsal root ganglion which at this level is still separate from the motor root, and finally the postganglionic composite spinal nerve. Pressure exerted on the "root" may trigger different neurodysfunctional phenomena, depending on which of the components of the root is compromised. Even though the term "root" is short, concise, and established, its complex composition of structural and neurophysiologically dissimilar elements may be better designated by terms such as "root complex" or "root bundle."

In its long course through the root canal, the root sleeve, ganglion, and nerve cannot yield superiorly because the root lies in a deep oblique furrow at the anterior aspect of the superior articular process (Fig. 5). In degenerative conditions such as spondylosis and unco-vertebral arthrosis, the uncinate process becomes sclerotic and hypertrophic (Fig. 7) and sometimes curves posteriorly. This immobilizes and encases the root bundle from anteriorly and superiorly. Compromise of the vertebral canal size and compression of the spinal cord have been observed when the lower endplate carries spondylotic spurs and ridges, especially when the spine is extended and when ossification of the posterior longitudinal ligament is present (7,8,9,10,12,15,16) (Figs. 9 and 10).

Numerous fractures and traumatic soft tissue injuries of the cervical spine have been studied in great detail (1,5). A few pathomorphological features in fracture dislocations of the elderly are shown in Figure 11. The clinical, diagnostic, and pathoanatomical data of the case presented in Figure 12 have been previously reported in detail (17). A traumatic disc herniation is shown in Figure 13. Our recent investigations include systematic assessment of cervical spinal injuries associated with skull fractures and detailed examinations of fractures and metastases of the cervical spine in which surgical decompression and/or stabilization had been conducted (11,12,13,16,18).

Only the diligent examination of spines of deceased patients in which surgery had been performed can render the immediate and vital feedback to the clinician which is necessary for both improvement of surgical techniques and the improvements of accuracy and specificity of the expensive computerized imaging modalities.

Acknowledgments and references follow on page 928.

→

FIG. 1 (opposite page). Mid-sagittal section through the upper cervical spine of a 34-year-old male. The odontoid process (1) is the most prominent structure. Only that and the posterior arch (2) are seen. The true synovial joint between the anterior arch (3) of the atlas and the dens is degenerated in this specimen. Arrows indicate the transverse portion of the cruciate ligament which holds the odontoid process posteriorly. The "transverse ligament" is covered by the tectorial membrane which constitutes a reinforcement of a parietal blade of the dura mater and which is continuous with the dura mater of the skull (pachymeninx). In addition, the thin apical ligament of the dens directly anchors the tip of the dens to the clivus portion (4) of the foramen magnum.

Posteriorly, the thin atlanto-occipital membrane connects the posterior arch of the atlas (5) with the rim of the foramen magnum. In the angle between the pons (6), the medulla oblongata (7), the cerebellar tonsils the posterior wall of the vertebral canal the cisterna magna is located (8).

Figures 2, 3, and 4 follow on pages 913–915.

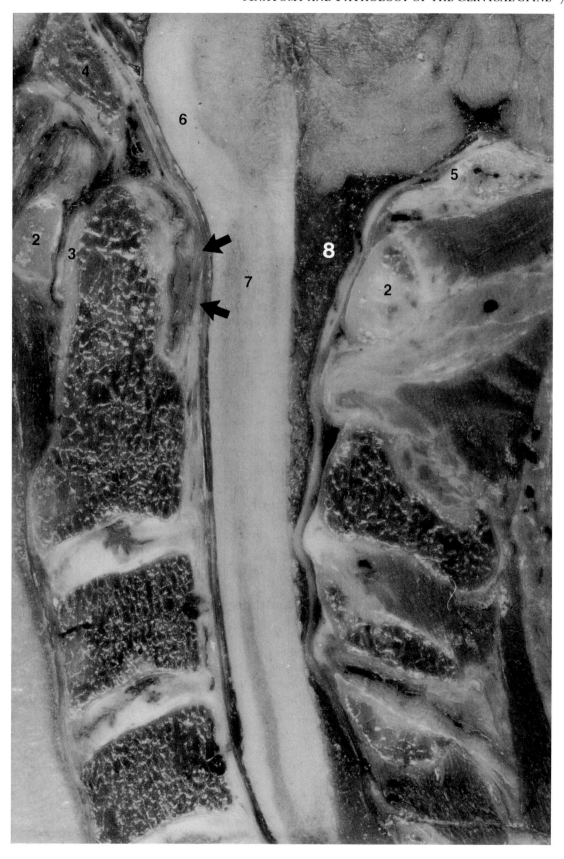

FIG. 2 (opposite page). Axial section through the superior portion of the atlas at the level of the tip of the odontoid process (1) lateral of which the strong alar ligaments (2) insert into notches at the anterior-inferior aspect of the occipital condyles (3). Richly vascularized areolar fat tissue (4) occupies the angles between the dens and the anterior arch of the atlas (5). Laterally the vertebral arteries (6) present as they curve posteriorly immediately after having left the transverse foramina of the atlas. A few millimeters cranial to this section the vertebral arteries (7) have pierced the atlanto-occipital membrane into the vertebral canal and are also traversing the thecal sac to become the intrathecal constituents of the basilar artery which forms by merging of these arteries anterior to the medulla oblongata in the midline. Posterior to the round lower medulla oblongata (8) the CSF compartment of the cisterna magna expands (9). Small intrathecal rootlets are located lateral to the medulla, thicker posterior root filaments are separated from thinner anterior root filaments by the suspensory dentate ligament. Anterior to the atlas lies the longus colli muscle. At their lateral aspect lie the internal carotid arteries (10) posterior to which the vagus nerve and the sympathetic trunk are located.

FIG. 3 (overleaf). Axial section of the atlas at the level of the lateral masses and the posterior arch and immediately inferior to the anterior arch. The mid-portion of the odontoid process displays articular cartilage anteriorly and also posteriorly where it articulates with the transverse ligament. Lateral to the dens loose areolar tissue with a rich supply of blood vessels and lymphatics is located (1). The lateral masses (2) are composed of strong cancellous bone whereas the arches contain more cortical bone. The vertebral arteries (3) are about to enter the transverse foramina of the atlas. They are surrounded by a rete of veins which is continuous with the venous sinusoids which surround the nerve roots in the root canals (periradicular venous plexus) and with the wide sinusoids which surround the thecal sac (epidural veins, internal vertebral venous plexus). These venous compartments display black on cadaveric sections because they are filled with cruor mortis. Note that these epidural veins constitute wide vascular compartments with relatively few septa rather than a serpiginous rete of veins. The thecal sac is oval and renders ample space for the spinal cord which clearly displays the anterior median fissure and the posterior median sulcus. A great number of rootlet filaments emerging from the anterolateral and posterolateral sulcus stepwise merge intrathecally to larger dorsal and ventral roots. The butterfly configuration of the gray matter is clearly outlined.

FIG. 4 (overleaf). Axial section through the C5-C6 motion segment of a normal cervical spine which was positioned and frozen in situ in moderate flexion. The osseous elements are the lower endplate of C5 (1) which on the right also displays the uncovertebral cleft (arrows), the inferior articular processes of C5 (2), and the upper articular processes of C6 (3). The oblique orientation of the articular facets of the cervical spine (see Fig. 5) causes a translatory anterior movement of C5 in relation to C6, considerably widening the sagittal diameter of the vertebral canal as well as the long osseoligamentous intervertebral conduits which commonly are referred to as neuroforamina but which rather constitute radicular or root canals of more than 2 cm length from the offset of the root sleeve from the dura to the tubercles of the transverse process. The thecal sac, the root sleeves, and the vertebral arteries are surrounded by one large continuous venous compartment which is subdivided only by a few thin membranes and septa.

The thecal sac is almost round, posteriorly bordered by (but not attached to) the arcade of the interlaminar ligamentum flavum. Anteriorly the dura is firmly affixed to the posterior longitudinal ligament which "fans out" as it approaches the endplates and the disc, firmly attaching the dura anteriorly at each motion segment. The flexion causes the spinal cord to move anteriorly in the thecal sac. Tension variations of the roots in various postures and the denticulate ligament control the movements of the spinal cord. Note the anterior and posterior spinal arteries and veins on the surface of the spinal cord and a free artery in the subarachnoid space (arrow).

Figures 5, 6, and 7 follow on pages 917–919.

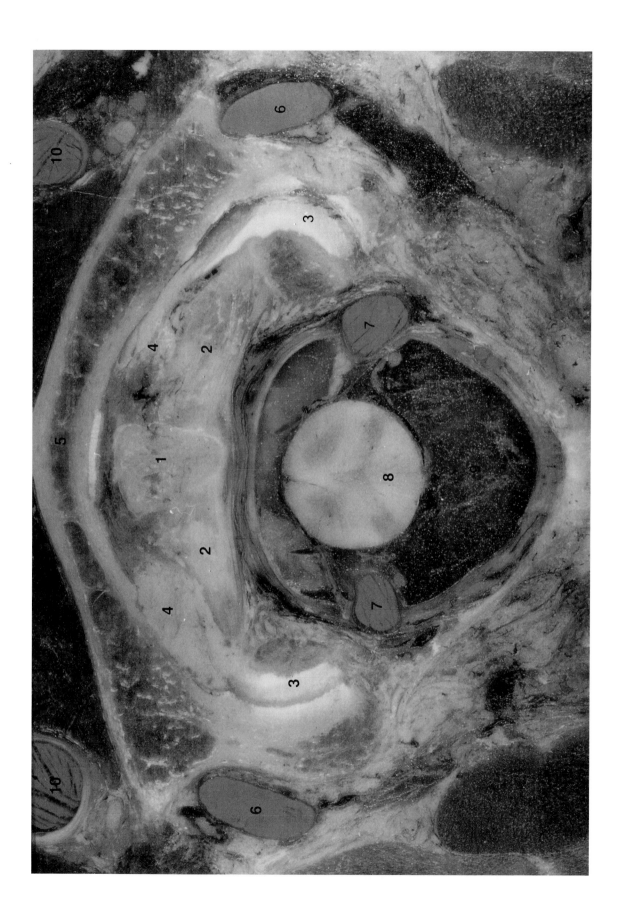

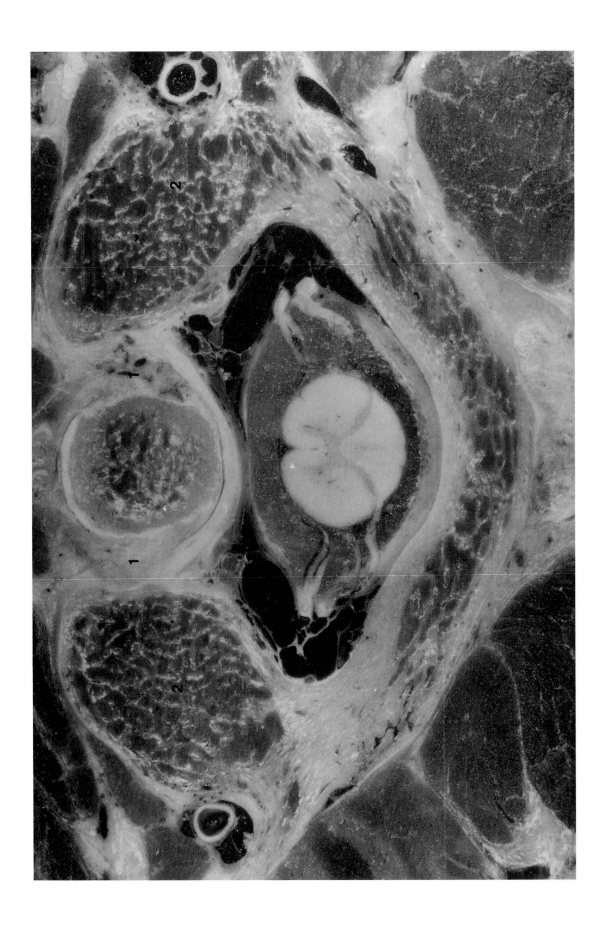

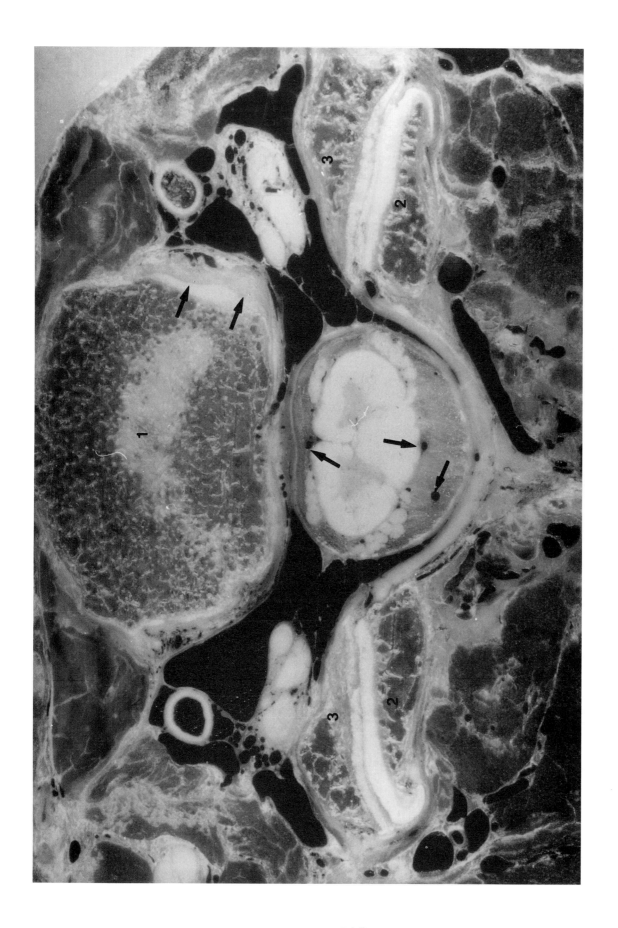

FIG. 5 (opposite page). Sagittal section through the lateral portion of the articular pillar of a normal mid-cervical spine. The articular masses are roughly rhomboid and carry obliquely sloping articular facets dorso-superiorly and ventro-inferiorly into which circumferential meniscoid synovial folds (tags) project (arrows). Anterior to the upper articular process deep notches accommodate the root sleeve, ganglion portion of the root, and the postganglionic cervical spinal nerve. This section also displays the vertebral artery (here black) running through the transverse foramina of the vertebrae. Anteriorly the artery is bounded by the thin bony shell of the rib anlage portion of the composite transverse process (see text).

FIG. 6 (overleaf). Coronal section through a severely degenerated lower cervical spine of a 70-year-old female who had neck pain but no history of radiculopathy or vertebral artery insufficiency. The spondylosis (degeneration between the vertebral bodies, i.e., the "disc joint") encompasses severe degeneration of the intervertebral discs and endplate sclerosis especially in the uncovertebral pseudojoints at which reactive degenerative bone apposition entails ridging which segmentally displaces the vertebral arteries laterally, causing them to take an undulating serpiginous course. On both sides the segmental nerves emerge behind the vertebral artery (see Fig. 5).

FIG. 7 (overleaf). Close-up view of a severely degenerated upper cervical spinal motion segment in axial section displaying advanced uncovertebral spondylosis and slight facet joint arthrosis. The uncinate process (1) has a sagittal orientation and is sclerotic and thickened, projecting laterally towards the vertebral artery (see also Fig. 6) and posteriorly into the root canal (foramen). Medially in the canal the motor root and the radicular arteries are compressed (arrows). The cylindrical and darker dorsal root ganglion (2) is buttressed against the superior articular process and its notch (see Fig. 6). Note the location of the vertebral artery (3) immediately anterior to the ganglion. The epidural and periradicular veins are small in this specimen. The orientation of the uncinate process and its relationships to the radicular structures and its contribution to neurovascular compromise is essential for the surgical strategy in decompressive procedures such as uncoforaminotomy. Most degenerated specimens displayed significant "anterior" encroachment emanating from the uncovertebral region. Facet joint osteophytes were usually small and rarely projected into the root canals.

Figures 8–12 follow on pages 921–925.

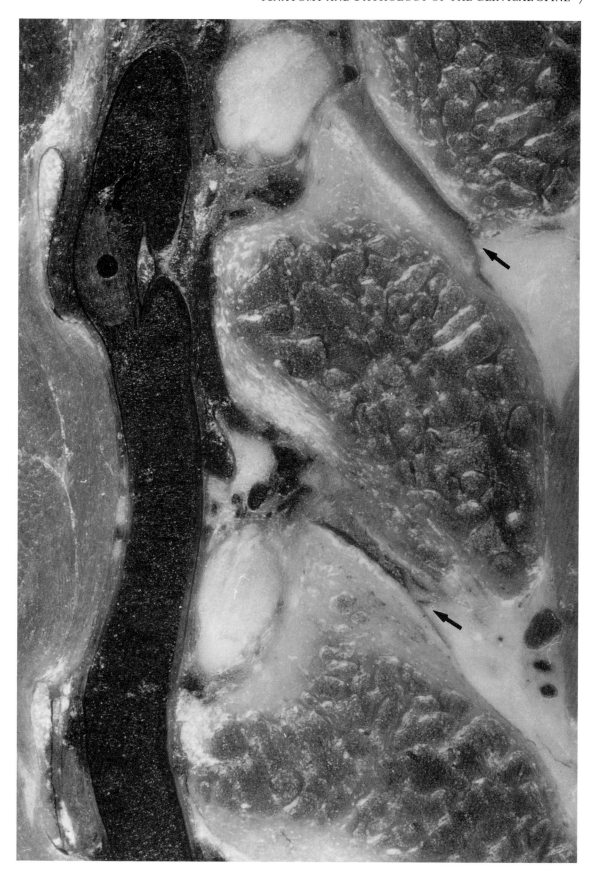

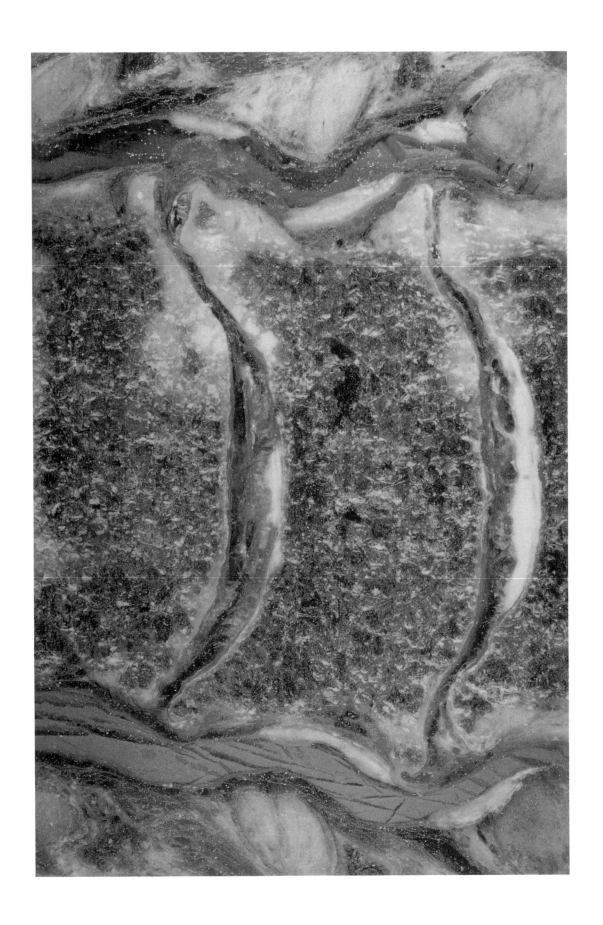

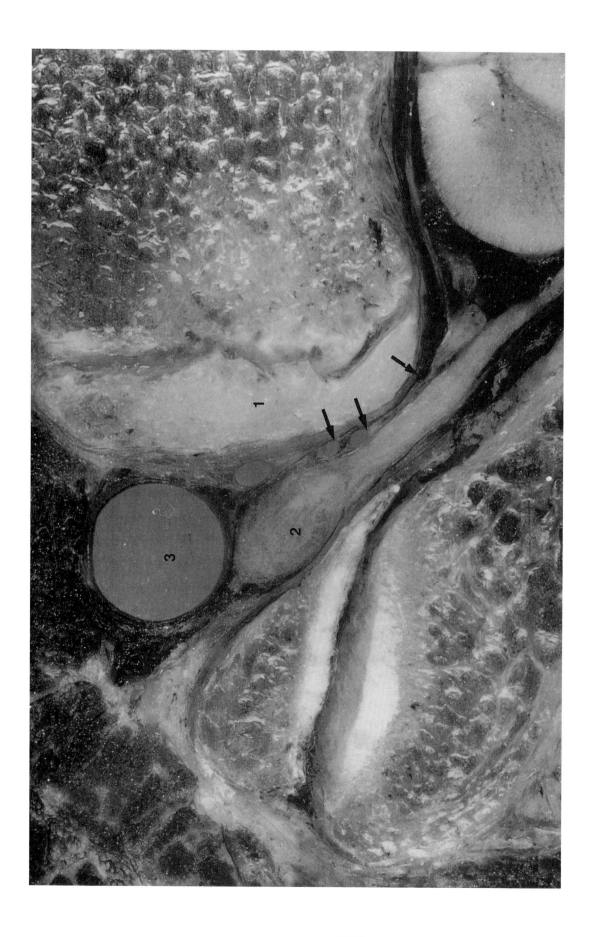

919

FIG. 8 (opposite page). Mid-sagittal section through the midthoracic spine of a 64-year-old female cadaver. The spine portion had been frozen in situ during routine autopsy in the supine position. The veins posterior to the spine are engorged as a result of rigor mortis; yet the spinal cord closely follows the vertebral bodies. All discs show degenerative changes, the disc between T9 and T10 is completely resorbed, and the cartilaginous endplates have fused. In the most spondylotic segments the anterior longitudinal ligament is thicker than in the less degenerated segments. Normally, thoracic discs have a perfectly straight posterior margin, even in extension they do not bulge into the vertebral canal. Of particular surgical interest is the relationship of the laminae to the intervening ligamentum flavum. The long slender spinous processes as well as the flat wide laminae overlap like obliquely sloping shingles, completely hiding the ligamentum flavum. The latter attaches to the adjacent laminae in a consistent fashion: It inserts into the anteriorly and slightly inferiorly directed surface of the suprajacent lamina and into the upper rim (margin) of the infrajacent lamina. Viewed from the spinal canal (anteriorly) only a narrow band of bone is visible; the posterior wall of the spinal canal thus is predominantly elastic-ligamentous, yet shielded by the "hidden" lamina portion. Note that the veins behind the dura (belonging to the posterior internal venous plexus) are invariably located at the level of the bony lamina, not the ligamentum flavum.

FIG. 9 (overleaf). Sagittal close-up view of two severely degenerated cervical spinal segments (C4-C5 and C5-C6) from a middle-aged woman who had suffered a significant "whiplash" injury 12 years before she died. All other discs had a normal appearance. At C4-C5, the disc is completely resorbed and the endplates are sclerotic. The disc space is occupied by gelatinous slightly hemorrhagic tissue. Posteriorly, endplate ridges project into the spinal canal. At the C5-C6 level, the anterior portion of the disc is reasonably intact whereas the central and posterior portions are liquified. In the upper endplate of C6 two large Schmorl's nodes communicate through defects of the bony endplate with the disc space. Note also the anterior endplate flanges which render the normally trapezoid sagittal cross-section of the cervical spinal vertebra an hourglass-shape. This close-up section shows the arrangement of the cancellous bony trabeculae and the dark gray bone marrow compartments.

FIG. 10 (overleaf). Mid-sagittal section through the "sub-axial" cervical spine (from C3 to T1) of an elderly deceased who had a history of occasional neck pain but no neurological symptoms. At C5-C6, and even more pronounced at C6-C7, there are severe spondylotic changes. Anteriorly, the circumferential flanges present as a "spur" on this sectional image. At C5-C6 these flanges are ridging anteriorly and have almost fused by ossification of the anterior annulus fibrosus. The dark texture in most vertebral bodies represents cancellous bone with normal hematopoetic bone marrow. This contrasts to the lighter portions posteriorly in the bodies of C6 and C7 which represent eburnation (sclerosis) of the cancellous bone. The posterior ridging of the endplates renders a waist shape to the vertebrae and also entails a thickening of the anterior wall of the dura mater in the degenerated segments. Note that the dura in normal segments (e.g., C7-T1) is barely discernible. Since the height of the discs in this specimen is reasonably preserved, there is no infolding of the ligamentum flavum. The segmental narrowing caused by this multilevel spondylosis is an almost exclusively anterior phenomenon where "beaks" formed by the sclerotic endplate flanges and the intervening hard remnant of the posterior annulus segmentally indent the dura. Motion between these "beaks" and the thecal sac probably accounts for the reactive thickening of the dura. This thickening is a common observation during surgery in spondylotic spines.

FIG. 11 (overleaf). A 63-year-old male was rendered tetraplegic after a traffic accident. He was operated on a C5-C6 fracture dislocation with posterior wiring and bone grafting but without anterior decompression and died two weeks post-operatively from respiratory and cardiovascular collapse. This paramedian sagittal close-up section shows sclerosis of the upper and lower endplate at the fracture level (1) and marked compression of the lateral portion of the spinal cord and the anterolateral and posterolateral intrathecal root filaments. Note the inveterated intramedullary hematoma. Spinal cord compression is caused anteriorly by a more than 2 cm wide spondylosis ridge (2) which is firmly attached to the vertebra by periosteum and peripheral annulus fibrosus lamellae. Posteriorly, the ruptured ligamentum flavum has retracted and is curled up under the lamina, abutting the anterior osseous compression by the bony flange (3). Especially the anterior bone fragment may be overlooked. If it cannot be removed, a hemicorpectomy or vertebrectomy may become necessary. Behind the lamina the wound hematoma and a bone graft are seen.

FIG. 12 (overleaf). Lower cervical spine of a young male adult who sustained a complete fracture dislocation with complete tetraplegia in a motor vehicle accident. He died after several closed reduction attempts from aspiration of massive stress ulcus hemorrhage. This paramedian sagittal section shows the anterior subluxation of the upper vertebra from which the annulus fibrosus and the periosteum and posterior longitudinal ligaments are stripped along the entire posterior surface of the vertebra, forming a triangular pouch into which large hinged disc fragments are dislodged. A small triangular ridge from the lower posterior endplate of the upper vertebra (arrow) effectively traps the disc fragments. Axial traction obviously would increase the compression of the cord. Note also the hemorrhage posteriorly in the disc above the fracture and the complete rupture of the interlaminar ligamentum flavum.

Figure 13 follows on page 927.

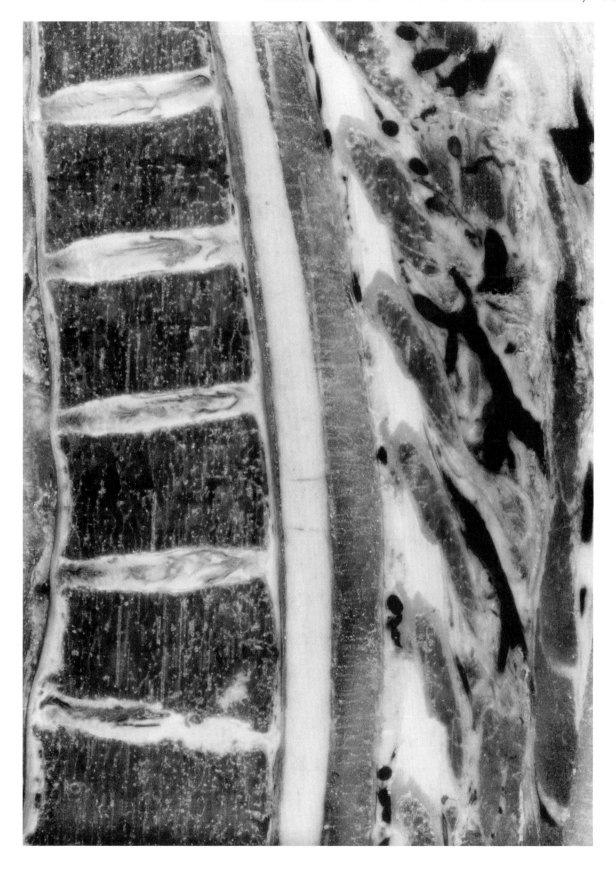

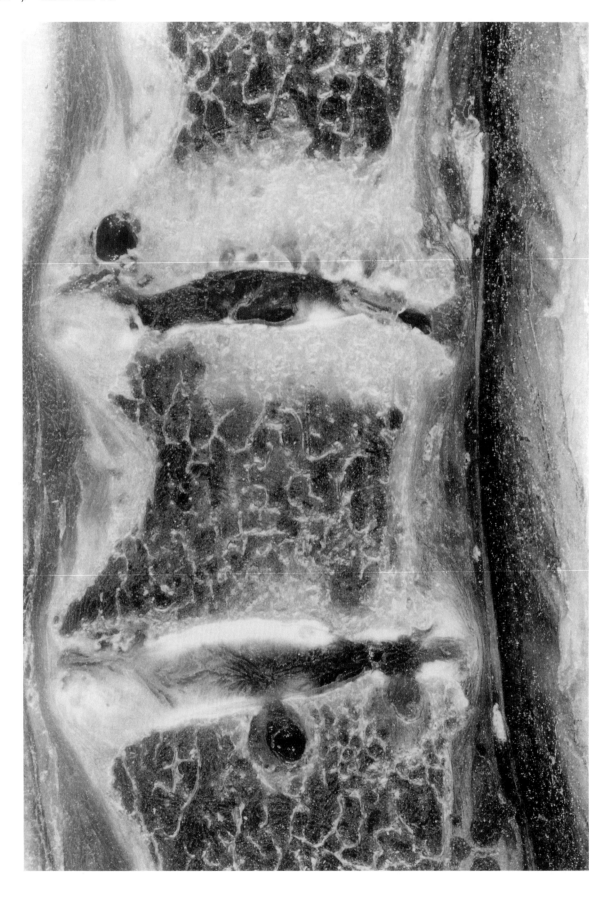

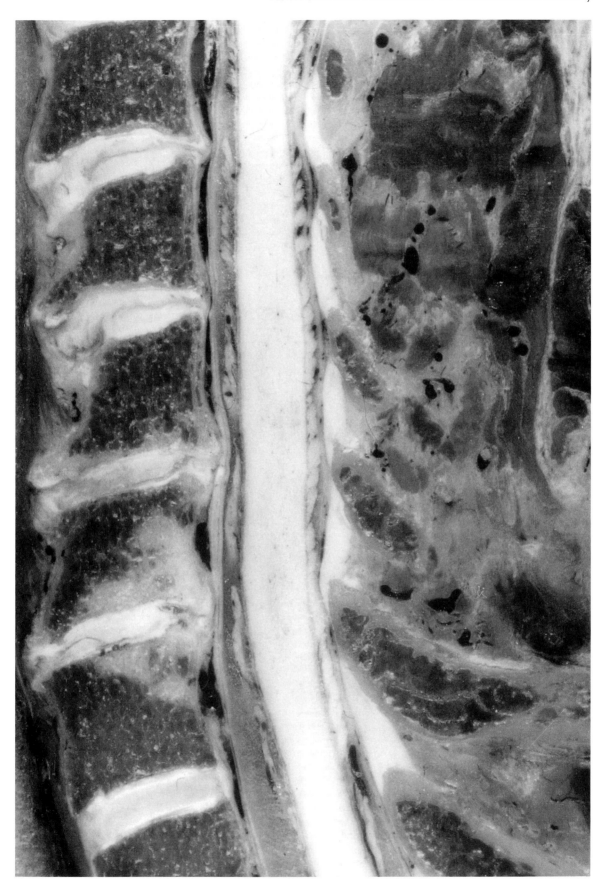

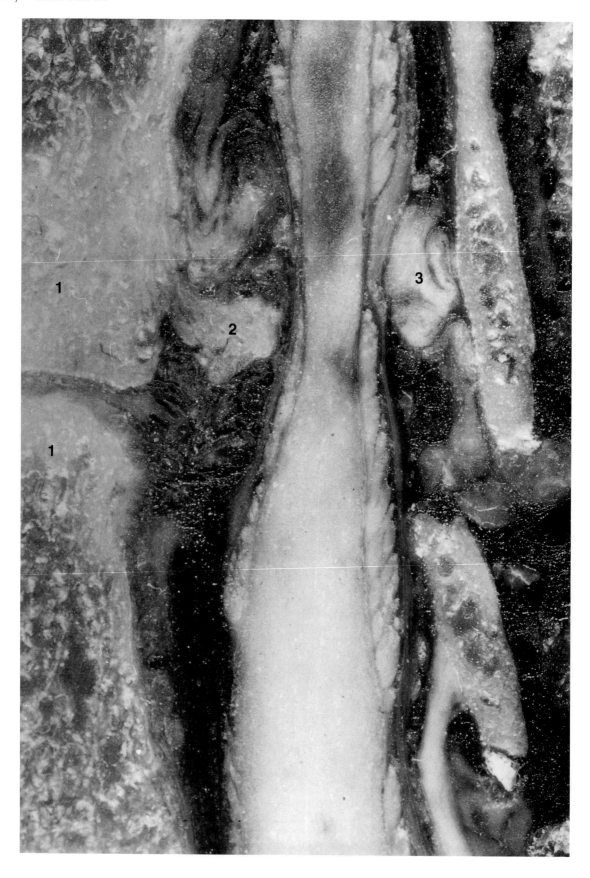

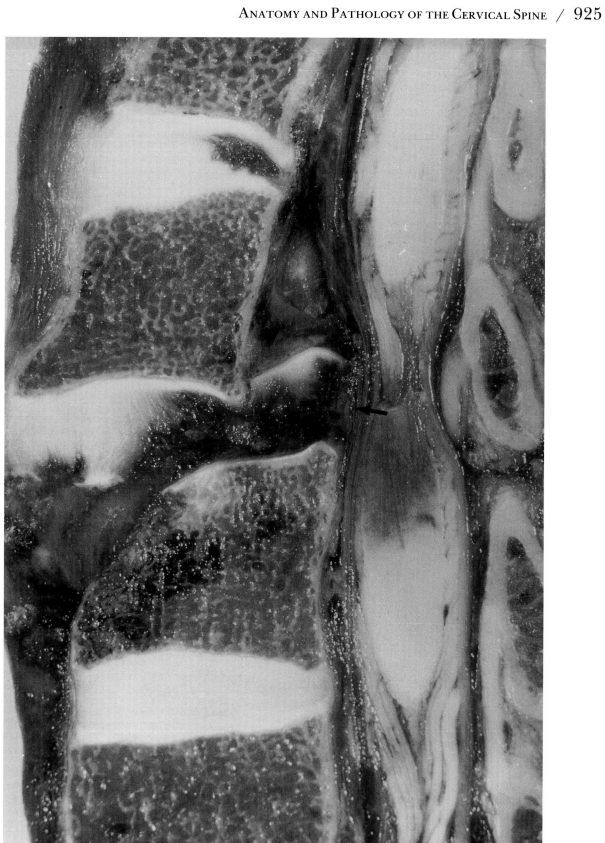

FIG. 13 (opposite page). Sagittal close-up view of a fresh, traumatic disc herniation in the cervical spine of a 23-year-old male who was run over by a car. During forensic autopsy, severe fractures of the facial skeleton as well as a fracture of the skull base were found, but no lesions of the cervical spine were seen. Plain AP, lateral, and oblique x-rays of the specimen were perfectly normal. Cryoplaning revealed a large herniation of the nucleus pulposus through a wide transverse rupture of the posterior annulus at its insertion into the apophyseal ring of C5. The herniation extended from the center of the spinal canal to the left side. Above and below the pedunculated disc fragment the venous sinuses are enlarged and engorged. The thecal sac at the level of the disc herniation is emptied of CSF and pushed posterior against the lamina. The anterior aspects of the dura and of the spinal cord are indented. The discs above and below this level both showed small ruptures of the posterior annulus fibrosus.

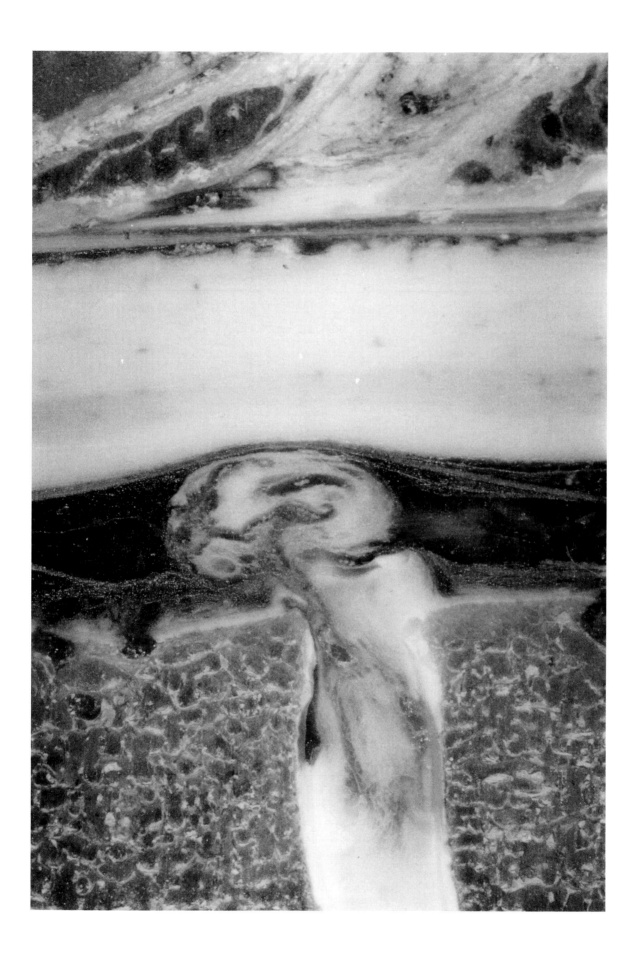

ACKNOWLEDGMENTS

The author wishes to thank the Swedish Medical Research Council, the Swedish Cancer Research Foundation, and the Trygg Hansa Insurance Company, Stockholm.

Halldór Jónsson, Jr., M.D., contributed Figure 13 in this chapter.

REFERENCES

1. Bohlman HH, Eismont FJ (1981): Surgical techniques of anterior decompression and fusion for spinal cord injuries. *Clin Orthop* (154):57–67.

2. Flannigan BD, Lufkin RB, McGlade C, Winter J, Batzdorf U, Wilson GH, Rauschning W, Bradley WG (1987): MR imaging of the cervical spine: Neurovascular anatomy. *Am J Neuroradiol* 8:27–32.

3. Ghoshaajra K, Rao KC (1980): CT in spinal trauma. *J Comput Tomogr* 4:309–318.

4. Gonsalves CG, Hudson AR, Horsey WJ, Tucker WS (1978): Computed tomography of the cervical spine and spinal cord. *Computerized Tomography* 2:279–293.

5. Green BA, Callahan RA, Klose KJ, De La Torre J (1981): Acute spinal cord injury: Current concepts. *Clin Orthop* (154):125–135.

6. Grieve GP (1981): *Common vertebral joint problems.* New York: Churchill Livingstone.

7. Hadley LA (1961): Anatomico-roentgenographic studies of the posterior spinal articulations. *Am J Roentgenol* 86:270–276.

8. Hohl M, Baker HR (1964): The atlanto-axial joint. Roentgenographic and anatomical study of normal and abnormal motion. *J Bone Joint Surg* [Am] 46:1739–1752.

9. Holt S, Yates PO (1966): Cervical spondylosis and nerve root lesions. Incidence at routine necropsy. *J Bone Joint Surg* [Br] 48:407–423.

10. Jones RT (1966): Vascular changes occurring in the cervical musculoskeletal system. *S Afr Med J* 40:388–390.

11. Jónsson H, Rauschning W, Petrén-Mallmin M, Andréasson I (1988): Pathoanatomy of cervical spine tumors and fractures studies with surface cryoplaning and correlations with CT and MRI. Cervical Spine Research Society Annual Meeting, Marseilles. *Orthop Transact* 12:454.

12. Payne EE, Spillane JD (1957): The cervical spine. An anatomico-pathological study of 70 specimens (using a special technique) with particular reference to the problem of cervical spondylosis. *Brain* 80:571–596.

13. Petrén-Mallmin M, Jónsson H Jr, Bring G, Sahlstedt B, Rauschning W (1989): Occult cervical spinal lesions in craniocerebral trauma. 75th Meeting of the Radiological Society of North America, Chicago. *Radiology* 173(Suppl):29.

14. Rauschning W (1983): Computed tomography and cryomicrotomy of lumbar spine specimens. A new technique for multiplanar anatomic correlation. *Spine* 8:170–180.

15. Rauschning W (1985): Detailed sectional anatomy of the spine (chapter 3). In: *Multiplanar CT of the spine,* SLG Rothman, WV Glenn, eds. Baltimore: University Park Press, pp. 33–85.

16. Rauschning W, Jónsson H Jr, McAfee P (1989): Pathoanatomical and surgical findings in cervical spinal injuries. *J Spinal Disorders* 2:213–222.

17. Rauschning W, Sahlstedt B, Wigren A (1980): Irreponible Luxationsfraktur der unteren Halswirbelsäule. Eine pathologisch-anatomische Studie mit der Gefrierschneidemethode. *Chirurg* 51:529–533.

18. Sahlstedt B, Bring G, Rauschning W, Jónsson H (1989): Radiographically occult cervical spinal lesions in fatal head injuries. *Acta Orthop Scand* (Suppl 231)60:41.

The Adult Spine: Principles and Practice,
J. W. Frymoyer, Editor-in-Chief.
Raven Press, Ltd., New York © 1991.

CHAPTER 45

Biomechanics of the Cervical Spine

Including Bracing, Surgical Constructs, and Orthoses

Martin H. Krag

Knowledge of the biomechanics of the cervical spine provides an essential framework for understanding the consequences of injury and other disorders, as well as intelligent planning for operative procedures and conservative treatment with orthoses. In this chapter the anatomy of the cervical spine will be reviewed from the biomechanical perspective, including the issues of kinematics and instability. The biomechanics and classification of cervical injury then will be reviewed, followed by analysis of surgical constructs and orthoses.

M. H. Krag, M.D.: Associate Professor, McClure Center for Musculoskeletal Research, Department of Orthopaedics and Rehabilitation, University of Vermont, Burlington, Vermont, 05405.

SPINAL COMPONENT BIOMECHANICS

Vertebrae

Lower Cervical

The lower cervical vertebrae are usually considered to include C3-C7, although T1 and even T2 to some extent function largely as if they were cervical. Each vertebra basically is made up of a cylindrical body with a group of "posterior elements" attached by means of the pedicles (Fig. 1). The body primarily serves as a compressive load-bearing element, and is significantly smaller than that of the thoracic or lumbar vertebrae. For example the antero-posterior diameter of the body of C4 is slightly less than half that of L4 [46% according to Anderson (11)], which reflects the smaller loads imposed on the cervical vertebrae. The uncus or uncinate process (131),

A

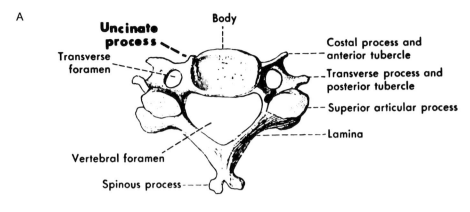

Uncinate process

Body

Transverse foramen

Costal process and anterior tubercle

Transverse process and posterior tubercle

Superior articular process

Lamina

Vertebral foramen

Spinous process

B

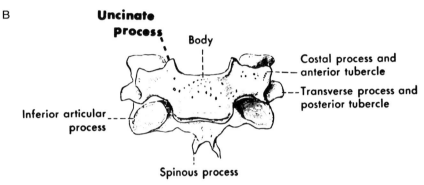

Uncinate Process

Body

Costal process and anterior tubercle

Transverse process and posterior tubercle

Inferior articular process

Spinous process

FIG. 1. Typical vertebra between C3 and C7. **A:** Superior view. **B:** Anterior view.

also known as the neurocentral lip (99), serves to modify the basic cylindrical shape of the body. It consists of a ridge oriented antero-posteriorly and slightly curved along each side of the upper end plate and is present from C3 to T1 (30). This functions as a rail (30) to provide resistance to lateral shifting, which would tend to happen with lateral loading of the superjacent vertebra. The region between the uncinate process and the superjacent vertebra is referred to as the uncovertebral joint or neurocentral joint of Luschka (138). Although there is some argument to the contrary it does not seem to be a synovial joint (84,131,205,219,284).

The posterior elements function primarily as "handles" or levers for producing and controlling the vertebral motion. Various muscles attach to each of the individual processes; virtually the only site at which muscles do not attach to the vertebrae is the anterior part of the body. This absence has clinical utility. During the anterior approach to the cervical spine, the non-muscular "gap" between right and left longus colli muscles is a helpful landmark.

The spinous processes increase in length between C3 and T1 or T2 consistent with the increase in torque along the spine needed to resist a given load on the head (Fig. 2). The longer the spinous process, the greater the leverage that the attached muscle has available to produce torque. However, if they protruded too far posteriorly in the midline, adjacent spinous processes would hit each other during extension of the neck. To prevent this contact and yet maintain length, the spinous processes of the

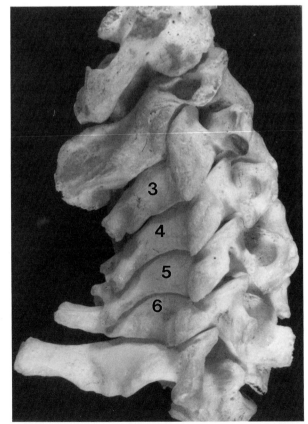

FIG. 2. Spinous process length gradually increases caudally. Synovial joint orientation at C1-C2 is transverse while below this is oblique. Bifid spinous processes "nest" together to allow extension without decrease in spinous process length.

central cervical vertebrae are bifid. These processes "nest" together in extension, which allows a greater range of motion than would otherwise be possible (see Fig. 2).

The articular processes, which make up the facet joints, provide major resistance to anterior shifting (translation) of each vertebra on its subjacent vertebra. Additional resistance is also provided by muscles whose orientation results in a component of anterior-posterior pull. The facet joint is a major determinant of the intervertebral motion (90), although by no means is it the only one. This will be discussed further in "Kinematics" (see page 936).

The orientation of the articular surfaces is different in the cervical region than in either the thoracic or lumbar regions, and is also different within the cervical region itself (Fig. 3). The articular plane is almost transverse at C1-C2, but at C2-C3 abruptly steepens to 55 to 60 degrees above the plane of the inferior end plate, or 45 degrees to the longitudinal axis of the spinal canal (30,63,143) and then remains approximately constant to C7-T1. At and below C3-C4, the facet joint planes are perpendicular to the sagittal plane, which allows easy visualization of the articular "space" by lateral view x-ray. At C2-C3, however, the joint planes also slope downward laterally by 10 to 20 degrees (30) and thus

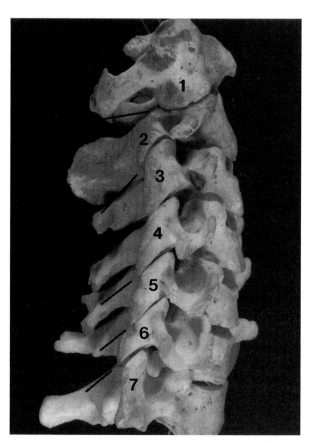

FIG. 3. The facet orientation and its change at different anatomic levels.

normally are not as clearly seen on lateral view x-ray. The transitional nature of C2-C3 (i.e., between C1-C2 and C3-C4) has been detailed by Mestdagh (188).

The transverse processes provide an important basis for attachment of various neck muscles, both anteriorly and posteriorly. The vertebral arteries pass through the foramina of the transverse processes. The C7 transverse process typically has neither foramen nor any scalene muscle origination.

The foramina formed between adjacent pedicles and continued anterolaterally by the transverse processes on each side are all oriented approximately parallel when the neck is in the neutral position. The orientation of the foramina is anterolaterally 45 degrees and anterocaudad 15 degrees. Either axial rotation of the head relative to the thorax or shifting of the head forward (capital protraction) will cause the foraminal axes to no longer be parallel. If oblique films are obtained with the x-ray source located posteriorly and the patient upright (central beam 45 degrees medially, 15 degrees caudad; plate perpendicular to central beam), there is a tendency for both axial rotation and capital protraction to occur, resulting in poor visualization of the foramina. If instead the oblique films are taken anteriorly (central beam 45 degrees medially, 15 degrees cephalad), there is less tendency for these malpositions to occur.

Anterior oblique films may be accomplished either with the patient upright, which allows the cassette easily to be perpendicular to the central beam and thus gridded, or with the patient supine and the cassette horizontal at 45 degrees to the central beam and thus non-gridded. The supine technique is particularly useful in assessing the traumatized patient, since no movement is needed. The absence of a grid and the "smearing out" from cassette angulation present minimal problems in film interpretation.

Upper Cervical

The occipito-atlanto-axial (or Oc-C1-C2) complex is a highly specialized articulation to provide a relatively large range of motion between the head and torso. The special nature of this region (Figs. 4A–D) is reflected by the absence of any intervertebral discs. All the articulations are synovial joints. For this reason, the majority of cervical spine problems caused by rheumatoid arthritis is in this upper region, most commonly C1-C2 subluxation or Oc-C1 settling. The complexity of this structure requires quite elaborate embryologic development (267), including the theft of the C1 vertebral body by C2 to form the odontoid. Not surprisingly, a variety of abnormalities can occur (138) such as various degrees of hypoplasia of the posterior arch of C1 or of the odontoid. An extensive treatise on this region has been published by Von Torklus and Gehle (291), and this topic is addressed in Chapter 44.

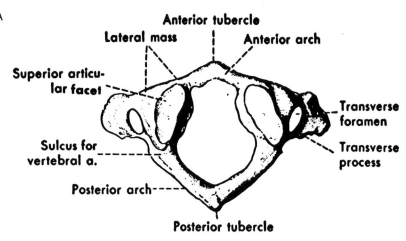

A

Anterior tubercle

Lateral mass

Superior articular facet

Anterior arch

Transverse foramen

Sulcus for vertebral a.

Transverse process

Posterior arch

Posterior tubercle

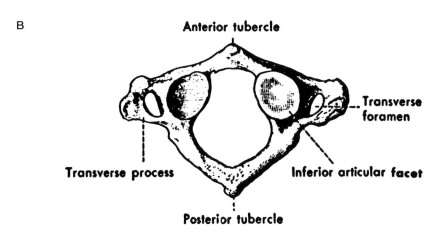

B

Anterior tubercle

Transverse foramen

Transverse process

Inferior articular facet

Posterior tubercle

FIG. 4. C1 and C2 vertebrae. A: C1 superior. B: C1 inferior. C: C2 superior. D: C2 anterior.

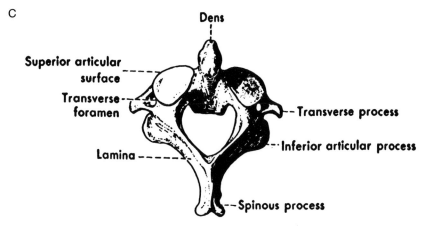

C

Dens

Superior articular surface

Transverse foramen

Transverse process

Inferior articular process

Lamina

Spinous process

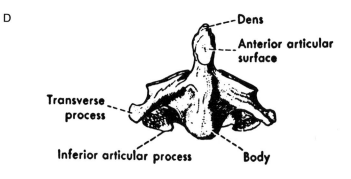

D

Dens

Anterior articular surface

Transverse process

Inferior articular process

Body

The basic structure of the Oc-C1-C2 complex is a biconcave ring (C1) interposed between two convex structures: the occipital (Oc) condyles from above and the upper facets of the C2 lateral masses from below. In addition, the odontoid (or dens) projects upwards from C2 to provide a post to which are anchored both the C1 ring and the occiput. The major ligamentous connections of the Oc are not to C1 but instead directly to C2, as detailed below. The occipital condyles are oriented approximately antero-posteriorly but converge somewhat anteriorly, and fit into corresponding concavities on the upper surface of the C1 lateral masses. The right and left portions of this joint are similar to a miniature version of the medial and lateral portions of the knee joint. The C1-C2 articulation consists of three joints: one between the odontoid and C1 anterior arch, and two (right and left) between the lateral masses of C1 and of C2.

Discs

As mentioned previously, there is no disc between the occiput and C1 or between C1 and C2. The discs from C2-C3 and below are very similar in structure, consisting of an outer fibrous ring (annulus fibrosus) and a central semi-solid core (nucleus pulposus). One characteristic of this specialized structure is its ability to transmit compressive loads throughout a range of motion yet prevent excessive stress concentration from occurring. This seems to be accomplished by posterior shifting of the nucleus with flexion and anterior shifting during extension (159,160) in the lumbar spine; presumably the same mechanism occurs in the cervical spine. Similar to the lumbar spine, herniations of the cervical nucleus pulposus tend to occur posterolaterally, where the rate of curvature of the annulus fibrosus is the greatest. This leads to stress concentration and fiber breakdown (313) which weaken the annulus and may allow herniation to occur. Unfortunately, the very site where herniations occur most often is the site at which the nerve root is the most closely applied to the annulus, setting the stage for the clinical problem of cervical radiculopathy from either disc herniation or osteophyte formation.

Ligaments

Ligaments may be considered as spanning across either multiple motion segments or only a single motion segment. The only significant ligament in the first category is the ligamentum nuchae, which usually is a dense, fibrous posterior midline band which runs from the external occipital protuberance to the spinous process of C7; the attachments to C2-C6 are much less substantial (136). Perhaps this is the reason why "clay shoveler's" fractures (262) (avulsion of the spinous process) typically occur at C7. This structure is generally considered to

provide a major constraint to excessive cervical flexion (33,35,37) although Halliday et al. (118) and Johnson et al. (139) have found this not always to be the case. Ligaments spanning across individual motion segments may be considered in two groups.

Lower Cervical

The major ligaments from front to back are the anterior longitudinal ligament (ALL), intertransverse process ligaments, posterior longitudinal ligament (PLL), facet joint capsules, ligamentum flavum, interspinous ligament, and supraspinous ligament (SL). Although the ALL, PLL, and SL span multiple levels, they attach at each individual vertebra, unlike the ligamentum nuchae. Careful and clinically relevant anatomic descriptions have been reported by various authors, for example Johnson et al. (139). Biomechanical testing (static and dynamic) of isolated bone-ligament-bone preparations of ALL and of ligamentum flavum has been reported by Yoganandan et al. (321). The rich innervation of facet joint capsules has been described by Wyke (320) who infers from this a possible proprioceptive role for the capsule. The effect of ligament damage on motion segment behavior is described later in "Hyperflexibility" (this chapter).

Upper Cervical

As mentioned previously, the odontoid of C2 provides a sturdy post to which are anchored both the occiput (Oc) and the ring of C1. The Oc is attached to the odontoid (Figs. 5A and 5B) by the alar ligaments (82) and the much less substantial apical ligament and the upper arm of the cruciform ligament. The C1 ring is attached to the odontoid by the quite sturdy transverse ligament (or transverse arms of the cruciform ligament) as well as the accessory C1-C2 ligaments (or C1-C2 portion of the alar ligament) (80) and C1-C2 facet capsules. Dvorak et al. (82) showed that the tensile strength of the transverse ligament was almost twice as strong (350 N) as that of the alar ligaments (200 N). The connection between the occiput and C1 is less substantial and is really limited just to the facet capsules.

Muscles and Tendons

The role of muscles and tendons in the neck is to produce motion and control position of the head relative to the thorax. The passive elements (bone, disc, ligaments, joints) exert important control over translations, as well as the location of the centers of rotation. However, the angles of rotation are controlled almost totally by the muscles, except perhaps at the end of the range of mo-

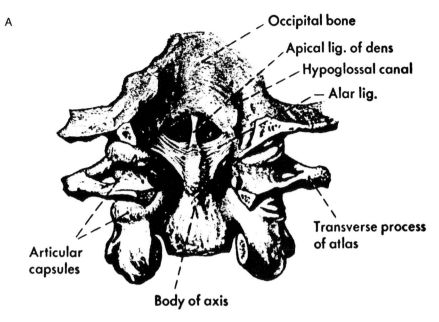

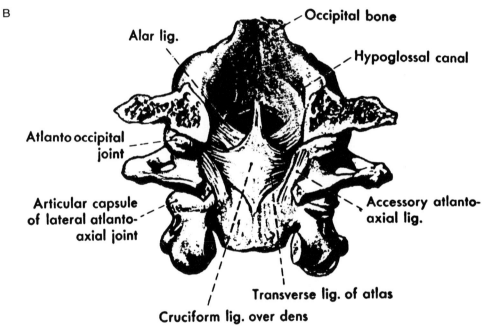

FIG. 5. Ligaments between occiput, C1 and C2 seen from dorsally. **A:** After removal of posterior elements and posterior longitudinal ligament. **B:** After removal of the cruciform ligament.

tion when ligaments dominate. The spinal column certainly does not function as a stiff rod which can support itself upright, but rather functions as a series of ball and socket joints which requires muscle action to prevent buckling collapse (304).

The general structure of these tissues in the neck is similar to that throughout the multi-segmented axial skeleton in that there are some "gross-function" muscles that span across many or a few motion segments, and other "fine-function" muscles which just cross one or

two segments. The gross-function muscles anteriorly are the longus colli, longus capitis, and scalenes which attach either to the vertebral bodies or to transverse processes. The fine-function anterior muscles are the intertransversarii, which span just one segment. Posteriorly, the gross function muscles attached to the spinous processes are the splenius capitis and semispinalis cervices; attached to the transverse processes are longissimus cervices and iliocostalis cervices. The posterior fine-function muscles are either between spinous processes (interspinals), between transverse processes (intertransversarii), or cross from spinous to transverse processes (long and short rotatores).

Another general feature of the neck muscles is the large extent to which their orientation is angulated "off-axis" or away from the longitudinal axis of the spine. Muscles oriented parallel to the longitudinal axis can efficiently produce the head rotations of flexion, extension, or lateral bendings, but it is the "off-axis" muscles which are needed to efficiently produce shifting (translation) of the head anteriorly, posteriorly, or laterally, as well as rotation about the longitudinal axis. For example, rotation of the head and upper cervical spine toward the right is caused by contraction of the right sternocleidomastoid and upper trapezius muscles as well as the left splenius capitis and longissimus capitis muscles. Quantitative detail of muscle site attachments and muscle forces in vivo and in vitro have been determined for purposes of neck biomechanical models (69,195,201). A recent functionally oriented review of muscle structure has also been reported by Parke and Sherk (218).

Muscle bulk in the neck is notably more massive posteriorly than anteriorly. This is related to the general tendency for the head to be positioned in such a way that its center of gravity is positioned anteriorly to the vertical support provided by the spinal column. This feature is obviously the case for quadrupeds, but is also true for bipeds. This feature, plus the much more extensive muscular attachment to the spinous processes than to the anterior aspect of the vertebral body, typically requires more muscular disruption during posterior surgical approaches than during anterior approaches.

The extent to which tendons are used within the cervical spine is fairly limited. Some of the small fine-function muscles tend to have a tendinous insertion to small attachment sites, such as the rotatores to the spinous processes. The role of tendons to allow a change in muscle direction around a pulley-like structure is only encountered in the neck with the omohyoid, the superior and inferior bellies of which are typically separated by a tendinous portion which passes through a fascial sling to the clavicle (162).

Cord, Dura, and Nerve Roots

Three major topics will be discussed, each of which has direct clinical relevance.

Effect of Neck Motion

Because the spinal cord is situated posteriorly to the centers of rotation for vertebral flexion and extension, it becomes longer and thinner with flexion, and shorter and thicker with extension. Breig (33–38) has written

extensively about this phenomenon. He performed dissections of cadavers and dynamic air myelograms of patients, and noted overall spinal cord length changes of 45 to 75 mm. More recently this phenomenon has been demonstrated by magnetic resonance scanning (60). An associated phenomenon is the longitudinal motion of the cord produced during flexion-extension relative to each vertebra. The "neutral point" at which no relative motion occurs between cord and vertebrae is at C5 [for humans (231)] or C4 [for primates (272)]. Maximum relative shifting of up to 18 mm occurred in the upper thoracic region (231).

Tensile forces in the cord produced by elongation are carried primarily by the dura (33,287) and the pia-arachnoid (288) rather than the cord itself, and are balanced by tensile forces not from the filum terminale but rather from the nerve roots (272). These forces are transmitted to the cord predominantly by the nerve root dural sheaths and dentate ligaments, rather than by the roots and rootlets themselves (33,231,288).

The effect of these mechanical changes on clinical findings or neurophysiological function was investigated extensively by Breig (33–38), who described patients with spondylitic myelopathy, acute trauma, or multiple sclerosis in whom flexion worsened neurological deficits or produced Lhermitte's sign (41,168). Because he observed a decrease in antero-posterior compression of the cord with flexion (decreased cord diameter and increased canal diameter), he reasoned by exclusion that the increased neurological dysfunction must be due to increased contact pressure against the anterior aspect of the cord, or caused by forward shifting of the cord, which in turn was produced by the flexion-induced tension. For cervical trauma or spondylosis, the local abnormality is outside the cord; for multiple sclerosis it is within the cord. The biomechanical analysis is essentially the same for both (34). This same author developed a surgical technique ("cervicolordodesis") which involved a connective tissue graft in the posterior aspect of the neck to limit flexion and reported favorable results in 21 patients (36,37). For acute trauma management Breig (38) recommended avoidance of flexion not only to prevent abnormal intervertebral motion, but also to prevent increased cord tension, which might cause or worsen neural damage.

Spinal Cord's Internal Stress/Strain

The relationship between internal stresses/strains and spinal cord injury production was investigated early on by McVeigh (187) who noted that axial compressibility was greater for the central gray matter than for the peripheral white matter. This topic is also contained in Ommaya's review of the earlier literature (203). A concentration of tissue damage centrally with external cord pressure was noted by others (46,178,257,258). The connection between these findings is clarified by the stress distribution that develops within spinal cord models, which has been reviewed and illustrated by Panjabi and White (214). Also related to this stress distribution is the viscoelastic behavior of the cord (264).

Experimental Cord Trauma

An experimental tool important for understanding pathophysiology and improving the treatment of cord trauma is the ability to create known, carefully controlled cord trauma. Allen's method (4) from 1911 was used for decades (71,73), but was flawed from a biomechanical viewpoint (73). Using a more appropriate measure for the mechanical injuring input (impulse rather than the Allen method of mass multiplied by drop distance), Dohrmann and co-workers (72) were able to establish a direct correlation between mechanical input and cord lesion volume. The experimental technique (207) also measured impact force over time and isolated cord deflection from thoracic deflection. Hung et al. (133) have also used a standardized impact load, and Somerson and Stokes (273) have developed an electromechanical injuring device. Most recently, Panjabi and Wrathall (217) have reported on the strong correlation between carefully controlled biomechanical input and in vivo functional outcome.

SPINAL COMPOSITE BIOMECHANICS

The components described above are the building blocks for the cervical spine. The manner in which they function together in the cervical spine has many different aspects. Three aspects which are particularly relevant clinically will be discussed here.

Kinematics

The motion or kinematics of the cervical spine is not determined solely by the passive elements (facets, disc, ligaments, bone) but is also influenced by the active elements (muscles and tendons). An obvious example is forward flexion of the head relative to the thorax. For any specified position of the head, there is an infinite number of different postures which may be assumed by the cervical vertebrae, each produced by different amounts of contraction of the various cervical muscles. A less obvious example is that even with forward flexion of a single motion segment, subtle variations in anterior-posterior or axial rotational position may occur. Resulting abnormal motion of the facet joints may be one cause of "snapping" noises in the neck. Because muscle action can affect the kinematics, interpretation of cadaveric biomechanical studies must be performed care-

fully, especially when multi-vertebral specimens are used.

To define the motion of an object in three-dimensional space requires six independent numbers, for example three coordinates (along the x, y, and z axes) to specify the location of the object and three angles (about the x, y, and z axes) to specify the rotation of the object. Such an object is thus said to have six "degrees of freedom." For two-dimensional space such as a cervical flexion-extension radiograph, only three independent numbers are needed to specify the motion of an object such as the image of a vertebra. In this circumstance only three degrees of freedom exist. Choosing which three independent numbers to use is a matter of convenience. One choice (Fig. 6A) would be to use the x and y components of translation of point 1 and the rotation angle A. The value of A will be the same regardless of where on the object it is measured; however, the x and y components will be different for each point (unless $A = 0$). Another choice (Fig. 6B) for these three independent numbers would be to use the x and y location of the center of rotation (CR), and again the angle A, which will be the same for the CR as for any other point "on" the object. The CR may be thought of as that one special point that has no translation (238).

Lower Cervical

A useful approximation of the range of motion at each motion segment between C2-C3 and C7-T1 is 10 degrees for each of the following: total excursion from flexed to extended, axial rotation to each side, and lateral bending to each side. There is a tendency for flexion/extension and axial rotation to be greatest in the mid-cervical region (decreasing both above and below this), and for lateral bending to be greatest at C2-C3, then to gradually decrease down the cervical spine (188). Also, there are fairly large variations in the values reported in the litera-

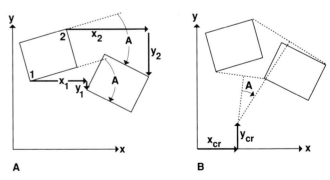

FIG. 6. Two different descriptions of planar vertebral motion, each of which requires three independent numbers. **A:** Motion x_1, y_1 of vertebral point 1 and vertebral rotation angle A. Note that motion x_2, y_2 at any other point 2 will be different than at point 1. **B:** Location x_{cr}, y_{cr} of center of rotation and vertebral rotation angle A. Note that only a single center of rotation occurs, and that the rotation angle is still A.

ture (93,174,303,304) and reviewed thoroughly by Dimnet et al. (70). Nonetheless, the above approximation is valid. Recent studies have carefully documented range of motion for all three axes in normal volunteers (9,190) or in cadavers (248). Computerized tomography (CT) scanning has been used to measure very accurately the axial rotational range of motion at each motion segment (81,221).

For flexion-extension the location of the CR for each pair of vertebrae is generally located within the body of the lower vertebra but gradually shifts from a position in the lower dorsal quadrant of C3 (for C2-C3 motion) to the middle of the upper end plate of C7 (for C6-C7 motion) (30,220). The CR is also approximately at the center of a circle passing through the articular surface of the facet joint. Although the CR appears to move for different steps of motion throughout the flexion-extension range, this motion (the tracing of which is known as the centrode) is relatively small compared to that in the lumbar spine (70). As flexion occurs, the amount of overlap or contact between the facets gradually decreases to the point that subluxation or actual dislocation can occur. As facet overlap changes, so also does the size of the neural foramina. Thus, full extension can cause enough foraminal closure to produce increased arm symptoms in a patient with disc herniation or osteophytic encroachment into the foramen.

For lateral bending, the CR for each pair of vertebrae is located not in the lower vertebral body but rather in the upper one because of the constraints imposed by the uncinate processes. For axial rotation, both the uncinate processes and the facet joints constrain the motion. Because the facet joint planes are perpendicular to the sagittal plane, these joints must either open up slightly (e.g., right joint opens with right axial rotation), or some lateral bending must occur. Probably it is the latter that most typically happens. The combination of these two movements is really equivalent to rotation of the neck about a vertical axis with the neck in a forward inclined position (220). This movement is very commonly used and allows minimal constraint to motion by the facet joints. In this circumstance the rotation axis is perpendicular to the articular plane, therefore the articular processes need only slide along and not separate from each other.

To date, abnormal kinematics have not been well characterized for cases in which obvious fracture or dislocation is absent, despite various efforts to accomplish this goal as reviewed by Dimnet et al. (70). The measurements are somewhat tedious and prone to error, and both inter- and intra-subject variability are problems. To control for this variability, comparison between the level above and level below the one in question is probably quite important. Widely accepted standards of abnormality for voluntarily produced movements have not yet been developed.

Abnormally large or small rotations are perhaps the most obvious and easily measured kinematic abnormalities, but they are not the only ones possible. Because planar motion (such as flexion-extension) has 3 degrees of freedom as described earlier, rotation angle measurement of the CR is also needed. If only the rotation is measured, a kinematic abnormality consisting of an abnormal CR location will be missed.

Upper Cervical

Basically the motion pattern in this anatomic area is the following: flexion-extension to some extent at both Oc-C1 and C1-C2, axial rotation at C1-C2 alone, and lateral bend only slightly at Oc-C1 alone (Table 1). This could be predicted from the arrangement of articular surfaces and ligamentous connections. Flexion-extension for Oc-C1 occurs about a CR approximately at the center of curvature of the occipital condyles. Flexion-extension for C1-C2 entails motion of the anterior arch of C1 cephalad and slightly posteriorly, facilitated by the curved anterior surface of the odontoid.

Axial rotation for Oc-C1 requires one occipital condyle to slide anteriorly on C1 and the contralateral one to slide posteriorly. The relatively deep fit of the condyles into the C1 upper articular concavity precludes this motion (221). In contrast, axial rotation is a major function for C1-C2, since approximately half of the maximum axial rotation for the entire neck occurs at this joint (221,297,303,304). Furthermore, within the central portion of this range, almost all the axial rotation is at C1-C2 (30,129). As C1 rotates toward the right, the anteromedial-most portion of the right lateral articular mass shifts posteriorly and laterally, while that of the left lateral articular mass shifts anteriorly and medially (the CR is posterior to these portions of the articular surfaces). An antero-posterior open-mouth x-ray will erroneously suggest subluxation laterally of C, on C2. Careful neutral positioning of both head and torso for x-ray exposure will prevent this misleading radiographic image.

Lateral bending occurs only to a small extent between Oc-C1. The strong alar ligaments force the rotation to be about the tip of the odontoid. This is allowed to occur by some lateral shifting of the C1 ring (30), which in turn requires some stretching out of the transverse ligament (transverse portion of the cruciform ligament). Lateral bending at C1-C2 is negligible.

TABLE 1. *Cervical motion*

	Oc-C1	C1-C2	C3-C7
Flexion-extension	Some	Some	Major
Axial rotation	No	Major	Some
Lateral bend	Slight	No	Major

No = none-slight.

Abnormal kinematics of the Oc-C1-C2 region is probably best illustrated by the C1-C2 subluxation which can occur by means of rheumatoid arthritic damage to the transverse ligament. This allows an abnormally large anterior translation of C1 on C2. Even though there may be no angular hypermobility, the CR can clearly be seen to be abnormally located. Abnormal kinematics can also occur with post-traumatic rotatory hypermobility ("instability"). This condition is probably underdiagnosed, especially in the adult, and has been elegantly studied with functional CT scanning by Dvorak and co-workers (79,81).

Instability

The most common mechanical definition of this term is that an abnormally or unexpectedly large motion occurs in response to an applied load. This may be illustrated by a simple example. If an average-sized individual (the load) sits on the edge of an "unstable" boat, it will tip by a large amount compared to a more stable boat, for which only a minimal tip occurs with the same load. A second closely related yet really very different meaning of instability is that any further load application beyond a certain "critical load" leads to increasing motion even without additional load increase. Subsequently, even if the load is removed the system does not return to its initial position, but remains in a new stable position. An example is a catamaran which is allowed to tip just a bit too far: even though the load is not increased, the boat will continue to tip more and more, flip over, and tend to remain in the new stable position.

In both of these examples it can be seen that assessment of stability depends on knowing not only the motion but also the loads involved. The problem is that in a clinical setting the loads acting upon the vertebrae are not known. Even when the external load on the neck is known (e.g., longitudinal traction as in the "stretch test") (216,256,304), the internal loads on the vertebrae or ligaments are not known. This is because there is load-sharing between these components and the muscles, and the loads taken by the muscles are not quantified.

Application of the term "stability" to spinal problems can thus be quite difficult. Loads are important in the true mechanical definition of stability and muscles are important in producing these loads, yet the magnitude of these loads is difficult to measure. Thus, the lack to date of an explicit, quantitative, agreed-upon definition of instability in the clinical literature is understandable.

Rather than continuing to struggle with this difficulty, perhaps the term "mechanical insufficiency" would be better than "instability." "Insufficiency" has a vagueness which accurately conveys the imprecision of our current knowledge, and "instability" as it is typically used clinically is often misleading and goes beyond today's knowledge. "Mechanical insufficiency" also has a breadth of meaning which could encompass various subtypes as our knowledge expands and terms become more precise. For example, "spinal dyskinesia" could be used to mean any abnormal motion even though the forces are not known, and "spinal segmental hypermobility" could mean a special type of dyskinesia, namely abnormally large motion at a single motion segment. "Hyperflexibility" (discussed below) could be used to describe situations both in which the loads and the displacements are known, as would result from use of the "stretch test" (216,256), and in which the displacements are large relative to the corresponding loads.

"Instability" could then be used in its true engineering sense, as in the catamaran example above. After all, the usual decision that needs to be made in a clinical setting is not really whether the spinal segment in question is "stable," but rather whether treatment of a particular type (e.g., internal fixation and grafting) will be helpful. Use of a less specific term such as "mechanical insufficiency" may allow a clearer focus on this clinical decision, without the distraction of imprecisely or unmeasurably defined "instabilities."

Hyperflexibility

Flexibility has to do with the ratio between loads and displacements. Strictly speaking, flexibility is the load required to produce a given displacement, whereas stiffness is the displacement produced from a given load. Panjabi et al. (212) tested human cadaveric motion segments from C2-C3 through C6-C7, used a full array of force types (anterior and posterior, right and left lateral, and tension and compression), and measured all six displacement components, i.e., translation along and rotation about each of the three axes. They defined a "neutral zone" in the load-displacement curves within which displacements occurred with very little load change.

Flexibility testing in vivo has been done only to a limited extent. Measurements of the effect of cervical traction have been done by various investigators. Goldie and Reichmann (112) used 150 N longitudinal distraction force and showed no disc widening in 47 of 54 discs in 15 normal subjects. Seven of 54 widened from 0.4 to 0.7 mm but this was unrelated to other radiographic features or to clinical findings. Schlicke et al. (256) applied traction equal to one third of body weight to normal volunteers in order to establish normal values for a diagnostic "stretch test." They found that the mean disc height increased 0.70 mm (SD = 0.50 mm) and the segmental extension angle increased 0.9 degrees (SD = 2.4 degrees). Some variation with vertebral level occurred (largest at C3-C4 and C4-C5, intermediate at C5-C6, and smallest at C2-C3).

The effect of deliberately produced structural abnormalities on flexibility has been investigated only using cadaveric specimens, of course. Panjabi et al. (215) investigated the response of human motion segments to an anteriorly directed force as ligaments were sequentially transected either from back to front or front to back. Eventually they reached a "pre-failure state" after which cutting one more ligament would produce complete dislocation. For this pre-failure state, the average amount of flexion was 11 degrees more than that present before any ligaments were cut. The average amount of anterior translation was 3.5 mm (measured at the inferior dorsal corner of the upper body relative to the superior dorsal corner of the lower body). Interestingly, this value is very close to the 3.5 mm mean maximum anterior displacement seen in intact cadaveric specimens subjected to an anteriorly directed force, as described above. Further ligament transection work was done by Moroney et al. (194) who subjected degenerated specimens and specimens with posterior elements removed to not only flexion/extension, but also to lateral bending and axial rotation.

The relationship of these ligament transection results to in vivo abnormal kinematics is far from clear for at least two reasons. The pattern of ligament disruption leading to abnormal motion in vivo is probably very different from sequential total transection of each ligament. In addition, the force distribution in vivo is not known and may be very different from that used in cadaver testing. Thus, use of these values for clinical decision-making remains to be validated.

Similar cadaveric work has been done using longitudinal traction instead of an anteriorly directed force (216) to help establish a normal basis for a clinical stretch test. One third body weight was applied, and ligaments were cut from front to back. The increased anterior disc height just prior to failure was 3.3 mm and the increase in extension angle was 3.8 degrees. For the posterior to anterior cutting sequence, spinous process spread increase was 27 mm and the increase in flexion angle was 30 degrees. Here again, the relation between these data and in vivo clinical problems has not been tested and remains to be established.

Wetzel et al. performed a corresponding study on rabbit spines (299) which demonstrated both important similarities to and differences from the human spine specimen results. They also documented for the first time in the cervical spine (299) the time course of healing after experimentally produced injuries (interspinous ligament sectioning, laminectomy, laminectomy and facet capsule excision, and sham operation).

Raynor et al. (230) have shown in human cadaveric fresh and embalmed specimens the effect of various degrees of facetectomy. For specimens in which the medial 50% of each facet joint was excised, only one of five failed by articular process fracture when subjected to an anterior shear load (four of five specimens failed by pulling away from their mounting). After 70% of each facet joint was excised, four of four specimens failed by articular process fracture.

TRAUMA

To facilitate communication about the wide variety of injuries that can occur in the cervical spine, various injury types have been defined and various classification schemes proposed. We will focus here only on the "indirect" injuries, defined as those produced by forces applied to the head either by contact with another object (e.g., diving into shallow water) or by acceleration/deceleration (whiplash). "Direct" injuries such as gunshot or knife wounds are excluded here and are discussed in Chapter 40. Two basically different approaches to the naming and classification of indirect injuries have been followed: a) radiographic appearance (29), or b) mechanistic (5,30,122,123,234), according to the direction and/or location of the force presumed to have caused the damage.

The first approach has the advantage of being very direct: the bony structural damage or malposition can be visualized by x-ray and the associated ligamentous structural damage can be reasonably well inferred. The injury type is derived directly from the X-ray appearance. Since treatment largely involves repairing or compensating for the structural damage, only a small step is needed to go from diagnosis to treatment. For example, if the x-ray shows a bilateral facet subluxation, one infers a torn interspinous ligament and facet joint capsules, and may treat this by "replacing" the torn interspinous ligament with a wire loop for temporary stabilization and by bone graft for permanent fusion.

The disadvantage of this radiographic approach is that the biomechanics get "lost." Mechanically important relationships between injury types are not clearly apparent within the classification. Very different structurally-defined injuries may be caused by the same force, e.g., both Jefferson fractures and burst fractures of C5 are caused by a compressive force with the neck in the neutral position. The reverse situation can also occur; that is, similar structural damage may be caused by very different forces. For example, bilateral C5 laminar fractures may be caused by forward flexion (in association with C4-C5 interspinous ligament failure and C5-C6 bilateral facet capsule failure), or may be caused by a compressive force acting on an already extended neck (causing the C4 inferior articular processes to be forced downward and the C5 lamina to fracture in hyperextension). As a result, x-ray appearance is not a very reliable predictor of mechanical damage or "instability," as noted by many authors (158,208).

To overcome these and other related disadvantages, the mechanistic approach to naming and classification has been used by a number of authors. An early method was that of Roaf (234) who proposed to classify injuries as flexion, compression, extension, lateral bend, and rotation. As a more detailed understanding of injury subtypes has evolved and a wider range of treatment options has been developed, this classification scheme has become too simple for many purposes. Largely because of a gradually improved understanding of injury biomechanics, more useful classification schemes are now available.

Such a scheme for the lower cervical spine was described by Allen et al. (5,6) and represents a major advance. The scheme consists of six categories: compressive flexion, vertical compression, distractive flexion, compressive extension, distractive extension, and lateral flexion. These terms, however, present certain problems. First, flexion is always associated with some compression of anterior elements and distraction of posterior elements. Thus "compressive flexion" and "distractive flexion" are somewhat confusing, since it is not clear what it is that is being compressed or distracted. This same problem is presented by the terms "compressive extension" and "distractive extension." Second, by "distractive flexion" the authors really mean flexion without any external compressive loads, but that absence does not really constitute distraction. Third, spinal compression usually is considered to mean a force acting downward along the longitudinal axis of the spine. In this context "vertical compression" is confusingly redundant.

In an effort to build on the substantial conceptual advance of this system and also to clarify the terminology, a modified system has been developed (Table 2). Each injury category is defined by two items: the force type that is applied to the head, named for the dominant motion which that force tends to produce, and the posture of the neck at the instant structural failure occurs. There are five force types (flexing, compressing, extending, distracting, and lateral bending) and five neck postures (flexed, neutral, extended, axially rotated, and laterally bent).

Many of the 25 possible combinations need not be considered. Some combinations do not occur because neck postural change is produced before significant damage; e.g., a flexing force will move the neck from a neutral or extended posture to the flexed posture before significant injury occurs. By similar reasoning, the combinations of extending and flexed, extending and neutral, or lateral bending and neutral also do not occur. Distraction in any posture other than extended does not occur because a distracting force can only be applied to the head anteriorly, i.e., to the mandible (except in the special case of hanging). Other combinations probably do not result in clinically distinguishable injuries: compressing and axially rotated; extending and axially rotated or laterally bent; lateral bending and flexed; extended or axially rotated.

After excluding these types from the 25 possible combinations, only 10 remain. These can be used to classify the full range of both upper and lower cervical injuries in a mechanistically clear manner. These are presented below, in the same order as they appear in Table 2 (Fig. 7).

Flexing/Flexed

A variety of radiographically different injuries are all produced in the flexing/flexed (FF) manner, and thus fall together in this category. Occipital-C1 dislocations are usually anterior (122,225,304) and apparently involve a flexing force, although the exact mechanism is not known. Usually these injuries are fatal and involve high energy input by contact with the head or are associated with multiple other injuries which make assessment difficult.

There are no typical C1 fractures known to be produced by this mechanism, although Mouradian et al. (197) found that an anteriorly directed pull on the occiput resulted in bilateral posterior arch fractures in 2 of 15 cadaveric specimens.

Acute traumatic C1-C2 subluxations (transverse ligament ruptures) presumably are produced by this same

TABLE 2. *Injuries categorized by force types and neck postures*

Load type	Neck posture				
	Flexed	Neutral	Extended	Axially rotated	Laterally bent

Flexing	Dens
	Spinous process
	Bilateral facet
	  dislocation
				Unilateral facet
				  dislocation
					Unilateral facet
					  dislocation

Compressing	Wedge
	Tear drop
		Jefferson
		Split
		Burst
			Spinous process
			Hyperextension
			  fracture/dislocation
					Lateral wedge
					Articular
					  compression
					Horizontal facet

Extending			Dens Avulsion		
Distracting			Hangman's		
Lateral Bending					Lateral wedge Articular compression Horizontal facet

mechanism but are usually fatal (94) and thus are not encountered often in clinical practice. Fielding et al. (94) found that the atlanto-dens interval was 3 to 5 mm just prior to failure from an anterior pull on C1 with C2 fixed. Thus, subluxation forward of more than 5 mm provides a strong argument that the transverse ligament is disrupted when there is a history of trauma in an otherwise normal patient.

Unilateral or "rotatory" dislocations apparently may occur by this FF mechanism (30) or may occur in a flexing/axially rotated (FA) or flexing/laterally bent (FL) manner.

Dens fractures have been conjectured to be caused by this mechanism, and Mouradian et al. (197) produced cadaveric specimen fractures in this manner. However, as will be discussed in the "Compressing/Flexed" section (this chapter), it appears more likely that some significant compressing component is needed as well.

Bilateral pars interarticular fractures of C2 (so called "hangman's fracture": see "Extending/Extended," this chapter) are more frequently reported to be caused with the neck extended, but flexing/flexed has also been described (66,282) based on the history and associated occipital scalp injuries. This probably is an uncommon occurrence.

In the lower cervical spine, spinous process fractures may occur. These may belong in the FF injury category, but may also be caused by an extending/extended (EE) mechanism. There has also been conjecture that these injuries may be caused by a lateral pull (304).

Also occurring in the lower cervical spine, bilateral facet subluxations or dislocations seem to be in this FF category. Bauze and Ardran (19) have produced this injury with anteriorly offset axial compression alone. However, the spinal specimen was immobilized in a manner somewhat different than usual, which raises some questions as to the clinical relevance of their result.

Various patterns of structural damage can occur. For example, a C4-C5 bilateral facet dislocation can occur either by failure of the C4-C5 interspinous ligament or by failure of the C3-C4 interspinous ligament plus bilateral laminar fractures of C4. Which of these occurs may well be influenced by subtle variations in the relative strength of the two different interspinous ligaments, rather than by the details of the force applied to the head.

Flexing/Axially Rotated and Flexing/Laterally Bent

The FA and FL categories probably may be combined because they do not produce clinically distinguishable spinal damage. Both involve asymmetric loading, and can result in unilateral facet fracture subluxation or dislocation on the side opposite to that toward which the axial rotation or lateral bending occurred.

Presumably a unilateral facet dislocation could also occur even without any asymmetric forces. For this to happen there must be sufficient asymmetry in facet joint capsular strength and the injuring force must be strong enough to tear the weaker but not the stronger facet capsule. In these circumstances, the upper vertebra flexes forward and axially rotates about the stronger facet joint as the weaker facet joint dislocates. Thus, it is possible for a unilateral facet dislocation to be produced by loads other than an applied axial torque.

Compressing

Four injury categories are grouped together here. The force type for each is the same (compressing), but the neck posture for each is different. One special feature of this group of injury categories is that the injuring force almost always results from contact between the head and some object. Forces arising from momentum of the head during deceleration are usually not great enough to produce such injuries. Another special feature is that the injuring force passes along the spine close to or directly through the injury site. This is in contrast to all the other force types that generally lie approximately in the transverse plane of the head and are thus relatively far from the typical mid or lower cervical injury site. Thus, even a small change from the neutral position into flexion, extension, or lateral bending will cause the compressing force vector to fall anteriorly, posteriorly, or laterally to the vertebral bodies. Each of these postures will in turn result in structurally quite different injuries (Fig. 16) (208,322).

This effect of neck posture on injury pattern produced by compressive loading has been shown by various investigators (7,184,208,322) who have studied experimental injuries in cadaveric spine specimens. An anterior movement of the upper cervical spine of only 1 cm was enough to convert the buckling pattern from extension to flexion in axially compressed cadaveric specimens (184).

To understand this effect it may be helpful to consider separately the externally applied force (compressing) and the internally derived forces resulting from neck posture (Fig. 7). For example, the flexed posture produces compression at the front of the vertebral body and tension posteriorly (Fig. 7A). A superimposed compressing force will further increase the compressive loads anteriorly, but will neutralize and reverse the posterior tensile loads to produce small compressive loads posteriorly. As a result, no tensile failure occurs posteriorly and compressive failure is worst anteriorly (wedge fracture).

Compressing/Flexed

In the upper cervical spine, dens fractures can be caused either by compressing/flexed, compressing/extended, or compressing/laterally bent mechanisms.

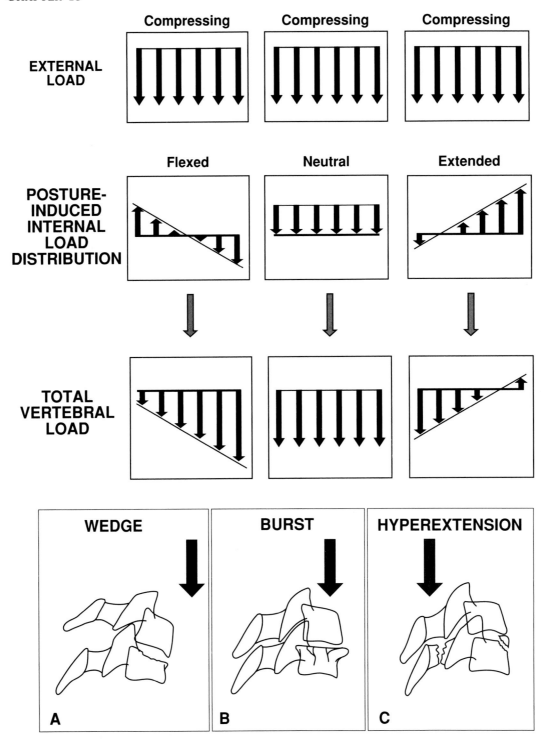

FIG. 7. Effect of neck posture on total vertebral loads during compression injuries. **A:** Compressing/flexed: Anteriorly, large compressive loads are present which cause vertebral compression. Posteriorly, the loads are also compressive, which prevents tensile failures. **B:** Compressing/neutral: Uniform load distribution results in a burst fracture. **C:** Compressing/extended: Anteriorly, only slight tensile loads occur, causing an avulsion fracture. Posteriorly, the compressive loads cause laminar fractures.

These three mechanisms of injury have been demonstrated by Althoff (7) in carefully performed impact loadings of cadaveric specimens. The key feature is the presence of a compressing force passing near to the dens. This is contrary to the various clinically based conjectures of pure flexion, extension, or shear mechanisms without a compressive component (7) which simply are not borne out by experimental injury production. The only other major report of experimentally produced dens fractures was by Mouradian et al. (197) who found that flexing/flexed or lateral bending/laterally bent mechanisms could produce dens fractures. However neither Althoff (7) nor Blockey and Purser (23) could produce injuries in this manner. The probable explanation is that Mouradian et al. (197) held the C2 vertebra fixed during injury production, which is quite different from the in vivo situation. Neither of the other reports used this technique.

Indirect evidence in support of these experimentally based compression mechanisms is the clinical observation that forceful contact with the head is required. Momentum of the head alone during decelerations (e.g., flexing/flexed or extending/extended) is not sufficient to produce this injury (10,55,134,206).

Both compressing/flexed and compressing/extended seem to be more common causes than the compression/laterally bent mechanism. Of 25 cases of dens fractures in which the mechanism of injury seemed fairly clear, Mouradian et al. (197) found that 16/20 were struck from behind, while 4/20 were struck from in front. Corresponding values in the review by Blockey and Purser (23) were 8/51 and 6/51 (with 37/51 not clear). White and Panjabi (304) state that an extension mechanism is more common, but no supportive data are provided.

It should be kept in mind that the residual displacement for an injury as hypermobile as a dens fracture may be very different from, even opposite in direction to, the displacement at the instant of injury. For example, even though a dens fracture may be caused by an extending force resulting in transient posterior displacement, the initial x-ray may show anterior residual displacement. Although anterior residual displacement is clearly more common than posterior displacement (23,55,134), the injury mechanism cannot necessarily be inferred from this observation.

It is not clear what determines whether an anteriorly directed force will produce a transverse ligament tear or a dens fracture. Only the former were produced by anterior loading applied to the ring of C1 (94), while both injury types (nine specimens with dens fractures, three with ligament tears) were produced by anterior loading applied to the occiput (197). This probably is an example of the way in which subtle relative variations in strength determine injury pattern: if the dens is slightly weaker than the transverse ligament, a fracture will occur and vice versa, even though the force direction and magnitude are constant (158).

In the lower cervical region, the combination of the external compressing force and the internal force distribution from the flexed posture tends to produce a wedge fracture initially (Fig. 7A), and a "tear-drop" fracture (with its typical sagittal plane component) if the compressing force is large enough. The rate of load application may also be important in determining which of these injuries occurs. The name "tear drop" is vague and

has meant very different things to different authors. Harris (122) summarizes the major literature and uses the terms "flexion tear-drop fracture-dislocation" and "extension tear-drop fractures" to distinguish between two very different types of tear drop. The former designation is that originally described by Schneider and Kahn (258) and used by others (2,20,21,100,103,224,234,242). This generally is a very "unstable" injury. The latter designation (Fig. 8) involves avulsion of the anterior-inferior corner of the vertebral body (130,227,246).

The displacement associated with the less extensive wedge fracture is not usually sufficient to cause severe disruption of the interspinous ligament or facet capsules. In addition, the posterior body height is usually maintained and the inferior end plate is intact. The more severe "flexion tear-drop fracture-dislocation" involves inferior end plate disruption both anteriorly and posteriorly and often bilateral facet subluxation as well. The interspinous ligament may also be torn.

Compressing/Neutral

In the upper cervical spine, the compressing/neutral combination results in a Jefferson fracture. Jefferson's contribution (137) was to call attention to two features of this injury: it is by no means necessarily fatal, and the mechanism of injury is tensile failure of the C1 ring, produced by an axial compressive force acting on the wedge-shaped lateral masses. It is interesting that none of Jefferson's own four cases and only three of the 25 cases described in his comprehensive literature review had four-part fractures (most were two-part fractures). Fur-

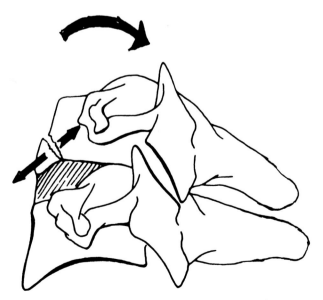

FIG. 8. Extension tear-drop fracture mechanism.

thermore, Jefferson did not attach any special significance to the number of fractured parts of the C1 ring. Thus "Jefferson fracture" should refer not only to four-part, but also to two- or three-part C1 fractures. Landells and Van Peteghem (161) have described a classification of these injuries.

If the resulting spread between the two lateral masses becomes too great, the transverse portion of the cruciform ligament will become torn, allowing anterior subluxation of C1 on C2. Spence et al. (275) tested 10 cadaveric Oc-C1-C2 specimens and showed that transverse ligament rupture occurred at a mean of 6.3 mm (range 4.8–7.6 mm) increased C1 lateral diameter. The tensile strength of this ligament is quite large: 350 N according to Dvorak et al. (82).

In the lower cervical spine, this injury mechanism produces a force distribution across the superior end plate that is fairly uniform (Fig. 6B). Because the uncinate processes support the inferior end plate along its lateral edges, vertebral body failure may occur along the sagittal plane where the stresses are highest. This may be the explanation for the "vertical compression fracture" (24,30,163,232,242), which is also one component of the true "tear-drop fracture-dislocation" described above.

With higher forces, burst fractures occur with typically extensive fragmentation of the entire vertebral body, but usually without much disruption to the facet capsules. There is no consensus on the relation of burst fractures to "tear-drop fracture-dislocation." Some authors have regarded these terms to mean significantly different injuries (53,103,122,224,234,258), while others have considered the tear drop to be a specific type of burst or to be synonymous with burst (20,21,130,242). Until the definitions are made more explicit and the mechanical characteristics of each are established, it is not clear whether this distinction is important.

Compressing/Extended

In the upper cervical spine, dens fractures can be produced in the compressing/extended manner, as discussed in the "Compressing/Flexed" section above (this chapter). This mechanism also may produce a bilateral pars interarticularis fracture of C2, as suggested by Cornish (62). For example, this may occur to an inadequately restrained driver in a deceleration automobile accident whose forehead strikes against the windshield with the upper neck in extension. This same injury can also be caused by the extending/extended and flexing/flexed mechanisms. Williams (315) emphasized the difference between these mechanisms and those occurring in a judicial hanging in which distraction is also present.

In the lower cervical spine, the extended posture results in compression along the posterior annulus and tension along the anterior annulus. Even with the superimposed compressing force, small tensile forces may re-

main anteriorly, with large compressive forces occurring posteriorly. In the lower cervical spine, the resulting injury does not have a widely agreed-upon name but has been described by Forsyth (97) as a hyperextension fracture-dislocation, and even more clearly by Allen et al. (5,6) as a subtype of a "compressive extension" injury. The injury includes tensile failure anteriorly and bending failure posteriorly of both lateral masses and/or laminae, or of the spinous process.

Compressing/Laterally Bent and Lateral Bending/Laterally Bent

Clear separation between the compressing/laterally bent (CL) and lateral bending/laterally bent (LL) injury mechanisms is not presently feasible in terms of the structural damage produced. Dens fractures were produced by Althoff (7) by this mechanism, as discussed in the "Compressing/Flexed" section above (this chapter). In the lower cervical spine, lateral wedge fractures involve asymmetric collapse of the upper end plate. Unilateral articular process compression may produce a triangular rather than diamond-shaped lateral mass (312) seen on lateral x-ray, or may fracture the pedicle and lamina which allows the entire lateral mass to rotate (97). Brachial plexus injuries can often be associated with these injuries (233).

Extending/Extended

Occipital dislocations in the posterior direction are placed into the extending/extended (EE) category, although these occur more commonly in an anterior direction. Bilateral C1 laminar fractures, either in isolation or in combination with a C2 bilateral pars interarticularis fracture, probably result from an extension mechanism (92,304), although the details are not clear and this injury certainly can be produced experimentally by a flexing/flexed injury mechanism (197). Perhaps the Oc-C1 joint is extended enough so that the capsular ligaments of these joints force the C1 arch down against the C2 spinous process. Alternatively, since the Oc-C1 joint extends posteriorly to the C1-C2 joint, perhaps instead it is a downward and backward thrust of the occipital condyles that causes the C1-C2 hyperextension. Another speculation is that the compression of the C1 arch between the occiput and C2 arch during hyperextension is the cause (270). White and Panjabi (304) conjecture that the hyperextending occiput may push downward on the arch of C1, while C1-C2 motion is blocked.

Dens fractures appear to require a compressing force component for their causation either in the extended, flexed, or laterally bent postures (discussed above). The major point to be made here is that these can be very unstable injuries and the method of reduction is determined by the residual displacement, not necessarily by the mechanism of injury.

Bilateral pars interarticularis fractures of C2 can be caused by an extending/extended mechanism, but also by flexing/flexed, compressing/extended, or distracting/extended mechanisms as discussed further in the respective sections (this chapter). Various authors report injuries involving force applied to the face or chin without apparent compressing or distracting force (179,259,282). There appear to be no well-documented reports concerning frequency of these different injuring mechanisms, but those involving an extended posture of the upper cervical spine seem to be more common.

In the lower cervical spine bony failure may occur in the form of an avulsion injury of the antero-inferior part of the body (180) (Fig. 8), or by a bending failure of a spinous process to strike the one below it. Typically the spinous process fragment remains slightly tipped up (312), which distinguishes this injury from a clay shoveler's fracture (FF injury type). Extension sufficient to cause substantial cord damage may occur even when there is no spinous process fracture or any other apparent spinal column disruption (227). This cord injury can result from shortening and inward bulging of the ligamentum flavum and shortening and thickening of the cord itself, since both of these structures are located behind the center of rotation (see "Spinal Cord, Dura, and Nerve Roots," this chapter).

Distracting/Extended

Cervical spine injuries do not often occur in the distracting/extended (DE) manner because it is only under very special circumstances that a longitudinal distracting force can be applied to the neck. An upward blow to the chin can produce quite forceful extension, but only a modest longitudinal force. Backward motion of the head tends to cause loss of further contact with the injuring object, preventing further distraction. The obvious exception is judicial hanging (with the knot under the chin) in which the circumferential noose allows application of substantial distracting force as well as extension. The resulting injury is a bilateral pars interarticularis fracture, or so-called hangman's fracture (318). Because this name so vividly conveys the sense of a distracting force and because none of the other causes of this injury involve significant distraction (i.e., flexing/flexed, compressing/extended, extending/extended), the name "hangman's fracture" should be reserved for injuries resulting from this one very special mechanism.

MECHANICAL SUPPORT BY INTERNAL FIXATION

Development of surgically implanted devices for mechanical support of the cervical spine extends back almost a century to Hadra's use of posterior spinous process wiring in 1891 (116,117) and has continued to the present at an increasingly rapid rate. Along with internal fixation, bone graft has come to be used almost universally as well, based on the recognition that over time implant loosening is highly likely without solid bone fusion. It is almost prophetic that in Hadra's original case, in which no bone graft was used, the wire slipped "after some weeks" and reoperation was performed. Thus, very few recent series have been reported in which bone graft was not used, although there certainly have been some, both for trauma (75,132,149,186,271,286), rheumatoid arthritic upper cervical spine subluxation (32,149), and spinal tumors (see "Polymethylmethacrylate" below, this chapter).

An integral part of spinal implants has been our improved understanding of spinal and implant biomechanics. Summaries of this topic are contained in various recent works (267,300,304).

Upper Cervical Spine

Wires

Wiring of C1-C2 has been attempted through a wide variety of posterior techniques. The forerunner of these was use of a "stout braided silk . . . passed about (the C1) posterior arch . . . [and] firmly anchored by tying the silk band about the [C2] spinous process . . ." by Mixter and Osgood (192). Willard and Nicholson (314) used a strip of fascia lata and both ends were pulled through a loop passed around the arch of C1 (Fig. 9A). Although this pattern is widely attributed to Gallie, neither of Gallie's early works (101,102) make any mention of vertebral levels or the wiring pattern used. Although at least one standard textbook (64) refers to Mixter and Osgood (192) for the method, those authors used only a single strand of silk suture passed once around the C1 lamina and under the C2 spinous process. Rogers (239), who really popularized wire fixation for trauma management, described two cases involving C1. In both cases, only a single strand of wire was passed around the C1 arch. Thus it appears that the "Gallie" wiring pattern should really be attributed to Willard and Nicholson (Fig. 9A).

In response to a fairly high non-union rate with these previous wiring patterns, a number of other techniques were developed in the last twenty years which were intended to provide improved motion control. A bone graft was incorporated under the single loop of wire by McGraw and Rusch (185) (Fig. 9B). Variations of this technique were described by a number of authors (8,68,95,173,319). Two separate grafts (one on each side) contoured to fit between the laminae were wired into place using either one loop (42,274) (Fig. 9C) or two loops (114) of wire on each side (Fig. 9D). Presumably

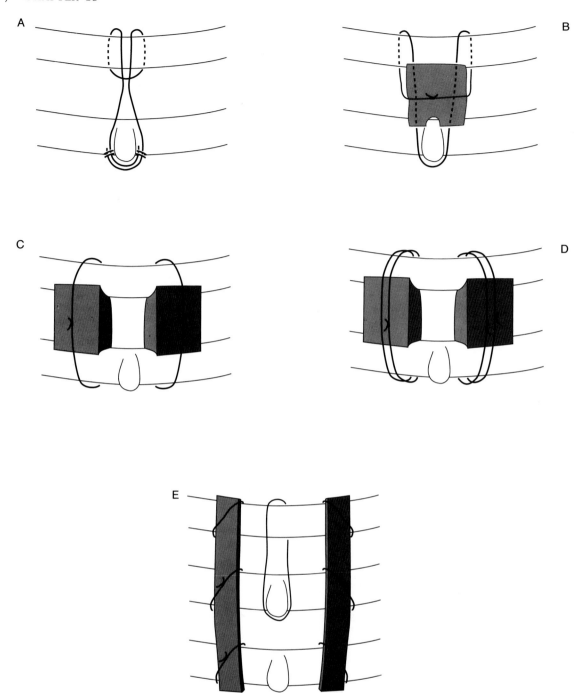

FIG. 9. Posterior wiring and bone graft methods for C1-C2. **A:** Willard and Nicholson, 1941 (314), the so-called "Gallie." **B:** McGraw and Rusch, 1973 (185). **C:** Brooks and Jenkins, 1978 (42). **D:** Griswold et al., 1978 (114). **E:** Forsyth et al., 1959 (98).

due to the improved motion control gained by the latter two methods, fusion rates of 94% and 97%, respectively, were achieved.

In order to obtain or maintain reduction of a C1 anterior subluxation, a posteriorly directed force would be the most effective. None of the C1-C2 wiring and grafting techniques described above are particularly strong in this regard because the graft and wire can flex forward by

rotating about the lamina of C2. To overcome this, Forsyth et al. (98) used rib allograft anchored by circumlaminar wires at C2 and at C3 (Fig. 9E). The C1 wire is thus able to provide anterior-posterior position control in a more secure manner. The effectiveness of this compared to other techniques is hard to judge because most reports of C1-C2 techniques do not describe the residual subluxation after graft healing.

Instead of C2 and C3, another alternative is to use C2 and the occiput for provision of the two "anchor points" for anterior-posterior control of C1. A variety of wiring methods for this technique exist and have been reviewed elsewhere (67,113,250). In the first of these occipital holes for wire fixation were used, as described in 1960 (236). Various graft patterns have been used, e.g., a single unicortical iliac plate (67,250) or bilateral bicortical iliac strips (113).

Because of the greater mobility at Oc-C1 than at C2-C3 and because of the greater difficulty in attaching to the occiput than to C3, the C1-C2-C3 method seems preferable to the Oc-C1-C2 method. Crellin et al. (63) refer to persistent symptoms if the Oc-C1 joint is not included (for rheumatoid arthritis patients), but many studies have had good results by fusing only C1-C2 without including the occiput. There have been no studies comparing these various techniques.

Screws

The attachment of C1 to C2 by posterior wires is prevented if the C1 lamina is hypoplastic, fractured, or surgically removed. To handle such cases, screws may be placed across the C1-C2 articular surfaces on each side. This can be accomplished using two screws oriented approximately in the coronal plane, inserted using a lateral approach on each side of C1 (17,77,269) as shown in Figs. 10A and 10B. Magerl (176) described another method used through a single posterior incision (Fig. 10C). Each screw enters one of the C2 inferior articular processes from below, angles upward and forward across the C1-C2 joint, crosses the lateral mass of C1 obliquely, and just penetrates through its anterior cortex. This Magerl technique is significantly stronger and stiffer than the so-called Gallie wiring, as shown by mechanical testing of cadaveric spine specimens (120). Supplemental posterior wiring can be done in combination with the screws. Magerl and Seeman have had favorable results with this technique in 23 patients (176), all of whom fused without any reduction loss. Neither this nor the Barbour lateral screw fixation are simple techniques, however, and one should have a solid understanding of the anatomical details before attempting them (see Chapters 44 and 46).

A fractured dens can be reattached to the C2 body by means of a screw or screws placed from below (Figs. 11A and 11B). This method apparently was first reported in 1982 (26,199) and has been used by others since then (88). Knöringer (151) devised a screw which has no head, but rather a second short segment of somewhat larger diameter threads, in an effort to reduce soft tissue irritation or C2-C3 disc damage. Although clinical results have been encouraging, this is a technically demanding close-tolerance procedure, and its risk to benefit ratio relative to that of other methods of treating dens mechanical insufficiency remains to be well established.

Plates and Rods

In an effort to improve on the security of wired-in bone grafts for fusions between the occiput and the upper cervical spine, metallic implants have been tried. These have been attached to the cranium either by wires in various ways [Luque rods (135), Luque rectangles (40,181,228), Harrington rods (198)] or by screws (91,128,246). Opinions vary as to whether the occipital screws should penetrate the inner cortex (246) or not (128).

For C1-C2 fusions, various types of clamp and rod systems have been described, such as the "Halifax clamp" (132,286) and others (191,241). Anterior plates in the upper cervical region have a very limited application: the only report seems to be that of Streli (278–280) who used a cruciate plate for C1-C2-C3 fixation of dens fractures.

Lower Cervical Spine

Spinous Process and Laminar Wires

As mentioned previously, Hadra (116,117) appears to have performed the earliest cervical wiring. Details of the method are not given except that the wire was passed "four to five times around [the C6-C7 spinous processes] in a figure of 8." Details of the revision, after the wire slipped off, are not given. Gallie (101,102) also gives no details of his method except that "the spines of the two vertebrae involved" were fastened "together with fine steel wire." Details were first presented by Ryerson and Christopher (249) in their case report. At first the wire went through the middle of the spinous process of C6 and of C7 in a simple loop and no bone graft was used. After the C6 spinous process fractured at nine weeks, the wire was repositioned around the C6 lamina and under the C7 spinous process; this time a bone graft was used.

The first series of patients was reported by Rogers (239). Forsyth et al. (98) simplified and strengthened the wiring pattern by placing it under the entirety of the lower spinous process and through the upper spinous process, in particular "near the top of [its] base," thereby decreasing the likelihood of spinous process failure. Bohlman (28) modified the Rogers technique by adding two additional transverse wires to hold unicortical bone graft plates against the spinous processes. Other methods have also been reported (255,265).

No clear differences between these wiring methods have been shown in terms of clinical outcome. The Forsyth pattern is probably the simplest to perform and has the largest amount of the upper spinous process enclosed

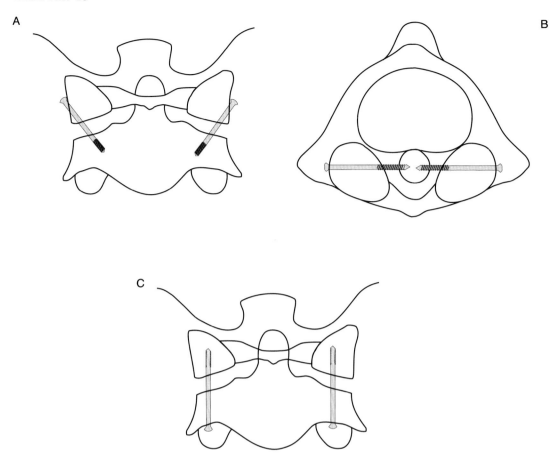

FIG. 10. Screw fixation of C1-C2. **A and B:** Barbour, 1971 (17): anterior and cephalad views. **C:** Magerl et al., 1987 (175).

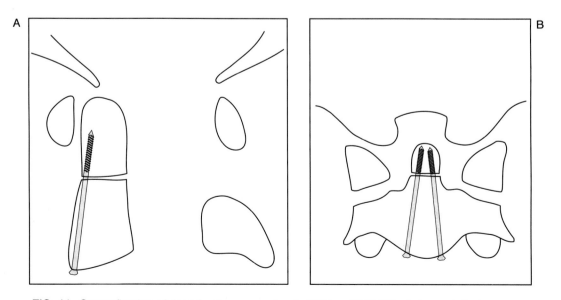

FIG. 11. Screw fixation of dens fracture according to Böhler, 1982 (26). **A:** Lateral. **B:** Anterior.

within the wire loop. The additional neurological risks of wire passage around the lamina instead of the spinous processes (30,89) seem unnecessary and ill advised unless spinous process fractures are present.

Concerning the diameter of the wire, Rogers (239) used "Babcock stainless steel #24 wire," Forsyth et al. (98) used "20 gauge wire," and McAfee (183) used 20 gauge for the main wire and 24 gauge for the transverse wires. Robinson and Southwick (235) preferred two strands of 24 or 26 gauge wire twisted together since its lower flexural rigidity allowed easier handling (304). Wang et al. (294) have shown that twisting the wire ends together is not as strong as knotting. Despite this, the convenience, adjustability, and very low failure rate of twisting is probably why it has been used in all the methods described above.

Articular Process ("Facet") Wires

Wires passed through the inferior articular process (perpendicular to the articular surface) provide a useful vertebral attachment when the laminae are absent (e.g., fractured or excised). Robinson and Southwick (236) first described the method in which multiple laminectomized vertebrae are tethered to a lower cervical spinous process. This was later modified (49) so that the articular process wires were tied around a longitudinal tricortical iliac graft on each side. Recently, others have tied these wires around Harrington compression rods instead (106,198). This construct has been shown (111) in vitro to restrict cervical spine motion to approximately 20% of that seen in the intact spine. This technique is safe and effective for dealing with difficult multi-level laminectomies. Although it may not provide as much rigidity as posterior plates, the graft bed is not obstructed as much and the risk of screw penetration through the anterior cortex of the lateral mass is entirely eliminated.

Articular process wires are also useful for dealing with superior articular process fractures (48). The wire passes obliquely from the intact inferior articular process of the superjacent vertebra, down and around the spinous process of the fractured vertebra. This provides a "de-rotating" force to prevent axial rotation and unilateral forward subluxation. This may be reinforced by an additional wire around both spinous processes. Articular process oblique wiring alone is useful even if the spinous process or lamina of the upper vertebra is fractured or excised.

Hooks and Rods

In 1963 Tucker (286) began using an implant very much like a miniature Harrington compression rod. The hooks were shaped to fit around the upper or lower laminar edges, and were connected by a threaded bolt. A large clinical series of trauma patients was reported by Holness et al. (132) from Halifax. In neither series was bone graft used. Although in two of the 51 patients the clamp slipped soon after surgery, there were no late failures. Patients were followed 1 to 10 years, and spontaneous bone fusion was present in all 32 of the patients who were followed for longer than 4 years.

No clinical or mechanical comparison between this implant and spinous process wires appears to have yet been made; the relative usefulness of these two can thus be conjectured only. The rod surely is stronger than a standard 20 gauge wire loop, which probably would fatigue fracture before spontaneous bone fusion occurred if no bone graft were placed. On the other hand, Halifax clamp placement requires dissection into the spinal canal and the implant is larger than a wire and may cause soft tissue irritation.

Load-Bearing Bone Grafts

Although not strictly implants, anterior interbody grafts do function in a load-bearing capacity. An inlay graft was first used in 1952 at the University of Michigan (15). This graft was $\frac{1}{2}''$ wide and $\frac{3}{16}''$ deep and thus did not have large load-bearing capacity. In 1954 Robinson and Smith (234a) at Johns Hopkins University began the use of a tricortical or "horseshoe" graft placed between adjacent vertebrae. A smaller loss of interbody height was noted when the end plates were left intact than when they were removed. Cloward in 1956 began the use of a unicortical, dowel-shaped graft (57). Simmons and Bhalla used a trapezoidal tricortical "keystone" graft (268) and Whitecloud and Larocca (307) used a fibular graft.

Mechanical testing (300) has shown that the dowel graft is 82% and the inlay graft is only 64% as strong as the tricortical graft in compression testing. Failure occurred mainly by the graft's sinking into the upper or lower vertebra. Thus the tricortical construct graft was stronger primarily because the end plates were left intact.

Anterior displacement of the graft has occasionally been a problem, both for the Cloward (146) and the tricortical patterns (143). One solution to this problem is to use a "double mortise and tenon" graft (277), the upper and lower tabs of which prevent displacement (Figs. 12A and 12B).

Posterior Plates

These have been used since the 1950s, according to Roy-Camille and Saillant (243) who have developed an extensive set of flat plates for use throughout the cervical spine (244–246). The screws are placed through holes 13 mm apart, enter the middle of the lateral mass at the most dorsally prominent location, and are directed 10

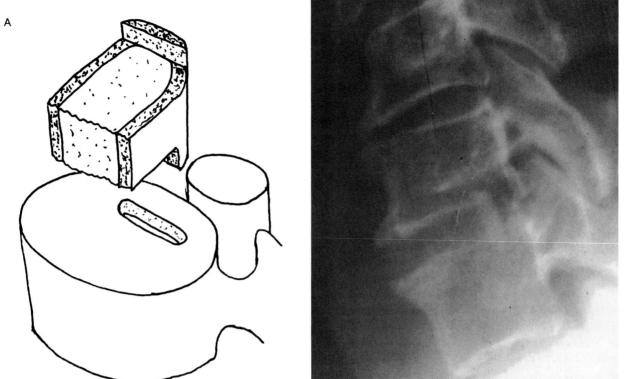

FIG. 12. A: Displacement prevented by "mortise and tenon" graft. B: Lateral x-ray of "mortise and tenon" graft.

degrees laterally to avoid the vertebral artery. Because spontaneous fusion was seen to occur, Roy-Camille does not use a bone graft (246). He claims no post-operative displacement in 85%, and 5 degrees or greater displacement in only 6 of 221 patients. Details of follow-up and measurement method are not given. Other authors (61,74,83,254) report favorable experience with this method, and additional information on other systems is also available (172,252).

A "hook plate" was described by Magerl et al. (175) (Fig. 13), the lower end of which hooks under the lamina, just medial to the facet joint. The upper end is attached by a screw oriented parallel to the facet joint (Fig. 13B) and anterolaterally 10 degrees (Fig. 13C), which is intended to be placed through the anterior cortex of the lateral mass. The advantages of this system are that there are two fewer drill holes to be made and the screws are oriented obliquely upward and through the anterior cortex of the lateral mass, which presumably strengthens the screw attachment.

Montesano and Juach (193) compared two different screw placement methods using the same plate with each: 20 to 22 mm screws placed obliquely (parallel to the articular facets), and 12 to 14 mm screws directed anteriorly. The former method was stiffer and failed by plate bending, whereas the latter failed by screw pullout. Issues remaining to be studied include determining

whether the anterior cortex should be penetrated, and the safest insertion method for avoiding a nerve root or vertebral artery.

Anterior Plates

Initial efforts began in 1964 (25) and used plates that were not specifically designed for the cervical spine (39,127). In 1971 the first specially designed plates began to be used, both by Senegas and Gauzere (164) and by Oroszco and Tapies (27). Both early designs have apparently evolved to a virtually identical five-hole "H" plate in use since 1975 (27). Other plate designs have also evolved, e.g., those by Caspar (51), Oliveira (202), Fuentes et al. (100), and Streli (279). Some of these have been reviewed elsewhere (296).

One of the big concerns regarding use of these plates is screw loosening and resultant esophageal irritation or loss of fixation. The rate of screw loosening with the early plate designs, which allowed only one screw per vertebra, was higher according to Weidner (296) than the new plates which allow two screws per vertebra. A summary of results from reports on the latter is in Table 3: the overall loosening rate is 3%, which is quite low. Irritation from the plate itself has not been reported. Cadaveric testing by Sandor and Antal (251,253) showed that

A

B

C

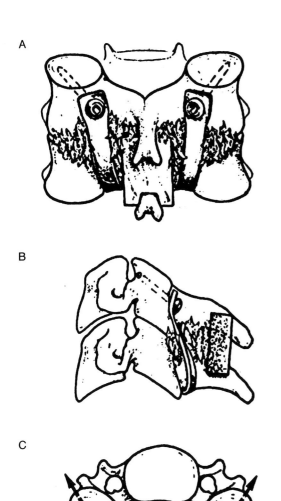

FIG. 13. Hook plate. **A:** Posterior. **B:** Lateral. **C:** Screw orientation in axial view.

screw torque fall-off with 10,000 flexion-extension cycles was quite small, which is consistent with the clinical experience.

How important is it to insert the screw through the posterior cortex? As shown in Table 3, the overall loosening rate for screws not through the posterior cortex (43,47,164) is 2.4% (4/166 patients). For screws that do penetrate the posterior cortex (27,51,202,283), the rate is a virtually identical 2.9% (4/139). Thus, penetrating the posterior cortex does not seem to provide an advantage. This comparison should only be made cautiously, however, because these studies varied in patient diagnosis, post-operative bracing regimen, and follow-up length.

In order to further reduce the screw loosening, modified screws have been designed. Lesoin et al. (165) developed an "expansion screw," the diameter of the dorsal end of which could be increased by a set screw. Morscher et al. (196) have taken a similar approach, although the set screw expands the ventral end of the screw against the hole in the plate, rather than the dorsal end against bone. In addition, the Morscher screw is hollow and fenestrated to allow bony ingrowth, and is made of titanium.

The other big concern with these plates is spinal cord damage by drill bit or screw, especially if the posterior cortex is deliberately penetrated. Drill guides and image intensifiers should be used very carefully to prevent overpenetration. It is encouraging that in none of the reported 318 patients (Table 3) was there any apparent cord damage.

Although the exact role that these plates have in cervical spine surgery remains to be further defined, they clearly can be useful for high-grade mechanical insufficiency, and may prevent the need for a second posterior procedure. The reported non-union rate of 0% (Table 3) is a bit difficult to completely believe, but if true is certainly an improvement over non-plated anterior graftings. In addition, graft extrusions have been virtually eliminated because the plate prevents anterior shifting, and the screw into the graft prevents posterior shifting.

TABLE 3. *Use of plates: Study results*

Reference	Posterior cortex	Plate type	Post-operative bracing	No. of patients	Increased deficit	Screws loose	Non-union
Bohler (27)	Through	Oroszco "H"	No casts	21	0	0	0
Caspar (51)	Through	Caspar	None	50	0	8 (4/50)	0
Tippets (283)	Through	Caspar	None	28	0	0	0
Oliveira (202)	Through	Oporto "H"	Collar	40	0	0	?
				139		2.9%	
Lesoin (164)	14 mm	Senegas "H"	Collar	145	0	1 (2/145)	?
Brown (43)	Not into	Oroszco "H"	Minerva	13	0	15 (2/13)	0
Cabanela (47)	To, not through	Oroszco "H"	Halo vest	8	0	0	0
				166		2.4%	
Gassman (107)	?	Oroszco "H"	Various	13	0	8 (1/13)	0
Weidner (295)	?	Oroszco "H"	None	62	0	5 (3/62)	10 (6/62)
				75		5.3%	

The header "Percent of patients with" spans the columns: Increased deficit, Screws loose, Non-union.

Comparative Mechanical Testing

Only a few studies have been done which compare a number of different fixation devices in vitro. All of these studies are limited by the usual factors affecting in vitro studies such as absence of muscles, lack of knowledge of in vivo load values, unknown relevance of the experimental "injury" to in vivo injuries, and absence of any healing processes. These limitations must be kept clearly in mind for accurate interpretation of these studies, and caution should be exercised to prevent "overinterpretation."

Gill et al. (109) compared interspinous process wiring (Forsyth pattern), Halifax clamps, 1/3 semi-tubular plates with unicortical screws and these same plates with bicortical screws. Individual intact motion segments were tested in flexion or extension using one at a time of each of three different implants per specimen. There was no statistically significant difference among any of the four implants.

Ulrich et al. (289) studied a posterior injury model at C5-C6 using an anterior "H" plate, a Magerl posterior hook plate, circumlaminar wiring, and various combinations of these, and found that the hook plates gave superior results, although their loading method (pull upward on the upper spinous process) may not be very relevant for the in vivo situation. Similar testing (252) compared posterior Roy-Camille type plates to combined anterior and posterior plating, and found little difference in terms of screw torque fall-off with 10,000 flexion-extension cycles.

The most extensive testing has been done by Coe et al. (58) on human specimens and, in a related study on bovine specimens in the same lab, by Sutterlin et al. (281). The former study compared intact specimens to those with extensive posterior damage: this consisted of cutting all connective tissue from posteriorly up through the dorsal half of the disc. The specimens were instrumented sequentially with: a) circumlaminar wires, b) Rogers spinous process wiring, c) Bohlman triple wiring, d) Roy-Camille posterior plates, e) Magerl posterior hook plate, f) Magerl posterior hook plate and Caspar anterior plate, and g) Caspar anterior plate alone. Six specimens were tested using each of five different load or displacement types. Quite low load values were used in order to prevent specimen damage, so multiple devices could be tested on each specimen. The major findings were the following: a) there were no significant differences between implants for many of the outcome measures (compression-induced anterior strain, axial rotational stiffness, flexion stiffness, extension stiffness, and fatigue flexion-load–induced flexion stiffness and anterior strain); b) circumlaminar wires were no better than spinous process wires; and c) the anterior plate alone was significantly less satisfactory than all other implants for compression- or flexion-induced posterior strain.

Polymethylmethacrylate

Broadly speaking, three approaches have evolved for the use of polymethylmethacrylate (PMMA) since its initial application to spinal problems (150). The most controversial of these is to use PMMA without bone graft in patients who do not have a short life expectancy. Kelly and co-workers (31,149,271) have reported a very favorable experience in treating otherwise healthy trauma patients with circumlaminar wires and PMMA, with follow-up of up to nine years. Duff (75) described the use of lateral mass bicortical screws linked longitudinally by PMMA in 26 trauma patients, eight of whom were followed for five years. A noteworthy report is that by Whitehill et al. (309). Twenty post-traumatic patients treated by posterior wiring and PMMA alone had their surgeries performed by the Department of Neurosurgery and their follow-ups performed by the Department of Orthopaedics. Eleven were found by x-ray not to be solid; four of these underwent further "stabilizing" surgery.

The second approach is to use PMMA in combination with bone grafting, for those situations in which additional strength is believed to be desirable, e.g., to forego post-operative bracing in a patient with severe rheumatoid arthritis. Brattström and Granholm (32) performed Oc-C1-C2 surgery for rheumatoid C1-C2 subluxation. They placed PMMA over the Oc-C1-C2 wire on one side and bone graft on the other side. In 28 patients there were two infections, two C2 spinous process fractures, and two broken wires. Bryan et al. (44) used a similar approach for 11 patients with complex rheumatoid deformities. They reported four instances of wound dehiscence, two of which were infected.

The third approach has been to use PMMA as a stop-gap measure in patients with very short life expectancies. The rationale is that death will occur before the potential long-term benefit of a solid bony fusion can be achieved, and thus the morbidity of bone graft harvest and the inconvenience of orthosis wear is not worth incurring. Scoville et al. (263) first used PMMA in this fashion to supplement occipito-cervical wiring for upper cervical metastases. Dunn (76) collected cases among members of the Cervical Spine Research Society and reported on 24 cases, all but four of whom were able to be mobilized by the third post-operative day with either no or minimal orthosis wear. A more recent series (153) of 18 patients has also demonstrated the utility of this approach, as have a number of other reports, some of which have also described use of bone graft with PMMA (52,54,119, 121,229). Various technical details concerning PMMA placement have been described including use of a metal spacer and a mold for PMMA containment (204).

There is fairly strong consensus concerning this third approach, less so for the second, and much less so for the first. The basic argument against the first approach

(PMMA and no bone graft in normal life expectancy patients) is that the bone-PMMA (or bone-metal-PMMA) interface will eventually weaken and lead to problems, either because of inadequate connective or bony tissue healing, or because of irritation to surrounding tissue due to motion. In addition, there is concern over an increased rate of infection, either post-operatively or from late hematogenous seeding. These concerns have been highlighted by a report of 24 cases (183) in which significant complications were encountered with the use of PMMA without bone grafting: 15 (14 cervical) for trauma and nine (eight cervical) for metastatic disease. The most common complication was loss of fixation, which occurred at a mean of 208 days (range 1–730 days), all instances of which were in posterior constructs. There were six deep wound infections, three of which occurred at more than four months post-operatively, one of which clearly occurred by hematogenous seeding after a dental procedure.

Whitehill et al. (308,311) studied PMMA fusions in dogs at various time points. They have clearly shown the ingrowth between PMMA and bone of a fibrous layer which weakened the overall construct, causing weakening of the PMMA-bone interface during the first month post-operatively. In contrast, the bone grafted spines were stronger by two months relative to normal spines. The postmortem mechanical testing by Panjabi et al. (207,209) is consistent with these experimental observations.

MECHANICAL SUPPORT BY ORTHOSES

A wide variety of designs has evolved and various classifications (124,141,142,316) for describing these orthoses have been suggested. Many of the terms have been based on certain structural characteristics (e.g., "4 poster") or place of origin (e.g., "Philadelphia collar"), which unfortunately conveys little meaning about the actual or intended function. Orthoses for the limbs have come to be named by the body parts they contact or immobilize: the same method is also useful for the spine. Wolf and Johnson (316) use the categories of cervical, head-cervical, head-cervical-thoracic, and halo devices. A somewhat different system (Table 4) is used here because a) the term "head" covers too wide a range and is too non-specific, and b) "halo devices" gets right back to using structural features for naming the device and thus departs from the principle of using the involved body parts for classifying the orthosis.

Certain basic principles should be kept in mind regarding orthoses and evaluations of their function. First, voluntarily produced neck motion (whether by normal or patient volunteers) is not necessarily the same as the motion occurring during activities of daily living. For example, soft foam rubber collars can easily be deformed

through almost a full normal range of motion (141), yet patients wearing a collar often actually move far less than this allowable range. Another example involving the halo vest shows that cervical spine flexion-extension motion was found to be significantly larger between lying down and sitting up (152,170,171) than between voluntarily produced flexed and extended postures in seated volunteers (22,141,189).

A second principle is that the relationship between motions and loads (forces or moments) in the neck is quite complex. Radiographic measures of motion alone do not give a full understanding of the load distributions, and ultimately it is the latter that produces, for example, a loss of reduction or undesired intervertebral motion.

A third principle is that muscle forces probably are important in determining outcomes with orthoses (306). This is illustrated by the observation that patients seem to seldom "hang" on their orthoses, even halo vests. Its importance remains to be studied.

A final principle is that short-term biomechanical performance outcomes are not necessarily the same as longer-term clinical outcomes, such as maintaining reduction, obtaining fusion, or preventing neurological deficit increase. No studies appear to have been done comparing devices in terms of clinical outcome.

Categories of Upper Spinal Orthoses

Cervical

These orthoses (Fig. 14) commonly referred to as neck collars derive little or no support from either the occiput or mandible above, or from the thorax below. They are made of various materials, ranging from soft foam rubber to fairly non-compressible polyethylene. Probably more than any other orthoses, these devices function as "reminders" to restrict motion, rather than to actually mechanically prevent or block motion (8,59,141).

Occipito-Mandibular-Cervical

These orthoses extend cephalad to contact and restrict motion of the mandible (especially the chin) and/or the

TABLE 4. Cervical orthoses

Category	Example
Cervical	Collar
Occipito-mandibular-cervical	Collar and chin piece
	Queen Anne collar
Occipito-mandibular-high thoracic	Philadelphia
	4-poster
Occipito-mandibular-low thoracic	Extended Philadelphia
	SOMI
Cranio-thoracic	Minerva
	Halo vest

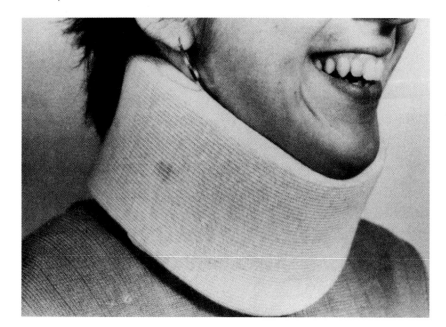

FIG. 14. Cervical orthosis (soft collar).

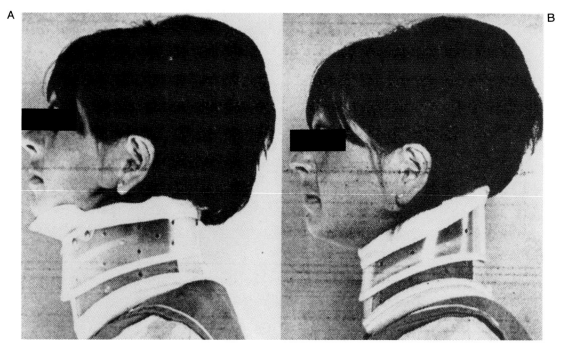

FIG. 15. Occipito-mandibular-cervical orthoses. **A:** Collar with chin extension. **B:** Queen Anne collar.

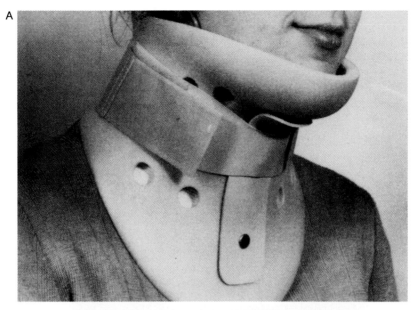

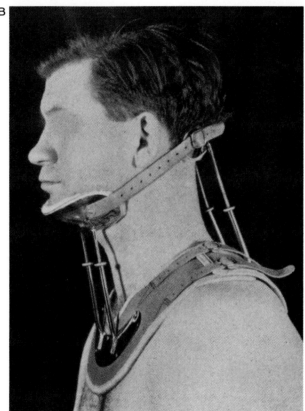

FIG. 16. Occipito-mandibular-high thoracic orthoses. **A:** Philadelphia collar. **B:** Thomas collar (''4 poster'').

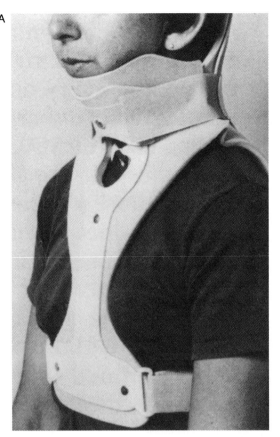
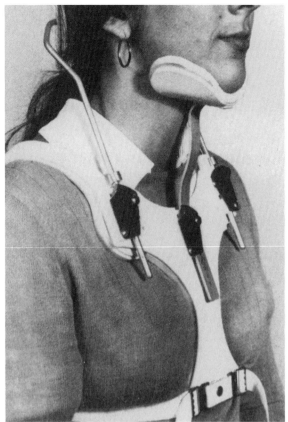

FIG. 17. Occipito-mandibular-low thoracic orthoses. **A:** Extended Philadelphia collar. **B:** Sternal-Occipital-Mandibular Immobilizer (SOMI).

occiput to a greater or lesser extent depending on the material stiffness. The thorax is not gripped to a significant extent. Examples of these are the collar with chin piece (Fig. 15A) and Queen Anne collar (Fig. 15B), motion restriction by which was reported by Colachis et al. (59).

Occipito-Mandibular-High Thoracic

These extend caudally to the upper portion of the sternum and interscapular region. Addition of a chin cup restricts axial motion as well as flexion. Examples include the semi-rigid Philadelphia collar (Fig. 16A) and the much stiffer "4-poster" (141), also known as an adjustable Thomas collar (239), shown in Fig. 16B. The straps connecting front and back halves on both of these designs are flexible.

Occipito-Mandibular-Low Thoracic

These extend along the length of the sternum anteriorly and along much or all of the thoracic spine posteriorly. The extended Philadelphia collar (Fig. 17A), "Yale brace" (140), SOMI (sternal occipital mandibular immobilizer) (Fig. 17B), and "cervico-thoracic orthosis" (124,141) are examples.

Cranio-Thoracic

The cephalad attachment for these includes (or in the case of the halo vest is limited to) the cranium. The Minerva cast contacts almost the entirety of the head, including occiput and mandible. The thermoplastic Minerva jacket (22,189) is not clearly described in terms of occipital or mandibular contact, but includes a circumferential head band. To prevent obstruction of mandibular motion (to allow emergency airway management) and yet maintain good cranial control, Rubin et al. (247) designed a Minerva-like device which uses pads under and in front of both zygomatic arches.

The vest portion of the halo vest originally was made of plaster (200,223) as shown in Fig. 18A. In the 1970's it was made from plastic (Fig. 18B), but without a major design change. Recently it has undergone substantial redesign to improve its grip on the thorax (154), as shown in Fig. 18C and described further below.

Quantitative Evaluation of Orthotic Function

Some of the earlier studies used cineradiography to visualize cervical motion within an orthosis (125,144). However, the difficulty in quantifying cineradiography has restricted the usefulness of these reports.

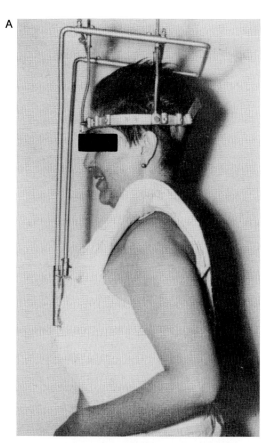

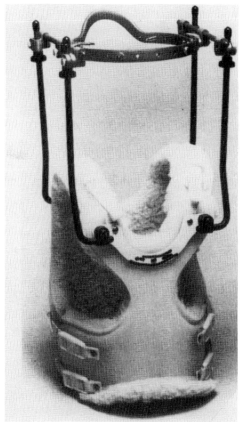

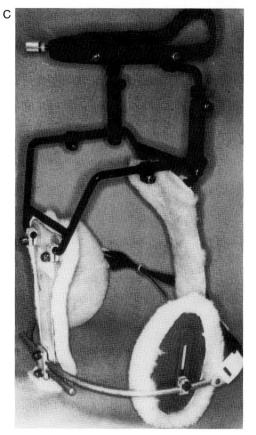

FIG. 18. Cranio-thoracic orthoses. **A:** Original halo-vest made from plaster. Note absence of contact between over-the-shoulder "straps" and top of shoulders. Also note absence of contact with upper thoracic spine and presence of contact with abdomen. **B:** Traditional plastic halo-vest. This provided a major advance in terms of skin care and access for hygiene. Vest design was basically unchanged. **C:** Four-pad halo-vest. Total absence of contact with shoulders and epigastrium avoids undesired force application by these structures. Contact with upper thoracic spine and multi-directional adjustability provides improved grip on thorax.

Colachis et al. (59) had normal subjects forcibly flex and extend while wearing no orthosis, a soft collar, a collar with chin piece, then a "Queen Anne" collar. Lateral view flexion-extension radiographs were taken to assess motion. They noted that the soft collar only slightly restricted extension and that the chin piece and occipital extension restricted flexion and extension, respectively, to a moderate extent. No statistical analysis was provided.

Fisher et al. (96) studied more rigid devices, namely the polyethylene collar with chin and occipital pads, Philadelphia collar, 4-poster, and SOMI. They also used normal subjects and voluntarily produced maximum flexion and extension efforts. Important methodological improvements consisted of standardizing the pressure under chin or occiput during flexion and extension, respectively, and statistical analyses of their results. They showed that: a) for C3-C4 to C6-C7 the Philadelphia and polyethylene collars reduced motion to approximately two thirds of normal, whereas the SOMI and 4-poster reduced motion to approximately one third of normal, a statistically significant difference; b) for C2-C3 all four designs restricted motion almost totally; and c) for Oc-C2 all four designs produced "paradoxical" motion, i.e., with forward rotation of the head and neck, local extension occurred at the upper cervical spine, more so for the Philadelphia and polyethylene collars than for the other two orthoses.

Althoff and Goldie (8) examined rheumatoid arthritis patients in each of the following: soft collar, Philadelphia collar, SOMI, and 4-poster. Lateral x-rays were used to assess flex-extension range at C1-C2 and C2-C4 as well as the atlanto-dens interval (ADI) in the flexed and extended positions. The major findings are: a) the C1-C2 flexion-extension range was only restricted from between 20% (soft collar) and approximately 45% (4-poster), and b) ADI increase with flexion was only restricted slightly compared to unbraced (4% by the soft collar up to approximately 20% by the 4-poster).

In the most thorough works on this topic, Johnson and co-workers (140,141) studied both flexion-extension and lateral bend radiographically, as well as axial rotation photographically. Orthoses tested were the cervical collar, Philadelphia collar, Philadelphia collar with rigid extensions (Yale brace), SOMI, 4-poster, a "cervico-thoracic orthosis," and halo vests. All were tested on normal volunteers except the halo vest which was used on patients. The major results from the study are the following: (a) the longer and stiffer devices generally do a better job at immobilization; (b) the non-halo devices are quite varied in their restriction of flexion-extension (13%–74% of normal range) and lateral bending (18%–83%), but none of them do a very good job for axial rotation (51%–92%); (c) the simple-to-fabricate "Yale brace" functions very much like the more complex "cervico-thoracic orthosis" or 4-poster; (d) the upper cervical spine is not well-immobilized by any of the non-halo devices; (e) even the typical halo vest allows motion in the lower cervical spine comparable to that seen with the 4-poster or "cervico-thoracic orthosis"; and (f) although clearly superior in the upper cervical spine, the typical halo vest still allows approximately 20% of the normal range of flexion-extension motion at both Oc-C1 and C1-C2, some of which is a "paradoxical" or "snaking" motion (upper cervical extension with lower cervical flexion and vice-versa). The authors emphasize that performance of orthoses on normal volunteers may not be directly applicable to patients.

Benzel et al. (22) compared the thermoplastic Minerva orthosis described by Millington et al. (189) to a standard halo vest by means of flexion-extension lateral x-rays of 10 patients. They found identical overall motion (occiput to C6 or to C7) with both orthoses: 5.2 degrees. The Minerva, however, allowed less "snaking" (upper cervical flexion with lower cervical extension, and vice versa), as measured by adding together the absolute values of the motion at each motion segment, the mean value of which was 23.4 degrees for the halo vest but only 14.8 degrees for the Minerva. Since cervical "snaking" is produced by capital protraction and retraction, its prevention requires control of antero-posterior motion between the orthosis and thorax. Differences in this feature between the halo vest and the Minerva orthosis probably explain the results. Unfortunately, no details concerning this are described or discussed by the authors.

Although halo vests represent a major step forward for cervical orthoses, there remain certain problems (reviewed more thoroughly elsewhere) (18,154). The first problem is the surprisingly large range of motion that can occur. Koch and Nickel (152) found 31% of the normal cervical range of motion occurring between various postures of daily living in patients fitted with Ace halo vests using basically the same vest design and a larger number of activities of daily living. Lind et al. (170,171) found greater motion occurring: approximately 70% of the full normal range. Wang et al. (293) using a modified vest apparently found even more motion than did Lind et al. These are all in contrast to Johnson et al. (141) who report only 4% of the normal flexion-extension motion. However, the latter study involved voluntary flexion/extension efforts in normal subjects rather than activities of daily living in patients.

The second problem is the loss of reduction during halo vest wear certainly can occur, as reported by various authors (45,86,126,147,152,167,290,310). Bucci et al. (45) and Whitehill et al. (310) have described this problem particularly clearly. Despite this, it should be kept in mind that excellent results have been reported with halo vest treatment of cervical spine trauma (154,170,171).

The third problem is that surprisingly high loads may be applied unintentionally by the wearer to the vest, and thus through the uprights to the neck. Koch and Nickel (152) measured peak distraction forces (mean ± SD) of 75 ± 40 N (16.8 ± 9.0 lbs) during flexion, and 65 ± 66 N (14.5 ± 14.8 lbs) during shoulder shrug. Ersmark et al. (87) reported distraction forces up to 50 N (11.2 lbs) during coughing. Lind et al. (170,171) showed much larger distraction forces (mean ± SD) of 159.6 ± 72.4 N (35.9 ± 16.3 lbs) during shoulder shrug and 122.9 ± 40.5 N (27.6 ± 9.1 lbs) during deep inspiration. Walker et al. (292) studied anterior-posterior and medial-lateral forces as well, and found the former comparable in magnitude to the distraction-compression forces.

The fourth problem is that the vest clearly contributes to pressure sore development (by covering over the scapulae) and may contribute to cranial pin loosening by allowing shoulder and abdominal motion to transmit undesired forces to the pins through the vest and uprights (154,200,222,292,317).

Finally, by covering a large portion of the thorax and abdomen, the vest can be uncomfortably warm, and dressing or washing underneath is difficult.

In response to one or more of these problems, various halo vest improvements or alternatives have been investigated. Appleby et al. (12) replaced the vest with a skeletal fixation framework attached by screws to the clavicles and scapulae. Movement of the clavicle and scapula with respect to the thorax and the cervical spine remained a predictable major and insurmountable problem. Garfin et al. (105) designed and tested a variety of skull pin tips to decrease loosening. Wang et al. (293) measured the effect of vest length on voluntarily produced neck motion in normal subjects. The vest extended down to either nipple line, twelfth rib, or iliac crest. There was no difference between the three designs in terms of motion restriction for C4-C5 and above. Below this level the results were mixed: surprisingly, at C6-C7 the longest vest worked the least well. Krag and Beynnon (154) reported the rationale and biomechanical test results of a fundamentally different vest design (Fig. 18C), which avoids contact with the shoulder girdle or abdomen and provides thorough adjustability to allow close fitting to nonmobile portions of the thorax. The biomechanical testing compared the mobility of each of seven standard and one experimental vest designs on each of four normal volunteers in response to each of nine load types. The mean rank order values (across load types and subjects) varied from 6.77 (most mobile) for the DePuy vest down to 3.22 (least mobile) for the experimental vest.

The reduced mobility in the experimental vest should provide improved cervical spine positional control as well, which presently is being evaluated. Thus, this vest addresses all five of the above-mentioned problems: motion is better controlled which in turn should lead to better reduction maintenance (currently being evaluated); and the absence of shoulder or abdomen contact precludes force transmission to neck, helps to avoid pressure sore development, and makes wear cooler and more convenient (154,155).

REFERENCES

1. Aebi M, Etter C, Coscia M (1989): Fractures of the odontoid process: Treatment with anterior screw fixation. *Spine* 14:1065–1070.
2. Alem NM, Nusholtz GS, Melvin JW (1984): Head and neck response to axial impacts. Proceedings of the 28th STAPP Car Crash Conference, Society of Automotive Engineers, Warrendale, Pennsylvania.
3. Alexander E Jr (1980): Decompression and fixation in cervical spine fractures: Indications and techniques. *Clin Neurosurg* 27:401–413.
4. Allen AR (1911): Surgery of experimental lesion of spinal cord equivalent to crush injury of fracture dislocation of spinal column: Preliminary report. *JAMA* 57:878–880.
5. Allen BJ Jr (1989): Recognition of injuries to the lower cervical spine. In: *The cervical spine, 2nd ed.*, Bailey RW, Sherk HH et al., eds. Philadelphia: J. B. Lippincott, pp. 283–298.
6. Allen BJ Jr, Ferguson RL, Lehmann TR, O'Brien RP (1982): A mechanistic classification of closed, indirect fractures and dislocations of the lower cervical spine. *Spine* 7:1–27.
7. Althoff B (1979): Fracture of the odontoid process. *Acta Orthop Scand* [Suppl] 177:1–95.
8. Althoff B, Goldie F (1980): Cervical collars in rheumatoid atlantoaxial subluxation: A radiographic comparison. *Ann Rheum Dis* 39:485–489.
9. Alund M, Larsson S-E (1990): Three dimensional analysis of neck motion: A clinical method. *Spine* 15:87–91.
10. Anderson LD, D'Alonzo RT (1974): Fractures of the odontoid process of the axis. *J Bone Joint Surg* [Am] 56:1163–1174.
11. Anderson RJ (1883): Observations on diameters of human vertebrae in different regions. *J Anat* [London] 17:341–344.
12. Appleby DM, Fu FH, Mears DC (1984): Halo-clavicle traction. *J Trauma* 24:452–455.
13. Babcock JL (1976): Cervical spine injuries. Diagnosis and classification. *Arch Surg* 111:646–651.
14. Bailey RW, Sherk HH et al., eds. (1974): *The cervical spine, 2nd ed.* Philadelphia: Lea & Febiger.
15. Bailey RW, Badgley CE (1960): Stabilization of the cervical spine by anterior fusion. *J Bone Joint Surg* [Am] 42:565–594.
16. Bailey RW, Sherk HH et al., eds. (1989): *The cervical spine, 2nd ed.* Philadelphia: J. B. Lippincott, pp. 1–881.
17. Barbour JR (1971): Screw fixation in fractures of the odontoid process. *South Austr Clin* 5(1):20–24.
18. Barr J Jr, Krag MH, Pierce DS (1989): Cranial traction and the halo orthosis. Chapter 6. In: *The cervical spine, 2nd ed.*, Bailey RW, Sherk HH et al., eds. Philadelphia: J. B. Lippincott, pp. 299–311.
19. Bauze RJ, Ardran GM (1978): Experimental production of forward dislocation in the human cervical spine. *J Bone Joint Surg* [Br] 60:239–245.
20. Beatson TR (1963): Fractures and dislocation of the cervical spine. *J Bone Joint Surg* [Br] 45:21–35.
21. Bedbrook GM (1971): Stability of spinal fractures and fracture-dislocations. *Paraplegia* 9:23–32.
22. Benzel EC, Hadden TA, Saulsbery CM (1989): A comparison of the Minerva and halo jackets for stabilization of the cervical spine. *J Neurosurg* 70:411–414.
23. Blockey NJ, Purser DW (1956): Fractures of the odontoid process of the axis. *J Bone Joint Surg* [Br] 38:794–817.
24. Blumensaat C (1953): Zum Problem der sagittalen Langsbrüche der Halswirbelkörper. *Chirurg* 24:193–195.
25. Böhler J (1967): Sofort- und Frühbehandlung traumatischer Querschnittlähmungen. *Zeitschr Orthopäd Grenzgebiete* 103:512–528.
26. Böhler J (1982): Anterior stabilization for acute fractures and non-unions of the dens. *J Bone Joint Surg* [Am] 64:18–27.
27. Böhler J, Gaudernak T (1980): Anterior plate stabilization for fracture-dislocations of the lower cervical spine. *J Trauma* 20:203–205.

28. Bohlman HH (1985): Surgical management of cervical spine fractures and dislocations. *Am Acad Ortho Surg Instruct Course Lectures* 34:163–186.

29. Bohlman HH, Boada E (1989): Fractures and dislocations of the lower cervical spine. In: *The cervical spine, 2nd ed.* Baily RW, Sherk HH et al., eds. Philadelphia: J. B. Lippincott, pp. 368–373.

30. Braakman R, Penning L (1971): Injuries of the cervical spine. Amsterdam: Excerpta Medica Pub., pp. 1–262.

31. Branch CL Jr, Kelly DL Jr (1987): Failure of stabilization of the spine with methylmethacrylate. A retrospective analysis of twenty-four cases (letter). *J Bone Joint Surg* [Am] 69:1108–1110.

32. Brattström H, Granholm L (1976): Atlanto-axial fusion in rheumatoid arthritis: A new method of fixation with wire and bone cement. *Acta Orthop Scan* 47:619–628.

33. Breig A (1960): Biomechanics of the central nervous system. Some basic normal and pathological phenomena concerning spine, discs and cord. Stockholm: Almqvist & Wiksell.

34. Breig A (1970): Overstretching of and circumscribed pathological tension on the spinal cord—A basic cause of symptoms in cord disorders. *J Biomech* 3:7–9.

35. Breig A (1972): The therapeutic possibilities of surgical bioengineering in incomplete spinal cord lesions. *Paraplegia* 9:173–182.

36. Breig A (1973): Pathological stress in the pons-cord-tissue tract and its alleviation by neurosurgical means. *Clin Neurosurg* 20:85–94.

37. Breig A (1978): Adverse mechanical tension in the central nervous system. Stockholm: Almqvist & Wiksell.

38. Breig A, El-Nadi AP (1966): Biomechanics of the cervical spinal cord. Relief of contact pressure on and overstretching of the spinal cord. *Acta Radiol Diagn (Stockh)* 4:602–624.

39. Bremer AM, Nguyen TQ (1983): Internal metal plate fixation combined with anterior interbody fusion in cases of cervical spine injury. *Neurosurgery* 12:649–653.

40. Bridwell KH (1986): Treatment of a markedly displaced hangman's fracture with a Luque rectangle and a posterior fusion in a 71 year old man. Case report. *Spine* 11:49–52.

41. Brody IA, Wilkins RH (1969): Lhermitte's sign. *Arch Neurol* 21:338–340.

42. Brooks AL, Jenkins EB (1978): Atlanto-axial arthrodesis by the wedge compression method. *J Bone Joint Surg* [Am] 60:279–284.

43. Brown JA, Havel P, Ebraheim N, Greenblatt SH, Jackson WT (1988): Cervical stabilization by plate and bone fusion. *Spine* 13:236–240.

44. Bryan WJ, Inglis AE, Sculco TP, Ranawat CS (1982): Methylmethacrylate stabilization for enhancement of posterior cervical arthrodesis in rheumatoid arthritis. *J Bone Joint Surg* [Am] 64:1045–1050.

45. Bucci MN, Dauser RC, Maynard FA, Hoff JT (1988): Management of post-traumatic cervical spine instability: Operative fusion versus halo vest immobilization. Analysis of 49 cases. *J Trauma* 28:1001–1006.

46. Bucy PC, Heimburger RF, Oberhill HRO (1948): Compression of the cervical spinal cord by herniated intervertebral discs. *J Neurosurg* 5:471–492.

47. Cabanela ME, Ebersold MJ (1988): Anterior plate stabilization for bursting teardrop fractures of the cervical spine. *Spine* 13:888–891.

48. Cahill DW, Bellesarrisue R, Ducker TB (1983): Bilateral facet to spinous process fusion: A new technique for posterior spinal fusion after trauma. *Neurosurgery* 13:1–4.

49. Callahan RA, Johnson RM, Margolis RN, Keggi KJ, Albright JA, Southwick WO (1977): Cervical facet fusion for control of instability following laminectomy. *J Bone Joint Surg* [Am] 59:991–1002.

50. Cantore G, Ciappetta P, Delfini R (1984): New steel device for occipitocervical fixation. Technical note. *J Neurosurg* 60:1104–1106.

51. Caspar W (1987): Anterior stabilization with the trapezial osteosynthetic plate technique in cervical spine injuries. In: *Cervical spine I*, Kehr P, Weidner A, eds. New York: Springer-Verlag, pp. 198–204.

52. Chadduck WM, Boop WC Jr (1983): Acrylic stabilization of the cervical spine for neoplastic disease: Evolution of a technique for vertebral body replacement. *Neurosurgery* 13:23–29.

53. Cheshire DJE (1969): The stability of the cervical spine following the conservative treatment of fractures and fracture-dislocations. *Paraplegia* 7:193–203.

54. Clark CR, Keggi KJ, Panjabi MM (1984): Methylmethacrylate stabilization of the cervical spine. *J Bone Joint Surg* [Am] 66:40–46.

55. Clark CR, White AA III (1985): Fractures of the dens: A multicenter study. *J Bone Joint Surg* [Am] 67:1340–1348.

56. Cloward RB (1961): Treatment of acute fractures and fracture dislocations of the cervical spine by vertebral body fusion: A report of 11 cases. *J Neurosurg* 18:201–209.

57. Cloward RB (1958): The anterior approach for removal of ruptured cervical disks. *J Neurosurg* 15:602–617.

58. Coe JD, Warden KE, Sutterlin CE III, McAfee PC (1989): Biomechanical evaluation of cervical spinal stabilization methods in a human cadaveric model. *Spine* 14:1122–1131.

59. Colachis SC Jr, Strohm BR, Ganter EL (1973): Cervical spine motion in normal women: Radiography study of effect of cervical collars. *Arch Phys Med Rehab* 54:161–169.

60. Condon BR, Hadley DM: Quantification of cord deformation and dynamics during flexion and extension of the cervical spine using MR imaging. *J Comput Assist Tomogr* 12:947–955.

61. Cooper PR, Cohen A, Rosiello A, Koslow M (1988): Posterior stabilization of cervical spine fractures and subluxations using plates and screws. *Neurosurgery* 23:300–306.

62. Cornish BL (1968): Traumatic spondylolisthesis of the axis. *J Bone Joint Surg* [Br] 50:31–43.

63. Crellin RQ, MacCabe JJ, Hamilton EBD (1970): Severe subluxation of the cervical spine in rheumatoid arthritis. *J Bone Joint Surg* [Br] 52:244–251.

64. Crenshaw AH (1971): *Campbell's operative orthopaedics, 5th ed.* St. Louis: C. V. Mosby, p. 628.

65. Davis D, Bohlman H, Walker AE, Fisher R, Robinson R (1971): The pathological findings in fatal cranio-spinal injuries. *J Neurosurg* 34:603–613.

66. De Lorme TL (1967): Axis-pedicle fractures. *J Bone Joint Surg* [Am] 49:1472.

67. de Groote W, Vercauteren M, Uyttendaele D (1981): Occipitocervical fusion in rheumatoid arthritis. *Acta Orthop Belg* 47:685–698.

68. de los Reyes RA, Malik GM, Wu KK, Ausman JI (1981): A new surgical approach to stabilizing C1-2 subluxation in rheumatoid arthritis. *Henry Ford Hospital Medical J* 29:127–130.

69. Deng YC, Goldsmith W (1987): Response of a human head/neck/upper torso replica to dynamic loading. II. Analytical/numerical model. *J Biomech* 20:487–497.

70. Dimnet J, Pasquet A, Krag MH, Panjabi MM (1982): Cervical spine motion in the sagittal plane: Kinematics and geometric parameters. *J Biomech* 15:959–969.

71. Dohrmann GJ (1972): Experimental spinal cord trauma: A historical review. *Arch Neurol* 27:468–473.

72. Dohrmann GJ, Panjabi MM (1976): "Standardized" spinal cord trauma: Biomechanical parameters and lesion volume. *Surg Neurol* 6:263–267.

73. Dohrmann GJ, Panjabi MM, Banks D (1978): Biomechanics of experimental spinal cord trauma. *J Neurosurg* 48:993–1001.

74. Domenella G, Berlanda P, Bassi G (1982): Posterior-approach osteosynthesis of the lower cervical spine by the R. Roy-Camille technique. (Indications and first results). *Ital J Orthop Traumatol* 8:235–244.

75. Duff TA (1986): Surgical stabilization of traumatic cervical spine dislocation using methylmethacrylate: Long term results in 26 patients. *J Neurosurg* 64:39–44.

76. Dunn EJ (1977): Role of methylmethacrylate in the stabilization and replacement of tumors of the cervical spine: A project of the Cervical Spine Research Society. *Spine* 2:15–24.

77. Dutoit G (1976): Lateral atlantoaxial arthrodesis: A screw fixation technique. *South Afr J Surg* 14:9–12.

78. Dvorak J, Grob D, Baumgartner H, Gschwend N, Grauer W, Larsson S (1989): Functional evaluation of the spinal cord by magnetic resonance imaging in patients with rheumatoid arthritis and instability of upper cervical spine. *Spine* 14:1057–1064.

79. Dvorak J, Hayek J, Zehnder R (1987): CT-functional diagnostics of the rotatory instability of the upper cervical spine. II. An evalua-

tion on healthy adults and patients with suspected instability. *Spine* 12:726–731.

80. Dvorak J, Panjabi M (1987): Functional anatomy of the alar ligaments. *Spine* 12:183–189.

81. Dvorak J, Panjabi M, Gerber M, Wichmann W (1987): CT-functional diagnostics of the rotary instability of upper cervical spine. I. An experimental study on cadavers. *Spine* 12:197–205.

82. Dvorak J, Schneider E, Saldinger P, Rahn B (1988): Biomechanics of the craniocervical region: The alar and transverse ligaments. *J Orthop Res* 6:452–461.

83. Ebraheim NA, An HS, Jackson WT, Brown JA (1989): Internal fixation of the unstable cervical spine using posterior Roy-Camille plates: Preliminary report. *J Orthop Trauma* 3:23–28.

84. Ecklin U (1960): Die Alterveränderungen der Halswirbelsäule. Berlin: Springer-Verlag.

85. Ehni G (1984) *Cervical arthrosis: Diseases of the cervical motion segments.* Chicago: Yearbook Medical Publishers, pp. 1–285.

86. Ekong CEV, Schwartz ML, Tator CH, Rowed DW, Edmonds VE (1981): Odontoid fracture: Management with early mobilization using the halo device. *Neurosurgery* 9:631–637.

87. Ersmark H, Kalén R, Löwenhielm P (1988): A methodical study of force measurements in three patients with odontoid fractures treated with a strain gauge-equipped halo-vest. *Spine* 13:433–455.

88. Etter C, Coscia M, Ganz R, Aebi M (1989): Bone screw osteosynthesis of dens fractures. Technical surgical aspects and results. *Unfallchirurg* 92:220–226.

89. Fairbank TJ (1971): Spinal fusion after laminectomy for cervical myelopathy. *Proc Soc Med* 64:634–636.

90. Fick R (1904–1912): *Handbuch der Anatomie und Mechanik der Gelenke unter Berücksichtigung der bewegenden Muskeln.* Jena: G Fischer, pp. 1904–1912.

91. Fidler MW (1986): Posterior instrumentation of the spine: An experimental comparison of various possible techniques. *Spine* 11:367–372.

92. Fielding JW (1983): The atlanto axial joint. In: *Surgery of the musculoskeletal system,* vol. 2. CM Evarts, ed. New York: Churchill Livingston.

93. Fielding JW (1964): Normal and selected abnormal motion of the cervical spine from the second cervical vertebra to the seventh cervical vertebra based on cineroentgenography. *J Bone Joint Surg* [Am] 46:1779–1781.

94. Fielding JW, Cochran GVB, Lawsing JF III, Hohl M (1974): Tears of the transverse ligament of the atlas: A clinical and biomechanical study. *J Bone Joint Surg* [Am] 56:1683–1691.

95. Fielding JW, Hawkins RJ, Ratzan SA (1976): Spine fusion for atlanto-axial instability. *J Bone Joint Surg* [Am] 58:400–407.

96. Fisher SV, Bowar JF, Awad EA, Gullickson G Jr (1977): Cervical orthoses effect on cervical spine motion: Roentgenographic and goniometric method of study. *Arch Phys Med Rehabil* 58:109–115.

97. Forsyth HF (1964): Extension injuries of the cervical spine. *J Bone Joint Surg* [Am] 46:1792–1797.

98. Forsyth HF, Alexander EA, Davis CH, Underdal RG (1959): Advantages of early spine fusion in the treatment of fracture-dislocations of the cervical spine. *J Bone Joint Surg* [Am] 41:17–36.

99. Frazer JE (1958): *Anatomy of the human skeleton, 5th ed.* AS Breathnach, ed. London: J. A. Churchill, p. 22.

100. Fuentes JM, Blancourt J, Vlahovitch B, Castan P (1983): Tear drop fractures. Contribution to the study of its mechanism and os osteo-disco-ligamentous lesions. *Neurochirurgie* 29:129–134.

101. Gallie WE (1937): Skeletal traction in the treatment of fractures and dislocations of the cervical spine. *Ann Surg* 106:770–776.

102. Gallie WE (1939): Fractures and dislocations of the cervical spine. *Am J Surg* 46:495–499.

103. Garber WN, Fisher RG, Holfman HW (1969): Vertebrectomy and fusion for "tear-drop" fracture of the cervical spine. *J Trauma* 9:887–893.

104. Garfin SR, Botte MJ, Centeno RS, Nickel VL (1985): Osteology of the skull as it affects halo pin placement. *Spine* 10:696–698.

105. Garfin SR, Lee TQ, Roux RD, et al (1986): Structural behavior of the halo orthosis pin-bone interface: Biomechanical evaluation of standard and newly designed stainless steel halo fixation pins. *Spine* 11:977–981.

106. Garfin SR, Moore MR, Marshall LF (1988): A modified technique for cervical facet fusions. *Clin Orthop* 230:149–153.

107. Gassman J, Seligson D (1983): Anterior cervical plate. *Spine* 8:700–707.

108. Gershon-Cohen J, Budin E, Glauser F (1954): Whiplash fractures of cervicodorsal spinous processes: Resemblance to shoveler's fracture. *JAMA* 155:560–561.

109. Gill K, Paschal S, Corin J, Ashman R, Bucholz RW (1988): Posterior plating of the cervical spine: A biomechanical comparison of different posterior fusion techniques. *Spine* 13:813–816.

110. Goel VK, Clark CR, Harris KG, Kim YE, Schulte KR (1989): Evaluation of effectiveness of a facet wiring technique: An in vitro biomechanical investigation. *Ann Biomed Eng* 17:115–126.

111. Goel VK, Clark CR, Harris KG, Schulte KR (1988): Kinematics of the cervical spine: Effects of multiple total laminectomy and facet wiring. *J Orthop Res* 6:611–619.

112. Goldie IF, Reichmann S (1977): The biomechanical influence of traction on the cervical spine. *Scand J Rehabil Med* 9:31–94.

113. Grantham SA, Dick HM, Thompson RC Jr, Stinchfield FE (1969): Occipitocervical arthrodesis, indications, technique and results. *Clin Orthop* 65:118–129.

114. Griswold DM, Albright JA, Schiffman E, Johnson R, Southwick WO (1978): Atlanto-axial fusion for instability. *J Bone Joint Surg* [Am] 60:285–292.

115. Grob M, Magerl F (1987): Operative stabilisierung bei Frakturen von C1 and C2. *Orthopäde* 16:46–54.

116. Hadra BE (1981): Wiring of the spinous process in injury and Potts' disease. *Trans Am Orthop Assoc* 4:206.

117. Hadra BE (1975): The classic: Wiring of the vertebrae as a means of immobilization in fractures and Potts' disease. *Clin Orthop* 112:4–8.

118. Halliday DR, Sullivan UR, Hollinshead WH, Bahn RC (1964): Torn cervical ligaments: Necropsy examination of normal cervical region. *J Trauma* 4:219–232.

119. Hansebout RR, Blomquist GA Jr (1980): Acrylic spine fusion: A 20 year clinical series and technical note. *J Neurosurg* 53:606–612.

120. Hanson P, Sharkey N, Montesano PX (1988): Anatomic and biomechanical study of C1-C2 posterior arthrodesis techniques. Proc Cerv Spine Res Soc 16th Ann Mtng, Key Biscayne, FL, pp. 100–101.

121. Harrington KD (1981): The use of methylmethacrylate for vertebral-body replacement and anterior stabilization of pathologic fracture dislocation of the spine due to metastatic malignant disease. *J Bone Joint Surg* [Am] 63:36–46.

122. Harris JH Jr (1978): *The radiology of acute cervical spine trauma.* Baltimore: Williams & Wilkins, pp. 1–116.

123. Harris JH Jr, Edeiken-Monroe B, Kopaniky OR (1986): A practical classification of acute cervical spine injuries. *Orthop Clin North Am* 17:15–30.

124. Hart DL, Johnson RM, Simmons EF, Owen J (1978): Review of cervical orthoses. *Phys Ther* 58:857–860.

125. Hartman JT, Palumbo F, Hill BJ (1975): Cineradiography of the braced normal cervical spine: A comparative study of five commonly used cervical orthoses. *Clin Orthop* 109:97–102.

126. Haw DW (1982): Collapse of cervical spine treated by Down's Ace mark III halo assembly. *Br Med J* 285:410.

127. Herrmann HD (1975): Metal plate fixation after anterior fusion of unstable fracture dislocations of the cervical spine. *Acta Neurochir (Wien)* 32:101–111.

128. Heywood AWB, Learmonth ID, Thomas M (1988): Internal fixation for occipito-cervical fusion. *J Bone Joint Surg* [Br] 70:708–711.

129. Hohl M, Baker HR (1964): The atlanto-axial joint, roentgenographic and anatomical study of normal and abnormal motion. *J Bone Joint Surg* [Am] 46:1739–1752.

130. Holdsworth FW (1963): Fractures, dislocations and fracture-dislocations of the spine. *J Bone Joint Surg* [Br] 45:6–20.

131. Hollinshead WH (1969): *Anatomy for surgeons, vol. III: The back & limbs, 2nd ed.* Chapter 2, The back. New York: Harper & Row, pp. 79–206.

132. Holness RO, Huestis WS, Howes WJ, Langille RA (1984): Posterior stabilization with an interlaminar clamp in cervical injuries:

Technical note and review of the long term experience with the method. *Neurosurgery* 14:318–322.

133. Hung TK, Lin HS, Albin MS, Bunegin L, Jannetta PJ (1979): The standardization of experimental impact injury to the spinal cord. *Surg Neurol* 11:470–477.

134. Husby J, Sorensen KH (1974): Fractures of the odontoid process of the axis. *Acta Orthop Scand* 45:182–192.

135. Itoh T, Tsuji H, Katoh Y, Yonezawa T, Kitagawa H (1988): Occipito-cervical fusion reinforced by Luque's segmental spinal instrumentation for rheumatoid diseases. *Spine* 13:1234–1238.

136. Janes JM, Hooshmand H (1965): Severe extension-flexion injuries of the cervical spine. *Mayo Clin Proc* 40:353–369.

137. Jefferson G (1920): Fracture of the atlas vertebra: Report of 4 cases and a review of those previously recorded. *Br J Surg* 7:407–422.

138. Jeffreys E (1980): *Disorders of the cervical spine.* London: Butterworth Publ., pp. 1–147.

139. Johnson RM, Crelin ES, White AA III, Panjabi MM, Southwick WO (1975): Some new observations on the functional anatomy of the lower cervical spine. *Clin Orthop* 111:192–200.

140. Johnson RM, Hart DL, Owen JR, Lerner E, Chapin W, Zeleznik R (1978): The Yale cervical orthosis: An evaluation of its effectiveness in restricting cervical motion in normal subjects and a comparison with other cervical orthoses. *Phys Ther* 58:865–871.

141. Johnson RM, Hart DL, Simmons EF, Ramsby GR, Southwick WO (1977): Cervical orthoses: A study comparing their effectiveness in restricting cervical motion in normal subjects. *J Bone Joint Surg* [Am] 59:332–339.

142. Johnson RM, Owen JR, Hart DL, Callahan RA (1981): Cervical orthoses: A guide to their selection and use. *Clin Orthop* 154:34–45.

143. Johnson RM, Southwick WO (1975): Surgical approaches to the spine. In: RH Rothman, FA Simeone, eds. *The Spine,* Philadelphia: W. B. Saunders, pp. 98–103.

144. Jones MD (1960): Cineradiographic studies of the collar-immobilized cervical spine. *J Neurosurg* 17:633–637.

145. Karlström G, Ölerud S (1987): Internal fixation of fractures and dislocations in the cervical spine. *Orthopaedics* 10:1549–1558.

146. Keblish PA, Keggi KJ (1967): Mechanical problems of the dowel graft in anterior cervical fusion. *J Bone Joint Surg* [Am] 49:198.

147. Kelly EG (1981): Loss of reduction in cervical fracture-dislocations managed in the halo cast. Proc Am Acad Ortho Surg Ann Mtng.

148. Kelly EG, Stauffer ES, Mazur JM, Mears DC (1983): Surgical techniques in the cervical spine. In: DC Mears, ed. *External skeletal fixation,* Baltimore: Williams & Wilkins, pp. 521–552.

149. Kelly DL Jr, Alexander E Jr, Davis CH Jr, Smith JM (1972): Acrylic fixation of atlanto-axial dislocations. Technical note. *J Neurosurg* 36:366–371.

150. Knight G (1959): Paraspinal acrylic inlays in treatment of cervical and lumbar spondylolysis and other conditions. *Lancet* 2:147–149.

151. Knöringer P (1987): Double-threaded compression screws in osteosynthesis of acute fractures of the odontoid process. In: *Disease in the cranio-cervical junction,* D Voth, O Glees, eds. New York: de Gruyter, p. 217.

152. Koch RA, Nickel VL (1978): The halo vest: An evaluation of motion and forces across the neck. *Spine* 3:103–107.

153. Kostuik JP, Errico TJ, Gleason TF, Errico CC (1988): Spinal stabilization of vertebral column tumors. *Spine* 13:250–256.

154. Krag MH, Beynnon BD (1988): A new halo-vest: Rationale, design and biomechanical comparison to standard halo-vest designs. *Spine* 13:228–235.

155. Krag MH, Beynnon BD, Gill K, Levine A, Weinstein J (1986): A new halovest: Initial clinical experience and comparison to a "standard" halovest. Proc Cerv Spine Res Soc, 14th Ann Mtg, West Palm Beach, Florida.

156. Krag MH, Byrt W, Pope MH (1989): Pull-off strength of Gardner-Wells tongs from cadaveric crania. *Spine* 14:247–250.

157. Krag MH, Monsey RD, Fenwick JW (1989): Cranial morphometry related to placement of tongs in the temporoparietal area for cervical traction. *J Spinal Disorders* 1:301–305.

158. Krag MH, Pope MH, Wilder DG (1986): Mechanisms of spine trauma and features of spinal fixation methods. Mechanisms of

injury. In: *Spinal cord injury medical engineering,* D Ghista, ed. Springfield, IL: Charles C Thomas.

159. Krag MH, Seroussi RE, Wilder DG, Pope MH (1987): Internal displacement distribution from in vitro loading of human lumbar spinal motion segments: Experimental results and theoretical predictions. *Spine* 12:1001–1007.

160. Krag MH, Trausch I, Wilder DG, Pope MH (1983): Internal strain and nuclear movements of the intervertebral disc. Proc Internat Soc Study Lumbar Spine 10th Ann Mtg, Cambridge, England.

161. Landells CD, Van Peteghem PK (1988): Fractures of the atlas: Classification, treatment and morbidity. *Spine* 13:451–452.

162. Langsam CL (1941): M. omohyoideus in American whites and Negroes. *Am J Phys Anthropol* 28:249–259.

163. Lee C, Kim KS, Rogers LF (1982): Sagittal fractures of the cervical vertebral body. *Am J Roentgenol* 139(1):55–60.

164. Lesoin F, Cama A, Lozes G, Servato R, Kabbag K, Jomin M (1982): Anterior approach and plates in lower cervical posttraumatic lesions. *Surg Neurol* 21:581–587.

165. Lesoin F, Jomin M, Viaud C (1983): Expanding bolt for anterior cervical spine osteosynthesis: Technical note. *Neurosurgery* 12:458–459.

166. Lesoin F, Viaud C, Jomin M (1985): Universal plate for anterior cervical spine osteosynthesis. *Acta Neurochirurg (Wien)* 70:60–61.

167. Levine AM, Edwards CC (1985): The management of traumatic spondylolisthesis of the axis. *J Bone Joint Surg* [Am] 67:217–226.

168. Lhermitte J (1929): Multiple sclerosis: The sensation of an electric discharge as an early symptom. *Arch Neurol Psych* 22:5–8.

169. Lhermitte J (1932): Étude sur la commotion de la moelle. *Rev Neurol* 39:210.

170. Lind B, Sihlbom H, Nordwall A (1988): Forces and motions across the neck in patients treated with halo vest. *Spine* 13:162–167.

171. Lind B, Sihlbom H, Nordwall A (1988): Halovest treatment of unstable traumatic cervical spine injuries. *Spine* 13:425–432.

172. Louis R (1982): *Posterior vertebral bone plates.* Paris: Ceprime.

173. Louis R (1983): *Surgery of the spine: Surgical anatomy & operative approaches.* New York: Springer-Verlag.

174. Lysell E (1969): Motion in the cervical spine. *Acta Orthop Scand* [Suppl] 123:1–61.

175. Magerl F, Grob D, Seemann P (1987): Stable dorsal fusion of the cervical spine (C2-T1) using hook plates. In: *Cervical spine I,* P Kehr, A Weidner, eds. New York: Springer-Verlag, pp. 217–221.

176. Magerl F, Seeman P-S (1987): Stable posterior fusion of the atlas and axis by transarticular screw fixation. In: *Cervical spine I,* P Kehr, A Weidner, eds. New York: Springer-Verlag, pp. 322–327.

177. Maiman DJ, Sances A, Myklebust JB, Larson SJ, Houterman C, Chilbert M, El-Ghatit AZ (1983): Compression injuries of the cervical spine: A biomechanical analysis. *Neurosurgery* 13:254–260.

178. Mair WGP, Druckman R (1953): The pathology of spinal cord lesions and their relation to the clinical features in protrusion of cervical intervertebral discs. *Brain* 76:70–91.

179. Marar BC (1975): Fractures of the axis arch. *Clin Orthop* 106:155–165.

180. Marar BC (1974): Hyperextension injuries of the cervical spine: The pathogenesis of damage to the spinal cord. *J Bone Joint Surg* [Am] 56:1655–1662.

181. Matsunaga S, Sakou T, Morizono Y, Yone K (1988): Occipito-atlanto-axial fusion utilizing a rectangular rod. Proc Cerv Spine Res Soc 16th Ann Mtg, Key Biscayne, Florida, pp. 106–107.

182. Mayfield FH (1966): Cervical spondylosis: A comparison of the anterior and posterior approaches. *Clin Neurosurg* 13:181–188.

183. McAfee PC, Bohlman HH, Ducker T, Eismont FJ (1986): Failure of stabilization of the spine with methylmethacrylate. *J Bone Joint Surg* [Am] 68:1145–1157.

184. McElhaney JH, Paver JG, McCrackin HJ, Maxwell GM (1983): Cervical spine compression responses. Proc 27th STAPP Car Crash Conference, Soc Automotive Engineers, Warrendale, Pennsylvania, pp. 163–177.

185. McGraw RW, Rusch RM (1973): Atlanto-axial arthrodesis. *J Bone Joint Surg* [Br] 55:482–489.

186. McLaurin RL, Vernal R, Salmon JH (1972): Treatment of frac-

tures of the atlas and axis by wiring without fusion. *J Neurosurg* 36:773–780.

187. McVeigh JF (1923): Experimental cord crushes; with a special reference to the mechanical factors involved and subsequent changes in the areas of the cord affected. *Arch Surg* 7:573–600.

188. Mestdagh H (1976): Morphological aspects and biomechanical properties of the vertebroaxial joint (C2-C3). *Acta Morphol Neerl Scand* 14:19–30.

189. Millington PJ, Ellingsen JM, Hauswirth BE, Fabian PJ (1987): Thermoplastic Minerva body jacket—A practical alternative to current methods of cervical spine stabilization. A clinical report. *Phys Ther* 67:223–225.

190. Mimura M, Moriya H, Watanabe T, Takahashi K, Yamagata M, Tamaki T (1989): Three-dimensional motion analysis of the cervical spine with special reference to the axial rotation. *Spine* 14:1135–1139.

191. Mitsui H (1984): A new operation for atlanto-axial arthrodesis. *J Bone Joint Surg* [Br] 66:442–445.

192. Mixter SJ, Osgood RB (1910): Traumatic lesion of the atlas and axis. *Ann Surg* 51:193–207.

193. Montesano PX, Juach E (1988): Anatomic and biomechanical study of posterior cervical spine plate arthrodesis. Proc Cerv Spine Res Soc Ann Mtg, Key Biscayne, Florida, pp. 39–40.

194. Moroney SP, Schultz AB, Miller JAA (1988): Analysis and measurement of neck loads. *J Orthop Res* 6:713–720.

195. Moroney SP, Schultz AB, Miller JAA, Andersson GBJ (1988): Load-displacement properties of lower cervical spine motion segments. *J Biomech* 9:769–779.

196. Morscher E, Sutter F, Jenny H, Ölerud S (1986): Die vordere Verplattung der Halswirbelsäule mit dem Hohlschrauben-Plattensystem aus Titanium. *Chirurg* 57:702–707.

197. Mouradian WH, Fietti VG Jr, Cochran GV, Fielding JW, Young J (1978): Fractures of the odontoid: A laboratory and clinical study of mechanisms. *Orthop Clin North Am* 9:985–1001.

198. Murphy MJ, Daniaux H, Southwick WO (1986): Posterior cervical fusion with rigid internal fixation. *Orthop Clin North Am* 17:55–65.

199. Nakanishi T, Sasaki T, Tokita N, Hirabayashi K (1982): Internal fixation for the odontoid fracture. *Orthop Trans* 6:176.

200. Nickel VH, Perry J, Garrett A, et al (1968): The halo. A spinal skeleton traction fixation device. *J Bone Joint Surg* [Am] 50:1400–1409.

201. Nolan JP Jr, Sherk HH (1988): Biomechanical evaluation of the extensor musculature of the cervical spine. *Spine* 13:9–11.

202. Oliveira JC (1987): Anterior plate fixation of traumatic lesions of the lower cervical spine. *Spine* 12:324–329.

203. Ommaya AK: Mechanical properties of tissues of the nervous system. *J Biomech* 1:127–138.

204. Ono K, Tada K (1975): Metal prosthesis of the cervical vertebra. *J Neurosurg* 42:562–566.

205. Orofino C, Sherman MS, Schechter D (1960): Luschka's joint—A degenerative phenomenon. *J Bone Joint Surg* [Am] 42:853–858.

206. Osgood RB, Lund CC (1928): Fractures of the odontoid process. *N Engl J Med* 198:61–72.

207. Panjabi MM, Dicker DB, Dohrmann GJ (1977): Biomechanical quantification of experimental spinal cord trauma. *J Biomech* 10:681–687.

208. Panjabi MM, Duranceau JS, Oxland TR, Bowen CE (1989): Multidirectional instabilities of traumatic cervical spine injuries in a porcine model. *Spine* 14:1111–1115.

209. Panjabi MM, Goel VK, Clark CR, Keggi KJ, Southwick WO (1985): Biomechanical study of cervical spine stabilization with methylmethacrylate. *Spine* 10:198–203.

210. Panjabi MM, Goel VK, Walter SD (1982): Errors in kinematic parameters of a planar joint: Guidelines for optimal experimental design. *J Biomech* 15:537–544.

211. Panjabi MM, Hopper W, White AA III, Keggi KJ (1977): Posterior spine stabilization with methylmethacrylate: Biomechanical testing of a surgical specimen. *Spine* 2:241–247.

212. Panjabi MM, Summer DJ, Pelker RR, Videman T, Friedlander GE, Southwick WO (1986): Three-dimensional load-displacement curves due to forces on the cervical spine. *J Orthop Res* 4:152–161.

213. Panjabi M, Summers DJ, Southwick W (1983): Cervical spine load displacement curves: A three-dimensional in vitro study. Advances in Bioengineering Winter Ann Mtg, Am Soc Mech Eng, Boston.

214. Panjabi MM, White AA III (1989): Biomechanics of nonacute cervical spinal cord trauma. In: *The cervical spine*, RW Bailey, HH Sherk et al, eds. Philadelphia: J. B. Lippincott, pp. 91–96.

215. Panjabi MM, White AA III, Johnson RM (1975): Cervical spine biomechanics as a function of transection of components. *J Biomech* 8:327–336.

216. Panjabi MM, White AA III, Keller D, Southwick WO, Friedlaender G (1978): Stability of the cervical spine under tension. *J Biomech* 11:189–197.

217. Panjabi MM, Wrathall JR (1988): Biomechanical analysis of experimental spinal cord injury and functional loss. *Spine* 13:1365–1370.

218. Parke WW, Sherk HH (1989): Normal adult anatomy. In: *The cervical spine, 2nd ed.* HH Sherk, et al, eds. Philadelphia: J. B. Lippincott, pp. 15–18.

219. Payne EE, Spillane JD (1957): The cervical spine. An anatomico-pathological study of 70 specimens (using a special technique) with particular reference to the problem of cervical spondylosis. *Brain* 80:571–596.

220. Penning L (1989): Functional anatomy of joints and discs. In: *The Cervical Spine, 2nd ed*, RW Bailey, HH Sherk, et al, eds. Philadelphia: J. B. Lippincott, pp. 33–56.

221. Penning L, Wilmink JT (1987): Rotation of the cervical spine: A CT study on normal subjects. *Spine* 12:732–738.

222. Perry J (1972): Halo in spinal abnormalities—Practical factors and avoidance of complications. *Orthop Clin North Am* 3:69–80.

223. Perry J, Nickel VL (1959): Total cervical spine fusion for neck paralysis. *J Bone Joint Surg* [Am] 41:37–60.

224. Petrie JG (1964): Flexion injuries of the cervical spine. *J Bone Joint Surg* [Am] 46:1800–1806.

225. Powers B, Miller MD, Kramer RS, Martinez S, Gehweiler JA Jr (1979): Traumatic anterior atlanto-occipital dislocation. *Neurosurgery* 4:12–17.

226. Prolo DJ, Runnels JB, Jameson RM (1973): The injured cervical spine. Immediate and long-term immobilization with the halo. *JAMA* 224:591–594.

227. Rand RW, Crandall PH (1962): Central spinal cord syndrome in hyperextension injuries of the cervical spine. *J Bone Joint Surg* [Am] 44:1415–1422.

228. Ransford AO, Crockard HA, Pozo JL, Thomas NP, Nelson IW (1986): Craniocervical instability treated by contoured loop fixation. *J Bone Joint Surg* [Br] 68:173–177.

229. Raycroft JF, Hockman RP, Southwick WO (1978): Metastatic tumors involving the cervical vertebrae: Surgical palliation. *J Bone Joint Surg* [Am] 60:763–768.

230. Raynor RB, Push J, Shapiro I (1963): Cervical facetectomy and its effect on spine strength. *J Neurosurg* 63:278–282.

231. Reid JD (1960): Effects of flexion-extension movements of the head and spine upon the spinal cord and nerve roots. *J Neurol Neurosurg Psychiatry* 23:214–221.

232. Richman S, Friedman RL (1954): Vertical fractures of the cervical vertebral bodies. *Radiology* 62:536–543.

233. Roaf R (1963): Lateral flexion injuries of the cervical spine. *J Bone Joint Surg* [Br] 45:36–38.

234. Roaf R (1960): A study of the mechanics of spinal injuries. *J Bone Joint Surg* [Br] 42:810–823.

234a. Robinson RA, Smith GW (1955): Anterolateal cervical disc removal and interbody fusion for cervical disc syndrome. *Bull Johns Hopkins Hosp* 96:223–224.

235. Robinson RA, Southwick WO (1960): Indications and techniques for early stabilization of the neck in some fracture-dislocations of the cervical spine. *South Med J* 53:565–579.

236. Robinson RA, Southwick WO (1960): Surgical approaches to the cervical spine. Am Acad Orthop Surg Instruct Course Lectures 27:299–316.

237. Robinson RA, Walker E, Ferlic DC, Wieckling DK (1962): Results of anterior interbody fusion of the cervical spine. *J Bone Joint Surg* [Am] 44:1569–1586.

238. Rodrigues O (1840): Des lois géométriques qui régissent les déplacements d'un système solide dans l'espace, et de la variation

des coordonées provenant de ces déplacements considérés in-
dépéndamment des causes qui peuvent les produire. *J Math
Pures Appl* 5:380–440.

239. Rogers WA (1942): Treatment of fracture-dislocation of the cervical spine. *J Bone Joint Surg* 24:245–258.

240. Rogers WA (1957): Fractures and dislocations of the cervical
spine. *J Bone Joint Surg [Am]* 39:341–376.

241. Roosen K, Travschel A, Grote W (1982): Posterior atlanto-axial
fusions: A new compression clamp for laminar osteosynthesis.
Arch Orthop Trauma Surg 100:27–31.

242. Rothman RH, Simeone FA, eds. (1975): *The spine.* Philadelphia:
W. B. Saunders, pp. 1–922.

243. Roy-Camille R, Saillant G (1972): Chirurgie du rachis cervical. 1.
Généralités. Luxations pures des articulaires. *Nouv Presse Med*
1(33):2330–2332.

244. Roy-Camille R, Saillant G (1972): Chirurgie du rachis cervical. 2.
Luxation-fracture des articulaires. *Nouv Presse Med* 1(37):2484–
2485.

245. Roy-Camille R, Saillant G (1972): Chirurgie du rachis cervical. 3.
Fractures complexes du rachis cervical inferieur; tetraplegies.
Nouv Presse Med 1(40):2707–2709.

246. Roy-Camille R, Saillant G, Mazel C (1989): Internal fixation of
the unstable cervical spine by a posterior osteosynthesis with
plates and screws. In: *The cervical spine, 2nd ed.* RW Bailey, HH
Sherk, et al, eds. Philadelphia: J. B. Lippincott, pp. 390–403.

247. Rubin G, Dixon M, Bernknopf J (1978): An occipito-zygomatic
cervical orthosis designed for emergency use—A preliminary report. *Bull Prosth Res,* Spring 1978, pp. 10–29.

248. Ruston SA (1984): Movements of the cervical spine measured by
biplanar photogrammetry. Thesis (Masters of Science), University of Strathclyde, Scotland.

249. Ryerson EW, Christopher F (1937): Dislocation of cervical vertebrae: Operative correction. *JAMA* 108:468–470.

250. Sadeghpour E, Noer HR, Mahinpour S (1981): Skull-C2 fusion in
rheumatoid patients with atlanto-axial subluxation. *Orthopaedics* 4:1369–1374.

251. Sandor L (1985): Primary stability of AO-plate osteosynthesis of
the lower cervical spinal column. II. Anterior spondylodesis with
H-plate osteosynthesis. *Z Exp Chir Transplant Kunstliche Organe* 18:93–101.

252. Sandor L (1985): Primary stability of AO-plate osteosynthesis of
the lower cervical spinal column. III. Posterior and combined
spondylodesis. Conclusions. *Z Exp Chir Transplant Kunstliche
Organe* 18:102–110.

253. Sandor L, Antal A (1985): Primary stability of AO-plate osteosynthesis of the lower cervical spinal column. I. Load-bearing capacity of the cervical vertebrae. *Z Exp Chir Transplant Kunstliche
Organe* 18:87–92.

254. Savini R, Parisini P, Cevellati S (1987): Surgical treatment of late
instability of flexion rotation injuries in the lower cervical spine.
Spine 12:178–182.

255. Schlicke LH, Schulak DJ (1981): Wiring of the cervical spinous
process. *Clin Orthop* 154:319–320.

256. Schlicke LH, White AA III, Panjabi MM, Pratt A, Kier L (1979):
A quantitative study of vertebral displacement and angulation in
the normal cervical spine under axial load. *Clin Orthop* 140:47–
49.

257. Schneider RC, Cherry G, Pantek H (1954): Syndrome of acute
central cervical spinal cord injury with special reference to the
mechanism involved in hyperextension injuries of the cervical
spine. *J Neurosurg* 11:546–577.

258. Schneider RC, Kahn EA (1956): Chronic neurologic sequelae of
acute trauma to the spine and spinal cord. Part I. The significance
of the acute-flexion or "tear-drop" fracture-dislocation of the cervical spine. *J Bone Joint Surg [Am]* 38:985–997.

259. Schneider RC, Livingston KE, Cave AJE, Hamilton G (1965):
"Hangman's fracture" of the cervical spine. *J Neurosurg* 22:141–
154.

260. Schneider RC, Thompson JM, Bebin J (1958): Syndrome of
acute central cervical spinal cord injury. *J Neurol Neurosurg Psychiatry* 21:216–227.

261. Schulte K, Clark CR, Goel VK (1989): Kinematics of the cervical
spine following discectomy and stabilization. *Spine* 14:1116–
1121.

262. Schultz RJ (1972): *The language of fractures.* Malabar FL: R. E.
Krieger, pp. 298–299.

263. Scoville WB, Palmer AH, Samra K, Chong G (1967): The use of
acrylic plastic for vertebral replacement or fixation in metastatic
disease of the spine: Technical note. *J Neurosurg* 27:274–279.

264. Scull ER (1979): The dynamic mechanical response characteristics of spinal cord tissue: A preliminary report. *Paraplegia*
17:222–232.

265. Segal D, Whitelaw GP, Gumbs V, Pick RY (1981): Tension band
fixation of acute cervical spine fractures. *Clin Orthop* 159:211–
222.

266. Sherk H, Nicholson J (1970): Fractures of the atlas. *J Bone Joint
Surg [Am]* 52:1017–1024.

267. Sherk HH, Parke WW (1989): Developmental anatomy. In: *The
cervical spine, 2nd ed.,* RW Bailey, HH Sherk, et al, eds. Philadelphia: J. B. Lippincott, pp. 1–7.

268. Simmons EH, Bhalla SK (1969): Anterior cervical discectomy
and fusion. Clinical and biomechanical study with 8 year follow-
up. *J Bone Joint Surg [Br]* 51:225–237.

269. Simmons EH, Dutoit G (1978): Lateral atlanto-axial arthrodesis.
Orthop Clin North Am 9:1101–1114.

270. Sinbert SE, Berman MS (1940): Fracture of the posterior arch of
the atlas. *JAMA* 114:1996–1998.

271. Six E, Kelly DL Jr (1981): Technique for C1, C2 and C3 fixation
in cases of odontoid fracture. *Neurosurgery* 8:374–376.

272. Smith CG (1956): Changes in length and position of the segments
of the spinal cord with changes in posture in the monkey. *Radiology* 66:259–266.

273. Somerson SK, Stokes BT (1987): Functional analysis of an electromechanical spinal cord injury device. *Exp Neurol* 96:82–96.

274. Sorenson KH, Husby J, Hein O (1978): Interlaminar atlanto-axial fusion for instability. *Acta Orthop Scand* 49:341–349.

275. Spence KF, Decker S, Sell KW (1970): Bursting atlantal fracture
associated with rupture of the transverse ligament. *J Bone Joint
Surg [Am]* 52:543–549.

276. Stauffer ES, Kelly EG (1977): Fracture-dislocation of the cervical
spine. Instability and recurrent deformity following treatment by
anterior interbody fusion. *J Bone Joint Surg [Am]* 59:45–48.

277. Stein A, Krag M, Hugus J (1987): Anterior cervical interbody
fusion: Description of a new technique with clinical follow-up of
the first 20 patients. Proc 15th Ann Mtg Cervical Spine Research
Soc, Washington, DC.

278. Streli R (1981): Kompressionsosteosynthese bei Frakturen und
Pseudarthrosen des Dens epistrophei. *Zeitschr Orthop* 119:675–
676.

279. Streli R (1987): Dens transfixation plate. In: *Cervical spine I,* P
Kehr, A Weidner, eds. New York: Springer-Verlag, pp. 239–243.

280. Streli R (1987): Double hole plate fixation of the lower cervical
spine. In: *Cervical spine I.* P Kehr, A Weidner, eds. New York:
Springer-Verlag, pp. 175–179.

281. Sutterlin CE III, McAfee PC, Warden KE, Rey RM Jr, Farey ID
(1988): A biomechanical evaluation of cervical spine stabilization
methods in a bovine model: Static and cyclical loading. *Spine*
13:795–802.

282. Termansen NB (1974): Hangman's fracture. *Acta Orthop Scand*
45:529–539.

283. Tippets RH, Apfelbaum RI (1988): Anterior cervical fusion with
the Caspar instrumentation system. *Neurosurgery* 22:1008–1013.

284. Töndury G (1959): The cervical spine—Its development and
changes during life. *Acta Orthop Belg* 25:602–626.

285. Transfeldt EE, Simmons EH (1981): Functional and pathological
biomechanics of the spinal cord: An in vivo study. Ann Mtg Scoliosis Res Soc, Montreal.

286. Tucker HH (1975): Technical report: Method of fixation of subluxed or dislocated cervical spine below C1-C2. *Can J Neurol Sci*
2:381–382.

287. Tunturi AR (1977): Elasticity of the spinal cord dura in the dog. *J
Neurosurg* 47:391–396.

288. Tunturi AR (1978): Elasticity of the spinal cord, pia and denticulate ligament in the dog. *J Neurosurg* 48:975–979.

289. Ulrich C, Wörsdorfer O, Claes L, Magerl F (1987): Comparative
study of the stability of anterior and posterior cervical spine fixation procedures. *Arch Orthop Trauma Surg* 106:226–231.

290. Van Peteghem PK, Schweigel JF (1979): The fractured cervical

spine rendered unstable by anterior cervical fusion. *J Trauma* 19:110–114.

291. Von Torklus D, Gehle W (1972): *The upper cervical spine: Regional anatomy, pathology and traumatology. A systematic radiological atlas and textbook* (translated by LS Michaelis). New York: Grune & Stratton.

292. Walker PS, Lamser D, Hussey RW, Rossier AB, Farberov A, Dietz J (1984): Forces in the halo-vest apparatus. *Spine* 9:773–777.

293. Wang GJ, Moskal JT, Albert T, Pritts ROT, Schuch CM, Stamp WG (1988): The effect of halo-vest length on stability of the cervical spine. *J Bone Joint Surg [Am]* 70:357–360.

294. Wang GJ, Reger SI, Jennings RL, McLaurin CA, Stamp WG (1981): Variable strengths of wire fixation. *Orthopaedics* 5:435–436.

295. Weidner A (1988): Complications and follow-up of instrumentation. Proc Cerv Spine Res Soc Ann Mtg, Key Biscayne, Florida.

296. Weidner A (1989): Internal fixation with metal plates and screws. In: *The cervical spine, 2nd ed.* RW Bailey, HH Sherk, et al, eds. Philadelphia: J. B. Lippincott, pp. 407–421.

297. Werne S (1957): Studies in spontaneous atlas dislocation. *Acta Orthop Scand [Suppl]* 23:1–150.

298. Wetzel FT, Panjabi MM, Pelker RR (1989): Biomechanics of the rabbit cervical spine as a function of component transection. *J Orthop Res* 7:723–727.

299. Wetzel FT, Panjabi MM, Pelker RR (1989): Temporal biomechanics of posterior cervical spine injuries in vivo in a rabbit model. *J Orthop Res* 7:728–731.

300. White AA III (1989): Clinical biomechanics of cervical spine implants. *Spine* 14:1040–1045.

301. White AA III, Johnson RM, Panjabi MM, Southwick WO (1975): Biomechanical analysis of clinical stability in the cervical spine. *Clin Orthop* 109:85–96.

302. White AA III, Jupiter J, Southwick WO, Panjabi MM (1973): An experimental study of the immediate load bearing capacity of three surgical constructions for anterior spine fusions. *Clin Orthop* 91:21–28.

303. White AA III, Panjabi MM (1978a): The basic kinematics of the human spine. *Spine* 3:12–20.

304. White AA III, Panjabi MM (1978b): *Clinical biomechanics of the spine.* Philadelphia: J. B. Lippincott.

305. White AA III, Panjabi MM (1984): The role of stabilization in the treatment of cervical spine injuries. *Spine* 9:512–522.

306. White AA III, Southwick WO, Panjabi MM (1976): Clinical instability in the lower cervical spine: A review of past and current concepts. *Spine* 1:15–27.

307. Whitecloud TS III, La Rocca H (1976): Fibula strut graft in reconstructive surgery of the cervical spine. *Spine* 1:33–43.

308. Whitehill R, Barry JC (1985): The evolution of stability in cervical spinal constructs using either autogenous bone graft or methylmethacrylate cement: A follow-up report on a canine in vivo model. *Spine* 10:32–41.

309. Whitehill R, Cicoria AD, Hooper WE, Maggio WW, Jane JA (1988): Posterior cervical reconstruction with methylmethacrylate cement and wire: A clinical review. *J Neurosurg* 68:576–584.

310. Whitehill R, Richman JA, Glaser JA (1986): Failure of immobilization of the cervical spine by the halo vest. A report of five cases. *J Bone Joint Surg [Am]* 68:326–332.

311. Whitehill R, Stowers SF, Fechner RE, Ruch WW, Drucker S, Gibson LR, McKernan DJ, Widweyer JH (1987): Posterior cervical fusions using cerclage wires, methylmethacrylate cement and autogenous bone graft: An experimental study of a canine model. *Spine* 12:12–22.

312. Whitley JF, Forsyth HF (1960): Classification of cervical spine injuries. *Am J Roentg* 83:633–644.

313. Wilder DG, Pope MH, Frymoyer JW (1988): The biomechanics of lumbar disc herniation and the effect of overload and instability. *J Spinal Disorders* 1:16–32.

314. Willard D, Nicholson JT (1941): Dislocation of the first cervical vertebra. *Ann Surg* 113:464–475.

315. Williams TG (1975): Hangman's fracture. *J Bone Joint Surg* 57:82–88.

316. Wolf JW Jr, Johnson RM (1989): Cervical Orthoses. In: *The cervical spine, 2nd ed.,* RW Bailey, HH Sherk, et al, eds. Philadelphia: J. B. Lippincott, pp. 97–105.

317. Wolf JW, Jones HC (1980): Comparison of immobilization of the cervical spine by halocasts versus plastic jackets. Proc Cerv Spine Res Soc Ann Mtng, Palm Beach.

318. Wood-Jones F (1913): The ideal lesion produced by judicial hanging. *Lancet* 1:53.

319. Wu KK, Malik G, Guise ER (1982): Atlanto-axial arthrodesis: A clinical analysis of 22 cases treated at Henry Ford Hospital. *Orthopaedics* 5:865–871.

320. Wyke B (1978): Clinical significance of articular receptor systems. *Ann R Coll Surg Engl* 60:137.

321. Yoganandan N, Pintar F, Butler J, Reinartz J, Sances A Jr, Larson SJ (1989): Dynamic response of human cervical spine ligaments. *Spine* 14:1102–1110.

322. Yoganandan N, Sances A Jr, Maiman DJ, Myklebust JB, Pech P, Larson SJ (1986): Experimental spinal injuries with vertical impact. *Spine* 11:855–860.

The Adult Spine: Principles and Practice,
J. W. Frymoyer, Editor-in-Chief.
Raven Press, Ltd., New York © 1991.

CHAPTER **46**

Surgical Approaches to the Craniocervical Junction

Arnold H. Menezes

The first anatomical descriptions of craniocervical junction abnormalities were reported in the early part of the nineteenth century (40). These autopsy examinations stimulated clinical interest; but confirmation of the diagnosis was lacking until death. With the advent of roentgenographic studies in the early part of the 20th century, craniocervical abnormalities, as well as trauma to this region, took new meaning. However, it was only after Chamberlain's (4) classic radiographic study of basilar invagination, that lesions at and around the craniocervical junction (CCJ) emerged from the realm of anatomical and pathological curiosity to the practical, clinical field of neuroscience. The post-mortem reports were replaced by clinical and radiographic studies of abnormalities in this region.

Recent advances in neurodiagnostic imaging and microsurgical instrumentation have increased our surgical armamentarium. Up to the early 1970s, anteriorly placed lesions at the craniocervical border were approached via a posterior decompression, and at times an associated fusion. The morbidity and mortality for such ventrally situated lesions were extremely high. A physiological approach to operative treatment that was based on an understanding of craniocervical dynamics, the stability of the craniovertebral junction, and the site of encroachment was adopted by the author at the University of Iowa Hospitals and Clinic in 1977 (44). Since then,

950 patients with craniocervical abnormalities were evaluated by the author, and 506 underwent treatment on the Neurosurgical Service at the University of Iowa Hospitals (Table 1). The pathology of these abnormalities is extensive. A thorough knowledge of the bony anatomy, embryology, and biomechanics at the craniocervical junction is necessary to understand the etiology of abnormalities in this area, and thus their treatment.

DIAGNOSIS OF CRANIOCERVICAL JUNCTION ABNORMALITIES

The symptoms and signs of craniocervical abnormalities stem from the osseous changes; brain stem, cervical cord, and cerebellar dysfunction; abnormal cerebrospinal fluid dynamics; and changes that occur in the vertebral basilar vascular tree (41,43). Perhaps the most interesting feature of this region's pathology is its diverse presentation.

Compromise of the cervicomedullary junction results in a multiplicity of symptoms and signs that may be indicated by brain stem and cervical myelopathy, cranial nerve and cervical root dysfunction, and the alterations of vascular supply to these structures (3,35,36,43). The symptoms may be insidious and present as a puzzling clinical condition with false localizing signs, or may be precipitated by minor trauma. In a significant number of patients there is a rapid neurological deterioration, which can be followed by sudden death.

A. H. Menezes, M.D.: Professor, Division of Neurosurgery, University of Iowa Hospitals, Iowa City, Iowa, 52242.

TABLE 1. *Summary of surgical treatment at the craniocervical junction in 506 patients (1977–1990)*

Stability	Compression	Approach	Post-operative stability	Posterior fusion
A. Reducible 244		Immobilization 34		210
B. Irreducible 262	Ventral 166	Anterior	Stable 29	
			Unstable 137	137
	Dorsal 96	Posterior	Stable 35	
			Unstable 61	61

METHOD OF APPROACH

Factors influencing specific treatment are (44):

1. Reducibility—whether the bony abnormality can be "reduced" to normal position and relieve compression of the cervicomedullary junction. This also implies restoration of anatomical relationships of the craniospinal axis.
2. The etiology of the lesion; whether bony or soft tissue. Vascular abnormalities, syrinx, and Chiari malformations fall within this category.
3. Presence of ossification centers and epiphyseal growth plates in certain congenital lesions, e.g., warfarin syndrome.
4. The mechanics of compression and the direction of encroachment.

The primary treatment for reducible craniocervical lesions is stabilization (Table 2). Surgical decompression is performed in patients with irreducible pathology. When irreducible lesions are encountered, the decompression is performed in the manner in which encroachment occurs. If a ventral encroachment is present, a transoral-transpalatal-pharyngeal decompression is made; with dorsal compression, a posterior decompression is mandated. If instability exists following either situation, a posterior fixation is required.

NEURORADIOLOGICAL INVESTIGATIONS

The factors influencing specific treatment are thus determined by plain radiographs, pleuridirectional tomography with associated dynamic studies to include the flexed and extended positions, computed tomography of the craniocervical area to include cerebrospinal fluid enhancement with Iohexol, and magnetic resonance imaging (3,37,41,56). The effects of cervical traction must be documented. The earlier chapters on diagnostic procedures have outlined the usefulness of each of these investigative modalities. Each of these techniques has important features and provides complementary information about the craniocervical junction and the presence of any incidental and pathological changes in the normal and abnormal relationships (Figs. 1A, 1B, 1C, and 1D).

With the advent of magnetic resonance imaging

TABLE 2. *Treatment of craniocervical abnormalities*

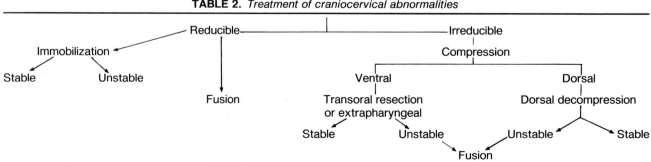

(MRI) over the past 6 years, there has been a gradual trend to make this the only neurodiagnostic procedure, apart from plain radiographs of the craniocervical border (41). However, the MRI fails to completely visualize the osseous pathology and is unable to delineate the true extent of congenital and developmental lesions in this region. Imaging of the craniocervical junction should start with outlining the bony pathology with pleuridirectional tomography in the frontal and lateral planes, from facet to facet. In addition, this is done with dynamic imaging in the flexed and extended positions, and subsequently with cervical traction. This defines the bony pathology and acts as a pre-operative assessment of stability in both the anterior-posterior and vertical dimensions. Magnetic resonance imaging follows in the axial, sagittal, and coronal planes. Dynamic views of the flexed and extended position are obtained in the mid-sagittal plane. Cervical traction via an MRI-compatible Halo is subsequently used to determine stability of the lesion (38,39) (Figs. 2A, 2B, 2C, and 2D). In selected patients, CT myelotomography is essential to identify and locate the abnormality in relationship to the subarachnoid space and its proximity to the vertebro-basilar vascular system. At times vertebral angiography is necessary to locate the position of abnormal vessels and to see the effects of head rotation in the flexed and extended position, should this be present in the symptomatology.

APPROACHES TO THE CRANIOCERVICAL JUNCTION

The term "craniocervical junction" refers to the occipital bone surrounding the foramen magnum and the atlas and axis vertebrae. Most approaches to this region are via either the ventral route or the dorsal routes. The lateral approach is limited (15,16,17,53,55).

Anterior approaches to the CCJ encompass the median route and the anterolateral approach (Table 3). The common denominator is the transoral-transpalatal-pharyngeal approach to the craniocervical junction, and to a much lesser extent the anterolateral-transcervical-extra-

TABLE 3. *Anterior approaches to the craniocervical junction*

I. Median
  A. Transoral-transpalatal-pharyngeal
    (7,9,11,13,18,21,22,31,44,48,65)
  B. Median labiomandibular glossotomy (1,19,25,27,47)
  C. Sublabial LeFort I maxillary osteotomy with maxillary "down-fracture" (2,60)
  D. Lateral rhinotomy (10,32,51)
    (B, C, and D are frequently combined with A.)
II. Anterolateral
  Transcervical extrapharyngeal (8,29,30,34,58,62)
III. Lateral
  Infratemporal fossa transzygomatic with resection/rotation of the condylar process (15,16,17,53,55)

pharyngeal operation. The dorsal approach has been used by the author for decompression, as well as fusion. The ensuing chapter will deal with these subjects.

Transoral-Transpalatal-Pharyngeal Approach

The transoral-transpalatal-pharyngeal approach to the craniocervical junction provides a safe, effective, and rapid exposure to the median 4.5 cm of the craniocervical junction from the mid-clivus to the C2-C3 interspace (Fig. 3). Further inferior access may be gained by median labial mandibular glossotomy (1,9,19,25,27,47). Rostral extension of the exposure may be provided by limited resection of the caudal hard palate (37,39) or by a sublabial LeFort I maxillary osteotomy with maxillary "down fracture" (2,60). An option is a lateral rhinotomy combined with the transoral-transpalatal-transpharyngeal approach (10,32,51).

The main indication for a transoral operation is irreducible ventral compression on the cervicomedullary junction due to osseous pathology, neoplasm, or inflammatory lesions. Bony tumors and chordomas have been approached in this manner (37,41,60). Meningiomas and schwannomas, which are primary intradural lesions, are best approached by the dorsal route, since they reside within the subarachnoid space. However, should this not be possible, a ventral operative approach may be essential (45). Similarly, midline vertebral basilar artery aneurysms have been clipped via this route with exposure through the clivus, when no other route would suffice (11,21,22,31,48,64). Even though there appears to be host immunity to the oropharyngeal flora, the main indication for an anterior transoral midline operative procedure is an extradural lesion. It is important to bear in mind that even though lesions may appear to be irreducible, the stabilization of cervical traction is essential during the ventral transoral procedure.

Pre-Operative Assessment

The nutritional status of symptomatic patients must be evaluated. The achievement of a high caloric intake is feasible in some individuals only via nasogastric feeding or intravenous hyperalimentation (7,41,53). This is an important part of the pre-operative and peri-operative management, since oral intake is not permitted during the first week after operation.

In circumstances such as rheumatoid arthritis affecting the temporomandibular joint, the ability to open the mouth may be limited (18,37). It is important to obtain a working distance of 2.5 to 3 cm between the upper and lower incisor teeth. If this is not possible, an alternative route may be sought. If not, a median mandibular split with midline glossotomy is essential to the transoral operation (1,39).

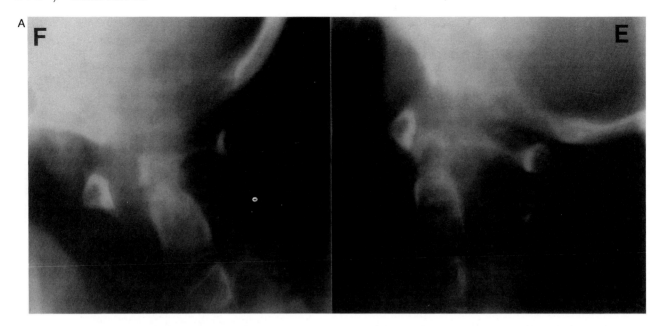

FIG. 1A. Case D.M. Midline pleuridirectional tomograms of the craniocervical junction (CCJ) in the flexed (**left**) and extended (**right**) positions. This 42-year-old rheumatoid was known to have a reducible atlanto-axial luxation for several years. Recent loss of arm and hand function prompted further evaluation.

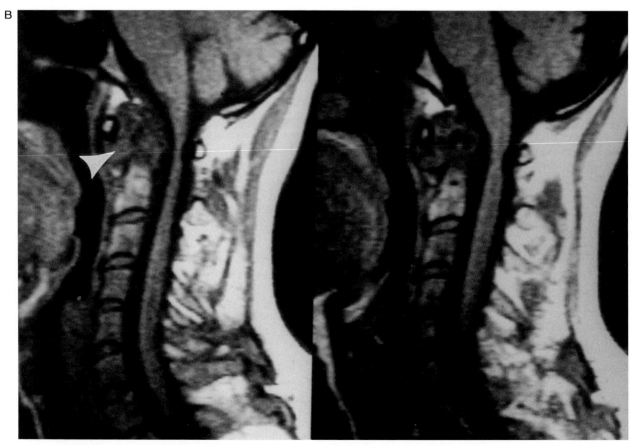

FIG. 1B. Case D.M. Mid-sagittal T1-weighted MRIs of the CCJ reveal a large mass (arrowhead) enveloping the entire odontoid process with ventral cervicomedullary (CM) neural compression. (Figs. 1C–1D follow.)

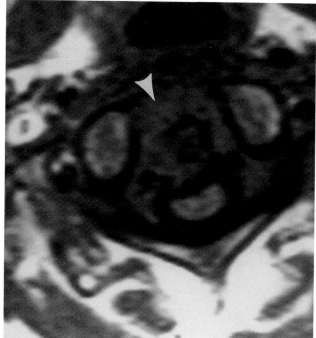

FIG. 1. *Continued.* **C: Case D.M.** Axial T1-weighted MRI at CCJ outlines pannus (arrowhead) surrounding the odontoid process with ventral cervicomedullary junction compression.

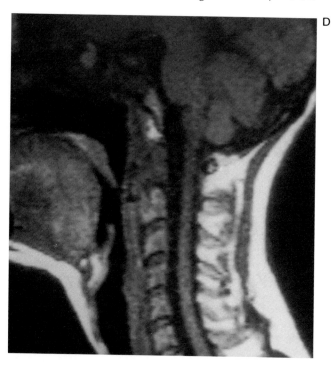

FIG. 1. *Continued.* **D: Case D.M.** Mid-sagittal T1-weighted MRI in Halo traction, 6 days after transoral operation for CM compression. Note the odontoid and pannus resection and the normal neural structures.

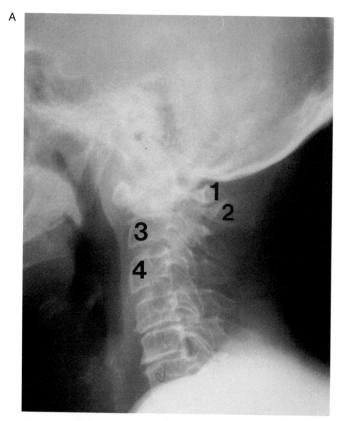

FIG. 2A. **Case M.T.** Lateral skull and cervical radiograph in a 67-year-old patient with long-standing rheumatoid arthritis. There is ''cranial settling.'' The anterior atlantal arch has telescoped down to the C2-C3 interspace, while the dorsal C1 arch is within the spinal canal.

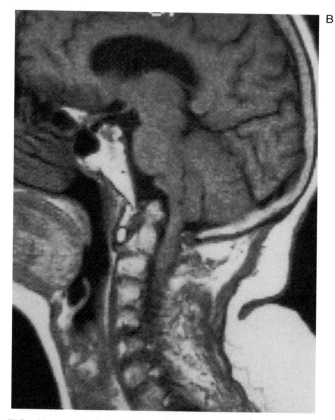

FIG. 2B. **Case M.T.** Mid-sagittal T1-weighted MRI of the CCJ. The odontoid has migrated into the ventral aspect of the posterior fossa compressing the medulla oblongata. (Figs. 2C–2D follow.)

C

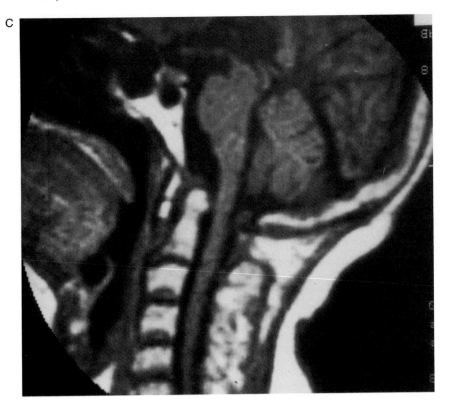

FIG. 2. *Continued.* **C: Case M.T.** Mid-sagittal T1-weighted MRI in Halo traction at 8 lbs. There is marked reduction in the odontoid invagination into the medulla.

D

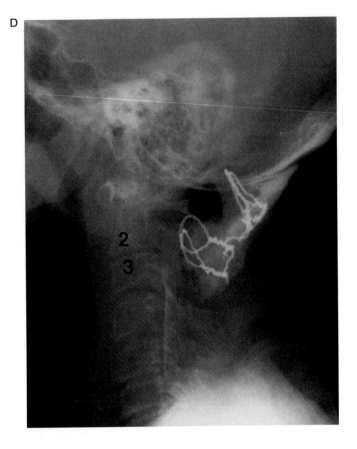

FIG. 2. *Continued.* **D: Case M.T.** Lateral cervical spine radiograph made 1 week after C1 posterior decompression and dorsal occipitocervical fusion with rib graft, wire, and methylmethacrylate. Note the reduction of the "cranial settling."

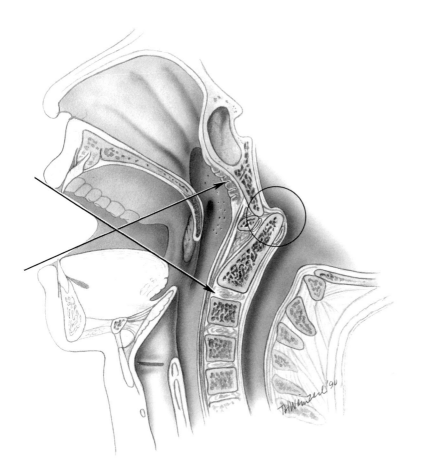

FIG. 3. Illustration of the extent of exposure (between arrows) via the transoral-transpalatal route to the craniocervical junction.

Pre-operative oral-pharyngeal cultures are obtained three days prior to a surgical procedure. No antibiotics are given unless pathological flora are present.

Should the lower cranial nerves be compromised, it is imperative that pre-operative assessment of the swallowing mechanism, as well as respiratory function, be made. At times this will mandate whether a tracheostomy is needed at the time of transoral operation.

Operative Procedure

The patient is transported to the operating theater on a fracture bed with skeletal traction applied via an MRI-compatible Halo at 7–8 pounds. Topical and regional block anesthesia facilitates an awake fiber-optic oral tracheal intubation. The patient is then examined awake to ensure that no change in neurological status has occurred due to positioning. A nasotracheal intubation is to be avoided, as this tends to disrupt the integrity of the high naso-pharyngeal mucosa, which is the avenue of approach to the craniocervical region. The patient is then positioned supine with the head resting in a Mayfield horseshoe head holder. Traction is maintained during the operation with mild extension of the neck. Once it is established that no neurological deficit has occurred,

general endotracheal and intravenous anesthesia is accomplished.

A tracheostomy is performed when the operation involves the craniocervical junction and structures rostral to it (41). In situations in which there is brain stem compromise, a tracheostomy is performed after the intubation. Following the intubation or tracheostomy, a gauze packing is placed to occlude the laryngopharynx and prevent secretions and blood from draining into the stomach.

A modified Dingman self-retaining mouth retractor secures the armored endotracheal tube and allows for exposure of the oral cavity, as well as the pharynx. In operative procedures involving the clivus and foramen magnum, it is essential to split the soft palate to provide the necessary exposure. The operating microscope provides magnification in a concentrated light source. The oral cavity is cleansed with 10% povidone-iodine (PVP) and hydrogen peroxide and rinsed with saline. A midline incision is made into the soft palate extending from the hard palate to the base of the uvula and deviating to one side (Fig. 4). Stay sutures are applied to the incised soft palate, retracting the soft palate flaps to either side, exposing the high posterior nasopharynx down to the C3 vertebral level. The posterior pharyngeal wall is anesthetized with topical 2.5% cocaine and the median raphe

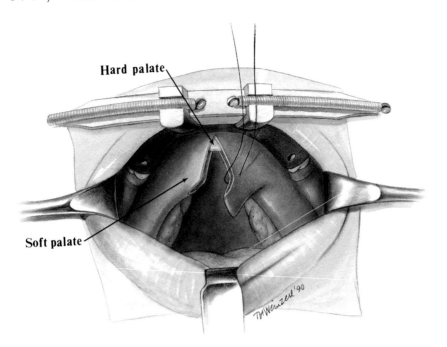

Hard palate

Soft palate

FIG. 4. Illustration of operative procedure. The mouth retractor is in position and the soft palate incision made.

infiltrated with .5% xylocaine with 1/200,000 epineph-rine (Fig. 5A). The midline posterior pharynx is now incised. The posterior pharyngeal flaps are then retracted to either side with stay sutures, exposing the clivus down to the upper border of C3. The pre-vertebral fascia and longus colli muscles are dissected free of their osseous and ligamentous attachment to expose the axis vertebra, the atlas, and the caudal clivus. The ligaments are now swept away to expose the midline anterior arch of the atlas from one lateral mass to the other, the caudal clivus, and the axis body and the base of the dens.

Lateral exposure is limited to 2 cm to either side of the midline to preserve the integrity of the eustachian tube orifice and to prevent injury to the hypoglossal nerve and the vertebral arteries.

The anterior arch of the atlas is removed with a high-speed drill, as is the caudal clivus (Fig. 5B). The soft tissue ventral to the odontoid process is now resected with rongeurs. Removal of the odontoid process is carried out in a rostral-caudal dimension using a high-speed drill with a diamond burr (Fig. 5C). Pannus encountered indicates the chronic instability. This has to be resected (Fig. 5D). Division of the odontoid process at its base and downward traction have been advocated by some (7,18). This endangers the patient and is fraught with difficulty. This is especially so if the pannus is tough and the odontoid has now achieved a subarachnoid location. After removal of the tectorial membrane (Fig. 5E), the surgeon is assured of adequate bony decompression by the pulsatile dura protruding into the decompression site (Fig. 5F).

Median nerve sensory evoked responses are utilized during the operation to record the brain stem latencies (54,57,64). Change in this latter parameter requires judicious handling of tissues and minimizing compression on the neural structures. This is especially important in patients with severe cervicomedullary compromise (Figs. 6A and 6B).

In the event of tumor being encountered, such as chordoma, direct visualization of the tumor extent is possible. Piecemeal removal is necessary without undue traction in case of dural penetration of the tumor. In situations in which an intradural lesion is encountered, a midline incision of the ventral dura must be made starting inferiorly and then proceeding upwards. Resection of an intradural lesion requires relieving the CSF turgidity by having previously placed a lumbar subarachnoid drain. The dura is opened in a midline fashion extending up as high as necessary into the ventral posterior fossa. A cruciate dural incision is made by converting the vertical incision to a cruciform one below the foramen magnum, thus avoiding the circular sinus. Once the intradural operation is completed, it is essential to bring the dural leaves together in as watertight a closure as possible. In a situation in which the dura has been violated, it is important to harvest external oblique aponeurosis for fascia to be laid against the dural closure. This must be reinforced with a fat pad prior to closure of the operative wound.

The longus colli muscles are approximated in the midline with subsequent anatomical closure of the posterior pharyngeal musculature and the posterior pharyngeal mucosa. Each of these layers is approximated with interrupted sutures of polyglycolic.

In the event the opening into the clivus is large, a pharyngeal pack is utilized for compression at the high nasopharynx with traction tubes brought out through the nostrils.

Closure of the soft palate is done by bringing the nasal mucosa together with interrupted sutures. The muscularis and oral mucous membrane of the soft palate are

A–C

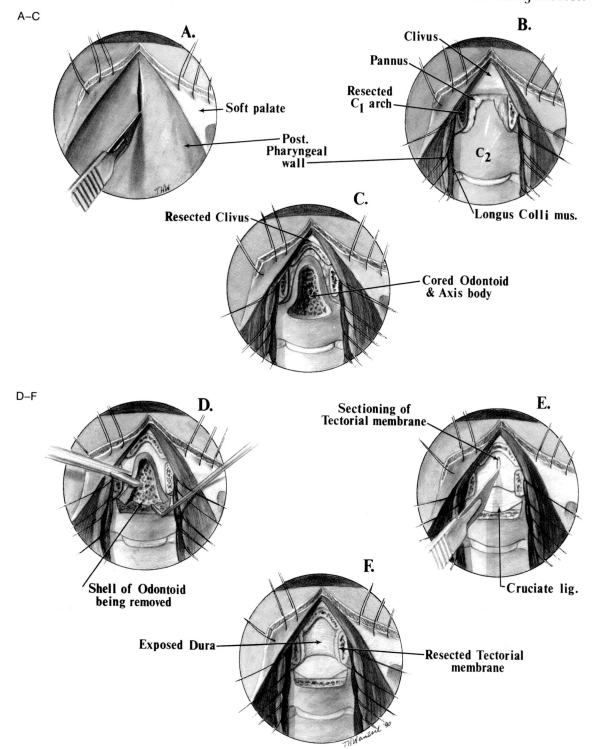

FIG. 5. Views through operating microscope. **A:** Incision of posterior pharyngeal wall. **B:** Resection of anterior atlas arch and caudal clivus brings the invaginated odontoid process into relief. **C:** The odontoid is cored out. **D:** The odontoid shell is being removed. **E:** The tectorial membrane is incised. **F:** Dural decompression.

approximated with interrupted vertical mattress sutures of similar strength.

In situations in which surgery is necessary through the clivus, or in patients with a foreshortened clivus and platybasia, the hard palate is exposed and the posterior 7

to 10 mm is resected. This allows high nasopharyngeal exposure without splitting the mandible or doing a median glossotomy. The patient is maintained in 5 to 7 pounds of skeletal traction after operation. Intravenous hyperalimentation is continued for 5 to 6 days, and no

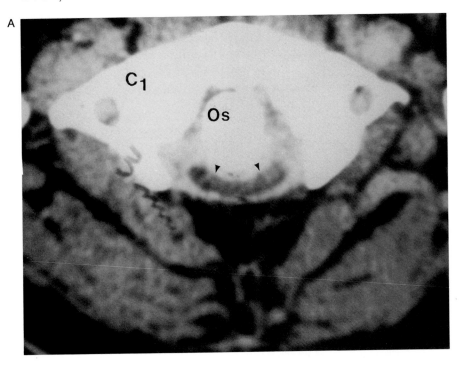

FIG. 6A. Case D.P. Axial view of CT myelogram at C1 level. This 23-year-old quadriparetic male worsened neurologically after dorsal C1-C3 laminectomies for os odontoideum with spinal cord compression. The ventrally located os odontoideum still causes cord compromise despite the posterior decompression.

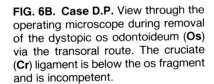
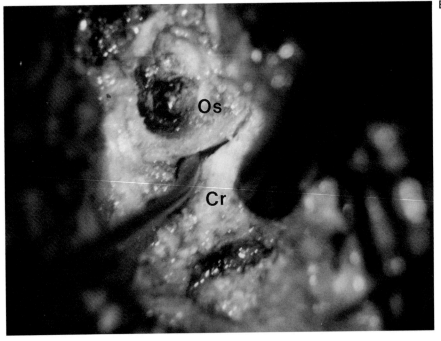

FIG. 6B. Case D.P. View through the operating microscope during removal of the dystopic os odontoideum (**Os**) via the transoral route. The cruciate (**Cr**) ligament is below the os fragment and is incompetent.

oral intake is permitted. This is then followed by a gradual increase in feeding to a regular diet by the end of 15 to 18 days.

In the event that the dura was opened, intravenous antibiotics (Cefotaxime, flagyl, and Methicillin) and spinal drainage are maintained for 10 days after the operation. The tracheostomy is discontinued only if a stabilization procedure is not required. In the event that no tracheostomy was performed, the armored endotracheal tube is left in place for the first 48 hours to counteract any lingual swelling or pharyngeal edema.

The post-operative stability is evaluated with pleuridirectional lateral tomography obtained one week after the transoral operation. This is done in the flexed and extended positions, as well as with and without traction, to assess vertical stability. An offset at the lateral occipito-atlanto-axial articulation during these studies, or vertical displacement of the craniospinal axis, is indicative of instability. Magnetic resonance imaging is performed at this time to assess the decompression (Fig. 1D). Should instability exist at the craniocervical junction, an occipitocervical fixation becomes mandatory. Of the 166 patients who underwent a ventral decompression, 137 required a dorsal fixation procedure (Table 1).

Neurological improvement was seen in all the author's patients who underwent a transoral operation. Table 4 outlines the pathology encountered during this operation. The patients who were ventilator dependent following previous primary posterior fossa decompression from a dorsal route had resolution of their neurological symptoms and signs (41). More importantly, patients with a Chiari malformation and basilar invagination who underwent primary ventral decompression had resolution of their symptoms. In addition, the syrinx, if present, showed objective regression on magnetic resonance imaging (40).

An intradural pathology was encountered in 18 individuals (Figs. 7A and 7B). This was handled in the manner previously described. In the author's own series, there were no episodes of meningitis, and a lumboperitoneal shunt was never required, nor was a septomucoperiosteal flap or a pharyngeal flap needed for clo-

TABLE 4. *Pathology encountered using the transoral-transpalatal-pharyngeal approach to the craniocervical junction (1977–1990)*

87	Primary basilar invagination
33	Rheumatoid "irreducible cranial settling"
12	Dystopic os odontoideum
6	Basilar invagination after malunion, O-C1-C2 dislocation
6	Odontoid fracture segment migration
6	Granulation mass
4	Calcium pyrophosphate mass
8	Chordoma clivus—C1
2	Osteoblastoma
2	Down's syndrome with cranial settling
166	Total

sure of the posterior pharyngeal wall or the dura (7,22,25,26,65). In the author's series, a 79-year-old male, with rheumatoid arthritis and cranial settling, succumbed to a myocardial infarction four weeks after his dorsal fixation operation. One patient had wound dehiscence in the post-operative period. This required intravenous hyperalimentation and intravenous antibiotics for 10 days. It is thus evident that the complications associated with this operation make one feel that there is host immunity to the existing flora within the oral cavity. The unfortunate morbidity and mortality attached to the earlier reported series by Fang et al. (13) are still quoted in recent publications as reason to avoid the transoral approach (34,62).

Transcervical Extrapharyngeal Approach

The anterior retropharyngeal approach to the upper cervical spine has been described by several authors (29,30,34,58,62). This approach provides anterior access to the neural elements from the clivus to the third cervical vertebra without entrance into the oral cavity, and allows for a ventral fusion procedure. The author has used a modification of this procedure for exposure from the clivus to the lower cervical spine.

The patient is intubated via a nasal endotracheal route using a fiber-optic awake intubation. The oral cavity is kept free of any tubes. The same precautions are taken as with the transoral route regarding the anesthesia and intubation. The cervical incision starts behind the ear, over the mastoid process, extending 1.5 cm below the angle of the mandible towards the midline above the hyoid bone. An inferior extension of this converts the transverse incision to a "T." This is done at the level of the omohyoid muscle and brought down over the sternomastoid. The head is turned to the left considering the right-handed surgeon. The extent of the vertical limb of the incision is dependent upon the amount of cervical spine that needs to be exposed. The incision traverses the subcutaneous tissue and the platysma. Subcutaneous dissection allows for mobilization in a subplatysmal plane of the superficial fascia. The inferior division of the facial nerve is identified. The superficial draining veins into the jugular vein are dissected free and ligated prior to their entrance into the common facial or the jugular vein. The superficial branches of the facial nerve are now protected by staying deep to this. The deep fascia at the anterior border of the sternomastoid is incised, allowing for visualization of the carotid sheath. Dissection is made anterior to this. The submandibular salivary gland may be elevated. However, resection of the submandibular salivary gland has no consequences if its duct is sutured properly to prevent a salivary fistula. The nodes in the carotid and the digastric triangle are now removed. The posterior belly of the digastric is traced to its tendon where it is transsected and transfixed with a suture for

A

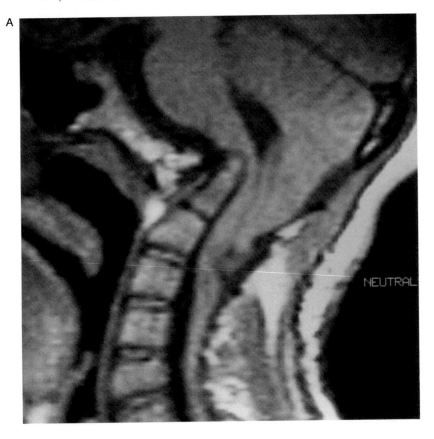

FIG. 7A. Case M.T. Mid-sagittal T1-weighted MRI at the CVJ. This 24-year-old male had previously undergone posterior fossa and upper cervical decompression for Chiari malformation. He had difficulty swallowing, sleep apnea, and couldn't walk. There is severe odontoid invagination into the ventral aspect of the medulla, atlas assimilation, and Chiari malformation.

B

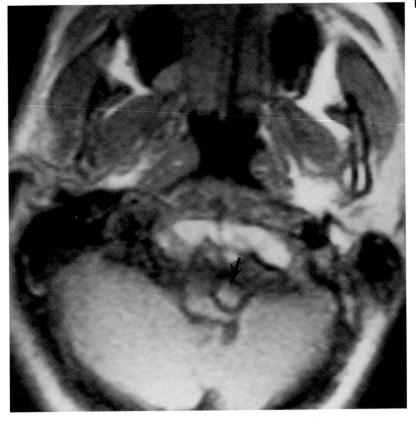

FIG. 7B. Case M.T. Axial T1-weighted MRI made 1.5 cm above the foramen magnum. The odontoid process (arrow) is intradural in location, abutting the 4th ventricle. This was successfully excised via the transoral route.

subsequent reapproximation. The stylohyoid muscle is now divided, allowing for medial retraction of the laryngopharynx. Care is taken to identify the hypoglossal nerve as it swings between the internal and external carotid arteries at the greater cornu of the hyoid bone. This is then mobilized superiorly, taking care to preserve the descendens hypoglossi. The retropharyngeal space is now achieved with blunt dissection. Any veins crossing the operative field into the jugular vein have to be sectioned.

The pre-vertebral fascia is incised in a vertical manner to expose the longus colli muscles. These are detached from their medial origin so as to expose the anterior arch of the atlas. Retractor care must be taken to prevent injury to the hypoglossal nerve as it emerges from the condylar foramen. Orientation to the midline must be maintained at all times. The osseous ligamentous structures are now swept away to visualize the caudal clivus and the upper cervical vertebrae in their anterior aspect.

Anterior decompression is accomplished using the high-speed drill, and the procedure is carried out as described with the transoral operation. Once decompression has been accomplished, fusion may be carried out using a tricorticate iliac crest graft or a fibular strut interposed between the caudal clivus and the inferior aspect of the axis vertebra (8).

Anterior fusion utilizing methylmethacrylate has been described by Lesoin et al. (30). This exposure may be carried inferiorly by extension of the vertical limb of the skin incision.

Closure of the cervical wound is first accomplished by approximating the longus colli muscles in the midline with 00 polyglycolic sutures. The digastric tendon is then approximated with 000 neurolon sutures. The deep fascia at the anterior border of the sternomastoid is approximated, as is the platysma. Skin approximation is done in a standard fashion. No drains are utilized.

The author has utilized this procedure infrequently due to the high risk of hypoglossal nerve injury and difficulty in visualizing deep midline structures at the true craniocervical border. However, this approach is ideal for extradural lesions at the axis and subaxial levels. The post-operative care requires placement into a Halo vest by the third or fourth day. This is maintained until fusion has been documented. The anterior fusion has been rightly called by McAfee et al. (34) as "conferring compressive stability only," and the patient should be kept in skull traction until posterior stabilization is achieved if the pathological process has made the spine unstable.

This approach requires a fair amount of dissection of the carotid sheath and structures at the carotid bifurcation. It is mandatory that the carotid system be scanned for plaques prior to embarking on such a procedure, as intra-operative stroke with embolization is a very real possibility.

Reducible Lesions Requiring Posterior Fusion

The majority of the author's patients required skeletal traction for a few days to achieve realignment of the craniocervical junction (5,6,12,14,35,42,61,63,66). This occurred in 80% of patients with cranial settling (36,43), thus obviating the need for an anterior decompressive procedure in addition. In other reducible lesions, such as Down's syndrome, os odontoideum, and atlas assimilation with instability, the traction was initiated at 7 pounds and followed by graded increases to a maximum of 15 to 18 pounds. The author has been unsuccessful in realigning the craniovertebral junction by cervical traction in those patients with rheumatoid arthritis, in whom the odontoid process had invaginated more than 20 mm into foramen magnum, or who had a fracture at the base of the dens. Reduction was not possible in those individuals with complete separation of the anterior and posterior arches of the atlas and basilar invagination. Granulation tissue at the sites of instability fixed the odontoid process to the atlas-clivus junction. This was especially true in patients with atlas assimilation who were over 16 years of age.

Skeletal traction is maintained via a Halo ring throughout the maneuvers of anesthetic induction. An awake fiber-optic, oral or nasal, endotracheal intubation is made. Following this, the patient is placed prone on the operating table with skeletal traction being maintained and the face and Halo ring resting on a padded Mayfield horseshoe headrest. The position of the head and neck is dictated by the pre-operative studies that showed the least neural compromise (Figs. 8A and 8B). The chest is elevated on laminectomy rolls or a Wilson frame. The neurological status is assessed, and a lateral radiograph documents the optimal position for reduction. This position is guided by the pre-operative dynamic films. After radiographic studies have been performed and position adjustments made, oral endotracheal and intravenous anesthesia ensues. Cervical traction is maintained over a pulley bar so as to allow for dynamic changes during the operation. A fixed head position with the pinned headrest, or the Halo vest, allows changes in alignment between the prone and supine positions. This is obviated by using a constantly moving mobile traction force that adapts to the patient's position.

The posterior scalp and cervical regions are prepared, as is the area for harvesting of donor bone, the iliac crest or the posterior-inferior rib cage. Cephalothin sodium (Keflin) 1 gm every 6 hours is administered 12 hours prior to the start of the procedure and maintained for 48 hours after the operation.

A midline incision from the external occipital protuberance to the spinous process of the fifth cervical vertebra is made. A subperiosteal exposure is obtained of the

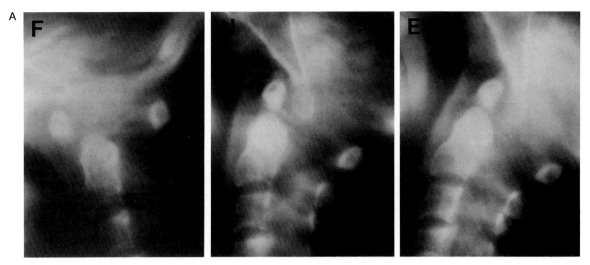

FIG. 8A. Case V.D. Composite of midline polytomograms of CCJ in the flexed (**F**), neutral (**N**), and extension (**E**) positions. This 15-year-old gymnast suffered sudden hemiparesis on the parallel bars. There is craniocervical instability secondary to a dystopic os odontoideum.

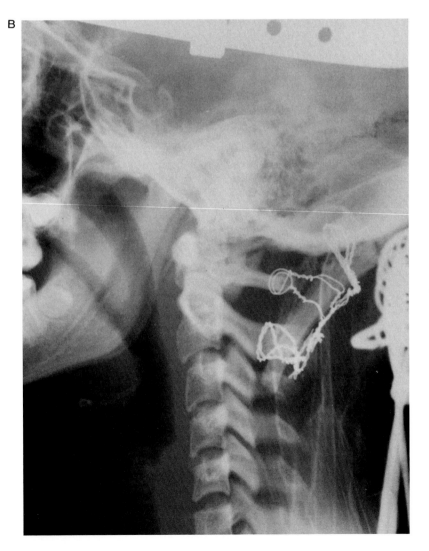

FIG. 8B. Case V.D. Plain lateral cervical x-ray made in Halo vest immobilization 1 week after C1 decompression and occipitocervical fusion.

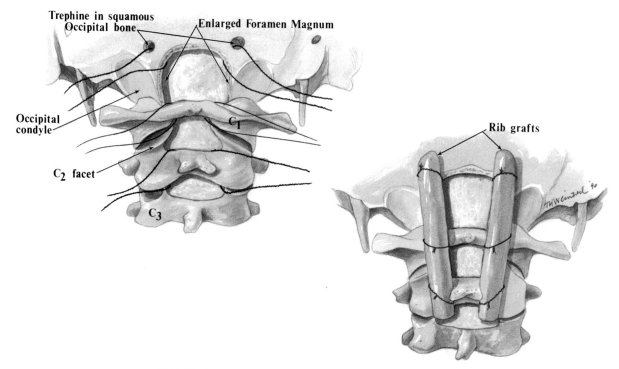

FIG. 9. Illustration of dorsal occipitocervical fusion technique.

squamous occipital bone and the posterior arches of the upper three cervical vertebrae using sharp dissection. If gross instability is present, a towel clip is passed through the spinous process of the axis for stabilization (14,61,66). This is likewise done to the posterior arch of the atlas when muscle dissection is performed. Stabilization of the operative exposure can be obtained by placing the D'Errico or Miskimon retractors at 90° to each other (42). This placement stretches and fixes the bone-muscle relationship so as to prevent motion of the occipito-cervical and atlanto-axial joints. In those patients with occipito-atlanto-axial instability, the fusion must include the occiput in addition to the atlas and axis vertebrae.

The posterior rim of foramen magnum is excised using Kerrison punch rongeurs and bone preserved for utilization in the construct. A craniectomy is made to excise the posterior rim of foramen magnum and ascend upwards for about 1.5 cm (Fig. 9). This is essential to remove the exoccipital bony ridge to facilitate easy passage of wire from a laterally placed trephine towards the midline (20). Trephines are made 2.5 cm to either side of the midline and 2 cm above foramen magnum. Epidural braided #20 or #22 wire is passed from the occipital trephine opening to the midline craniectomy. Similarly braided #20 or #22 wire is passed beneath the lamina of the axis vertebra individually (59). An unbraided #20 wire is used beneath the lamina of C1. This is to prevent saw-like cutting of the posterior arch of the atlas, which in many circumstances is thin. The donor bone is harvested from the rib or ilium. The author has consistently

utilized full thickness rib, removed close to the head of the rib to provide for the contour and approximation between the occiput and the dorsal surface of the atlas and axis vertebrae. Decortication of the spinous process and laminae is essential to the recipient site, and also at the occiput. The donor bone is secured to the occiput, atlas, and axis vertebrae by passing the wire through the graft to anchor them into position. Matchstick-sized slivers of bone are then packed into the remaining crevices at the donor-recipient site.

The patient is maintained in skeletal traction for 3 to 4 days after operation prior to immobilization in a Halo vest. Immobilization is required for 3 to 4 months for atlanto-axial fusions and 6 months for occipito-atlanto-axial arthrodesis (5,24,42,43). In the latter circumstance, less prolonged immobilization may result in non-union, union in an abnormal position, or in those patients with rheumatoid arthritis additional cranial settling with subsequent increased neurological deficit (6,28,35, 49,50,61).

In severely disabled patients, such as those with rheumatoid arthritis, immediate internal stabilization can be obtained by supplementing the bone fusion construct with acrylic and wire fixation (5,12). In this situation, the wires anchoring the bone graft are preserved for a length of 2 cm. These are then converted into hooks to act as pegs for the oncoming acrylic onlay. Methylmethacrylate is fashioned in a horseshoe-shaped manner, with the horizontal connecting limb being molded to the occiput and the vertical stripes cascading over the bone graft,

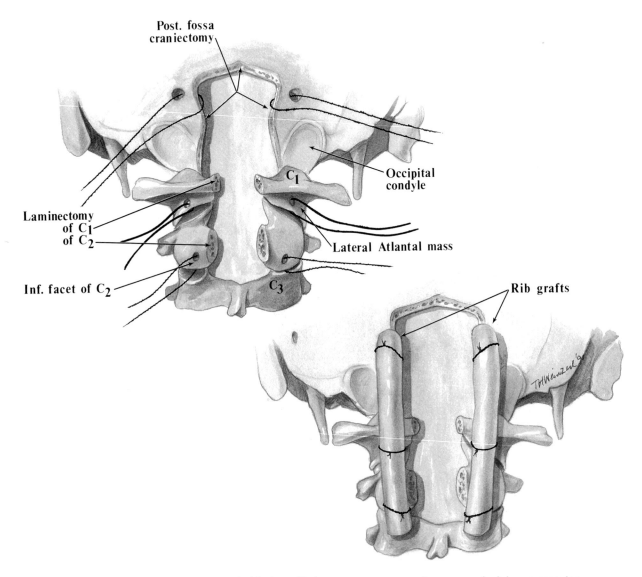

FIG. 10. Illustration of occipitocervical fusion with foramen magnum and upper cervical decompression.

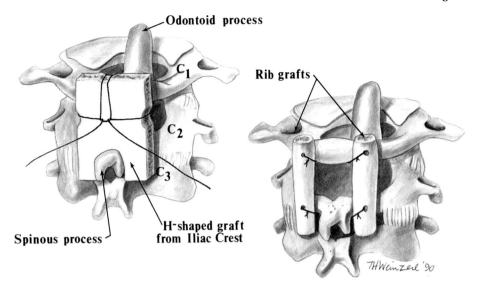

FIG. 11. Illustration of dorsal C1-C2 fusion.

enveloping the wire pegs, but staying free of the lateral surface of bone. This allows for muscle approximation over the bony construct, thus providing for vascularization.

In those circumstances in which a posterior decompression of the atlas arch and posterior fossa may be essential prior to fixation, the fusion is modified (Fig. 10). Unbraided #22 wire is passed through small trephines made in the inferior facet of C1 and C2 and a lateral occipitocervical fusion accomplished.

Posterior Decompression of the Craniocervical Junction

The procedures for positioning the patient and the induction of anesthesia, as well as the operative exposure, are identical to those described earlier. The craniectomy is done to include the posterior and lateral bone surrounding foramen magnum. Pre-operative investigations determine the exact amount of decompression required of the squamous occipital bone, foramen magnum, and upper cervical spine (Fig. 10). Should a situation such as a Chiari malformation exist or achondroplasia, the upper cervical decompression may be necessary. In addition, in situations in which intradural surgery is necessary in the posterior fossa, this is first completed. Dural closure must be accomplished primarily or with fascial graft. If a fusion is required, the amount of squamous occipital bone to be resected is limited so as to allow placement of the bone grafts away from the site of the decompression. Should stabilization be necessary subsequent to the posterior decompression and laminectomy, a lateral facet fusion technique is utilized.

Dorsal Occipito-Atlanto-Axial Instrumentation

Several instrumentation procedures have now been introduced into the armamentarium of atlanto-axial and occipito-cervical fusion. These include clamps, screws, rods, and contoured loops (7,23,46,49,50,52,55). The success of any fusion construct is ultimately dependent on achieving a solid bony fusion. This must be achieved prior to stress fatigue; hence there is always a race to achieve osseous integration prior to construct fatigue. For this reason, post-operative immobilization is mandatory. The placement of instrumentation only serves for the immediate post-operative period, until the osseous fusion has occurred. Clamp devices that approximate the atlas to the axis or in the Gallie-type fusion will only worsen a situation such as cranial settling in the rheumatoid patient (46). The ideal atlanto-axial arthrodesis should maintain spacing, prevent rotation, and accommodate flexion and compressive forces (Fig. 11). The utilization of the previously described procedure (limited to the atlanto-axial level) allows for this.

RESULTS

In no circumstance in the author's series has there been an increase in neurological deficit. The incidence of non-union in 310 occipito-cervical fusions and 98 atlanto-axial fusions has been 1%. This is attributed to the design of the fusion construct, the extent of immobilization, and removing the anterior compressive pathology at the craniocervical junction prior to posterior fixation (14,20,33,43,59,61). There was one wound infection. The post-operative follow-up has been throughout the 13 years of this series.

REFERENCES

1. Arbit E, Patterson RH Jr (1981): Combined transoral and median labiomandibular glossotomy approach to the upper cervical spine. *Neurosurgery* 8:672–674.
2. Archer DJ, Young S, Uttley D (1987): Basilar aneurysms: A new transclival approach via maxillotomy. *J Neurosurg* 67:54–58.
3. Bundschuh C, Modic MT, Kearney F, Morris R, Deal C (1988): Rheumatoid arthritis of the cervical spine. Surface-coil MR imaging. *AJR* 151:181–187.
4. Chamberlain WE (1939): Basilar impression (platybasia): A bizarre developmental anomaly of occipital bone and upper cervical spine with striking and misleading neurological manifestations. *Yale J Biol Med* 11:487–496.
5. Clark CR, Goetz DD, Menezes AH (1989): Arthrodesis of the cervical spine in rheumatoid arthritis. *J Bone Joint Surg* [Am] 71:381–392.
6. Conaty JP, Mongan ES (1981): Cervical fusion in rheumatoid arthritis. *J Bone Joint Surg* [Am] 63:1218–1227.
7. Crockard HA, Pozo JL, Ransford AO, Stevens JM, Kendall BE, Essigman WK (1986): Transoral decompression and posterior fusion for rheumatoid atlanto-axial subluxation. *J Bone Joint Surg* [Br] 68:350–356.
8. DeAndrade JR, MacNab I (1969): Anterior occipito-cervical fusion using an extra-pharyngeal exposure. *J Bone Joint Surg* [Am] 51(8):1621–1626.
9. Delgado TE, Buckhert WA (1983): Surgical management of tumors in and around the clivus via the transoral approach. *Contemporary Neurosurg* 4(20):1–6.
10. Derome PJ (1977): The transbasal approach to tumors invading the base of the skull. In: Schmidek HH, Sweet WH, eds. *Current techniques in neurosurgery.* New York: Grune and Stratton, pp. 223–245.
11. Drake CG (1981): Progress in cerebrovascular disease. Management of cerebral aneurysm. *Stroke* 12:273–283.
12. Eismont FJ, Bohlman HH (1981): Posterior methylmethacrylate fixation for cervical trauma. *Spine* 6(4):347–353.
13. Fang HSY, Ong GB (1962): Direct anterior approach to the upper cervical spine. *J Bone Joint Surg* [Am] 44:1588–1604.
14. Feilding WJ, Hawkins RJ, Ratzan SA (1976): Spine fusion for atlantoaxial instability. *J Bone Joint Surg* [Am] 58(3):400–407.
15. Fisch U, Matton D (1988): Infratemporal fossa approach. In: Fisch U, Matton D, eds. *Microsurgery of the skull base.* New York: Thieme, pp. 136–281.
16. Fisch U, Pillsbury HC (1979): Infratemporal fossa approach to lesions in the temporal bone and base of the skull. *Arch Otolaryngol* 105:99–107.
17. Gates GA (1988): The lateral facial approach to the nasopharynx and infratemporal fossa. *Otolaryngol Head and Neck Surg* 99(3):321–325.
18. Hadley MN, Spetzler RF, Sonntag VK (1989): The transoral approach to the superior cervical spine. A review of 53 cases of extradural cervicomedullary compression. *J Neurosurgery* 71:16–23.
19. Hall JE, Denis F, Murray J (1977): Exposure of the upper cervical spine for spinal decompression by a mandible and tongue-splitting approach. *J Bone Joint Surg* [Am] 59(1):121–123.
20. Hamblen DL (1967): Occipitocervical fusion. Indications, technique and results. *J Bone Joint Surg* [Br] 49:33–45.
21. Hashi K, Hakuba A, Ikuno H, et al. (1976): A midline vertebral artery aneurysm operated via transoral transclival approach. *Nishinkei Geka-Neurological Surgery* [Japan] 4:183–189.
22. Hayakawa T, Kamikawa K, Ohnishi T, et al. (1981): Prevention of postoperative complications after a transoral transclival approach to basilar aneurysms. *J Neurosurg* 54:699–703.
23. Itoh T, Tsuji H, Katoh Y, Yonezawa H, Kitagawa H (1988): Occipito-cervical fusion reinforced by Luque's segmental spinal instrumentation for rheumatoid disease. *Spine* 13:1234–1238.
24. Johnson RM, Hart DL, Simmons EF, et al. (1977): Cervical orthoses. A study comparing their effectiveness in restricting cervical motion in normal subjects. *J Bone Joint Surg* [Am] 59:332–339.
25. Krespi YP (1988): Transmandibular exposure of the skull base. *Abstracts of International Symposium on Cranial Base Surgery.* Pittsburgh, Pa., Sept.
26. Krespi YP, Har-El G (1988): Surgery of the clivus and anterior cervical spine. *Arch Otolaryngol Head Neck Surg* 114:73–78.
27. Krespi YP, Sisson GA (1984): Transmandibular exposure of skull base. *Am J Surg* 148:534–538.
28. Larsson SE, Toolanen G (1986): Posterior fusion for atlanto-axial subluxation in rheumatoid arthritis. *Spine* 11:525–530.
29. Lesoin F, Jomin M, Pellerin P, Pruvo JP, Carini S, Servato R (1986): Transclival transcervical approach to the upper cervical spine and clivus. *Acta Neurochir (Wien)* 80(3–4):100–104.
30. Lesoin F, Pellerin P, Thomas CE 3rd, et al. (1984): Acrylic reconstruction of an arthritic cervical spine using the transcervical-transclival approach. *Surg Neurol* 22:329–334.
31. Litvak J, Sumners TC, Barron JL, Fisher LS (1981): A successful approach to vertebrobasilar aneurysms. Technical note. *J Neurosurg* 55:491–494.
32. Malis LI (1985): Surgical resection of tumors of the skull base. In: Wilkins RH, Rengachary SS, eds. *Neurosurgery.* New York: McGraw-Hill, pp. 1010–1021.
33. McAfee PC, Bohlman HH, Ducker T (1986): Failure of stabilization of the spine with methyl methacrylate. *J Bone Joint Surg* [Am] 68:1145–1157.
34. McAfee PC, Bohlman HH, Riley LH, Robinson RA, Southwick WO, Nachlas NE (1987): The anterior retropharyngeal approach to the upper part of the cervical spine. *J Bone Joint Surg* [Am] 69:1371–1373.
35. Meijers KA, Cats A, Kremer HP, Luyendijk W, Onvlee GJ, Thomeer RTW (1984): Cervical myelopathy in rheumatoid arthritis. *Clin Exp Rheumatol* 2:239–245.
36. Menezes AH (1984): "Cranial settling" in rheumatoid arthritis. *Contemporary Neurosurgery* 6(16):1–8.
37. Menezes AH (1990): Anterior approaches to the craniocervical junction. In: *Clinical Neurosurgery: Proceedings of the Congress of Neurological Surgeons.* New York: Williams and Wilkins, in press.
38. Menezes AH (1990): Problems and complications of craniocervical junction and upper cervical spine surgery. In: Caimins M, O'Leary P, eds. *Disorders of the Cervical Spine.* New York: Williams and Wilkins, in press.
39. Menezes AH (1990): Transoral approach to the clivus and upper cervical spine. In: Wilkins R, Rengachary S, eds. *Neurosurgery Update.* New York: McGraw-Hill, pp. 306–313.
40. Menezes AH, Smoker WRK, Dyste GN (1990): Syringomyelia, chiari malformations and hydromyelia. In: Youmans J, ed. *Neurological surgery, 3rd ed.* Philadelphia: W. B. Saunders, pp. 1421–1459.
41. Menezes AH, VanGilder JC (1988): Transoral-transpharyngeal approach to the anterior craniocervical junction. 10-year experience with 72 patients. *J Neurosurg* 69:895–903.
42. Menezes AH, VanGilder JC (1990): Abnormalities of the craniovertebral junction. In: Youmans J, ed. *Neurological surgery, 3rd ed.* Philadelphia: W. B. Saunders, pp. 1359–1420.
43. Menezes AH, VanGilder JC, Clark CR, El-Khoury G (1985): Odontoid upward migration in rheumatoid arthritis. An analysis of 45 patients with "cranial settling." *J Neurosurg* 63:500–509.
44. Menezes AH, VanGilder JC, Graf CJ, McDonnell DE (1980): Craniocervical abnormalities: a comprehensive surgical approach. *J Neurosurg* 53:444–455.
45. Miller E, Crockard HA (1987): Transoral transclival removal of anteriorly placed meningiomas at the foramen magnum. *Neurosurg* 20:966–968.
46. Mitsui H (1984): A new operation for atlanto-axial arthrodesis. *J Bone Joint Surg* [Br] 66(3):422–425.
47. Moore LJ, Schwartz HC (1985): Median labiomandibular glossotomy for access to the cervical spine. *J Oral Maxillofacial Surg* 43:909–912.
48. Pasztor E, Vajda J, Piffko P, et al. (1984): Transoral surgery for craniocervical space-occupying processes. *J Neurosurg* 60:276–281.
49. Ranawat CS, O'Leary P, Pellicci P, Tsairis P, Marchisello P, Dorr L (1979): Cervical spine fusion in rheumatoid arthritis. *J Bone Joint Surg* [Am] 61:1003–1010.
50. Ransford AO, Crockard HA, Pozo JL, Thomas NP, Nelson IW (1986): Craniocervical instability treated by contoured loop fixation. *J Bone Joint Surg* [Br] 68(2):173–177.

51. Robin PE, Powell DJ (1981): Treatment of carcinoma of the nasal cavity and paranasal sinuses. *Clin Otolaryngol* 6:401–414.
52. Roosen K, Trauschel A, Grote W (1982): Posterior atlanto-axial fusion. A new compression clamp for laminar osteosynthesis. *Arch Orthoped and Traumatic Surg* 100:27–31.
53. Sekhar LN, Schramm VL Jr, Jones NF (1987): Subtemporal preauricular infratemporal fossa approach to large lateral and posterior cranial base neoplasms. *J Neurosurg* 67:488–499.
54. Selman WR, Spetzler RF, Brown R (1981): The use of intraoperative fluoroscopy and spinal cord monitoring. *Clin Orthop* (154):51–56.
55. Simmons EH, DuToit G Jr (1978): Lateral atlanto-axial arthrodesis. *Orthop Clin North Am* 9(4):1101–1114.
56. Smoker WR, Keyes WD, Dunn VD, Menezes AH (1986): MRI versus conventional radiologic examinations in the evaluation of the craniovertebral and cervicomedullary junction. *Radiographics* 6:953–994.
57. Sollazzo D, Bruni P (1985): Brainstem auditory evoked potential (BAEP) abnormalities in subjects with craniovertebral malformations. *Ital J Neurol Sci* 6:185–189.
58. Stevenson GC, Stoney RJ, Perkins RK, Adams JE (1966): A transcervical transclival approach to the ventral surface of the brain stem for removal of a clivus chordoma. *J Neurosurg* 24:544–551.
59. Taitsman JP, Saha S (1977): Tensile strength of wire-reinforced bone cement and twisted stainless steel wire. *J Bone Joint Surg* [Am] 59(3):419–425.
60. Uttley D, Moore A, Archer DJ (1989): Surgical management of midline skull base tumors: A new approach. *J Neurosurg* 71:705–710.
61. Wertheim SB, Bohlman HH (1987): Occipitocervical fusion. Indications, technique, and long-term results in thirteen patients. *J Bone Joint Surg* [Am] 69:833–836.
62. Whitesides TE Jr (1983): Lateral retropharyngeal approach to the upper cervical spine. In: *The Cervical Spine.* The Cervical Spine Research Society. Philadelphia: Lippincott, pp. 517–527.
63. Winfield J, Cooke D, Brook AS, Corbett M (1981): A prospective study of the radiological changes in the cervical spine in early rheumatoid disease. *Ann Rheum Dis* 40:109–114.
64. Yamada T, Ishida T, Kudo Y, et al. (1986): Clinical correlates of abnormal P14 in median SEP's. *Neurology* 36:765–771.
65. Yamaura A, Makino H, Isobe K, Takashima T, Nakamura T, Takemiya S (1979): Repair of cerebrospinal fluid fistula following transoral transclival approach to a basilar aneurysm. Technical note. *J Neurosurg* 50:834–838.
66. Zoma A, Sturrock RD, Fisher WD, Freeman PA, Hamblen DL (1987): Surgical stabilisation of the rheumatoid cervical spine. A review of indications and results. *J Bone Joint Surg* [Br] 69:8–12.

The Adult Spine: Principles and Practice,
J. W. Frymoyer, Editor-in-Chief.
Raven Press, Ltd., New York © 1991.

CHAPTER 47

Anterior and Posterior Surgical Approaches to the Cervical Spine

Thomas S. Whitecloud III, and Lee A. Kelley

The surgical approaches to the cervical spine have been developed and modified by numerous surgeons. Generally, these make use of natural anatomical planes and are relatively bloodless and relatively safe if the surgeon has a thorough knowledge of surgical anatomy of the region. This chapter describes the approaches to the anterior spine from C3 to C7, anterior approach to C1 and C2, three different types of anterior extrapharyngeal approaches to the upper cervical spine, and the standard posterior approaches to the upper cervical and lower cervical spine.

ANTERIOR APPROACH

Skin Landmarks and Fascial Planes

The skin on the anterior portion of the neck is highly mobile, thin, and highly vascular. In the lower portion of

T. S. Whitecloud III, M.D., Professor and Acting Chairman;
L. A. Kelley, M.D.: Department of Orthopaedic Surgery, Tulane University School of Medicine, New Orleans, Louisiana, 70112.

the neck, the anterior skin creases run transversely, and then course obliquely in the more cephalad portion near the mandible. Skin incisions should be placed in these skin creases so that the surgical wound heals with minimal cosmetic compromise. Relatively small horizontal incisions on the anterior portions of the neck are possible for one- and two-level anterior fusions because retraction of the mobile skin affords excellent exposure through these relatively small incisions. Various palpable landmarks may be a clue to identifying vertebral levels about the anterior aspect of the neck. The arch of the atlas is generally located at the level of the hard palate. The C1-C2 interspace is generally at the level of the angle of the mandible, while the lower border of the mandible is generally at the level of C2-C3. The hyoid bone correlates to the level of C3, and the upper border of the thyroid cartilage generally correlates to the level of C4-C5. The cricoid cartilage is usually at the level of the C6 vertebral body, and this may be confirmed by palpation of the carotid tubercle (Chassaignac's tubercle), which is the tubercle on the anterior transverse process of the C6 vertebral body. Despite the anatomic landmarks, a lateral roentgenogram of the neck prior to incision can help ensure accurate placement of the skin incision. The skin

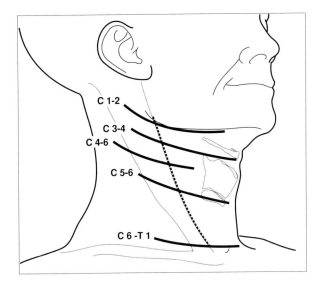

FIG. 1. Placement of skin incision for various levels in the cervical spine. Note that transverse incisions course from midline to the medial border of the sternocleidomastoid muscle. The oblique incision for multiple level exposure courses along the medial border of the sterno-cleidomastoid muscle.

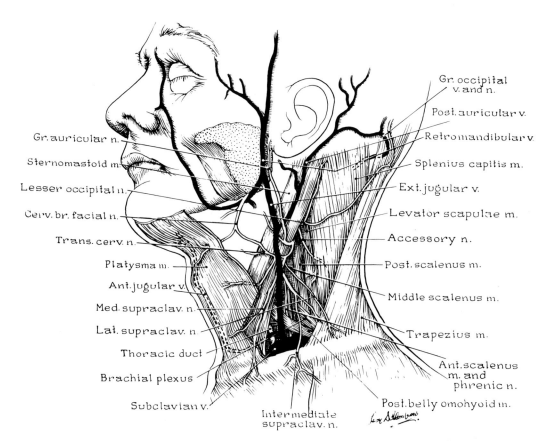

FIG. 2. Cutaneous nerves of the neck in relation to the sternocleidomastoid muscle. Short transverse incisions will usually encounter small terminal branches of these nerves, but large trunks may be encountered with oblique or longitudinal incisions.

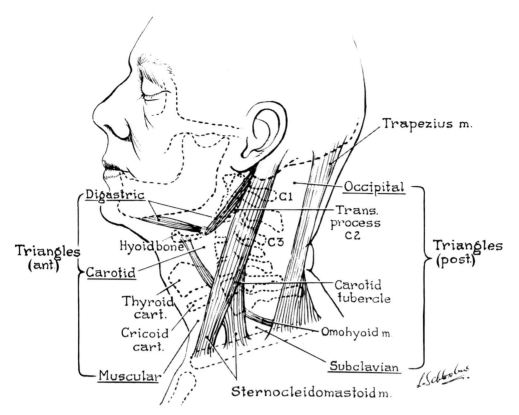

FIG. 3. Triangles of the neck.

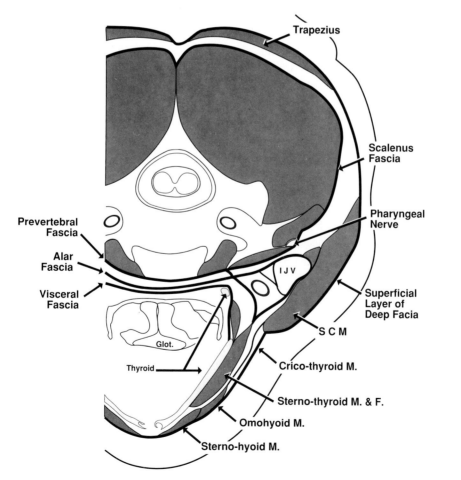

FIG. 4. Cross section of the fascial compartments of the neck at the level of the thyroid cartilage.

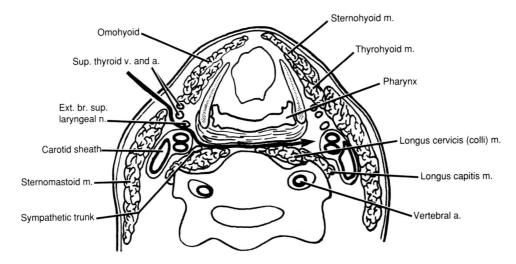

FIG. 5. Order of transection of cervical fascial layers in the anteromedial approach to C3-C7.

incision should be placed in relation to the patient's shoulder as visualized on the lateral roentgenogram of the neck (Fig. 1).

Just beneath the skin is the superficial fascia, which contains the platysma muscles anteriorly. The platysma muscles are paired muscles of variable development that extend from the lower border of the mandible to the superficial fascia over the chest. The mediolateral extent of the muscles is generally from midline to the lateral border of the sternocleidomastoid muscle. These are innervated by the cervical branch of the facial nerve (cranial nerve VII). These muscles are pierced by the anterior cutaneous nerves as these course to innervate the skin. The muscle fibers of the platysma may be transected in the transverse plane during the course of an approach or may be split longitudinally in line with their fibers. These are usually closed as a separate layer at the conclusion of an anterior approach to the cervical spine.

Just deep to the superficial fascia lies the first layer of the deep cervical fascia. Within this layer are the four nerve trunks of the cutaneous nerves of the neck, which emanate from the posterior border of the sternocleidomastoid muscle near its midpoint. The most superior of these nerves is the lesser occipital nerve, which is derived from the second cervical nerve root and courses to the posterior aspect of the neck to supply the skin over the lateral occipital region. The great auricular nerve arises from the second and third cervical roots and may be seen to emanate just caudal to the lesser occipital nerve. This nerve crosses superficial to the sternomastoid and is parallel to the external jugular vein, supplying the area over the parotid gland and some of the skin about the ear. The anterior cervical cutaneous nerve arises from the second and third roots as well. It crosses superficial to the sternocleidomastoid muscle and supplies the region of skin about the hyoid bone. The fourth nerve is the supraclavicular nerve, which arises from the third and fourth

cervical roots and divides into three main branches that supply the skin about the clavicle and anterior trapezius muscle. Injury to any of these nerves in the course of an anterior or lateral approach to the neck will result in areas of cutaneous sensory deficit. However, in the standard anterior approach using short transverse incisions in the anterior cervical triangle, only the terminal branches of these sensory nerves are generally encountered. When longitudinal incisions in the anterior triangle are used or transverse incisions posterior to the sternocleidomastoid muscle are used, the larger nerve trunks are vulnerable and may result in larger areas of cutaneous sensory deficit should they be transected (Fig. 2).

Deep to the superficial fascia and platysma muscles, the anterior and posterior triangles, divided by the large sternocleidomastoid muscle, are encountered. The anterior and posterior cervical triangles are then subdivided by the digastric and omohyoid muscles into smaller triangles, which are named for their local anatomic features (digastric, carotid, or subclavian triangles). These are useful in anatomic description of various approaches; however, the most common anterior approach is entirely within the anterior cervical triangle (Fig. 3).

The fascial layers of the neck were described by Grodinsky and Holyoke (6) and have proven to be very useful as guides to dissection throughout the neck (Fig. 4). In performing the anterior approach, detailed knowledge of these fascial planes is essential to avoid injury to the contiguous viscera and neurovascular structures in the neck. The cervical fascia is divided into one superficial and four deep layers. The superficial fascia, as previously mentioned, is that portion of the fascia that contains the platysma muscle in its deeper portion. This layer of fascia is noted to surround the entire neck at the level of the subcutaneous tissue. Deep to the superficial fascia lies the superficial layer of the deep cervical fascia, the first of the four components of the deep cervical fascia. It surrounds the neck and encloses the sternocleidomastoid and trapezius muscles. The next three layers of deep fascia are considered to be the middle layers of the deep fascia. The first of these layers encloses the strap muscles and the omohyoid muscle in the anterior cervical region, then extends laterally to the scapula. The deepest component of the middle layer is the visceral fascia, which surrounds the larynx, trachea, esophagus, and thyroid. The recurrent laryngeal nerve is also enclosed within the visceral fascia. Care should be taken to avoid entering this fascial plane so that the enclosed structures as mentioned above will not be injured. The fourth portion of the deep fascia is the alar fascia, which spreads like wings (hence its name) behind the esophagus and surrounds the carotid sheath structures laterally. The deepest layer of fascia in the neck is the prevertebral fascia, which surrounds the vertebral bodies in the paraspinous muscles. Also enclosed in this layer are the phrenic nerve and the scalene muscles. It is noted to be continuous with the lumbodorsal fascia in its caudal-most extent. The prevertebral fascia and alar fascia are both considered portions of the deepest layer of the deep fascia. The alar fascia is noted to blend with the prevertebral fascia at the level of the transverse processes, but generally does not have connections with the prevertebral fascia in the midportions of the neck. When performing a standard anteromedial approach to the cervical spine, the fascial layers are transected as follows: The superficial fascia is transected in conjunction with the platysma muscle; the superficial layer of the deep fascia is transected sharply at the medial border of the sternocleidomastoid muscle; the middle layer of the deep fascia is transected just anterior to the anterior border of the carotid artery, generally by finger dissection; and the alar fascia and prevertebral fascia are transected sharply directly in the midline to obtain access to the vertebral bodies and discs of the anterior cervical spine (Fig. 5).

Anteromedial Approach to the Vertebral Bodies and Intervertebral Discs from C3 Through C7

This approach has been previously described by Robinson, Southwick, and Riley (9,10,12) and is the standard approach to the anterior cervical spine from C3 through C7. This approach allows the discs between C2-C3 and C7-T1, and all intervening discs, to be exposed in a relatively easy manner.

There has been considerable discussion whether the approach is more advantageous on the right or left side of the midline. The rationale for approaching on the left side of the midline is that the recurrent laryngeal nerve ascends in the neck on the left side between the trachea and the esophagus, having branched off from its parent nerve, the vagus, at the level of the arch of the aorta. The right recurrent laryngeal nerve travels alongside the trachea in the neck after passing beneath the right subclavian artery. In the lower part of the neck, the right recurrent laryngeal nerve is vulnerable to damage as it crosses from the subclavian artery to the tracheoesophageal groove. Its course in relation to the groove is more variable on the right than on the left and, therefore, the right recurrent laryngeal nerve is slightly more vulnerable to injury than the left. The approach from the left side has the possibility of injuring the thoracic duct, which enters the jugular vein–subclavian vein junction at the base of the neck on the left. However, many surgeons prefer to perform the incision and approach to the right of the midline if they are right-handed, believing that this facilitates both orientation and technical performance in the procedure. Still others feel that the incision should be made on the side of the predominant pathology. However, due to the fact that generous exposure of the anterior cervical spine can be obtained from either side, the surgical approaches should be done on the side that is most comfortable to the surgeon.

The operation may be performed through a transverse or longitudinal skin incision. In general, the transverse skin incision is sufficient to expose three consecutive vertebral bodies and two consecutive intervertebral discs. If more than two intervertebral discs must be exposed and a prolonged segment of the cervical spine needs to be accessed, such as would be needed in multiple vertebrectomy and strut grafting, then an oblique incision should be made paralleling the anterior border of the sternocleidomastoid muscle. A transverse skin incision should extend to the midline and be centered over the anterior border of the sternocleidomastoid muscle overlying the segment of the spine to be exposed (Fig. 6). Generally, the fifth, sixth, and seventh cervical segments should be approached through a transverse incision placed two to three finger breadths superior to the clavicle; and the third, fourth, and fifth cervical segments should be approached through a transverse skin incision placed three to four finger breadths superior to the clavicle. As previously mentioned, a lateral roentgenogram made prior to the initiation of the incision will help ensure proper placement of the incision. A longitudinal or oblique incision should be made overlying the medial border of the sternocleidomastoid muscle and may extend from the tip of the mastoid process to the superster-nal notch if this degree of exposure is necessary.

Once the skin incision is made, the platysma muscle is sharply incised at the level of the lateral limb of the transverse incision or at the caudal limb of the longitudinal or oblique incision. It may then be bluntly separated from the underlying structures by passing an instrument deep to the muscle. This is important to prevent inadvertent incision of the underlying structures, which would include the sternocleidomastoid muscle at the lateral-most extent of the transverse incision or at the caudal extent of

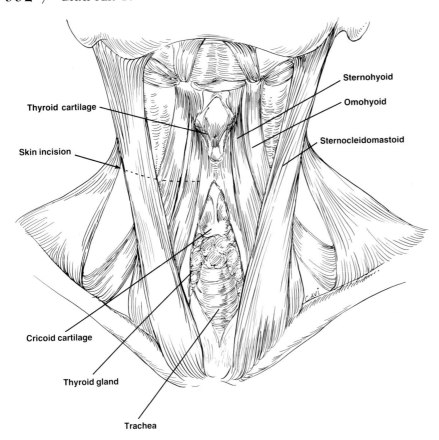

Thyroid cartilage

Skin incision

Cricoid cartilage

Thyroid gland

Trachea

Sternohyoid

Omohyoid

Sternocleidomastoid

FIG. 6. Transverse and longitudinal incision in relation to underlying muscles of the neck. The head should be placed in neutral position prior to making a transverse incision. The authors prefer to make both types of incisions on the right side.

an oblique incision. On the medial aspect of the incision, the thyroid gland may be vulnerable to injury during the course of transecting the platysma muscle. The anterior border of the sternocleidomastoid muscle is clearly identified once the platysma muscle has been transected. The fascia investing the sternocleidomastoid muscle should be sharply incised at the medial border of the sternocleidomastoid muscle so that it may be retracted laterally. The middle layer of the cervical fascia is now well demonstrated, and the omohyoid muscle will be seen to cross the field in the mid portion of the neck, generally just above the level of the sixth cervical vertebral body. This muscle may be mobilized and retracted inferiorly or superiorly, or divided and retracted to provide adequate exposure. The external jugular vein may be encountered deep to the sternocleidomastoid muscle, and both the external jugular vein and the anterior jugular vein may require division and ligation if these interfere with adequate exposure.

It is in the layer of the middle portion of the deep cervical fascia that the vessels and nerves coursing from lateral to medial are generally located. Palpation beneath the sternocleidomastoid muscle for the carotid pulse will identify the contents of the carotid sheath. The sternocleidomastoid muscle and the carotid sheath should be retracted together laterally, and the middle cervical fascia should be transected by finger dissection during the course of the lateral retraction of these structures. The

following structures should be identified in the middle layer of the deep cervical fascia. The digastric muscle, hypoglossal nerve, and glossopharyngeal nerve are found in the superior-most portion of this exposure. These should be retracted superiorly. The superior thyroid artery and vein and the superior laryngeal nerve are the next structures encountered inferiorly. These should be identified and retracted as necessary. The middle thyroid vein courses from lateral to medial below the thyroid vessels and may be transected and ligated if necessary. The inferior thyroid vein and artery are the inferior-most vascular structures during this approach and may be retracted inferiorly or superiorly, according to the level being exposed.

Once the deep layer of the middle cervical fascia is traversed by blunt dissection and the appropriate structures retracted, palpation of the anterior surface of the cervical spine is usually possible. At this point, the viscera and the midline should be inspected. The esophagus may be seen just posterior to the trachea, and more superiorly, it lies posterior to the larynx. The esophagus is often thin and ribbon-like and should be retracted with care to avoid perforation. A blunt retractor such as a Cloward retractor is ideal for medial retraction of the esophagus, trachea, and thyroid gland (Fig. 7).

The prevertebral fascia may then be incised longitudinally in the midline of the neck and retracted to either side. This fascia must be incised as close to the midline of

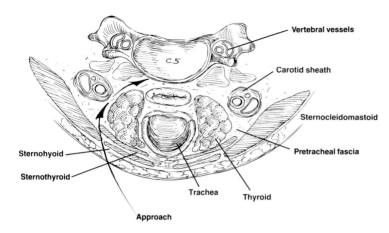

FIG. 7. The midline musculovisceral column may be bluntly retracted medially as a unit. The lateral structures include the sternocleidomastoid muscle and the contents of the carotid sheath.

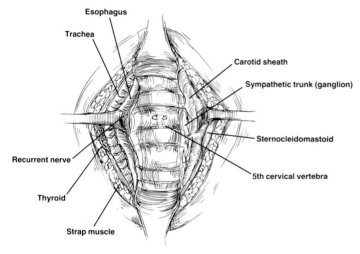

FIG. 8. Once the prevertebral fascia is visualized by appropriate retracting of medial and lateral structures, it should be incised as close to the midline as possible to minimize damage to contiguous structures.

the cervical spine as possible to avoid injury to the other structures in the neck (Fig. 8). It has been emphasized that one must not mistake the palpable anterior tubercles of the transverse processes for the vertebral bodies. Otherwise, an incision that was intended to be made through the prevertebral fascia in the midline of the cervical spine may be made instead through the longus colli muscle, which lies immediately lateral to the midline of the cervical spine. This can result in possible damage to the cervical sympathetic chain or to the vertebral artery that lies deep in the longus colli muscle and may also result in excessive bleeding. Once the prevertebral fascia is incised in the midline, the longus colli muscles may be sharply elevated from the intervertebral disc and the vertebral bodies. They are then retracted laterally to allow more complete exposure to the entire segment of the vertebral bodies and intervertebral disc. Before elevating the longus colli muscle, its medial edge should be coagulated. This will prevent unnecessary bleeding. At this point, there should be adequate exposure of the vertebral bodies and disc spaces for performing a variety of proce-

dures, including discectomy, corpectomy, biopsy, or fusion.

Consequences of Injury to the Neurovascular Structures During the Anterior Approach

The vertebral artery is at risk for injury during the anterior approach. This can occur during excision of a cervical disc when the dissection is carried posterior lateral to the joints of Luschka. The vertebral arteries pass through the transverse foramen at each cervical level from C6 cephalad to C1. Once the vertebral artery reaches the first cervical vertebra, it curves posteriorly immediately over the lateral masses between C1 and C2 and then follows a groove in the posterior arch of the atlas to pass into the foramen magnum. The vulnerability of these vessels at this location will be discussed in the next section on the posterior approaches. At each level, the cervical nerve root passes directly behind the vertebral artery. Thus, the roots are also in jeopardy if the vertebral artery is tied blindly when surgical injury occurs. If the artery is injured and bleeding cannot be controlled by tamponade, it must be exposed in the region of the transverse foramen and controlled proximally and distally prior to ligation. In young individuals, it is usually safe to ligate one vertebral artery, but this may result in cerebral or cerebellar ischemia in older individuals. This is due to one vertebral artery being compromised by spurring about the foramen and also may be due to traumatic disruption or occlusion of one vertebral vessel. In these circumstances, surgical compromise of the contralateral vessel results in significant ischemia.

Injury to neural structures during the approach can include damage to the cervical sympathetic chain, which is a deep structure located near the longus colli muscles. The sympathetic chain lies deep in a reflection of the carotid sheath along the anterior surface of the lateral masses and prevertebral muscles. It extends from the second cervical vertebra downward and exhibits three gangliotic enlargements: the superior ganglion in front of the second and third cervical vertebrae, the middle ganglion in front of the sixth cervical vertebra, and the inferior ganglion, frequently fused with the first thoracic ganglion just below the seventh cervical vertebra, called the stellate ganglion. Injury to the cervical sympathetic chain can result in a Horner's syndrome.

Other nervous structures vulnerable to injury include the pharyngeal and superior laryngeal branches of the vagus nerve, which run deep to the carotid and superior thyroid arteries. These supply the trachea muscles of the back of the pharynx and sensory innervation to the larynx and the cricothyroid. These are generally retracted

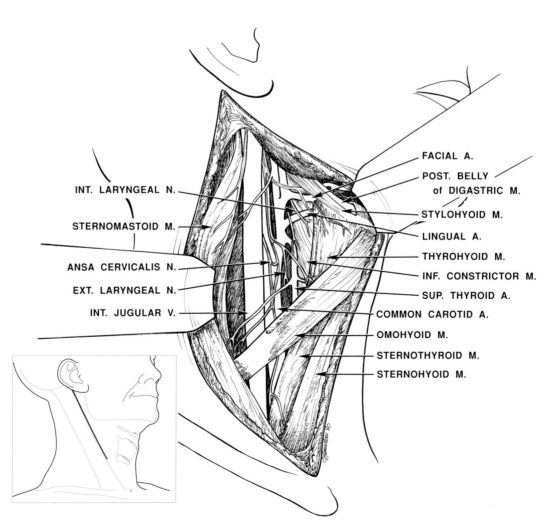

INT. LARYNGEAL N.

STERNOMASTOID M.

ANSA CERVICALIS N.

EXT. LARYNGEAL N.

INT. JUGULAR V.

FACIAL A.

POST. BELLY
of DIGASTRIC M.

STYLOHYOID M.

LINGUAL A.

THYROHYOID M.

INF. CONSTRICTOR M.

SUP. THYROID A.

COMMON CAROTID A.

OMOHYOID M.

STERNOTHYROID M.

STERNOHYOID M.

FIG. 9. Neurovascular structures encountered in the anteromedial approach.

with the viscera, and since they run in a longitudinal oblique course, they are not damaged as part of usual exposures.

The recurrent laryngeal nerve arises from the vagus at the level of the subclavian artery on the right and recurs below the subclavian artery and then ascends between the trachea and esophagus, protected by the visceral fascia. The left recurrent laryngeal nerve arises at the level of the aortic arch and passes around the arch to ascend in a similar manner as on the right. Retraction may cause temporary paralysis of the recurrent laryngeal nerve during the anterior approach, but this is less likely to happen with a left-sided approach due to the fact that the recurrent laryngeal nerve is more frequently located in the tracheoesophageal groove on the left than on the right. The nerve gives branches to all muscles of the larynx except the cricothyroid. It communicates with the internal laryngeal nerve and supplies sensory filaments to the mucous membrane of the larynx below the level of the vocal cords. It also carries afferent fibers from the stretch receptors in the larynx. Injury to both recurrent laryngeal nerves causes the vocal folds to be motionless in the same position they are normally found in tranquil respiration. When only one recurrent laryngeal nerve is injured, the vocal fold of the same side is motionless. The function in the fold of the opposite side will allow phonation to be possible, but the voice will be altered and weak in timbre. Injury to the superior laryngeal nerve will result in anesthesia of the mucous membrane in the upper part of the larynx so that foreign bodies can readily enter the cavity. Since the nerve supplies the cricoid thyroid, the vocal folds cannot be made tense and the voice is deep and hoarse (17) (Fig. 9).

Anterior Approach to C1 and C2

This approach is attributed to Crowe and Johnson by Robinson and Southwick (10,12). However, Riley attributes this approach to Fang (5,9). Historically, this approach has been used primarily for drainage of retropharyngeal abscess and biopsy of the anterior arch of the first cervical vertebra and the body of the second cervical vertebra. A midline longitudinal incision is carried through the pharyngeal membrane and fascial planes directly to the mass or to the bone. The mid pharynx is usually avascular, and the small number of vessels that are cut may be ligated with absorbable sutures. Partial closure with interrupted gut sutures is usually used. When used to drain abscesses, this incision should not be closed. The transoral approaches have the obvious limitations of being small exposures with small spaces in which to work. However, with the use of the operating microscope, it is possible to perform such procedures as odontoid resection transorally. There is a reported high rate of infection using these exposures. For more extensive work in the upper cervical spine, alternative exposures should be considered (Figs. 10 and 11).

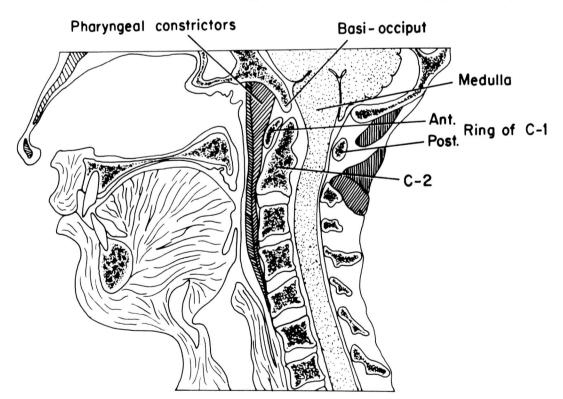

FIG. 10. Relationship of C1 ring and C2 body to the posterior pharynx. Note the relationship of the hard and soft palates to the atlanto-axial junction.

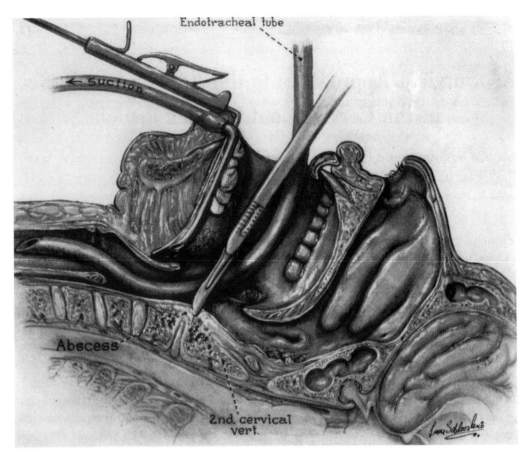

FIG. 11. Transoral pharyngeal approach for drainage of retropharyngeal abscess.

Anterior Extrapharyngeal Approaches to the Upper Cervical Spine

Three extrapharyngeal approaches to the upper cervical spine have been used as alternatives to transpharyngeal approaches. These include approaches described by De Andrade and Macnab (3) as well as the approach described by Riley (9), which requires anterior dislocation of the mandible on the side of the approach along with resection of the submaxillary gland with an extensive dissection of the anatomic structures in this area. Both of these approaches are medial to the carotid sheath. The lateral retropharyngeal approach to the upper cervical spine, as described by Whitesides et al. (15,16), is a modification of Henry's (8) approach to the vertebral artery and is carried anterior to the reflected sternocleidomastoid but posterior to the carotid sheath. The approach can then be extended medially into the retropharyngeal space, exposing all the vertebral bodies of C1 through C7.

The extrapharyngeal approaches may be used for treatment of a variety of problems in the cervical spine in which the upper cervical spine exposure is required. These include os odontoideum, fracture, non-union or mal-union, and post-laminectomy deformity. These may also be undertaken for purposes of stabilization in

problems relating to inflammatory and collagen diseases, such as rheumatoid arthritis, ankylosing spondylitis, scleroderma, and lupus erythematosus. Biopsy and treatment of tumor in the upper cervical spine are common reasons for utilizing this approach. Although infection may be treated by this approach, the transoral retropharyngeal approach may be used more commonly to approach the upper cervical spine in this situation.

Lateral Retropharyngeal Approach to the Upper Cervical Spine

Whitesides originally described the use of this approach for an anterior cervical fusion in a patient with neurofibromatosis who required extensive anterior fusion for a recurrent deformity (15,16). It may be performed with the neck in halo traction in slight extension and rotation to the contralateral side to be approached if possible. However, neither rotation nor extension is required to successfully approach the anterior cervical spine by this method. Due to potential respiratory problems from swelling after extensive retropharyngeal dissection, elective tracheostomy may be performed prior to commencing the procedure. If this is not anticipated, then nasotracheal intubation may be carried out in order to allow the mandible to be unobstructed during the

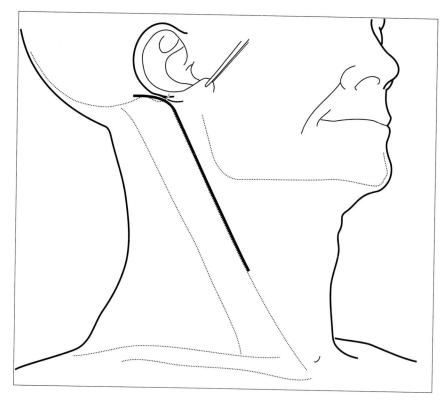

FIG. 12. Incision for lateral retropharyngeal approach (Whitesides technique).

course of the procedure. It is helpful to prep the ipsilateral ear inside and out and sew the earlobe anteriorly to the cheek in order to facilitate the exposure of the sternocleidomastoid insertion through the posterior limb of the hockey stick incision. The hockey stick incision is the initial horizontal portion of the incision, which begins just posterior to the tip of the mastoid process and is carried across the tip of the mastoid process anteriorly until the anterior border of the sternocleidomastoid

muscle is reached, and then the incision is turned inferiorly in an oblique fashion along the anterior border of the sternocleidomastoid muscle (Fig. 12). Once the skin is incised, the greater auricular nerve should be identified and may be retracted cephalad. However, if retraction is not possible and this structure impedes further exposure, it may be divided and ligated, resulting in a minor sensory deficit in the distribution of the terminal portion of the greater auricular nerve. At this point, the

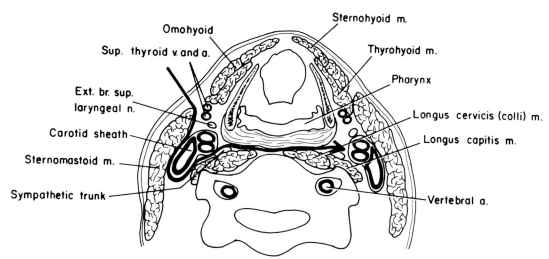

FIG. 13. Plane of dissection in lateral retropharyngeal approach is anterior to the sternocleidomastoid muscle and posterior to the carotid sheath.

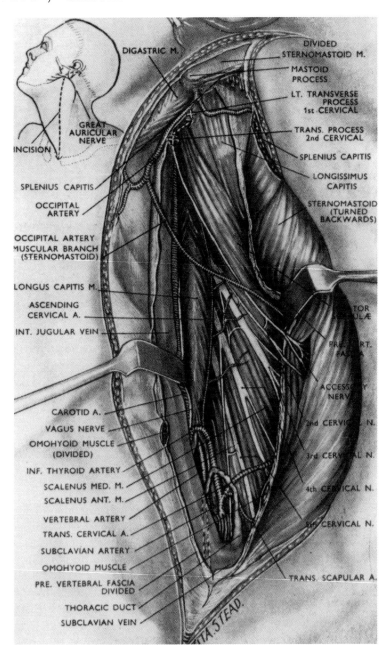

FIG. 14. Nerves and vessels in retropharyngeal approach.

platysma muscle is divided along the oblique portion of the incision just anterior to the sternocleidomastoid muscle, and the deep fascia along the medial border of the sternocleidomastoid muscle is divided sharply. The interval between the sternocleidomastoid muscle and the contents of the carotid sheath may then be developed by finger dissection in the cephalad portion of the wound. If only the upper portion of the cervical spine need be approached, the sternocleidomastoid muscle may be retracted posterolaterally and the carotid sheath contents retracted anteromedially and the dissection continued in this interval. However, if the sternocleido-

mastoid muscle is well developed, or if exposure of both the upper and lower cervical spine is required for the procedure, the sternocleidomastoid muscle will be divided at its insertion along the mastoid process. Prior to dividing the sternocleidomastoid muscle at its insertion, the entrance of the spinal accessory nerve into the sternocleidomastoid muscle should be visualized. The spinal accessory nerve generally enters the sternocleidomastoid muscle two to three centimeters caudal to the tip of the mastoid process. Care should be exercised in retraction of the sternocleidomastoid muscle posterolaterally after the division of its insertion so that exces-

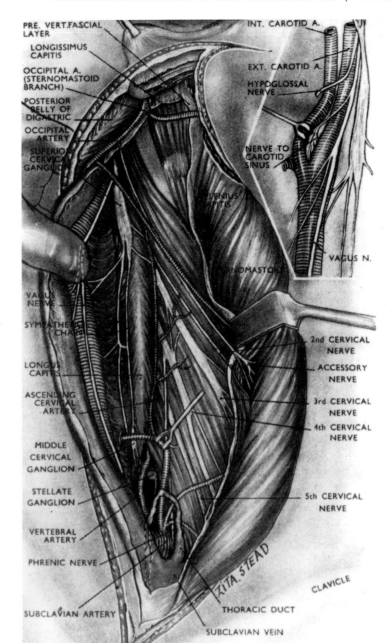

FIG. 15. Cervical sympathetic chain demonstrated.

sive traction is not placed on the spinal accessory nerve. It may be necessary to dissect the spinal accessory nerve from the jugular vein in the direction toward the jugular foramen in order to effect safe lateral retraction with the sternocleidomastoid muscle. After reflection of the sternocleidomastoid muscle, the interval just posterior to the carotid sheath contents is developed by finger dissection, and the prominent transverse process of C1 is palpated. It should be noted that if the patient's head is turned toward the contralateral side of the body, then the transverse process of C1 will be rotated away from the transverse process of C2.

Henry's original description of this approach involved access to the vertebral artery for ligation (8). A portion of the vertebral artery extending between the transverse foramen of C2 and the transverse foramen of C1 was a cephalad extent of Henry's second stage of the vertebral artery, and since there is a relatively larger interval between the C2 transverse foramen and the C1 transverse foramen compared to the other contiguous transverse foramina of the cervical spine, this site is accessible for ligation of the vertebral artery (Figs. 14 and 15).

As the dissection is carried medially from the transverse processes of the upper cervical vertebral bodies, the sagittal fascial band, which binds the midline viscera to the prevertebral fascia (the fibers of Charpey), may be divided in order that the anterior musculovisceral column may be retracted anteromedially; thus the retropharyngeal space is entered with the prevertebral fascia being visible along the anterior cervical vertebral bodies and the longus colli and longus capitus muscles evident in the more anterolateral aspect of these vertebral bodies. Sharp transection of the prevertebral fascia may be performed after coagulation of the edges of the muscle fibers in the area. Subperiosteal dissection may then be performed to expose the anterior cervical vertebral bodies and their intervening disc spaces. The anterior cervical muscles down to the level of the upper thoracic region may be removed during the course of this anterior subperiosteal exposure if such exposure is required.

This approach may be used for simultaneous exposure of the right and left lateral C1-C2 articulations for procedures such as screw fixation, as described by Barbour (1,4,11). Other uses for this exposure include vertebrectomy and incision of the odontoid, biopsy of lesions in all areas of the anterior cervical spine, fusion of C1 to T1, and exposure of a small amount of the basiocciput for fusion to that area when necessary. Once the procedure is concluded, the sternocleidomastoid muscle may be reapproximated to its origin at the mastoid tip using ab-

sorbable suture, and a drain should be allowed to remain deep within the wound. The platysma is closed using absorbable suture and the skin approximated with a subcutaneous stitch. External immobilization with a halo vest may be required for certain types of fusion in this area.

Complications associated with the approach have included facial nerve palsy, which may be secondary to retraction on the digastric muscle and subsequent injury to the seventh cranial nerve. Also, there is potential to injure the spinal accessory nerve, which would denervate the sternocleidomastoid muscle. Obviously, it is important to positively identify the jugular vein in the course of dissecting posterior to the contents of the carotid sheath so that this structure may not be injured during the course of this dissection. Infection rate has been acceptably low, especially as compared to the transoral approach. In Whiteside's series, a 2.5% incidence of infection was reported (16). In general, this approach offers a safe, effective means of exposing both the upper cervical spine and the combined exposure of the upper and lower cervical spine.

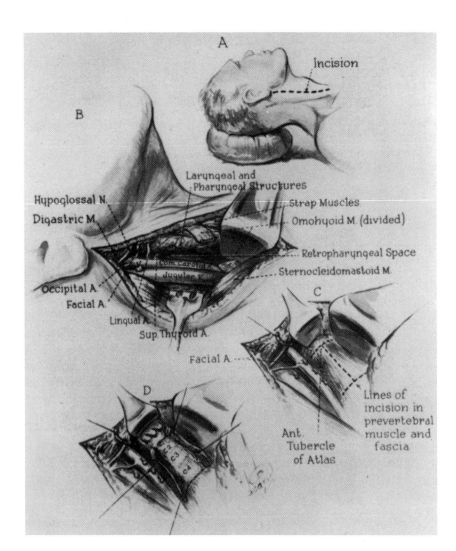

FIG. 16. Anteromedial retropharyngeal approach as described by DeAndrade and Macnab (3).

Anteromedial Retropharyngeal Approach to the Upper Cervical Spine and Basiocciput

This approach was described by De Andrade and Macnab in order to gain access to the basiocciput in order to accomplish occipitocervical fusion (3). As described, it is a cranial extension of the approach popularized by Smith and Robinson and Bailey and Badgley. It involves extending the oblique incision just along the medial border of the sternocleidomastoid muscle as used in the anteromedial approach cephalad to the angle of the mandible. The platysma muscle and deep cervical fascia are divided sharply and the lower cervical spine approached by the same dissection as used in the anteromedial approach. The branches of the external carotid artery, which prevent access to the retropharyngeal space in the upper cervical spine, are divided and ligated to facilitate this portion of the exposure. These include the superior thyroid, lingual, and facial arteries. The other structures that hinder access to the retropharyngeal space in the upper cervical and craniocervical junction are the digastric muscle and hypoglossal nerve, which are retracted during the course of the procedure, and the pharyngeal and laryngeal branches of the vagus nerve, which are also retracted during the course of the procedure. The traction on the pharyngeal and laryngeal

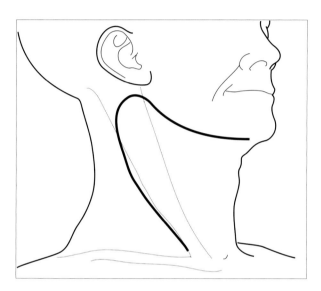

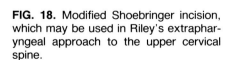

FIG. 17. Neck incision in Riley's anteromedial retropharyngeal approach.

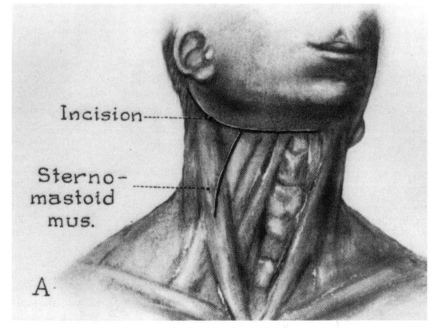

FIG. 18. Modified Shoebringer incision, which may be used in Riley's extrapharyngeal approach to the upper cervical spine.

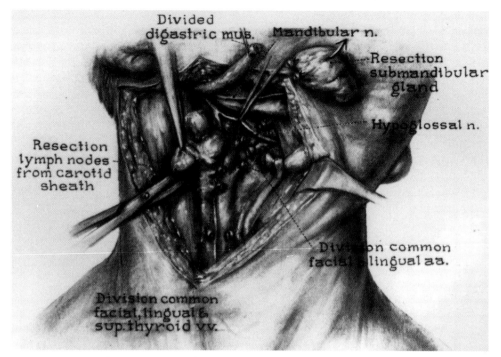

FIG. 19. Excision of submaxillary gland to improve exposure.

branches of the vagus nerve may result in temporary or permanent hoarseness and other problems related to the timbre of the voice (Fig. 16).

Anteromedial Retropharyngeal Approach to the Upper Cervical Spine (Riley's Technique)

This technique (9) is essentially an alternative means of extending the standard anteromedial approach cephalad to the C1-C2 vertebral bodies. The two major differences involve the use of a modified Shoebringer incision and the excision of the submaxillary gland and anterior dislocation of the temporomandibular joint to improve access to the upper cervical spine. The incision is begun in the submandibular area, just inferior to the edge of the mandible and carried posteriorly in a horizontal fashion to the angle of the mandible. The incision is then carried inferiorly in an oblique fashion, just at the posterior edge of the sternocleidomastoid muscle. At the lower third of the sternocleidomastoid muscle the incision is then gently curved anteriorly and inferiorly to cross the clavicle and terminate near the suprasternal space (Figs. 17 and 18). The deeper part of the incision involves transecting the subcutaneous tissue and platysma muscle in the same line as the incision and then retracting skin, subcutaneous tissue, and platysma as a single flap medially exposing the underlying sternocleidomastoid muscle at the lateral border of the dissection and the musculovisceral column medially. Superiorly the mandible and submaxillary fascia will be visible. At this point

the mandibular branch of the facial nerve should be identified just inferior to the angle of the mandible and should be protected throughout the course of the dissection. The sternocleidomastoid muscle is then freed along its medial and lateral borders and retracted laterally. The omohyoid muscle is divided in its portion, which lies just deep to the sternocleidomastoid muscle, and then retracted superiorly and inferiorly. The blunt dissection through the middle layer of the cervical fascia is then carried medially to the carotid sheath toward the prevertebral fascia. The medial musculovisceral column may then be retracted medially and the contents of the carotid sheath retracted laterally with the sternocleidomastoid muscle. This will provide access to the vertebral bodies from the C2-C3 disc space to the C7-T1 disc space.

The superior development of the dissection to access C1 and C2 involves identifying the superior thyroid artery, which crosses the field horizontally from lateral to medial as it exits the external carotid artery en route to the thyroid gland. The superior thyroid artery may be divided and ligated in order to proceed superiorly to the superior laryngeal neurovascular bundle and the hypoglossal nerve. Both of these structures should be identified and protected during the course of the superior dissection. The stylohyoid muscle and digastric muscle are then identified, divided, and retracted. As the larynx and pharynx are retracted medially and the external carotid artery laterally, the floor of the submaxillary triangle will then be visualized. This may be retracted superiorly in order to visualize the base of the skull and anterior arch of C1. At this point the exposure may be improved by

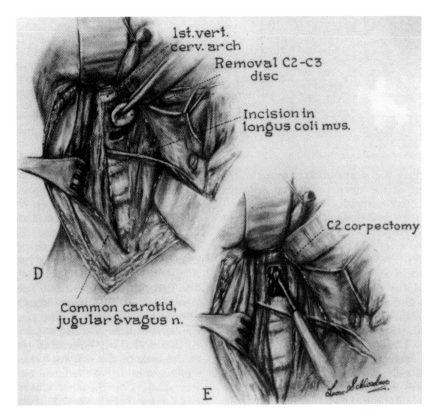

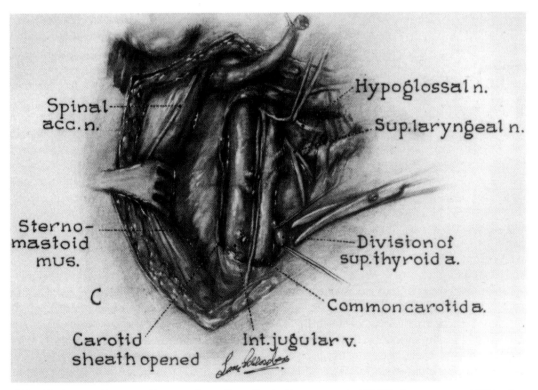

FIG. 20. Top and bottom: Deeper dissections illustrating access to C2-C3 disc space and C2 body.

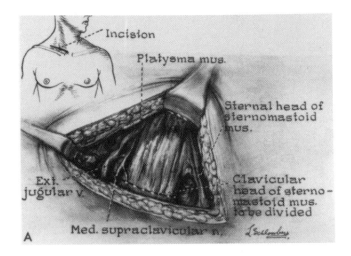

FIG. 21. Incision for supraclavicular approach.

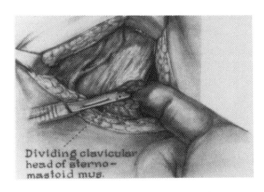

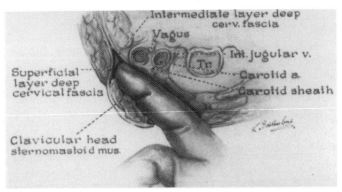

FIG. 22. Transection of clavicular head of sternocleido-mastoid muscle and plane of dissection.

excising the submaxillary gland and by manual anterior dislocation of the temporomandibular joint (Fig. 19). The mandible may then be rotated out of the field of dissection, which improves the superior retraction of the floor of the submaxillary triangle to expose the base of the skull and the entire anterior aspect of C1. This allows adequate access to C1-C2, and the vertebral arteries are visualized in the course of this approach and may be controlled as necessary. Subperiosteal dissection of the longus colli muscle in a lateral direction will expose the transverse processes and the vertebral artery. Closure may be accomplished by relocating the dislocated temporomandibular joint and repairing the digastric and stylohyoid tendons. A suction drain should be placed deep within the wound and the platysma muscle reapproximated throughout the course of the incision. A subcuticular absorbable suture is used for closure of the skin (Fig. 20).

The disadvantages of this approach involve not only the need to excise the submaxillary gland and the potential problems with dislocation of the temporomandibular joint, but also the same risk as in the approach described by De Andrade and Macnab. The hypoglossal nerve and superior laryngeal nerve remain vulnerable to injury during this procedure, since they must be retracted as work is performed through this interval.

Supraclavicular Approach to the Lower Cervical Spine

This approach was also described by Riley as a means of accessing the lower cervical spine through an anterolateral approach (9). It provides excellent access to the transverse processes, pedicles, and vertebral artery.

A transverse incision is placed one finger breadth above the clavicle extending from the midline of the neck to just beyond the posterior border of the sternocleidomastoid muscle (Fig. 21). Transection of the platysma muscle is then performed in line with the skin incision, and the medial and lateral borders of the sternocleidomastoid muscle are defined by blunt and sharp dissection. The sternocleidomastoid muscle should then be separated from its underlying structures by blunt dissection, and the anterior jugular vein and external jugular vein identified and ligated if necessary. The sternocleidomastoid muscle is then divided by incising it from its lateral border to its medial border, taking special care to avoid the internal jugular vein. The muscle is then retracted superiorly and inferiorly to access the area of the middle cervical fascia. The omohyoid and sternohyoid muscles should then be visualized. The middle cervical fascia is bluntly dissected lateral to the carotid sheath in order to access the surface of the anterior scalene muscle (Fig. 22). The omohyoid muscle may be divided and retracted in a fashion similar to the sternocleidomastoid muscle to improve access to this area. The phrenic nerve should be identified lying on the surface of the anterior scalene muscle. It crosses from lateral to medial in its superior to inferior course. The phrenic nerve may be retracted medially after it is gently freed from the surface of the anterior scalene muscle. The cords of the brachial plexus will be noted to emerge from beneath the lateral border of the anterior scalene muscle, and these should be visualized and protected throughout the course of the dissection. The anterior scalene muscle is then sharply divided approximately one inch inferior to the side of the desired exposure. The entire superior portion of the muscle may be excised; however, it should be noted that the slips of origin of the anterior scalene muscle emanate from the anterior tubercles of the cervical transverse processes so that the vertebral arteries are vulnerable to injury as they pass between the bony foramen and the transverse processes of the cervical vertebrae as these slips are being resected (Fig. 23). The standard approach involves lateral retraction of the carotid sheath; however, if possible, the internal jugular vein and carotid sheath may be retracted medially. Also, the anterior scalene muscle may be retracted laterally rather than resected if possible. The close relationship of the anterior scalene muscle to the perital pleura should be noted. The deep surface of the anterior scalene muscle is covered by a continuation of the prevertebral fascia known as Sibson's fascia, and the deep surface of Sibson's fascia is formed by the apex of the perital pleura and lung. Care

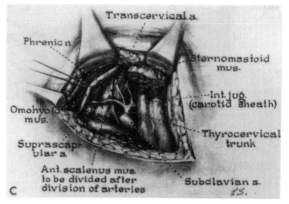

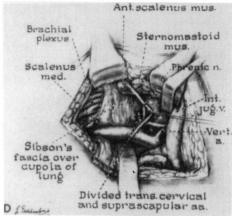

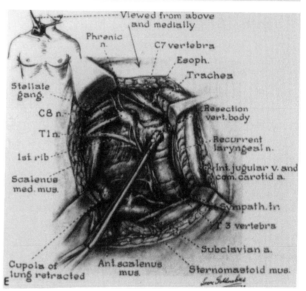

FIG. 23. Deeper dissection in supraclavicular approach.

should be taken not to violate this fascial plane, as this would involve entering the thoracic cavity. Sibson's fascia may then be followed medially toward the transverse processes of the cervical vertebrae, where it may be incised and bluntly retracted inferiorly (Fig. 24). The recurrent laryngeal nerve should be retracted medially with the carotid sheath and the medial musculovisceral column. The prevertebral fascia may then be sharply tran-

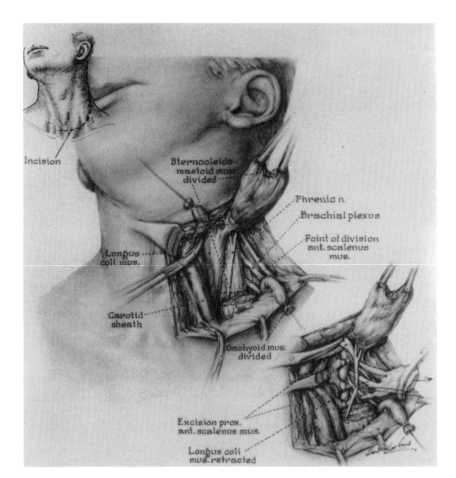

FIG. 24. Exposure of transverse process by retraction of divided sternocleidomastoid muscle and resection of the cephalad portion of anterior scalene muscle.

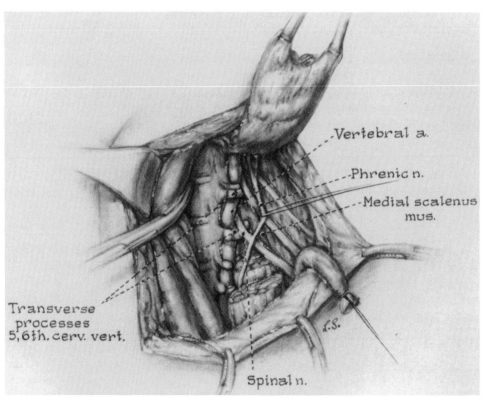

FIG. 25. Reflection of longus colli muscle improves access to vertebral bodies, neural foramina, and vertebral artery.

sected in the midline, and subperiosteal dissection of the fascial attachment and longus colli muscle may then be performed. The dissection may then be carried superiorly to expose vertebral bodies up to the C2-C3 disc space. If the transverse processes, pedicles, or neural foramina are to be exposed, then the longus colli muscle may be reflected medially (Fig. 25).

As previously mentioned, a left-sided approach places the thoracic duct vulnerable to injury. During the course of this approach, if it is performed from the left side, the thoracic duct should be carefully sought at its junction with the internal jugular-subclavian vein complex. If injury to this structure is noted during the course of the dissection it may be tied proximally and distally to prevent formation of a chylothorax. The other potential complications involve pneumothorax as previously mentioned and injury to the cervical sympathetic chain as it ascends along the longus colli muscle.

Direct Anterior Approach to the Upper Cervical Spine

This approach was described by Fang and Ong in order to gain access to the first four cervical vertebrae and their intervertebral discs, including the atlanto-axial and atlanto-occipital joints (5). The transthyrohyoid approach involves making a transverse incision along the uppermost crease of the neck at a level between the hyoid bone and thyroid cartilage and extending it laterally to the level of the carotid sheath. The platysma muscle is then transected in line with the transverse incision. The sternohyoid muscles are in the next layer, and these are isolated near their attachment to the hyoid bone and sharply divided, which exposes the underlying thyrohyoid muscles. This next layer of muscle may also be delineated and divided near its attachment to the hyoid bone. The thyrohyoid membrane then comes into view. This structure is detached from the lower edge of the hyoid bone from the greater cornu on either side, with care to avoid cutting the epiglottis, which lies immediately deep to this structure. The most important structures exposed during the course of this dissection are the internal laryngeal nerves and the superior laryngeal arteries at their entrance on either side of the thyrohyoid membrane. The mucous membrane lining the valleculae is then exposed and the pharynx is entered by cutting through it. Retraction of the hyoid bone and epiglottis with a self-retaining retractor exposes the posterior pharyngeal wall, which lies immediately superficial to the second, third, and fourth cervical vertebral bodies. A midline incision may then be made straight down to bone in order to expose these vertebral levels. The soft tissues are then dissected by subperiosteal dissection laterally on either side of the midline, and long sutures may be used to maintain the retraction of these flaps. If care is taken to perform electrocautery along the edges of these subperiosteal flaps prior to raising them, there will be little bleeding during the course of the dissection. Once the procedure is completed, the posterior pharyngeal walls may be closed in three layers using O-chromic catgut. The thyrohyoid membrane may be reattached and the thyrohyoid and sternohyoid muscles repaired to their tendinous attachments at the hyoid bone. A drain is placed at this level, and the platysma muscle and skin are sutured as separate layers to complete the closure. As previously mentioned, all of the approaches that violate the pharynx have a high incidence of post-operative infection.

If wider exposure is necessary, this may be achieved through the anterolateral open-mouth approach. The mandibular-tongue-pharynx splitting approach offers direct anterior wide exposure of the cervical vertebral bodies from the clivus to C6. This was described by Stauffer and has been used successfully by him for a variety of procedures in this area (2). A vertical incision is made from the center of the lower lip and carried inferiorly to the prominence of the chin, where the incision turns posteroinferiorly to the posterior aspect of the chin (Fig. 26). The mucous membrane is then divided longitudinally and the mandible is pre-drilled to facilitate closure. The mandible is then cut in a step-cut fashion to facilitate accurate approximation of the bone during the closure (Fig. 27). The tongue is divided longitudinally through its central raphe, and the two portions of the mandible and the tongue are each retracted laterally away from midline, exposing the posterior structures of the epiglottis and palate. Palpation through the posterior pharyngeal wall will allow location of the bony prominences of the C1-C2 vertebral bodies (Fig. 28). A longitudinal incision then transects the posterior pharyngeal wall and mucosa in the midline; this incision may be carried down through the periosteum to the bone of the upper cervical segments. Subperiosteal dissection may then be performed after electrocoagulating the edges of the flaps and raising a subperiosteal flap to the lateral aspect on either side (Fig. 29). Extending this exposure cephalad allows exposure to the level of the clivus. The inferior extent of the exposure may go down to C6. Closure is then performed by reapproximating the tongue with absorbable sutures and repairing the mandible through the pre-drilled holes with wire suture. The skin should be repaired with fine interrupted nonabsorbable sutures for optimal cosmesis.

Post-operatively, a halo jacket will usually be required for immobilization, as this will supplant any orthosis that would place pressure on the underside of the mandible. The halo jacket will also facilitate the patient's respiration through tracheostomy, which will have been performed prior to the commencement of the procedure. Stauffer has reported a minimal post-operative morbidity, which he feels is acceptable when compared with the safety of the improved exposure of the upper cervical spine and neural canal.

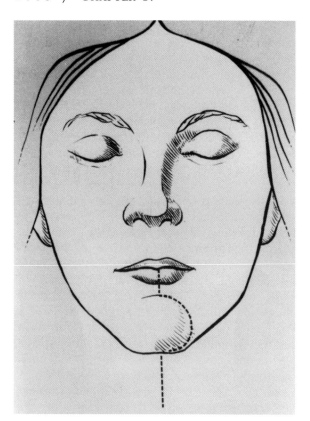

FIG. 26. Incision for mandibular-tongue-pharynx splitting approach to upper cervical spine.

FIG. 27. Step-cut the mandible to facilitate closure.

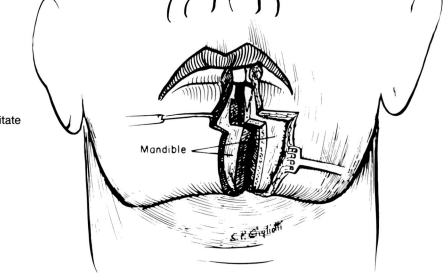

Mandible

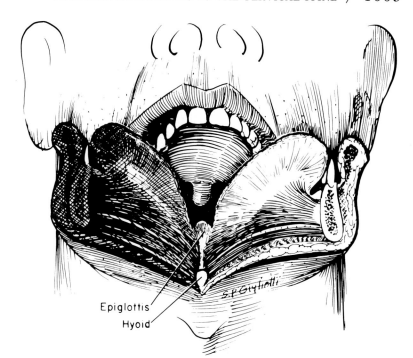

FIG. 28. The tongue is split down its central raphe exposing the epiglottis and palate.

Epiglottis

Hyoid

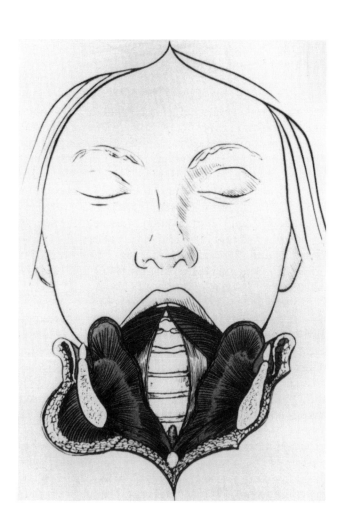

FIG. 29. A midline longitudinal incision transects the posterior pharyngeal wall and mucosa exposing the upper cervical segments.

POSTERIOR APPROACHES

Posterior Approach to C1-C2

The posterior approach to C1-C2 is used for fusions involving both the C1-C2 articulations and the occipitocervical articulations. The exposure may be extended cephalad to include the occiput and caudad to include the lower cervical spine.

The patient is prone on the operating table, and the head may be supported with either a headrest or self-retaining head fixation device that is attached to the table. The standard incision for a C1-C2 posterior fusion involves a midline incision from the caudal aspect of the occiput to the C3 spinous process. This is carried through the skin with a scalpel blade, and deeper dissection may be carried out with either a scalpel blade or electrocautery. The midline avascular structure, the median raphe or the ligamentum nuchae, follows a tortuous course; this generally prevents dissection in a straight line from posterior to anterior if this plane is to be followed. Care should be taken to remain within this raphe, as straying into the paraspinous muscle masses will cause unnecessary bleeding. The dissection may be carried down to the occiput in the cephalad extent into the spinous processes in the caudal portion of the exposure. In children, exposure of unnecessary levels should be avoided in order to avoid spontaneous fusion at levels adjacent to those necessary for the procedure. The ligamentous attachments to C2 are most prominent in this area, and dissection may begin at the C2 spinous process using either electrocautery or a subperiosteal elevator. The dissection then proceeds from the C2 spinous process out on to the lamina of C2 in a lateral direction. The dissection will often be carried caudal to the C2 level in order to provide adequate exposure. The exposure of the C2 and C3 laminae should extend to the medial one third of the facet joint at the base of the laminae, but should not extend beyond the facet joints during the course of the lateral exposure. The occiput may be subperiosteally exposed in a similar fashion. The intervening area will contain the ring of C1, which may be very deep with respect to C2. The posterior tubercle of C1 is usually palpable in the midline, and subperiosteal dissection using a small subperiosteal elevator may proceed from the posterior tubercle of C1 laterally.

Care must be taken during the course of this dissection to avoid excessive pressure on the C1 ring, as it may be thin and easily fractured. Slipping off of the C1 ring in a cephalad direction during the course of subperiosteal dissection may cause penetration of the atlanto-occipital membrane and injury to the underlying structures. In the case of atlanto-axial instability, direct pressure of the C1 ring against the dura may leave the dura vulnerable to injury during the course of dissection. The dura may be penetrated on both the superior and inferior edges of the ring of C1, so care must be taken during the course of this portion of the dissection, and the pathology involved must be taken into account during the course of this dissection as well.

The lateral extent of exposure at C1 is approximately 1.5 centimeters. The lateral landmark at the ring of C1 is the second cervical ganglion, which lies approximately 1.5 centimeters on the lamina of C1 in the area of the groove for the vertebral artery. The medial aspect of the groove for the vertebral artery must be carefully identified, as this is found on the superior border of the C1 ring. The vertebral vein is usually visualized first and noted by its bluish color. Care must be taken in this area to avoid damage to the vertebral artery as it courses from the slightly posteriorly placed foramen transversarium of C1 in a posterior medial direction to enter the foramen magnum just above the ring of C1. The vertebral artery and vein, then, are vulnerable not only in the groove at C1, but also as the artery passes from the foramen transversarium of C2 to the foramen transversarium of C1, where it is in close lateral and posterior proximity to the joint (Fig. 30). The vertebral vein will be encountered first as the dissection is carried from medial to lateral along the lamina. Penetration of the atlanto-occipital membrane just off the superior border of the ring of C1, more medial than the usually safe 1.5-centimeter margin from the midline, may also result in damage to the vertebral artery. It is therefore imperative that these relationships be known in exposure of the C1, C2, and occipital portions of the upper cervical spine. Self-retaining retractors are useful in maintaining retraction of the cervical paraspinous muscles during procedures in the upper and lower cervical spine. If a more lateral approach to the C1-C2 facet joint is desired, the vertebral artery between the C1 and C2 articulation must be identified. It should be noted that in rotatory dislocations of the C1-C2 articulation, the artery is stretched tightly across the joint on the side that C1 is anterior to C2 and is easily damaged.

It should be noted that the position of the head is important during all posterior cervical spine procedures, and the head is generally held in as close to neutral alignment as possible. Flexion will often aid in the exposure by bringing the occiput away from the C1-C2 articulations in a cephalad direction. However, the pathology being treated must be considered, in that flexion of the occiput may not be possible in order to retain reduction of the C1-C2 articulation. The ultimate position of the cervical spine must be evaluated with a lateral x-ray prior to commencing any surgical incision. This should be assessed for both position of the neck with respect to the procedure to be performed and radiographic accessibility to the areas undergoing surgery, so that evaluation of the procedure may be performed radiographically during the course of the procedure.

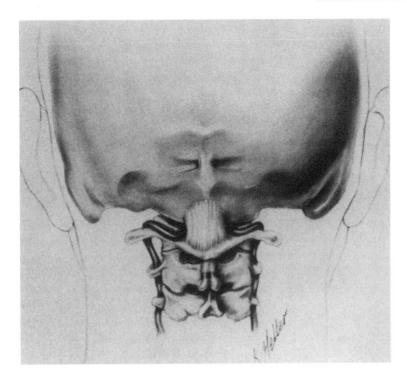

FIG. 30. The relationship between the C1 ring, C2 posterior elements, atlanto-occipital membrane, and the vertebral artery.

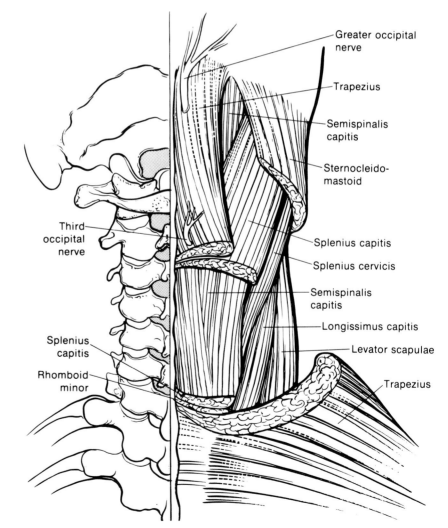

FIG. 31. Posterior cervical muscles: superficial layer.

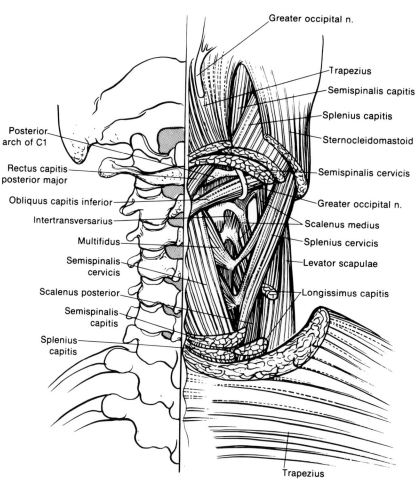

Greater occipital n.

Trapezius

Semispinalis capitis

Splenius capitis

Sternocleidomastoid

Semispinalis cervicis

Greater occipital n.

Scalenus medius

Splenius cervicis

Levator scapulae

Longissimus capitis

Trapezius

Posterior arch of C1

Rectus capitis posterior major

Obliquus capitis inferior

Intertransversarius

Multifidus

Semispinalis cervicis

Scalenus posterior

Semispinalis capitis

Splenius capitis

FIG. 32. Posterior cervical muscles: deeper layer.

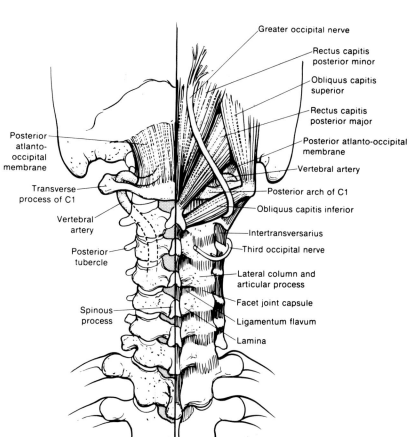

Greater occipital nerve

Rectus capitis posterior minor

Obliquus capitis superior

Rectus capitis posterior major

Posterior atlanto-occipital membrane

Vertebral artery

Posterior arch of C1

Obliquus capitis inferior

Intertransversarius

Third occipital nerve

Lateral column and articular process

Facet joint capsule

Ligamentum flavum

Lamina

Posterior atlanto-occipital membrane

Transverse process of C1

Vertebral artery

Posterior tubercle

Spinous process

FIG. 33. Muscle attachments of upper cervical spine.

Posterior Exposure of the Lower Cervical Spine

In exposure of the lower cervical spine, the prominent C7 spinous process should be palpated to determine the level and length of the midline posterior cervical incision. Once again, it is important to remain within the ligamentum nuchae during the course of the procedure to keep bleeding from the paraspinous muscles to a minimum. Once the skin and subcutaneous tissues are transected with a scalpel blade, the trapezius fascia is incised and retraction of the muscle mass on the side of the lesion is then performed. Subperiosteal dissection of the cervical paraspinous muscles can then be performed. These muscles include the splenius, the semispinalis capita, the lower semispinalis cervicis, and the multifidus. Dissection of these muscles may be performed using Bovie electrocautery, which is the method preferred by some. If not indicated, the extensor muscular insertions at C2 should not be removed to preserve both function and stability. Exposure of the laminae in the lower cervical spine is therefore performed with relative impunity and may be carried laterally to expose the medial two thirds of the zygapophyseal joints. Dissection beyond the zygapophyseal joints may result in denervation of the paraspinous muscles; this may also make the vertebral artery vulnerable to injury, should the dissection be carried beyond the joint and slightly anterior to the crossing of the vertebral artery between the foramen transversarium of two adjacent bodies (Fig. 31).

Just as in exposure of the upper cervical spine, a lateral roentgenogram taken prior to commencing the surgical prep is of paramount importance (Figs. 32 and 33).

REFERENCES

1. Barbour JR (1971): Screw fixation in fractures of the odontoid process. *S Australian Clin* 5:20–24.
2. The Cervical Spine Research Society, Editorial Committee (1989): *The cervical spine, 2nd ed.* Philadelphia: J.B. Lippincott, pp. 805–807.
3. De Andrade JR, Macnab I (1969): Anterior occipito-cervical fusion using an extra-pharyngeal exposure. *J Bone Joint Surg* [Am] 51:1621–1626.
4. Du Toit G (1976): Lateral atlantoaxial arthrodesis. A screw fixation technique. *S African J Surg* 14:9–12.
5. Fang HSY, Ong GB (1962): Direct anterior approach to the upper cervical spine. *J Bone Joint Surg* [Am] 49:1588–1604.
6. Grodinsky M, Holyoke EA (1938): Fascial and fascial spaces of the head, neck and adjacent regions. *Am J Anat* 63:367.
7. Hall JE, Denis F, Murray J (1977): Exposure of the upper cervical spine for spinal decompression by a mandible and tongue-splitting approach. *J Bone Joint Surg* [Am] 59:121–123.
8. Henry AK (1973): *Extensile exposure.* New York: Churchill Livingston.
9. Riley LH (1973): Surgical approaches to the anterior structures of the cervical spine. *CORR* 91:16–20.
10. Robinson RA, Southwick WO (1978): Surgical approaches to the cervical spine. *AAOS Instructional Course Lecture* 17:299–330.
11. Simmons EH, du Toit G (1978): Lateral atlantoaxial arthrodesis. *OCNA* 9(4):1101–1113.
12. Southwick WO, Robinson RA (1976): Surgical approaches to the vertebral bodies in the cervical and lumbar regions. *J Bone Joint Surg* [Am] 39:631–644.
13. Watkins RG (1983): *Surgical approaches to the spine.* New York: Springer-Verlag.
14. Whitecloud TS, LaRocca H (1976): Fibular strut graft in reconstructive surgery of the cervical spine. *Spine* 1(1):33–43.
15. Whitesides TE Jr, Kelly RP (1966): Lateral approaches to the upper cervical spine for anterior fusion. *Southern Med J* 59:879–883.
16. Whitesides TE Jr, McDonald AP (1978): Lateral retropharyngeal approach to the upper cervical spine. *OCNA* 9(4):1115–1127.
17. Williams PL, Warwick R, eds. (1980): *Gray's anatomy 36th ed.* Philadelphia: W.B. Saunders.

The Adult Spine: Principles and Practice,
J. W. Frymoyer, Editor-in-Chief.
Raven Press, Ltd., New York © 1991.

CHAPTER **48**

Congenital Bony Anomalies of the Cervical Spine

Henry H. Sherk and Gurvinder S. Uppal

UPPER CERVICAL SPINE

Congenital malformations of the upper cervical spine include the following:

1. Basilar impression
2. Accessory occipital vertebra
3. Occipitalization of the atlas (congenital atlanto-occipital fusion)
4. Malformations of the atlantal ring
5. Malformations of the dens
6. Congenital spondylolisthesis of the axis
7. Spina bifida and iniencephaly.

The development of the skull base and upper cervical spine is slightly more complicated than elsewhere and a brief review of the phases of embryologic and fetal development helps to understand these lesions. The occiput forms from the fusion of the five most rostral somites and the atlas derives from the mesenchymal cells which grow ventrally and dorsally from the hypochordal bow.

   H. H. Sherk, M.D.; G. S. Uppal, M.D.: Department of Orthopaedic Surgery, Medical College of Pennsylvania, Philadelphia, Pennsylvania 19129.

In more distal segments in humans, below the atlas, the hypochordal bow forms the thick portion of the anterior longitudinal ligament. At C1 it forms an ossified ring about the dens. The dens itself develops from the C1 somite, and the body of the axis forms the fusion of the caudal half of the C1 somite and the rostral half of the C2 somite. Disruption of this normal developmental process can give rise to the congenital malformations described here (25) (Fig. 1).

BASILAR IMPRESSION

Failure of formation or fusion of the occipital somites results in basilar impression. This is a term used to describe a condition in which the odontoid process is displaced upward into the base of the skull in the region of the foramen magnum. It is a condition which can be congenital or acquired. In the congenital variety, occipital hypoplasia is usually associated with various other malformations in the skull base, as well as the upper cervical spine and brain stem. Acquired basilar impression is usually due to a disease process which weakens the skull base, such as Paget's disease, rickets, osteoporo-

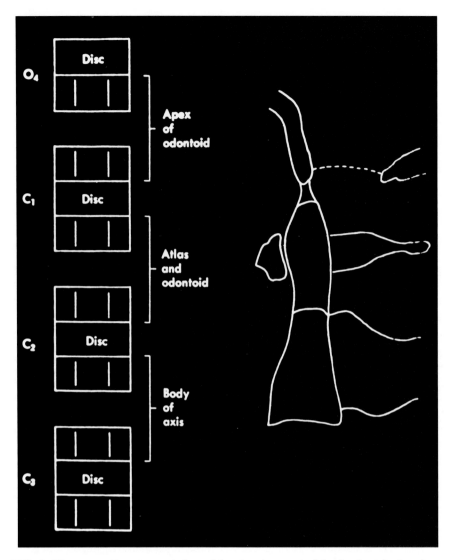

FIG. 1. Diagrammatic representation of the development of the basi occiput and upper cervical spine.

sis, or rheumatoid arthritis. In these conditions, the skull can be thought of as sagging down about the cervical spine which consequently pushes up into the posterior fossa (Fig. 2).

Basilar impression can be detected and measured by using several lines. Chamberlain's line (2), for example, is drawn from the hard palate to the posterior rim of the foramen magnum. If the upper tip of the dens is 5 mm above the line, the patient is considered to have basilar impression. McGregor's line extends from the hard palate to the most caudal part of the occipital curve, and the upper tip of the dens should be less than 7 mm above this line. Chamberlain's line best measures congenital basilar impression while McGregor's line is more likely to be abnormal in acquired basilar impression. The reason for this difference is that the softening of the skull base that occurs in secondary basilar impression pushes in the occiput, but the dens and atlas may remain below the fora-

men magnum. Their position might not appear altered in reference to the lines extending backwards to the foramen magnum (11,14) (Fig. 3).

Basilar impression is not platybasia. The latter term describes an increase in the basal angle of the skull, which is determined by a line drawn along the plane of the sphenoid and another drawn along the clivus, as seen on the lateral x-ray of the skull. Flattening of the skull base was described by nineteenth century anthropologists and is probably meaningless from the clinical standpoint.

ACCESSORY OCCIPITAL VERTEBRA

Accessory occipital vertebra occurs when the most distal occipital somite fails to fuse correctly to the more rostral occipital segments. An occipital vertebra can

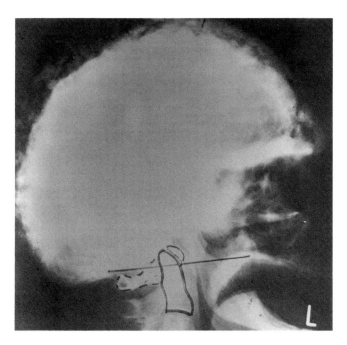

FIG. 2. Lateral roentgenogram of the skull and upper cervical spine showing basilar impression secondary to Paget's disease.

manifest itself as a complete vertebral ring, or accessory atlantal arches, or as accessory paracondylar masses. These lesions can be unilateral or bilateral. They are often associated with narrowing and crowding of the foramen magnum as well as with other bony and neural malformations.

OCCIPITALIZATION OF THE ATLAS

Occipitalization of the atlas (19) or congenital atlanto-occipital fusion is one of the more common anomalies of the upper cervical spine and was found in 25% of a group of patients who presented with congenital malformations of the foramen magnum. Most often fusion occurs as a coalition of the anterior arch of the atlas through the anterior rim of the foramen magnum. Occasionally there is some segment of the posterior arch and lateral masses present. These lesions also produce a situation in which a single lateral atlantal mass results in a severe and progressive torticollis. These lesions can be much more complex than single level fusions and may involve several or multiple subjacent vertebrae. Occipitalization of the atlas occurs frequently in conjunction with other

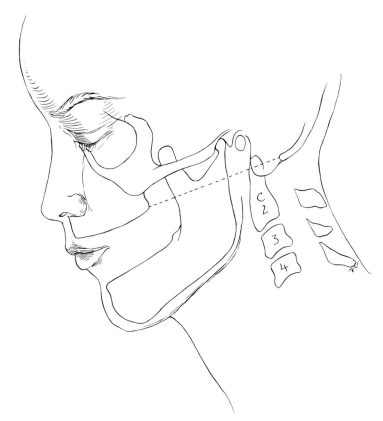

FIG. 3. Diagrammatic representation of Chamberlain's line (2), a line drawn from the hard palate to the posterior rim of the foramen magnum, which should lie just above the tip of the odontoid process.

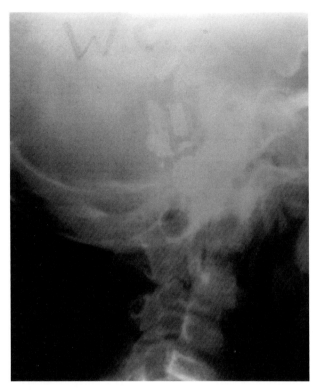

FIG. 4. Lateral roentgenogram of skull and upper cervical spine showing occipitalization of the anterior arch of the atlas and basilar impression.

malformations, such as an abnormally large or malpositioned odontoid process, and these combinations can have significant adverse consequences for the neurologic structures contained therein (Figs. 4 and 5).

MALFORMATIONS OF THE ATLANTAL RING

Malformations of the atlas are very common and often are picked up on roentgenograms taken for other purposes (18). Partial or complete absence of the posterior arch and failure of closure of the anterior arch are common findings and usually have no clinical significance. They result from failure of fusion of the synchondroses, normally present in the cervical spines of infants and children. Absence of the posterior arch of the atlas may have unexpected significance, however, if the surgeon attempts a C1-C2 fusion only to find that the posterior arch of C1 is absent. A normal variant occasionally seen in the atlas is Kimmerle's anomaly also known as the foramen arcuale or posterior ponticulus (6). This is an arch of bone which extends over the vertebral artery and suboccipital nerve where they ascend behind the lateral mass of the atlas over the posterior arch of C1. This is probably an anomalous ossification center that occurs in the posterior atlanto-occipital membrane. It has no clinical significance. It has numerous variations and can be unilateral, bilateral, partial, or complete (Fig. 6).

MALFORMATIONS OF THE DENS

Malformations of the odontoid process include:

1. Absence
2. Hypoplasia
3. Duplication
4. Isolated C1 vertebral body
5. Condylicus tertius
6. Os terminale
7. Os odontoideum.

Absence, hypoplasia, and odontoid fragments unattached to the axis may result from trauma and thus are not really congenital malformations. There are a number of reports of children who had normal x-rays on an initial examination who were found to have one of these lesions in later years. The assumption is made that an injury to the blood supply of the dens through the arcades of the vertebral artery resulted from trauma and that avascular necrosis of the dens or non-union of a fracture resulted. Clearly this does occur in some patients but a prospective review of dens fracture in children failed to reveal any of these lesions and these lesions also do occur with other congenital malformations. Absence of the dens, hypoplasia, os odontoideum, and os terminale, therefore, are probably both congenital and traumatic in origin. These lesions are often quite unstable and may have catastrophic consequences for the patient (Fig. 7).

The condylicus tertius syndrome, however, occurs when a large abnormal dens articulates with a third occipital condyle on the anterior rim of the foramen magnum. This lesion is not necessarily unstable but produces cord involvement because of narrowing of the foramen magnum with brain stem compression (Fig. 8). Duplication of the dens usually results from derangements of normal segmentation and is associated with deformity or hypoplasia of an attached lateral mass. These patients most often present with torticollis.

CONGENITAL SPONDYLOLISTHESIS OF THE AXIS

Congenital spondylolisthesis of the axis manifests itself as bilateral defects in the pedicles or neural arches of the axis. The lesion is similar to the hangman's fracture and is a cause of anterior displacement of the upper cervical spine and cord damage. It requires stabilization either anteriorly with a dowel graft at C2-C3 or a posterior fusion from C1 to C3 (Fig. 9).

SPINA BIFIDA AND INIENCEPHALY

Spina bifida and encephalocele, cervical meningocele, iniencephaly, and anencephaly are rare lesions which

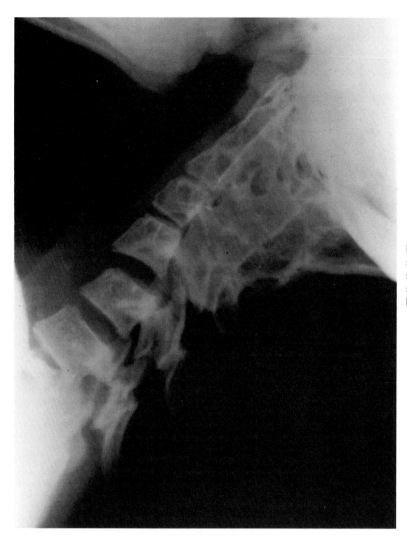

FIG. 5. Lateral roentgenogram of the base of the skull and the upper cervical spine showing massive atlanto-occipital fusion extending from the skull base to the mid cervical spine. The patient has a dangerous motion segment below fusion.

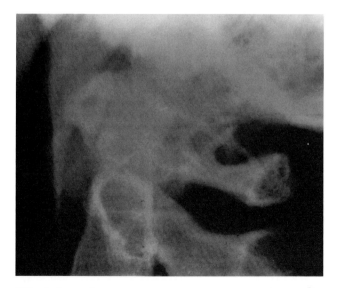

FIG. 6. Lateral roentgenogram of basi occiput C1 and C2 showing a posterior ponticulus.

have a wide range of presentation and manifest varying degrees of severity. Iniencephaly is probably more common than recognized and consists of posterior defects in the skull base and upper cervical spine with hyperextension contracture of the upper neck and often a cervical meningocele. Usually, also, these patients have multiple congenital cervical fusions. The lesion has been known to exist for a number of years and descriptions still appear from time to time in the medical literature (8) (Fig. 10).

From the clinical standpoint, congenital malformations of the upper cervical spine can cause (a) deformity of the upper neck, or (b) they may be associated with central nervous system lesions. The central nervous system lesions themselves may be primary developmental malformations or they can develop as a result of the osseous malformations. Various other congenital malformations and conditions occur with upper cervical spine lesions and these include vertebral artery anoma-

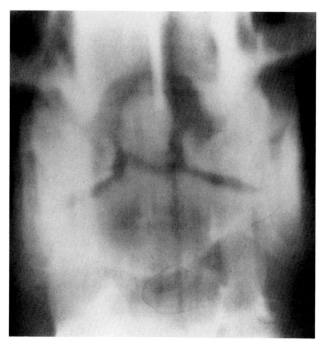

FIG. 7. AP tomogram of basi occiput of C1 and C2 revealing a defect at the base of the odontoid. The defect is smooth and is classifiable as an os odontoideum.

lies and vascular lesions such as hemangiomas. These patients also can present with associated dermoid tumors, frontonasal dysplasia, and malformations of the petrous pyramids with congenital deafness and vertigo (14).

Torticollis may be caused by congenital anomalies of the atlas. Dubousset (3) described 17 such patients in whom torticollis was caused by isolated hemi atlas, partial aplasia of the atlas, partial atlanto-occipital fusion, and asymmetry of the lateral mass of the atlas. Dubousset noted that these malformations produced a severe and progressive torticollis. He observed, however, that when the patients were still young children the neck was flexible despite the deformity and could be passively corrected. He reported that gradual straightening of the deformity in a halo cast followed by posterior occipito-cervical fusion produced lasting and satisfactory correction.

The fixed retroflexion deformity of the head in iniencephaly is also amenable to this type of treatment. We have corrected this type of deformity by performing a posterior release followed by gradual correction of the hyperextension in a halo cast. A posterior occipital fusion has appeared to maintain satisfactory alignment.

CENTRAL NERVOUS SYSTEM LESIONS

Central nervous system lesions are probably the most important consideration relative to bony abnormalities of the upper cervical spine. These can be caused by (a)

brain stem and upper cord compression due to static encroachment, (b) upper cord compression due to instability, and (c) primary central nervous system lesions. Basilar impression, elevation of the dens, shortening of the clivus, invagination of the occipital condyles, narrowing of the foramen magnum, and elevation of the petrous pyramids can all cause encroachment on the brain stem and upper cord. Dural bands in these lesions form across the posterior rim of the foramen magnum and compress the upper cord and block the normal flow of cerebral spinal fluid. If blockages of the foramina of Lushka and Magendi occur, these patients can experience distension of the central canal of the cord with the formation of hydromyelia. If the ependymal lining of the central canal fails to restrain the elevated cerebral spinal fluid, pressure within the central canal may push out into the cord parenchyma to form a cyst or syrinx within the cord substance. Once such a lesion has formed, coughing, sneezing, or straining by increasing the pressure in the spinal canal compresses the cord and forces the syringomyelia to track down into the lower cord or up into the medulla in which case it is called a syringobulbia. These lesions can reach enormous size and result in very significant neurologic deficits (Fig. 11). Other spinal deformities, particularly scoliosis, can result from

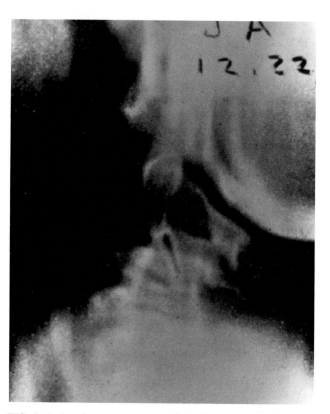

FIG. 8. Lateral roentgenogram of skull base and upper cervical spine showing occipitalization of C1 and a large condyle on the anterior rim of the foramen magnum to which the odontoid process articulates. This is known as the condylicus tertius.

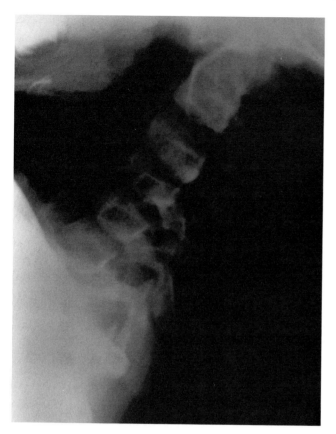

FIG. 9. Lateral roentgenogram of the upper cervical spine in flexion showing anterior displacement at C2-C3 secondary to a pars defect of C2.

these. Disruption of the spinalthalmic tract can also result in development of neurotrophic joints, especially in the upper limb. The presence of a Charcot joint in the upper extremity therefore should alert one to the possibility of malformations of the upper cervical spine (24).

Lesions of the Odontoid Process

Instability of the upper cervical spine produces a different type of cord lesion. This is the situation that usually occurs with lesions of the odontoid process especially os odontoideum and absence of the dens. Juhl and Seerup (13) described symptoms in 3 groups of patients seen with an os odontoideum:

1. Post-traumatic neck pain
2. Gradually worsening signs of medullary compression
3. No symptoms.

Treatment based on this classification, however, might be misleading since some patients with these lesions develop very severe signs of upper cord and brain stem compression after only minor trauma (16). Nevertheless, most patients who are asymptomatic, or whose symptoms are limited to neck pain, have a good progno-

sis without fusion. Patients with gradually worsening symptoms and neurologic signs, on the other hand, have a poor prognosis and can be expected to worsen neurologically without treatment. A small group of these patients have vertebral artery compression at or just below the foramen magnum. They may present with confusing symptoms which may lead to incorrect diagnoses.

Arnold-Chiari Lesions

The third reason for central nervous system involvement in these patients is the presence of a primary central nervous system malformation, the most common being the Arnold-Chiari malformation. There are four subgroups of Arnold-Chiari malformations which really only define the degree and direction of displacement of neural structures from the posterior fossa. In Type I, the cerebellar tonsils are displaced downwards into the cervical canal. In Type II, the cerebellar tissue and part of the medulla are displaced through the foramen magnum. In Type III deformities, portions of the cerebellum and the lower medulla, including at least part of the fourth ventricle, are displaced downwards into the cervical canal. In Type III lesions, there is usually a kinking of the medulla over the more distal cervical segments. It should

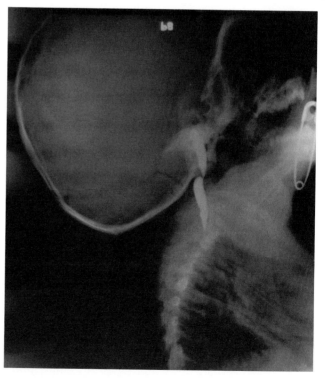

FIG. 10. Lateral roentgenogram of skull and cervical spine showing findings of iniencephaly. There is fixed retroversion of skull, contact between the inion and the spinous processes of T1, and a large defect in the skull base. The cervical vertebrae are fused and there is a herniation of the contents of the posterior fossa into the upper cervical canal.

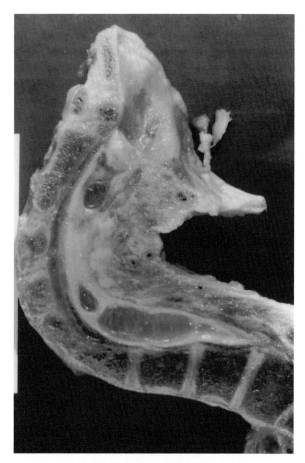

FIG. 11. Sagittal section of the skull base, cervical spine, and upper thoracic spine showing very severe cervical lordosis and thoracic kyphosis. The contents of the posterior fossa had been herniated into the cervical canal. There is a huge cyst in the substance of the spinal cord (syringomyelia).

also be noted that Type III Arnold-Chiari lesions are almost always associated with hydrocephalus and myelomeningocele (5). In Type IV Arnold-Chiari lesions, the contents of the posterior fossa are herniated upwards through the falx cerebri. This lesion is also called the Dandy-Walker syndrome.

Patients with an Arnold-Chiari lesion often develop disruption of cerebral spinal fluid mechanics with dilation of the central canal of the cord with the formation of hydromyelia or a syringomyelia.

DIAGNOSIS

The diagnosis (17) of upper cervical spine malformations begins with a history and physical examination. These lesions are not usually painful. Patients can present with an obvious deformity such as torticollis but more often they have symptoms and findings related to neurologic involvement and the upper cervical spine malformation is found either serendipitously or as a re-

sult of a careful diagnostic work-up. Adult onset scoliosis, or very rapidly progressing and unusual curve patterns in children, might suggest such a lesion. Charcot joints in the upper limbs should also suggest them. Occasionally, these patients have bizarre and unusual complaints (23) and findings and are thought initially to be hysterics or malingerers (20).

In general, symptoms and findings depend on the site of neural compression. The cerebellar involvement of the Arnold-Chiari syndrome produces nystagmus, ataxia, and loss of coordination. Posterior compression of the upper cord from a narrowed foramen magnum or dural band causes posterior column symptoms and signs such as a loss of deep pressure sensation as well as loss of vibration and proprioception. Anterior upper cord compression resulting from atlanto-axial instability or posterior displacement of the dens produces pyramidal tract signs. These patients manifest spasticity, hyper-reflexia, pathologic reflexes, weakness, and ataxia. All of the foregoing may be associated with vertebral artery insufficiency and the complaints and findings of the Wallenberg syndrome.

The diagnosis is based on plain x-rays, MRI, and CT with myelography. Chamberlain's line and McGregor's line are two useful measurements in defining basilar impression and have already been described. These have the disadvantage, however, of using the line of the hard palate as the reference. Since the hard palate is not part of the skull base and may vary in position due to a facial malformation or high arched palate, some authors suggest that the position of the dens should be referenced to the line connecting either the digastric grooves or the tips of the mastoid processes (7).

The space available for the cord or the SAC is a critical measurement in these cases and can be determined at the level of the foramen magnum by measuring the sagittal diameter of the foramen from the anterior to the posterior rims. McCrae reported that patients with less than 19 mm of space available at the level of the foramen magnum had symptoms and findings related to upper cord and brain stem compression. One should also measure the sagittal diameter from the posterior aspect of the dens to the nearest posterior structure, which is usually the posterior arch of the atlas. In some patients, in whom the posterior arch of the atlas is absent, however, the nearest posterior structure may be the posterior rim of the foramen magnum (11).

Currently there appears to be some debate about the relative usefulness of MRI and CT myelography. Because of its superior soft tissue contrast resolution, MRI permits the visualization of spinal cord lesions with excellent delineation of the Arnold-Chiari malformation, hydromyelia, and syringomyelia. MRI is probably superior to CT and myelography therefore in screening in the diagnosis of the neurologic disorders associated with upper cervical spine malformations (Fig. 12). In fact, it now

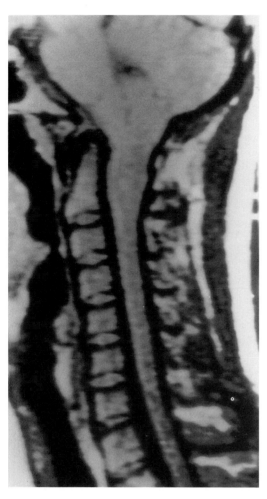

FIG. 12. Sagittal MRI of the skull and upper cervical spine posterior fossa and spinal cord showing an Arnold-Chiari malformation.

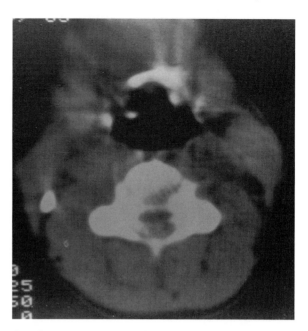

FIG. 13. Myelogram and CT of the upper cervical canal showing a double shadow consistent with a Type III Arnold-Chiari malformation. The medulla is displaced distally into the cervical canal and there is dorsal over-riding of the upper cervical cord by the medulla.

appears that these lesions are more common than heretofore recognized since so many patients are now being demonstrated to have them due to the wider use of MRI. MRI is currently limited because of relatively long data acquisition times and the possible degradation of the image by physiologic motions. This is especially important in the neck due to the pulsations of the vertebral and carotid arteries as well as involuntary swallowing by some patients. It seems, therefore, that MRI is the sensitive study which should be done first in these patients. Myelography and CT (1) make it possible to localize precisely levels at which encroachment on the neural elements occurs and these studies should be done prior to surgery as the specific test to localize the abnormality (Fig. 13).

TREATMENT

Treatment of malformations of the upper cervical spine depends on the type of symptoms and their sever-

ity. Deformity can be managed by traction and fusion as has already been discussed. With regard to the management of patients with neurological involvement, it is important to recognize that many patients have multiple and complex malformations. In cases of static encroachment on the brain stem and upper cord by basilar impression, occipital vertebrae, or atlanto-occipital fusion, suboccipital decompression and C1 and possibly C2 laminectomy may be necessary. The destabilization of the upper cervical spine by this type of surgery should be considered, however, and fusion may also be necessary. Posterior decompression may not suffice in cases in which an enlarged odontoid process or third occipital condyle on the anterior rim of the foramen magnum compresses the anterior aspect of the brain stem and cord. In these cases, anterior decompression may also be indicated (4,9,10).

Malformations of the odontoid probably do not require treatment if the lesion is relatively stable and the space available for the cord is not compromised. These patients probably should be followed very closely, however, since several reports of sudden death after only minor trauma indicated that these lesions do have the potential for developing sudden catastrophic instability.

Patients who have decreased space available for the cord of less than 13 mm and a history of myelopathy should have a posterior fusion. If the upper cervical spine is grossly unstable and can easily be reduced, pre-operative traction is not required and a standard Gallie or

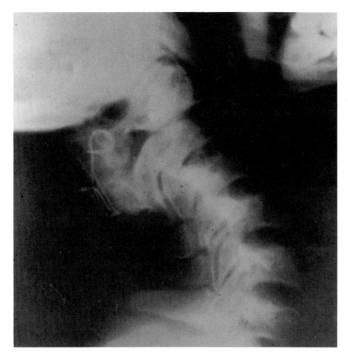

FIG. 14. Lateral roentgenogram of the skull and cervical spine showing congenital malformation of C1. The odontoid process has developed into an isolated C1 vertebral body and is incorporated into the atlas vertebrae. The resulting instability caused severe neurological findings. A Gallie type of posterior C1-C2 fusion stabilized the spine although a slight degree of anterior displacement remains.

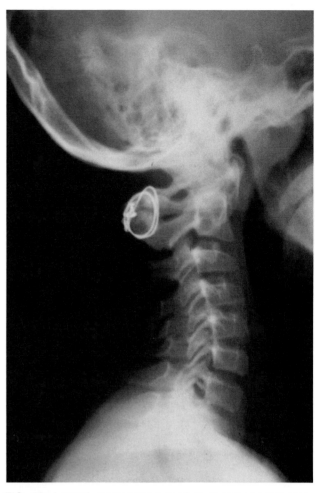

FIG. 15. Lateral roentgenogram of skull and cervical spine showing the final result of a Brooks fusion to stabilize the C1-C2 displacement caused by an os odontoideum. The wires have been passed sublaminarly at C1 and C2.

Brooks type of fusion can be performed. If passive manipulation does not correct the atlanto-axial displacement, a period of skeletal traction is advisable. If the displacement can be corrected with the traction, passing sublaminar wires is probably safe and a Gallie or Brooks type of fusion can be carried out. If, however, the C1-C2 displacement cannot be corrected by pre-operative traction, passing sublaminar wires under the arch of the atlas can be too hazardous. In these cases, one should perform an in situ fusion over the arch of C1 from the occiput to C2. This will, of course, leave the patient with narrowing of the upper spinal canal but the stability provided by the fusion may cause the symptoms of the myelopathy to resolve. Should this not occur, one should consider an anterior cord decompression with either retropharangeal or an open mouth approach (10,15) (Figs. 14 and 15).

Treatment of the Arnold-Chiari malformation with hydromyelia and syringomyelia usually does not fall into the realm of the orthopedist. Surgery done for these lesions, however, may be done by the neurosurgeon and orthopedic surgeon working together to decompress the brain stem and upper cord and stabilize the upper cervical spine. Treatment of these lesions is complex and hazardous. It requires well planned and well executed surgical strategies combining the skills of orthopedics, neurosurgery, and radiology (4,21,22).

REFERENCES

1. Agnoli L (1983): Computer-tomographic investigation in malformations of the occipito-cervical junction. *Neurosurgical Rev* 6:177–185.
2. Chamberlain WE (1939): Basilar impression (Platybasia): A bizarre developmental anomaly of the occipital bone and upper cervical spine with striking and misleading neurologic manifestations. *Yale J Biology Med* 11:487–496.
3. Dubousset J (1986): Torticollis in children caused by congenital anomalies of the atlas. *J Bone Joint Surg* [Am] 68:178–188.
4. Elies W (1984): Surgery in craniocervical dysplasia. *Otolaryngologic Clin N Am* 17:553–563.
5. Emery JL (1986): The cervical cord of children with meningomyelocele. *Spine* 11:318–322.
6. Erickson LC, Greer RO Jr (1984): Ponticulus posticus, an anomaly of the first cervical vertebra as seen on the cephalometric head film. *Oral Surgery, Oral Medicine, Oral Pathology* 57:230.
7. Fischgold H, Metzger J (1952): Etude radiotomographique de l'impression basilaire. *Rev Rheum* 19:261–264.
8. Gardner WJ (1979): Klippel-Feil syndrome, iniencephalus, anencephalus, hindbrain hernia, and mirror movements: Overdistention of the neural tube. *Childs Brain* 5:361–379.
9. Georgopoulos G, Pizzutillo PD, Lee MS (1987): Occipito-atlantal instability in children. *J Bone Joint Surg* [Am] 69:429–436.

10. Hensinger RN (1986): Osseous anomalies of the craniovertebral junction. *Spine* 11:323–333.
11. Hinck VC, Hopkins CE, Savara BS (1961): Diagnostic criteria of basilar impression. *Radiology* 76:572–585.
12. Hinck VC, Hopkins CE, Savara BS (1962): Sagittal diameter of the cervical spinal canal in children. *Radiology* 79:97–108.
13. Juhl M, Seerup KK (1983): Os odontoideum: A cause of atlantoaxial instability. *Acta Orthop Scand* 54:113–118.
14. Kane RJ, O'Connor AF, Morrison AW (1982): Primary basilar impression: An aetiological factor in Meniere's disease. *J Laryngol Otol* 96:931–936.
15. Koop SE, Winter RB, Lonstein JE (1984): The surgical treatment of instability of the upper part of the cervical spine in children and adolescents. *J Bone Joint Surg* [Am] 66:403–411.
16. Krone A (1983): Traumatic tetraparesis in craniocervical dysplasia. Case report. *Neurosurgical Rev* 6:235–237.
17. Kumar A, Jafar J, Mafee M et al (1986): Diagnosis and management of anomalies of the craniovertebral junction. *Annals Otol Rhinol Laryngol* 95:487–497.
18. Mace SE (1986): Congenital absence of the C-1 vertebral arch. *Am J Emergency Med* 4:326–329.
19. McRae DL, Barnum AS (1953): Occipitalization of the atlas. *Am J Roentgenol* 70:23–46.
20. Michie I, Clark M (1968): Neurological syndromes associated with cervical and craniocervical anomalies. *Archives Neurol* 18:241–247.
21. Nagashima C, Kubota S (1983): Craniocervical abnormalities. Modern diagnosis and a comprehensive surgical approach. *Neurosurgical Rev* 6:187–197.
22. Pia HW (1983): Craniocervical malformations. *Neurosurgical Rev* 6:169–175.
23. Rosamoff HL (1986): Occult respiratory and automatic dysfunction in craniovertebral anomalies and upper cervical spinal disease. *Spine* 11:345–347.
24. Sherk HH, Charney E, Pasquariello PA, et al (1986): Hydrocephalus, cervical cord lesions and spinal deformity. *Spine* 11:340–342.
25. Spillane JD, Pallis C, Jones AM (1957): Developmental abnormalities in the region of the foramen magnum. *Brain* 80:11–48.

LOWER CERVICAL SPINE

HISTORICAL OVERVIEW

In 1912, Klippel and Feil presented a unusual case report regarding a patient without a neck (l'homme sans cou). They described a triad of findings in this patient which consisted of a low posterior hairline, very short and in fact apparently absent neck, and marked loss of motion of the cervical spine. The syndrome they described has been called the Klippel-Feil anomaly since that time. Strictly speaking, osseous malformations of the cervical spine should be called the Klippel-Feil anomaly only if their triad is present, but virtually any congenital osseous malformation of this area has gone by that term since their report was published.

Osseous malformations of the cervical spine have been extensively reviewed. In 1965, Gray et al. reviewed all of the available reports of patients with congenital fusions of the cervical spine (27). They were able to locate 462 cases from the world literature. They noted that congenital cervical fusions of the cervical spine have been recognized since 500 BC and that anatomical descriptions of the anomaly were present in the sixteenth and eighteenth centuries AD. The advent of the roentgen ray made recognition possible in living patients and the anomaly has subsequently been extensively annotated. In their definitive review, Gray et al. noted that congenital fusions of the cervical spine can occur at any level. They are most common in the upper cervical spine, however, and 75% involve at least one of the first three cervical vertebrae. Half of the patients with congenital cervical fusions in their study had involvement of three or fewer levels. Twenty-five percent of the fusions were at the occiput-C1 level but the joint between the second and third cervical vertebrae was the single most frequently fused level (Fig. 1). Fusions involve the entire circumference in about half of the cases, anterior only in 18%, posterior 9%, and laterally only in about 3% of patients.

Gray, Avery, and other authors noted that the osseous malformations were only "the tip of the iceberg" in these patients and that the multiple associated malformations involving many other systems are usually of greater clinical significance than the bony malformations themselves (3,33,45). Thus the existence of an osseous malformation of the lower cervical spine is probably most significant as an important indicator of the possible presence of other system involvement.

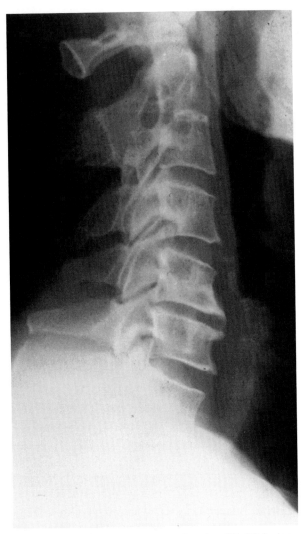

FIG. 1. Lateral roentgenogram showing C2-C3 fusion.

RELEVANT EMBRYOLOGY

The subaxial cervical spine develops normally according to the sequence outlined in many papers and texts (80). The embryonic phase lasts from conception to approximately six weeks of embryonic life. During this period, the notochord extends rostrally from the primitive streak on the embryonic disc, and the mesenchymal cells on each side of the notochord organize themselves into somites which give rise to the myodermatomes and sclerotomes. The cells of the sclerotome migrate ventrally to surround the notochord during this period, while at the same time the neural crests fold together to form the neural tube. The completion of the formation of the neural tube and somites immediately precedes the process of resegmentation in which the cranial portion of one somite fuses with the caudal portion of the adjacent somite to form a vertebra. The intervertebral disc develops from clusters of cells in the central portion of the somite, which in turn differentiate into nucleus pulposus

and annulus fibrosis. Resegmentation with formation of the vertebral column is associated with continued migration of mesenchymal cells dorsally over the neural tubes to enclose that structure in rudimentary laminae and related dorsal bony elements.

Mesenchymal cells from the newly formed vertebrae also migrate laterally and ventrally to form the costal processes in the cervical spine and ribs in the thoracic spine. At the end of the somite phase, the developing individual is no longer an embryo and can be referred to as a fetus. The importance of this event is that the individual no longer significantly changes its structure. It is now recognizable as a human fetus in which tissues and organs grow and differentiate but do not materially change morphologically. In the spine, differentiation proceeds from the mesenchymal phase to that of chondrification and then ossification in which the mesenchymal model of a vertebra first changes over to a cartilaginous structure and finally into one that is ossified. It has become the convention to describe the development of the embryo as occurring in "horizons." These correspond to stages of maturation with given crown-rump lengths and gestational ages. At each horizon of development the various systems are expected to have evolved in a relationship to each other in a predictable way (72). Disruption of the normal process, therefore, can often be anatomically and temporally defined by referring to these horizons.

The physical proximity of various other developing tissues to the spinal column results in a number of other systems being involved when pathologic processes disrupt the normal sequence of events. For example, the branchial arches arise from the intermediate mesoderm adjacent to the cervicothoracic somites. Thus derangement of the somites or developing vertebrae can be associated with malformations of the structures which arise from the branchial arches such as the ear, maxilla, and mandible (74). Similarly the pronephros originates at the level of the lower cervical spine and teratogenic factors at those levels can be associated with the abnormal development of the genitourinary system (15). The very close proximity of the developing spinal cord to the osseous structures in the cervical spine is obvious and it is no surprise that malformations of the central nervous system can co-exist with the congenital osseous lesions in this area (61).

The etiology of osseous malformations in the subaxial cervical spine is probably multifactorial (8). Autosomal dominant inheritance of cervical ribs has been reported (70) and the congenital cervical fusions occurring in such abnormalities as Apert's and Crouzon's syndromes are probably based on autosomal recessive and autosomal dominant inheritance respectively (77).

Genetic inheritance does not account for many such lesions, however, and there is strong evidence to suggest that congenital malformations of the cervical spine and related structures result from vascular occlusions. Bavrinck and Weaver (5) suggested a "subclavian artery supply disruption sequence" (SADS) to explain the pathogenesis not only of the Klippel-Feil anomaly but also the Poland and Mobius anomalies, isolated absence of the pectoralis major with breast hypoplasia, isolated terminal transverse limb deficits, and the Sprengel anomaly. They suggested that these anomalies resulted from hypoxia caused by interruption of the embryonic circulation of the subclavian artery and its branches with the specific pattern of the anomaly depending on the location, timing, and severity of the vascular disruption. It was proposed that interruption of blood flow at a critical time in embryologic development, before the embryo could achieve a compensatory collateral circulation, would result in an ischemia, lack of development, and degeneration of the structures supplied by specific blood vessels. Bavrinck and Weaver believed that cervical vertebral fusions resulted from disruption of intersegmental vessels arising from the vertebral arteries at the time of resegmentation of the sclerotomes. They hypothesized that the many anomalies that are associated with the Klippel-Feil defect result from associated vascular insults. They worked out a scheme to define mechanisms that would cause the SADS, citing mechanical, embryologic, and environmental factors causing ischemia, hypoxia, edema, hemorrhage, and blistering in the developing embryonic tissues (8).

Rather specific refinements of this scheme have been suggested by other authors. Treadwell and Smith (86) noted that cervical spine anomalies occurring as a result of the fetal alcohol syndrome have an association with cardiac defects more often than genitourinary malformation. The fetal alcohol syndrome variant of the Klippel-Feil lesion is always associated with a single level of congenital fusion in contrast to a 20% single level fusion in other cases of the Klippel-Feil lesion. Treadwell and Smith collected 50 such cases and presented them as a definable subset related to a specific teratogenic insult, occurring at the 24th to 28th day of embryonic life.

Vascular occlusion, however, may be only one of several causes of congenital malformations of the cervical spine. Causon (9) described anatomic specimens in which failure of development of the zygoapophyseal joint appeared to cause vertebral body fusions ("blocked vertebrae"). He cited evidence that suggested that the dorsal arch of each cervical vertebra arises from the adjacent caudal sclerotomes. In his specimens, these "blocked vertebrae" contained two independent vertebral arches including pedicles, transverse processes, laminae, articular processes, and a spinous process. The arches and invertebral bodies had developed normally but were fused together. He suggested that their fusion, apparently after normal development, showed that the fusion event occurred at the time of facet joint differentiation during the phase of chondrification of the mesen-

chymal vertebral anlage. It was hypothesized that this event was in turn caused by abnormalities of the neuraxis. Since the neuraxis has the inductive capacity to promote and stabilize chrondrification of the vertebrae, lesions of the neuraxis could be expected to result in spinal column malformations, due to failure of differentiation of vertebrae from mesenchyme to cartilage (37).

KLIPPEL-FEIL SYNDROME

Musculoskeletal Deformities

Deformities associated with osseous malformations of the cervical spine include torticollis, scoliosis, kyphosis, lordosis, and associated musculoskeletal deformities.

Many patients with congenital malformations of the cervical spine have symmetrical fusions or blocked vertebrae and so present with no obvious deformity of the neck. Indeed if the fusion exists at one or two levels only, these individuals may not even be aware of the existence of the congenital fusion and are surprised when it is revealed by x-rays taken for unrelated causes such as after a minor rear-end collision.

Other individuals, however, may have much more obvious deformity. Torticollis, defined as a "wry neck" with a lateral deviation of the head associated with rotational misalignment, is more likely to be associated with lesions of the upper cervical spine, particularly hemi-vertebrae of C1, and deformities of the subaxial cervical spine are more properly termed scoliosis.

Cervicothoracic scoliosis is most often associated with hemi-vertebrae at C7 or T1. Winter (92–94) noted that patients with this malformation can develop progression of the deformity and require fusion. Most mid-cervical curves do not progress and usually do not require treatment. Progression of cervicothoracic scoliosis results in head tilt and loss of level eye position if compensatory curves above and below the cervicothoracic curve do not develop. Worsening deformity with flexible curves can probably be treated with bracing but in a younger patient, this might mean many years of using a cervicothoracic orthosis or even a cervicothoracic lumbosacral orthosis if congenital or idiopathic curves are present in lower levels.

Under these circumstances a posterior fusion with autologous iliac bone should be done. The fusion should extend to the uppermost level of the cervicothoracic curve. Post-operatively the head should be held in the best alignment possible in an orthosis or plaster minerva jacket until the fusion is solid. A halo might be necessary in some patients in whom these devices cannot control position but in most instances one would prefer not to use a halo on young patients. The reasons for this are that (a) the thinness of the cranium increases the chance of penetration, and (b) traction across the rigid cervical spine deformity may cause cord injury. Fusion of the cervicothoracic spine is a fairly straightforward procedure usually requiring no internal fixation. The surgeon should evaluate the curve pre-operatively with CT to determine if a spina bifida exists in the area to be fused. Mistaking one side of an incomplete spinous process or lamina for an intact posterior arch would lead the surgeon into the spinal canal, possibly causing unintended and otherwise avoidable cervical cord injury.

Cervical lordosis is part of the deformity associated with iniencephaly and will be discussed in that context. Congenital cervical kyphotic deformity is rare (Fig. 2). Winter and Moe (94) reviewed 123 patients with congenital kyphosis and did not define this entity as such. They did note that upper thoracic kyphotic deformities tended to be more sharply angulated than those malformations

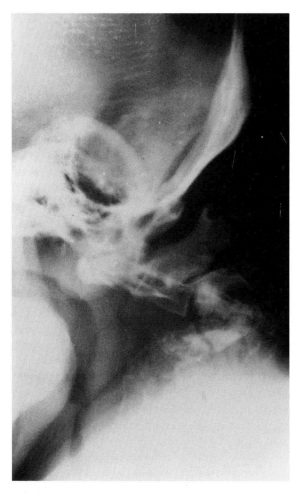

FIG. 2. Lateral roentgenogram of severe congenital kyphotic deformity of the cervical spine. The patient had multiple congenital fusions with posterior angulation at approximately C3. Clinically there was a very short neck with a low posterior hairline but no neurological deficits.

lower in the spinal column, presumably because they were of the Type 1 variety, which occurs because of localized failures of vertebral body formation. The same authors noted that high thoracic kyphotic deformities were more likely to be associated with paraplegia and cardio-respiratory deficiencies.

James (35) reviewed 5 patients with cervicothoracic kyphoscoliosis. Three of these were congenital and the other 2 were thought to be acquired. Three patients became paraplegic. James noted that "one limb of the kyphosis is the cervical spine" in these patients and described a number of other malformations such as anomalous ribs and hemi-vertebrae in these individuals. Treatment of this type of deformity is difficult. Non-operative therapy with a halo brace or a cervicothoracic orthosis has not been successful in the face of progressive deformity. Posterior fusion for kyphotic deformities under 50 degrees prevents progression of deformity in most patients but for those with more severe deformity a combined anterior and posterior exposure is deemed necessary. In upper thoracic kyphotic deformities, which also involved the lower cervical spine, the surgeon must use both a standard anterior approach and a high thoracic approach. The latter requires a third rib thoracotomy and the cervicothoracic spine is exposed by developing these two approaches from above and below. The anterior longitudinal ligament is divided, the disc spaces curetted, permitting correction of the deformity, and either anterior strut grafting or interbody grafting is utilized. The anterior procedure should probably be combined with the posterior fusion either at the same sitting or, if operative morbidity is considered to be too great, at a second procedure two weeks later.

The use of spinal instrumentation to achieve correction in such cases is open to question. New cervical spine fixation devices are currently under development for stabilization of the cervical vertebrae after trauma, rheumatoid arthritis, and loss of position due to tumors.

Congenital elevation of the scapula or Sprengel's deformity is one of the more common anomalies associated with Klippel-Feil syndrome (9,32). About one third of the patients with Sprengel's deformity have an associated omovertebral bone (Figs. 3 and 4). This is a band of bone tissue which extends from the spinous processes, laminae, or transverse processes of the mid-cervical vertebrae to the superior angle of the scapula. The Sprengel's lesion manifests itself in a variety of ways such as partial or complete synostosis joining the scapula to the cervical spine, or an incompletely developmental band of bone, cartilage, and fibrous tissue replacing the levator scapulae muscle. A costovertebral bone has also recently been described in which a bar of bone extended from the spinous process of C6 to the third rib (26). The costal vertebral bone appeared to be the cause of a cervicothoracic scoliosis noted in the patient who had the lesion. Congenital elevation of the scapula can be of varying

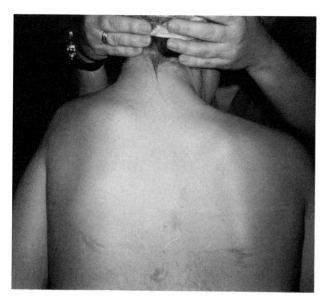

FIG. 3. Photograph of patient with Sprengel's deformity (congenital elevation of the scapula). There is also a low posterior hair line and short neck consistent with Klippel-Feil syndrome.

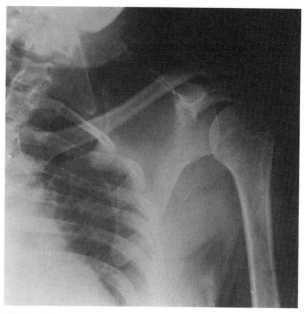

FIG. 4. AP roentgenogram of patient with Sprengel's deformity with omovertebral bone extending from the cervical spine to the scapula.

degrees of severity ranging from a barely perceptible deformity to extreme elevation of the shoulder in which the superior angle of the scapula is near the occiput. The Woodward operation is the most commonly used corrective procedure at this time for the Sprengel's lesion. The goal of the procedure is to lower the scapula by detaching the trapezius, rhomboid, and levator scapulae muscles from their origins on the vertebrae and transferring them distally. Prior to the muscle transfer it is necessary to osteotomize the distal clavicle and excise the omovertebral bone or prominent superior angle of the scapula.

Another common malformation associated with the Klippel-Feil syndrome is pterygium colli. The lesion consists of webbing of the skin on the lateral side of the neck, usually on each side (24). Z-plasties have been recommended as a means of lengthening the webs and it has been suggested that this be done between the ages of 1 and 6 years (43). The Z-plasty type of repair, however, does not provide for a natural hairline and leaves patients with noticeable scars on the side of the neck. The low posterior hairline in these patients is often also associated with thick hair growth laterally so that one limb of the Z-plasty must be hair bearing. The transposition of this limb anteriorly distorts the hairline still more and does not provide a pleasing cosmetic correction of the skin web. Better correction of pterygium colli is achieved by a posterior surgical approach in which redundant skin is mobilized through T-shaped or Y-shaped incisions. By rotating the flaps, the webs can be eliminated. Excess skin is excised and the flaps sutured together. The posterior approach is successful particularly in patients with Turner's syndrome where skin is loose and mobile. In other patients, however, the skin may be thicker, more

rigid, and less mobile and in these individuals correction of the pterygium might be more difficult to achieve (11,22,73).

Iniencephaly

Iniencephaly is a term used to describe an unusual disorder of the cervical spine consisting of congenital cervical synostoses, fixed retroflexion of the head, severe cervical lordosis, and varying degrees of incomplete posterior closure (47,75,76,80,91). Most individuals with this combination of deformities do not survive and several authors have noted that patients with this condition rarely live into adult life. Earlier reports classified iniencephaly into several stages depending on the presence or absence of meningocele or encephalocele and the severity of the deformity. Patients who do survive and who remain functional can be handicapped by the cervical lordosis and hyperextension of the head. This posture makes it impossible for such individuals to see straight ahead without flexing the low back and the hips. We found it possible to correct this type of deformity in one patient, by performing a posterior suboccipital release followed by gradual flexion of the head over a period of 6 weeks. The patient was placed in a high profile halo cast. The posterior turn buckles were positioned to pull upwards on the occiput and anterior turn buckles were placed so as to depress the frontal bone. Minimal daily correction was achieved and over the 6 week period a 70 degree extension contracture of the head was brought to a neutral straight ahead alignment. A posterior occipitocervical fusion permitted most of the correction to be maintained over a follow-up period of 5 years.

Iniencephaly, anencephaly, encephalocele, and cervical meningocele possibly differ from each other only in degree, and certainly there is a significant variation in the degree of deformity noted in iniencephaly. In those patients with iniencephaly who survive, deformity must be more mild and in some instances correctable as described. In more severely deformed individuals, the inion may be extremely deformed with hyperextension severe enough to cause the inion and gluteal muscles to merge. These grotesque malformations are too severe to permit survival and thus are rarely if ever seen by clinicians treating older patients. The severity of the deformities associated with iniencephaly has led to the development of techniques of prenatal diagnosis to permit subsequent termination of the pregnancy. It is postulated that iniencephaly is a neural tube defect and that determination of the alphafeto protein from the amniotic fluid should be carried out when the malformation might occur. It has a recurrency risk of about 5% in each successive pregnancy in women who have a prior history of children with similar lesions. The alphafeto protein level should be determined by amniocentesis in pregnancies with this background. Ultrasonography at 16 to 20 weeks should reveal absence of normal parietal bones, absence of brain tissue, retroflexion, and a myelomeningocele and thereby confirm the diagnosis of iniencephaly, anencephaly, encephalocele, or meningocele.

Neurological Disorders

The disruption of the normal embryologic development that produces bony deformities of the cervical spine can also cause neurological abnormalities and in the recent past a number of papers have documented many of these. Krishnaswany et al. (39), for example, described a case of schizophrenia associated with Klippel-Feil syndrome. Other authors (33,52,64) have noted cranial nerve palsies, Arnold-Chiari malformations, Horner's syndrome, syringomyelia, and various other central nervous system lesions. Holliday and Davis (34) described a patient with multiple meningiomas of the cervical cord associated with the Klippel-Feil syndrome. They postulated that the meningiomas were a forme fruste of neurofibromatosis. Meningomatosis, multiple meningiomas, and solitary meningiomas all originate from mesodermal tissues and they suggested that a focal mesodermal dysplasia limited to the cervical spine may have existed in their patient. The congruity of the extent of the meningiomas with the extent of the bony abnormality in their patient apparently led to this conclusion.

Mirror movement (synkenesia) has been recognized for a number of years as being a common finding in patients with Klippel-Feil syndrome (33). These patients are unable to dissociate movements of the two hands. In some patients, the association is obligatory and individuals so afflicted cannot perform activities requiring separate hand use such as knitting or playing the piano. Synkenesia is demonstrable electromyographically and the EMG may be useful in confirming the presence of synkenesia when the finding is subtle and difficult to detect on physical examination.

Synkenesia should suggest the presence of significant central nervous system abnormalities. Autopsy studies on patients with Klippel-Feil syndrome and synkenesia have shown malformations of the spinal cord consisting of fibrous diastematomyelia, duplication of the cord, flattening and cord dysplasia with dorsal malfusion and prominent lateral columns, separated by a deep anterior median fissure. More central lesions in these patients consisted of an abnormally thin or absent corpus callosum. The common and unifying aspect of these lesions is the existence of a central nervous system abnormality that would lead to an impairment of inter-hemispheric transmission and disruption of the crossover of the pyramidal tracts. There is, therefore, a failure of function of the motor inhibitory center and failure of suppression of bilateral motor cortical activity (4,30,90).

Less severe forms of central nervous system deformity, however, may exist without the patient manifesting synkenesia (2). Nagib et al. (53) described the case of the 31-year-old woman with transient neurologic findings whose myelogram and CT revealed neuroschisis of the upper and mid-cervical cord in which the neural tube failed to closed. Levine (42) also described the demonstration of cervical diastematomyelia with computerized tomography.

The Klippel-Feil syndrome also puts the cervical cord at risk on the basis of a mechanical abnormality. Congenital fusions over several spinal segments reduce the ability of the cervical spine to compensate for excessive forces in flexion, extension, rotation, and lateral bending, and stresses that might be tolerated by a normal neck are not safe for a cervical spine with limited mobility. Forces applied to the neck develop movements at each motion segment and if only one or two motion segments exist where there should be eight, the force may exceed the strength of the restraining ligaments. The resultant dislocation can produce injury to the cervical cord, especially if that structure is abnormal to begin with. In the reports of these patients that are available, it is of interest that frequently the trauma is minor or indirect and the x-rays show little other than the presence of congenital fusions. It appears, therefore, that the abnormal motion imposed on a single motion segment may cause a dislocation that often self-reduces but which can place significant stresses on the cervical spinal cord (17,74,82,89).

Congenital spinal stenosis is another feature of the Klippel-Feil syndrome which may increase the risk of even minor stress applied to the cervical spine. Epstein and Epstein (18) and Prusick and Samberg (62) both described patients with Klippel-Feil syndrome and congenital spinal stenosis. The patient described by Epstein and Epstein (18) had complained of upper limb paresthesias prior to injury but developed a transient quadriplegia after sustaining a hyperextension injury while body surfing. This patient had a congenital C2-C3 fusion with the stenosis but x-rays after the injury showed no evidence of a fracture or dislocation. The authors postulated that the excessive motion at C3 superimposed on the narrow spinal canal at C3-C4 compressed the cord to a degree sufficient to cause injury without causing a fracture or demonstrable dislocation. In the case described by Prusick and Samberg (62) congenital fusions at C2-C3 and C6-C7, with congenital occipitalization of the atlas, were associated with a narrow spinal canal with a mid-cervical AP diameter of less than 9 mm. These authors suggested that the inherent hypermobility at levels between fused segments could lead to spondylotic changes which would narrow the canal still further. The consequences of even minor injuries could be considerable loss of function of the spinal cord and indeed their patient required an open door laminoplasty for decompression.

Nagib et al. (53) reviewed a group of patients with Klippel-Feil syndrome in an effort to identify those who were at higher levels of risk for a neurologic injury. They suggested a new classification for patients at neurological risk as follows: group 1, patients with an unstable fusion pattern; group 2, patients with craniocervical anomalies; and group 3, patients with fusions associated with spinal stenosis (Fig. 5). They found that the stenotic segment or segments may occur above, below, or at the level of fusion.

Patients in group 1 were advised to avoid contact sports and to have spinal stabilizations if they developed neurological symptoms or progressive deformity. Patients in group 3 were advised to have decompression and stabilization if they became symptomatic. Upper cervical spine lesions (group 2) are described in Part A of this chapter.

The definition of stenosis requires some explanation. The average canal diameter is approximately 17 mm as measured in the mid-cervical spine from the posterior aspect of a vertebral body to the anterior aspect of the lamina at the same level. This measurement is taken from a lateral roentgenogram with a focus grid distance of 72 inches. If the AP canal diameter is less than 10 mm, there is probably sufficient narrowing of the canal present to permit compression of the spinal cord with extension of the neck. The canal diameter increases slightly with flexion but decreases in extension as the ligamentum flavum folds in onto the cervical cord. In addition, the cord moves up and down with neck motion, migrating 2 mm to 3 mm, thus angulating the nerve roots at

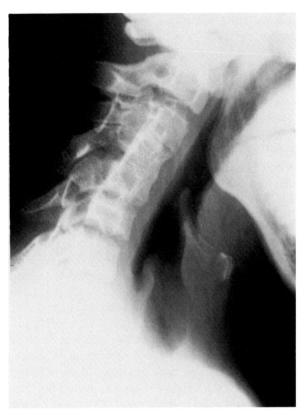

FIG. 5. Lateral roentgenogram showing congenital fusion of C3-C4-C5 with a motion segment at C5-C6. There is relative narrowing of the spinal canal of C5-C6. The combination of a motion segment with stenosis puts the patient at risk for cord injury.

their foraminae. Thus canal diameter becomes a determinant of neurologic compromise (16).

An additional factor in the production of symptoms due to cord involvement in cervical spinal stenosis is the ratio of the anterior posterior diameter to the transverse diameter of the cervical canal. Anteroposterior narrowing is usually associated with a relatively higher transverse diameter of the canal, and cervical cord involvement appears to be in good correlation with developmental narrowing of the canal as determined by the anteroposterior compression ratio. A more convenient ratio to measure, however, is the spinal canal to vertebral body ratio. This ratio is determined by measuring the anteroposterior diameter of the vertebral body and the cervical canal at the same level. The ratio of these measurements should be approximately one to one but when the canal is relatively narrower with a ratio of less than 0.8, the cervical cord is at risk and cervical spinal stenosis may be said to be present. The importance of the ratio lies in the fact that the numerical measurement of the spinal canal may be erroneous if the focus grid distance is not correct. The ratio eliminates this possible error and makes it unnecessary to rely on numerical determinations which may not be measurable accurately if a technical error is made in taking the roentgenogram (24,84).

Deafness, Ear Deformities, and Facial Malformations

The proximity of the cervical somites and branchial arches during embryologic development permits a localized teratogenic event to have an effect both on the cervical spine and the structures arising from the mesenchyme of the branchial arches. These structures include the outer ear, ossicles, semicircular canals, mandible, and part of the maxilla and hyoid bone. Since the extent of injury and the timing of injury may vary, several types of ear and facial malformations and syndromes can occur in common with various types of cervical spine malformations (47).

For example, cervical spine malformations are noted with frontonasal dysplasia, maxillonasal dysplasia, and duplication of mandibular rami (23,40,60). These rare anomalies, however, are less common than the syndromic malformations described below. A review of these syndromic facial malformations (such as Apert's, Crouzon's, Treacher-Collins, and Goldenhar's syndromes, Fig. 6) revealed that patients with Apert's and Crouzon's tended to have craniocervical abnormalities or "blocked cervical vertebrae" without significant neck deformity. Patients with Treacher-Collins syndrome did not manifest neck deformities in this series. Patients with Goldenhar's syndrome had cervicothoracic scoliosis associated with a hemi-facial microsomia with severe ear deformities frequently being noted. Apert's, Crouzon's, and Treacher-Collins syndromes are inherited as autosomal recessive, autosomal dominant, and autosomal recessive traits respectively. Goldenhar's syndrome, however, is multifactorial and its occurrence may in part depend on localized injury to developing embryonic structures. The unilateral hypoplasia or absence of the ear in Goldenhar's syndrome is associated with mandibular hypoplasia, macrostomia, and an ocular dermoid, and fused vertebrae or hemi-vertebra usually in the lower cervical and upper thoracic levels (77).

Hearing impairment in these patients is predictable. Even in the absence of obvious malformations of the face and ear, hearing loss is common in patients with Klippel-Feil syndrome, occurring in up to 30% of Klippel-Feil syndrome patients (46). The deafness is more often on the basis of sensorineural impairment and is less often a conductive or mixed hearing loss. Occasionally, however, malformations of the ossicles in the middle ear will cause these structures to be fixed to the oval window resulting in a conductive hearing impairment which may require surgical correction. Mobilization of the stapes may be hazardous, however, because deformities of the oval window and semicircular canals may co-exist with a fistula connecting the reservoirs of cerebral spinal fluid and perilymph contained in the labyrinth. Removing the stapes from the oval window may result in a "stapes gusher" in which the perilymph gushes uncontrollably from the window. Repair and closure of the gusher may be difficult and may result in worsening of the hearing deficit. In addition, the resultant stapedial foot plate fistula exposes the perilymph and CSF to colonization by microorganisms, possibly resulting in recurrent meningitis (13,59,66).

Wildervrank's syndrome, or cervico-oculo acousticus syndrome, has recently received a considerable amount of attention in the literature. Patients with this combination of malformations have congenital cervical fusions, abducens paralysis with retraction of the eyeballs, and a congenital deafness which may be sensorineural or conductive. Patients with this syndrome have been reported to manifest lens subluxations, facial paralysis, pseudopapilledema, and occipitomeningocele (11,71,74).

Thoracic Outlet Syndrome

Thoracic outlet syndrome comprises cervical rib syndrome, scalenus anticus syndrome, hyperabduction syndrome, pectoralis minor syndrome, costoclavicular syndrome, and first thoracic rib syndrome.

The essential feature of this syndrome is compression or irritation of the brachial plexus or subclavian vessels at the region of the thoracic outlet proximal to the insertion of the pectoralis minor. Fifteen percent of patients with Klippel-Feil syndrome have accessory cervical ribs and most of these are females (64). In the general population, cervical ribs occur in 1% of individuals and they are usually (80%) bilateral. These ribs, most often present at C7, compress or irritate the brachial plexus and subclavian vessels (65) (Fig. 7).

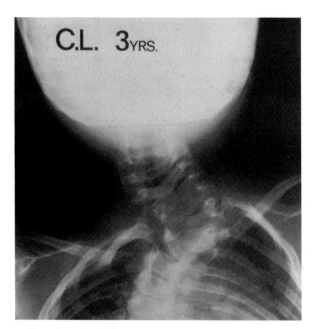

FIG. 6. AP roentgenogram showing the cervicothoracic scoliosis with multiple congenital malformations of the lower cervical spine as seen in Goldenhar's syndrome.

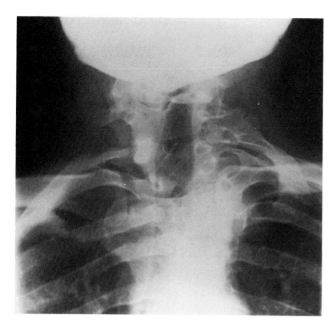

FIG. 7. AP roentgenogram showing multiple congenital malformations of the cervical spine with cervical ribs.

Symptoms of the thoracic outlet syndrome may be neurologic or vascular. Pain, radiating in either the ulnar and median nerves distribution or up into the shoulder and neck, is the most common symptom (83). While the pain is continuous, it may be exaggerated by turning the head toward the side affected, or by forcefully pulling the shoulder downward. Hyperesthesia, paresthesia, and anesthesia may present after strenuous upper extremity exertion. Late presentation of brachial plexus compression

is muscular atrophy. On electromyographic testing, the median nerve motor branch has less than 50% conduction amplitude as compared to the normal contralateral limb. The amplitude of conduction in the ulnar nerve sensory branch may also be reduced by 50%. If both of these amplitudes of conduction are reduced, the site of plexus compression distal to C8 is excluded because nerve fibers common to both nerves are contiguous only in the medial cord of the brachial plexus (64).

Vascular symptoms may result from compression of the subclavian artery, organic changes in the subclavian artery, or sympathetic nervous system disturbances. These include:

1. inability to exercise with the upper extremity
2. inability to lift heavy objects
3. presence of edema and cyanosis
4. gangrene of the digits.

Diminution of the radial pulse caused by the head turning toward the affected side while the arm is abducted (Adson's test), by retraction of the arm backward and downward (costoclavicular compressive maneuver), or by hyperabduction of the arm are subjective tests for positional subclavian arterial compression (95). Objectively, arteriography with the arm at the side and in abduction may reveal a region of compression. Plethysmographic changes in digital flow with the arm abducted may non-invasively demonstrate arterial compression (68) (Fig. 8).

Haggart and Nelson reported that conservative treatment consisting of anti-inflammatory medication and exercises to strengthen the shoulder girdle muscles re-

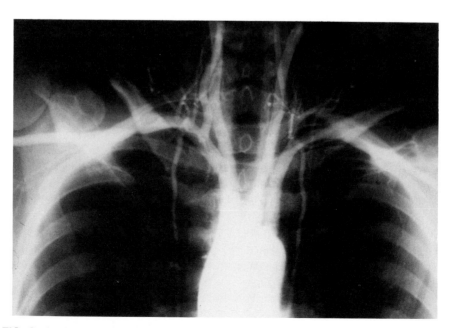

FIG. 8. Aortogram showing a cervical rib on the right with stenosis of the subclavian artery as it passes over the cervical rib. There is post-stenotic dilation serving as a source of emboli to the fingers in this patient.

lieved symptoms in 70% of patients with thoracic outlet syndrome (31). Changing sleeping habits to prevent hyperabduction of the arm and repeated injections with lidocaine in the scalenus anterior region may also relieve symptoms. Scalenotomy and cervical rib resection relieved symptoms in 60% of patients while scalenotomy alone has been successful in 30% of patients (79). The surgical approach most commonly used for a cervical rib resection or a scalenotomy is a transaxillary approach. Takagi and Yamage (83) studied 43 patients who had incapacitating pain after 3 to 6 months of conservative therapy. Resection of the cervical rib and partial scalenotomy, through a transaxillary approach, resulted in a 55% excellent, a 25% good, and a 20% poor result in pain relief.

Urologic, Cardiac, and Gastrointestinal Disorders

Genitourinary anomalies have been associated with Klippel-Feil syndrome and, in fact, the original patient described by Drs. Klippel and Feil died of uremia (33). Gray et al. (27) reported 8 urogenital anomalies in 418 patients with Klippel-Feil syndrome, Hensinger et al. (33) reported the association to be 35%, and Moore et al. (48) reported it to be 64%.

The most common anomaly is unilateral renal agenesis occurring more frequently in Klippel-Feil syndrome patients than in the normal population. The second most common renal anomaly is malrotation of a normal functioning kidney. Renal pelvic and ureteral duplication occurs more often in Klippel-Feil syndrome patients than in the general population. This occurs as a result of ureteral bud splitting and usually results in normal renal function. Renal ectopia is also a reported anomaly which does not alter renal function. The kidney is usually unilaterally involved and most often located in the pelvis with no preponderance toward right or left side. Renal dysgenesis with subnormal renal function is a rare anomaly occurring 40 times more than in the general population (48). These patients are at risk of developing uremia. Thus serial renal function monitoring is necessary. It is because of these associated anomalies that an ultrasonic study of the renal system is essential in complete evaluation of patients with Klippel-Feil syndrome (33). If anomalies are discovered, an intravenous pyelogram is indicated for complete functional analysis. If renal malformations are present, an ultrasonic study of the ovaries, fallopian tubes, and uterus is also indicated. Hypospadias, cryptorchidism, and vaginal agenesis are reported with greater frequency than in the general population (1). Conversely, whenever these anomalies are discovered, presence of co-existing renal anomalies must also be ruled out.

A distinctive association of Mullerian duct aplasia, renal agenesis or aplasia, and cervical and thoracic spine dysplasia is described as the MURCS association (28). It is theorized that the association occurs because there is an intimate spatial relationship at four weeks of embryologic development (blastoma phase) between the lower cervical and upper thoracic spine somites and pronephric duct (which in turn induce Mullerian duct development). A teratogen would alter all three of these structures and their subsequent development. Duncan (15) reported that in MURCS association patients, 80% have involvement of two to four vertebrae, 88% have renal agenesis or ectopia, and 96% have uterine hypoplasia or aplasia. Additionally, most cases of MURCS association appear sporadically, although there are reports of families with multiple siblings afflicted.

The VATER association (6), consisting of vertebral defects and atresia, tracheoesophageal fistula, and radial limb diplegia, has also been recognized as a combination of anomalies occurring in a non-random manner. The MURCS association and VATER association seem to overlap, however, and each contains elements seen in the other. The importance of lumping a group of anomalies into an "association" therefore seems to lie in the recognition that none of the malformations cited are likely to occur as an isolated event and that recognition of one should lead a physician to search for all the others.

Patients with Klippel-Feil syndrome have a higher risk of associated congenital heart disease (4.2%) than the general population (21). Even though cervical deformities are present equally in both sexes, congenital heart disease is more prevalent in females with Klippel-Feil syndrome (49). No single lesion is characteristic, but a ventricular septal defect is most often reported (8 of 20). These patients may additionally have associated pulmonary hypertension, patent ductus arteriosus, anomalous pulmonary veins, and atrial septal defects. Dextrocardia was reported to be the next most frequently occurring anomaly. This may occur in association with situs inversus, pulmonary stenosis, aortic stenosis, double outlet right ventricle, and ostium primum defect. The symptoms resulting from cardiac anomalies are (in order of decreasing frequency) cyanosis, dyspnea, short stature, and fingernail clubbing (49,57). Digoxin can control cardiac failure.

Anesthetic considerations during surgery of these patients are not isolated to cervical spine instability although patients are at high risk for spinal cord injury during laryngoscopy, intubation, and positioning (55). Sudden rotatory movements have been reported to precipitate syncopal attacks. A large occipital encephalocele makes it impossible to align the head and body in supine position thus making intubation possible only in the semilateral position. Anticipation of a difficult intubation should preclude the use of muscle relaxants during anesthesia induction as this prevents adequate visualization of the vocal cords. Awake intubation may precipitate a hypertensive or tachycardic episode which can be avoided by intravenous lidocaine administration prior to intubation. Maintenance anesthesia using halothane should be avoided because of direct myocardial depression and hypotension. A persistent ductus provides a site for infective endocarditis development and thus prophylactic antibiotics are indicated prior to any surgical procedure.

Although reported gastrointestinal defects include duplication, congenital megacolon, neurenteric cysts, and accessory lobes of the liver, their exact pathogenesis has not been discovered (7,19). There is evidence that in the presomite embryo, adhesions forming between the ectodermal and endodermal germ layer may split or deviate the developing notochord. Veenklaas theorized that incomplete separation of the notochord from the endoderm allows a diverticulum of endodermal tissue to be withdrawn from the primitive foregut forming a cyst (88). Attachment of the cyst to the developing notochord could prevent complete fusion of vertebral bodies. The resulting anomalies include anterior or posterior spina bifida and alimentary system duplication cysts in the posterior mediastinum or between the layers of mesentery, or in both. Because there is an intimate spatial arrangement between the rod of notochordal cells, the somites that later form the vertebral bodies, and the ectodermal and endodermal adhesions, there may be a failure of segmentation of the vertebrae adjacent to the adhesions. This is the proposed "split notochord" theory proposed by Feller and Sternberg (20). This may explain the association of fused vertebrae, as in Klippel-Feil syndrome, and enteric cysts.

Severe dyspnea in infancy may be secondary to an intra-thoracic enteric cyst. Generally percutaneous aspiration of these cysts may result in leakage of acidic gastric secretions into the thorax resulting in a chemical pneumonitis. Lowry and Moorman found that if aspiration is done emergently to relieve the dyspnea and cyanosis, the aspirate should be evaluated for gastric fluid to demonstrate the presence of active gastric epithelium lining the cyst wall (44). Leahy and Butsch advocated early surgical resection of these cysts (41) because occasionally these cysts have eroded into the lung from the mediastinum producing massive and often fatal hemoptysis. Enteric cysts may be mediastinal, abdominal, or both. Abdominal enteric cysts which erode into the bowel may produce melena, therefore chest and spinal radiologic examination are indicated in a patient with tarry stools. Additional thoracic anomalies such as extra lobes of lung or failure of lobe differentiation, although asymptomatic, have been reported (19).

It is obvious that the presence of a congenital fusion of a lower cervical vertebra should alert the physician to a myriad of associated abnormalities. Many will probably be diagnosed and treated in childhood, but surgeons treating adults with congenital cervical fusion should be aware of other possible congenital anomalies.

REFERENCES

1. Ashley DJB, Mostley FK (1960): Renal agenesis and dysgenesis. *J Urol* 83:211–230.
2. Anand HK (1985): Cervical diastomatomyelia: Uncommon presentation of a rare congenital disorder. *Comp Radiology* 9:45–49.
3. Avery LW (1936): The Klippel-Feil syndrome: A pathological report. *Archives Neurol Psychiatry* 36:1068–1076.
4. Baird PA (1967): Klippel-Feil syndrome: A study of mirror movement detected by electromyography. *Am J Disease Child* 113:546–551.
5. Bavrinck ON, Weaver DD (1983): Subclavian artery supply distribution sequence: Hypothesis of a vascular etiology for Poland, Klippel-Feil syndrome, and Mullerian anomalies. *Am J Med Genetics* 23:903–918.
6. Beals RK, Rolfe B (1989): VATER Association. *J Bone Joint Surg* [Am] 71:948–950.
7. Beardnoire HE, Wiglesworth FW (1958): Vertebral abnormalities and alimentary duplication. *Ped Clin N Am* 5:457.
8. Brill CB (1987): Isolation of right subclavian artery with subclavian steal in a child with Klippel-Feil anomaly: An example of subclavian artery supply distribution sequence. *Am J Med Genetics* 26:933–940.
9. Causon S (1987): Failure of articular process joint development as a cause of vertebral fusion (block vertebrae). *J Anatomy* 153:55–62.
10. Cox HE (1984): Computed tomography of absent cervical pedicle. *J Comput Assist Tomography* 8:537–539.
11. Cremers CW (1984): Hearing loss in the cervico-oculo-acoustic syndrome. *Archives Otolaryngol* 110:54–57.
12. Cronin TD (1977): Deformities of the cervical region. In: *Reconstructive plastic surgery,* JM Carverse, ed. Philadelphia: Saunders, pp. 1659–1664.
13. Danilidis J, Maganoris T (1978): Stapes gusher and Klippel-Feil syndrome. *Laryngoscope* 88:1178–1183.
14. Dolan KD (1977): Developmental anomalies of C-spine below the axis. *Radiol Clin N Am* 15:167.
15. Duncan PA (1977): Embryologic pathogenesis of renal agenesis associated with cervical vertebral anomalies (Klippel-Feil phenotype). *Embryology and pathogenesis of prenatal diagnosis.* The National Foundation March of Dimes birth defects original article series, vol. 13, no. 3D. D Bergsma, RB Lowry, eds. New York: Alan R Liss, pp. 91–101.
16. Edwards WC, La Rocca H (1983): The developmental segmental sagittal diameter of the cervical spinal canal in patients with cervical spondylosis. *Spine* 8:20–27.
17. Elster AD (1984): Quadriplegia after minor trauma in the Klippel-Feil syndrome: A case report and review of the literature. *J Bone Joint Surg* [Am] 66:1473–1474.
18. Epstein NE, Epstein JA (1984): Traumatic myelopathy in a seventeen year old child with cervical spinal stenosis (without fracture or dislocation) and C2-C3 Klippel-Feil fusion. *Spine* 9:344–347.
19. Fallon M, Gordon ARG (1954): Mediastinal cysts of foregut origin associated with abnormalities. *Br J Surgery* 41:520.
20. Feller A, Sternberg H (1929): Zur Kenntnis der Fehibildungen der Wirbelsaule. Die Wirbelkorperspalte und ihre formale Genese. *Virchows Arch Path Anat* 272:613.
21. Forney WR, Robinson SJ, Pascoe DJ (1966): Congenital heart disease, deafness, and skeletal malformations: A new syndrome. *J Ped* 68:14–26.
22. Foucar HO (1948): Pterygium colli and allied conditions. *Can Med Assoc J* 59:251.
23. Fragoso R (1982): Frontonasal dysplasia in the Klippel-Feil syndrome: A new associated malformation. *Clin Genetics* 22:270–273.
24. Frawley JM (1925): Congenital webbing. *Am J Disease Child* 29:799–809.
25. Gilobach J (1983): Transoral operation for craniospinal malformations. *Neurosurg Review* 6:199–209.
26. Goodwin CB, Simmons EH, Taylor I (1984): Cervical vertebralcostal process—a prevously unreported anomaly. *J Bone Joint Surg* [Am] 66:1477–1479.
27. Gray SW, Romaine CB, Pascoe DJ (1965): Congenital fusion of the cervical vertebrae. *Surg Gyn Obst* 118:373–385.

28. Greene RA (1986): MURCS association with additional anomalies. *Human Pathol* 17:88–91.
29. Grimer RJ (1983): Thoracic outlet syndrome following correction of scoliosis in a patient with cervical ribs. A case report. *J Bone Joint Surg* [Am] 65:1172–1173.
30. Gunderson CH, Solitaire GB (1968): Mirror movements in patients with Klippel-Feil syndrome. *Arch Neurol* 18:675–679.
31. Haggart GE, Nelson (1948): Value of conservative management in cervicobrachial pain. *JAMA* 137:508.
32. Haurnau N (1986): Congenital elevation of the scapulae and Brown-Sequard syndrome. *Clin Neurol Neurosurg* 88:289–292.
33. Hensinger RN, Lang JR, MacEwen GD (1974): Klippel-Feil syndrome: A constellation of associated anomalies. *J Bone Joint Surg* [Am] 56:1242–1253.
34. Holliday PO, Davis C (1984): Multiple meningiomas of the cervical cord associated with Klippel-Feil syndrome. *Neurosurg* 14:353–357.
35. James JP (1955): Kyphoscoliosis. *J Bone Joint Surg* [Br] 77:414–426.
36. Kinipers F, Wieberdink J (1953): An interthoracic cyst of enterogenic origin in a young infant. *J Ped* 42:603.
37. Kosher RA (1976): Inhibition of "spontaneous" notochord induced and collagen induced in vitro somite corrogenesis by cyclic AMP derivatives and theophylline. *Developmental Biol* 53:265–276.
38. Krieger AJ, Rosomoff HL (1969): Occult respiratory dysfunction in craniovertebral anomalies. *J Neurosurg* 31:15.
39. Krishnaswany S et al (1985): A case of schizophrenia with the Klippel-Feil syndrome. *Med J Malaysia* 40:330–332.
40. Lawrence TM (1985): Congenital duplication of mandibular rami in Klippel-Feil syndrome. *J Oral Med* 40:120–122.
41. Leahy LJ, Butsch WL (1949): Surgical management of respiratory emergencies during the first few weeks of life. *Arch Surg* 59:466.
42. Levine RS (1985): C.T. demonstration of cervical diastoematomyelia. *J Comput Assist Tomography* 9:592–594.
43. Lindsay WK (1986): *Congenital defects of the skin, muscles, connective tissue, tendons, and hands.* Welsh KJ, Randolph JG, Ravitch MM, O'Neil JH, Rowe MI, eds. Chicago: Yearbook Medical, p. 1484.
44. Lowry T, Moorman LJ (1938): Accessory stomach in the right thorax. *Am Review TB* 38:27–31.
45. MacEwen GD, Winter RB (1972): Evaluation of kidney anomalies in congenital scoliosis. *J Bone Joint Surg* [Am] 54:1451.
46. Milner LS, Daridge-Pitts KJ (1983): Recurrent meningitis due to round window fistula in Klippel-Feil syndrome. A case report. *South African Med J* 64:413–414.
47. Morcy I (1986): Prenatal diagnosis and pathoanatomy of iniencephaly. *Clin Genetics* 30:81–86.
48. Moore WB, Mathews TJ, Rabinowitz R (1975): Genitourinary anomalies associated with Klippel-Feil syndrome. *J Bone Joint Surg* [Am] 57:355.
49. Morrison S (1968): Congenital brevicollis (Klippel-Feil syndrome) and cardiovascular anomalies. *Am J Disease Child* 115:614.
50. Myamato RT (1983): Klippel-Feil syndrome and associated ear deformities. *Am J Otol* 5:113–119.
51. Nagib MG (1984): Management of Klippel-Feil syndrome: Correction [letter]. *J Neurosurg* 61:1161.
52. Nagib MG, Maxwell RE, Chou SN (1985): Klippel-Feil syndrome in children: Clinical features and management. *Child Neurol System* 1:255–263.
53. Nagib MG, Larson DA, Maxwell RE (1987): Neuroscoliosis of the cervical spinal cord in a patient with Klippel-Feil syndrome. *Neurosurg* 20:629–631.
54. Nagib MG, Maxwell RE, Chou SN (1984): Identification and management of high-risk patients with Klippel-Feil syndrome. *J Neurosurg* 61:525–530.
55. Naguib M, Faray H (1986): Anesthetic considerations in Klippel-Feil syndrome. *Can Anesthesia Society J* 33:66–70.
56. Negenbogen L (1985): Cervico-oculo-acoustic syndrome. *Ophthalmic Paed Genet* 6:183–187.
57. Nora JJ (1961): Klippel-Feil syndrome with congenital heart disease. *Am J Disease Child* 102:110.
58. Ogino H, Tada K (1983): Canal diameter, anteroposterior compression ratio, spondylotic myelopathy of the cervical spine. *Spine* 8:1–15.
59. Olitani I (1985): Oral anomalies in the Klippel-Feil syndrome. *Am J Otol* 6:468–471.
60. Olow-Nardenram MA (1984): Maxillo-nasal dysplasia (Binder syndrome) and associated malformations of the cervical spine. *Acta Radiol* 25:353–360.
61. Payne EE (1957): The cervical spine: An anatomico-pathological study of 70 specimens using a special technique with particular reference to the problem of cervical spondylosis. *Brain* 80:571–596.
62. Prusick VR, Samberg LC (1985): Klippel-Feil syndrome associated with spinal stenosis. A case report. *J Bone Joint Surg* [Am] 67:161–164.
63. Ramsay J, Bliznak J (1971): Klippel-Feil syndrome with renal agenesis and other anomalies. *Am J Roentgenol* 113:460.
64. Resnick D (1988): Additional congenital or heritable anomalies and syndrome. In: *Diagnosis of bone and joint disorders.* Resnick D, Niwayama, eds. Philadelphia: Saunders, ch. 89.
65. Roos D (1976): Congenital anomalies associated with thoracic outlet syndrome: Anatomy, symptoms. *Am J Surg* 132:771.
66. Sakai M, Shinkawa A (1983): Klippel-Feil syndrome with conductive deafness and histologic findings of removed stapes. *Annals Otol Rhinol Laryngol* 92:202–206.
67. Sakou T (1983): Congenital absence of pedicle in the cervical spine. A case report. *Clin Orthop* (175):51–55.
68. Sanders RJ, Monsour JW, Gerber WF (1979): Scalenectomy versus first rib resection for treatment of the thoracic outlet syndrome. *Surgery* 85:109.
69. Sandliam A (1986): Cervical vertebral anomalies in cleft lip and palate. *Cleft Lip and Palate J* 23:206–214.
70. Schapera J (1987): Autosomal dominant inheritance of cervical ribs. *J Clin Genetics* 31:386–388.
71. Schild JA (1984): Wildervanck syndrome—the external appearance and radiologic findings. *Int J Ped Otorhinolaryngol* 7:305–310.
72. Sensenia EC (1949): The early development of the vertebral column. *Contributions to Embryology* 33:21–51.
73. Shearin JC, DeFranyo AJ (1980): Butterfly correction of webbed-neck deformity in Turners syndrome. *Plastic Reconstr Surg* 66:129–133.
74. Sherk HH, Nicholson JT (1977): Cervico-oculo-acoustices syndrome: Case report of death caused by injury to abnormal cervical spine. *J Bone Joint Surg* [Am] 54:1776–1778.
75. Sherk HH, Schut L (1976): Correction of neck deformities in iniencephaly. *Jefferson Orthop J* 5:51–55.
76. Sherk HH, Schut L, Chung S (1974): Iniencephalic deformity of the cervical spine. *J Bone Joint Surg* [Am] 56:1254.
77. Sherk HH, Whittaker LT, Pasquariello PD, Cohen ML (1980): Facial malformations and spinal anomalies. A predictable relationship. Proceedings of the cervical spine research society. Orthopaedic Transactions. *J Bone Joint Surg* 4:47.
78. Sholam Z, Cospi B (1988): Iniencephaly: Prenatal ultrasonographic diagnosis—a case report. *J Prenatal Med* 16:139–143.
79. Silver D (1975): The thoracic outlet syndrome. In: *Practice of surgery.* Lewis, ed. New York: Harper and Row.
80. Stephens TD (1980): *Atlas of human embryology.* New York: Macmillan.
81. Strax TE, Baran E (1975): Traumatic quadriplegia associated with Klippel-Feil syndrome: Discussion and case report. *Arch Physical Med Rehab* 56:363–365.
82. Strisciuglio P, Raia V (1982): Wildervancks syndrome with bilateral subluxation of lens and facial paralysis. *J Med Genet* 20:72–73.
83. Takagi K, Yamage M (1987): Management of thoracic outlet syndrome. *Arch Orthop Trauma Surg* 106:78.
84. Thurston SE (1984): The association of spinal and gastroesophageal anomalies. A case report and review. *Clin Ped* 23:652–654.
85. Torg JS, Pavlor H (1986): Neuropraxia of the cervical spinal cord with transient quadriplegia. *J Bone Joint Surg* [Am] 68:1354–1370.
86. Treadwell SJ, Smith DF (1982): Cervical spine anomalies in fetal alcohol syndrome. *Spine* 7:331–334.

87. VanDyk, Aryn R (1987): The absent cervical pedicle syndrome. *Neuroradiol* 29:69–72.

88. Veenklaas GMH (1952): Pathogenesis of intrathoracic gastrogenic cysts. *Am J Disease Child* 83:500.

89. Weisy GM (1983): Trauma to the anomalous cervical spine. *Spine* 8:225–227.

90. Whittle IR, Besser M (1983): Congenital neural abnormalities presenting with mirror movements in a patient with Klippel-Feil syndrome. *J Neurosurg* 59:891–894.

91. Wilson WG (1985): Palctol anteversion as part of the iniencephaly malformation sequence. *J Craniofacial Genetic Devel Biol* 5:5–10.

92. Winter RB (1983): *Congenital deformities of the spine.* New York: Thieme, pp. 302–304.

93. Winter RB, Moe JH (1984): The incidence of Klippel-Feil syndrome in patients with congenital scoliosis and kyphosis. *Spine* 9:363–366.

94. Winter RB, Moe JH (1973): Congenital kyphosis. *J Bone Joint Surg* [Am] 55:223–256.

95. Wright IS (1945): The neurovascular syndrome produced by hyperabduction of the arms: The immediate changes produced in 150 normal controls, and the effects on some persons of prolonged hyperabduction of the arms, as in sleeping, and in certain occupations. *Am Heart J* 29:1.

The Adult Spine: Principles and Practice,
J. W. Frymoyer, Editor-in-Chief.
Raven Press, Ltd., New York © 1991.

CHAPTER 49

Diagnosis and Treatment of Congenital Neurologic Abnormalities Affecting the Cervical Spine

Francis W. Gamache, Jr.

There are congenital neurologic abnormalities that may affect the structure or function of the cervical spine, and the one that concerns the clinician most often is Arnold-Chiari malformation and syringomyelia. The higher bony deformities are all discussed in other chapters. In those diseases, there are abnormalities found on neurologic examination and radiographic characteristics. This chapter is intended to provide a practical update of the more common disorders of the nervous system.

DIAGNOSIS

Clinical (Neurologic) Exam

Unfortunately, there are no neurological findings on examination that are pathognomonic for a congenital spinal cord disorder. The clinician must integrate the information from the patient's history and physical with the findings obtained from diagnostic testing. Table 1 provides a simplified summary of neurological findings that may be helpful in localizing the level of the problem affecting the cervical spine. The C1 and C2 nerve roots usually have no disc component ventral to them. All the remaining cervical roots are susceptible to encroach-

ment by disc herniation or degenerative changes. Disc herniations most frequently occur at C7, followed by C6, followed by C8, in that order (54). Multi-level disc herniation is distinctly uncommon in the neck and compression of roots by degenerative (spondylotic) disease is two to three times as frequent as disc compression (54). While the clinician is faced frequently with the common problems of disc herniation and degenerative disease of the neck, these facts must be kept in mind when patients present in a fashion involving multiple levels or in a manner where spondylosis is an unlikely explanation for the patient's problem. Pain in the area of the back of the head has been attributed to the greater occipital nerve and referred to as "occipital neuralgia." Operations directed at relieving this condition with occipital neurectomy generally have not been successful. On the other hand, unilateral painful arthrosis of the atlantal axial joint may present with ipsilateral suboccipital pain and point tenderness over the area of the abnormality, with limited motion of the neck. This condition is frequently relieved by a small amount of local anesthesia applied to the posterior aspect of the atlantal-axial joint.

Cervical roots 5, 6, 7, and 8 as well as the first thoracic root supply the arm and hand via the anterior primary divisions of the spinal nerves and brachial plexus. The paraspinal muscles are innervated by the posterior divisions of these spinal nerves. Irritation of any of these

F. W. Gamache, Jr., M.D.: The New York Hospital-Cornell Medical Center, New York, New York 10021.

TABLE 1. *Summary of neurologic findings*

Root	Area of sensation affected	Major muscle affected	Comments
C1	Usually no sensory component	Nuchal	Not susceptible to disc encroachment
C2	Face bordering trigeminal skin zone to "high collar" area	Nuchal/strap	
C3-C4	Side of neck to corner of shoulder, clavicle-shoulder	Diaphragm/nuchal strap, rhomboids	Single root lesion, generally causes no significant motor loss
C5	Biceps, radial arm	Supraspinatus, infraspinatus, deltoid, biceps	Decrease of biceps reflex, pain may mimic angina
C6	Thumb, index finger	Extensor carpi rad brachioradialis	Decrease of biceps/brachioradialis reflexes
C7	Index, middle finger	Triceps, latissimus dorsi, pectoralis maj, ext. carpi ulnaris, ext. digitorum	Decrease in triceps reflex
C8	Fourth, fifth fingers	Wrist/finger flexors, intrinsic hand muscles	

lower cervical roots produces pain in the base of the neck, scapular region, and shoulder (19). Thus, the precise level of involvement usually may not be determined simply by noting the distribution of pain, muscle tenderness, or neck position. Of note, lesions involving the T1 root may produce weakness of intrinsic hand muscles as well as ptosis, miosis, or anhydrosis.

Neurophysiologic Testing

EMG/nerve conduction velocity (EMG/NCV) testing may help confirm findings on a neurologic examination. Abnormalities in these tests frequently require days (NCV) or weeks (EMG) of neurologic dysfunction before the test patterns become frankly abnormal. Many weeks must pass once an offending lesion is removed before the EMG pattern may return to normal. Similarly, in senior citizens who routinely harbor degenerative changes in the neck, mild baseline abnormalities in EMG/NCV should be anticipated. Particularly in these patients or patients with an old injury, another pathological process beginning in the cervical spine will make interpretation of EMG/NCV findings difficult. The EMG/NCV changes frequently are not pathognomonic.

Routine somatosensory evoked potentials may not be able to localize a neurological problem to the cervical spinal cord. At times it is difficult electrophysiologically to pinpoint the level of dysfunction between the brachial plexus, cervical spinal cord, or medulla. Emerson and Pedley have suggested the use of additional recording electrodes and recording points to delineate cervical cord pathology (20). A normal somatosensory evoked potential response does not rule out anterior spinal cord pathology.

Radiographic Evaluation

Plain films of the spine are still quite useful in providing information regarding basic anatomical abnormalities involving the cervical spine such as spina bifida, mal-formed vertebrae, fused vertebrae (a single unit or in blocks), and the presence or absence of malalignment. AP, lateral, and oblique films provide basic information about structure but not about motion of the spine (17). As a result, voluntary gentle flexion-extension views are frequently useful, particularly where congenital abnormalities such as Klippel-Feil syndrome, Down's syndrome, or neurofibromatosis may cause abnormal motion segments in the cervical spine.

Computed tomography (CT) of the cervical spine with or without myelography has been the radiographic cornerstone for the diagnosis and evaluation of bony malformations, meningoceles, or parenchymal spinal cord pathology. In the case of cavitary lesions of the cervical spine, myelography with post CT frequently is necessary (60).

Magnetic resonance (MR) scanning is especially useful in the diagnosis of abnormalities of the nervous system at the skull base and cervical spine. This diagnostic modality, however, is frequently not available on an emergency basis and is still not available to all clinicians on demand. Where available, MR scanning has replaced myelography and CT in many instances. With CSF appearing bright on T2-weighted images, T2 views are especially useful for documenting spinal cord compression. T1-weighted images provide better morphologic detail about the cord helping to provide useful patho-anatomic information such as cyst formation. Many radiologists believe good quality MRI scans in combination with plain films make CT and/or myelography unnecessary. The exception to this rule, however, would be the evaluation of syringomyelia or neurofibromatosis with an associated curvature (i.e., scoliosis), where MR images are deformed. In this situation, myelography with post-myelography CT through individual segments of the cervical scoliosis provides useful information. Where issues of instability are concerned, MR images taken in rapid sequence with the patient flexing or extending the neck ("dynamic MRI") are being utilized and provide extremely useful information.

Surgical Exploration

A clear cut diagnosis of a problem may not always rest with simply ascertaining the presence of an abnormality on the above mentioned radiographic studies. Occasionally, tumor is suggested in the spinal canal from a vague abnormality found with one of the above-mentioned imaging techniques. In these instances, surgical exploration may become necessary to confirm or refute the diagnosis. In some cases, tumor may have been suspected but not found at surgical exploration; the cause of which can only be speculative. On the other hand, over-interpretation of an MRI finding may lead to unnecessary surgical exploration (i.e., negative exploration for a lesion which did not exist). One is thus cautioned about proceeding with surgical procedures based on minimal radiographic documentation of such lesions. While MR exams are extremely useful, the meaning of many findings remains to be elucidated. It is frequently useful to have other confirmatory imaging information and compelling clinical reasons before proceeding with a surgical "exploration." However, in certain and undoubtedly rare circumstances, the ultimate diagnostic test may have to rest in such an exploratory approach.

DISEASES

Syringomyelia

Syringomyelia is a condition defined by the presence of a fluid-filled cavity within the substance of the spinal cord. The condition may develop subsequent to traumatic injury to the spinal cord, may be related to the presence of tumor in the spinal cord, or may follow arachnoiditis. Most commonly the condition is associated with congenital malformations such as meningomyelocele, Chiari malformation, or may develop idiopathically. In Chapter 48 the four types of Arnold Chiari malformation are presented. A large percentage of *non-traumatic* syrinxes appear to communicate with the fourth ventricle, especially those associated with the various Chiari malformations. But, in the case of posttraumatic syrinx, the cavity within the spinal cord usually does not communicate with the fourth ventricle. Because of the variety of anatomical locations in which syrinxes begin within the spinal cord, as well as the variation with time and anatomical direction in which they grow, patients may present with a variety of complaints or neurologic symptoms. Classical teaching has been that because of the central location of the cavitation within the spinal cord, commonly in the cervical area, the lesion interrupts ascending pain and temperature pathways from each side of the body. A resultant loss of pain and temperature sensibility in a segmental distribution in the upper extremities thus follows. Proprioception and simple touch are usually spared. As the disease progresses and extends to the anterior gray horns of the spinal cord, weakness and atrophy of muscles innervated by the involved anterior horns will be demonstrated. A pattern of muscle wasting in the upper extremities, with cape-like sensory loss in the upper extremities as well, thus has been considered diagnostic of syringomyelia.

Presently, with the widespread use of MR scanning of the head and neck, the classical findings are no longer being reported by clinicians because the diagnosis is made earlier. Motor and sensory symptoms remain frequent (5,71) but pain is a common complaint early in the disease in many patients (5,35,36,44). The mean age of presentation is approximately 32 with patients complaining of diffuse pain rather than a radicular pain.

On neurologic examination, the combination of pain and sensory dysfunction in a syringomyelic pattern has been found in approximately 50% to 80% of patients (6,9,12,36,44,48,65,70). An associated scoliosis is often present early in the disease but is frequently centered in the upper thoracic spine (12,35). It is not unusual for sensory and motor findings to develop subsequent to the observation of the scoliosis.

Previously, radiologic evaluation has involved myelography with delayed CT scanning performed approximately 12 to 24 hours after myelography (2,60). Since the advent of the MR scanner, MRI of the spine has generally become the neurodiagnostic imaging study of choice. Plain film examination of the cervical spine should always be obtained. In those individuals with scoliotic curves, where an MR image may be deformed, myelography with delayed CT remains the standard for neuroradiographic evaluation.

Multiple surgical procedures have been advocated for the treatment of syringomyelia. Included among these procedures is posterior fossa decompression by suboccipital craniectomy with some form of duraplasty. The decision to perform additional procedures in the posterior fossa such as tonsillectomy, fourth ventricular shunting, or other diversionary procedures remains controversial (6,12,23,29,45,61). Laminectomy and myelotomy remain other primary procedures employed for the treatment of syringomyelia. Percutaneous aspiration of the syrinx has been found to provide temporary relief in nearly 40% of cases, although the explanation for this remains unclear (61).

Various shunting procedures of the syrinx itself, (syringo-subarachnoid (SS) shunt, syringo-pleural shunt, syringo-peritoneal (SP) shunt) have also gained recent favor (42,43,59,68). Indirect shunting of the syrinx by means of ventricular shunting (VS) was introduced in 1969 by Krayenbuhl (9). This has not gained widespread favor, however, and the follow-up reported in 1974 was generally very brief (40).

In patients with hind brain malformation, primary shunting of the syrinx has been considered by some to be contraindicated because of the possibility of precipitating additional hind brain herniation. Wisoff and Epstein, however, have not found this to be a problem when utilizing syringo-pleural shunts as their primary procedure in dysraphic children presenting with hydromyelia (71). Tator has had the same experience and recently has commented that "drainage of the syrinx should be the primary surgical procedure" (68).

The natural history of untreated syringomyelia remains unclear (6,10,44). This is probably due to the generally short period of follow-up for those patients with this diagnosis. One series with excellent long-term follow-up is that of Boman and Iivanainen; they reported on 55 patients, some of whom were followed for 40 years (11). Just under half of those patients were stable with regard to their disease for periods of up to 10 years. On the other hand, more than half of the patients had gradual progression of symptoms over a period of 2 to 45 years. Of the 55 patients, 43 had changes in the anatomy of their spine, such as scoliosis (11). Thus, length of follow-up contributes in a major way to the clinical definition of the neurologic implications of syringomyelia (1). Brief follow-up may falsely suggest arrest of syringomyelia (5).

Probably because of the variation in follow-up, one may find various surgical series treating hydromyelia with Chiari malformations with rates of improvement or stabilization ranging from 10% to 90% (6,23,29,44,45, 48,61,65,68).

Curiously, patients may remain remarkably neurologically intact despite considerable distortion of spinal cord observed on computed tomography or MRI scanning. Perhaps earlier diagnosis and treatment may lead to more satisfactory results. Nevertheless, in view of the variation of the natural history, anatomy, treatment, and follow-up periods reported to date, very few firm conclusions regarding syringomyelia may be drawn. Generally, no single surgical procedure predictably remedies syringomyelia for the long term. Frequently multiple procedures are required. Direct treatment of the syrinx cavity certainly makes intuitive sense, particularly for those syrinxes that do not communicate with the fourth ventricle. In view of the fact that a syrinx cavity may be septated, a complete drainage may require attention to more than one area of the lesion.

To complete the frustrating nature of the problem, even when the syrinx cavity may be totally drained, not all of the patient's symptoms necessarily clear. The ultimate treatment for syringomyelia thus remains to be defined. A recent review may be consulted for additional details regarding the neurological and surgical aspects of syringomyelia (27).

Klippel-Feil Syndrome

Klippel-Feil syndrome refers to patients with congenital fusion of cervical vertebra. It is a bony anomaly, as discussed in Chapter 48, that heads the neurologic prob-

lems (4,37,38,39,47). In this, the bony problem may include two segments or the entire cervical spine.

The neurologic symptoms are generally localized to the head, neck, and arms as a result of irritation or impingement of the cervical nerve roots (32). With time, the neural-foraminae become compromised by osteophytes. This may be compounded by instability of the motion segment because of repetitive trauma over time. Findings range from cervical radiculopathy with mild spasticity in the lower extremities to hyporeflexia and frank myelopathy muscular weakness in the upper extremities with gross spasticity in the lower extremities secondary to spinal cord and root compression.

Patients with a mild degree of fusion of the cervical spine should be expected to lead a normal life (4). On the other hand, those patients with severely involved spines have a better prognosis if early preventive measures are taken to avoid the complications resulting from undue stress or compression of the nervous system. The associated scoliosis and renal abnormalities, if treated early on, also promote longer life. The role of prophylactic surgical stabilization in the asymptomatic patient remains controversial. In a small percentage of patients, however, when instability is documented, reduction of misalignment and surgical stabilization are appropriate. Either the anterior or posterior approach to myelopathy, outlined in Chapters 56 and 57, are appropriate.

Surgical intervention, however, may be dangerous if other associated abnormalities of the brain stem and spinal cord have not been considered during the patient's work-up. This involves a team effort of neurologists, neurosurgeons, and orthopedists working together (62).

Medical treatment for the hidden and often unrecognized associated anomalies, including scoliosis, renal abnormalities, cardiac abnormalities, and hearing abnormalities may provide more benefit to the patient than preoccupation with the cervical fusion itself (3,25,49, 52,53,56,57).

Congenital Atlantoaxial Instability

This problem is discussed in Chapter 46. However, the bony anomalies can be associated with other anomalies. Congenital scoliosis, Down's syndrome, bone dysplasias, osteogenesis imperfecta, and neurofibromatosis are all capable of producing significant degrees of atlantoaxial instability. In Down's syndrome, approximately 20% of patients have been found to have laxity of the transverse atlantal ligament (TAL) (46,67). These patients appear to have attenuation or rupture of the transverse ligament with reduction of the space available to the spinal cord. As long as the alar ligaments remain intact, they may limit movement of the odontoid process and help to prevent spinal cord compression. With time and chronic stress, however, the alar ligaments may become incompetent and cord compression develops. Similar findings occur in neurofibromatosis and the other disorders listed above.

Patients may present neurologically with a puzzling clinical picture characterized by intermittent pain, numbness, and weakness in the arms or legs. Should the medulla be indented by the odontoid, the patient may present with cranial nerve palsies and/or respiratory difficulties. Should the vertebral arteries be compressed, a clinical picture of syncopy may develop.

While the normal space seen on the lateral roentgenogram between the anterior aspect of the dens and the posterior aspect of the anterior ring of the atlas (ADI) is usually no more than 3 mm in the adult, patients with chronic atlantoaxial instability (AAI) (e.g., congenital anomalies, rheumatoid arthritis, Down's syndrome, neurofibromatosis) may present with a larger ADI. Because of these conditions, the odontoid is frequently found to be hypermobile, particularly in flexion. Surprisingly, however, few patients are symptomatic (16). This is because the more important space for the spinal cord is the space available between the posterior aspect of the odontoid and the posterior arch of the atlas. Since this distance may change with flexion or extension, flexion-extension views should be performed routinely in a gentle manner on each patient suspected of having AAI. For those patients with formation of abnormal bone, a computed tomogram may be useful in this regard. With the advent of MRI scanning, radiolucent soft tissue masses posterior to the odontoid, such as those occurring in rheumatoid arthritis, may be well imaged and help to explain what otherwise might be neurologic dysfunction in a seemingly "adequate" size canal. Anatomic studies by McRae (50) and Greenberg (33) reveal that spinal cord compression invariably occurs when this distance is 14 mm or less. Where soft tissue masses may exist, and MRI scanning is not available, myelography with post-myelography CT may be extremely useful in further identifying intra-canalicular anatomy.

The role of prophylactic surgical stabilization in patients with documented congenital atlantoaxial instability is reviewed in Chapter 48. If marked instability is demonstrated or the patient is frankly symptomatic neurologically, there is general agreement that surgical fusion (posterior) of C1 and C2 is appropriate and sufficient. Since respiratory dysfunction occurs more frequently in these patients than anticipated (31,41), pulmonary function testing pre-operatively is well advised. In addition, attention should be addressed to compromise of lower cranial nerve function since pre-operative tracheostomy may also be necessary. Prior to surgical intervention, reduction of the atlantoaxial malalignment is best achieved by traction (24,28). Operative reduction has been associated with an increased morbidity and mortality (66,69). The patient should be left in the reduced position pre-operatively until improvement or stabilization of the neurologic condition has been observed. Should no neurologic improvement appear, ad-

ditional neurologic work-up may be necessary. For those cases where an abnormality in C1 may also be associated with TAL abnormality, an occiput to C2 stabilization may be necessary.

Scoliosis is a well recognized feature of Von-Recklinghausen's neurofibromatosis, occurring in approximately one quarter of such patients. While the spine deformity in neurofibromatosis may lead to the neurological problems described above, the scoliotic deformity infrequently involves the cervical spine. As a result, a more detailed description of neurofibromatosis and scoliosis will be found in Chapter 65.

Chiari Malformation

In the late 1800s, Chiari described an anomaly of the hind brain involving the upper cervical spine, which eventually was subdivided into different types (14,15) (reviewed in detail in Chapter 48). Abnormalities of the skull and cervical spine associated with a Chiari malformation are common. The Chiari malformation, while congenital, may remain silent and be discovered accidentally by routine computed tomography or MRI studies of the cranial cervical junction performed for evaluation of other problems. In a review by Garcin and Oeconomos, 60% of their cases were documented between the second and third decade of life (30). Perhaps the delay in the appearance of neurologic dysfunction is a reflection of slow, progressive, restructuring of the foramen magnum. Perhaps progressive ligamentous distraction develops with atlantoaxial instability resulting. A water hammer effect of cerebrospinal fluid (CSF) on posterior fossa structures also may be important when free egress of CSF from the fourth ventricle is not possible as with Chiari anatomy.

Seemingly minor trauma may be responsible for bringing a Chiari malformation to medical attention, since relatively insignificant flexion injuries to the neck may bring out atlantoaxial instability.

When hydrocephalus is present, the evidence of increased intracranial pressure or symptoms of normal pressure hydrocephalus prompt the diagnosis of Chiari malformation.

In the case of compression of the cerebellum and medulla, patients may present with dizziness, vertigo, nystagmus, and/or ataxia. If high cervical spinal cord compression is the primary problem, patients may present with spastic quadriparesis, proprioceptive abnormalities, with perhaps weakness and paresthesias greater in the upper extremities than the lower extremities. Cranial nerve palsies may present as compromise in gagging, coughing, or swallowing. Many times, however, the symptoms are rather vague and the diagnosis difficult to make until imaging studies prompt the diagnosis.

The advent of MR scanning has made arteriography and myelography generally unnecessary. MRI nicely

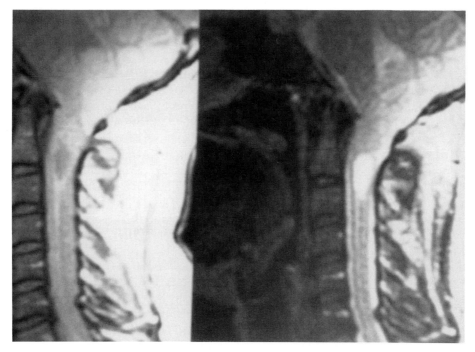

FIG. 1. Sagittal MRI demonstrating Chiari malformation with cerebellar tonsil displacement through foramen magnum down to C1-C2 and associated C2-C3 cord syrinx.

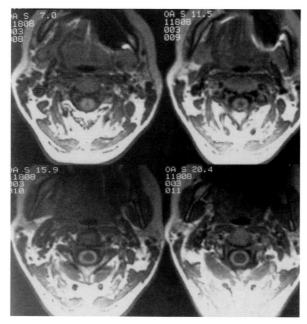

FIG. 2. Axial cut of same patient shows large syrinx within the center of the spinal cord. The fluid density is the same as CSF.

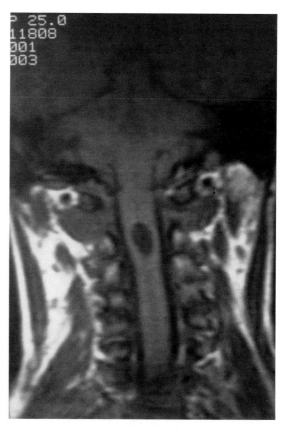

FIG. 3. Coronal view of same patient who had been completely worked up for headaches and diffuse hyper-reflexia with loss of coordination shows syrinx in the middle of the cord with the cerebellar tonsil displaced laterally through foramen magnum.

demonstrates hind brain abnormalities as well as those of the cervical spinal cord (Figs. 1, 2, and 3). Bony abnormalities, however, remain better demonstrated with plain skull and cervical spine films augmented by computed tomography where necessary. In view of the association of syringomyelia with a Chiari malformation, MRI also satisfactorily describes the anatomy of the syrinx without the need for myelography and post-myelography CT. A CT or MR scan of the brain also should be performed in Chiari patients in view of the association with hydrocephalus.

Treatment is directed at hydrocephalus, if it exists, with decompression of the posterior fossa and upper cervical cord, if symptoms derive from compression of neural structures at that level, and stabilization of the cervical spine, if spinal instability exists.

A posterior decompression of the upper cervical spine and posterior fossa usually involves a laminectomy beginning below the level of the herniated tonsils and extending up to a suboccipital craniectomy with a duraplasty of some kind. This provides adequate space for the cerebellum and kinked spinal cord. Unnecessarily wide laminectomy should be avoided in order to reduce the likelihood of post-operative spinal instability. In the case of cerebellar ectopia, or when the foramenae of the fourth ventricle are closed by arachnoidal adhesions, these adhesions should be opened. The question of tonsillectomy or other diversionary procedures between the fourth ventricle and the subarachnoid space remains controversial, since a certain number of patients experience progressive deterioration despite multiple procedures (18,61).

The Chiari malformation may be associated with other abnormalities of the brain such as hydrocephalus (mentioned above), forking of the aqueduct, malformation of the thalamus, and microgyria, and this material is covered in Chapter 48. The Chiari malformation is also associated with congenital anomalies of the spinal cord, meningomyelocele being the most common. Syringomyelia and diastematomyelia have also been associated. Paul et al. (58), in evaluating a group of patients with Chiari I malformations, observed an instance of 32% syringomyelia in their patients. Milhorat (51) found hydrocephalus in 65% of the Chiari cases he reviewed.

Cervical Myelomeningocele

While approximately one third of myelomeningoceles occur in the thoracic or thoracolumbar spine, it is well known that the spinal cord above the involved area frequently shows considerable anatomic variation with associated intraspinal abnormalities (13,21,22). A review of the distribution of myelomeningocele by one author revealed that approximately 3% occur in the cervical region (26). The vertebrae in the affected area generally

describe a wider but shallower spinal canal with deformation of the pedicle and virtual absence of the lamina. Clinicians recognize that bony spina bifida generally exceeds the level of the skin deficiency (7). With myelomeningocele occurring up in the cervical area, a Chiari malformation and hydrocephalus should be anticipated as well.

MR evaluation of the head and cervical spine would be the most practical way for examining hydrocephalus, hind brain abnormalities, and the cervical meningocele. This may be supplemented with plain spine films of the neck to assess bony abnormalities in the neck.

With such high level of spinal cord dysfunction, satisfactory motor and sensory function below the level of the lesion is not likely and a high mortality rate during early life is to be anticipated.

Congenital curves and structural abnormalities of the vertebrae such as failure of formation or segmentation at or above the level of the myelomeningocele are common. The instance of congenital scoliosis in myelomeningocele is approximately 30% and usually progresses with time (63).

CONCLUSIONS

A few congenital neurologic abnormalities affecting the cervical spine in the adult may be prevented by genetic counseling. Most of these disorders described in the last three chapters develop idiopathically. With earlier diagnosis and therefore earlier treatment, which requires a team effort between obstetricians, pediatricians, neurologists, neurosurgeons, and orthopedists, the overall outcome from these problems may improve. Currently, the treatment of many disorders remains unsatisfactory, requiring multiple procedures over several years. In several cases the cervical bony and neurologic problems are less important than the associated multi-system anomalies. Such anomalies, if not followed and treated expectantly, may in fact cause more difficulty for the patient than the primary problem involving the neck. MR scanning has provided a non-invasive technique for imaging the spinal cord. This technique not only aids diagnosis but also provides a simple means of following these patients over years. A new technique of "dynamic MR scanning" in flexion and extension augments information regarding stability and spinal cord compression. By gathering more information about the natural history of the disease processes, perhaps effective treatment will follow.

REFERENCES

1. Aboulker J (1979): La syringomyelie et les liquides intrarachidiens. *Neurochirurgie* 25(Suppl 1):1–144.
2. Aubin ML, Vignaud J, Jardin C, et al (1981): Computed tomography in 75 clinical cases of syringomyelia. *AJNR* 2:199–204.
3. Baga N, Chusid EL, Miller A (1969): Pulmonary disability in the

Klippel-Feil syndrome. A study of two siblings. *Clin Orthop* (67):105–110.

4. Baird PA, Robinson GC, Buckler WS (1967): Klippel-Feil syndrome. A study of mirror movement detected by electromyography. *Am J Dis Child* 113:546–551.

5. Barbaro NM, Wilson CB, Gutin PH, et al (1984): Surgical treatment of syringomyelia. Favorable results with syringoperitoneal shunting. *J Neurosurg* 61:531–538.

6. Barnett HJM, Foster JB, Hudgson P (1973): *Syringomyelia*. Philadelphia: Saunders.

7. Barson AJ (1970): Spina bifida: The significance of the level and extent of the defect to the morphogenesis. *Develop Med Child Neurol* 12:129–144.

8. Bauman GI (1932): Absence of the cervical spine; Klippel-Feil syndrome. *JAMA* 98:129–132.

9. Benini A, Krayenbuhl H (1969): Ein neuer chirurgischer Weg zur Behandlung der Hydro und Syringomyelie. *Schweiz Med Wschr* 99:1137–1142.

10. Bertrand G (1973): Chapter 26. Dynamic factors in the evolution of syringomyelia and syringobulbia. *Clin Neurosurg* 20:322–333.

11. Boman K, Iivanainen M (1967): Prognosis of syringomyelia. *Acta Neurol Scand* 43:61–68.

12. Cahan LD, Bentson JR (1982): Considerations in the diagnosis and treatment of syringomyelia and the Chiari malformation. *J Neurosurg* 57:24–31.

13. Cameron AH (1957): Malformations of the neuro-spinal axis, urogenital tract and foregut in spina bifida attributable to disturbances of the blastopore. *J Path Bact* 73:213–221.

14. Chiari H (1891): Ueber Veranderungen des Kleinhirns infolge von Hydrocephalie des Grosshirns. *Deutsch Med Wschr* 17:1172–1175.

15. Chiari H (1895): Uber die Veranderungen des Kleinhirns, der Pons und der Medulla oblongata infolge von congenitaler Hydrocephalie des Grosshirns. *Denkschr Akad Wissensch Wien* 63:71–117.

16. Davidson RG (1988): Atlantoaxial instability in individuals with Down Syndrome: A fresh look at the evidence. *Pediatrics* 81:857–865.

17. Dolan KD (1977): Expanding lesions of the cervical spinal canal. *Radiol Clin North Am* 15:203–214.

18. Dyste GN, Menezes AH, VanGilder JC (1989): Symptomatic Chiari malformations. *J Neurosurg* 71:159–168.

19. Ehni G (1982): Extradural spinal cord and nerve root compression from benign lesions of the cervical area. In: Youmans JR, ed. *Neurological surgery*. Philadelphia: Saunders, p. 2595.

20. Emerson RG, Pedley TA (1986): Effect of cervical spinal cord lesions on early components of the median nerve somatosensory evoked potential. *Neurology* 36:20–26.

21. Emery JL, Lendon RG (1972): Clinical implications of cord lesions in neurospinal dysraphism. *Develop Med Child Neurol* [Suppl] 27:45–51.

22. Emery JL, Lendon RG (1973): The local cord lesion in neurospinal dysraphism (meningomyelocele). *J Path* 110:83–96.

23. Faulhauer K, Loew K (1978): The surgical treatment of syringomyelia. Long-term results. *Acta Neurochir* 44:215–222.

24. Fielding JW, Hawkins RJ, Ratzan SA (1976): Spine fusion for atlanto-axial instability. *J Bone Joint Surg* [Am] 58:400–407.

25. Forney WR, Robinson SJ, Pascoe DJ (1966): Congenital heart disease, deafness, and skeletal malformations: A new syndrome? *J Pediatr* 68:14–26.

26. French BN (1982): Midline fusion defects and defects of formation. In: Youmans JR, ed. *Neurological surgery*. Philadelphia: Saunders, p. 1248.

27. Gamache FW, Ducker TB (1990): Syringomyelia: A neurological and surgical spectrum. *J Spinal Disorders*.

28. Garber JN (1964): Abnormalities of the atlas and axis vertebrae: Congenital and traumatic. *J Bone Joint Surg* [Am] 46:1782–1791.

29. Garcia-Uria J, Leunda G, Carrillo R, et al (1981): Syringomyelia: Long-term results after posterior fossa decompression. *J Neurosurg* 54:380–383.

30. Garcin R, Oeconomos D (1953): *Les aspects neurologiques des malformations congenitales de la charniere cranio-rachidienne*. Paris: Masson.

31. Grantham SA, Dick HM, Thompson RC Jr, et al (1969): Occipito

32. Gray SW, Romaine CB, Skandalakis JE (1964): Congenital fusion of the cervical vertebrae. *Surg Gynecol Obstet* 118:373–385.

33. Greenberg AD (1968): Atlanto-axial dislocations. *Brain* 91:655–684.

34. Gunderson CH, Greenspan RH, Glaser GH, Lubs HA (1967): Klippel-Feil syndrome: Genetic and clinical reevaluation of cervical fusion. *Medicine* 46:491–512.

35. Hall PV, Holden RW, Matthews TJ (1981): Syringomyelia. *Contemp Neurosurg* 3:1–6.

36. Hankinson J (1978): The surgical treatment of syringomyelia. In: Krayenbuhl H, ed. *Advances and technical standards in neurosurgery, vol. 5*. New York: Springer-Verlag, pp. 127–151.

37. Hensinger RN, Lang JE, MacEwen GD (1974): Klippel-Feil syndrome: A constellation of associated anomalies. *J Bone Joint Surg* [Am] 56:1246–1253.

38. Hensinger RN, MacEwen GD (1982): Congenital anomalies of the spine. In: Rothman RH, Simeone FA, eds. *The spine*. Philadelphia: Saunders, pp. 188–315.

39. Jalladeau J (1936): Malformations congenitales associees au syndrome de Klippel-Feil. *Theses de Paris*.

40. Krayenbuhl H (1974): Evaluation of the different surgical approaches in the treatment of syringomyelia. *Clin Neurol Neurosurg* 2:110–128.

41. Krieger AJ, Rosomoff HL, Kuperman AS, et al (1969): Occult respiratory dysfunction in a craniovertebral anomaly. *J Neurosurg* 31:15–20.

42. Laha RK, Malik HG, Langille RA (1975): Post-traumatic syringomyelia. *Surg Neurol* 4:519–522.

43. Lesoin F, Petit H, Thomas CE III, et al (1986): Use of the syringoperitoneal shunt in the treatment of syringomyelia. *Surg Neurol* 25:131–136.

44. Levy WJ, Mason L, Hahn JF (1983): Chiari malformation presenting in adults: A surgical experience in 127 cases. *Neurosurgery* 12:377–390.

45. Logue V, Edwards MR (1981): Syringomyelia and its surgical treatment. An analysis of 75 patients. *J Neurol Neurosurg Psychiatry* 44:273–284.

46. Martel W, Tishler JM (1966): Observations on the spine in mongoloidism. *Am J Roentgenol* 97:630–638.

47. McElfresh E, Winter R (1973): Klippel-Feil syndrome. *Minn Med* 56:353–357.

48. McIlroy WJ, Richardson JC (1965): Syringomyelia: A clinical review of 75 cases. *Can Med Assoc J* 93:731–734.

49. McLay K, Maran AG (1969): Deafness and the Klippel-Feil syndrome. *J Laryngol Otol* 83:175–184.

50. McRae DL (1953): Bony abnormalities in the region of the foramen magnum: Correlation of the anatomic and neurologic findings. *Acta Radiol* 40:335–355.

51. Milhorat T (1972): *Hydrocephalus and the cerebrospinal fluid*. Baltimore: Williams and Wilkins.

52. Moore WB, Matthews TJ, Rabinowitz R (1975): Genitourinary anomalies associated with Klippel-Feil syndrome. *J Bone Joint Surg* [Am] 57:355–357.

53. Morrison SG, Perry LW, Scott LP 3d (1968): Congenital brevicollis (Klippel-Feil syndrome) and cardiovascular anomalies. *Am J Dis Child* 115:614–620.

54. Murphey F, Simmons JC, Brunson B (1973): Chapter 2. Ruptured cervical discs, 1939–1972. *Clin Neurosurg* 20:9–17.

55. Naik DR (1970): Cervical spinal canal in normal infants. *Clin Radiol* 21:323–326.

56. Nora JJ, Cohen M, Maxwell GM (1961): Klippel-Feil syndrome with congenital heart disease. *Am J Dis Child* 102:858–864.

57. Palant DI, Carter BL (1972): Klippel-Feil syndrome and deafness. A study with polytomography. *Am J Dis Child* 123:218–221.

58. Paul KS, Lye RH, Strang FA, et al (1983): Arnold-Chiari malformation. Review of 71 cases. *J Neurosurg* 58:183–187.

59. Phillips TW, Kindt GW (1981): Syringoperitoneal shunt for syringomyelia: A preliminary report. *Surg Neurol* 16:462–466.

60. Resjo IM, Harwood-Nash DC, Fitz CR, et al (1979): Computed tomographic metrizamide myelography in syringohydromyelia. *Radiology* 131:405–407.

61. Rhoton AL Jr (1976): Microsurgery of Arnold-Chiari malformation in adults with and without hydromyelia. *J Neurosurg* 45:473–483.

62. Rothman R, Simeone F, eds. (1982): *The spine.* Philadelphia: Saunders, pp. 216–233.

63. Rozen MJ (1977): Pathophysiology and spinal deformity in myelomeningocele. In: McLaurin RL, ed. *Myelomeningocele.* New York: Grune & Stratton, pp. 565–579.

64. Russell DS, Donald C (1935): The mechanism of internal hydrocephalus in spina bifida. *Brain* 58:203–215.

65. Schlesinger EB, Antunes JL, Michelsen WJ, et al (1981): Hydromyelia: Clinical presentation and comparison of modalities of treatment. *Neurosurgery* 9:356–365.

66. Sinh G, Pandya SK (1968): Treatment of congenital atlanto-axial dislocations. *Proc Aust Assoc Neurol* 5:507–514.

67. Spitzer R, Rabinowitch JY, Wybar KC (1961): A study of the abnormalities of the skull, teeth and lenses in mongolism. *Can Med Assoc J* 84:567–572.

68. Tator CH, Meguro K, Rowed DW (1982): Favorable results with syringosubarachnoid shunts for treatment of syringomyelia. *J Neurosurg* 56:517–523.

69. Wadia NH (1967): Myelopathy complicating congenital atlanto-axial dislocation (a study of 28 cases). *Brain* 90:449–472.

70. West RJ, Williams B (1980): Radiographic studies of the ventricles in syringomyelia. *Neuroradiology* 20:5–16.

71. Wisoff JH (1988): Hydromyelia: A critical review. *Childs Nerv Syst* 4:1–8.

Traumatic Disorders
of the Cervical Spine

The Adult Spine: Principles and Practice,
J. W. Frymoyer, Editor-in-Chief.
Raven Press, Ltd., New York © 1991.

CHAPTER 50

Cervical Sprain Syndrome

Diagnosis, Treatment, and Long-Term Outcome

Henry La Rocca

SCOPE OF THE PROBLEM

Acceleration injury of the neck is this author's preferred term for that cluster of clinical problems attendant upon the sudden application of a propulsive force to the head and neck complex, in which tissue damage occurs directly as the result of the propulsion. This is in contradistinction to contact injury in which an object impacting the head or neck (whether a swinging beam, or the bottom of a swimming pool) imparts a compressive or translatory force which creates internal loading to failure. The acceleration injury is variously called neck sprain, neck strain, whiplash (4), or soft tissue neck injury, all of which share the inference of tissue stretching. Contact injuries, on the other hand, encompass the spectrum of fracture and dislocation of the vertebral column itself. The diagnostic and therapeutic approaches to the management of the effects of these two mechanisms of injury are substantially different. However, the frequency with which acceleration injury continues to occur mandates as probing an explication of this topic as is generally afforded contact injury, which often is conceptually more simple.

A wide variety of clinical problems occurring following acceleration injury have been reported, as discussed below. They are tabulated in Table 1. The first major report of acceleration injuries of the neck was that of Gay and Abbott in 1953 (7). They described a clinical syndrome produced generally by rear-end motor vehicle collisions in which oscillations of the head and neck into flexion and extension are induced, resulting in a variety of pathological states. In 1955, Severy, Mathewson, and Bechtol described a precise experimental study of the rear-end collision as they reported an investigation of related engineering and medical phenomena (28). Their work established that there is a significantly forceful deflection and acceleration of the head and upper torso upon impact because the head and neck projected above the seat of automobile models in use at that time. This observation, furthered by other studies, led to the proposition that neck injuries due to rear-end collision could be minimized by restraining the head and neck with altered seat design, an eminently reasonable and even obvious conclusion. Regrettably, as recently as 1987, with contemporary automotive design, Deans et al., reported that 62% of 137 patients attending a hospital following a motor vehicle accident suffered pain in the neck at some time following their accident; 5 had continuous pain one year later (5). Balla reports an estimated 900 new cases of acceleration injury occurring per year in the state of Victoria, Australia alone (1). Further, Olney and Marsden found no statistically significant reduction in injuries when a head restraint was part of the motor vehicle seat (21). Clearly acceleration injury remains an important medical and engineering challenge.

CLINICAL ISSUES

The report of Gay and Abbott of 1953 (7) described the clinical characteristics of the syndrome which fol-

H. La Rocca, M.D.: Clinical Professor of Orthopaedic Surgery, Tulane University School of Medicine, New Orleans, Louisiana 70115.

TABLE 1. *Clinical problems arising from acceleration injury*

Spinal symptoms:
1. Diffuse neck pain with non-radicular radiation and normal radiographs
2. Diffuse neck pain with or without radicular symptoms, and with radiographic evidence of pre-existing cervical spondylosis of varying extent
3. Cervical radiculopathy
4. Cervical myelopathy
5. Lumbar pain syndromes, including herniated nucleus pulposus

Central nervous system:
1. Cerebral concussion
2. The Barre syndrome (sympathetic dysfunction)
3. Multiple cranial nerve dysfunction
4. Chronic headache (including migraine)
5. Cognitive impairment

Psychiatric symptoms:
1. Mood and personality change
2. Sleep disturbance
3. Psychoneurotic reaction
4. Depression
5. "Litigation neurosis"

Other:
1. Temporomandibular joint derangement
2. Esophageal laceration with or without mediastinitis

lowed acceleration injury. The authors noted that about 15% of vehicular accidents which resulted in death, injury, or property damage were caused by a rear-end collision. They noted that a paradox existed in that seemingly inconsequential trauma resulted in a clinical problem of extraordinarily lengthy duration. Ninety percent of the cases they described followed upon a rear-end collision in which the victim was typically seated in an unmoving vehicle which was struck from the rear by another traveling at low velocity. Unlike other types of trauma, 70% of the victims were women instead of men. In parallel with this observation, the occupations of the victims of rear-end collisions tended to be light regarding physical demands. There were no heavy laborers in the group, and the victims were housewives, skilled laborers, managers, clerks, or professionals. The age distribution was between 30 and 50 years of age. None of the patients had received a direct blow to the head or neck, and the presenting symptoms included neck pain, limited neck motion, with spasm and tenderness of the cervical musculature. Pain was accentuated by motion. The physical examination detected paracervical spasm and tenderness with extension into the interscapular region and into the shoulder girdles. The neurological examination was generally normal. The authors noted that the patient "showed marked hyper-tonicity of the neuromuscular system and general nervous symptoms."

Gay and Abbott described five different clinical presentations:

1. Cervical radiculitis was described in 70% of cases who experienced cervical pain which radiated to the occiput, jaw, shoulders, upper anterior chest, and upper extremity. Transient reflex or sensory abnormalities were noted in this group.
2. Sixty-one percent of cases had experienced a cerebral concussion and were initially bewildered, stunned, dazed, or dulled by the accident. Members of this group complained of persisting headache and a variety of anxiety related symptoms including tension, restlessness, irritability, poor concentration, insomnia, and mood changes. They also experienced vasomotor instability and vertigo.
3. Twenty-six percent of cases demonstrated evidence of intervertebral disc herniation with symptoms similar to the group with cervical radiculitis but with more severe spasm and restricted motion. Changes in the deep tendon reflexes and in sensory disturbance were more persistent.
4. Fifty-two percent of the patients were considered seriously handicapped by persisting psychoneurotic reactions arising from circumstances inherent in the mechanism of injury involving a sudden violent and unexpected jolt which constituted a disturbing experience. Medical evaluation following the accident generally detected little by way of injury and treatment recommendations were minimal. However, with the passage of time, the physical symptoms worsened and provoked the development of apprehension, anxiety, and neuromuscular tension. Cervical muscular hypertonicity, aggravated by anxiety, aggravated the clinical problem. Later, social factors such as institution of litigation stimulated a self-perpetuating cycle of pain and anxiety.
5. Thirty percent of cases experienced an associated low back injury with lumbar and lower extremity pain problems.

In this series, radiographic examination demonstrated no abnormality in half of the 50 patients. In the remainder, there were some with manifestations of degenerative disease. A subluxation was noted in one patient, and a fractured lamina in one other. Hence, major vertebral column disruption was apparent in only 2 of 50 patients.

Because of the intensity of symptoms, especially when the injury was associated with concussion, approximately half of the patients required temporary treatment in the hospital. Following that, a variety of conservative measures were employed in treating the persisting symptoms, which included the use of neck collars, cervical traction, and various physical modalities. Response to treatment was slow, and the authors determined that the whiplash injury is a chronic condition often associated with some form of psychoneurotic reaction.

In 1980, Balla reported on the late whiplash syndrome

(1), and defined it as a collection of symptoms and disabilities seen more than six months after a neck injury from a motor vehicle accident. In three hundred cases studied, late whiplash syndrome persisted in 88% of the cases more than one year after the injury, and in 64% more than two years afterwards. Balla noted that there was no real difference in symptomatology between the groups seen either at six months or two years following injury. Women victims outnumbered men by nearly 2 to 1. The majority were in the age range of 21 to 50 years. Nerve root pain occurred at some point in the clinical course in only 14 cases (5%), and a clear sensory disturbance in an anatomical distribution was observed only in 13 cases (4%). Two of the 300 cases (0.7%) had a reflex loss. The complex of headache, neck pain, and stiffness was present in nearly all patients, and at some stage almost 40% complained of arm pain. A high proportion of patients complained of anxiety, irritability, depression, and sleep disturbance. Some reduction in work capabilities occurred in two-thirds of cases, and 10% were not expected to return to work. Correlation of plain-film radiological changes with symptoms was poor. Thirty-nine percent of cases exhibited mild degenerative changes, while the remainder were considered normal. Balla's data confirmed the observation of Gay and Abbott that the occupations of the victims of the late whiplash syndrome were the less physically demanding types of employment. Balla concluded that in the late whiplash syndrome there is an interaction between the physical, psychological, and sociological factors producing the disease state.

Norris and Watt addressed the issue of prognosis of neck injuries resulting from rear-end collisions in 1983 (19). They noted that there had been no simple method of estimating prognosis at, or soon after the time of injury owing to the heterogeneous and miscellaneous nature of the published reports. Their effort was to establish a simple prognostic classification system which might be of utility in estimating future disability and the likelihood of litigation. A collection of 61 patients was appraised, and each was placed into one of three groups based upon the symptoms and signs at the time of initial presentation. The maximum time elapsing between the injury and the evaluation was seven days. Group 1 patients complained of symptoms but had no abnormality on physical examination. Group 2 patients had symptoms along with a reduced range of motion of the cervical spine but no neurological abnormality. Group 3 patients had symptoms, reduced range of motion, and evidence of objective neurological deficit. Of the 61 patients studied, 27 patients were assigned to Group 1, 24 to Group 2, and 10 to Group 3. Patient gender and age distribution were the same in each group. All complained of pain and stiffness in the neck with occipital headache being the second most common symptom. All patients in Group 3 had complaints of paresthesia, but

less than half of the Group 1 and Group 2 patients had this symptom. There were no other symptoms which were more common in any specific group. Symptom onset was not immediate in every case, but was delayed from three to forty-eight hours in approximately 20% of the patients in each of the three groups. The proportion of patients wearing seatbelts or head restraints was comparable among the three groups, and comprised between 38% and 48%. The overwhelming majority of patients in the three groups were seated in stationary vehicles at the time of impact.

Follow-up averaged nineteen months for the Group 1 patients, twenty-three months for Group 2, and twenty-four months for Group 3. The time off work was two weeks in Group 1, four weeks in Group 2, and ten weeks in Group 3 on average. Only 10% of patients in Group 3 were entirely free of symptoms at follow-up, compared to 19% in Group 2, and 56% in Group 1. Of those with persisting neck pain, 20% in each group were disabled from work. Of those with persisting symptoms in Group 3, there was interference with recreational activity as well. While neck pain was the most common complaint, headache was also often noted. It affected 70% of patients in Group 3 and 37% in Groups 1 and 2. A notable observation was the absence of headache at follow-up in the seven patients who had been using a head restraint at the time of accident.

Claims of personal injury were filed by 56% of patients in Group 1, 67% in Group 2, and 100% in Group 3. At long-term follow-up there was no statistical difference among the groups regarding improvement of symptoms following settlement. All patients in Group 3 had residual neck pain in comparison with 57% of patients in Group 1.

Norris and Watt also considered the effect of radiographic findings in their 61 patients. Entirely normal radiographs were found in 30% of patients in Group 1, 12.5% of patients in Group 2, but in none of the patients in Group 3. Spondylosis was the commonest abnormality, present in 26% of patients in Group 1, 33% in Group 2, and 40% in Group 3. Normal lordotic curves were found in 74% of Group 1 patients but only 30% of Group 3 patients. Conversely, straight cervical spines were observed in 60% of Group 3 patients and 18.6% of Group 1 patients. Kyphosis was observed in 7.4% of Group 1, 12.5% of Group 2, and 10% of Group 3.

The authors expressed regret that it was impossible to obtain an accurate estimate of the speed of impact since clearly the energy of the impact can reasonably be assumed to be proportionate to the injuries produced. However, no definite trend could be established. On the other hand, the groupings of the patients did prove to have merit. The higher grouping had a poorer prognosis, with greater time off work, and persistence of symptoms grave enough to affect recreation. Legal claims were also greater in Group 3 suggesting that litigation is more dependent upon the severity of injury than upon some neurotic tendency since the patients were all classified within seven days of injury before any legal action had been taken. Persistent headache was more likely to be associated with filing legal claims than was residual neck pain. Group 1 patients were either improved after the settlement of the claim or were no worse. On the other hand, in Group 3 only two patients were improved following settlement. These findings suggest to Norris and Watt that litigation itself has little influence on symptoms, and persons with milder syndromes are less likely to file a claim. Those with more serious injuries (Group 3) all filed claims, but most failed to show any improvement after settlement. Lastly, Norris and Watt suggest that pre-existing degenerative changes in the cervical spine, however slight, do alter the prognosis adversely. Further, abnormal curves in the cervical spine reflective of spasm of the neck muscles are more common in patients with a poor outcome.

Deans et al., attempted to learn the true incidence of pain in the neck following motor vehicle accidents. They studied 137 patients between one and two years after they had presented to a hospital following a motor vehicle accident (5). Eighty-five patients (62%) complained of pain in the neck following their accident. In 36 (26%) the pain persisted longer than one year. Five patients (3.7%) had severe and continuous pain. Only 10 of the 137 patients (7%) had experienced pain in the neck before their accident. Most accident victims (77%) experienced the onset of pain within twelve hours of injury, but 7% noted no symptoms until after forty-eight hours. The authors conclude that when an individual in a motor vehicle accident sustains an injury sufficiently severe to cause him to attend a hospital, he or she has a 62% chance of suffering neck pain, which may have a delayed onset after leaving the hospital. Twenty-six percent of cases are likely to continue to experience neck pain one year after the incident. Nygren reported permanent disability in approximately 10% of rear-end collision victims and 4% of front or side impact victims who suffered neck injury (20).

In the data of Deans et al., the 62% incidence of pain in the neck following vehicular collisions is nine times greater than that which occurs spontaneously in the community (7%). Regarding the direction of impact, their data confirm that pain in the neck occurs after impact from any direction but is disproportionately frequent following rear-end collision, with impact from that direction causing pain almost twice as frequently as front-end collisions.

A finding of great significance is that which was observed by Rutherford et al., in 1985 (25). They had shown that the compulsory requirement to wear seatbelts in Great Britain was followed by a rise in the number of neck injuries. Deans et al., confirmed that there were more sprains in the neck in those wearing seatbelts

than those not doing so, a finding not adequately understood (5). In any case, they conclude that soft tissue injury of the neck is a very common result of automobile accidents and the clinical problems which result may be quite protracted over time and seriously impair the work and social activities of the victims.

Certainly the commonest syndrome arising following acceleration injury is the complex of neck, interscapular, and arm pain with associated occipital headache. Frank disc herniation may be induced (Fig. 1). However, other types of syndromes have been reported and merit mention. Rosa et al., described a case report of multiple cranial nerve palsies due to hyperextension injury of the neck in a patient without other evidence of central nervous system injury (24). The patient in their case report showed signs of a unilateral injury to the sixth cranial nerve as well as bilateral injury to the lower cranial nerves from IX through XII. These palsies were proposed to be the result of severe stretching occurring with hyperextension of the neck. Scher has emphasized once again that hyperextension trauma to the neck in the elderly may give rise to a central cord syndrome as the result of indirect cervical spine trauma to a neck with advanced spondylosis (27).

Internal derangement of the temporomandibular joint was encountered in 25 whiplash patients reported by Weinberg and Lapointe in 1987 (30). They proposed that shear stress is applied to the intra-articular disc and this results in loss of synchronization of the disc and the mandibular condyle that progresses to the classical syndrome of internal derangement of the temporomandibular joint with clicking and pain. Arthrographic examina-

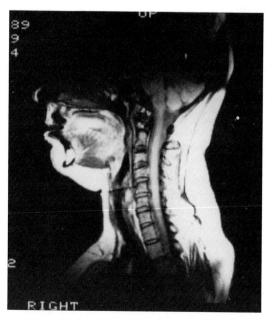

FIG. 1. Magnetic resonance scan of the cervical spine of a 37-year-old woman following acceleration injury demonstrating frank herniation of the disc at C5-C6.

tion of the joint in 25 of the patients demonstrated anterior disc displacement of varying degrees. Surgical treatment was required in ten of the patients, and the arthrographic findings were confirmed intra-operatively in each case with anterior disc displacement being noted. This displacement is considered to be produced by hyperextension of the neck in which the mandible moves posteriorly less quickly than the cranium resulting in downward and forward displacement of the disc-condyle complex relative to the cranial base. Stretching and tearing of the posterior attachment and synovial tissues along with loosening or tearing of the discal attachment to the condylar poles occurs. After the hyperextension, reactive flexion occurs in the head and neck and the attachment tissues are crushed between the mandibular condyle and the glenoid fossa of the temporal bone. After the injury, muscle spasm may produce additional displacement of the disc and perpetuate the temporomandibular joint syndrome.

A graver injury that can be produced by hyperextension of the neck is perforation of the esophagus (29), which may even lead to cervical sepsis and a descending mediastinitis (25). Presumably, the perforation results from impingement of the esophagus against an exostosis on the edge of a vertebral body, or entrapment of the esophageal wall between the vertebral bodies in the recoil flexion phase of the event.

Among the most taxing and challenging of the features of acceleration injury of the neck is the Barre syndrome (2). In this constellation, there are complaints of suboccipital headache, vertigo, tinnitus, intermittent aphonia and hoarseness, fatigue, temperature changes, and dysesthesias of the hands and forearms provoked by emotion, temperature, humidity, or noise. Cranio-facial complaints also occur with associated pain, numbness, nausea, vomiting, and even diarrhea. Objective neurological findings are generally absent, although there may be an absent corneal reflex. These symptoms are generally considered to arise from hypertonia of the sympathetic nervous system. This may result from stretch injury and hemorrhage within the sympathetic ganglia, or by irritation of the ventral nerve roots from C5–T1, all of which contain sympathetic fibers. Various arterial structures including the carotid plexus, the external carotid artery, the external maxillary, lingual, occipital, postauricular, superficial temporal, and internal maxillary arteries could be induced into vasospasm giving rise to the bizarre symptom complexes described. Sympathetic blocks and surgical sympathectomies have occasionally resulted in relief of the Barre syndrome thus lending credence to the sympathetic hypertonia theory. Chrisman and Gervais have reported symptoms of the Barre syndrome in 6 of 29 patients (20%) with cervical acceleration injury, and in contrast, 13 of 33 cases (40%) with cervical spondylosis (3) also had this syndrome.

There is also a relationship between whiplash injury and migraine headache, as reported by Winston (36). He described five cases of women who had suffered acceleration injury to the neck and argued that whiplash is trauma-precipitated cervical migraine. Symptoms arise following trauma of the acceleration variety and include headache, cervical symptoms, tinnitus, vertigo, scotomata, and upper extremity complaints as well. Winston proposed that there had been trauma to the brain in these cases as a result of an acceleration injury. Neck pain, stiffness, and muscular tenderness were common features, aggravated by motion. The five patients responded well to the variety of drugs customarily administered for migraine.

The recent report of Rajanov, Dvorak, and Valach (23) describes the occurrence of cognitive deficit in patients suffering acceleration injury of the neck. Fifty-one such patients underwent clinical and psychometric examination. There was formal testing of self-estimated cognitive impairment, as well as auditory and visual information processing. The results indicated the existence of two different syndromes. The first, termed cervicoencephalic syndrome was characterized by headache, tiredness, dizziness, poor concentration, disturbed accommodation, and impaired adaptation to light intensity. The second, termed lower cervical spine syndrome, is accompanied by neck and arm pain. In the first syndrome there was demonstrated abnormality of auditory information processing, while visual information processing was reduced to an equal degree in both syndromes. The authors assume that there is reduced processing of working memory as a result of the acceleration injury which they consider may be responsible for more global cognitive problems as well as secondary neurotic reaction (23).

Considering all of the foregoing, acceleration injury of the neck presents multiple diagnostic and therapeutic challenges. Symptoms vary from short-lived discomfort in the neck all the way to both sympathetic and central nervous system dysfunction. Psychological and sociological factors play important contributing roles in many cases. The clinician is best advised not to prejudge and categorize victims of acceleration injury but instead to approach each one with an informed awareness of the possibilities at hand.

EFFECTS OF LITIGATION

In Gay and Abbott's series of 50 cases, 66% had entered legal action in connection with their accidents, underscoring a special feature of the whiplash syndrome (7). Gotten noted the problem of wide divergence among surgeons regarding the severity of the injury and the future prognosis when the surgeons were called upon to give expert testimony in legal disputes (8). He also notes a prevalence of psychoneurotic symptoms so great as to preclude a proper evaluation of these patients and permit unanimity of the surgeons' opinions. These dilemmas prompted an investigation of whiplash injuries limited to cases in which all litigation had been settled. One hundred patients were reviewed. Of these, 88% had recovered, 54% without residual symptoms and 34% with only trivial symptoms not requiring treatment. Twelve percent continued to have severe symptoms. Work absence occurred in 41% of the patients before settlement, but in only 7% after settlement.

Gotten also evaluated the issue of satisfaction with the legal settlement as a potential modifier of the clinical course. Of 49 satisfied patients 29 had no residual symptoms, whereas 30 of 39 dissatisfied patients continued to have physical complaints. These considerations led him to conclude that there were "indications that the injury was being used by the patient as a convenient lever for personal gain, so to speak, though not necessarily on a conscious level." Such personal gain might be financial or psychosocial. He also concluded that "the evidence indicates the great difficulty in evaluating whiplash type of injuries due to the complicating factor of monetary compensation."

Macnab also reviewed 145 patients two or more years after settlement of litigation, and found that 121 were still having symptoms which, in the majority were "a continuing nuisance rather than a significant disability" (15). Of an overall series of 266 cases, 45% continued to have symptoms after settlement of claims. With such a large number he was not content to dismiss these patients as hysterical, neurotic, or dishonest. He pointed out that patients who experienced forward flexion or lateral flexion stresses rarely suffered discomfort, but those whose head-neck complex was deflected into hyperextension constituted nearly the entire group with chronic pain. In forward or lateral flexion, the neck merely goes through a normal range of motion, with motion terminating as the chin strikes the chest or the ear strikes the shoulder. In hyperextension stresses the normal range of motion is greatly exceeded as the occiput strikes the upper posterior thorax.

A further observation is that patients with neck injuries of this type often have associated extremity injuries which healed on schedule and did not become sources of chronic complaints. If the causes of neck complaints were purely psychoneurotic, why would the extremity injuries be excluded from the neurotic disorder?

Macnab commented, "If neck pain following acceleration injuries is purely neurotic in origin, it is difficult to understand why patients commonly become neurotic if their head is thrown backward but rarely institute litigation if it is jolted forward or sideways" (16). He postulated therefore that hyperextension beyond the normal range produced damage, not well defined at that time, which was the cause of the lingering symptomatology.

Norris and Watt demonstrated that there was no statistical significance in improvement in symptoms or the lack thereof following settlement of claims (19). DePalma et al., had earlier also concluded that litigation did not influence the outcome of anterior cervical fusion (6).

Litigation following acceleration injury is so common that it may even be considered a part of the syndrome, and must be accepted as a fact of life. The litigant often has serious injury even if there are psychosocial factors at play, and medical evaluation and treatment should not be denied. The physician is the only professional who can establish the fact and the extent of physical injury, and, utilizing the psychologist consultant, determine the degree to which psychological factors are affecting the clinical problem. With contemporary technology, there is little excuse for the hostility which pervaded earlier times.

EXPERIMENTAL STUDIES

Much of the information needed to understand what happens in vehicular collisions to produce acceleration injury has long been available; Severy and associates conducted elegant studies of such collisions and described their results as long ago as 1955 (28). The work deserves far greater currency than it has received. These authors produced controlled rear-end collisions and measured the forces and deflections which resulted, using accelerometers and motion picture technique (Fig. 2). Human volunteers participated in some of the runs, and anthropomorphic models were used in the others. A front car was placed in a stationary position and was impacted from the rear by a second car moving at basically low rates of speed, approximately 10 miles per hour. The impact imparts energy to the stationary vehicle, causing it to accelerate forward. These forces are applied to the seat on which the unrestrained subject is seated. The subject's torso and shoulders accelerate with the seat, but because the head is not supported by the seat, there is a delay in its acceleration owing to its translational and rotational inertia, since it is propelled from below its center of rotation. Hence, the magnitude of acceleration of the head is greater than the peak acceleration of the car body since the delayed reaction results in a shorter time interval to overcome the differential velocity between head and car. Enormous forces are thus applied to the head and neck complex, even with low speed impact. Typical head accelerations of eleven times gravity were recorded resulting in the application of traction forces in excess of one hundred pounds to the head-neck complex. The initial direction of deflection was into hyperextension, and head action continued until a maximum extension of 122 degrees was reached, far in excess of the normal extension of 60 degrees. After extension ceases,

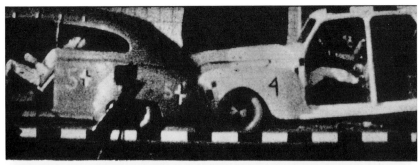

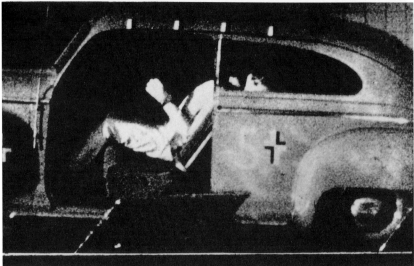

FIG. 2. Photograph of an experimental collision conducted by Severy et al. (28) showing marked hyperextension of the neck of the subject in the front car in response to acceleration imparted by a rear-end collision.

there is rebound into flexion, and several oscillations may occur (Fig. 3). These data demonstrate conclusively that a low speed rear-end collision is capable of applying seriously damaging forces to the head and neck, especially in anterior neck structures.

Animal experimentation has been conducted to investigate the pathology which results from the application of such forces. Macnab performed experiments in which monkeys were exposed to gravitational forces resulting in hyperextension strain (15). Anatomical dissection after the experimental injuries demonstrated a variety of pathological lesions, ranging from tears of the sternocleidomastoid muscles to ruptures of the longissimus colli muscles with associated retropharyngeal hematoma, all consistent with destructive elongation of these anterior structures from the excessive excursion of the neck into extension. Also observed were esophageal injury and disruption of the cervical sympathetic plexus. In some animals there was disruption of the anterior longitudinal ligament, and, most importantly, avulsion of the upper surface of the intervertebral disc from the vertebral body above (Fig. 4). Hence, a pathoanatomical basis for cervical intervertebral disc injury from hyperextension strain was established which is different from classical disc herniation. Avulsion of disc from bone deprives it of its normal nutritional pathway, and disc degeneration becomes preordained. A living human verification of this pathology was established surgically by Harris et al., who operated upon a patient with intractable symptoms following a whiplash injury and found separation of the C6–C7 disc from bone, with an inspissated fragment of end plate cartilage located within degenerated disc tissue (9).

Wickstrom and associates conducted a variety of studies of the whiplash injury in hares and primates which lend additional lucidity to the understanding of the etiology of protracted symptomatology (31,33–35). These exhaustively detailed experiments yielded a profusion of data which can only be briefly summarized here. In Belgium hares, the injuries sustained in acceleration injury included retrobulbar hemorrhage and hemorrhage into the ventricles, epidural space, and about the spinal cord (33). Disruption of the anterior longitudinal ligament was observed at C5–C6, and of the intertransverse ligament at C6–C7. Some animals developed tears of the atlanto-occipital ligaments and fractures of the upper cervical transverse processes. Disruption of the vertebral artery at the upper edge of C1 was also noted. More subtle abnormality was subperiosteal hemorrhage and hemorrhage under the posterior longitudinal ligament in the lower cervical vertebrae. The rabbit, however, was not found to be the most appropriate animal for comparison

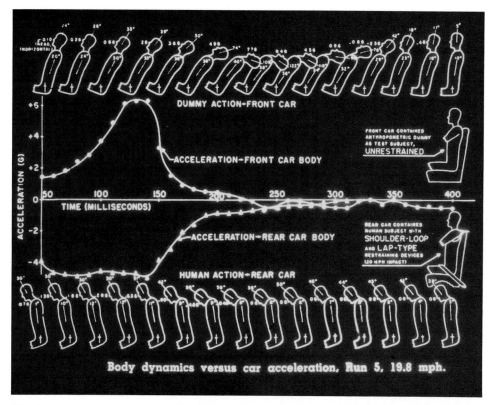

FIG. 3. This figure from the experimental studies of Severy et al. (28) is an illustration of details of the effect of acceleration on the neck in an unrestrained anthropomorphic dummy in the unmoving front car and a restrained human volunteer in the striking rear car which was traveling at 19.8 mph. Note the severe delayed hyperextension of the neck of the upper figure. Note further that the lower figure flexes the neck only within its normal range of motion.

with humans owing to the extreme flexibility of its neck and the proportionately lighter weight of its head in contrast to that of humans.

A more appropriate subject for comparison proved to be the monkey, and a number of experiments were conducted with this animal as subject (31,34,35). Inventory of tissue injury produced in primates detected brain damage in 32%, spinal cord damage in 5%, and nerve root damage in 0.7%. Ligamentous injury concentrated between C4 and C7 was noted in 11%, and intervertebral disc damage in 2.3% of the animals. Other pathologic changes included retropharyngeal hemorrhage, laryngeal hyperemia, and hemorrhage beneath the posterior longitudinal ligament or within the paraspinous muscles.

The skeletal injuries observed often involved apophyseal joint damage, inapparent on x-ray examination. Such changes included capsular tearing, cartilage fissuring with degenerative changes, and subchondral bone fracture, explaining a possibility for posterior column injury as a source of pain.

Following upon Wickstrom's initiative, Liu and associates studied electroencephalographic changes in rhesus monkeys after acceleration injury (14). EEG recordings were made from both scalp electrodes and chronically implanted electrodes. Wickstrom's earlier work had shown that scalp electrodes were a poor indicator of nervous tissue injury (31). With the use of implanted electrodes, Liu et al., were able to demonstrate epileptiform activity in the brain following experimental whiplash (14). Heath had shown that epileptiform discharges which met certain specific requirements were associated with "gross behavioral aberrations in the form of impaired emotionality and reduced awareness which progressed to catatonia" (10). Liu et al., proposed that the EEG spiking exhibited by whiplash primates "might be considered as a subclinical form of post-traumatic epilepsy." Whether or not these animal findings have relevance to the human whiplash syndrome, they certainly provoke thought, especially addressing Macnab's observation: "As the months roll by, it becomes increasingly apparent that the patient is grossly emotionally disturbed" (16). Leopold and Dillon had reviewed 47 patients with whiplash injury and found no relationship between post-traumatic emotional disorder and previously existing psychological disease (13). These considerations allow a justifiable, although tentative, conclusion that the effects of whiplash injury may include tissue damage in the brain as well as the skeleton.

Complementing all of these experimental studies is

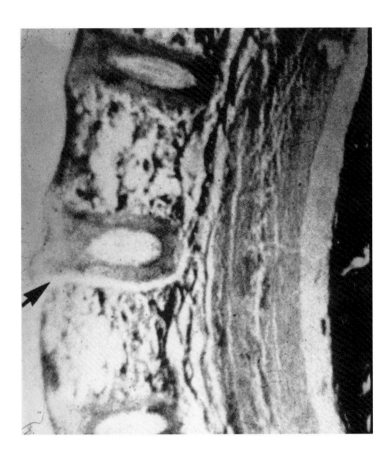

FIG. 4. A photomicrograph of one of Macnab's animal studies (15) showing avulsion of the disc from bone of the vertebral body above (arrow).

the report of Hohl who reviewed 146 patients at a mean time of 7 years following acceleration injury (11). None of the victims had evidence of pre-existing degenerative changes on acute phase radiographic examination, but at follow-up 39% demonstrated such changes, a frequency more than six times the expected 6% frequency for this age group. More detailed statistical analysis revealed that persons with more severe injury demonstrated a follow-up frequency of degenerative change of 60%. These included individuals who (a) were rendered unconscious by the injury, (b) demonstrated restricted motion at one level on dynamic lateral roentgenograms, or (c) were required to wear a collar for symptom control for three months or longer following injury.

The prognostic significance of radiologic abnormalities following acceleration was analyzed in a group of 73 patients by Miles et al. (18). Radiographs were evaluated for specific changes, and then the clinical situation at two years following injury was assessed. Patients who had degenerative changes at the time of initial presentation were significantly more likely to have persisting problems at follow-up, while those with angular deformities at presentation had a better prognosis regarding symptom persistence two years later. They found no late effect related to the presence of prevertebral soft tissue swelling in the absence of bony injury.

These data indicate that the intervertebral disc injury

found in the various laboratory experiments is probably a significant and frequent component of the human acceleration injury as well, and if so, helps explain why the clinical course is often protracted. Unfortunately, plain-film radiography does not demonstrate the development of degenerative changes for many years, and even magnetic resonance imaging will not do so until a damaged disc has had time to dessicate. If the severity of the problem is grave enough, provocative radiologic techniques including discography and/or facet blocking may be the only way to identify the source of peripheral nociception.

MANAGEMENT

Precise, detailed history elicitation is the essential beginning of management of any victim of an acceleration injury, for it provides the best measure of the magnitude of force to which the head-neck complex has been exposed. The greater the magnitude, the more ominous is the prognosis. Physical examination also can provide prognostic information, as established so well by Norris and Watt (19). Radiographic study is imperative, including flexion and extension laterals (36). Should there be straightening of the cervical curve (Fig. 5), acute cervical reversal on dynamic study (11), or pre-existing degenera-

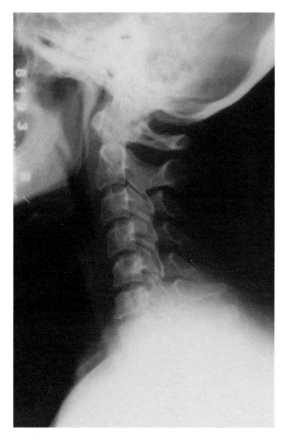

FIG. 5. Lateral radiograph of the cervical spine of a 35-year-old woman taken within hours of an acceleration injury, demonstrating straightening of the vertebral column and degenerative changes at C6-C7, which pre-existed the event. Symptoms have persisted in excess of 18 months, in spite of conservative therapy.

tive changes, again the prognosis is not favorable for early recovery.

Which therapeutic modalities are appropriate in a given case is determined by the severity of the problem (12). The customary conservative measures of orthopedics and neurosurgery are indicated, and include the use of cervical collars, physical therapy modalities, and anti-inflammatory, muscle relaxant, and analgesic medications. Although these are generally administered on an out-patient basis, if symptoms are too intense, a brief hospitalization may be required. The role of epidural injection of a narcotic and steroid has not been systematically evaluated, but based on anecdotal experience, may be reasonably considered to interrupt the "pain-spasm" cycle. The application of the mobilization principles of sports medicine has been reported to show promise in treatment of acceleration injuries (17).

Surgery is reserved for the more severe and intractable cases. Definite and certainly progressive neurologic deficits may demand decompression early on. Disc avulsion injuries with attendent disc degeneration may require

disc excision and fusion, if they persist in provoking intolerable symptoms for six to twelve months in spite of acceptable conservative therapy.

A more suitable approach than management of injury remains prevention of the injury in the first place. Ever since the report of Severy et al., it has been known that the most injurious aspect of acceleration injury is hyperextension of the head-neck complex (28). It would seem that better automotive design could minimize the disorder, but the report of O'Neill et al., is most discouraging, indicating that the requirement for head restraints has not appreciably reduced the frequency of whiplash injuries, estimated to be in excess of one million per year in the United States (22). The fault is not in the concept, but in its application, for if the restraint is improperly positioned, it either does not restrain or serves as a more vicious fulcrum. Olney and Marsden were unable to show a significant reduction in neck injuries when head restraints were in place (21), and attribute this largely to improperly positioned restraints, usually placed too low or too far posterior to the driver's head. They recommend that the head should be as close as possible to the restraint before impact, 25 mm or less. This should restrict head propulsion enough to eliminate damaging forces. Depending upon how sanguine one's view of humanity is, there does remain the possibility that the epidemic of acceleration injury can be eliminated through the transfer of scientific information into the public domain, generating both better automotive design and increased driver awareness.

REFERENCES

1. Balla JI (1980): The late whiplash syndrome. *Aust NZ J Surg* 50:610–614.
2. Bland JH (1987): *Disorders of the cervical spine.* Philadelphia: W.B. Saunders, pp. 224–225.
3. Chrisman OD, Gervais RF (1962): Otologic manifestations of the cervical syndrome. *Clin Orthop* 24:34–39.
4. Crowe HD (1958): Whiplash injuries in the cervical spine. Proc. insurance negligence and compensation law. American Bar Association, pp. 176–184.
5. Deans GT, Magalliard JN, Kerr M, Rutherford WH (1987): Neck sprain—a major cause of disability following car accidents. *Injury* 18(1):10–12.
6. DePalma AF, Rothman RH, Lewinnek GE, Canale ST (1972): Anterior interbody fusion for severe cervical disc degeneration. *Surg Gynecol Obstet* 134:755–758.
7. Gay JR, Abbott KH (1953): Common whiplash injuries of the neck. *JAMA* 152:1698–1704.
8. Gotten N (1956): Survey of one hundred cases of whiplash injury after settlement of litigation. *JAMA* 162:865–867.
9. Harris WH, Hamblen DL, Ojemann RG (1968): Traumatic disruption of cervical intervertebral disk from hyperextension injury. *Clin Orthop* 60:163–167.
10. Heath RG (1972): Physiologic basis of emotional expression: evoked potential and mirror focus studies in rhesus monkeys. *Biol Psychol* 5:15–31.
11. Hohl M (1974): Soft-tissue injuries of the neck in automobile accidents. *J Bone Joint Surg* [Am] 56:1675–1682.
12. La Rocca H (1978): Acceleration injuries of the neck. *Clin Neurosurg* 25:209–217.

13. Leopold RL, Dillon H (1960): Psychiatric considerations in whiplash injuries of the neck *Pa Med* 63:385–389.
14. Liu YK, Chandran KB, Heath RG, Unterharnscheidt F (1984): Subcortical EEG changes in rhesus monkeys following experimental hyperextension-hyperflexion (whiplash). *Spine* 9:329–338.
15. Macnab I (1964): Acceleration injuries of the cervical spine. *J Bone Joint Surg* [Am] 46:1797–1799.
16. Macnab I (1969): Acceleration-extension injuries of the cervical spine. In: *Symposium on the Spine.* St. Louis: C.V. Mosby, pp. 10–17.
17. Mealy K, Brennan H, Fenelon GC (1986): Early mobilization of acute whiplash injuries. *Br Med J* [*Clin Res*] 292:656–657.
18. Miles KA, Maimaris C, Finlay D, Barnes MR (1988): The incidence and prognostic significance of radiological abnormalities in soft tissue injuries to the cervical spine. *Skeletal Radiol* 17:493–496.
19. Norris SH, Watt I (1983): The prognosis of neck injuries resulting from rear-end vehicle collisions. *J Bone Joint Surg* [Br] 65:608–611.
20. Nygren A (1984): Injuries to car occupants—some aspects of the interior safety of cars. *Acta Otolaryngol (Stockh)* 395(Suppl.):1–164.
21. Olney DB, Marsden AK (1986): The effect of head restraints and seat belts on the incidence of neck injury in car accidents. *Injury* 17:365–367.
22. O'Neill B, Haddon W Jr, Kelley AB, Sorenson WW (1972): Automobile head restraints—frequency of neck injury claims in relation to the presence of head restraints. *Am J Public Health* 62:399–406.
23. Rajanov BP, Dvorak J, Valach I (in press): Cognitive deficits in patients after soft tissue injury of the cervical spine. *Spine.*
24. Rosa L, Carol M, Bellegarrique R, Ducker TB (1984): Multiple cranial nerve palsies due to a hyperextension injury to the cervical spine. *J Neurosurg* 61:172–173.
25. Rotstein OD, Rhame FS, Molina E, Simmons RL (1986): Mediastinitis after whiplash injury. *Can J Surg* 29:54–56.
26. Rutherford WH, Greenfield AA, Hayes HRM (1985): *The medical effects of seat-belt legislation in the United Kingdom.* London: HMSD.
27. Scher AT (1983): Hyperextension trauma in the elderly: an easily overlooked spinal injury. *J Trauma* 23:1066–1068.
28. Severy DM, Mathewson JH, Bechtol CO (1955): Controlled automobile rear-end collisions; an investigation of related engineering and medical phenomena. *Can Serv Med J* 11:727–759.
29. Stringer WL, Kelly DL Jr, Johnston FR, Holliday RH (1980): Hyperextension injury of the cervical spine with esophageal perforation. *J Neurosurg* 53:541–543.
30. Weinberg S, Lapointe H (1987): Cervical extension-flexion injury (whiplash) and internal derangement of the temporomandibular joint. *J Oral Maxillofac Surg* 45:653–656.
31. Wickstrom J, La Rocca H (1975): Management of patients with cervical spine and head injuries from acceleration forces. In: Ahstrom JP Jr, ed. *Current practice in orthopaedic surgery.* St. Louis: CV Mosby, pp. 83–98.
32. Wickstrom JK, Martinez JL, Johnston D, Tappen NC (1965): Acceleration-deceleration injuries of the cervical spine in animals. In: Proceedings of the seventh stapp car crash conference. Springfield: Thomas, pp. 284–301.
33. Wickstrom JK, Martinez J, Rodriguez R (1967): Cervical sprain syndrome, experimental acceleration injuries of the head and neck. In: Proceedings of the symposium on the prevention of highway injury. Ann Arbor: The University of Michigan Press, pp. 182–187.
34. Wickstrom JK, Martinez JL, Rodriguez R, Haines DM (1970): Hyperextension and hyperflexion injuries to the head and neck of primates. In: Gurdjian ES, Thomas IM, eds. *Neckache and Backache.* Springfield: Thomas, pp. 108–117.
35. Wickstrom JK, Rodriguez RP, Martinez JL (1968): Experimental production of acceleration injuries of the head and neck. In: *Accident pathology.* Washington DC: US Government Printing Office, pp. 185–189.
36. Winston KR (1987): Whiplash and its relationship to migraine. *Headache* 27:452–457.

The Adult Spine: Principles and Practice,
J. W. Frymoyer, Editor-in-Chief.
Raven Press, Ltd., New York © 1991.

CHAPTER 51

Cervical Spine Trauma

Paul C. McAfee

Traumatic injuries to the cervical spine, a common cause of death and disability, range in severity from simple soft tissue injuries to fractures with paralysis or death. These injuries are often seen in the emergency room and must be carefully evaluated to minimize adverse long-term sequelae to the patient. Early diagnosis, restoration and preservation of spinal cord function, and stabilization are the keys to successful management.

Up to one third of cervical spine injuries result from motor vehicle accidents, one third from falls, and a final third from injuries sustained in athletics or from falling objects or fired projectiles (5,17). The majority of injuries occur in young, active individuals during adolescence and early adulthood. The second largest group comprises individuals in their sixth and seventh decades. Pre-existing canal stenosis and cervical spondylosis predispose this age group to severe neurologic injuries when a small amount of force is imparted to the cervical spine.

The formation of spinal cord injury centers has significantly improved emergency, medical, and surgical care and rehabilitation of the patient who has sustained a

P. C. McAfee, M.D.: Associate Professor, Departments of Orthopaedic Surgery and Neurosurgery, The Johns Hopkins Hospital, Baltimore, Maryland; Chief of Spinal Surgery, St. Joseph's Hospital Spinal Center, Towson, Maryland; Orthopaedic Associates, P.A., Baltimore, Maryland, 21202.

spine and spinal cord injury. Bohlman (5), Ducker (18), Stauffer (45), and the National Acute Spinal Cord Injury Study Group (7), among others, have made advances in the pathophysiologic basis of spine and spinal cord injuries that have allowed improved non-operative and operative approaches, including internal fixation of the injured spine. It has been recognized that a team approach is essential to the care of the spinal-cord-injured patient to obtain the optimum result (6). Whereas mortality from cervical injuries was 80% just 50 years ago (24), the current mortality rate with spine injury centers is now 6% (7). The initial therapeutic goals are to preserve life, maintain neurologic function or restore cord and nerve root function through appropriate decompression, provide stabilization of the cervical spine, and allow optimum rehabilitation. These goals are attainable if proper care is provided.

PRINCIPLES OF TREATMENT

Emergency Resuscitation

Care for a patient with a possible cervical spinal injury should begin at the scene of the accident. McGuire (32) determined the most effective means of immobilizing the cervical spine and allowing extraction of a victim from a motor vehicle accident. A Philadelphia halo immobilizer proved to be the most effective orthosis and was specifically designed for this purpose. It can immobilize the head, cervical spine, and upper thoracic spine, whether the patient is found initially in the prone or supine position. The patient can be kept in the Philadelphia halo immobilizer throughout the entire emergency room and radiographic evaluation. Care should be taken to prevent further injury, which can be caused by inadvertent axial load, flexion, extension, distraction, or rotation forces or the application of overzealous traction (Figs. 1 and 2). If a Philadelphia halo immobilizer is not available, the patient's neck should be placed in a Philadelphia collar and the head supported with sand bags until a significant cervical injury can be assessed by spinal radiographs. Upon arrival in the emergency department, resuscitation should be performed with the usual priority for airway, breathing, and circulation. In the process of securing an airway, care should be taken to prevent further cervical injury. In the event severe facial swelling prevents intubation without cervical manipulation, a cricothyroidotomy should be performed. A useful technique is to insert a 14-gauge angiocath needle through the cricothyroid membrane. The outside housing on a 5 cc syringe is then attached to the 14-gauge angiocath, and the syringe is then connected to the supe-

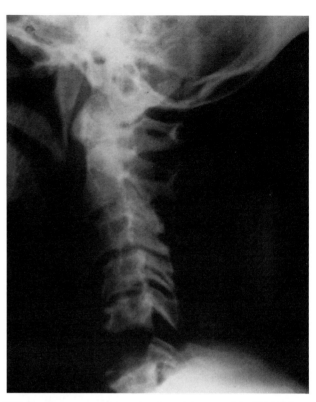

FIG. 2. Gross overdistraction is evident as this C5-C6 fracture dislocation was treated in 40 pounds of halo traction. This magnitude of weight is well within the general guidelines of 5 pounds traction per level down to the level of injury. However, with 3-column injuries (anterior, middle, and posterior osteoligamentous longitudinal columns) check x-rays must be obtained after each 5 pounds of sequential weight.

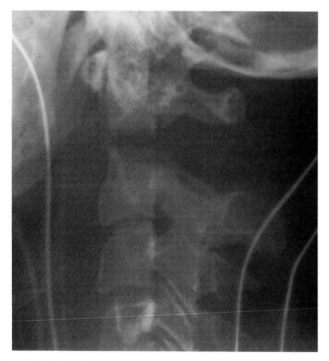

FIG. 1. Overdistraction can unfortunately occur in the upper cervical spine. Above is a 20-year-old white male who sustained a Type II odontoid fracture. With only 10 pounds of traction, the fracture has grossly overdistracted. Particularly with traumatic injuries superior to the C2-C3 disc space, a maximum of 5 pounds, and usually 3 pounds, is recommended for initial reduction.

rior end of a Shierly-7 endotracheal tube. This technique allows the airway apparatus to be connected to an Ambu bag or directly to a ventilator. One hundred percent oxygen can be administered, which is sufficient to provide a patient with oxygenation for approximately 35 minutes. This greatly increases the time in which a tracheostomy can be successfully performed. Intravenous access should also be established for fluid resuscitation.

An initial history must be obtained from the patient, paramedics, or witnesses to determine the mechanism of injury. A history of a loss of consciousness or paralysis at the scene of the accident is important. The patient who has a spinal cord concussion may have no objective findings at the time of evaluation in the emergency department. Thus, important neck injuries may be overlooked.

In Bohlman's (5) evaluation of 300 cervical spinal injuries, 100 were initially missed at the time of presentation. Delay in diagnosis ranged from 1 day to 1 year. The common causes for lack of initial recognition were closed head injuries, polytrauma, alcohol intoxication, and initial misdiagnosis such as cerebrovascular accidents. An alteration in the level of consciousness contributed to the lack of proper evaluation and failure to take appropriate radiographs. These patients often do not complain of neck pain, particularly in the presence of facial and skull lacerations. Bohlman (5) found a high correlation between head and neck injuries in patients; thus, any evidence of head trauma increases the suspicion of a cervical spine injury.

While a history is being obtained, a general physical examination can be performed (9). As noted, the presence of craniofacial trauma can be important in the assessment of the mechanism of injury (8). If the patient is conscious, the anterior and posterior cervical structures can be gently palpated to determine local pain and soft tissue swelling. The posterior elements can be palpated along the midline posteriorly—particular attention should be paid to an increase in the interspinous distance. The anterior vertebral bodies can be palpated in the interval between the sternocleidomastoid and the trachea.

In addition to a general physical examination, a detailed neurologic examination must be performed. The general state of consciousness must be specifically assessed, as must the respiratory state of the patient. The diaphragm is innervated by cervical level C3 to C5. Complete transection of the cord above the level of C5 can lead to respiratory failure. If the patient is conscious, a detailed motor and sensory examination of the upper and lower extremities is performed. In all patients reflex activity must be tested and rectal tone determined. If the patient shows signs of spinal cord shock or if the bulbocavernosus reflex is absent in a patient with a neurologic deficit, a Foley catheter should be inserted. All patients with a spinal cord injury should have a nasogastric tube and Foley catheter in place, as well as a large-bore intravenous line for access; consideration should also be given to a central venous line. The presence or absence of sacral sparing or the bulbocavernosus reflex should be repeatedly monitored in light of its prognostic significance to later return of neurologic traction.

Radiographic Evaluation

As the initial evaluation proceeds, the radiographic examination of the cervical spine must be planned and executed. A lateral view of the cervical spine must include visualization of the entire cervical spine, including the anterior and posterior elements of C3 to C7. A swimmer's view, tomography, or CT scan may be necessary to delineate the C7-T1 relationship if manual distraction of the shoulders is not sufficient. After the lateral view is examined, the anteroposterior and oblique views can be

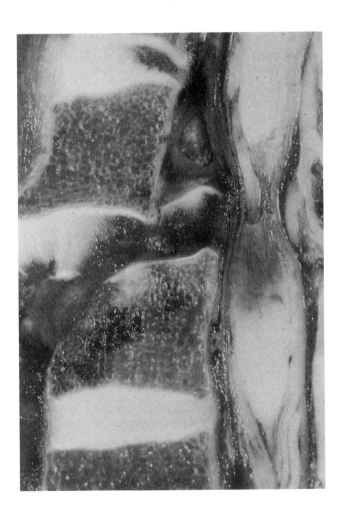

FIG. 3. This paramedian sagittal section is taken from a 25-year-old man thrown from his automobile. On admission he was tetraplegic below C6. Two attempts were made at closed reduction under anesthesia which were unsuccessful, and the partial reduction obtained could not be maintained. Note the anterior upper portion of the C6 body is crushed, C5 is subluxed anteriorly, and the annulus has avulsed a bony endplate ridge from the posterior lower endplate of C5. The periosteum and posterior longitudinal ligament have been stripped off the posterior surface of C5, resulting in a triangular subperiosteal pocket into which large fragments of ruptured disc have dislodged. If attempts at posterior reduction or wiring were made, or increased axial load applied, this would force the disc posteriorly, further compressing the spinal cord. If narrowing of the intervertebral disc is seen on plane lateral radiographs, an MRI should be obtained rather than simply increasing the amount of skeletal traction (with permission from ref. 37).

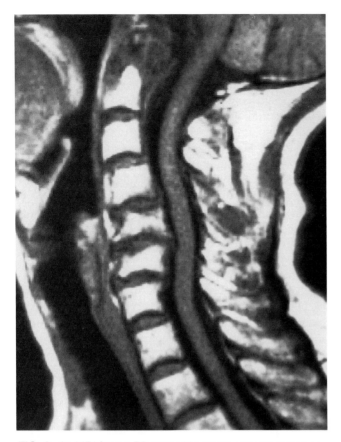

FIG. 4. An MRI from a 75-year-old patient with cervical spondylitic myelopathy stemming from avulsion of a C5 posterior marginal vertebral body osteophyte. A C5-C6 anterior decompression must include a hemicorpectomy at C5 and C6 to remove the offending osteophytes in order to accomplish an adequate spinal decompression.

obtained in succession. If substantial osseous injury is found on the AP and lateral views, then pillar views should be obtained in a caudal to cranial angle of 30 degrees so that the facets can be visualized without turning the head. An open-mouth view is necessary to assess the odontoid and C1-C2 relationship.

A water-soluble contrast enhanced CT scan is helpful in defining injured structures and the presence of bone or soft tissue fragments in the space available for the cord, as well as areas in need of decompression. A C1-C2 puncture with insertion of water-soluble contrast can be performed by an experienced neuroradiologist without turning the patient. The available radiographic data must be interpreted carefully to assess osseous fracture and displacement. In addition, the retropharyngeal space must be examined to look for the presence of swelling, which lends further evidence to the presence of osseous or ligamentous injury (47). In addition, MRI is gaining increased popularity, and there is some evidence that it may be a better predictor of the potential for neurologic recovery (16), as well as predict risks for neurologic injury with certain fractures, and fracture/dislocations (Figs. 3 and 4). A lesion, as shown in Figure 3, is at risk for increased neurologic deficit with increasing traction or attempted posterior reduction and fusion, shown clinically by Eismont et al (21). MRI is essential to delineate the true nature of the pathology in such cases.

After the initial views are interpreted, one can assess the clinical stability of the spine using the biomechanical criteria of White and Panjabi (49) (Table 1). Before assessing stability, it is important to determine the fracture pattern. The anterior, posterior, and lateral elements can be involved solely or in combination.

TABLE 1. *Guidelines for biomechanical interpretation of radiographs*

Element	Point value
Anterior elements destroyed or unable to function	2
Posterior elements destroyed or unable to function	2
Relative sagittal plane translation > 3.5 mm	2
Relative sagittal plane rotation > 11°	2
Positive stretch test	2
Spinal cord damage	2
Nerve root damage	1
Abnormal disc narrowing	1
Dangerous loading anticipated	1

Total of 5 or more = unstable

With permission from ref. 49.

FRACTURES AND DISLOCATIONS FROM THE BASE OF THE SKULL TO C3

Functionally, flexion and extension occur largely as a function of the occiput to C1 joint, and approximately 50% of rotation occurs at C1-C2 (34). One way to classify these injuries is shown in Figure 5. When rotation is forced between the skull and C1, a rare but serious occipitocervical dislocation occurs. Either the left or the right lateral masses of C1 are forced posteriorly or anteriorly on the occipital condyles. This dislocation, if the patient survives, may go undetected despite bizarre angulation of the skull unless good quality tomograms or CT scans are obtained. This is an extremely unstable injury and should be treated with a posterior occiput to C2 fusion and wire stabilization. The patient should also be managed in a halo for approximately 3 months. Eismont and Bohlman (20) reported a case of posterior dislocation of the occiput sliding off posteriorly on the supporting masses of C1. The tip of the odontoid was avulsed by the alar ligament. It is common for these cases to be misdiagnosed, and their case was no exception.

JEFFERSON'S FRACTURE

The Jefferson's fracture is a bursting of the ring of C1 as a result of axial loading directly downward on the ring of C1, causing multiple fractures of the ring and usually accompanied by a spreading of fragments (Figs. 6A–6E). An anteroposterior film generally shows widening of the distance between the odontoid and lateral masses of C1. Spence's rule is that the overhang from the lateral masses of C1 on each side should not total more than 6.9 mm. In addition, a lateral view may show anterior subluxation of C1 on C2, indicating a disruption of the attachments of the transverse odontoid ligament (35–38). The advent of CT scanning made the diagnosis of Jefferson's fracture and follow-up of the healing process easier and more accurate. In addition, congenital anomalies of the arch of C1, such as agenesis of a posterior ring of C1, are commonly observed in patients with traumatic injuries.

An additional condition that may occur in upper cervical spinal injuries is avulsion of the superior aspect of the odontoid secondary to avulsion of the alar ligaments. The fragment can migrate superiorly into the foramen magnum, resulting in compression of the base of the brain at the pontomedullary junction. It is not possible to remove a fractured odontoid fragment from a posterior approach. If the patient has a neurologic deficit, consideration should be given to a transoral approach to the neck or an anterior retropharyngeal approach.

A combination of Jefferson's fracture and fracture of the odontoid is fairly common. The traditional treatment is to manage the patient in a halo vest or halo cast until the Jefferson's fracture heals. Once it has healed, and if the odontoid fracture progresses to delayed nonunion, a posterior C1-C2 arthrodesis can be performed.

The current state of the art for treatment of a combined Jefferson's fracture and odontoid fracture is anterior open reduction and internal fixation of the odontoid using two 4.0 mm AO/ASIF screws placed in an oblique direction starting at the inferior anterior edge of C2 and aiming in a cephalad direction to engage the odontoid process. As an alternative, Magerl (27) recommends a posterior open reduction accompanied by internal fixation C1-C2 arthrodesis. Two screws are placed in an oblique position starting at the inferior edge of the lamina of C2, which cross the C1-C2 facet joints between the vertebral artery laterally and the spinal cord medially. However, North American investigators have very little experience with this technique.

Vertebrobasilar injuries have also been reported with atlanto-occipital dislocations. Although total disruption of the vertebrobasilar system causes death, there are more than 20 cases in the literature of less severe injuries to the vertebrobasilar system produced by mechanisms such as chiropractic manipulation, yoga exercises, overhead work, and cervical traction. The mechanism of injury is cervical hyperextension accompanied by excessive rotation. Severely diminished blood flow through the vertebral artery may lead to occlusion of the posterior inferior cerebellar artery on that side, resulting in Wallenberg's syndrome. The syndrome is characterized by ipsilateral loss of cranial nerves V, IX, X, and XI; cerebellar ataxia; Horner's syndrome; and contralateral loss of pain and temperature sensation.

Suspected vertebrobasilar injury should be diagnosed or confirmed by subtraction angiography. Arteriography also helps to assess the adequacy of collateral circulation. Treatment consists of immediate anticoagulation with Heparin to prevent further extension of thrombosis and administration of oxygen to maintain cerebral oxygenation.

TRAUMATIC SPONDYLOLISTHESIS OF THE AXIS

The best review and classification of hangman's fracture were reported by Levine and Edwards (26) in 1985 on a series of 52 patients. Type I injuries have a fracture through the neural arch with no angulation and as much as 3 mm of displacement. Type II fractures have significant angulation and/or significant displacement. Type IIA fractures show minimum displacement, but there is severe angulation; apparently the vertebral bodies remain hinged together through the anterior longitudinal ligament. Type III axis fractures combine bilateral facet dislocation between the second and third cervical vertebrae with a fracture of the neural arch. Angulation between C2 and C3 is measured by the Cobb technique, and anterior translation is measured as the distance between two lines drawn, one parallel to the posterior margin of the body of the third cervical vertebra and the second parallel to the posterior margin of the body of the second cervical vertebra at the level of the C2-C3 space. According to Levine and Edwards (26), Type I fractures are stable injuries and are adequately treated with collar protection. Most Type II injuries require reduction with the patient in halo traction, followed by immobilization in a halo vest. Type IIA injuries show increased displacement in traction and are best reduced with very gentle extension followed by compression in a halo vest. Type III injuries are grossly unstable and require surgical stabilization through a posterior approach. Type I injuries result from hyperextension and axial loading forces; Type II injuries from an initial hyperextension-axial loading force followed by severe flexion; Type IIA injuries from flexion/distraction; and Type III injuries from flexion/compression. In any case, the severity of instability of the hangman's fracture is dependent on the ligamentous stability of the C2-C3 intervertebral disc space. It is extremely important to recognize unstable hang-

Text continues on page 1075.

FIG. 5. Craniocervical trauma with injuries around the C1-C2 complex.

In injuries high in the cervical spine, there are a series of fractures that occur depending on the major vector of the traumatic force. As represented in this clock of injuries, the vector of force at 12 o'clock is distraction, while 3 o'clock is forced extension, 6 o'clock is compression, and 9 o'clock is forced flexion. When these vectors cause trauma at the C1-C2 complex, including the cranial junction, there are known injury patterns.

If the resultant injury is severe with marked malalignment, the majority of the patients are killed instantaneously or die soon afterwards for lack of respiration and cardiovascular support. Such injuries, which cause complete cord damage, give not only paralysis, but also give a complete sympathectomy and destroy all drive for respiration including the phrenic nerve function. However, many injuries through this area give an incomplete cord injury or do hardly any damage to the nervous system at all. Each of these injuries is discussed separately in this chapter. This diagram is simply to give the reader an overall view of the injury patterns. These diagrams will help us understand the treatments. Diagrams were developed for teaching purposes by Doctors Thomas B. Ducker and Paul C. McAfee, and many of these diagrams have been used in teaching materials by the American College of Surgeons as well as the medical schools.

At 12 o'clock, there is primarily a distraction injury wherein the condyles of the occiput are pulled from the C1-C2 complex. This particular injury is more likely to be seen on the lateral skull x-ray as opposed to a lateral cervical spine x-ray. Also, it can occur in young children, where the head is much bigger in proportion to the body. It is also commonly reported in those patients sustaining an injury who are killed in the accident wherein there is no other obvious reason for death.

At 2 o'clock, the extension injury may cause a high fracture of the odontoid process itself. There is usually retrolisthesis of the C1 complex on the C2 vertebral body and its surrounding lamina and spinous process.

At 3 o'clock, the extension injury often causes fractures through the lamina of C1 and C2. If the fracture through C2 comes more anteriorly, then it will cause traumatic spondylolosis. Even on rare occasions, the odontoid may be fractured as well.

At 4 o'clock, one sees a typical Hangman's fracture with a traumatic spondylolosis between the facet area of C2 and the major body of C2. The line of trauma will separate the body of C2 with all of C1, leaving behind the C2 lamina and spinous process, which are in turn attached to the C3 vertebra. The Hangman's fracture can truly occur with hangings, but one will rarely see that clinically. More commonly, it is associated with a vehicular accident where there is forced extension of the head and upper part of the spine on the mid and lower part of the cervical spine.

At 5 o'clock, one is more likely to see a compression fracture into the body of C2. This may be a form of the Type III odontoid fracture where there is a burst in the body.

At 6 o'clock, there tend to be two types of fractures. When the C1 vertebra alone is involved, some form of a Jefferson ring fracture is apparent. Or, in some lesions the ring of C1 will be maintained and there will be a burst fracture of C2. Admittedly, the latter is rare, but has been documented. This would be marked as a very severe Type III odontoid fracture in select cases, but there is bursting of the body below.

At 7 o'clock, there are various types of Type II and Type III odontoid fractures. If the force is considerably anterior as well as compressed, there will be a form of the Type III fracture. However, as the force becomes more pure flexion, more likely the patient will suffer a Type I fracture. On rare occasions, one can see the trauma as depicted at 8 o'clock, usually with a devastating outcome to the patient. There is marked displacement on a Type II fracture with disruption of the anterior ligaments.

At 9 o'clock, one typically sees the Type II dens fracture with displacement of the C1 vertebra along with the dens of C2 anteriorly.

At 10 o'clock, there can be disruption of the ligaments from the C1 vertebral body which holds the peg of the C2 dens in alignment. This rupture of the cruciate ligament can lead to anterior displacement of C1 with all the bony elements of C2 being maintained.

At 11 o'clock, there is the rare Type I dens fracture. This is an avulsion fracture. It is rarely documented. Clinically we have seen only one case. We feel the mechanism is probably a function of twisting, flexion, and some distraction.

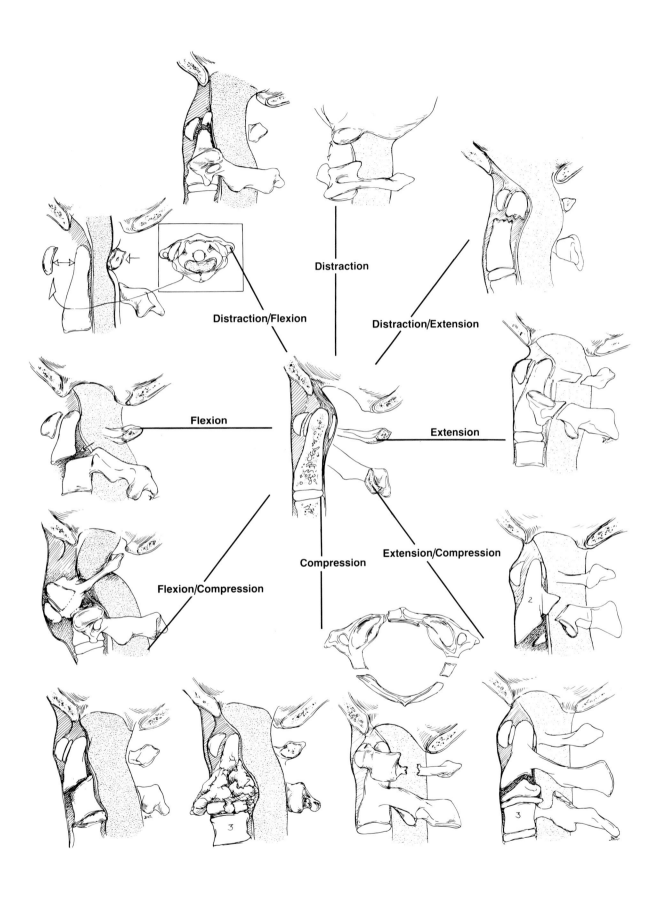

A

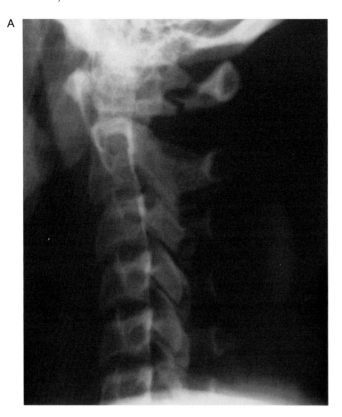

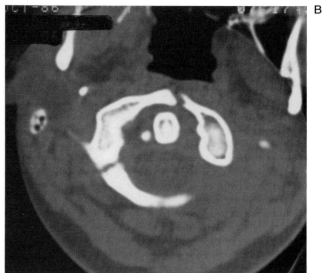

B

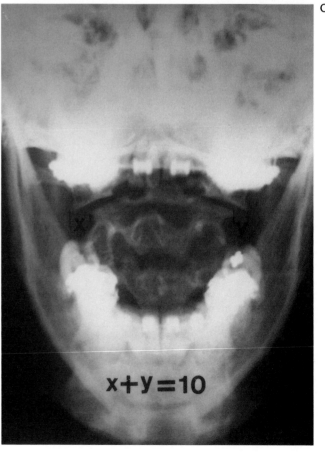

C

FIG. 6. An 18-year-old girl sustained a Jefferson's fracture, as well as an unstable C1-C2 subluxation secondary to avulsion of the lateral mass of C1 from the transverse odontal ligament. **A:** The lateral radiograph demonstrates the Jefferson's fracture. **B:** An axial CT image demonstrates avulsion of the lateral mass of C1 from the left hand attachment of the transverse ligament. Also evident is the anterior and left posterolateral portions of the Jefferson's fracture. **C:** This view demonstrates Spence's rule which is that the overhanging distance of the C1 lateral masses on C2 should never total more than 6.9 mm. X + Y in this patient's example is 10 mm and therefore demonstrates a displaced Jefferson's fracture. (Figs. 6D–6E follow.)

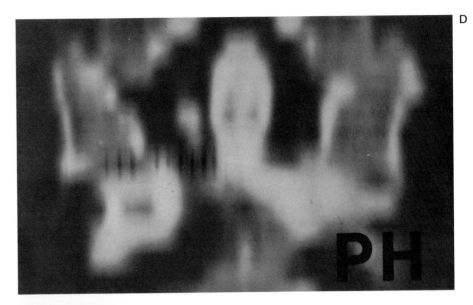

D

FIG. 6. *(Continued)* **D:** A reconstructed coronal multiplanar CT scan demonstrates the odontoid, as well as the fleck of bone which has avulsed from the lateral mass of C1.

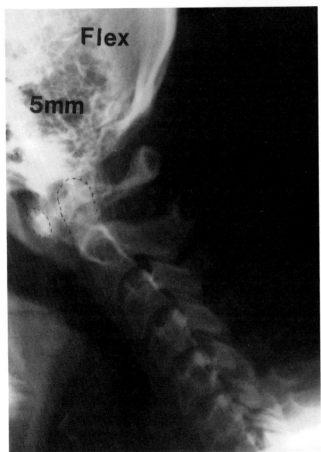

E

Fig. 6. *(Continued)* **E:** Following 6 months of treatment in a halo the patient still demonstrated C1-C2 anterior instability of 5 mm. For this reason, a posterior fusion at C1-C2 was performed. Two years after surgery the C1-C2 arthrodesis was solid. The initial treatment of the patient in the halo obviated the need for posterior fusion and stabilization to extend to the occiput.

A 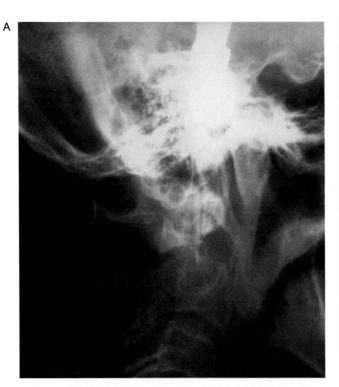 B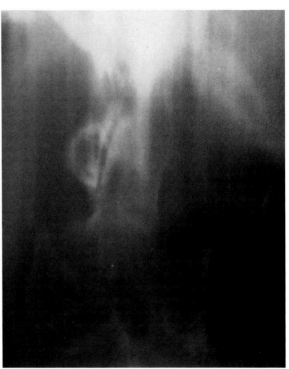

FIG. 7. This 72-year-old woman sustained a posteriorly displaced Type II odontoid fracture and was neurologically intact. Original lateral radiograph **(A)** taken in 5 pounds of Gardner-Wells tongs shows that the fracture is still unreduced and displaced the entire diameter of the odontoid. As a general rule, slight flexion with traction aids the reduction of these injuries (which are much more unstable than the usual anteriorly-displaced odontoid fracture). A lateral tomogram **(B)** demonstrates the large degree of anterior bone loss due to the comminution of the C2 vertebral body. (Figs. 7C-7E follow.)

C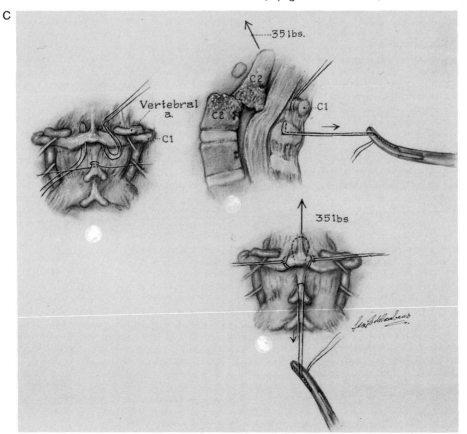

FIG. 7. *(Continued)* **C:** Open reduction and internal fixation through a posterior approach were required in this patient. By placing a wire through and around the junction of the base of the spinous process of C2 and the lamina of C2, a posteriorly directed force on the C2 vertebra could be applied. Two wires were then placed through and around the posterior C1 arch. The patient was placed in 35 pounds of intra-operative traction and near-anatomic reduction of the fracture was achieved. (Figs. 7D-7E follow.)

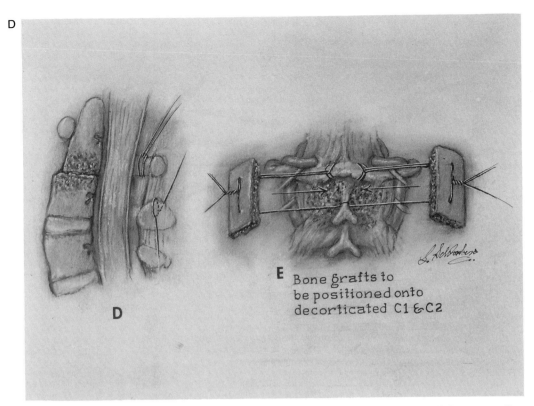

FIG. 7. *(Continued)* **D:** Posterior triple wire fixation and fusion were obtained (*D*) utilizing two cortico-cancellous bone struts (*E*) harvested from the iliac crest.

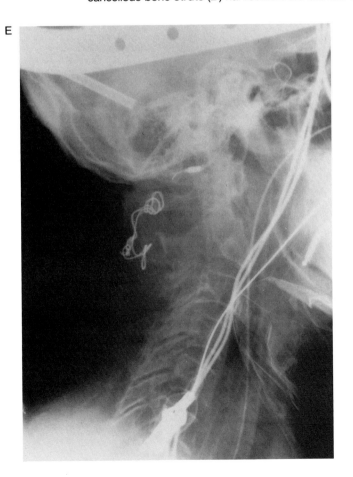

FIG. 7. *(Continued)* **E:** An intra-operative lateral radiograph demonstrates near anatomic reduction of the fracture with posterior C1-C2 stabilization.

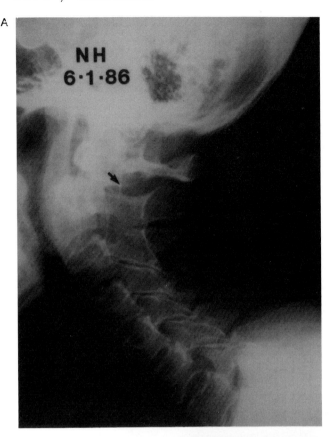

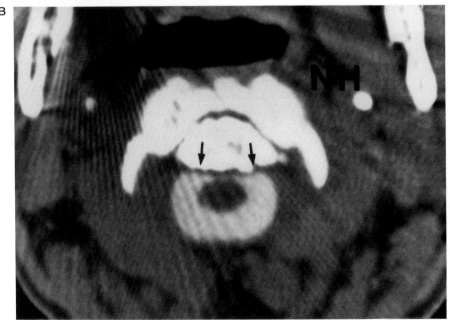

FIG. 8. This is a middle-aged woman who was treated in a halo for 1 month following a posteriorly displaced C1-C2 injury. In contrast to the case in Figure 7, the fracture could not be reduced at the time of referral to us, as early healing had occurred. The patient had hyperactive reflexes and spasticity, as well as bilateral ankle clonus. **A:** The arrow demonstrates the site of neurologic compression. **B:** An axial CT myelogram demonstrates anterior compression of the spinal cord secondary to the posteriorly displaced odontoid fragment. (Figs. 8C-8D follow.)

C

D

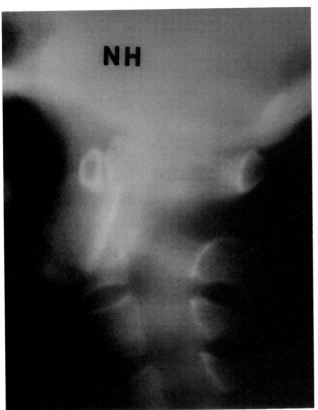

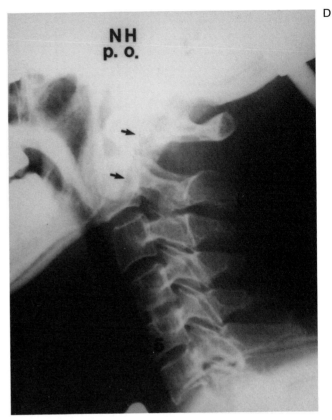

FIG. 8. *(Continued)* This injury required anterior extraoral decompression of the odontoid fracture secondary to the fixed nature of the deformity. The tomogram **(C)** outlines the posterior aspect of an iliac strut graft which has been wedged from the odontoid remnant and the inferior aspect of the C2 vertebral body. An excellent anterior decompression of the spinal canal was achieved. Three months following anterior extraoral decompression and fusion **(D)**, the patient was neurologically intact and a solid arthrodesis is evident.

man's fractures, as only 5 pounds of traction will cause gross overdistraction of the cervical spine and can lead to neurologic injury (Fig. 1).

FRACTURES OF THE ODONTOID PROCESS OF THE AXIS

In 1974, Anderson and D'Alonzo (3) reported a series of 60 patients with fractures of the odontoid process treated at the Campbell Clinic from 1964 through 1972. Forty-nine of these patients were followed for a minimum of 6 months.

After reviewing the roentgenograms of each of these patients carefully, they identified three distinct types of fractures based on the anatomical location of the fracture line. This classification has served as the "gold standard" for the diagnosis and treatment of odontoid fractures. Type I fractures have an oblique fracture line through the upper part of the odontoid process and probably represent an avulsion fracture at the alar ligament attachment. Type II is a fracture occurring at the junction of the odontoid process and the body of the axis, but

this does not represent an epiphyseal injury. The neuro central synchondrosis of the axis fuses at age 3 to 6 years. It is located approximately midway down the body of the C2 vertebra. Fielding and Hawkins (22) described a high association of os odontoideum with patients giving a history of previous cervical trauma. There is a growing, but still controversial, belief that os odontoideum is in reality a non-union of Type II odontoid fractures. Type III is a fracture that extends down into the cancellous bone of the body of the axis and, in fact, is a fracture through the body of C2.

Type I fractures are rare stable injuries that have a good prognosis and require only minor treatment. Type II fractures, the most common type, tend to be unstable and have a high rate of non-union when treated by conservative methods, with an approximate one-third non-union rate when treated in a halo (2) (Figs. 7A–7E). The apical paired alar and accessory ligaments all attach to the proximal enlargement in this fracture and explain its potential instability. Furthermore, if a halo vest is not meticulously applied, distraction forces can be placed across the Type II fracture, further adding to the risk of non-union. Type III fractures, because of their large can-

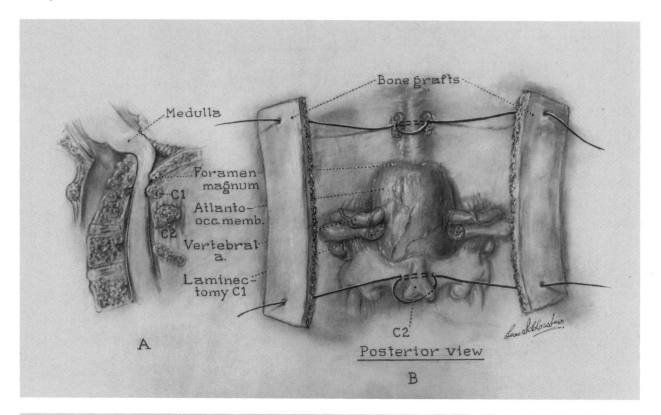

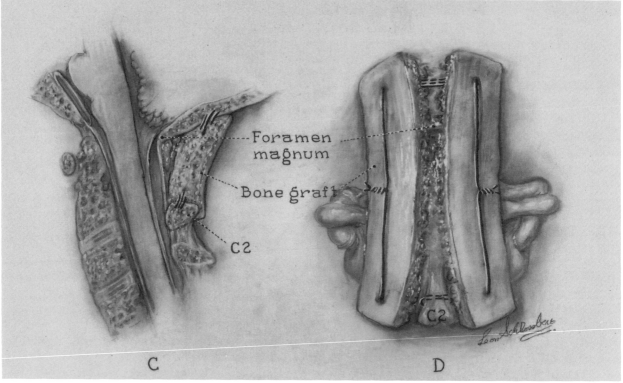

FIG. 9. Posterior triple wire stabilization for occipitocervical dislocations and C1-C2 instability with agenesis or fracture of the posterior C1 vertebra can be accomplished by posterior occipitocervical fusion. **Top:** Penetrating the inner table of the skull is not required. A burr is used to penetrate the outer table of the occipital cortex. A wire is passed through and around the cortical ridge of bone present over the posterior occiput **(A).** Two iliac strut grafts **(B)** are then wired in place spanning the posterior fractured arch of C1 or the spina bifida occulta of C1. **Bottom:** Extra cancellous pieces of iliac bone graft are then packed between the two iliac struts **(C and D).** The posterior axial height from C2 to the occiput is maintained by the strut grafts. In our experience, all patients need to be stabilized for 3 months in a halo cast or halo vest in order to achieve a solid arthrodesis following traumatic C1-C2 or occipitocervical traumatic injuries (with permission from ref. 46).

cellous surfaces, are more stable and have a better prognosis for union with non-operative treatment. Various explanations have also been offered regarding the blood supply to the odontoid in distinguishing the different fusion rates of Type II and Type III injuries.

The mechanism of injury of odontoid fractures is either flexion or extension. The fractures have been extremely difficult to produce in vitro using cadaveric material. In addition to the direction of the force, the various ligaments play an important role. In flexion injuries the strong transverse ligament is forced against the posterior odontoid process and causes it to fracture the body with anterior displacement. Conversely, with extension injuries the posterior aspect of the ring of the atlas is forced against the anterior odontoid, causing it to fracture and displace posteriorly. The most serious of odontoid fractures, flexion/anterior displacement injuries, outnumber extension/posterior displacement odontoid fractures by a ratio of 6 or 7 to 1. Clark and White (13) report a large series of odontoid fractures gathered from the membership of the Cervical Spine Research Society. Sixty-one percent of Type II and 87% of Type III fractures were anteriorly displaced. Thus, it appears that flexion is a much more common cause of odontoid fractures than is extension. In the less common group of patients with posteriorly displaced odontoid fractures, traction must be applied with the head in the flexed position. These injuries also tend to be more unstable than the flexion type (Figs. 7 and 8). Others recommend the technique for posterior C1-C2 and occipital to C2 arthrodesis. Posterior triple-wire stabilization for occipital cervical dislocations and C1-C2 instability can be performed (Fig. 9). Posterior triple-wire stabilization is a versatile technique and can be performed for either occipital dislocations or C1-C2 instability.

For occipital cervical dislocations, the patient is placed in a halo at the start of the operative procedure and somatosensory-evoked spinal cord potentials are monitored throughout the procedure. The use of fiber-optic intubation has greatly diminished the morbidity of posterior arthrodesis and stabilization, as manipulation of the neck is not required. A standard posterior approach is undertaken from the occiput to C2 as subperiosteal dissection. A high-speed burr is used to penetrate the outer occipital cortex approximately 2.5 cm superior to the edge of the foramen magnum. Penetrating the inner table of the skull is not required. A 20-gauge wire is passed through and around the cortical ridge of bone present over the posterior occiput. Two iliac strut grafts are then wired in place spanning the posterior fractured arch of C1 down to C2. For C1-C2 arthrodesis, two 22-gauge wires are passed around the C1 arch. In cervical fusions, this is my only indication for the passage of a sublaminal wire. Two iliac strut grafts are then wired in place from C1 to C2. An intra-operative x-ray, as well as an x-ray in the recovery room, are necessary to be sure displacement of the occipital of the C2 complex has not occurred. In occiput to C2 and C1 to C2 fusions, the patient is managed 3 months post-operatively in a halo vest or a halo cast.

CRITERIA FOR STABILITY OF THE LOWER CERVICAL SPINE

White and Panjabi (49) have defined clinical instability as the loss of the ability of the spinal elements to maintain a relationship between the vertebral segments under physiologic loads. This loss leads to irritation or damage of the spinal cord or nerve roots, and the structural changes resulting from instability may lead immediately or later to deformity or pain. The anatomy of the spine is critical in the maintenance of stability. The annulus fibrosus is the most important anterior structure. Sharpey's fibers form strong attachments to the vertebral bodies. The well-developed posterior longitudinal ligament also provides considerable strength and stability, but the posterior elements, facet joints, and capsules are the most important source of tensile and rotational stability. The ligamentum flavum provides stability in the extremes of motion.

When considering an injured lower cervical spine, it is important to note that 10% of all non-surgically treated unstable lower cervical spine fractures will dislocate. Unilateral facet dislocations associated with neurologic damage or facet fracture must be considered unstable. A facet dislocation with an intact annulus and yellow ligament may be considered stable. Bilateral facet dislocations are often associated with neurologic damage and are unstable. Burst fractures are unstable and highly correlated with spinal cord injury. Multiple-level laminectomy, with or without facetectomy, may lead to instability. The presence of facetectomy or laminectomy with discectomy will further increase the potential loss of cervical stability.

A number of factors must be considered in the radiographic assessment of stability. Translation of a superior vertebra that exceeds 3.5 mm at a level under clinical suspicion implies instability when the tube to film distance is 1.83 meters (72 inches). Angulation of greater than 11 degrees between segments also indicates instability. The presence of arthritic changes must also be considered (35–38). Osteophytes along the posterior longitudinal ligament can compromise the spinal cord with an extension injury and result in a subsequent central cord syndrome (35–38).

Clinical evidence of spinal cord injury is a strong indicator of instability. Nerve root injury, secondary to foraminal encroachment, may be present in a stable unilateral facet dislocation where the motion segment has not been rendered unstable.

Disc space narrowing of the involved levels is suggestive of disruption of the annulus fibrosus in a young person (35–38). The physiologic load requirements of the injured spine must be considered in the post-injury period. This factor can further influence the treating physician's decision to implement a particular mode of therapy.

CLASSIFICATION OF CLOSED FRACTURES AND DISLOCATIONS OF THE LOWER CERVICAL SPINE

Historically, a variety of classifications were proposed for cervical injuries (Fig. 10). In 1982, Allen et al. (1) presented a universally accepted classification for lower cervical spine fractures and dislocations. They described a study of 165 cases demonstrating the various spectra of injury, called phylogenies, and developed a classification based on the mechanism of injury. The first type is compressive flexion injury with stages I through V. As the fracture becomes progressively severe, increased comminution of the vertebral body occurs with a tear-drop-type fragment. The vertebral arch characteristically remains intact. However, a beak fragment on the anterior portion of the vertebral body is a characteristic of this fracture pattern. The major injury vector in this phylogeny is a compressive force directed obliquely downward and posterior in the sagittal plane with stress concentration at the anterosuperior margin of the vertebral body. The second type of phylogeny is vertical compression injury with stages I through III. Because the major force vector is in the axial direction, both vertebral end plates are fractured with cupping deformities. There may be fracture lines through the centrum of the vertebral body, depending on the amount of force. The characteristic burst fracture of the cervical spine is in this phylogeny. Distractive flexion injuries are the third phylogeny described by Allen et al. (1), and they are the most common cervical spinal injuries. Distraction flexion injuries range from stage I to stage IV. In distractive flexion stage III injuries, there is bilateral facet dislocation at approximately 50% anterior displacement of the vertebral body. Distraction stage IV injury is grossly unstable, as the superior vertebra is displaced anteriorly the full diameter of a vertebral body and gives the appearance of a "floating vertebra." Compressive extension phylogeny ranges in stages from I through V. In this injury there is no comminution of the vertebral bodies, but because the forces are directed posteriorly, there is comminution of the posterior elements. In addition, there can be disruption of the vertebral disc space and anterior translation of the upper cervical spine. The last two types of injury are distractive extension injuries and lateral flexion injuries. In the literature and in the practical management of cervical spinal injuries, it is difficult to remember all the

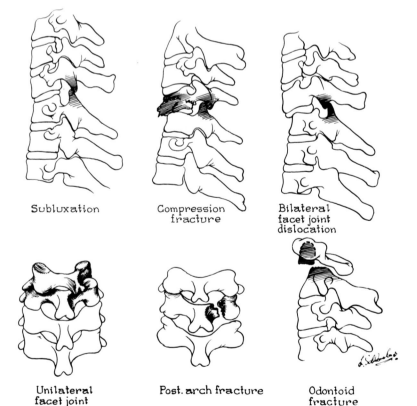

Subluxation

Compression fracture

Bilateral facet joint dislocation

Unilateral facet joint dislocation

Post. arch fracture

Odontoid fracture

FIG. 10. From Robinson and Southwick's original report (1960) discussing the classification of cervical spinal injuries (with permission from ref. 41).

various stages of Allen's classification. Therefore, Ducker's and McAfee's clock of studying the resultant force at the time of injury for both lower cervical and upper cervical spinal injuries may be a more practical method (Fig. 11).

TREATMENT OF LOWER CERVICAL SPINAL INJURIES

Spinal alignment can be corrected after the patient is medically stabilized. If there is compression of neurologic tissue, vertebral fractures or dislocations must be reduced to minimize ischemia and edema formation. Reduction can be accomplished with skull traction, and this is the determinant for the long-term outcome of the patient. Recent evidence also suggests improved neurologic outcomes if methylprednisone is given within 8 hours in a bolus of 30 mg/kg body weight followed by infusion of 5.4 mg/kg body weight for 23 hours (7).

When tongs are required to obtain alignment of a fracture dislocation, they should be left in place with the patient in bed with the head of the bed elevated 30 degrees to reduce disorientation and to reduce cervical edema and subsequent airway problems. Cervical dislocations are associated with substantial disruption of anterior posterior ligamentous structures and clinical instability (Fig. 12). Patients who are undergoing re-alignment and traction must be constantly monitored and examined to prevent iatrogenic injury to the neural elements resulting from stretching across injured segments.

Unilateral facet dislocation may be difficult to reduce (Fig. 13). We perform an open reduction and posterior fusion if closed reduction fails when 40 pounds of traction are applied. After the tongs are placed in a sterile manner, 15 to 20 pounds of traction are initially applied, preceded by appropriate sedation, and a lateral radiograph is obtained. Weight is then added in 5-pound increments with a lateral radiograph following each change until a reduction is documented radiographically. Our preference is to utilize Gardner-Wells tongs initially, because they can be easily applied by one person in an emergency room setting. Although Trippi-Wells tongs are easy to apply, pin site selection is limited. We prefer to apply a halo later under elective surgical circumstances with multiple-skilled individuals present after the fracture dislocation has been reduced and a thorough radiographic evaluation is complete. Some surgeons prefer to apply the halo first because they believe it facilitates closed reduction, allows better quality radiographs, and is also MRI compatible.

If a unilateral facet dislocation cannot be reduced within the first 24 hours, the patient is taken to the operating room for reduction and stabilization under general or local anesthesia. After reduction, posterior triple-wire stabilization and fusion with iliac bone graft are performed. A post-operative orthosis such as a 2-poster brace or a reinforced Philadelphia collar is used until fusion occurs, usually within 8 to 12 weeks. The results with this treatment are superior to those obtained if the dislocation is not reduced (42).

In patients in which there is no compression of the neural elements and the stability of the spine has not been jeopardized, a course of bracing in a rigid orthosis for 6 to 12 weeks may be appropriate. Follow-up radiographs must be obtained at regular intervals to assess healing. Isolated fractures of the posterior and lateral elements may be stable injuries and can be treated in a rigid orthosis. If there is an associated dislocation or neurologic deficit, operative stabilization fusion is indicated.

Axial loading fractures with mild compression of the anterior elements also can be treated in a rigid orthosis for 8 to 12 weeks. At the end of the treatment, radiographs must illustrate evidence of healing before discontinuing therapy. However, severe axial compression is an unstable injury and requires stabilization and sometimes decompression if bony fragments have compressed the spinal cord. Posterior kyphosis cannot be prevented if a burst fracture with posterior ligamentous disruption is treated in a rigid orthosis. In this situation, we prefer to perform a posterior wiring first and then do an anterior decompression and fusion (28).

INDICATIONS FOR EARLY OPERATIVE THERAPY

The criteria for urgent early operation in patients who have sustained cervical spinal cord injuries are: (a) progression of neurologic signs and (b) complete block of a subarachnoid space on myelography. A cervical root may require decompression to allow the patient increased function and independence. Acute anterior spinal cord injury requires operative intervention. Open fractures and penetrating injuries require irrigation and debridement. Acute cervical tear-drop fracture dislocations and facet fracture dislocations may cause anterior cord compression and instability. Locked unilateral or bilateral facet dislocations may not reduce with traction and require early surgical interventions.

The absolute indication for urgent operation is myelographic evidence of spinal cord compression by hematoma, bone, or disc elements after alignment has been optimized. Our clinical experience over the last 6 years at the Johns Hopkins Hospital continues to demonstrate the value of early decompression in optimizing neurologic recovery and stabilization.

POSTERIOR OPERATIVE PROCEDURES

The mainstay of operative treatment is posterior fusion. If the posterior elements are compromised or a facet dislocation cannot be reduced, posterior stabiliza-

Text continues on page 1083.

FIG. 11. Mid and Lower Cervical Spinal Fractures.

Mid and lower cervical spinal fractures involve the vertebrae 3 through 7 and do follow a common pattern. This clock of injuries (see also Fig. 5) again shows 12 o'clock with distraction, 3 o'clock with extension, 6 o'clock with compression, and 9 o'clock with flexion injuries. The original clocks showing these fractures were developed by Doctors Roberto Bellegarrigue and Mark Carol, while working with Dr. Ducker at the University of Maryland Shock Trauma Unit. This teaching material has since been used by the American College of Surgeons. These new drawings represent that work, along with the fine work of Dr. Benjamin Allen (1). Each of these injuries is described in the text of this chapter by Dr. McAfee.

At 1 or 2 o'clock, extension injuries in the mid cervical spine can cause disruption of the anterior longitudinal ligament with some posterior displacement of the superior and/or cephalad vertebrae on the more caudal vertebrae. When there is some forced extension, like in the 3 o'clock injury, there may be fracture of the spinous process, and even the lamina. This is to be differentiated from a stress fracture, referred to as Clay Shoveler's fracture, which occurs on the C7 spinous process.

The 4 o'clock injury represents a forced extension injury, wherein there is some form of fracture through the facet area, like an incomplete spondylolosis which is seen in the lumbar spine or seen at C2. All the injuries at 2 o'clock, at 3 o'clock, and at 4 o'clock, can occur in the elderly population where there is pre-existing cervical spondylytic stenosis. When the injuries occur in the elderly patient, there is buckling of the disc and joint space anteriorly into the canal, and buckling of the inner spinous ligament and the ligamentum flavum posteriorly to squeeze the spinal canal and squeeze the spinal cord to give the central cord syndrome.

With further compression injuries, as seen at 6 o'clock, the patient typically suffers a burst fracture. If there is a strong vector posteriorly, the bones may be displaced posteriorly. If there is a strong vector more anteriorly, the bones can be displaced and malaligned anteriorly. With the bursting of the fracture, the bone segments are in many pieces. Typically, bone is fractured back into the spinal canal to compress the spinal cord.

At 7 and 8 o'clock, there is a combination of flexion and compression. The vertebral body anteriorly will fracture. There is permanent compression anteriorly. There may be posterior disruption of the inner spinous ligaments. If these injuries are mild, the neurologic deficit is not great, and the disc material may not be ruptured back into the canal, although that can occur.

At 9 o'clock, the flexion injury causes either a unilateral or bilateral facet dislocation. There may be various fractures of the facet. In these injuries, the disc material is often disrupted. There is always a fear that the disc may be dislodged back in the canal with alignment.

At 10 and 11 o'clock, there may be forced distraction injuries where the posterior elements are torn and the vertebral bodies themselves are intact, along with the disc space. In some of these patients, the muscle spasm will cause the spine to realign, yet the neurologic injury may be quite devastating. In other cases, the muscle spasms will cause the spine to malalign with either a unilateral or bilateral facet dislocation. In these patients, the neurologic deficit is often severe and often will ascend above the level of the trauma.

Finally, the 12 o'clock injuries, which are seen where there are separations of C4-C5, are usually only documented after a forced flexion injury with traction maintained at a joint where there was complete ligamentous disruption. Obviously these lesions are very unstable. More likely, the distraction injuries will occur higher in the cervical spine.

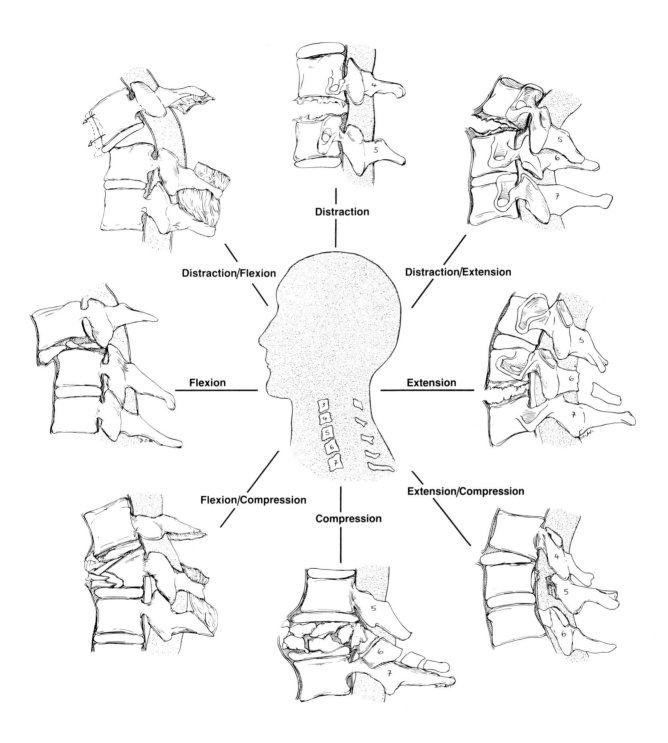

Distraction

Distraction/Extension

Distraction/Flexion

Flexion

Extension

Flexion/Compression

Compression

Extension/Compression

A

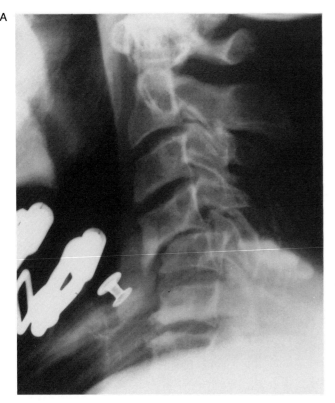

B

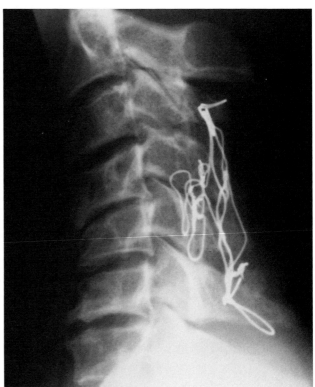

C

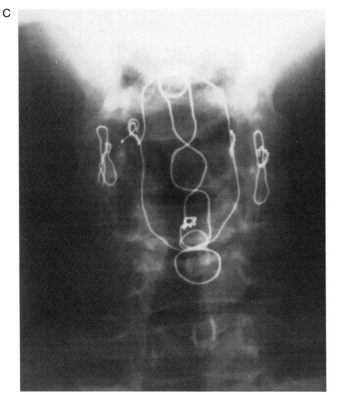

FIG. 12. This 40-year-old lumberjack had a log fall on the back of his neck. He sustained a C4-C5 flexion/compression injury and was neurologically intact. **A:** The fracture has subluxed despite adequate treatment with a meticulously applied halo. This is a severe 3-column injury and a well-fitting halo vest was unable to secure adequate stabilization. **B:** Anatomic reduction has been achieved following posterior wire fixation and fusion. **C:** Due to posterior comminution of the 2 involved levels of injury, bilateral facet wires were applied at the subluxed facets in a Southwick manner. The patient remained neurologically intact and was able to return to work in the logging industry 5 months post-operatively.

A

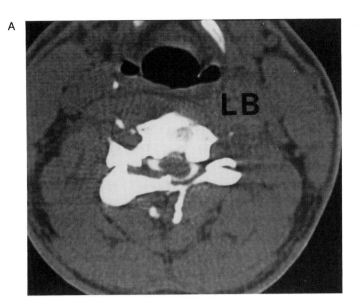

B

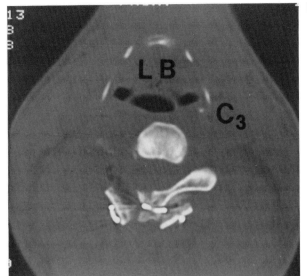

C

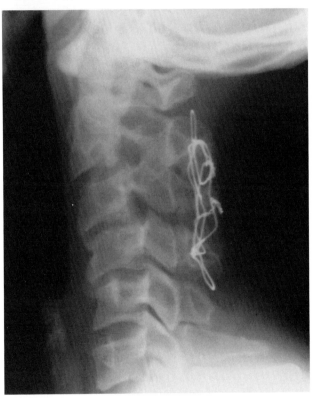

FIG. 13. A 30-year-old male sustained a diving injury and had left C4 radicular symptoms. **A:** The axial CT myelogram demonstrates comminution of the C3-C4 facet joint as well as posterior compression of the spinal cord from an angulated laminar fracture. **B:** The patient was treated with posterior decompression of the C3 laminar fracture and posterior triple wire stabilization and fixation from C2 to C4. The adequacy of posterior decompression is evident. **C:** The lateral radiograph demonstrates a solid fusion from C2 to C4 3 months following injury. It should be noted that posterior decompression for acute cervical spinal injuries is decidedly uncommon in comparison to the need for anterior decompressions for compressive lesions. Once spinal alignment has been achieved, a good quality contrast-enhanced CT scan is the imaging study of choice in evaluation of acute cervical traumatic injuries.

tion may be necessary. After the patient has been resuscitated and placed in tongs, the patient is placed in a spine turning frame (Stryker, Foster, Hess, or hydraulic operative wedge frame) for traction and surgery (31). In general, I prefer the Bohlman triple-wire technique (Fig. 14).

Satisfactory general anesthesia is obtained with fiberoptic intubation, and the patient is placed in a prone position. The shoulders of the longitudinal traction are pulled towards the end of the bed and held with adhesive tape. The posterior aspect of the neck is prepped with Betadine; the neck and iliac crest are prepared with anti-

septic solution and towels are sewn in place to prevent interference with the intra-operative radiographs. Cervical spinous processes can be palpated in the midline. A posterior midline incision is made and the cautery is used freely to minimize blood loss. The use of a cell saver is usually not required for posterior cervical spinal surgery. A midline superiorosteal dissection is performed, and the Cobb elevators are used more for retraction rather than dissection. Blunt force and trauma to the posterior neural elements are avoided. If there is question about the spinal level, an intra-operative radiograph

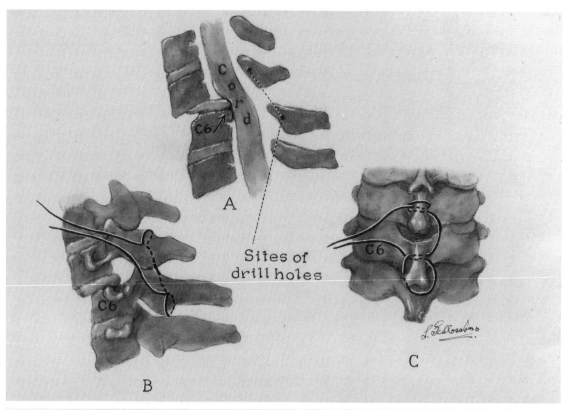

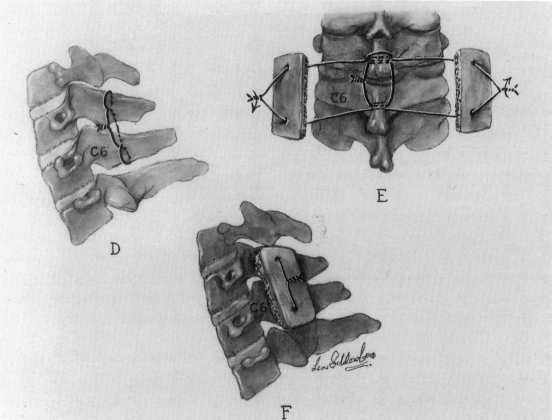

FIG. 14. Bohlman's triple wire fixation technique for a C5-C6 bilateral facet dislocation. The procedure can be performed under local anesthetic in patients with severe medical complications. **Top:** Through a posterior midline cervical incision **(A)**, a midline tethering wire is placed through and around the spinous processes of C5 and C6. With the patient in Gardner-Wells tong traction **(B)**, the facets are reduced. After the midline 20-gauge tethering wire has been securely tightened **(C)**, initial stability should be evident intra-operatively. **Bottom:** Two corticocancellous iliac strut grafts are wired in place from C5 to C6 using 22-gauge wires **(D)**. The addition of the posterior strut grafts adds to rotational stability **(E)**, as well as increasing the speed of fusion due to the compressive effect of the cancellous bone against the posterior aspect of the vertebrae **(F)** (with permission from ref. 46).

is obtained. For reduction of a unilateral or bilateral facet dislocation, a high-speed burr is used to remove a small portion of the superior articular process, which blocks the reduction. It is helpful to use motor or somatosensory-evoked potentials (spinal cord monitoring) throughout the reduction. After confirming the levels of fusions and obtaining a reduction, a 20-gauge wire is placed through a hole and placed in the junction of the spinous process and lamina. The use of the wire through and around the base of the spinous process prevents a cheese-cutter effect of the wire cutting out through osteoporotic bone. One midline tethering wire of 20-gauge stainless steel is passed through and around the involved spinous processes. At this point, a 20-gauge wire is then passed through and around the superior-most and inferior-most spinous processes. Full-thickness corticocancellous bone struts are then wired in place across the site of injury. Before the graft is placed, all the soft tissue covering the lamina of the spinous process must be removed, and the bone surface is roughened with a burr to allow fusion. The grafts are oriented to maximize bone-to-bone contact and the wires are tightened, thus compressing the cancellous bone of the graft against the can-

cellous bone of the lamina. Although this is a highly useful technique, occasionally the results may be compromised by unsuspected pathology (Fig. 15). If additional rotational stability is required and if the posterior lamina and spinous processes are fractured, wires can be easily passed through the posterior facets as originally described by Robinson and Southwick (40). As an alternative, facet joint screws and plates can be inserted according to the recommendations of Magerl (27) or Roy-Camille (43).

An anatomic comparison of the Roy-Camille and Magerl technique for screw fixation of the lower cervical spine was presented by Heller et al. (25) at the Cervical Spine Research Society in December 1989. Ten fresh human cadaveric spines from C1 to T4 were dissected and 3.5 mm cortical screws were inserted from C3 to C7. The Magerl method was used on one side and the Roy-Camille method on the other. A three-zone anatomic rating system was devised to evaluate whether or not the screw trajectory was correct or in danger of jeopardizing the underlying nerve roots. The results of careful direct examination of the specimens as well as radiographic evaluation showed that 96% of the Roy-Camille screws

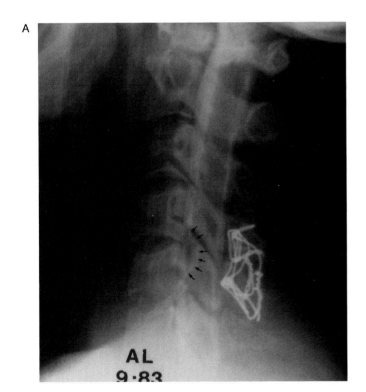
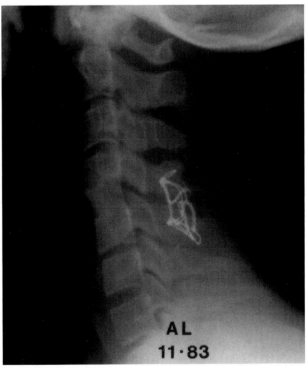

FIG. 15. A traumatic disc herniation that became more symptomatic following posterior wiring and fusion. This 19-year-old man sustained a C4-C5 unilateral facet subluxation following a high speed bicycle accident. After reduction, posterior stabilization, and fusion, his profound right-sided Brown-Sequard syndrome failed to improve. The metrizamide myelogram **(A)** shows retropulsion of the C4-C5 intervertebral disc (arrows) causing spinal cord compression. The herniated disc was removed by anterior cervical discectomy and the two vertebrae were fused. A lateral radiograph taken 2 months post-operatively **(B)** shows restoration of the spinal canal dimensions and solid fusion. The patient had complete neurologic recovery with the exception of Grade 4/5 intrinsic muscle strength.

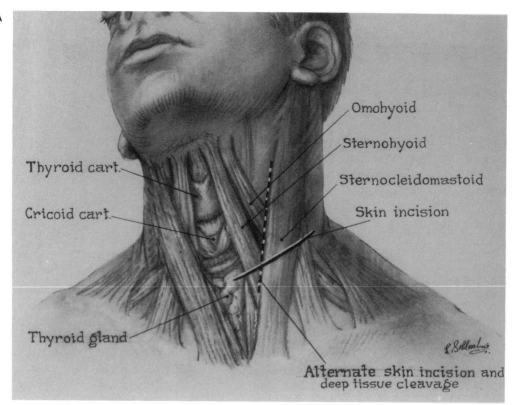

A

Thyroid cart.

Cricoid cart.

Thyroid gland

Omohyoid

Sternohyoid

Sternocleidomastoid

Skin incision

Alternate skin incision and deep tissue cleavage

FIG. 16. The Smith-Robinson anterior cervical approach used for either discectomies or corpectomies as required in Figure 24. **A:** After a transverse or vertical incision is made through the skin and platysma, the superficial layer of deep cervical fascia is dissected off the anterior border of the sternocleidomastoid muscle (Figs. 16A–16C with permission from ref. 44).

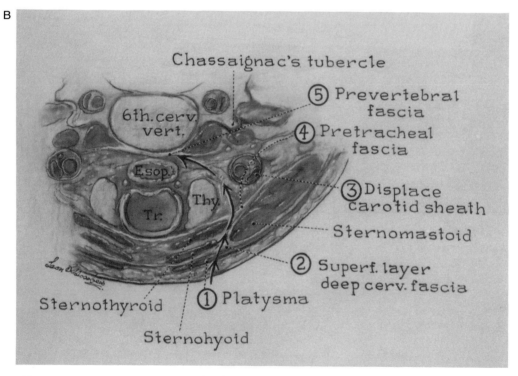

B

Chassaignac's tubercle

6th. cerv. vert.

Esop.

Tr.   Thy.

Sternothyroid

Sternohyoid

① Platysma

⑤ Prevertebral fascia

④ Pretracheal fascia

③ Displace carotid sheath

Sternomastoid

② Superf. layer deep cerv. fascia

FIG. 16. *(Continued)* **B:** Cross-sectional view of the level of Chassaignac's tubercle on the C6 cervical vertebra. In traumatic lesions, particularly with disruption of the intervertebral disc, it is much easier to get into the vertebral arteries, as compared to anterior approaches for degenerative conditions. Furthermore, it is necessary to use a small amount of traction, usually between 10 and 20 pounds, during the anterior approach. One should be careful of using larger amounts of traction secondary to the fact that the patient's muscles are relaxed under general anesthesia. (Fig. 16C follows.)

C

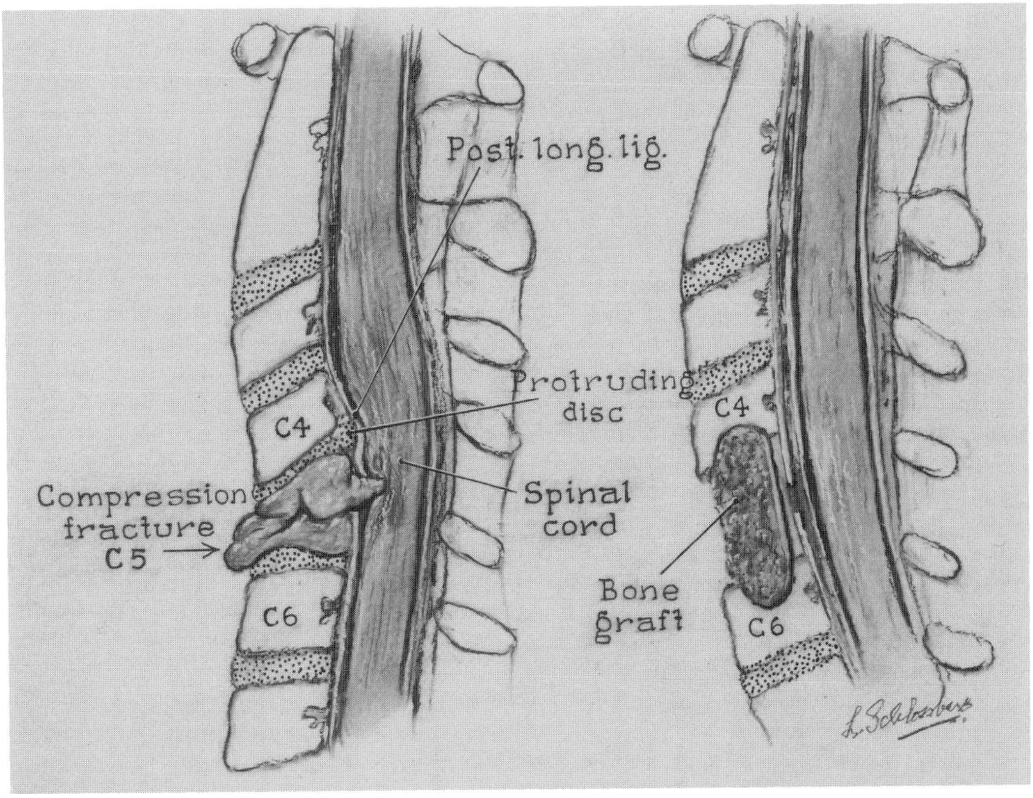

FIG. 16. *(Continued)* C: The C4-C5 and C5-C6 discectomies are performed first, as these can be performed with very minimal blood loss. After thorough discectomies, and with the posterior longitudinal ligament visualized, corpectomy is performed. A high speed burr is used to remove the C5 vertebral body. Performing the disc removal before removing the fractured vertebral body fragments allows the operative surgeon to be correctly oriented as to the depth of the spinal canal and compromised spinal cord. The drawing on the right demonstrates that an iliac bone strut has been wedged between the C5 and C6 vertebral bodies with the posterior cortex in alignment with the middle osteoligamentous column of the spine (with permission from ref. 8).

were in the proper zone, whereas only 42% of the Magerl screws were in the correct zone. In other words, excellent bone stock is available in the posterior facet joints for fracture fixation. The greatest degree of safety occurs if the screws are placed in a direct transverse orientation (the Roy-Camille method versus angling superiorly in a direction parallel with the facet joint cartilage—Magerl's method). These innovative techniques are only beginning to gain popularity and experience in North America. The biomechanical advantages of posterior screw and plate fixation are examined later in this chapter.

ANTERIOR DECOMPRESSION AND FUSION

In May 1953, Robinson revolutionized the treatment of cervical spinal injuries by first performing an anterior cervical approach to the spine. He later reported his results (39,41). Currently, the Robinson anterolateral approach between the carotid sheath and the esophagus is optimally suited for access to cervical levels C3 through C7 (Figs. 16, 17, and 18). Modifications of the technique, such as the anterior retropharyngeal approach described

by McAfee et al. (30), allow exposure as far superior as the clivus (Figs. 19 and 20). With exacting technique, one can reach as high as the C2 vertebra without taking down the stylohyoid or posterior belly of the digastric muscle. In addition, exposure can be made as low as the T2-T3 intervertebral disc space through a Robinson-Smith approach (39). In fracture management, the approach is suited for decompression of herniated disc material and decompression of retropulsed fragments of compressed vertebral bodies.

After the patient has been placed in the appropriate cervical traction, anesthesia is administered through a nasotracheal or endotracheal tube with assistance of fiber-optic equipment. When approaching the cervical spine below C3, the incision is usually made on the left-hand side of the neck, but for the anterior retropharyngeal approach we recommend making the incision on the right-hand side of the neck (Fig. 19). The lower cervical spine can be approached by a transverse incision placed two finger breadths above the clavicle. The incision extends from the midline to the border of the sternocleidomastoid. The longitudinal incision can be used for approaching the entire cervical spine; however, this author has not found a longitudinal incision necessary for reconstruction of traumatic deformities.

The platysma muscle is identified and elevated with Metzenbaum scissors and it is transversely incised. The superficial layer of deep cervical fascia is dissected along the anterior border of the sternocleidomastoid in a longitudinal direction. This is the key step in allowing mobility and exposure superiorly and inferiorly along the cervical spine. The omohyoid muscle can be cut if it traverses the field. The carotid artery with its investing sheath is identified by palpation of an arterial pulse. The carotid sheath is then retracted with the index finger laterally. The middle layer of deep cervical fascia is then dissected just medial to the carotid sheath. An appendiceal or long Richardson retractor is used to retract the trachea and esophagus medially. This identifies the alar fascia, which is the first layer of the deep cervical fascia. The alar fascia is a wispy layer and can be easily dissected free using a blunt dissector. The prevertebral layer is the deepest of the deep layer of cervical fascia and needs to be incised sharply with Metzenbaum scissors in a longitudinal direction. With the esophagus safely retracted medially with a blunt Richardson retractor and a thyroid retractor gently retracting the carotid sheath laterally, the longus colli muscles are dissected off the anterior surface of the spine using cautery (8). There is usually a venous plexus along the anterior border of the longus

Text continues on page 1094.

A

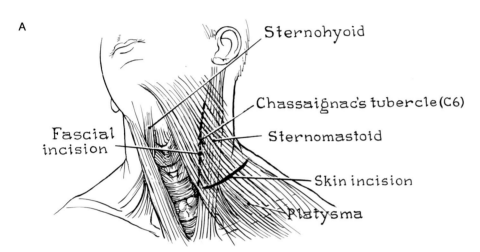

FIG. 17. For more extensive injuries, multiple level corpectomies may be required. **A:** For multiple level corpectomies, the same anterior approach of Smith-Robinson (see Fig. 16) is undertaken. However, most patients with more than two levels of cervical instability, regardless of the degree of neurologic compromise, will already have needed a posterior wire stabilization and fusion.

FIG. 17. *(Continued)* **B:** The superficial layer of deep cervical fascia is dissected for a much longer distance across the anterior border of the sternocleidomastoid. An anterior approach exposing C3 to C7 can be easily achieved through a transverse rather than a longitudinal skin incision. In the author's experience, it has never been necessary to use a longitudinal cervical spinal incision to achieve exposure from the C3 vertebra down as low as the T2-T3 intervertebral disc space. (Figs. 17C-17D follow.)

B

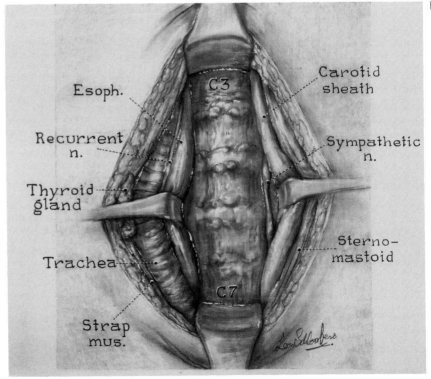

C

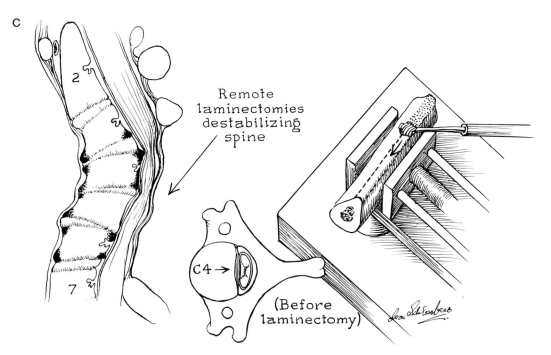

FIG. 17. *(Continued)* **C:** After anterior corpectomies, which are performed following C3-C4, C4-C5, and C5-C6 anterior discectomies, an increase in skeletal traction can be applied while visualizing the spinal cord through the corpectomy defect. Because injuries of the cervical spine involving two or more vertebral levels have a large degree of kyphosis, overdistraction of the cervical spine in correction of a kyphosis should not be performed. Distraction across fixed kyphosis will cause compression of the anterior spinal cord unless the offending vertebral body fragments are thoroughly decompressed first.

D

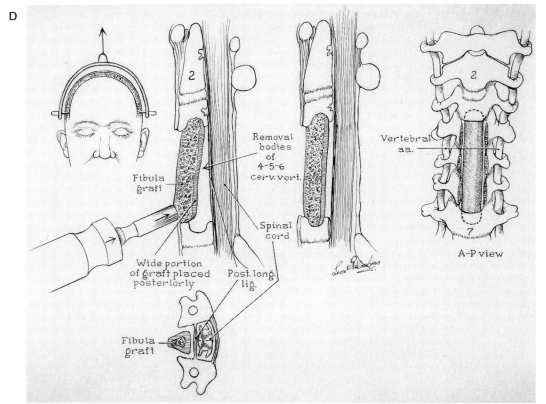

FIG. 17. *(Continued)* **D:** After corpectomies at C4, C5, and C6, a fibular strut is inserted from C3 to C7. It should be noted that the maximum number of vertebrae that can be spanned with an iliac crest is two. If more than two vertebrae need to be resected, then the use of a fibula is recommended.

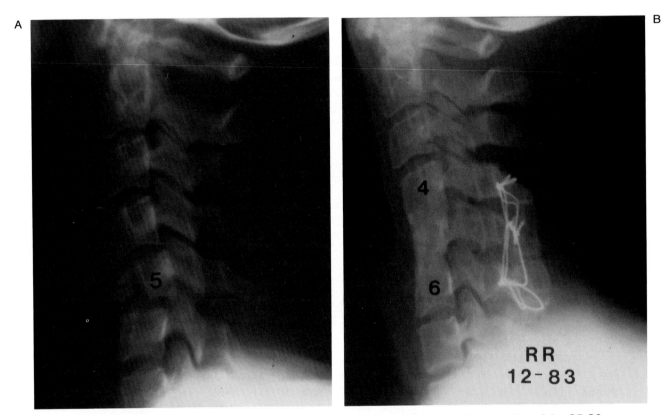

FIG. 18. This is a 17-year-old woman who sustained a C5 burst fracture with disruption of the C5-C6 posterior ligaments. **A:** The patient was Frankel Grade B on presentation 20 months after injury. She had a C5 anterior corpectomy with C4-C5 and C5-C6 anterior discectomies. This was augmented with a posterior triple wire arthrodesis from C4 to C6 and the patient recovered to Frankel Grade D. **B:** Fifty-five months post-operatively, solid arthrodesis is evident, there is no encroachment on the spinal canal, and the spinal malalignment has been corrected.

A

B

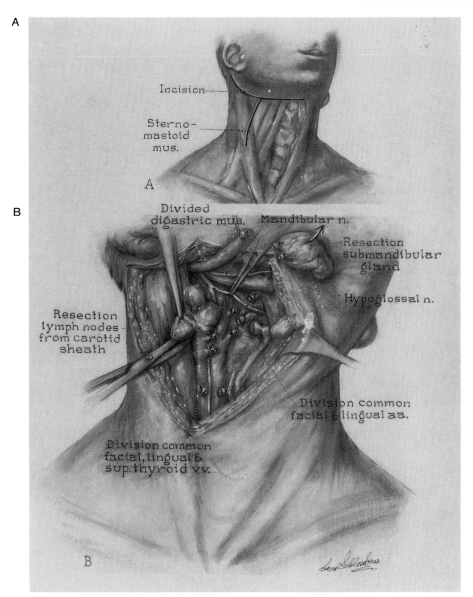

FIG. 19. The anterior retropharyngeal approach to the upper cervical spine. **A and B:** Key features of the extramucosal anterior approach to the atlas and axis. Through a submandibular incision on the right side, the submandibular gland is resected and the digastric tendon is divided. It should be noted that the lower limb of the incision is not used unless concomitant exposure to the mid-cervical levels is required (with permission from ref. 30). (Figs. 19C–19F follow.)

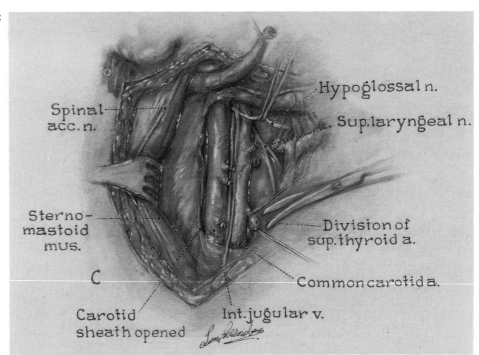

FIG. 19. *(Continued)* **C:** As the superficial layer of the deep cervical fascia is incised along the anterior border of the sternocleidomastoid, the superior thyroid artery and vein are divided. The hypoglossal and superior laryngeal nerves are mobilized. Additional branches of the carotid artery and internal jugular vein are ligated to allow mobilization of the contents of the carotid sheath laterally as the hypopharynx is mobilized medially.

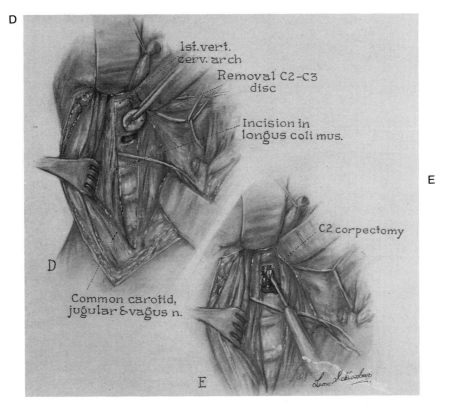

FIG. 19. *(Continued)* **D:** The first step of the anterior spinal decompression is the meticulous removal of the disc between the second and third cervical vertebrae. The longus colli muscle is dissected in a lateral direction, exposing the second cervical vertebral body and the anterior arch of the atlas. Removal of the body of the second cervical vertebra can then be performed with a high speed burr. **E:** Fractures of the second cervical vertebral body often have comminuted fragments in the vicinity of the vertebral artery. The advantage of the anterior retropharyngeal approach to the upper cervical spine as opposed to Whiteside's more lateral approach to the C2 vertebral body is that both vertebral arteries can be ligated and controlled in the former approach. Usually strut grafts are wedged between the anterior arch of the atlas after subperiosteal dissection and decortication. (Fig. 19F follows.)

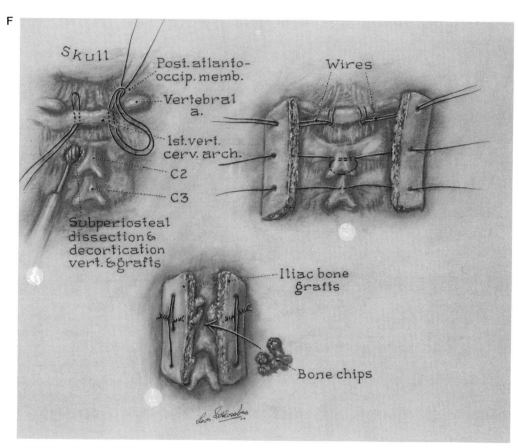

FIG. 19. *(Continued)* **F:** After anterior decompression, posterior wiring and fusion is performed from the first to the third cervical vertebrae to provide a circumferential spinal fusion. This was necessary in 11 of our series of 17 patients.

A

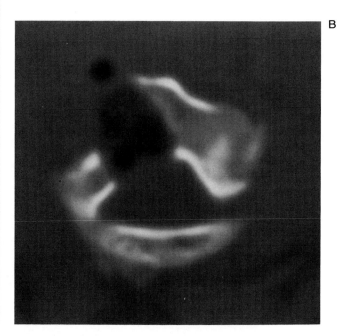

B

FIG. 20. This 42-year-old white male had sustained a Hangman's fracture with a profound Brown-Sequard syndrome secondary to a malunited displaced fragment on the left C2 lateral mass. **A:** The CT axial image shows spinal cord compression from a malunited fragment of bone from the C2 lateral mass. **B:** A Whiteside's lateral approach (52) was undertaken to the C2 vertebra to accomplish an anterolateral decompression. Because the surgery was performed 6 months after injury, a fusion was not required. Gelfoam was placed intra-operatively in the area of decompression and is visualized on the post-operative transaxial CT image. The adequacy of the lateral decompression performed through Whiteside's approach can be appreciated. The patient improved two grades of motor strength in his corresponding lower extremity major muscle groups.

colli muscle. The anterior portion of the spine can be safely dissected laterally without injury to the sympathetic chain, provided the dissection is not carried farther than the superior edge of the uncovertebral joint. Useful landmarks include the anterior carotid tubercle (Chassaignac's tubercle), which is palpated over the lateral mass of the sixth vertebra. An intra-operative radiograph can be obtained to confirm the level of injury. After the investing anterior longitudinal ligament has been identified, it is opened with a #15 blade to permit access to the intervertebral disc adjacent to the injured vertebral body. A curette is used to loosen the disc material, which is then removed with pituitary forceps. Complete excision of the intervertebral disc is essential to provide orientation to the proper depth of the posterior longitudinal ligament. If bone fragments are compressing against the spinal cord, a corpectomy is performed. When performing a corpectomy, it is advised to always perform thorough discectomies above and below the corpectomy. Aside from identifying the correct depth of

FIG. 21. One-stage anterior cervical decompression and posterior stabilization with circumferential arthrodesis for traumatic injuries. **Opposite page, top:** Typical appearance **(A)** of a patient with a fixed post-traumatic flexion deformity that does not correct with skeletal traction. There are anterior compressive fractures **(B)** at the fourth, fifth, and sixth cervical levels. The posterior facet joints are subluxed at the fourth and fifth and at the fifth and sixth cervical levels, with disruption of the capsules of the facets and tearing of the interspinous ligaments. A sagittal cross-section **(C)** demonstrates that the fifth cervical vertebra causes the most severe neurologic deficit, but the compression of the spinal cord actually extends from the caudad aspect of the fourth cervical vertebra to the cephalad aspect of the sixth cervical vertebra due to the kyphosis.

Opposite page, bottom: After anterior discectomies at C3-C4, C4-C5 and C5-C6, skull traction can be increased, if necessary, to reduce the kyphosis. A Cobb elevator **(D)** is wedged between the vertebral bodies at the apex of the gibbus to loosen the shortened fibrotic ligaments. An anterior intervertebral distractor **(E)** is used to help lock in tricortical iliac crest grafts **(F)** in performing an anterior arthrodesis at the third through sixth cervical levels. (with permission from ref. 28). (Figs. 21G-21I follow.)

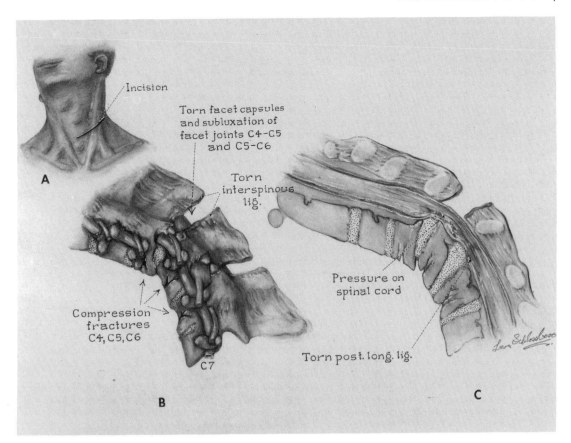

A

Incision

Torn facet capsules
and subluxation of
facet joints C4-C5
and C5-C6

Torn
interspinous
lig.

Compression
fractures
C4, C5, C6

C7

B

Pressure on
spinal cord

Torn post. long. lig.

C

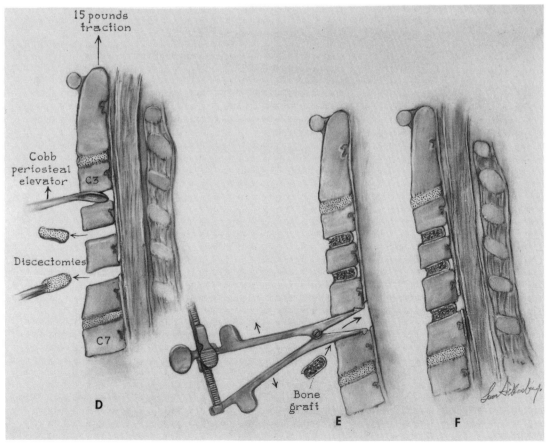

15 pounds
traction

Cobb
periosteal
elevator

C3

Discectomies

C7

Bone
graft

D

E

F

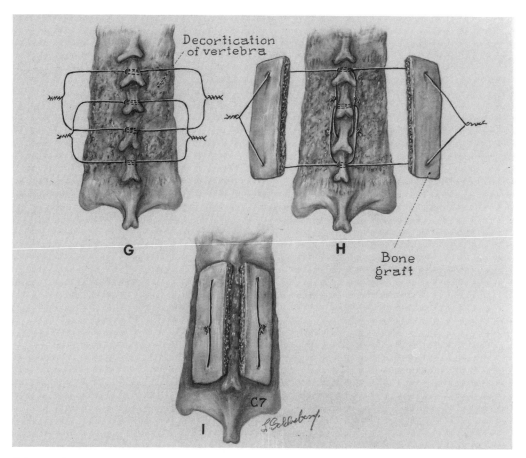

FIG. 21. *(Continued).* With the kyphosis reduced by cervical tong traction, the patient is turned in the prone position on an operative wedge or Stryker frame. Posterior stabilization is performed using the triple wire technique **(G)**, with 20-gauge wires inserted through and around the junction of the lamina and base of the spinous processes from the third through the sixth cervical levels, comprising the midline tethering wire. Two 22-gauge wires **(H)** are inserted at the end vertebra to compress two thick corticocancellous iliac grafts against the lamina at the third through the sixth cervical levels. This construct **(I)** provides enough immediate stability for the patient to be allowed out of bed wearing a two-poster cervical orthosis on the second post-operative day; a halo is not needed. (with permission from ref. 28). (Figs. 21J-21M follow.)

the posterior longitudinal ligament, this also greatly reduces blood loss. The bulk of comminuted vertebral bone fragments can be removed with a high-speed burr, but the posterior cortex is usually removed with a curved triple "0" curette. Injury to the spinal cord is minimized because retraction of the neural elements is not necessary, and the retropulsed fragments are removed under direct vision. The lateral cortices are left intact to protect the vertebral arteries.

When the acute injury is very unstable or there is a fixed post-traumatic deformity, a one-stage anterior decompression may be combined with posterior stabilization (Fig. 21).

REVERSED SMITH-ROBINSON GRAFT

Herniated disc material must be removed in the inferior end plate of the level above the injury, and the superior end plate of the level below must be exposed. This will permit placement of a full-thickness iliac crest graft with inferior and superior pegs to provide for maximum stability and to minimize migration. The increased fixation and decrease in incidence of graft migration have been found by the author since utilizing the reversed Smith-Robinson graft. The cortical part of the tricortical iliac crest is driven in first so that the strongest aspect of the graft is in line with the middle osteoligamentous col-

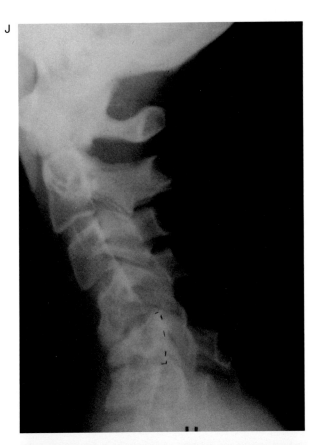

FIG. 21. *(Continued)* **J:** This 18-year-old lifeguard dove into a wave and hit his head on the sand sustaining an unstable C5 burst fracture. This was treated initially for 3 months with a halo and the kyphosis increased. The patient developed right deltoid and biceps weakness during the third month following injury.

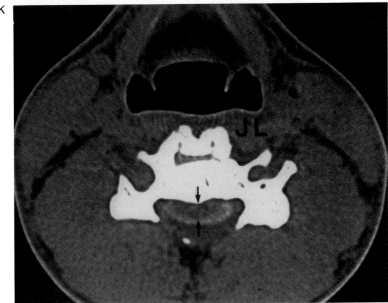

FIG. 21. *(Continued)* **K:** The contrast-enhanced CT image through the C5 vertebral body demonstrates flattening of the spinal cord due to posterior retropulsion of the C5 vertebral body and kyphosis. (Figs. 21L–21M follow.)

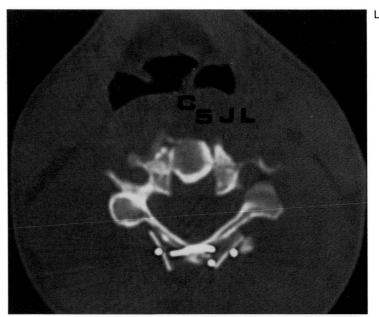

FIG. 21. *(Continued)* **L:** The patient underwent anterior cervical corpectomy, iliac strut grafting, and one-stage posterior wire stabilization and fusion. Following the combined one-stage procedure, excellent decompression of the spinal cord is demonstrated.

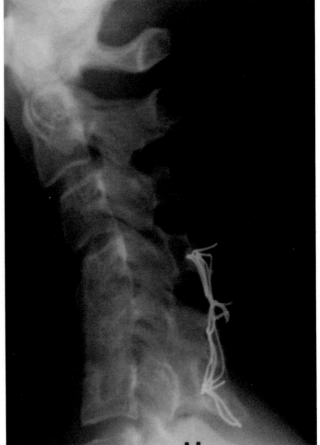

FIG. 21. *(Continued)* **M:** One year after one-stage anterior and posterior reconstructive surgery, the kyphosis has been corrected and a solid circumferential arthrodesis of the spine is shown. The patient had full neurologic recovery and was swimming competitively at a major southern university.

umn. In our 150 anterior cervical fusions performed for degenerative disease as well as trauma, we have not had a graft lose position. The pseudarthrosis rate is comparable with other techniques and in our hands is 2%. A fibular strut graft is necessary when fusing and spanning more than two vertebral bodies. It does not give as large an area of surface contact and may allow further collapse because of the decreased surface area of the end plates over which the axial forces can be distributed. After placement of the graft it is mandatory to obtain a lateral radiograph not only to assess decompression but also to judge the position of the bone graft. It is sometimes useful to double-check the stability of the graft by having the anesthetist remove the weight off the patient's traction—the neck can then be flexed and extended while the surgeon looks at the graft under direct visualization. If the graft does not move, the weight is placed back on the patient's traction and the wounds are closed in a routine fashion.

CERVICAL INSTRUMENTATION

The most stable biomechanical technique in reconstructing the anterior and middle columns of the spine has been the use of the Caspar anterior plate (Figs. 22 and 23) (4,10,11,12,33). This technique requires meticulous fluoroscopic control. A trapezoidal plate is placed across the vertebral bodies spanned by the anterior cervical fusion. Two screws are placed in each vertebral body. Each vertebral body needs to be drilled with a 3.5 mm drill, then tapped with a 4.5 mm tap; two screws are then inserted. The drill bits are penetrated to a depth of an average of 22 mm, which corresponds to the average diameter of the vertebral body. For maximum stability it is necessary to obtain penetration of the posterior vertebral cortex and to actually enter the spinal canal. The surgeon has three checks for position: (a) fluoroscopic control, (b) palpation of the decrease in resistance as one enters the spinal canal, and (c) an adjustable hex nut on the drill bit that prevents further penetration into the spinal canal. The technique is very exacting as it requires a minimum of four cortical screws placed into the vertebral bodies. Furthermore, because of the continuous use of fluoroscopy, it is necessary to use self-retaining retractors in the cervical spine, which often have teeth. The position of the retractors must be continuously monitored to prevent laceration of the esophagus or contents of the carotid sheath. As presented later in this chapter, the advantages of the biomechanical stability of the Caspar anterior plate need to be weighed against the increased technical difficulty and potential complications.

In our hands, it is much easier and less time-consuming to augment an anterior corpectomy graft with a one-stage posterior stabilization and fusion rather than adding an anterior trapezoidal plate (28). Even in the best surgeon's hands, the use of an anterior cervical plate simply serves as a tension band. In other words, the anterior trapezoidal plate acts most effectively in extension injuries in preventing cervical spinal distraction or tension across the intervertebral disc. An anterior plate is at a biomechanical disadvantage in preventing splaying apart of the facet joints. Because distractive flexion injuries are the most common phylogeny of cervical injuries, the majority of patients would be better served by one-stage posterior wiring and stabilization rather than augmenting an anterior decompression and fusion with anterior internal fixation.

In my experience over the past 7 years at Johns Hopkins Hospital and at St. Joseph's Hospital in Baltimore, an anterior Caspar instrumentation has been used in only 15 patients. I have found it much easier and biomechanically stronger to perform a one-stage combined anterior decompression and posterior stabilization (28). We reported 24 cases of one-stage anterior decompression–posterior stabilization and have had no infections, no iatrogenic neurological deficits, and no progressive kyphosis or loss of fixation.

BIOMECHANICS OF CERVICAL FIXATION DEVICES

In our laboratory (46), a bovine model was developed for biomechanical evaluation of surgical procedures, stabilizing traumatic cervical injuries disrupting the anterior and posterior spinal column. As flexion distraction injuries are the most common cervical spinal injuries, bilateral facet fracture dislocations were created in bovine spines at the C4-C5 level. Cyclical testing was performed to compare the following stabilization methods: (a) the intact cervical spine; (b) Rogers posterior wiring method; (c) Bohlman's triple-wire technique (31), which utilizes a midline tethering wire and bilateral 22-gauge wires that fix an iliac strut against the posterior aspect of the facet joints; (d) sublaminar wiring; (e) anterior Caspar cervical plate stabilization (Fig. 23); and (f) Magerl posterior hook plate stabilization (Fig. 24). The results of cyclical testing showed that anterior cervical plate instrumentation proved inadequate and was the least rigid with axial and flexural loading (p < .05) (Fig. 25). There was no significant difference among the three posterior wiring methods, and all generally restored stability equal to that of the uninjured intact cervical spine. Posterior hook plating with an interspinous bone graft serving as an extension block was a most effective method in reducing flexural stress across the injured C4-C5 segment (p < .05). Cyclical in vitro testing was the most sensitive method in highlighting mechanical differences among instrumentation systems, particularly with "on-line" continuous measurement of anterior and posterior strains. Anterior cervical plate stabilization did not appear to confer enough stability in cervical facet injuries to obviate the need for posterior cervical stabilization

A

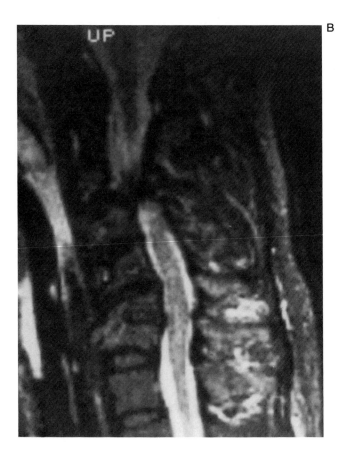

B

C

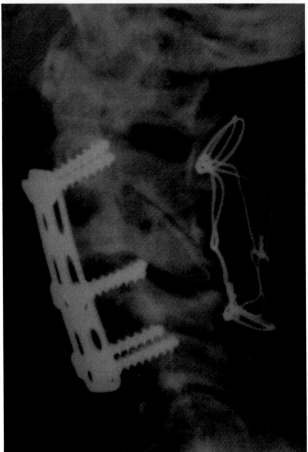

FIG. 22. One-stage anterior Caspar plate instrumentation and posterior stabilization. **A:** This middle-aged female had sustained an incomplete quadriparesis secondary to a fall due to athetoid cerebral palsy. The MRI, which had to be performed under general anesthesia due to her athetosis, shows anterior and posterior spinal cord compression. The compression on the anterior aspect of the spinal cord is due to a herniated disc at C2-C3 and the compression of the posterior aspect of the spinal cord is due to 5 mm of forward subluxation at C2-C3. **B:** A more magnified sagittal MR image illustrates the spinal cord compression in greater detail. During anterior cervical discectomy at C2-C3, retropulsion of disc material was documented. Due to the patient's athetosis and continued cervical spinal movement, anterior instrumentation was chosen to augment stability. During the same general anesthetic, the patient was turned posteriorly and had a posterior triple wire stabilization and fusion from C2 to C4. **C:** The patient is currently 2 years post-operative and has developed full neurologic recovery secondary to her traumatic injury. The anterior Caspar plate enhanced stability, thereby increasing the chances of successful fusion at the C2-C3 and C3-C4 iliac crest bone grafts. Note that with Caspar instrumentation for optimum stability, penetration of the posterior vertebral body cortex is necessary from the screws which are placed under fluoroscopic control.

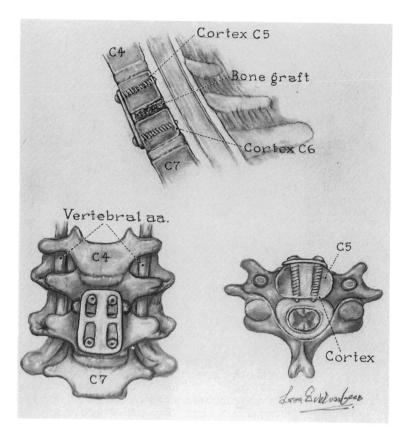

FIG. 23. The Caspar trapezoidal anterior plate stabilization technique. A Robinson tricortical iliac bone graft replaces the disrupted intervertebral disc at the level of subluxation. Care should be taken to insure that all cortical screws obtain maximum stability by obtaining purchase of the posterior vertebral body cortexes, actually entering the spinal canal as recommended. The drilling of the posterior cortex, the insertion of a depth gauge, the use of a tap, and the final insertion of the screw should all be done using lateral fluoroscopic control (with permission from ref. 46).

procedures (48). The recently developed posterior hook plate technique's mechanical advantages must be weighed against the greater technical precision needed for insertion and the increased potential for neurologic and vascular complications.

In 1989, Coe et al. (14) from our laboratory corroborated the previous study on the bovine calf spine but used cadaveric cervical segments. Distractive flexion stage III injuries were created at the C5-C6 level. With flexural and torsional testing, the stability of eight cervical stabilization constructs was tested cyclically and nondestructively. The Roy-Camille posterior plate fixation technique, the AO posterior hook plate fixation technique, and the anterior Caspar plate fixation techniques were compared to traditional wiring methods. Biomechanical testing demonstrated no significant differences in any of the posterior stabilization methods tested. There was little biomechanical justification for the use of potentially dangerous sublaminar wire fixation and posterior plating methods in these biomechanical studies.

METHYLMETHACRYLATE IN CERVICAL SPINE TRAUMA

Methylmethacrylate should not be used in the treatment of acute or chronic traumatic injuries of the spine. The use of methacrylate is justified only in pathologic cervical spinal fractures (19). Dunn, in a multicenter study sponsored by the Cervical Spine Research Society,

found that there has been almost unanimous agreement on the indications for methylmethacrylate stabilization of the cervical spine. This would include the patient with metastatic or unresectable primary tumor with a limited life span, yet who could be expected to withstand surgery and who is troubled by severe neck pain and/or progressive deformity or instability likely to lead to or already producing a neurologic deficit. McAfee et al. (29) reported that 24 patients had major complications after attempted stabilization of the spine with methylmethacrylate (Figs. 26, 27, 28, and 29). In none of the cases was the methylmethacrylate augmented with bone graft, despite the fact that 15 patients had acute traumatic injuries. The complications were as follows: 11 patients had a progressive neurologic deficit, 6 patients had a deep wound infection. Loosening and failure of fixation was the most common complication, and it occurred in 12 of the 15 patients who had a traumatic lesion. Salvage operations after failed methylmethacrylate are extremely difficult, particularly in the presence of infection.

Coe et al. (15), in a basic scientific study, developed a rat model studying the characteristics of the interface between bone and methacrylate when it is placed in the dorsal elements of the spine. They found a layer of fibrous tissue morphologically similar to tissue found in dogs when methylmethacrylate was used in the spine (51). The tissue synthesized several basement membrane components (Type IV collagen, laminin, and fiberonectin). These cells synthesized an extracellular matrix protein that was capable of degrading Type I collagen. In

A

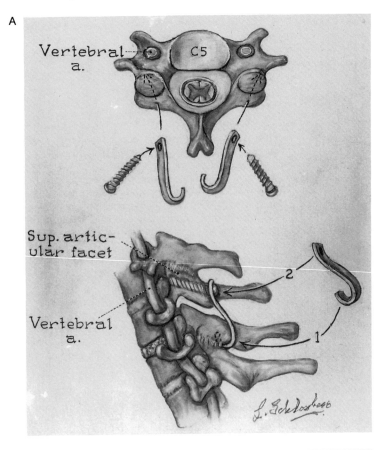

Vertebral a.

C5

Sup. artic-ular facet

Vertebral a.

2

1

B

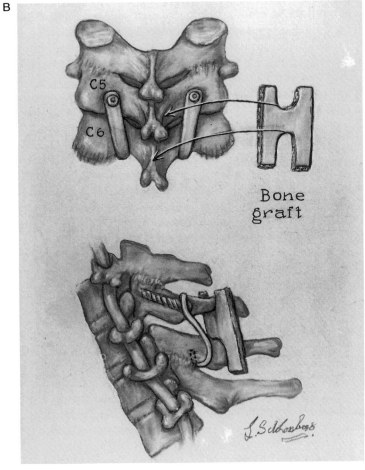

C5

C6

Bone graft

FIG. 24. The posterior AO hook plate technique advocated by Dr. Magerl (27) requires the placement of 2 cortical screws and a posterior interspinous bone block. The recommended angle of insertion is parallel with the posterior facet joints and requires engagement of the anterior cortex. The exit point of the screws is adjacent to the foramen transversarium, in close proximity to the vertebral arteries. Note that the posterior bone block prevents extension of the injured segment. The posterior hook plate, on the other hand, acts as a posterior tension band and prevents flexion (with permission from ref. 46).

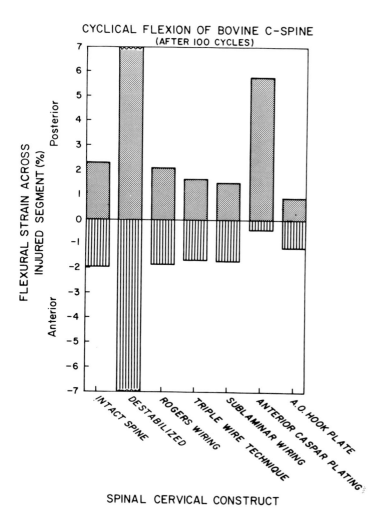

CYCLICAL FLEXION OF BOVINE C-SPINE
(AFTER 100 CYCLES)

FIG. 25. Summary of the long-term cyclical tests of the major spinal fixation systems. The flexural strains across the C4-C5 bovine vertebrae are demonstrated. The anterior column strains are compressive (striped bars) and the posterior column strains (solid bars) are tensile. Overall, the most successful construct in reducing anterior and posterior strains with flexion loads was the AO hook plate followed by all three posterior C4-C5 wiring techniques ($p < 0.05$). Caspar anterior plating was actually the most effective in reducing anterior strain because the plate and the anterior bone graft act as a block preventing compression. However, Caspar anterior plate instrumentation permits unacceptably high tensile strain to be transferred to the posterior elements. (In other words, the posterior elements can still distract apart in bilateral and unilateral facet injuries.) (With permission from ref. 46.)

FIG. 26. Methylmethacrylate was originally advocated in the neurosurgical literature for fracture stabilization. This lateral radiograph made 12 days post-operatively shows a 70 degree acute gibbus with lateral displacement of the massive cement and a Kirschner wire. Fortunately, no loss of neurologic function occurred. However, this acute 70 degree kyphosis is unacceptable.

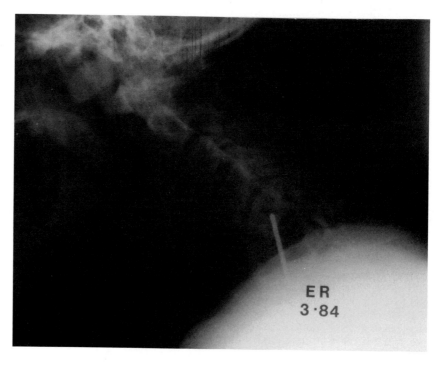

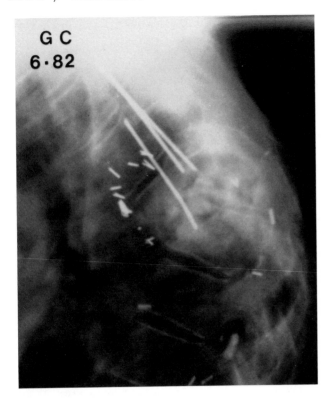

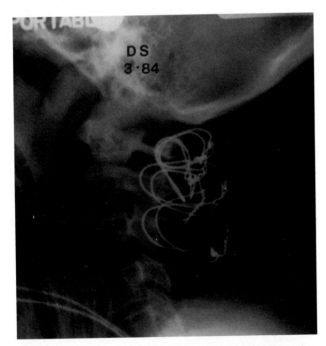

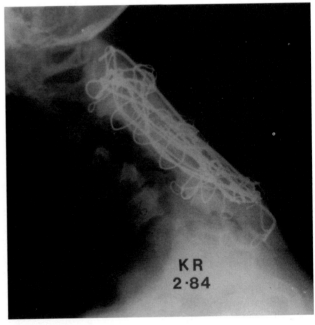

FIG. 27. This is a 27-year-old female who had migration of K wires into the spinal canal. Common with any methylmethacrylate construct used without fusion, the bone cement interface loosens and the wire material can migrate. This case demonstrates the occurrence in the thoracic spine although the same biomechanical considerations pertain to the cervical spine.

FIG. 28. This 70-year-old male sustained an unstable odontoid fracture and was treated with sublaminar wires from C1 to C3 with radiolucent methylmethacrylate from C1 to C3. As soon as the patient's Gardner-Wells tongs were removed, instability recurred and he developed a progressive myelopathy. Sublaminar wires should not be used below the C1 spinal level: previous biomechanical studies indicate no increased stability with the use of sublaminar wires rather than wires passed through the base of the spinous processes outside the spinal canal.

FIG. 29. This 47-year-old female had extreme kyphosis despite the use of posterior wire and methylmethacrylate which spanned the cervical spine from C2 to T1. Methylmethacrylate is particularly ineffective in the posterior column of the spine as it does not provide stability in tension.

A

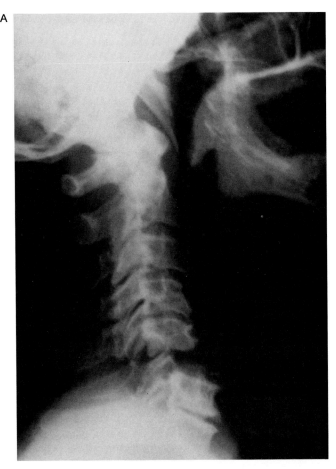

B

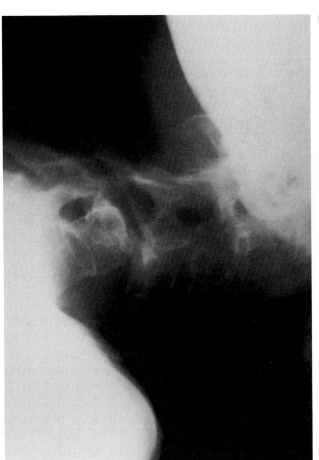

FIG. 30. Patients with ankylosing spondylitis should be treated with traction in the direction of the pre-existing deformity. Attempts to use the usual axial traction in line with the thoracolumbar spine can result in catastrophic neurologic loss. **A:** Patient with spondylitic spine treated in so much extension that the posterior facet joints have subluxed in a posterior direction. **B:** Patient with ankylosing spondylitis with complete dislocation of C4 on C5 with anterior translation the entire diameter of the vertebral body. To preserve neurologic integrity, this patient would require very gentle amounts of traction applied in line with the C5 and C6 vertebrae rather than axial traction in a Stryker frame. Patients with ankylosing spondylitis are also prone to develop neurologic deficits from acute epidural hemorrhage.

other words, when methylmethacrylate is used in the cervical spine for trauma or for any other indication, it can be anticipated that with any degree of microscopic loosening a tissue will be developed that has the capability of resorbing bone and degrading collagen. Even in patients with aseptic loosening of methylmethacrylate in the cervical spine, the resorption of bone and surrounding soft tissue inflammation can cause scarring. It is our opinion that methylmethacrylate is contraindicated in patients with traumatic injuries of the spine for this reason.

FRACTURES IN ANKYLOSING SPONDYLITIS

Fractures that occur with ankylosing spondylitis present spinal problems. Because of the fracture, instability sometimes presents the pre-existent deformity. This may present pitfalls, particularly with the use of traction (Fig. 30). This topic is discussed in greater detail in Chapter 36.

REFERENCES

1. Allen BL Jr, Ferguson RL, Lehmann TR, O'Brien RP (1982): A mechanistic classification of closed, indirect fractures and dislocations of the lower cervical spine. *Spine* 7:1–27.
2. Anderson LD, Clark CR (1989): Fractures of the odontoid process of the axis. In: Sherk HH, ed. *The cervical spine.* The Cervical Spine Research Society. Philadelphia: J.B. Lippincott.
3. Anderson LD, D'Alonzo RT (1974): Fractures of the odontoid process of the axis. *J Bone Joint Surg* [Am] 56:1663–1674.
4. Bohler J, Gaudernak T (1980): Anterior plate stabilization for fracture dislocations of the lower cervical spine. *J Trauma* 20:203–205.
5. Bohlman HH (1979): Acute fractures and dislocations of the cervical spine. An analysis of three hundred hospitalized patients and review of the literature. *J Bone Joint Surg* [Am] 61:1119–1142.
6. Bracken MB, Hildreth N, Freeman DH Jr, Webb SB (1980): Relationship between neurological and functional status after acute spi-

nal cord injury: An epidemiologic study. *J Chronic Dis* 33:115–125.

7. Bracken MB, Shepard MJ, Collins WF, et al. (1990): A randomized, controlled trial of methylprednisolone or naloxone in the treatment of acute spinal cord injury. *N Eng J Med* 322:1405–1411.

8. Carroll C, McAfee PC (1988): Cervical spinal fractures and dislocations. In: Chapman MW, ed. *Operative orthopaedics*. Philadelphia: J.B. Lippincott.

9. Carroll C, McAfee PC, Riley LH (1986): Objective findings for the diagnosis of "whiplash" injuries. *J Musculo Med* 3:57–76.

10. Caspar W (1982): Advances in cervical spine surgery. First experiences with the trapezial osteosynthetic plate and a new surgical instrumentation for anterior interbody stabilization. *Orthopaedic News, U.S.A.* 4(6).

11. Caspar W (1984): Anterior cervical fusion and interbody stabilization with the trapezial osteosynthetic plate technique. Tuttlingen: Aesculap-Wissenschaftliche Informationen in Selbstverlag der Aesculap-Werke AG.

12. Caspar W (1984): Die Ventrale Interkorporale Stabilisierung mit der HWS-Trapex-Osteosyntheseplatte. Indikation, Technik, Ergebnisse. Tagung fur Orthopadie und Traumatologie. *Z Orthop* 122 Stuttgart: F. Enke Verlag.

13. Clark CR, White AA 3rd (1985): Fractures of the dens. A multicenter study. *J Bone Joint Surg [Am]* 67:1340–1348.

14. Coe JD, Warden KE, Sutterlin CE 3rd, McAfee PC (1989): Biomechanical evaluation of cervical spinal stabilization methods in a human cadaveric model. *Spine* 14:1122–1131.

15. Coe MR, Fechner RE, Jeffrey JJ, Balion G, Whitehill R (1989): Characterization of tissue from the bone polymethylmethacrylate interface in a rat experimental model. Demonstration of collagen degrading activity and bone resorbing potential. *J Bone Joint Surg [Am]* 71:863–874.

16. Cotler HB, Kulkarni MV, Bondurant FJ (1988): Magnetic resonance imaging of acute cord trauma: Preliminary report. *J Orthop Trauma* 2:1–4.

17. Davis D, Bohlman H, Walker AE, Fisher R, Robinson R (1971): The pathological findings in fatal craniospinal injuries. *J Neurosurgery* 34:603–613.

18. Ducker TB (1990): Treatment of spinal cord injuries. *N Eng J Med* 322:1459–1461.

19. Dunn EJ (1977): The role of methyl methacrylate in the stabilization and replacement of tumors of the cervical spine. A project of the Cervical Spine Research Society. *Spine* 2:15–24.

20. Eismont FJ, Bohlman HH (1978): Posterior atlantooccipital dislocation with fractures of the atlas and odontoid process. *J Bone Joint Surg [Am]* 60:397–399.

21. Eismont FJ, Green BA, Arena JJ (1987): Intervertebral disk extrusion associated with cervical facet subluxation and dislocation. Presented at the Fifteenth Annual Meeting of the Cervical Spine Research Society, Washington, DC.

22. Fielding JW, Hawkins RJ (1976): Roentgenographic diagnosis of the injured neck. American Academy of Orthopaedic Surgeons Instructional Course Lectures 25:149–169.

23. Harris JH Jr, Edeiken-Monroe B, Kopaniky DR (1986): A practical classification of acute cervical spine injuries. *Orthop Clin N Amer* 17:15–30.

24. Hartwell JB (1917): Analysis of 133 fractures of the spine treated at the Massachusetts General Hospital. *Boston Med Surg J* 177:31–41.

25. Heller JG, Carlson G, Abitbol JG, Garfin S (1989): Anatomical comparisons of the Roy-Camille and Magerl techniques for screw fixation of the lower cervical spine. Presented at the Cervical Spine Research Society meeting, New Orleans.

26. Levine AM, Edwards CC (1985): The management of traumatic spondylolisthesis of the axis. *J Bone Joint Surg [Am]* 67:217–226.

27. Magerl F, Seemm P-S (1987): Stable posterior fusion of the atlas and axis by transarticular screw fixation. In: Kehr P, Werdner A, eds. *Cervical spine I.* Berlin: Springer-Verlag.

28. McAfee PC, Bohlman HH (1989): One stage anterior cervical decompression and posterior stabilization with circumferential arthrodesis. A study of twenty-four patients who had a traumatic or a neoplastic lesion. *J Bone Joint Surg [Am]* 71:78–88.

29. McAfee PC, Bohlman HH, Ducker T, Eismont FJ (1986): Failure

30. McAfee PC, Bohlman HH, Riley LH Jr, et al. (1987): The anterior retropharyngeal approach to the upper part of the cervical spine. *J Bone Joint Surg [Am]* 69:1371–1383.

31. McAfee PC, Bohlman HH, Wilson WL (1985): The triple wire fixation technique for stabilization of acute fracture-dislocations: A biomechanical analysis. *Orthop Trans* 9:142.

32. McGuire RA, Amundson G, Degnan G (1989): Evaluation of current extrication orthoses in immobilization of the unstable cervical spine. Presented at the Cervical Spine Research Society meeting, New Orleans.

33. Orozco DR, Llovet TJ (1971): Osteosintesis en las lesiones traumaticas y degenerativas de la columna vertebral. *Rev Traumatol Cirujia Rehabil* 1:45–52.

34. Pierce DS, Barr JS (1989): Fractures and dislocations at the base of the skull and upper cervical spine. In: Sherk HH, ed. *The cervical spine.* The Cervical Spine Research Society. Philadelphia: J.B. Lippincott.

35. Rauschning W (1983): Computed tomography and cryomicrotomy of lumbar spine specimens. A new technique for multiplanar anatomic correlation. *Spine* 8:170–180.

36. Rauschning W (1987): Normal and pathologic anatomy of the lumbar root canals. *Spine* 12:1008–1019.

37. Rauschning W, McAfee P, Jonsson H (1989): Pathoanatomical and surgical findings in cervical spine injuries. *J Spinal Disorders* 2:213–222.

38. Rauschning W, Sahlstedt B, Wigren A (1980): Irreponible luxationsfraktur der unteren halswirbelsaule. Eine pathologisch-anatomische studie met der gerfierschneidemethode. *Chirurg* 51:529–533.

39. Robinson RA, Smith GW (1955): Anterolateral cervical disc removal and interbody fusion for cervical disc syndrome. *Bull Johns Hopkins Hosp* 96:223–224.

40. Robinson RA, Southwick WO (1960): Indications and techniques for early stabilization of the neck in some fracture dislocations of the cervical spine. *South Med J* 53:565–579.

41. Robinson RA, Southwick WO (1960): *Surgical approaches to the cervical spine in instructional course lectures.* American Academy of Orthopaedic Surgeons. St. Louis: C.V. Mosby. 17:299–330.

42. Rorabeck CH, Rock MG, Hawkins RJ, et al. (1987): Unilateral facet dislocation of the cervical spine. An analysis of the results of treatment in 26 patients. *Spine* 12:23–27.

43. Roy-Camille R, Saillant G, Mazel C (1989): Internal fixation of the unstable cervical spine by posterior osteosynthesis with plates and screws. In: Sherk HH, ed. *The cervical spine.* Philadelphia: J.B. Lippincott.

44. Southwick WO, Robinson RA (1957): Surgical approaches to the vertebral bodies in the cervical and lumbar regions. *J Bone Joint Surg [Am]* 39:631–644.

45. Stauffer ES, Kelley EG (1977): Fracture-dislocations of the cervical spine. *J Bone Joint Surg [Am]* 59:45–48.

46. Sutterlin CE 3rd, McAfee PC, Warden KE, Rey RM Jr, Farey ID (1988): A biomechanical evaluation of cervical spinal stabilization methods in a bovine model. Static and cyclical loading. *Spine* 13:795–802.

47. Templeton PA, Young JW, Mirvis SE, Buddemeyer EU (1987): The value of retropharyngeal soft tissue measurements in trauma of the adult cervical spine. Cervical spine soft tissue measurements. *Skeletal Radiol* 16:98–104.

48. Ulrich C, Worsdorfer O, Claes L, Magerl F (1987): Comparative study of the stability of anterior and posterior cervical spine fixation procedures. *Arch Orthop Trauma Surg* 106:226–231.

49. White AA III, Panjabi MM (1978): *Clinical biomechanics of the spine.* Philadelphia: J.B. Lippincott, p. 223.

50. White AA, Southwick WO, Panjabi MM (1976): Clinical instability in the lower cervical spine. A review of past and current concepts. *Spine* 1:15.

51. Whitehill R, Drucker S, McCoig JA, et al. (1988): Induction and characterization of an interface tissue by implantation of methylmethacrylate cement into the posterior part of the cervical spine of the dog. *J Bone Joint Surg [Am]* 70:51–59.

52. Whiteside TE Jr, Kelly RP (1966): Lateral approach to the upper cervical spine for anterior fusion. *South Med J* 59:879–883.

The Adult Spine: Principles and Practice,
J. W. Frymoyer, Editor-in-Chief.
Raven Press, Ltd., New York © 1991.

CHAPTER 52

Late Complications of Cervical Fractures and Dislocations and Their Management

Michael J. Bolesta and Henry H. Bohlman

Tremendous progress has been made over the past decade to improve the care of trauma victims. Highly skilled emergency medical technicians stabilize the seriously injured and rapidly transport them to designated trauma centers. Once there, experienced personnel thoroughly evaluate, stabilize, reevaluate, and manage problems systematically. From beginning to end, refined protocols help identify all important injuries, but as Bohlman et al. have pointed out, cervical injuries often occur in association with other injuries, which can divert attention away from the neck (10,45). Despite the progress made, every spine surgeon still faces a number of problems after the acute phase. Early identification and appropriate management of cervical injuries under the best of circumstances can still be plagued by later complications. These are classified as instability, persistent neural compression, progressive loss of neurologic function, and a miscellaneous group of infections and failures of previous stabilizations.

M. J. Bolesta, M.D., Assistant Professor of Orthopaedics; H. H. Bohlman, M.D., F.A.C.S., Professor of Orthopaedics: Case Western Reserve University School of Medicine, The Reconstructive and Traumatic Spine Surgery Center, University Hospitals of Cleveland, Cleveland, Ohio 44106.

INSTABILITY WITH PAIN OR DEFORMITY

Etiology

White and Panjabi (55) defined instability as a loss of the ability of the spine under physiologic loads to maintain relationships between vertebrae in such a way that there is neither damage nor subsequent irritation to the spinal cord or nerve roots and, in addition, there is no development of incapacitating deformity or pain due to structural changes. In broad terms, stability is dependent on the integrity of the bones, joints, joint capsules, and ligaments of the spine. Trauma can render the cervical spine unstable by disrupting any or all of these components. The cervical musculature can splint the spine acutely, but cannot substitute for osteoligamentous integrity.

Bohlman (10) has documented that the torn posterior ligament complex in flexion injuries may not heal even following long rigid immobilization (Fig. 1). White and Panjabi (55) consider the atlanto-occipital joint to be relatively unstable, and injuries are usually fatal. Most are produced by a blow to the head.

Atlanto-axial stability depends on the integrity of the lateral joint capsules and, more importantly, on the

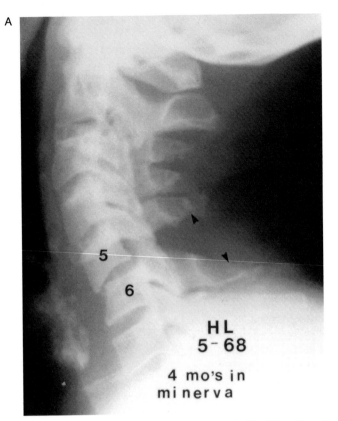 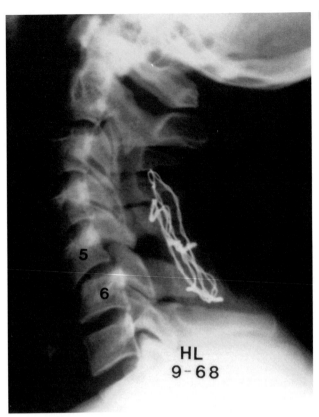

FIG. 1. A middle-aged man with C5–C6 subluxation treated in a Minerva jacket for 4 months. **A:** Lateral radiograph after 4 months of immobilization, showing persistent subluxation. **B:** Solid fusion after open reduction and internal fixation.

transverse portion of the cruciate ligament, although there are many secondary support structures. The transverse ligament may be ruptured with flexion or in association with a severe C1 burst injury (Jefferson fracture). Complete dislocation can occur with minor trauma in Down's syndrome (38). Depending on the amount of anterior stability, the late presentation is with cervical occipital pain, usually without a neurologic deficit. Approximately 12% of atlanto-axial injuries, treated operatively and non-operatively, will develop chronic pain; some have postulated a demyelinating process, since several of these patients describe L'Hermitte's phenomenon (25). A torticollis deformity is seen with rotary subluxation, which can occur with or without significant trauma.

Traumatic spondylolisthesis of the axis, or the hangman's fracture, occurs through the pedicles of the axis, and may be associated with disruption of the C2–C3 disc and ligament complex. In the Maryland series of 52 patients, early conversion of traction to halo vest was associated with significant residual deformity, which also correlated with the classification scheme (40). A larger series of 123 cases found no correlation between nonunion and time of bed rest, displacement, or angulation (28). Those patients were divided into three treatment groups: traction for 4 to 12 weeks, traction for 3 days to 3 weeks, or an orthosis alone. Irrespective of treatment method, only seven required an operation; six for nonunion and one for a painful kyphosis at C3–C4 after C2 healed.

Denis popularized the three-column concept of the thoracolumbar spine (21,22), relating this to stability. Similar concepts can be applied to the subaxial cervical spine. Although more complex, a mechanistic classification was proposed by Allen and Ferguson (1). Experimentally, White and Panjabi sequentially divided the soft tissue in cadaveric cervical spines from anterior to posterior or posterior to anterior trauma, eventually producing instability (54). The extent of this damage, as well as its location, will influence the timing of presentation. Severe trauma with neurologic deficit is unlikely to present late, unless there is an associated head injury or other multiple injuries that obscure the cervical fracture-dislocation. More subtle injuries will take time to manifest themselves, usually as persistent pain or deformity (35). The most common deformity is kyphosis secondary to flexion and axial loading injuries. This deformity can produce pain, probably secondary to muscle spasms as the patient attempts to maintain head position (41) or neural compression even without paralysis. There can be a rotary deformity in addition to the kyphosis with a unilateral facet injury. Although such deformity can be reduced closed in the early period, reduction may be lost, even with halo fixation (56).

Evaluation

A detailed history will cover details of the accident, catalog all associated injuries, and review the management to date. This will provide valuable information about the mechanism of injury by also documenting sites of head or facial injury. Physical examination will localize the portion of the cervical spine involved and document clinical deformity and loss of motion. A thorough neurologic examination is essential.

Plain radiographs provide information about the location of injury and the presence of malalignment or deformity. As in the acute situation, it is essential to visualize the body of C7 and ideally T1, which may require the use of arm traction or the swimmer's view. Oblique films should be obtained to evaluate the facet joints. The odontoid view provides information not present on the standard anteroposterior film. With rotary subluxation or dislocation, there is asymmetry between the dens and the lateral masses of the atlas as well as the atlanto-axial joint (Fig. 2). Goddard et al. classified these findings into two types. In Type I, which occurs in children and adults, the C1–C2 joints are fixed in partial rotation but not dislocated. On the anteroposterior view, the anteriorly rotated lateral mass of C1 appears to be widened, closer to the odontoid, and slightly elevated. In Type II, one inferior facet of C1 is anteriorly dislocated and locked, which they believed occurred only in children. On the AP view, again, the anteriorly rotated mass of C1 appeared widened, but appeared further from the odontoid and was tilted downward (30). When there is concern about the atlanto-occipital joint, a lateral view of the skull may give better detail of this region than the standard lateral of the cervical spine, and comparison should be made to films obtained at the time of injury when possible.

Abnormalities at the atlanto-occipital level prompt further diagnostic studies and may require stabilization. At the atlanto-axial level, the interval between the posterior or the anterior arch of C1 and the dens should not exceed 3 mm in adults and 5 mm in children. Of even greater importance is the distance between the dens and the posterior arch of C1, which in adults should normally measure 22 to 24 mm. Voluntary flexion/extension lateral radiographs are helpful in this evaluation of late instability in the subaxial spine. By White and Panjabi's criteria (54), greater than 3.5 mm of vertebral body translation or more than 11 degrees rotation connotes instability. A complete facet dislocation, either unilaterally or bilaterally, should be considered unstable because of the disruption of the facet capsules and ligaments.

Plain tomography is a valuable technique to define bony anatomy, particularly in the upper cervical spine as well as the lower cervical spine posterior elements.

Myelography, combined with computerized axial tomography, is used to assess the neural elements in patients with paralysis. They will identify associated disc herniation and posterior element fractures not readily appreciated on plain films. Water-soluble dye inserted at the atlanto-axial level is well tolerated, and the technology is readily available.

Magnetic resonance imaging has the advantage of direct sagittal imaging and is non-invasive. It is the modality of choice for diagnosing spinal cord lesions such as syringomyelia. However, it is not as widely available, and resolution of osseous structures is inferior to that of computerized tomography. Dynamic studies are possible and can be quite useful in the upper cervical spine.

Treatment

The patient who survives a traumatic dislocation of the atlanto-occipital joint requires occipital cervical fusion for stability. Wertheim and Bohlman describe a technique of posterior arthrodesis (53). A midline incision is used (Fig. 3A). A burr creates a ridge at the external occipital protuberance, preserving the inner table. Twenty-two gauge wire is passed through this, looped, and passed through the hole again. A sublaminar wire is passed at C1. A spinous process wire is placed at C2 (Fig. 3B). Large corticocancellous grafts are harvested through a separate incision (Fig. 3C) and secured by the wires (Fig. 3D). Additional cancellous bone is packed between the grafts and interstices between the grafts and underlying bone (Fig. 3E). Depending on the surgeon's assessment of pre-operative instability, the patient is immobilized for 8 to 12 weeks in either a halo or two-poster orthosis. Kahanovitz et al. described an unusual case in which the atlas dislocated and became fixed intracranially. This was missed because of significant intracranial trauma, which masked the dislocation. When recognized late, it was stable and did not require treatment (37).

For late atlanto-axial instability secondary to a torn transverse ligament or Type II odontoid fracture, posterior arthrodesis is the standard treatment (Fig. 4). A variety of techniques may be utilized, depending on the surgeon's preference. A modification of the Gallie technique is to place a sublaminar wire at C1 (Fig. 5A). A second wire is placed through and around the spinous process of C2. The cortical cancellous grafts are harvested and holes placed to accommodate the wires (Fig. 5B). Grafts are firmly secured by the wires. Cancellous bone is placed between the grafts and the bone (Fig. 5C). This technique is technically less demanding than the Brooks fusion, does not require a C2 sublaminar wire, and provides excellent, immediate stability and a high fusion rate.

Text continues on page 1114.

A

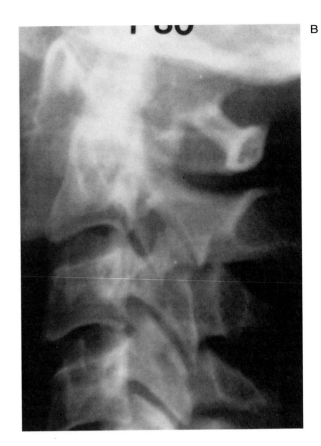

B

C

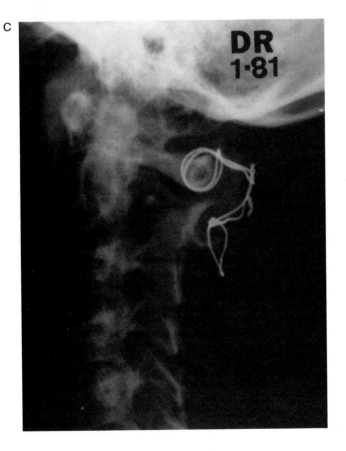

FIG. 2. A young woman with post-traumatic torticollis. **A:** AP odontoid view demonstrating offset between the lateral mass of the atlas and the superior facet of the axis. **B:** The lateral view reveals rotation of C1 as well as a fracture of the atlas. **C:** Lateral view showing a posterior atlanto-axial arthrodesis without reduction. Clinically there was resolution of the torticollis and pain.

A

B

C

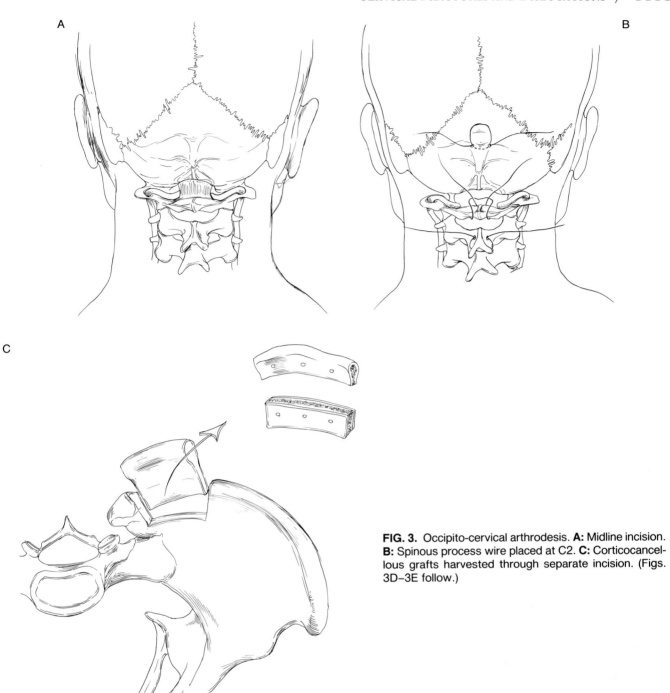

FIG. 3. Occipito-cervical arthrodesis. **A:** Midline incision. **B:** Spinous process wire placed at C2. **C:** Corticocancellous grafts harvested through separate incision. (Figs. 3D–3E follow.)

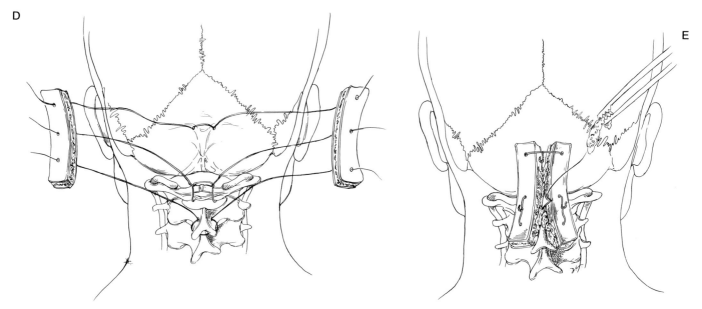

FIG. 3. *Continued.* **D:** Corticocancellous graft secured by wires. **E:** Additional cancellous bone.

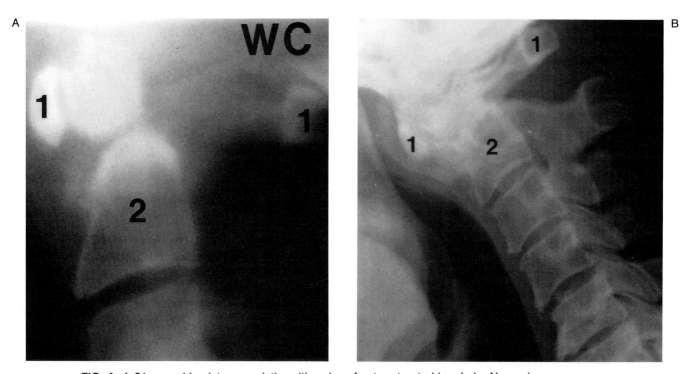

FIG. 4. A 61-year-old polytrauma victim with a dens fracture treated in a halo. Non-union was recognized, but surgical stabilization was delayed due to cardiac instability after anesthetic induction. He was later fused successfully. He was free of symptoms until dying from pneumonia 15 months later. **A:** Lateral tomogram demonstrating the nonunion. **B:** Anterior atlanto-axial instability with flexion. (Fig. 4C follows.)

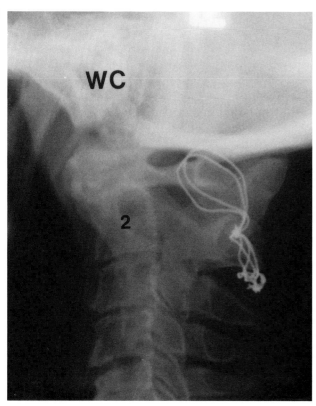

FIG. 4. *Continued.* **C:** Healed posterior atlanto-axial arthrodesis.

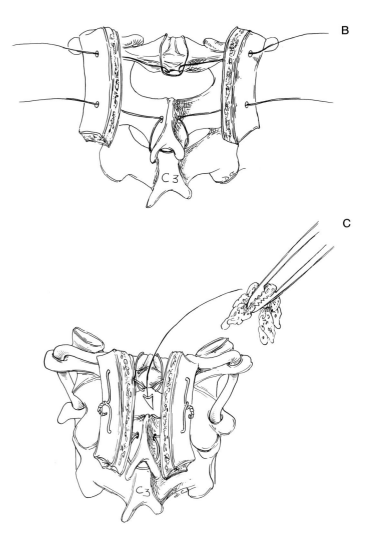

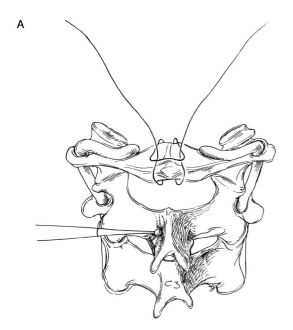

FIG. 5. Modified Gallie technique of posterior atlanto-axial arthrodesis. **A:** Sublaminar wire at C1. **B:** Cancellous grafts harvested and holes placed to accommodate wires. **C:** Cancellous bone between the grafts and the bone.

In the Brooks technique, wire or braided wire is passed beneath the arch of C1 and the lamina of C2. This is done bilaterally. A corticocancellous bone graft is placed between the arch of the atlas and the lamina of the axis and secured by the wire, which is tied posteriorly.

Although there have been trials of anterior screw fixation of dens fractures, this technique has not been applied to established non-unions. Facet fusions have also been described, but offer little advantage over the posterior technique described. Halifax clamps obviate the need to pass sublaminar wires at C1, but the bulky clamps do reduce the area available for fusion, and the

published follow-up has been short (19). Bohler described combined anterior and posterior fusion for dens non-unions in 13 patients (9).

In the unusual event that there is a congenitally absent posterior arch of the atlas with atlanto-axial instability, there are three options. First, screw fixation of the atlanto-axial facet joints may be performed through an anterior extraoral approach (31,44). A 2.5-cm screw is inserted through the lateral mass of C1 into the body of C2. With the head in neutral rotation, the drill is directed in the line from the mastoid process to the tip of the transverse process of C1. Because of the angle required,

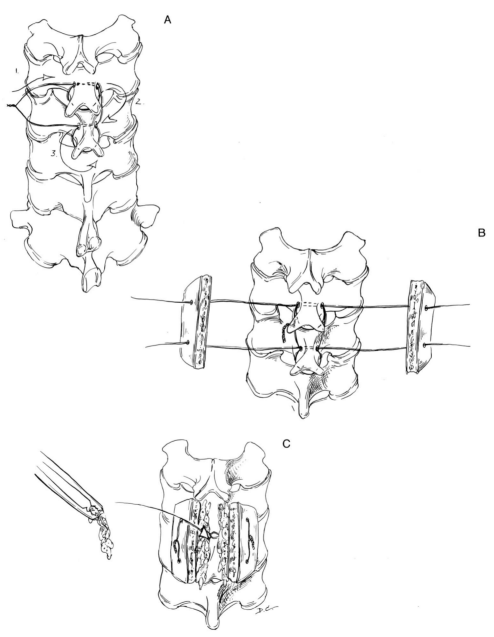

FIG. 6. Triple-wire technique of posterior cervical arthrodesis. A 20-gauge tethering wire (**A**) provides immediate stability, and 22-gauge wires are passed through and around the spinous processes (**B**) to secure corticocancellous grafts (**C**).

bilateral anterolateral exposure is required. Alternatively, facet screws may be placed via a posterior exposure. A longer incision than usual is made, which allows for far lateral exposure. If this technique fails, or the atlanto-occipital joint is diseased, or if these two approaches are too extensive for the patient, a posterior occipital cervical arthrodesis can be performed as described below.

If the pre-operative evaluation reveals cervical cord compression by the posterior arch of C1 that is fixed and cannot be reduced, then simple atlanto-axial arthrodesis is contraindicated, because there is not enough room to pass a sublaminar C1 wire (12). The arch of C1 is therefore resected, and an occipital cervical arthrodesis performed. If the compression is anterior, as with a dens malunion, posterior arthrodesis may be followed with anterior resection of the odontoid. The transoral approach has been described (2,26,48), as have several extraoral dissections (44). The latter have the distinct advantage of being less disfiguring and carrying a lower risk of infection and death.

In a series of 123 cases of traumatic spondylolisthesis of the axis, one patient developed a painful C3–C4 kyphosis below a healed C2 fracture. This responded to a C2–C4 posterior cervical fusion (28).

Pain and instability without kyphotic deformity in a subaxial spine are treated with posterior arthrodesis using a triple wire technique. After exposure through a midline incision, a 20-gauge tethering wire is placed through and around the spinous processes and tied to itself, providing immediate stability (Fig. 6A). Twenty-two gauge wires are passed through and around the spinous processes (Fig. 6B) and are used to secure corticocancellous grafts (Fig. 6C). Six to eight weeks in a two-poster orthosis is generally sufficient to assure a solid fusion.

Roy-Camille has developed alternative fixation with plates applied to the articular processes (23,33,47). Experience is limited in this country, but certain centers are investigating their use. One early report is that of Barquet and Pereyra (4). Alternatively, anterior cervical discectomy and fusion may be performed for posterior instability (46), but experimentally this is shown to be biomechanically inferior to posterior fixation (49). Bucci et al. (17) have advocated non-operative management of cervical instability with halo fixation, but eight (40%) of their patients so treated had persistent symptoms; five of them underwent delayed surgery, and two of these five had worsening of neurologic symptoms prior to the operation.

When there is significant late fixed kyphosis of the lower cervical spine an anterior approach is utilized. Corpectomies are performed followed by a strut fusion. Up to two bodies can be spanned by iliac crest, but longer fusions require the use of fibula. Intra-operative traction helps provide correction and intra-operative stability. Some investigators are utilizing anterior plates to fix the graft, but follow-up is short (16) and this fixation is unstable in flexion. Intra-operative evoked potential monitoring is routinely used. Depending on the status of the posterior column, posterior arthrodesis may also be indicated if there is associated torn ligament complex. This also affects the post-operative immobilization required. Depending on neurologic function, the patient may be maintained in traction or stabilized with a posterior arthrodesis and early mobilization in a halo (32).

In patients with ankylosing spondylitis, the fracture deformity may be corrected through the fracture with halo traction, but careful neurologic monitoring is necessary with slow gradual correction to avoid overdistraction and retrolisthesis.

PERSISTENT NEURAL COMPRESSION

Etiology

Unless obscured by other injuries, major neurologic deficit is generally apparent at the time of the injury. When the compression is milder, the deficit may be more subtle; in some cases, pain is the only manifestation of neural compression. Therefore, a careful pre-operative assessment, as described previously, is essential.

Spinal cord compression occurs as the result of a reduction in the size of the spinal canal for various reasons, including a herniated disc, a fractured vertebra, or dislocation. In a developmentally narrow spinal canal, a bulging disc without herniation can produce cord compression. Eismont et al. were able to correlate the severity of neurologic deficit to the size of the spinal canal (24) (Fig. 7). Instability also can produce cord compression (Fig. 8).

Anterior nerve root compression may result from a lateral disc herniation (Fig. 9), while fractures of the pedicles or fracture-dislocations of the facets may compromise the spinal nerves posteriorly.

Anterior spinal cord decompression facilitates recovery from incomplete nerve root or spinal cord injury, which has been demonstrated experimentally and clinically (10,13,42). In the patient with complete spinal cord injury, there is currently no way to restore distal cord function; however, root function may recover, with decompression resulting in significant improvement in activities of daily living (6,7). Late unreduced dislocations should be treated operatively.

Evaluation

Evaluation is very similar to that described for instability. Myelography with computerized tomography, magnetic resonance imaging, and plain tomograms help the surgeon localize and characterize the nature of the root or cord compression (43). This should be correlated with

Text continues on page 1121.

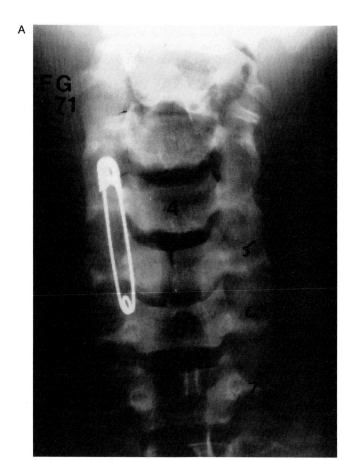

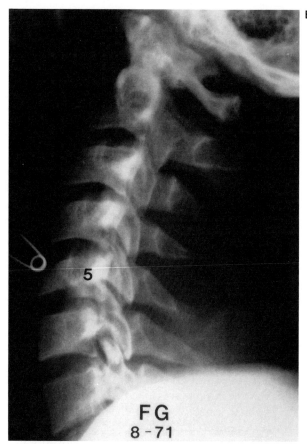

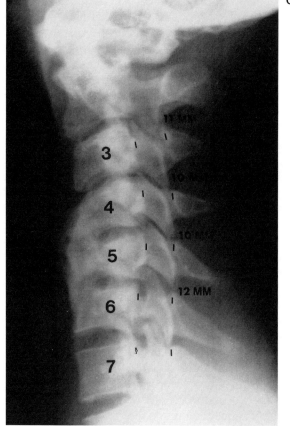

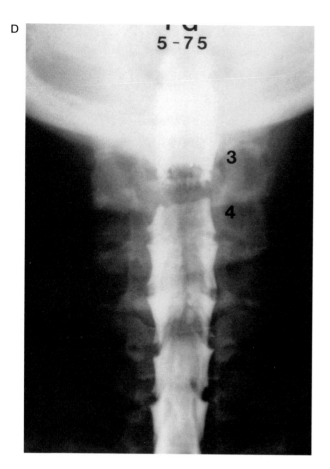

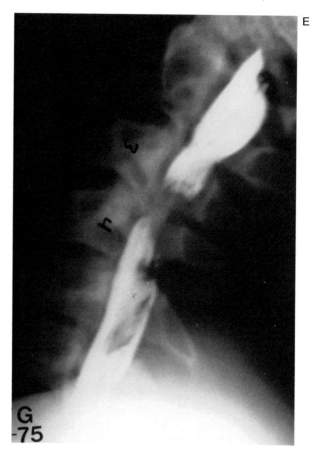

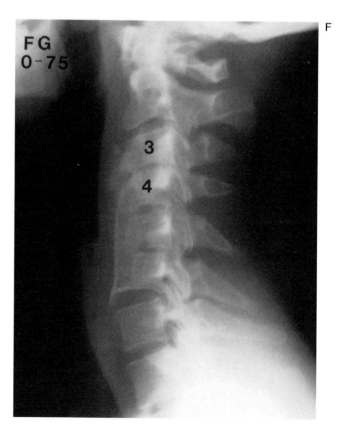

FIG. 7. A 20-year-old man with developmental stenosis who developed an anterior cord syndrome after a C5 fracture. He enjoyed complete recovery after an anterior fusion. Four years later, he again injured his neck and again developed anterior cord syndrome, secondary to a C3–C4 herniated disc above his fusion. After anterior discectomy and fusion, he recovered completely. **Opposite page:** AP (**A**) and lateral (**B**) radiographs of the original C5 compression fracture. One year later (**C**), there was healing of the anterior graft from C4 to C6. Note the marked narrowing of the cervical canal. **This page:** AP (**D**) and lateral (**E**) myelograms revealing C3–C4 disc herniation. Lateral radiograph (**F**) after C3–C4 discectomy and fusion.

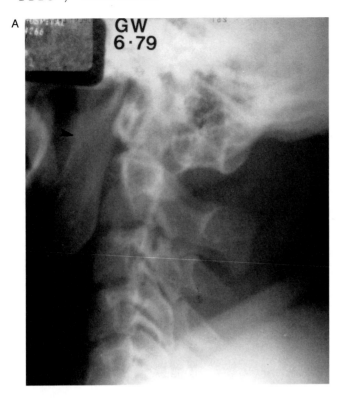

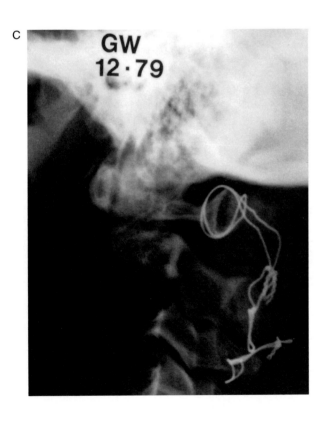

FIG. 8. Man with an unrecognized nondisplaced dens fracture who went on to unstable non-union and myelopathy. **A:** Lateral radiograph from the time of injury. Note the soft tissue swelling anterior to the upper cervical spine. **B:** Lateral tomogram revealing a displaced non-union. **C:** Lateral radiograph after posterior atlanto-axial arthrodesis. The patient's myelopathy improved significantly.

A

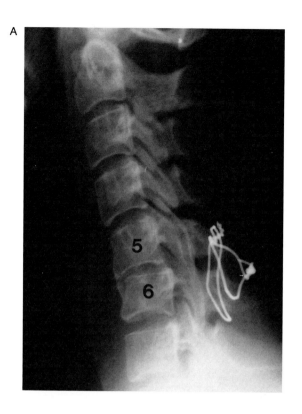

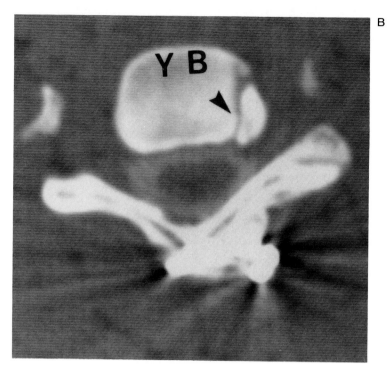

B

C

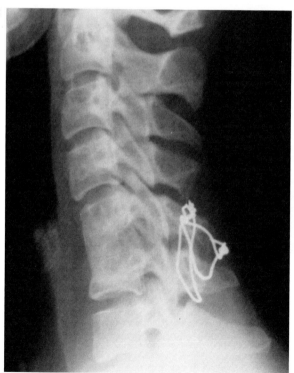

FIG. 9. Young woman who sustained a C5–C6 fracture-sub-luxation, treated with posterior cervical fusion. One year later, she presented with hypesthesia and weakness in the C6 distribution. **A:** Lateral radiograph 1 year after injury reveals a healed posterior fusion with mild residual C5–C6 subluxation. **B:** CT with contrast demonstrates unilateral root compression at the level of the uncovertebral joint. **C:** Lateral radiograph after anterior discectomy and fusion at C5–C6. The patient experienced complete resolution of radiculopathy.

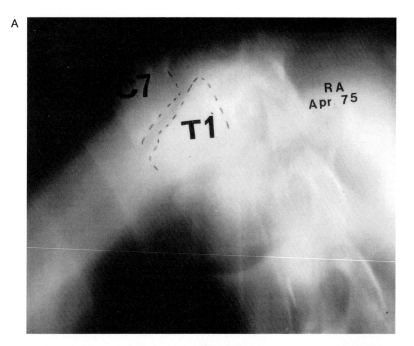

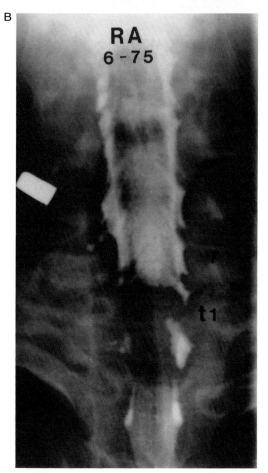

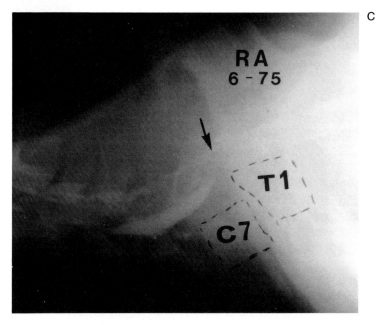

FIG. 10. Man with C7-T1 fracture-dislocation and anterior cord syndrome treated with laminectomy without reduction. He did not improve and was left with kyphotic deformity. **A:** Lateral tomogram demonstrating a C7–T1 dislocation and a healed compression fracture of T1. (Figs. 10B–10C, below.)

FIG. 10. *Continued.* AP (**B**) and lateral (**C**) myelograms revealing high-grade block at this level. (Fig. 10D, opposite page.)

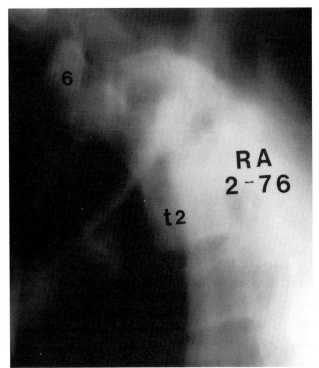

D

FIG. 10. *Continued.* **D:** Lateral tomogram after anterior corpectomy and strut grafting with iliac crest. The patient regained significant motor function.

the patient's symptoms and any neurologic deficit. It is also essential to identify any coexisting instability.

Treatment

In a patient with a healed malunion of an odontoid or axis body fracture and anterior cord compression with myelopathy, an anterior approach is indicated, which may be transoral (8) or, as we prefer, by the extrapharyngeal approach with arthrodesis (44).

In a patient presenting late with root compression from an unreduced facet subluxation, dislocation, or fracture, a posterior approach is utilized to remove the superior articular process with a power burr, which will facilitate a foraminotomy and reduction, followed by posterior arthrodesis as previously described. An unusual case of nerve compression was reported by Cartwright et al. in which a synovial cyst developed below anterior C5–C6 and posterior C2–C3 fusions for trauma, which was treated by resection (18).

Disc herniations are safely and reliably treated by anterior cervical discectomy and fusion (Fig. 7), and biomechanical studies have established the Robinson technique to be superior. An anterior approach should be used in all central and lateral disc herniations. Tamura has described the associated cranial symptoms with C4 root compression after trauma, postulating sympathetic involvement. These 40 patients had headaches, vertigo, tinnitus, or ocular problems. They responded well to discectomy and fusion (50).

When there is malunion of a vertebral body burst fracture with compression of the spinal cord or in the presence of a kyphotic deformity, corpectomies are necessary (Fig. 10). An anterior approach is again used. Discectomies are performed rostral and caudal to each involved body (Fig. 11A). Rongeurs or burrs are used to remove the central portion of the body (Fig. 11B). Lateral cortices are preserved, to avoid damage to the vertebral arteries. Enough disc is removed proximally and distally to identify the posterior longitudinal ligament. The posterior cortex of the body is removed with a diamond burr (Fig. 11C). Concavities are created in the remaining rostral and caudal vertebral bodies (Fig. 11D). A strut is fashioned from iliac crest or fibula, depending on the number of vertebral bodies resected. One or two corpectomies can be spanned with iliac crest (Fig. 11E); more than that require a fibula due to the curvature of the crest. The patient is maintained post-operatively for 6 to 12 weeks in an orthosis or halo, depending on the integrity of the posterior column. A posterior arthrodesis, utilizing the triple wire technique described above, may be necessary if there has been extensive damage to the posterior column. Facet wiring and fusion is employed if a laminectomy has been performed earlier.

PROGRESSIVE LOSS OF NEURAL FUNCTION

Etiology

Multiple studies have demonstrated the potential for neural recovery after decompression following cervical

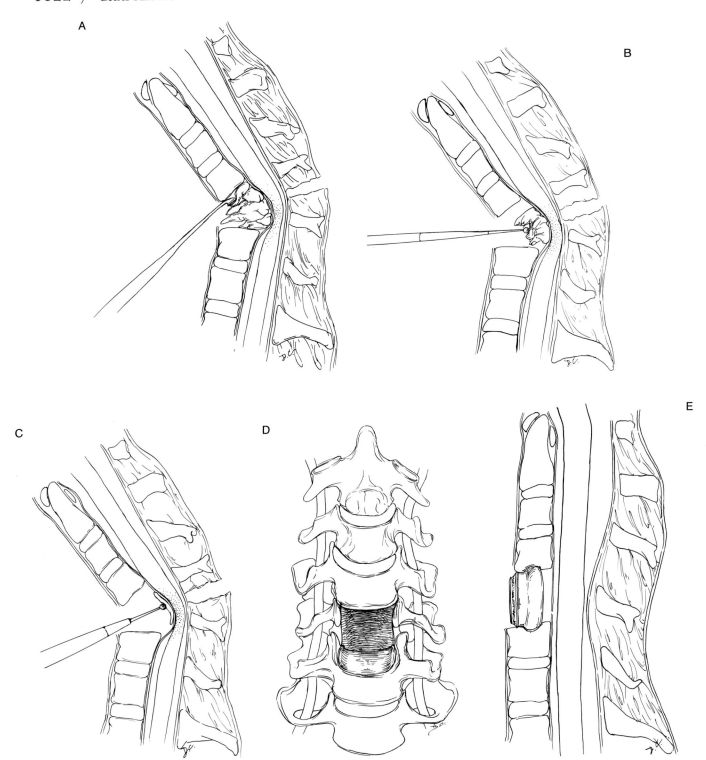

FIG. 11. Anterior corpectomy and strut arthrodesis. **A:** Discectomies rostral and caudal to each involved body. **B:** Rongeurs or burrs remove the central portion of the body. **C:** Diamond burr removes the posterior cortex of the body. **D:** Concavities in the remaining rostral and caudal vertebral bodies. **E:** Strut fashioned from iliac crest.

injury. This can occur even with delayed decompression. However, chronic persistent compression can result in late neurologic deterioration. The exact mechanism for this is unknown but may be due to chronic ischemia in the presence of mechanical neural compression. It may be a manifestation of the aging nervous system.

Post-traumatic cysts of the spinal cord, one type of syringomyelia, may present with pain or progression of a previously static neurologic deficit. The mechanism by which these cysts develop is unknown. They may result from liquefaction of necrotic cord, absorption of hematoma, or increased pressure within the central canal and may be found from months to years after trauma.

Evaluation

Assessment in the case of chronic persistent compression has been described, and is best accomplished with myelography, computerized tomography, and magnetic resonance imaging.

MRI is clearly the best modality for evaluating intrinsic cord pathology such as a post-traumatic cyst (14,15,29,36) by providing direct sagittal and transverse images (Fig. 12). It is non-invasive and can be repeated serially, which is useful when these cysts are small and when the correlation with clinical symptoms is equivocal. Worsening symptoms and ascending paralysis with a documented increase in size should prompt posterior cord decompression. In addition, the MRI is ideal in evaluating the success of a shunt in decompressing the spinal cord.

If magnetic resonance imaging is unavailable, delayed computerized tomography after the administration of intrathecal contrast may be used. As this is an invasive procedure, this cannot be as easily repeated as MRI. Furthermore, timing of the scan is critical; it is easier to

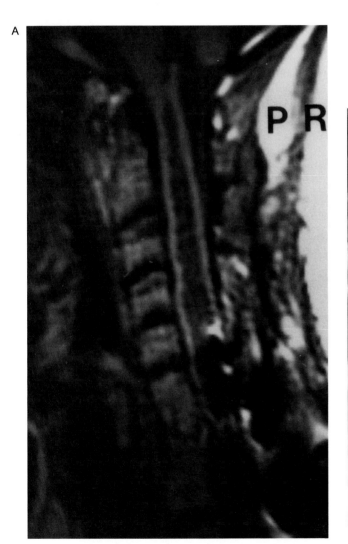
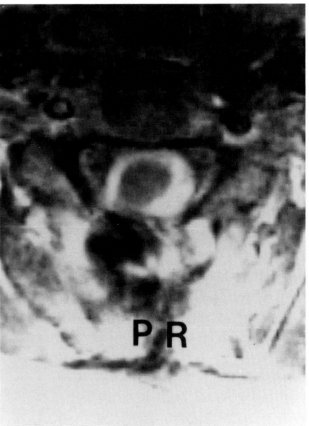

FIG. 12. Man with long-standing complete quadriplegia at the C7 level, treated with anterior decompression and fusion. He developed new pain and ascending weakness. Sagittal (**A**) and transverse (**B**) magnetic resonance imaging demonstrate a large post-traumatic cyst, which extends proximally within the cord. He experienced significant recovery with myelotomy and drainage.

underestimate the size of a cyst or miss it entirely using this technique.

Another less common neurologic manifestation of cord injury is reflex sympathetic dystrophy. Wainapel described two people with sympathetic dystrophy associated with central cord syndrome (52).

Treatment

The surgical treatment of persistent neural compression is detailed above.

Large post-traumatic cysts and those documented as increasing in size should be drained by a posterior expo-

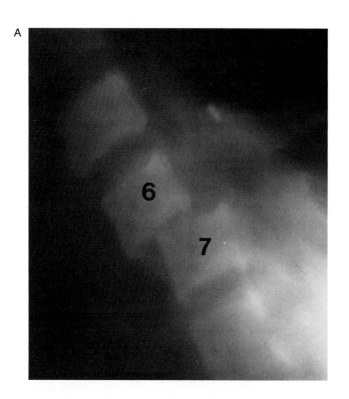

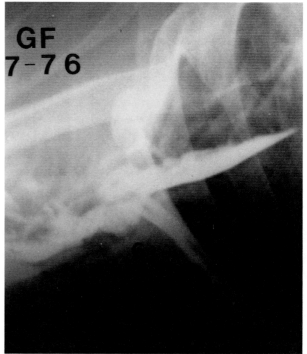

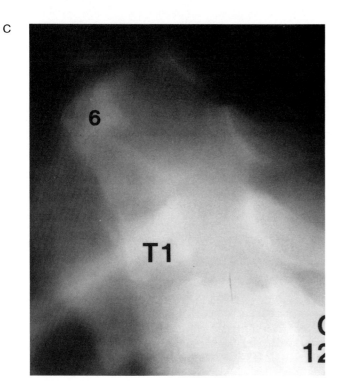

FIG. 13. Man with a C6–C7 dislocation that was never reduced. Lateral radiograph (**A**) demonstrating a 50% translation of C6 on C7 consistent with bilateral facet dislocation. Lateral myelogram (**B**) revealing a cord compression at the level of the dislocation. Lateral tomogram (**C**) after C7 corpectomy and C6–T1 anterior strut graft with iliac crest.

sure; microscopic myelotomy is performed and a tube is placed to shunt the cyst cavity into the subarachnoid space. Smaller cysts may be followed clinically with serial magnetic resonance imaging studies (see Chapter 23.)

OTHER COMPLICATIONS

Infection

Although rare, the esophagus can be injured at the time of initial insult (5,39,51). Patients sustaining cervical fractures and dislocations often have other injuries, so there is often a lag between the time of injury and resumption of oral feedings. Contamination of the neck can occur secondary to a ruptured esophagus. Cervical and often mediastinal abscess will generally present with sepsis. However, unsuspected abscesses have been encountered at the time of tracheostomy. A high index of suspicion is necessary to make the diagnosis. Esophagoscopy may not be possible because of the spinal injury. Contrast studies with a barium swallow followed by CT usually confirm the diagnosis. Adequate drainage and antibiotics are essential to the successful management of this potentially lethal complication.

Instability at Another Level

Careful initial evaluation and management will minimize this rare complication. When another more subtle level presents after treatment of a different cervical lesion, the same principles are used as described above. Decompression and/or arthrodesis are performed as indicated.

Non-Union and Malunion

Non-union of odontoid fractures may be painful with or without instability. These require posterior atlantoaxial arthrodesis. Os odontoideum likely represents disruption of the vasculature about the dens, secondary to a remote fracture altering odontoid growth, and results in late instability requiring arthrodesis (27,34).

Traumatic spondylolisthesis of the axis or hangman's fracture can usually be treated with traction and a halo. In the 123 patients of Francis et al. (28), 5.5% went on to non-union. This type of instability can be treated by anterior C2–C3 or posterior C1–C3 arthrodesis. In addition, that series included one posterior C2–C4 arthrodesis for a painful kyphosis at C3–C4 after the axis healed.

Malunion in the lower cervical spine can lead to loss of motion, pain, and perhaps neurologic deficit. Radiologic evaluation will define the pathology. Based on this, the appropriate fusion or decompression can be performed (Fig. 13).

Finally, non-union of a previous attempt at cervical fusion may be diagnosed by flexion/extension plain films and tomography. Myelography, computerized tomography, and magnetic resonance imaging should be used if there is suspicion of persistent neural compression. If present, this should be addressed at the time of revision fusion. If not, the surgeon may wish to consider anterior fusion for a failed posterior fusion and vice versa. The location of the persistent recurrent neural compression will usually dictate the operative approach required.

REFERENCES

1. Allen BL Jr, Ferguson RL, Lehmann TR, O'Brien RP (1982): A mechanical classification of closed, indirect fractures and dislocations of the lower cervical spine. *Spine* 7:1–27.
2. Ashraf J, Crockard HA (1990): Transoral fusion for high cervical fractures. *J Bone Joint Surg* [Br] 72:76–79.
3. Barbour JR (1971): Screw fixation in fracture of the odontoid process. *South Aust Clin* 5:20.
4. Barquet A, Pereyra D (1988): An unusual extension injury to the cervical spine. A case report. *J Bone Joint Surg* [Am] 70:1393–1395.
5. Benoit BG, Russell NA, Cole CW, Clark AJ, McIntyre RW (1983): Meningitis secondary to retropharyngeal abscess. Report of a case occurring in association with cervical spine fracture. *Spine* 8:438–439.
6. Benzel EC, Larson SJ (1986): Recovery of nerve root function after complete quadriplegia from cervical spine fractures. *Neurosurgery* 19:809–812.
7. Benzel EC, Larson SJ (1987): Functional recovery after decompressive spine operation for cervical spine fractures. *Neurosurgery* 20:742–746.
8. Blazier CJ, Hadley MN, Spetzler RF (1986): The transoral surgical approach to craniovertebral pathology. *J Neurosci Nurs* 18:57–62.
9. Bohler J (1982): An approach to non-union of fractures. *Surg Annu* 14:299–315.
10. Bohlman HH (1979): Acute fractures and dislocations of the cervical spine. An analysis of three hundred hospitalized patients and review of the literature. *J Bone Joint Surg* [Am] 61:1119–1142.
11. Bohlman HH (1986): Complications of treatment of fractures and dislocations of the cervical spine. In: Epps CH Jr, ed. *Complications in orthopaedic surgery, 2nd ed.* Philadelphia: J.B. Lippincott, pp. 897–918.
12. Bohlman HH (1985): Surgical management of cervical spine fractures and dislocations. *Instr Course Lect* 34:163–187.
13. Bohlman HH, Bahniuk E, Raskulinecz G, Field G (1979): Mechanical factors affecting recovery from incomplete cervical spinal cord injury: A preliminary report. *Johns Hopkins Med J* 145:115–125.
14. Bosley TM, Cohen DA, Schatz NJ, Zimmerman RA, Bilaniuk LT, Savino PJ, Sergott RS (1985): Comparison of metrizamide computed tomography and magnetic resonance imaging in the evaluation of lesions at the cervicomedullary junction. *Neurology* 35:485–492.
15. Bradway JK, Kavanagh BF, Houser OW (1986): Post-traumatic spinal cord cyst. A case report. *J Bone Joint Surg* [Am] 68:932–933.
16. Bremer AM, Nguyen TQ (1983): Internal metal plate fixation combined with anterior interbody fusion in cases of cervical spine injury. *Neurosurgery* 12:649–653.
17. Bucci MN, Dauser RC, Maynard FA, Hoff JT (1988): Management of post-traumatic cervical spine instability: Operative fusion versus halo vest immobilization. Analysis of 49 cases. *J Trauma* 28:1001–1006.
18. Cartwright MJ, Nehls DG, Carrion CA, Spetzler RF (1985): Synovial cyst of a cervical facet joint: Case report. *Neurosurgery* 16:850–852.

19. Cybulski GR, Stone JL, Crowell RM, Rifai MH, Gandhi Y, Glick R (1988): Use of Halifax interlaminar clamps for posterior C1–C2 arthrodesis. *Neurosurgery* 22:429–431.

20. Day GL, Jacoby CG, Dolan KD (1979): Basilar invagination resulting from untreated Jefferson's fracture. *Am J Roentgenol* 133:529–531.

21. Denis F (1983): The three column spine and its significance in the classification of acute thoracolumbar spinal injuries. *Spine* 8:813–831.

22. Denis F (1984): Spinal instability as defined by the three-column spine concept in acute spinal trauma. *Clin Orthop* 189:65–76.

23. Domenella G, Berlanda P, Bassi G (1982): Posterior-approach osteosynthesis of the lower cervical spine by the R. Roy-Camille technique. (Indications and first results). *Ital J Orthop Traumatol* 8:235–244.

24. Eismont FJ, Clifford S, Goldberg M, Green B (1984): Cervical sagittal spinal canal size in spine injury. *Spine* 9:663–666.

25. Ersmark H, Kalen R (1987): Injuries of the atlas and axis. A follow-up study of 85 axis and 10 atlas fractures. *Clin Orthop* 217:257–260.

26. Fang HSY, Ong GB (1962): Direct anterior approach to the upper cervical spine. *J Bone Joint Surg* [Am] 44:1588–1604.

27. Fielding JW, Hensinger RN, Hawkins RJ (1980): Os odontoideum. *J Bone Joint Surg* [Am] 62:376–383.

28. Francis WR, Fielding JW, Hawkins RJ, Pepin J, Hensinger R (1981): Traumatic spondylolisthesis of the axis. *J Bone Joint Surg* [Br] 63:313–318.

29. Gabriel KR, Crawford AH (1988): Identification of acute posttraumatic spinal cord cysts by magnetic resonance imaging: A case report and review of the literature. *J Pediatr Orthop* 8:710–714.

30. Goddard NJ, Stabler J, Albert JS (1990): Atlanto-axial rotatory fixation and fracture of the clavicle. *J Bone Joint Surg* [Br] 72:72–75.

31. Henry AK (1957): *Extensile exposure*. Baltimore: Williams and Wilkins, pp. 61–66.

32. Hershman EB, Bercik RJ, Allen SC, Fielding JW (1985): Correction of chin-on-chest deformity in ankylosing spondylitis through a fracture site. A case report. *Clin Orthop* 201:201–204.

33. Honnart F, Patel A, Furno P (1982): Fractures of cervical spine with neurological lesion treated by reduction and fixation with plates. *Ann Acad Med Singapore* 11:186–193.

34. Hukuda S, Ota H, Okabe N, Tazima K (1980): Traumatic atlantoaxial dislocation causing os odontoideum in infants. *Spine* 5:207–210.

35. Johnson JL, Cannon D (1982): Nonoperative treatment of the acute tear-drop fracture of the cervical spine. *Clin Orthop* 168:108–112.

36. Jourdan P, Pharaboz C, Ducolombier A, Pernod P, Desgeorges M (1987): Early syringomyelia following benign cervical injury. Contribution of postoperative MRI. *Neurochirurgie* 33:57–61.

37. Kahanovitz N, Mehringer MC, Johanson PH (1981): Intracranial entrapment of the atlas complicating an untreated fracture of the posterior arch of the atlas. A case report. *J Bone Joint Surg* [Am] 63:831–832.

38. Kobori M, Takahashi H, Mikawa Y (1986): Atlanto-axial dislocation in Down's syndrome. Report of two cases requiring surgical correction. *Spine* 11:195–200.

39. Krespi YP, Grossman BG, Berktold RE, Sisson GA (1985): Mediastinitis and neck abscess following cervical spinal fracture. *Am J Otolaryngol* 6:29–31.

40. Levine AM, Edwards CC (1985): The management of traumatic spondylolisthesis of the axis. *J Bone Joint Surg* [Am] 67:217–226.

41. Levine AM, Edwards CC (1986): Complications in the treatment of acute spinal injury. *Orthop Clin N Am* 17:183–203.

42. Maiman DJ, Barolat G, Larson SJ (1986): Management of bilateral locked facets of the cervical spine. *Neurosurgery* 18:542–547.

43. McAfee PC, Bohlman HH, Han JS, Salvagno RT (1986): Comparison of nuclear magnetic resonance imaging and computed tomography in the diagnosis of upper cervical spinal cord compression. *Spine* 11:295–304.

44. McAfee PC, Bohlman HH, Riley LH, Robinson RA, Southwick WO, Nachlas NE (1987): The anterior retropharyngeal approach to the upper part of the cervical spine. *J Bone Joint Surg* [Am] 69:1371–1383.

45. Reiss SJ, Raque GH Jr, Shields CB, Garretson HD (1986): Cervical spine fractures with major associated trauma. *Neurosurgery* 18:327–330.

46. Rifkinson-Mann S, Mormino J, Sachdev VP (1986): Subacute cervical spine instability. *Surg Neurol* 26:413–416.

47. Roy-Camille R, Saillant G, Mazel C (1989): Internal fixation of the unstable cervical spine by a posterior osteosynthesis with plates and screws. In: Sherk HH, et al, eds. *The cervical spine research society: The cervical spine, 2nd ed.* Philadelphia: J.B. Lippincott, pp. 390–403.

48. Sakou T, Morizono Y, Morimoto N (1984): Transoral atlantoaxial anterior decompression and fusion. *Clin Orthop* 187:134–138.

49. Sutterlin CE III, McAfee PC, Warden KE, Rey RM Jr, Farey ID (1988): A biomechanical evaluation of cervical spinal stabilization methods in a bovine model. Static and cyclical loading. *Spine* 13:795–802.

50. Tamura T (1989): Cranial symptoms after cervical injury. *J Bone Joint Surg* [Br] 71:283–287.

51. Tomaszek DE, Rosner MJ (1984): Occult esophageal perforation associated with cervical spine fracture. *Neurosurgery* 14:492–494.

52. Wainapel SF (1984): Reflex sympathetic dystrophy following traumatic myelopathy. *Pain* 18:345–349.

53. Wertheim SB, Bohlman HH (1987): Occipitocervical fusion. Indications, technique, and long-term results in thirteen patients. *J Bone Joint Surg* [Am] 69:833–836.

54. White AA III, Johnson RM, Panjabi MM, Southwick WO (1975): Biomechanical analysis of clinical stability in the cervical spine. *Clin Orthop* (109):85–96.

55. White AA III, Panjabi MM (1978): The problem of clinical instability in the human spine: A systematic approach. In: White AA III, Panjabi MM, eds. *Clinical biomechanics of the spine*. Philadelphia: J.B. Lippincott, pp. 191–192.

56. Whitehill R, Richman JA, Glaser JA (1986): Failure of immobilization of the cervical spine by the halo vest. A report of five cases. *J Bone Joint Surg* [Am] 68:326–332.

57. Zdeblick TA, Bohlman HH (1989): Cervical kyphosis and myelopathy. Treatment by anterior corpectomy and strut-grafting. *J Bone Joint Surg* [Am] 71:170–182.

The Adult Spine: Principles and Practice,
J. W. Frymoyer, Editor-in-Chief.
Raven Press, Ltd., New York © 1991.

CHAPTER 53

Post-Traumatic Syringomyelia

Thomas A. Zdeblick and Thomas B. Ducker

Improvement in emergency medical services as well as increased awareness of spine injuries in the trauma patient have led to an increase in the survival of the patient with an injured spinal cord. Neurologic deficit is primarily a result of the initial traumatic event. Neurologic worsening in the acute phase after injury has been thought to be due to either spinal cord edema or hemorrhage. However, untoward management events may also play a role in acute worsening (17).

Increasing neurologic deficit in the chronic phase following spinal cord injury may also occur. Spine instability with progressive deformity may lead to increasing neurologic deficit. However, the most common cause of late ascending neurologic loss is the development of a post-traumatic syringomyelia.

OVERVIEW

Syringomyelia was first described in 1827 by Ollivier, who felt that the spinal cord was distended by fluid from within (29). In 1871, Hallopeau described a cystic lesion of the spinal cord at autopsy in a patient who had suffered a spinal cord injury (10). In 1915, Holmes noted oval or cylindrical cavities in spinal cord specimens from patients with spinal gunshot wounds (11), and Freeman (1953) was the first to equate "ascending spinal paralysis" in the post-traumatic patient with syringomyelia (6).

T. A. Zdeblick, M.D.: Assistant Professor, Division of Orthopaedic Surgery, University of Wisconsin Hospital, Madison, Wisconsin 53792.
T. B. Ducker, M.D.: Department of Neurological Surgery, The Johns Hopkins University School of Medicine, Baltimore, Maryland 21205.

The development of a progressive neurologic deficit extending to previously uninvolved segments months or years after a spinal cord injury, and due to a syrinx, is uncommon. The incidence of post-traumatic syringomyelia has been estimated to be between 0.3% and 2.3% of spinal cord injuries (21,28). In a large series, Barnett found that 1.8% of spinal cord injured patients developed a symptomatic syrinx, compared to the incidence of idiopathic syringomyelia of 0.01% (3). Most authors state that thoracic and lumbar lesions are more common than cervical lesions (8,29).

SYMPTOMS

The presentation of a post-traumatic syrinx may be quite subtle. The classic signs are severe pain unrelieved by analgesics, an ascending disassociated sensory loss, or progression of an incomplete lesion. Pain is the most commonly reported symptom, and numerous authors have stressed the importance of pain that increases with coughing, straining, or sneezing (15,22,24,26,27). Occasionally, radicular pain is present, although axial pain is more common. Dissociate sensory loss describes a state where the patient has objective loss of sensation to pain and temperature but the preservation of touch sensation (4,15,24). This sensory loss may increase distal to the injury or, more commonly, ascend to previously unimpaired levels.

Signs of muscle wasting or lower extremity spasticity are also found, although less commonly. In incomplete lesions, progression of the motor paralysis may occur. In thoracic or lumbar level injuries, signs of cranial nerve involvement may occur rarely with syringomyelia (26).

In cervical level injuries that develop a syrinx, up to 25% will have bulbar signs (24). A much less common finding, and quite rare as a method of presentation, is the presence of a neuropathic joint (14,20). Charcot joints, particularly of the upper extremity, may be due to syringomyelia. Rarely, an increase in urinary dysfunction may herald the onset of a syrinx (25).

The onset of symptoms from a post-traumatic syrinx is often quite delayed from the time of injury. Delays from 6 months to 16 years have been reported (3,16,22). Typically, a syrinx will develop several years after the injury. Several studies have shown that syringomyelia presents earlier in patients with complete spinal cord lesions than in those with incomplete lesions. Lyons et al. (16) and Barnett et al. (3) both demonstrated an average delay of approximately 4 years in patients with complete lesions, compared to 9 years in patients with incomplete spinal cord injury. As noted earlier, there is a greater tendency for a syrinx to form in a thoracic or lumbar lesion than in a cervical lesion.

PATHOPHYSIOLOGY

The pathophysiology of post-traumatic syringomyelia is not completely understood. The etiology of spinal cord cavitation is probably multifactorial. Most syrinxes form in the gray matter between the dorsal horns and the posterior columns (28). Autopsy examination has shown the cavity to form in the partially damaged level of the cord, adjacent to an area of complete injury (5). Williams feels that the intramedullary hematoma, which forms at the time of injury, liquifies (28). This eventually leads to a cystic degeneration within the cord. Kao favors the theory that trauma leads to neural disruption and the formation of myelin microcysts (12). These microcysts then coalesce into an intramedullary cavity.

The mechanisms for extension of the cavity are better understood. The "slosh" mechanism of Williams states that hydrodynamic dissection of the spinal cord is caused by the rapid movement of fluid within the cavity in response to pressure changes in the subarachnoid cerebrospinal fluid space (29). This compression of the cerebrospinal fluid space may be due to pressure changes in the epidural venous plexus or direct changes due to coughing, straining, or sneezing. Syrinx fluid may accumulate due to continued cord necrosis, transudation of proteinaceous fluid, direct passage of fluid via diffusion through the cord, or "sucking" of fluid through the cisternae during pressure changes (7).

DIAGNOSIS

Confirmation of a syrinx by radiologic means is currently undergoing change. In the past, air or panto-paque contrast myelography demonstrated an enlarged cord at the level of injury as presumptive evidence of a syrinx. Water soluble myelography increased the visualization of the cord, and delayed contrast computed tomography scanning further refined the definition of the syrinx (8,19,24). Contrasted computed tomography (CT) is particularly helpful in following the post-operative course of a syrinx. Endomyelography, in which water soluble dye is injected within the cavity itself, is quite good at outlining the extent of a syrinx (24). This technique, however, may miss the multicentric cord cavitation.

Rarely, non-radiologic means are helpful in delineating a syrinx. Radioisotope ventriculography has been found to be useful (9). Electrodiagnostic studies will demonstrate normal nerve conduction velocities. Electromyography shows an increase in polyphasic spikes with an increase in motor unit action potential duration (4).

The best current method to diagnose post-traumatic syringomyelia is magnetic resonance imaging (MRI). This test is non-invasive and provides excellent visualization of the spinal cord and the cranio-vertebral junction. It has been shown to be as accurate as contrasted computed tomographic scanning in making the diagnosis (13,18). The low intensity intramedullary signal on T1 imaging, or a bright signal on T2 imaging is evidence of a syrinx. MRI, however, has some drawbacks. In patients with spinal instrumentation it is technically less helpful. False positives have been seen with MRI scanning; the low intensity signal of myelomalacia is indistinguishable from that of an intramedullary cyst (18). Examples of post-traumatic syrinx are shown in Chapter 23 and in Figure 1.

TREATMENT

The treatment of post-traumatic syrinx should be surgical. The natural history of an untreated syrinx is progressive. Vernon followed 40 symptomatic patients nonoperatively and found that all progressed and demonstrated an increase in severity and an ascending level of pain and sensory loss (26).

In 1892, Abbe first demonstrated the feasibility of syringostomy performed at autopsy (1). Freeman, in a series of experiments with cats and dogs, found that spinal cord trauma led to intramedullary cavities, and he proceeded to drain these cavities (6). In 1959, Freeman performed the first syringostomy in humans (22). Other early surgeons treated syringomyelia in patients with complete lesion by cord transection, allowing drainage of the syrinx. However, in both simple syringostomy and cord transection, the problem of resealing the opening leading to recurrent syrinx occurred (15,22).

Shunting procedures have the benefit of being minimally invasive and of keeping an open channel for de-

A
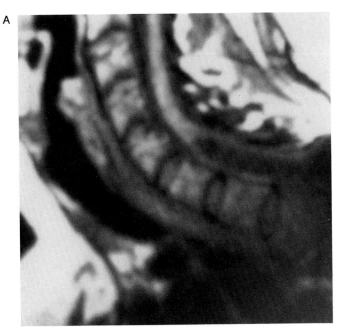

B
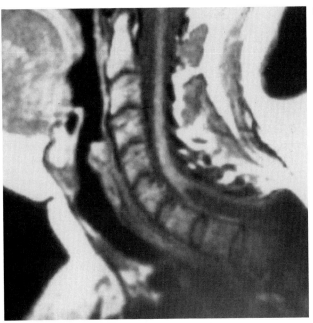

FIG. 1, A and B. This patient had a high thoracic fracture, and 8 years later developed a progressive syrinx going up into the spinal cord, causing numbness and weakness in the hands.

compression of the cavity. Both syringoperitoneal (SP) shunts and syringosubarachnoid shunts have been popularized (2,23,24). Suzuki et al. demonstrated that 22 of 29 patients treated with an SP shunt improved (23). Tator felt that SP shunting led to a higher complication rate, and treated 40 patients with syringosubarachnoid shunting (24). He had good to excellent results in 29 of 40 patients, with 10 of the 14 post-traumatic patients making an excellent recovery. Vernon demonstrated that pain or motor recovery can be expected in about 50% of patients treated with shunting, that sensory symptoms improve in 33%, and that the procedure failed to halt the progression of symptoms in 10% of patients (27).

The procedure of choice is probably the syringosubarachnoid shunt. When possible, the operation is performed with somatosensory evoked potential monitoring to assess cord function during surgery. Following laminectomy and durotomy, intra-operative ultrasonography is often helpful in locating the cystic cavity. A posterior midline myelotomy is then performed. Some surgeons first perform needle aspiration for localization. A small silastic catheter is then placed in the cavity, extended to the subarachnoid space, and sewn to the dura. The dura is then closed. Post-operative monitoring of the syrinx is then performed by physical exam, MRI, or contrasted CT scan.

In summary, the occurrence of post-traumatic syringomyelia is rare and its diagnosis often difficult. However, once found, surgical treatment can lead to improvement in a good proportion of cases.

REFERENCES

1. Abbe R, Coley WB (1892): Syringomyelia, Operation; Exploration of cord; Withdrawal of fluid. Exhibition of patient. *J Nerv Ment Dis* 19:512–520.
2. Barbaro NM, Wilson CB, Gutin PH, Edwards MS (1984). Surgical treatment of syringomyelia. Favorable results with syringoperitoneal shunting. *J Neurosurg* 61:531–538.
3. Barnett HJ, Jousse AT, Morley TP, Lougheed WM (1971): Post-traumatic syringomyelia. *Paraplegia* 9:33–37.
4. Benedetto MD, Rossier AB (1977): Electrodiagnosis in post-traumatic syringomyelia. *Paraplegia* 14:286–295.
5. Foo D, Bignami A, Rossier AB (1989): A case of post-traumatic syringomyelia. Neuropathological findings after one year of cystic drainage. *Paraplegia* 27:63–69.
6. Freeman LW, Wright TW (1953): Experimental observations of concussion and contusion of the spinal cord. *Ann Surg* 137:433–443.
7. Gardner WJ (1965): Hydrodynamic mechanism of syringomyelia: Its relationship to myelocele. *J Neurol Neurosurg Psychiatry* 28:247–259.
8. Griffiths ER, McCormick CC (1981): Post-traumatic syringomyelia (cystic myelopathy). *Paraplegia* 19:81–88.
9. Hall PV, Kalsbeck E, Wellman HN, Campbell RL, Lewis S (1976): Radioisotope evaluation of experimental hydrosyringomyelia. *J Neurosurg* 45:181–187.
10. Hallopeau FM (1871): Sur une faite de sclerose diffuse de la substance grise et strophie musculaire. *Gaz Med de Paris* 25:183.
11. Holmes G (1915): The Goulstonian lectures on spinal injuries of warfare. *Br Med J* 2:769–774.
12. Kao CC, Chang LW, Bloodworth JM Jr (1977): The mechanism of spinal cord cavitation following spinal cord transection. *J Neurosurg* 46:745–756.
13. Kokmen E, Marsh WR, Baker HL (1985): Magnetic resonance imaging in syringomyelia. *Neurosurgery* 17:267–270.
14. Kolawole T, Banna M, Hawass N, Khan F, Rahman N (1987): Neuropathic arthropathy as a complication of post-traumatic syringomyelia. *Brit J Radiol* 60:702–704.
15. Laha RK, Malik HG, Langille RA (1975): Post-traumatic syringomyelia. *Surg Neurol* 4:519–522.
16. Lyons BM, Brown DJ, Calvert JM, Woodward JM, Wriedt CHR

(1987): The diagnosis and management of post traumatic syringomyelia. *Paraplegia* 25:340–350.

17. Marshall LF, Knowlton S, Garfin SR, et al (1987): Deterioration following spinal cord injury: A multicenter study. *J Neurosurg* 66:400–404.

18. Pojunas K, Williams AL, Daniels DL, Haughton VM (1984): Syringomyelia and hydromyelia: Magnetic resonance evaluation. *Radiology* 153:679–683.

19. Quencer RM, Green BA, Eismont FJ (1983): Posttraumatic spinal cord cysts: Clinical features and characterization with metrizamide computed tomography. *Radiology* 146:415–423.

20. Rhoades CE, Neff JR, Rengachary SS, et al (1983): Diagnosis of post-traumatic syringohydromyelia presenting as neuropathic joints: Report of two cases and review of the literature. *Clin Ortho Rel Res* (180):182–187.

21. Rossier AB, Foo D, Shillito J, et al (1981): Progressive late post-traumatic syringomyelia. *Paraplegia* 19:96–97.

22. Shannon N, Symon L, Logue V, Cull D, Kang J, Kendall B (1981): Clinical features, investigation and treatment of post-traumatic syringomyelia. *J Neurol Neurosurg Psychiatry* 44:35–42.

23. Suzuki M, Davis C, Symon L, Gentili F (1985): Syringoperitoneal shunt for treatment of cord cavitation. *J Neurol Neurosurg Psychiatry* 48:620–627.

24. Tator CH, Briceno C (1988): Treatment of syringomyelia with a syringosubarachnoid shunt. *Can J Neurol Sci* 15:48–57.

25. Umbach I, Heilporn A (1988): Evolution of post-traumatic cervical syringomyelia: Case report. *Paraplegia* 26:56–61.

26. Vernon JD, Silver JR, Ohry A (1982): Post-traumatic syringomyelia. *Paraplegia* 20:339–364.

27. Vernon JD, Silver JR, Symon L (1983): Post-traumatic syringomyelia: The results of surgery. *Paraplegia* 21:37–46.

28. Williams B, Terry AF, Jones F, McSweeney T (1981): Syringomyelia as a sequel to traumatic paraplegia. *Paraplegia* 19:67–80.

29. Williams B, Weller RO (1973): Syringomyelia produced by intramedullary fluid injection in dogs. *J Neurol Neurosurg Psychiatry* 36:467–477.

The Adult Spine: Principles and Practice,
J. W. Frymoyer, Editor-in-Chief.
Raven Press, Ltd., New York © 1991.

CHAPTER 54

The Rehabilitation of the Patient with Neurologic Dysfunction as a Result of Cervical Trauma

E. Shannon Stauffer

The rehabilitation of a person with traumatic quadriplegia consists of prevention of metabolic complications, further neurologic deterioration, and musculoskeletal atrophy, followed by education to reenter family and social life at maximum functional capacity. The main determinants of the rehabilitation are the degree, vertebral level, and permanence of the neurologic injury. Rehabilitation planning begins with the initial evaluation of the patient by the physician, ideally in the emergency room within several hours of the accident. With a careful history and physical examination, the physician can determine the severity and level of the neurologic injury, initiate measures to prevent the metabolic complications that may be life threatening, develop a realistic prognosis for future recovery and function, and make plans for

realistic rehabilitation goals with the patient and his or her family.

PATIENT EVALUATION

History

It is important to determine whether the patient had a neurologic deficit when first seen at the scene of the accident. Were there any voluntary motions observed, and what were the patient's complaints? Were there any signs of decreasing neurologic function during transportation? Was the injury caused by a high- or low-energy impact?

Classification of Extent of Paralysis

A classification of the extent of paralysis is necessary to document degree of impairment and recovery rates and provide a uniform medium for communication.

E. S. Stauffer, M.D.: Professor and Chairman, Division of Orthopaedics and Rehabilitation, Southern Illinois University School of Medicine, Springfield, Illinois, 62708.

TABLE 1. *Frankel classification of spinal cord injury paralysis*

A.	Complete	No motor or sensory
B.	Incomplete	Sensory only
C.	Incomplete	Motor—useless
D.	Incomplete	Motor—useful
E.	Normal	Full recovery

The classification described by Frankel (1) is the most commonly accepted and quoted in the literature. Each patient should be classified at the time of injury and again at one-year follow-up to document improvement (Table 1).

Physical Examination

Prior to moving the patient from the emergency room table, a rapid neurologic examination is performed, specifically looking for areas of sharp and dull sensibility and the presence of voluntary muscle function. First observe the patient's breathing pattern. Is the patient breathing on his or her own without ventilatory assistance? Is the breathing by diaphragmatic inhalation only and passive exhalation? Is there any evidence of intercostal function with elevation of the chest on inspiration? Is there any evidence of abdominal function by abdominal muscle contraction on forced exhalation or coughing? If the patient is breathing on his or her own by the diaphragm, this places the patient at least at a cervical 4 functional level.

Beginning at the head, we document that the patient understands the commands by asking the patient to move his or her facial muscles as in a smile, frown, etc. We then examine the sternocleidomastoid function by asking the patient to turn his or her chin isometrically against resistance (cranial nerve 11). Next is to shrug the shoulders (cranial nerve 11). Next we determine whether there is any active power in shoulder abduction by palpating for a contraction of the deltoid and elbow flexion by palpating the biceps (cervical 5). We next examine for active wrist extensors (cervical 6), followed by active wrist flexors and triceps (cervical 7), followed by finger flexors to produce a grip (cervical 8), and finally by finger abduction to test for intrinsics (thoracic 1) (Fig. 1).

The level of voluntary muscle function designates the functional level of quadriplegia. We then ask the patient to take a deep breath and document the presence or absence of intercostal muscle activity. By palpating the abdominals during a cough, we assess voluntary abdominal muscle control. Moving to the lower extremities, we ask the patient to contract the quadriceps, plantarflex and dorsiflex the foot, and flex and extend the toes and document the muscle grade of any of these voluntary actions.

Following the muscle examination we proceed with sharp/dull discrimination sensibility testing, again beginning with the face and neck so that the patient understands the commands. We determine whether the patient can differentiate sharp/dull discrimination and/or deep pressure over the face (cranial 5), back of scalp (cervical 2), neck (cervical 3), infraclavicular area (cervical 4), deltoid and lateral arm (cervical 5), radial forearm, thumb, index finger (cervical 6), long finger (cervical 7), ring finger (cervical 8), and small finger (thoracic 1). This sensory examination will document the level of intact sensibility, which should coincide with the muscle functional level (Table 2).

It is important then to run the pinwheel across the trunk and down over the legs, particularly on the plantar

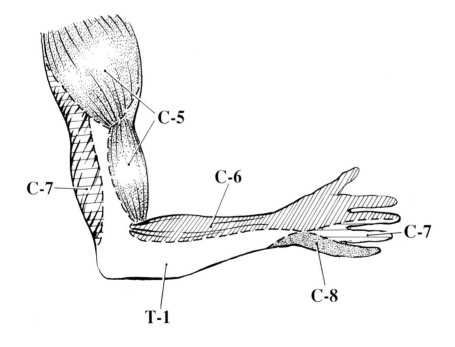

FIG. 1. Cervical nerve root functional levels.

TABLE 2. *Functional root level documentation*

	Sensibility	Motor
C5	Lateral arm	Deltoid—biceps
C6	Thumb index	Wrist extensors
C7	Ring finger	Triceps, finger extensors
C8	Small finger	Finger flexors
T1	Medial forearm	Intrinsics

surface of the foot, to look for any sparing of lumbar or sacral long tract transmission in the cervical spinal cord.

Rectal Examination

The examination of the perianal and rectal area is probably the most important single examination in determining the severity and permanency of a traumatic quadriplegia. Due to the far lateral positioning of the sacral tracts in the cervical spinal cord, these tracts are more likely to be spared following a traumatic impact than those more central. The perirectal examination consists of:

1. Careful examination to elicit any sensation that may be present around the rectum and perineum.
2. A rectal examination with a gloved finger to determine whether there is any active sphincter control.
3. A tug on the indwelling Foley catheter or a tap on the glans penis or mons pubis to detect the presence of a bulbocavernosus reflex.

DIAGNOSIS

Complete Lesions

If the patient has no active muscle control or sensibility below the zone of injury in the cervical spinal cord, specifically with no retained perianal sensation or sphincter or toe flexor muscle control, one may diagnose a "presumed" complete lesion quadriplegia. The patient may be in spinal shock, however, which is a short period of paralysis, insensibility, and absence of reflex activity following any severe traumatic injury to the spinal cord. This period rarely lasts more than several hours. The end of spinal shock is heralded by the presence of the bulbocavernosus reflex. Therefore, if the patient has no active muscle power and has no sensibility below the level of injury and the *bulbocavernosus reflex is present,* the patient has a "confirmed" complete spinal cord lesion. The significance of this is that the patient will make no significant functional recovery. The patient may gradually regain some vague sensibility and may possibly regain some minimal active spastic control of small muscles of the feet, but a clinical prediction can be made that the prognosis is a permanent functional quadriplegia.

Recovery of Motor Root Function

Since the nerve root at the level of the vertebral injury is injured at the neuroforamen after it exits from the intact spinal cord above the level of the cord lesion, the nerve root is likely to recover and upper extremity function is likely to improve during the first six weeks following an injury. Overall, approximately two thirds of patients will recover one additional nerve root level of function. With a C4-C5 level injury, only one third of patients will regain the fifth nerve root recovery. At the C5-C6 level (the most common level of injury), two thirds will have sixth root recovery. At the C6-C7 level, virtually all patients recover the seventh root level function (7) (Fig. 2).

Incomplete Lesions—Quadriparesis

If the patient has some retained sensibility or voluntary muscle control, however slight, distal to the zone of injury, this places him or her in the "incomplete lesion" category. This patient has a good potential for progressive recovery of neurologic function. There are three basic syndromes that can be identified, each with its own specific physical findings and prognostic implications.

Brown-Sequard Syndrome

If the patient has voluntary function and sensibility below the zone of injury and the muscle weakness is greater on one side and the loss of sensibility is greater on the opposite side, this places the patient in Brown-Sequard (hemicord injury) syndrome. This patient has an excellent prognosis for progressive recovery. Since one side of the body has good muscle function and the other side has good sensation, virtually all of these patients become ambulatory and regain bowel and bladder control (Fig. 3).

Central Cord Syndrome

This syndrome is characterized by the patient who has a severe quadriparesis, but has "sacral sparing." He or she can differentiate sharp/dull discrimination at least around the perineum and sometimes over other areas of the lower extremities. He or she has a dense muscle paralysis and may have no spared muscle function or just some weak sphincter control or toe flex or voluntary activity. With the presence of sharp/dull discrimination, the prognosis is good for functional recovery in 50% to 70% of these patients. A few patients (2% to 5%) may have virtually full recovery; however, the majority will have enough recovery to ambulate with walking aids, but will have a slow, spastic-type gait and permanent upper-

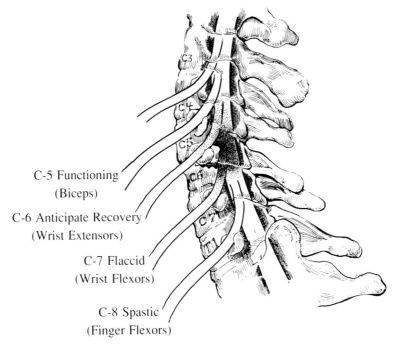

FIG. 2. Anticipated cervical nerve root recovery pattern of a complete C5-C6 quadriplegia. The patient has voluntary C5 muscle function. C6 muscles may be paralyzed, but are expected to recover function. C7 muscles have a permanent flaccid paralysis. C8 muscles have a permanent paralysis with reflex spasticity.

extremity weakness due to central cord grey matter destruction (7).

Anterior Cord Syndrome

The third syndrome consists of those patients who have retained deep pressure sensibility only, with no evidence of sharp/dull discrimination or voluntary muscle control. These patients have only a 10% to 20% chance of any functional recovery, and even these patients have virtually no chance of becoming "normal." The great majority (80% to 90%) will have no functional muscle recovery. They may develop some voluntarily controlled

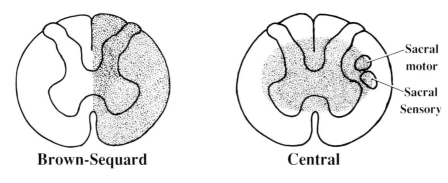

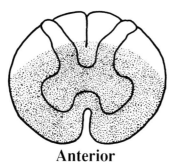

FIG. 3. Incomplete spinal cord injury syndromes.

spastic activity of the foot or leg muscles, which is of no value for functional activities or ambulation.

With this initial evaluation and the confirmation of the complete versus the incomplete lesion, the designation of the level, and the prognosis of root recovery, one can outline the rehabilitation goals for the traumatic quadriplegic.

Respirator-Dependent Quadriplegia

If the patient has a functional level above cervical 4, due to either a fracture of the cervical 3-4 level or an ascending deterioration of a lower initial quadriplegic level, the patient will be respirator dependent. Patients with a high cervical cord injury (C1-C2-C3) usually die at the scene of the accident due to respiratory paralysis; however, if there is respirator assistance available by either knowledgeable cardiopulmonary resuscitation or Ambu bag, the patient may arrive at the hospital dependent on ventilatory assistance. If there is no recovery of the cervical 4 nerve root, the patient remains ventilator dependent permanently. These patients have control only of their face, head, and mouth muscles. Their rehabilitation consists of being able to control an electric wheelchair using head and neck mobility.

Pentaplegia

If the patient has an injury of C1 or C2, which produces a complete spinal cord injury, the patient is not only respirator dependent but has lost the use of the head and neck muscles. He or she has sensation only over the face in a "hockey goalie mask" distribution and no voluntary control of the head other than facial muscles. These patients are completely respirator dependent and do not have enough neck function to operate a mouth-stick-driven electric wheelchair (8).

PRINCIPLES OF TREATMENT

Acute Period

In the acute period, the first principle of treatment consists of stabilizing the spine to prevent further cord or nerve root damage. This can be accomplished by skeletal traction, which may be followed by surgical stabilization. Early mobilization of the patient with a stabilized spine is an important adjunct to preventing metabolic complications and accomplishing early rehabilitation.

Organ System Complications

G.I. Tract. Virtually all patients with a significant spine or spinal cord injury will suffer an ileus of the intes-tinal tract. Nasal gastric suction must be continued until the period of spinal shock is over, the ileus has resolved, and active bowel sounds are heard. If the ileus is not treated, abdominal distension may aggravate the pulmonary problem by decreasing diaphragm excursion. Following a traumatic quadriplegia, especially at the higher levels, the patient will frequently develop a hemorrhagic gastritis. One must be aware of the possibility of an eroding gastric or duodenal ulcer. This complication has become less frequent with the routine administration of cimetidine prophylactically.

Pulmonary Complications. Complications of the pulmonary system are the most important of the early complications. They occur rapidly and may be lethal. They occur much more commonly with the higher lesions. Virtually every patient with a C4-C5 level lesion, most patients with a C5-C6 level lesion, and a few patients with a C6-C7 level lesion will develop significant pulmonary complications. These patients have only the diaphragm for respiratory function. The diaphragm contraction may provide approximately 50% of the expected vital capacity. However, without intercostal muscle stabilization of the rib cage, the patient's vital capacity can be predicted to be approximately 1,000 to 1,500 milliliters of air, or approximately 20% to 30% of normal. These patients cannot fully expand all the alveoli due to paralysis of the intercostals, and they cannot cough or forcibly exhale due to paralysis of the abdominal muscles. Therefore, respiration consists of voluntary inhalation of 1,000 to 1,500 ccs of air and a reciprocal relaxation to expel this amount of air. Patients are not able to expel the expiratory reserve. Secretions accumulate in the bronchial tree. The secretions become thick and may plug off bronchial tubules, resulting in atelectasis. Without treatment, this atelectasis will rapidly lead to pneumonia and the demise of the patient (Fig. 4).

Therefore, one must begin early with aggressive pulmonary toilet, daily chest x-rays, bronchoscopic removal of bronchial plugs, and tracheostomy if breathing becomes labored or the vital capacity drops below 1,000 ccs. Temporary ventilatory assistance is frequently required through either an endotracheal tube or a tracheostomy, depending on the aeroarterial blood gas analysis. Fortunately, pulmonary complications usually last only 3 to 4 weeks. Following this, the patient's vital capacity increases to 30% to 40% of predicted normal. The diaphragm is assisted by the neck accessory respiratory muscles. Repeated pneumonia attacks in the chronic period are not uncommon.

Skin Care

The greatest detriment to long-term function of the quadriplegic is pressure ulceration of the skin. Since the patient has no sensibility to warn him or her of impend-

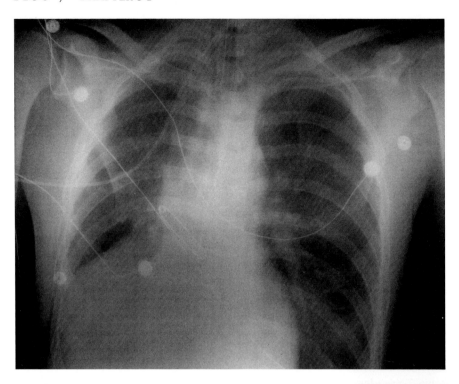

FIG. 4. Chest x-ray demonstrating RLL atelectasis following a C5 cord injury.

ing ulceration and insufficient muscle power to move in the lying and sitting positions, the skin over the bony prominences of the sacrum, trochanters, scapulae, occiput, and heels is likely to break down with pressure ulceration while the patient is in bed during the early phases of rehabilitation. This must be prevented by frequent repositioning of the patient and inspection of the skin. All bony prominences are kept free of pressure by bridging with soft pillows under the fleshy parts of the anatomy.

After the patient is sitting in a wheelchair, a custom wheelchair cushion must be manufactured to prevent excessive pressure over the ischial tuberosities. Frequent pressure-monitoring checks must be made to confirm that the skin/seat cushion interface does not exceed 50 to 70 milliliters of pressure over an hour (Fig. 5).

Urinary Tract Drainage

When the patient is first seen in the emergency room, a Foley catheter is inserted to drain the paralyzed bladder and monitor fluid output. Following the period of fluid retention (first 48 hours) and the period of diuresis (48 to 96 hours), intermittent catheterization every 6 hours is initiated on or about the fifth day to prevent urinary tract infection.

Muscle and Joint Contracture

As the peripheral reflexes return and the muscles begin involuntary spastic contractions, it is important to maintain range of motion of all the joints in the upper and

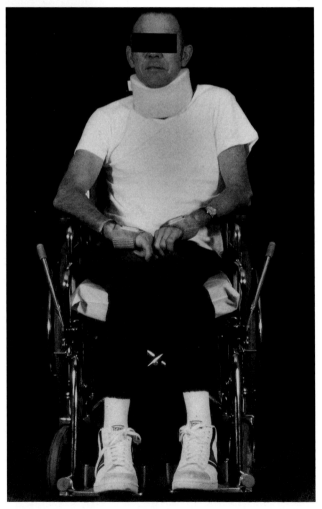

FIG. 5. Quadriplegic patient sitting in wheelchair with customized seat.

lower extremities by daily passive stretching exercises. If joint contractures are allowed to develop, they will prevent future function and cause increased spasticity. Positional hand splints are placed on the patient's hands within the first several days following surgery to maintain wrist extension, MP and IP flexion, and thumb adduction (Fig. 6).

Deep Vein Thrombosis and Pulmonary Embolism

The occurrence of lower extremity deep vein thrombosis is very high in patients with spinal cord injuries. The risk is greatest between 2 and 12 weeks following injury. Since the legs are anesthetic, there is no pain. The presenting signs are fever and swelling (9). The incidence is 10% to 15% if diagnosis is based on clinical presentation. The incidence is 40% to 80% if routine phlebography is used (2).

Pulmonary embolism occurs in 5% to 15% of patients Prophylactic use of anticoagulants decreases the DVT incidence to 1.3% (9).

Overall complication rates are greatly decreased by early admission to specialized spinal injury treatment centers. When days until admission to such centers are divided into three groups—30 days, 30 to 60 days, and 60 days—the incidence of urinary tract infections, spasticity, joint contractures, and heterotopic ossification is greatly increased in group 3 over group 1 (4).

Heterotopic Ossification

Heterotopic ossification (or para-articular ossification) occurs in approximately 20% of patients with a spinal cord injury (3). The etiology and when it actually begins to form are unknown. It begins as a thickening of the extra-periosteal, para-articular tissue anterior to the hip and extends from the anterior-superior spine of the ilium to the lesser trochanter. Early x-rays are negative, and it is frequently misdiagnosed as DVT. The swelling, however, is limited to the thigh and does not extend to the calf as it does in DVT. Gradual limitation of hip flexion, rotation, and extension becomes apparent. X-ray evidence of ossification becomes apparent at about 8 to 10 weeks following injury. The treatment of heterotopic ossification is controversial. As soon as the diagnosis is made, diphosphonate (Didrinel) is administered to retard the mineralization of the heterotopic ossification and passive range-of-motion exercises are continued by physical therapy to break up the ossification as it forms. As the ossification matures, if it is continually fragmented by exercises, motion will be preserved. If a continuous bony bar forms from ilium to femur, the joint will be essentially ankylosed and a later resection of the mature bone will be required.

REHABILITATION

Once the diagnosis and prognosis are established and the spine is stable, early mobilization begins—first by placing the patient on the tilt board until he or she can tolerate the upright position without syncope, and then mobilizing the patient to a wheelchair. The earlier this is done the easier it will be to mobilize the patient without cardiovascular complications (Fig. 5).

Activities of Daily Living

As soon as the patient is upright in a wheelchair, the occupational therapist begins training the patient in self-feeding, grooming, and bathing. Dynamic hand splints

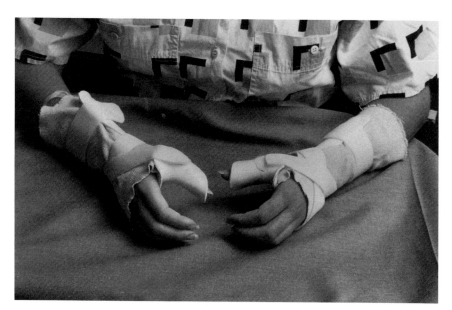

FIG. 6. Early positional hand splints to prevent contractures.

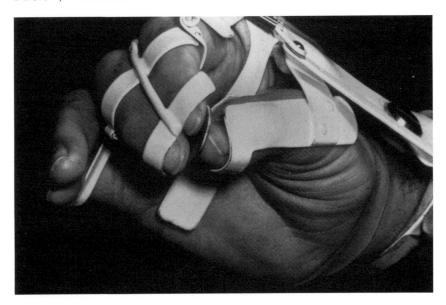

FIG. 7. Dynamic wrist extensor driven hand splint to provide prehension (for C6 and C7 quadriplegia).

are prescribed to provide pinch and grip function (Fig. 7). Passive closing ratchet locking hand splints may be used by the high (C4) quadriplegic for prehension (Fig. 8).

Communication

With the use of hand splints, patients can learn to write with a pencil or ballpoint pen and type using typing sticks. The advent of personal computers and word processors has greatly advanced communication, vocational, and avocational potential for quadriplegics. With these devices, quadriplegics can write, do calculations, and enter into interactive study programs using computers. Telephones and environmental controls are eas-

ily adapted with new electronics to allow quadriplegics greater independence (Fig. 9).

Functional Goals and Equipment

Incomplete Syndromes

Brown-Sequard. People with Brown-Sequard syndrome usually do not have any specific equipment requirements. Progressive recovery is the rule, and they are able to ambulate without assistant devices. A cane and an AFO on the weaker leg may be necessary temporarily.

Central Cord Syndrome. Those patients who have enough functional recovery to ambulate will require a pick-up walker for early walking training and will

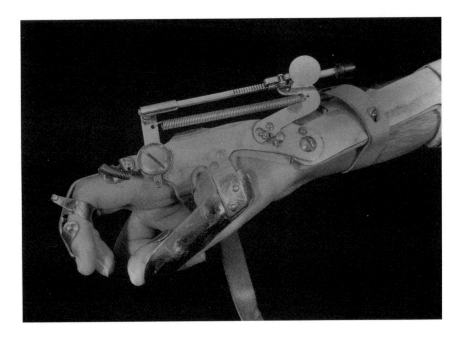

FIG. 8. Ratchet locking hand splint to provide passive prehension (for the high C4 quadriplegic patient).

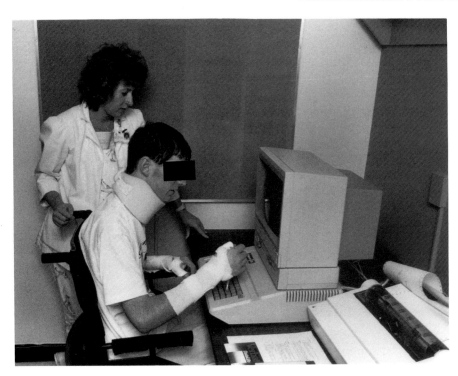

FIG. 9. Quadriplegic patient learning computer operation.

usually graduate to forearm crutches or two canes. They can be expected to use some type of aid indefinitely, however, due to lower extremity spasticity and persistent incoordination.

Anterior Cord Syndrome. Anterior cord syndrome patients will require the same equipment as complete lesion quadriplegics.

Complete Lesions

C1-C3 Respiratory Quadriplegics. These patients will require constant 24-hour attendant care, a mechanical respirator attached to a permanent tracheostomy, and an electric wheelchair with mouth-stick control. The patient with a very high lesion (C1-C2) that is above the phrenic nerve centers in the spinal cord may be a candidate for implanted phrenic nerve stimulators to allow respiration independent of a mechanical respirator. Most respiratory quads are at the C3-C4 level, however; due to destruction of the spinal cord centers, with resultant deterioration of the phrenic nerve fibers, they are not candidates for phrenic nerve stimulation.

C4 High Quadriplegics. These patients are breathing on their own; however, they have no active upper extremity muscle control, and therefore remain completely dependent in activities of daily living. They can be placed in electric wheelchairs, which they can power with a mouth control (Fig. 10).

C5 Quadriplegics. These patients have active deltoid and biceps, but no wrist or hand muscles. They require full-time attendants for care during the day for dressing,

transferring, and positioning in the wheelchair, and for positioning meals and other equipment for activities of daily living. They should be able to feed themselves with positional hand splints, which must be applied by an attendant. They will be dependent in bowel and bladder care, and must constantly be observed for skin pressure ulcers over bony prominences.

C6 Quadriplegics—Average Quads. The addition of active wrist extensor power allows these patients to put on and use flexor-hinge hand splints and be independent in dressing, feeding, wheelchair transfer, and wheelchair propulsion with specialized quad pegs on the wheelchair hand rims. They will need attendant help for housecleaning and some help in dressing and other daily living activities if they are going to school or functioning on a job. Strong C6 level quadriplegics are able to transfer in and out of a car and drive with hand control modifications (Fig. 11).

C7 Quadriplegics—Low Quadriplegics. These patients have wrist extensors, wrist flexors, triceps, and finger extensors, but no finger flexor function. They also require a flexor-hinge hand splint for prehension, but should be able to transfer in and out of bed to a wheelchair, dress themselves, propel the wheelchair, make their own meals, and be functionally independent except for furniture moving and housecleaning.

C8 Quadriplegics. These very low quadriplegics have finger flexors for grip, and therefore have essentially the same goals as a high paraplegic, which would be complete independence in wheelchair activities and transfer, and in activities of daily living.

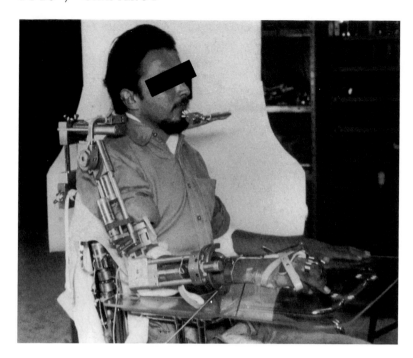

FIG. 10. Electric wheelchair with mouth controls.

Psychological Rehabilitation

There is a great amount of psychological adaptation that must be accomplished by the patients and their families. Often it is more difficult for the parents to accept the permanency of the injury than it is for the young patients. Patients and their families must be treated honestly. They must be advised of the severity of the injury, the realistic prognosis and prediction for recovery, and the aims of the rehabilitation measures.

People who suffer a sudden permanently disabling injury go through a predictable sequence of psychological stages. The first stage is *denial.* They know something seriously wrong has happened, but they are not able to accept the fact that this may be permanent. During the first several days following injury, the patients and families are informed that there is a serious paralysis that may be permanent. They are informed as to the necessity of the various rehabilitation procedures and that we must work with the functional abilities that are present at this time. As several weeks go by and the patients become mobilized in wheelchairs, they begin to realize that they

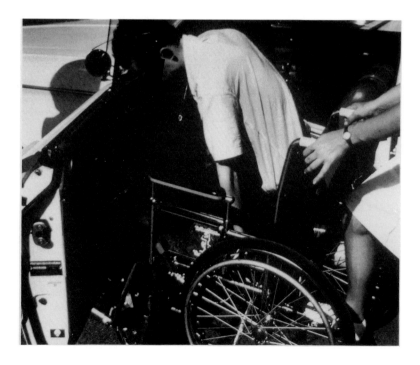

FIG. 11. C6 quadriplegic transferring into automobile.

may not recover and go through a period of *mourning* in which they mourn their former selves and may become angry at the world and the doctors and therapists for not curing their disability. The third phase is *bargaining*, in which the patients try to assert some control over their treatment and destiny by placing demands on the therapists who are in turn placing daily demands on them. The fourth period is *depression*. Unfortunately; this usually coincides with the time that patients are about to be discharged from the hospital, approximately 4 to 5 months following injury. They realize that the time is approaching when they are going to be going home and they are not cured. At this time, greater demands are going to be made on the family with the imminent discharge from the hospital. Once the patients get home it is very difficult for them to get out and around the community. They may not want to be seen in a wheelchair, and the friends who flocked to the hospital to visit become rather scarce. Patients begin to realize that they have to cope with this new life situation; only then can they make realistic plans regarding scholastic, vocational, and social activities. By the time one year has passed, the reality of the permanency is apparent and they know what abilities they have to cope with their new life situations.

Medical Social Work

During the hospitalization, the medical social worker works with the family and helps them adapt to the patient's disability, as well as discussing preparations for home modifications and financial assistance from insurance or government funds.

The goal of rehabilitation is to reintegrate patients into the family and social environment at about one year following injury without significant complications and to teach them how to make the most of their residual abilities.

FOLLOW-UP PERIOD—OUTPATIENT MANAGEMENT

After patients are discharged from the hospital, they must be seen periodically, usually at six-month intervals, for several years for early complication prevention, maintenance of infection-free urinary tract function, and possible further rehabilitation goal potential if neurologic improvement occurs. The specific problems that occur during the outpatient period are the ever-present danger of pressure sores; fever of unknown origin, which is usually due to urinary tract sepsis; and increasing uncontrollable muscle spasticity. After one year has passed following injury, patients may benefit by tendon surgery such as tendo-Achilles lengthening or adductor tenotomy to decrease spasticity. They may also be candidates for tendon transfers of the upper extremity to improve hand function. These are well-described by Moberg (5), Zancoli (10), and Smith (6).

REFERENCES

1. Frankel HL (1969): The value of postural reduction in the initial management of closed injuries of the spine. *Paraplegia* 7:179–192.
2. Grulia UF (1985): Prevention of thromboembolic complications in paraplegia. *Paraplegia* 23:124.
3. Hsu J (1975): Heterotopic ossification around the hip joint in spinal cord injured patients. *Clin Orthop* 112:165–169.
4. Jansen T (1988): Complications of spinal cord injuries. *Paraplegia* 26:50.
5. Moberg E (1987): The present state of surgical reconstruction of the upper limb in tetraplegia. *Paraplegia* 25:351–356.
6. Smith R (1987): *Tendon transfers for quadriplegia. Tendon transfers of the hand and forearm.* Boston: Little, Brown.
7. Stauffer ES (1984): Neurologic recovery following injuries to the cervical spinal cord and nerve roots. *Spine* 9:532–534.
8. Stauffer ES, Bell G (1978): Traumatic respiratory quadriplegia and pentaplegia. *Orthop Clinics North Am* 94:1081–1089.
9. Weingarten SI (1988): Fever and thromboembolic disease in acute spinal cord injury. *Paraplegia* 26:35–43.
10. Zancoli E (1979): *Structural and dynamic basis of hand surgery.* Philadelphia: J. B. Lippincott.

Degenerative Conditions of the Spine

The Adult Spine: Principles and Practice,
J. W. Frymoyer, Editor-in-Chief.
Raven Press, Ltd., New York © 1991.

CHAPTER **55**

Degenerative Conditions of the Spine

Differential Diagnosis and Non-Surgical Treatment

Charles R. Clark

Degenerative conditions of the cervical spine are very common. Schmorl and Junghann (106) reported that 90% of males over age 50 and 90% of females over age 60 have radiographic evidence of degeneration. Indeed chronic cervical degeneration is the most common cause of progressive spinal cord and nerve root deterioration (27). Cervical spondylosis is the term used to describe degeneration of the cervical spine. Primarily it is a process which involves the intervertebral disc. It progresses with age and often develops at multiple interspaces (62). Cervical spondylotic myelopathy is the most serious consequence of cervical intervertebral disc degeneration, especially when associated with a narrow cervical vertebral canal (73).

This chapter discusses cervical spondylosis including spondylotic radiculopathy as well as spondylotic myelopathy. It is important to differentiate between these two conditions not only when approaching a patient for treatment but when reviewing articles which discuss these topics. Many authors in the past have failed to differentiate between these two conditions which may affect the interpretation of their findings. In addition to describing the clinical diagnosis of cervical spondylosis, this chapter highlights the differential diagnosis of degenerative conditions. This encompasses intrinsic cervical conditions including inflammatory, neoplastic, infectious, and miscellaneous afflictions as well as extrinsic disorders affecting the upper extremity which often pose problems in differential diagnosis. The last section of this chapter will deal with principles of treatment. Although non-surgical approaches will be the main emphasis, surgical management will be briefly discussed in order to put it in its proper perspective in the overall management of patients with cervical degenerative disease.

CERVICAL SPONDYLOSIS

Cervical spondylosis can be divided into three primary groups of clinical manifestations. The first group of patients includes those that have radicular complaints, i.e., signs and symptoms primarily in the distribution of a nerve root. The second group of patients are those with myelopathy secondary to cervical spondylosis. Patients who present primarily with neck pain without a true radicular or myelopathic component comprise the third

C. R. Clark, M.D.: Professor of Orthopaedic Surgery, Director, Orthopaedic Spine Fellowship, University of Iowa College of Medicine, Iowa City, Iowa 52242.

group. Internal disc derangement is included in this group. These patients will be discussed under the subheading of cervical spondylotic radiculopathy for the purposes of discussion only.

The introduction notes the importance of differentiating cervical spondylotic radiculopathy from myelopathy. This is important not only in the clinical management of patients but when reviewing the medical literature. In general, the results of management of cervical spondylotic radiculopathy tend to be more favorable than those described for the treatment of myelopathy. If this distinction is not made and all patients are grouped together, the surgical outcome may be biased with the inclusion of a large group of one of these two types of patients. In addition to these two conditions, it is important to differentiate cervical spondylosis from intrinsic degeneration of the central nervous system (27). Epstein et al. (40) have pointed out the importance of recognizing patients with motor neuron disease, particularly amyotrophic lateral sclerosis (ALS), as well as multiple sclerosis. Indeed such intrinsic conditions may coexist with cervical spondylosis.

It is important to understand the natural history of cervical spondylosis. Gore et al., (49) reported a 10 year follow-up of patients with neck pain. They found that following this interval of time, 79% of patients had a decrease in their neck pain and 43% of patients actually had no pain. Thirty-two percent of patients, however, had residual moderate or severe pain. The authors concluded that patients with the most severe involvement appeared not to have improved. They also found that a significant number of patients did not respond to conservative treatment.

Myelopathy is common secondary to cervical spondylosis (127) and is the most serious consequence of intervertebral disc degeneration (73). Spondylotic myelopathy is the commonest cervical cord disorder during and after middle age (28). Patients with this myelopathy often have very long periods without the development of new or worsening signs and symptoms.

The early surgical results for the treatment of cervical spondylotic myelopathy described by Northfield (89) and Campbell and Phillips (17) did not differ significantly from the natural history of the condition, and therefore Lees and Turner (69) concluded that conservative treatment should be the rule. The natural history of 114 patients treated conservatively revealed that 36% actually improved while 64% showed no increase in symptomatology and only 26% of patients worsened. Therefore there is some evidence to justify a conservative approach to this group of patients (13,69,91,101). Surgical management may be particularly efficacious in selected patients and this will be discussed under surgical management, however understanding the natural history of this condition is a prerequisite for treatment.

Crandall and Batzdorf (27) described five categories of cervical spondylotic myelopathy based on the predominant neurological findings (in order of decreasing frequency):

1. Transverse lesion syndrome (corticospinal and spinothalamic tracts and posterior columns are involved).
2. Motor syndrome (primarily corticospinal or anterior horn cell involvement).
3. Central cord syndrome (motor and sensory involvement of the upper extremities greater than the lower extremities).
4. Brown-Sequard syndrome (unilateral cord lesion with ipsilateral corticospinal tract involvement and contralateral analgesia below the level of the lesion).
5. Brachialgia and cord syndrome (predominant upper limb pain in some associated long tract involvement).

This classification has been described in many subsequent papers and appears to be clinically useful particularly when comparing the results of various treatment modalities.

Pathophysiology

The pathophysiology of cervical spondylosis is multifactorial including anatomic, biomechanical, as well as electrophysiological factors. The blood supply of the spinal cord as well as canal size are important anatomic factors. Parke described in detail the blood supply of the spinal cord which consists of three major longitudinal arteries: A large ventral (anterior) spinal artery and two dorsolateral arteries which are fed by medullary vessels of segmental origin. The location of the anterior spinal artery makes it vulnerable to direct compression by osteophytes and degenerative disc material. In addition, medullary feeder vessels may be compressed as they traverse along the neuroforaminae to the midventral surface of the cord (23,93).

Canal size must also be considered. Organic narrowing of the spinal canal may either be congenital/developmental or acquired. The former group includes such conditions as Klippel-Feil syndrome, achondroplasia, spina bifida, spondylolisthesis, and congenital narrowing (12,120). Acquired conditions include degenerative disease (cervical spondylosis), rheumatoid arthritis, ankylosing spondylitis, inflammation, and tumors (12). Congenitally narrow canals per se are usually asymptomatic, however the spinal cord may be more vulnerable to additional encroachment (120). Further compromise may occur due to protrusion of disc material, subluxation of the vertebrae (96), buckling of the ligamentum flavum, and/or development of osteophytes (6,23).

Compression of the cord and interference with the blood supply may result.

Several parameters have been used to describe canal size. These include the sagittal diameter of the canal, as well as the cross-sectional area. The developmental sagittal diameter of the cord is measured at the mid level of the vertebral body and the spondylotic sagittal diameter is measured at the level of the intervertebral disc. This latter measurement takes into consideration the effect of osteophytes (37). Ratios have been developed and are useful since they eliminate the effect of image magnification present on plain radiographs. Pavlov's ratio compares the relationship between the sagittal diameter of the canal to the vertebral body (116). Plain radiographs are typically used to determine canal size and measurements will be discussed further in the section on clinical diagnosis. The CT scan is useful to quantitate the cross-sectional area of the cord. The magnetic resonance image provides perhaps the best appraisal of canal size because in addition to determining the area it details characteristics of the spinal cord as well as the degree of anterior and posterior defects on the subarachnoid space and neural structures (79). Batzdorf and Batzdorff (7) feel that spinal curvature is an additional important anatomic factor. They found no clear correlation between severity of myelopathy and degree of sagittal curvature. Severe myelopathy was present in patients with straight, lordotic, as well as hyperlordotic spines, however, neck pain was most severe in patients with reversed cervical curvature, and the degree of curvature seemed to correlate with post-operative results. Patients with normal curvature showed the greatest improvement in symptomatology following treatment. Spinal geometry is a factor in the selection of patients when surgical intervention is considered.

Panjabi and White described the biomechanics of the spine in cervical spondylotic myelopathy. Abnormal stresses and strains on the spinal canal are caused by static as well as dynamic factors. Static factors include those previously mentioned such as a small canal, osteophytes, disc herniation, hypertrophy of the ligamentum flavum, and apophyseal joint deformation. Dynamic factors include normal and abnormal motion, normal and abnormal loads applied, and the mechanical properties of the spinal cord and spinal column (23,92,124). Bohlman and Emery (11) reported that electrophysiological changes occur in the pathophysiology of this condition. They noted alterations of evoked potentials as the disease progresses. Intrinsic changes occur within the spinal cord. These include blockage of axoplasmic flow, distortion of cord tissue, and stretching of intrinsic transverse terminations of the spinal artery. These authors found that tissue destruction with demyelination of white matter occurs in severe cases and concluded that the pathological findings appear to correlate with clinical severity (11,23).

Cervical Spondylotic Radiculopathy

Cervical spondylosis may result in radicular pain (i.e., pain in a distribution of a nerve root). This may be the result of a herniation of nuclear material through the annulus fibrosis (soft disc) (Fig. 1) or encroachment on the neural foramina by osteophytes (hard disc). The most mobile segments of the spine are the most frequently involved levels in cervical degeneration (32). The C5-C6 interspace is the most commonly involved followed by C6-C7 and C4-C5 (16).

The anteromedial wall of the neuroforamen is formed by the uncovertebral joint and the posterolateral wall is formed by the apophyseal or facet joint. Osteophytes involving either of these articulations may compress the neuroforamina resulting in radicular pain. Soft disc herniation actually is a spectrum of entities ranging from tears of the annulus fibrosis with mild bulging of nuclear material to frank herniation with sequestration. The most common location of a soft disc herniation is posterolateral, however, herniation may also occur anteriorly or posteriorly (central herniation). Posterior herniations may produce myelopathy and will be discussed later. Anterior herniations may cause extrinsic compression of the esophagus. In addition, osteophytes along the anterior surface of the vertebral bodies may also compress the esophagus.

Dysphagia may result from anterior soft or hard disc encroachment upon the esophagus. Bony protuberances into the hypopharynx or esophagus may be accompanied by soft tissue inflammation resulting in increased symptoms (64). Dysphagia due to organic, anatomic narrowing of the gut lumen must be differentiated from muscular or neuromuscular disorders. Typically such anatomic dysphagia is worse for solid foods compared to liquids and there is no difficulty in expelling food from the pharynx to the hypopharynx (64). The diagnosis is confirmed by having the patient ingest barium-impregnated solids and obtaining lateral radiographs. Hyperostosis of the cervical spine is common but only a rare cause of dysphagia (57). The initial treatment of this condition is conservative since dysphagia may be magnified by local edema and in some cases treatment with nonsteroidal anti-inflammatory agents or steroids may be useful. Long term follow-up is necessary to determine the validity of surgical excisions of osteophytes in the treatment of this condition (57).

Internal disc derangement may be a source of neck pain and is included in this section, typically however, it does not produce radicular pain. Whitecloud and Seago (126) reported 34 patients who underwent cervical arthrodesis because of a positive discogram. Reproduction of the patient's symptoms at the time of disc space injection was used to determine the involved levels. The authors reported 70% good or excellent results utilizing their technique. They cautioned, however, that the cervi-

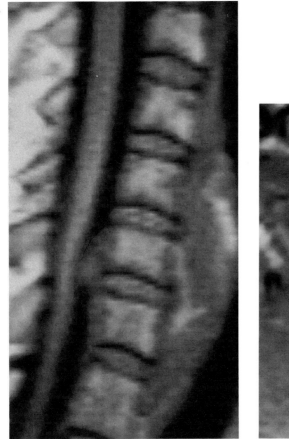

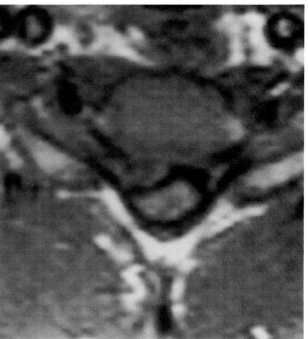

FIG. 1. Magnetic resonance images from a 35-year-old patient with an acute soft disc herniation at C6-C7. **A:** Sagittal image demonstrating the herniation with cord compression. **B:** Transverse image.

cal discogram should only be considered following a complete diagnostic workup including myelography, CT scan and/or MRI, and following a prolonged period of unsuccessful conservative management. They reported positive surgical results in approximately two-thirds of patients when the pain pattern is reproduced by the disc space injection and specific guidelines followed (23,126).

Cervical Spondylotic Myelopathy

Myelopathy secondary to cervical spondylosis is a fairly common problem, particularly in patients over the age of 55 (20). Typical neurological findings include lower motor neuron and reflex changes at the level of the lesion and upper motor neuron involvement below. The gait abnormality is often the most common clinical concern of the patient and Nurick classified cervical spondylotic myelopathy largely on the basis of gait (Table 1) (90,91,125).

The Japanese Orthopaedic Association (55) has devised an objective assessment scale to quantitate the degree of involvement secondary to spondylotic myelopa-thy. The scale involves four categories: motor dysfunction of the upper extremity, motor dysfunction of the lower extremity, sensory deficit, and sphincter dysfunction (Table 2). The maximum number of points is 17 (normal). Hirabayashi described a formula, based on the JOA score, to assess the recovery rate after surgical intervention in patients with myelopathy secondary to ossification of the posterior longitudinal ligament (Table 3) (20,55). This formula has also been used to quantitate recovery in patients with cervical spondylotic myelopathy.

TABLE 1. *Nurick's classification of disability in spondylotic myelopathy*

Grade 0	Root signs and symptoms
	No evidence of cord involvement
Grade I	Signs of cord involvement
	Normal gait
Grade II	Mild gait improvement
	Able to be employed
Grade III	Gait abnormality prevents employment
Grade IV	Able to ambulate only with assistance
Grade V	Chair bound or bedridden

With permission from ref. 90.

TABLE 2. *The assessment scale proposed by the Japanese Orthopaedic Association*

I. Motor dysfunction of the upper extremity
Score
0 = Unable to feed oneself
1 = Unable to handle chopsticks, able to eat with a spoon
2 = Handle chopsticks with much difficulty
3 = Handle chopsticks with slight difficulty
4 = None

II. Motor dysfunction of the lower extremity
Score
0 = Unable to work
1 = Walk on flat floor with walking aid
2 = Up and/or down stairs with handrail
3 = Lack of stability and smooth reciprocation
4 = None

III. Sensory deficit
A. The upper extremity
Score
0 = Severe sensory loss or pain
1 = Mild sensory loss
2 = None
B. The lower extremity, same as A
C. The trunk, same as A

IV. Sphincter dysfunction
Score
0 = Unable to void
1 = Marked difficulty in micturition (retention, strangury)
2 = Difficulty in micturition (pollakiuria, hesitation)
3 = None

With permission from ref. 55.

TABLE 3. *Recovery rate after surgery*

1. Maximum gain = maximum score − pre-operative score
2. Maximum rate of recovery (%) =
$$\frac{\text{maximum score} - \text{pre-operative score}}{17 \text{ (full score)} - \text{pre-operative score}} \times 100$$
3. Final gain = final score − pre-operative score
4. Final rate of recovery (%) =
$$\frac{\text{final final score} - \text{pre-operative score}}{17 \text{ (full score)} - \text{pre-operative score}} \times 100$$

With permission from refs. 20 and 55.

CLINICAL DIAGNOSIS

History and Physical Findings

As previously noted symptoms referable to cervical degenerative disease can be divided into three categories: neck pain, radicular symptoms, and myelopathic symptoms. An individual patient may manifest findings from one, two, or all three of these areas. The neck pain referable to cervical degenerative disease tends to be posterior, located in the paraspinous muscular region. Associated with this patients may have occipital headaches as well as interscapular pain. The pain may be exacerbated by neck motion as well as use of the arms in the over-shoulder position. Patients also tend to complain of neck stiffness with pain at the extremes of motion. The pain may be lessened or relieved with immobilization of the neck with a cervical orthosis.

Radicular symptoms secondary to cervical degenerative disease are characterized by proximal pain and distal paresthesias. In general, the symptoms are referable to an individual nerve root. Note however, that there is overlap between the dermatomes innervated by a particular nerve and it is rare to have findings strictly isolated to the distribution of a single dermatome. The upper extremity is primarily supplied by the C5 through C8

and T1 nerve roots. The sensory dermatomes of these roots follow a relatively simple pattern. If one thinks of the upper extremity with the arm positioned in the anatomic position (i.e., the palms supinated) the sensory dermatomes follow a circular pattern. The C5 dermatome provides sensation to the lateral arm. The C6 dermatome provides sensation to the lateral forearm including the thumb. The C7 dermatome includes the middle portion of the hand and middle finger. The C8 dermatome provides sensation to the medial forearm and the T1 dermatome provides sensation to the medial arm. There certainly is overlap of the innervation to the muscles in the upper extremity and this is also true of the reflexes. A helpful way to remember the nerve supply of the upper extremity muscles is to think of the primary joints innervated by a particular root. The C5 root involves the shoulder (deltoid-shoulder abduction). The C6 root primarily supplies the elbow flexors (biceps, brachialis) and the wrist extensors (extensor carpi radialis longus and brevis and extensor carpi ulnaris). The C7 root is basically the antagonist of the C6 root (elbow extension-triceps, wrist flexion-flexor carpi radialis and flexor carpi ulnaris) with the addition of finger extension at the metacarpal phalangeal (MP) joints. The C8 and T1 roots primarily supply the hand intrinsics with the C8 roots primarily responsible for flexion at the MP joints and T1 roots supplying the abductors and adductors of the fingers.

The reflex innervation is as follows: the biceps reflex is supplied by C5 and C6. The brachioradialis is primarily supplied by C6 and the triceps is primarily supplied by C7.

The cervical nerve roots exit above the corresponding vertebral body (i.e., the C5 root exists above the C5 vertebral body. Therefore, a disc rupture of C4-C5 will usually compress the C5 root. Since the C8 root comes out above the T1 body the relationship of the nerve root to the disc space is different below the cervical-thoracic junction.

As previously noted patients with cervical radiculopathy have a predominance of proximal pain and distal paresthesias. Therefore, a patient with cervical degeneration at C5-C6 with compression of the C6 root tends to have pain in the lateral arm with paresthesias in the lateral forearm down into the thumb. In addition, the patient may have weakness of the elbow flexors and wrist extensors with hyporeflexia of the biceps and/or brachioradialis reflexes.

The onset of symptoms with cervical radiculopathy secondary to a hard disc or degenerative disease is insidious in many cases. However, a patient often will ascribe the onset to a specific incident such as a lifting injury, a vigorous recreational activity or a household work project. Patients who present with the abrupt onset of symptomatology may have a soft disc rupture superimposed upon their cervical degenerative disease.

Patients with a ruptured cervical disc may have relief of pain with arm abduction. This maneuver is similar to bending the knee during Laseque's maneuver. Such relief however, is uncommon in patients with cervical radiculopathy secondary to spondylosis (8).

Myelopathy secondary to cervical spondylosis typically has an insidious onset, developing gradually over a long period of time (Fig. 2) (27,127). The most common clinical pattern involves short periods of worsening followed by long intervals of relative stability (69). The sudden onset of myelopathy may occasionally develop in the presence of cervical spondylosis. Severe hyperexten-

sion injuries, acute superimposed soft disc herniation, or torsion dystonia may cause an acute myelopathy (2,9,59,73). When the onset is acute and there is rapid deterioration a vascular etiology should also be considered (121). It is important to rule out motor neuron disease when considering the diagnosis of myelopathy secondary to spondylosis. Conditions such as multiple sclerosis and particularly amyotrophic lateral sclerosis must be excluded (40).

A deep aching pain and burning sensation is clinical evidence of spinal cord involvement (42). Patients often complain of loss of hand dexterity. Many will have painful dysesthesias and difficulty writing. Diffuse nonspecific weakness may be present. Patients also complain of difficulty walking and often loose their balance. The typical walking pattern is a broad-based gait. Bladder incontinence may also be present (20,112).

Patients with cervical spondylotic myelopathy tend to exhibit myelopathic findings more commonly than root symptoms; motor and reflex changes more commonly than sensory changes; and analgesia is more common than anesthesia, which is more common than proprioceptive loss (74).

The typical motor findings are lower motor neuron

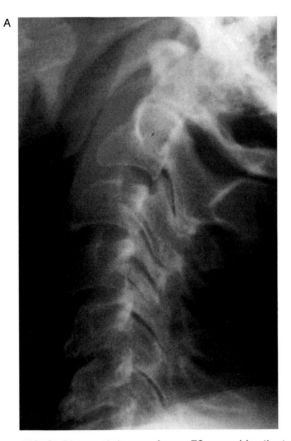
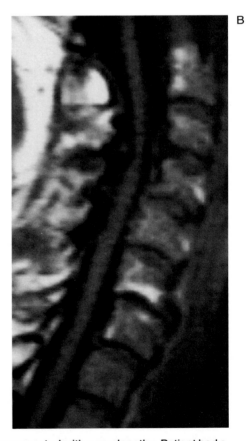

FIG. 2. Diagnostic images from a 72-year-old patient who presented with a myelopathy. Patient had a gradual onset over a period of several years. She had a broad-based unsteady gait. **A:** Lateral radiograph demonstrating multi-level cervical spondylosis. **B:** Sagittal magnetic resonance image demonstrating cord compression at multiple levels.

involvement at the level of the lesion and upper motor neuron manifestations below the level. This includes the lower levels of the upper extremities as well as the lower extremities. Upper extremity involvement tends to be unilateral while the lower extremities are affected bilaterally (20). Sensory findings are often variable because compression of sensory pathways occurs at several levels. Typically sensory findings occur at a level below the area of compression, touch sensation is often preserved, and pain and temperature may be diminished as well as proprioception and vibratory sense (20). Reflex changes usually follow the pattern of motor involvement, i.e., lower motor neuron findings (hyporeflexia) at the level of involvement and upper motor neuron (hyperreflexia) below. A positive Hoffmann and/or Babinski sign may be present indicating an upper motor neuron lesion.

As previously noted, Crandall and Batzdorff described five categories of presentation (transverse, motor, central, Brown-Sequard, and brachial cord) (27). This classification is useful when categorizing the clinical presentation of a patient with myelopathy. It may also relate to the prognosis of treatment.

High cervical spondylosis (C3–C5) may present with a distinctive clinical syndrome of "numb, clumsy hands" and stereoanesthesia of the hands (47). Such higher lesions cause a different syndrome compared to the more common lower lesions. This syndrome is characterized by paresthesia and proprioceptive loss in the hands with minimal sensory changes in the legs. This is similar to the central cord syndrome of Crandall and Batzdorf. The clinical picture of lower cervical involvement (C5–C8) typically includes spasticity as well as proprioceptive loss in the legs (39,47,50,75,81).

Physical findings include a positive Spurling's maneuver (present in 25% of patients) (27). Oblique extension with compression of the head and neck produces cervical root compression resulting in pain. A Lhermitte's sign is a shock like sensation in the trunk or limbs following quick extension or flexion of the neck. This sign is present in approximately 25% of patients with myelopathy secondary to cervical spondylosis (27). Spasticity is almost invariably present in these patients.

Imaging and Laboratory Investigation

Imaging modalities play a major role in the diagnosis and management of patients with cervical spondylotic myelopathy. Modic et al. (86), have outlined the advantages and disadvantages of the various studies used to image degenerative disease of the cervical spine. Plain x-rays are rapid and provide an inexpensive screen of osseous pathology, however, they are unable to directly visualize encroachment or compression of the neural structures. Water-soluble nonionic contrast myelography is able to image the entire cervical region except in cases of high grade stenosis. However, it is invasive and lacks diagnostic specificity. Computed tomography with intrathecal contrast provides excellent differential between bone and soft tissue lesions, directly demonstrates canal size and foraminal narrowing, is minimally operator dependent, and able to visualize abnormalities distal to severe narrowing or blockage (4,25,29,35,65,86, 87,107). The magnetic resonance image provides excellent, non-invasive evaluation of the spinal cord, other neural structures, and soft tissues. This operator-dependent study primarily reflects the physiology of the imaged area rather than the anatomy per se. Modic et al., feel that the MRI might now be the appropriate first test for the evaluation of the cervical spine in a patient with signs of symptoms referable to degenerative disease when therapeutic intervention is considered. The MRI is ideally suited to exclude intramedullary lesions of the central nervous system (79). The additional information provided by this study may compensate for its additional cost. It is important to understand however that the MRI may be positive in asymptomatic individuals with degenerative disease. Modic et al., have shown that disc protrusions are present in 20% of patients aged 45 to 55 and 57% of patients greater than age 64. In addition, spinal cord impingement may be present in 16% of patients less than age 64 and 26% of patients greater than age 64 (86). Certainly, diagnostic studies must be correlated with the patient's history and clinical findings prior to considering therapeutic intervention.

As noted earlier, several dimensions of the spine have clinical importance. These include the sagittal diameter of the spinal canal, the cross-sectional area of the canal, the mobility of the spinal cord, and spinal curvature (7). The sagittal diameter is most commonly assessed on a plain radiograph. Measurements should be determined on lateral radiographs with a focus-grid distance of 72 inches (102). Normally the spinal canal is oval shaped in the mid-cervical region and there is a sagittal diameter of 17 mm (130). The cervical cord diameter varies little from C1–C7 and averages 10 mm (102). The diameter of the spinal canal increases with flexion and decreases with extension. The spinal cord moves rostrally as much as 3 mm at C7 during flexion and extension and results in angulation of the nerve roots at their foramina (14).

The role of a narrow cervical spinal canal in relation to clinical syndromes was investigated by Edwards and La Rocca (37). They described several measurements (Fig. 3). The developmental segmental sagittal diameter (DSSD) is determined at the level of the pedicle. A perpendicular line is drawn to the posterior margin of the spinal canal as determined by the most anterior bony landmark for the segment. A second perpendicular line is drawn at the level of the disc indicating the spondylotic segmental sagittal diameter (SSSD). The difference between these two measurements is the spondylosis index (SI) and represents the amount of narrowing due to the

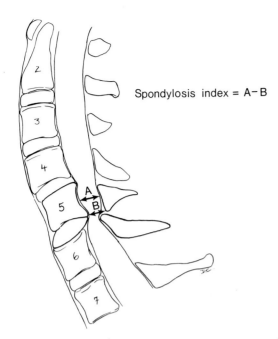

Spondylosis index = A − B

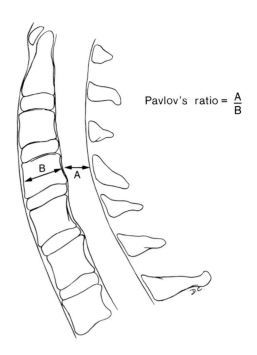

Pavlov's ratio = $\dfrac{A}{B}$

FIG. 3. Schematic diagram depicting the developmental segmental sagittal diameter (DSSD) (label A) and the spondylotic segmental sagittal diameter (SSSD) (label B). The spondylosis index (SI) is the difference between the DSSD and SSSD (see text for details) (with permission from ref. 37).

FIG. 4. Schematic diagram depicting the measurements made on a plain lateral radiograph to determine Pavlov's ratio. Pavlov's ratio = A/B (see text for details) (with permission from ref. 115).

disease process (15,37,38). Edwards and LaRocca stated that the ultimate significance of the developmentally narrow canal will depend on the amount of reserve space present within the canal and the rate of progression of the disease (37). They used mid-cervical (C4–C6) diameters as predictors. Patients with developmental diameters of 10 to 13 mm and spondylotic narrowing of 2 to 4 mm per segment were in the premyelopathic group. Patients with diameters greater than 13 mm were less prone to develop myelopathy however, and tended to have symptomatic cervical spondylosis. Patients with greater than 17 mm diameters tolerated spondylosis without significant symptoms. The authors found that, using a measurement of 17 mm as the normal cutoff between wide and narrow as determined by Wolf (130), patients with a narrow canal only tolerated a spondylosis index of 2.1 mm per segment compared to an index of 3.3 mm per segment for patients with a wide canal.

A concern about making absolute measurements on plain radiographs is the variability of magnification. Torg et al. (115), have described a ratio method (Pavlov's ratio) which eliminates this variable (Fig. 4). Their method involves determining the sagittal diameter of the spinal cord from the midpoint of the posterior aspect of the vertebral body to the nearest point on the corresponding spinolaminar line. This ratio compares the sagittal diameter of the spinal canal with the anteroposterior width of the vertebral body measured through the mid-

point of the body. Furthermore, these authors investigated neurapraxia of the cervical spinal cord with transient quadriplegia in athletes and found that the control group of normal individuals had a Pavlov's ratio of 1 or greater. They found statistically significant spinal stenosis (p < 0.0001) in patients with cord neurapraxia compared to controls. This group had a ratio of less than 0.8. They found, however, no evidence that the occurrence of neurapraxia of the spinal cord predisposed to permanent injury (115).

Patients with stenotic spinal canals are usually asymptomatic (120). However, they are more vulnerable to encroaching lesions such as herniated discs, protruding or bulging of the annulus fibrosis, osteophytes, and/or infolding of the ligamentum flavum.

Besides canal diameter, sagittal spinal curvature should be evaluated on lateral plain radiographs. As previously noted Batzdorf and Batzdorff found that neck pain was most severe in patients with a reversal of the cervical curve. Further, the degree of spinal curvature correlates with post-operative outcome. Patients with normal curvature show the greatest improvement in signs and symptoms following surgery. Spinal geometry should be considered in patient selection for surgery (7). Certainly the rationale for laminectomy includes dorsal migration of the spinal cord into the space developed by the removal of the ligamentum flavum and laminae (1,108). Posterior decompression allows the cord to migrate dorsally thereby decreasing axial tension and improving vascular profusion of the cord (41). If a patient has a significant kyphotic deformity, the majority of compression may be anterior to the cord. Such a deformity is a relative contraindication to a posterior approach (22).

Dynamic magnetic resonance images obtained in hyperflexion, neutral, and hyperextension are useful in the diagnosis of cord compression in patients with spinal stenosis and myelopathy (43). In addition, these studies are useful to determine the relief of cord compression following surgical intervention.

Electrodiagnostic studies play a limited role in the evaluation of cervical spondylotic myelopathy. Electromyography (EMG) may be less sensitive compared to somatosensory evoked potentials in detecting cervical root lesions (68). The greatest role for electromyography is the differentiation of radicular disease from peripheral involvement. In many cases nerve conduction velocities can rule out a peripheral nerve compression which may mimic cervical radiculopathy and/or myelopathy. Electrodiagnostic changes preferably in combination with mixed nerve sensory evoked potential testing may be important in evaluating cases with early cervical myelopathy (98). Leblhuber et al., evaluated the diagnostic value of different electrophysiologic tests in cervical disc prolapse (68). They found abnormal EMGs in 67% of patients and abnormal dermatomal somatosensory evoked potentials in 85%. Certainly the use of evoked potentials, particularly the motor evoked potential, is an evolving technology at the present time and holds promise for the future. Evoked potentials are primarily used investigationally to monitor the status of patients intra-operatively. With further refinement they will undoubtedly become routine during spinal surgery.

DIFFERENTIAL DIAGNOSIS

This section highlights the major clinical conditions which should be considered in the differential diagnosis of patients presenting with symptoms referable to the neck. It includes two major subheadings: intrinsic and extrinsic conditions. Intrinsic cervical conditions include inflammatory, neoplastic, infectious, and miscellaneous disease processes. Extrinsic conditions include degenerative, inflammatory, neoplastic, infectious, and miscellaneous conditions of the upper extremity which may have a clinical presentation similar to that of degenerative disease of the cervical spine and must be considered in the differential diagnosis. This section discusses these various disorders pointing out clinical features which differentiate these conditions from manifestations of cervical spondylosis. Indeed one must keep in mind that many of these conditions may coexist with cervical spondylosis.

Intrinsic Cervical Conditions

Inflammation: Rheumatoid Arthritis

Rheumatoid arthritis frequently affects the cervical spine and the majority of patients with this disease have cervical involvement. The pathophysiology of cervical involvement is similar to that in the peripheral joints. The primary disease process involves the synovium with resultant destruction of bone, cartilage, and ligaments. This may produce significant instability of the cervical spine with neurologic compromise. There are three common patterns of involvement: atlantoaxial subluxation (C1–C2), cranial settling (also known as atlantoaxial or occipital-atlantoaxial impaction), and subaxial subluxation (18). Any or all of these conditions may coexist in the same patient. Atlantoaxial subluxation results from loss of integrity of the transverse, alar, and/or apical ligaments and is present in 19% to 71% of patients (26,33,77,80,110,113). Instability is determined on lateral, flexion, and extension radiographs (Figs. 5 and 6). When the anterior atlantodental interval (ADI) is greater than 3 mm, integrity of the transverse atlantoaxial ligament is jeopardized and instability may be present. When the ADI is greater than 10 to 12 mm, all of the supporting ligaments of the atlantoaxial complex are disrupted and the segment is grossly unstable (44). Some patients may stabilize in the subluxed position, therefore, instability is considered present when *mobility* is demonstrated on flexion and extension radiographs. Cranial settling results from destruction of the occipitoatlantal and atlantoaxial joints with the dens protruding through the foramen magnum providing the potential for brain stem compression. This condition is present in 5% to 32% of patients with rheumatoid arthritis (33,80,97,99). Several parameters based on plain radiographs are used to determine and quantitate the degree of cranial settling (Fig. 7). The McGregor line (McG) is drawn from the posterior edge of the hard palate to the most inferior portion of the occiput. Normally the tip of the odontoid process should not protrude more than 4.5 mm above this line (53). The method of Redlund-Johnell involves determining the distance from the base of C2 to McGregor's line. Normally this distance is greater than 17 mm. Cranial settling is considered present when this interval is less than 15 mm in males and 13 mm in females (21). The simplest way to quickly screen for the possibility of cranial settling is to note the relationship of the anterior arch of C1 to C2. This parameter is known as the station of the atlas and was described by Clark (Fig. 8) (21). The station of the atlas is determined by dividing the axis into thirds along its sagittal plane. Normally the anterior arch of C1 is adjacent to the tip of the dens (station 1). As cranial settling progresses the anterior arch of C1 may be adjacent to the base of the dens

A

B

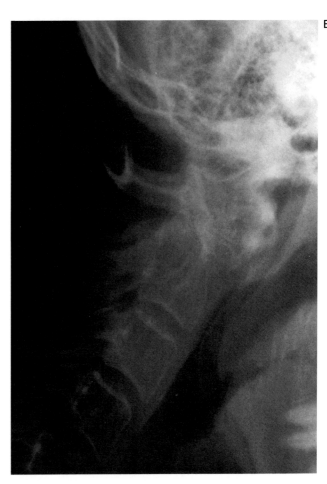

FIG. 5. Lateral flexion and extension radiographs from a rheumatoid patient with severe atlantoaxial subluxation. **A:** Extension view demonstrating reduction of the subluxation. **B:** Flexion view demonstrating significant mobile atlantoaxial subluxation.

(station 2). In cases of severe cranial settling the anterior arch of the atlas may be adjacent to the body of the axis (station 3) or even lower (21). The advantage of this parameter is that a determination can be made with relative ease on plain radiographs. Subaxial (below C2) subluxation may be present in 10% to 20% of patients (5,85,109). This condition may be present at one or several levels and results from synovitis of the apophyseal as well as uncovertebral joints with resulting ligamentous and capsular laxity.

The clinical presentation of patients with rheumatoid involvement of the cervical spine is varied. Patients may complain of neck pain, however, and many are asymptomatic. Such patients have multiple joint involvement and frequently suffer from chronic disease. Therefore, they may present with relatively few cervical complaints. Symptoms result from tissue inflammation, neurologic dysfunction, and/or vertebral artery insufficiency. Synovitis and mechanical instability may result in referred pain into the intrascapular area, the chest, shoulder,

and/or upper extremity. Neurologic dysfunction is present in 7% to 34% of patients and may include the brain stem, spinal cord, and/or nerve roots (26,97,113). Cranial settling may include impingement of the dens on the lower cranial nerves as well as cardiorespiratory center and pyramidal tracts. Atlantoaxial subluxation may cause cord compression with spasticity, pathologic reflexes, and urinary retention or incontinence. Vertebral artery insufficiency is the least common mode of presentation. Such patients may present with dysequilibrium, tinnitus, vertigo, visual disturbances, diplopia, dysphagia, and nystagmus (71).

The treatment of rheumatoid arthritis is somewhat controversial and certainly beyond the scope of this chapter. However, because of the likelihood of progressive instability, posterior arthrodesis should be considered when there is radiographic evidence of major instability and cord compression demonstrated on neuroradiographic studies. This may be necessary even in the absence of pain or neurological deficit (21).

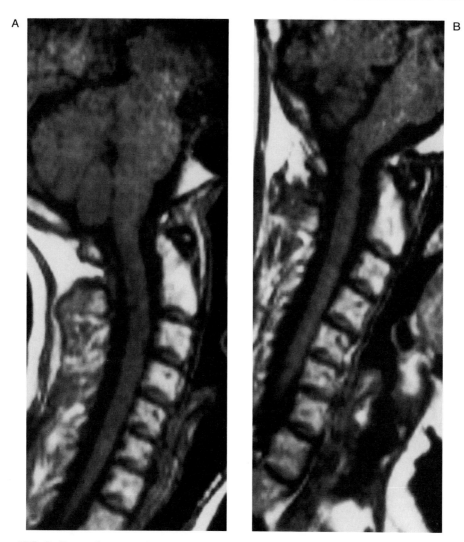

FIG. 6. Dynamic magnetic resonance images of the rheumatoid patient in figures with atlantoaxial subluxation. **A:** Extension image (C1-C2 reduced). **B:** Flexion image demonstrating significant kinking of the cord at the cervicomedullary junction.

Neoplastic Conditions

Primary cervical neoplasms are rare and account for approximately 1% of patients with primary bone tumors (112). Spinal lesions in older patients are most frequently malignant; spinal lesions in children and adolescents are usually benign (123). Benign primary cervical neoplasms include: hemangioma, osteochondroma, osteoid osteoma, osteoblastoma, and giant cell tumor of bone. Malignant primary cervical neoplasms are less common than the benign tumors and include chordoma, multiple myeloma, osteosarcoma and chondrosarcoma.

The spine is a common site for skeletal metastases irrespective of the primary tumor (108). Seventy-five percent of vertebral metastases originate from carcinoma of the breast, prostate, kidney, or thyroid, or from lymphoma, or myeloma (51).

The clinical presentation of patients with neoplastic disease includes localized pain in the area of involvement. Neck pain tends to be the most common presenting symptom (10). The pain tends to be unremitting. It is often more intense at night, at rest, or during times of inactivity. It may be associated with headaches and upper extremity pain. Neurologic abnormalities frequently develop in patients with primary cervical neoplastic disease. Radicular pain is common and the spinal cord level is usually discrete (3).

Intrinsic spinal cord tumors are extremely rare. Only a small percentage of primary central nervous system tumors are intraspinal. These tumors are classified as extradural, intradural-extramedullary, and intramedullary. Extradural tumors account for 22% of primary spinal cord tumors. The rest are intradural. Seventy-one percent of these are extramedullary with the most common tumors being meningiomas and schwannomas.

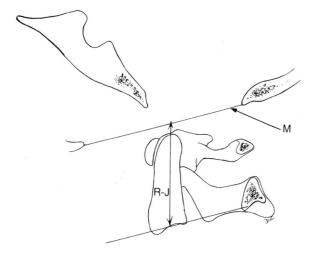

FIG. 7. Schematic diagram depicting McGregor's line (M) and the measurement of Redlund-Johnell (see text for details) (with permission from ref. 24).

Twenty-nine percent are intramedullary tumors and these include ependymomas and astrocytomas (72). The clinical presentation of spinal cord tumors includes nocturnal and rest pain. The pain may be local as well as referred and is often localized to a discrete neurologic level. Intradural-extramedullary lesions may produce asymptomatic myelopathic deficits. Extramedullary lesions produce radicular sensory and motor loss. Bladder dysfunction may also be present with these tumors (72).

Infections

Spinal sepsis constitutes only a small portion of all cases of skeletal infection due to pyogenic organisms (114). Of these, 3% to 4% occur in the cervical spine (47). This condition generally occurs in children and the elderly as well as medically compromised patients (46,58,70). Spread to the epidural space occurs in up to one-third of patients. Antecedent infection can be identified in only a minority of patients.

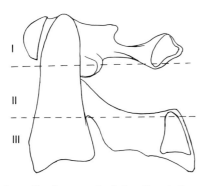

FIG. 8. Schematic diagram depicting the station of the atlas (see text for details) (with permission from ref. 21).

The clinical presentation includes tenderness, guarding, and limited spine motion. Pain is increased with axial compression or percussion of the spinal process of the involved vertebrae. Radiculopathy or myelopathy may be present if structural instability or epidural extension exists.

Although the spine is the most common site of tuberculous skeletal involvement, only 3% to 5% of cases of spondylitis involve the cervical spine (34,78). Neurological deficit may result from direct pressure of granulation tissue, abscess formation, extruded necrotic bone or disc material, or spinal instability. The clinical findings include progressive pain and neck stiffness. Pain may be referred to the shoulders, upper extremities, or occiput. When myelopathy is present there tends to be lower motor neuron findings at the level of infection and upper motor neuron findings distal to the level (60).

Miscellaneous Differential Conditions

Multiple sclerosis (MS) is often considered "the great imitator" in neurologic disease (94). MS has a prevalence of approximately 30 to 80 per 100,000 people in the northern United States and southern Canada (83). Because of the ubiquitous nature of this condition it must be considered in the differential diagnosis of patients presenting with cervical myelopathy. The average age of onset is 32 years (94). In the younger patient the clinical course tends to be one of remission and relapse however an older patient often has a chronically progressive course.

The clinical presentation involves acute loss of central vision in 16% to 30% of patients with slightly greater than 10% of patients complaining of diplopia. Incoordination, fatigability, dysarthria, dysphasia, urinary tract dysfunction, and acute loss of sensory and/or motor function in the upper or lower extremities may be present. Up to one-third of patients may have a positive Lhermitte's sign. Patients typically have reduced vibratory and position sense and approximately 30% exhibit absent deep tendon reflexes. Muscular atrophy is an infrequent finding (94).

Ossification of the posterior longitudinal ligament (OPLL) is a common cause of myelopathy in Oriental populations. However, this condition is being more frequently recognized in non-Oriental populations (82). The diagnosis is suspected on a clinical basis and frequently the ossification is easily seen on plain lateral radiographs, however, neuroradiographic studies may be required to confirm the diagnosis as well as to determine the extent of cord compression.

Patients who present with hyperextension/hyperflexion injuries of the cervical spine (the so-called "whiplash syndrome") will often present with neck and shoulder pain. These patients should be considered in the differential diagnosis. However, the history of preceding trauma often confirms the diagnosis. A hyperextension or hyperflexion injury may also aggravate a preexisting cervical spondylotic condition. This subject is discussed in greater depth in the chapter on the cervical sprain syndrome.

Pancoast tumors must be considered in the differential diagnosis of patients presenting with neck and upper extremity pain as well as neurological symptoms. These lesions constitute 5% of all bronchogenic tumors and arise in the apical parietal pleura (111). The tumor may invade the stellate ganglia of the sympathetic chain as well as elements of the brachial plexus resulting in Horner's syndrome as well as upper extremity symptoms. Early diagnosis is essential to successful management. About 60% of cases are surgically resectable with a 5 year survival of 31% and a 15 year survival of 22% (95). The clinical presentation includes local pain in the area of the scapula and shoulder. Pain may radiate into the ulnar distribution of the upper extremity. Wasting of hand intrinsics and Horner's syndrome may be present. Radiographs may reveal thickening of the apical pleura, destruction of the first to third ribs and erosions of the vertebral bodies (111). The tumor may be seen on the AP radiograph of the cervical spine if the lung fields are carefully scrutinized on this view (Fig. 9).

Syringomyelia may result from a congenital or developmental disorder or may be post-traumatic in origin. Generally, there is combined sensory and motor dysfunction (105). Patients typically present with paresthesias or dysesthetic pain producing a prickling or tingling sensation (128). Sensory loss is present in 90% of patients. Pain is present in only 20% and may be radicular and simulate nerve root compression. Thermal and pain modalities are affected more than proprioception and light touch. Motor weakness is present in the majority of patients. The characteristic cerebrospinal fluid findings include low protein (105).

Extrinsic Conditions: Upper Extremity

Shoulder

Extrinsic shoulder problems are perhaps the most common conditions which need to be differentiated from cervical pathology. Indeed conditions in both areas may coexist but typically one condition precedes the onset of the other. Primary cervical conditions which refer pain to the shoulder include cervical spondylosis with foraminal encroachment, acute soft disc herniation with nerve root compression and radicular pain, post-traumatic degeneration with foraminal compromise, and miscellaneous cervical conditions including tumors (52). Referred pain to the shoulder from the cervical spine can initiate the process of tendinitis in the shoulder with a resultant "frozen shoulder." The keys in differentiating cervical from shoulder conditions are the history and

physical examination. Clinically, patients with cervical spine disorders complain of neck pain and headaches. Pain is typically at the top of the shoulder, may be increased at night, and is often relieved with the use of a cervical orthosis. Pain secondary to shoulder impingement or rotator cuff problems is located predominantly over the deltoid insertion and is not relieved by a cervical orthosis (52).

When evaluating shoulder conditions it is helpful to separate those which limit passive glenohumeral motion from those which do not. Therefore, physical diagnosis is essential to determine a specific diagnosis. Conditions which typically do not limit passive shoulder motion will be discussed first.

Rotator cuff tendinitis results from impingement of the rotator cuff between the acromion and the humeral head. The coracoacromial ligament is also important in the pathophysiology of this condition. Neer identified three stages of impingement (88). Stage 1 consists of edema and hemorrhage of the rotator cuff. Stage 2 involves tendinitis, fibrosis, and calcification of the supraspinatus tendon; in addition there is thickening and fibrosis of the subacromial bursa. In Stage 3 rotator cuff tendinitis occurs with partial or complete rupture of the rotator cuff. The clinical presentation consists of an aching or gnawing pain in the deltoid region. Pain is often worse at night and exacerbated with overhead work. Abduction and external rotation against resistance increases symptoms. Impingement may be reproduced by forward elevation of the humerus against resistance. With a torn rotator cuff there is loss of active motion particularly in abduction or external rotation.

Bicipital tendinitis may develop secondary to inflammation of the rotator cuff. Typically patients complain of shoulder pain in the region of the bicipital groove. Increased symptoms result from resistance to forward flexion of the shoulder with the elbow in extension and the forearm supinated.

Calcific tendinitis of the rotator cuff occurs most frequently in the supraspinatus tendon. Calcification is a different pathologic process than impingement (84,118). Symptoms result from rupture of calcium deposits into the subacromial bursa producing an acute, extremely painful, crystal-induced bursitis. The clinical findings are characterized by an atraumatic, acute onset of pain in the region of the greater tuberosity. Diagnosis is confirmed by a positive radiograph.

Another important group of disorders which do not typically limit passive glenohumeral range of motion includes acromioclavicular (AC) joint problems. Such patients complain of pain in the region of the AC joint. Symptoms may be aggravated by adducting the affected upper extremity or extreme glenohumeral abduction.

Several intrinsic shoulder conditions limit full passive glenohumeral motion. Adhesive capsulitis generally results from immobilization for a painful condition such

A

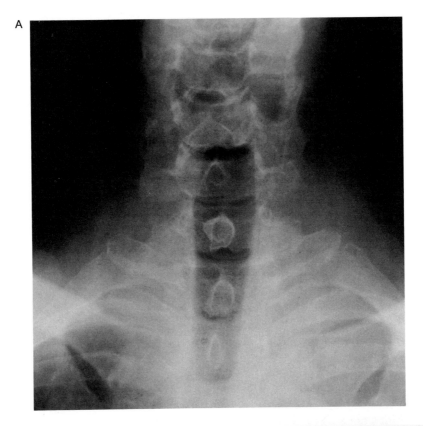

B

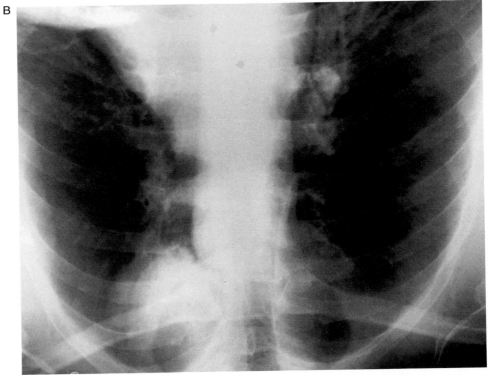

FIG. 9. Middle-aged patient with Pancoast tumor of the left upper lobe of the lung. Patient presented with neck and radicular pain in the C8-T1 distribution. He had a Horner's syndrome. **A:** Anteroposterior cervical radiograph suggesting a fullness in the apex of the left lung. **B:** Posteroanterior chest radiograph depicting the lesion at the apex of the left lung.

as rotator cuff inflammation, glenohumeral arthritis, pulmonary disease, or myocardial infarction. Clinically patients typically present with poorly localized intense pain about the shoulder. Pain may also be referred to the deltoid insertion. The earliest motion that is lost is that of external rotation. Disuse atrophy of the shoulder is often present.

Glenohumeral arthritis also tends to limit passive glenohumeral motion. Both inflammatory and degenerative disorders produce painful limitation of motion and a weakness of the shoulder girdle; crepitance is frequently present. The range of motion is limited due to capsulitis. Radiographic findings are characteristic and confirm the diagnosis.

Pyogenic arthritis of the glenohumeral joint must also be considered in the differential diagnosis. Clinically patients present with pain, swelling, and limitation of shoulder motion. Systemic manifestations are infrequent. The only abnormalities may be a mild elevation of temperature and leukocyte count.

Many extrinsic disorders result in referred pain to the shoulder region. These produce phrenic nerve irritation. Typically such patients present with pain in the supraclavicular or trapezial regions or at the superior angle of scapula. Disorders which may produce diaphragmatic irritation include pneumonia, pulmonary infarct, hepatobiliary disease, and subphrenic abscess.

Brachial plexitis is an inflammatory process of uncertain etiology. It may be viral in origin. The majority of patients have involvement of the upper plexus. Approximately one-third of patients recover from symptoms in one year and 90% are recovered in three years (117). Recovery is generally more rapid with lesions of the proximal plexus. Patients who have recurrent or prolonged pain and no sign of motor recovery after 3 months have a poor prognosis. The clinical presentation consists of acute onset of pain and tenderness in the region of the shoulder. Pain is maximal at the time of onset in three-fourths of cases. The pain may be sharp, stabbing, throbbing, or achy in character. Pain may radiate into the scapula or the upper extremity (31). Muscle weakness develops within the first 2 weeks of onset in approximately 70% of patients (117). The most frequent muscles involved include the deltoid, supraspinatus, infraspinatus, serratus anterior, biceps, and triceps (31).

Compressive Neuropathies

The suprascapular nerve originates from the first branch of the brachial plexus and is derived from the C5–C6 roots. Entrapment occurs at the suprascapular notch and produces atrophy of the supraspinatus and infraspinatus muscles. Patients typically exhibit weakness of glenohumeral external rotation and abduction.

The thoracic outlet syndrome may be the result of congenital, developmental, or post-traumatic abnormalities of osseous or soft tissue structures. Approximately 30% of cases are due to osseous abnormalities including first rib or clavicular fractures, cervical ribs, or osteochondromas of the clavicles (30). Approximately 70% are due to soft tissue problems including involvement of the scalenus anticus, scalenus medius and pectoralis minor muscles, and/or fibrous bands. Functional factors play an important role such as overuse, poor posture, and trauma. Clinical findings include pain in the neck, shoulder, or upper extremity. Paresthesias or weakness may be present. Less commonly there is vascular involvement. Provocative tests include adduction/external rotation, costoclavicular, and hyperabduction tests. Pulse obliteration with the arm and/or head in various positions (Adson's test) is a normal finding in the majority of asymptomatic people and has no relation to the etiology or presence of symptoms (103). Therefore it is not useful in diagnosing this condition. Patients with upper plexus involvement typically have tenderness with palpation in the region of the C5–C6 roots. Tilting of the head to the opposite side is painful. Patients may have weakness of the biceps, triceps, and wrist. In addition, they may have hypesthesia in the radial nerve distribution. Patients with lower plexus involvement tend to have tenderness in the supraclavicular area and along the course of the ulnar nerve and weakness of hand grip and interosseous muscles (104).

The median nerve may be compressed at several sites along its anatomic course producing various neuropathies. Anatomic sites include: the supracondylar process, Lacertus fibrosis, pronator teres, arch of the flexor digitorum superficialis, and the carpal tunnel. Carpal tunnel syndrome is the most common entrapment neuropathy of the upper extremity. Patients typically present with pain and paresthesias in the median nerve distribution of the hand. The pain tends to be worse at night and with use of the hand. Clinical examination may include a positive Tinel's sign, a positive Phalen's sign, thenar atrophy, and weakness with altered sensibility in the median nerve distribution of the hand. It is not unusual to find an increased incidence of cervical arthritis and diabetes in patients with carpal tunnel syndrome. The phenomenon of the "double-crush" syndrome has been suggested as an explanation of this association (119).

The ulnar nerve is typically compressed at two sites: the cubital tunnel and Guyon's canal. Symptoms include aching pain in the medial side of the proximal forearm and paresthesias within the ulnar nerve distribution. Sensory changes include the area supplied by the dorsal cutaneous branch of the ulnar nerve. Weakness of the intrinsic muscles of the hand may also be present.

Shoulder Hand Syndrome

This condition is a type of reflex sympathetic dystrophy (RSD). Typically it results from trauma to the shoulder or upper extremity or from pain due to a visceral lesion such as a stroke or myocardial infarction (67). The pathogenesis includes a "vicious cycle" of pain, immobility, edema, tissue reaction, and vasospasm leading to a stiff non-functional dystrophic extremity (66). Clinically, patients often present with adhesive capsulitis of the shoulder with pain, swelling, and limitation of motion. With time, pain and swelling develop particularly over the dorsum of the hand. Characteristic atrophy of the skin with irreversible flexion deformities of the fingers develop later in the disease process. The diagnosis is typically made on a clinical basis, however, nuclear diagnostic studies may be useful to confirm this condition. A diffusely positive late image on a three-phase bone scan, with all areas showing increased activity, is considered diagnostic of RSD, with both sensitivity and specificity greater than 95% (76).

PRINCIPLES OF TREATMENT

The treatment of a patient with cervical spondylosis should begin with the obvious: a careful clinical history and physical examination. This should be followed by an appropriate diagnostic evaluation to establish an accurate diagnosis. These factors are essential in the successful management of patients with spondylosis, however, they may be easily overlooked.

When considering management of patients with cervical spondylosis it is important to categorize patients according to the predominance of the signs and symptoms. Patients should be divided into three primary groups: neck pain alone, radiculopathy, and myelopathy. The role of surgical management of patients with neck pain alone is controversial and very limited. Certainly there is a role for non-operative management of patients with radiculopathy and/or myelopathy and the vast majority of patients are treated in this manner.

Several factors are very important when planning treatment. First of all the severity of neurological involvement needs to be considered. Secondly, the rate of progression is important. Patients with a rapidly progressive neurological deficit may be identified for prompt surgical management provided a vascular etiology is ruled out. Duration of symptoms should also be considered. There are several studies to suggest that patients with cervical spondylotic radiculopathy and/or myelopathy have the best prognosis following surgery when symptoms have been of relatively short duration (9,22,36,61).

Relative contraindications to operative management include a long history of non-progressive symptoms (22,36). Patients with profound neurological deficit may not respond well to surgical management. In addition, other disorders of the nervous system may coexist with cervical spondylosis and portend a poorer prognosis from surgical management (36). As mentioned earlier in this chapter the differential diagnosis must be considered to rule out other disorders that may have a similar clinical presentation. Amyotrophic lateral sclerosis and multiple sclerosis may mimic spondylotic myelopathy (22). In addition, patients with associated cerebral vascular disease, multiple strokes, or low pressure hydrocephalus may present in a similar manner (20,22,41).

The overall medical status of the patient needs to be considered when developing a treatment plan. Severe cardiac disease, diabetes mellitis, poorly controlled hypertension, as well as various psychological disorders may be contraindications to surgical intervention.

The cornerstone of successful non-operative management of patients with cervical spondylosis is accurate diagnosis. Many patients can be adequately managed with nonsteroidal anti-inflammatory medication, the short term use of a cervical orthosis, and judicious physical therapy modalities. Physical therapy tends to be most effective when used during acute exacerbations of symptoms. Such treatments include transcutaneous electrical nerve stimulation, ultrasound, neuroprobe, and cervical traction. Many of these treatment modalities are most effective when used for relatively short periods of time rather than relying on them over prolonged periods. Certainly, one of the most important components of non-operative treatment is the longitudinal follow-up of patients including a careful neurological examination to rule out the development and/or progression of neurological signs and symptoms. Since this disease process tends to be slowly progressive it is important to document the neurological status of patients at regular intervals to monitor for any insidious change.

Therapeutic injections may have a role in the treatment of patients with cervical spondylosis. Injections should be used judiciously and tend to work best when symptoms are acute. Trigger point and facet injections may provide prompt improvement of symptomatology. Cervical epidural steroid injections (CESI) may have a role in the non-operative management of patients with cervical pain with or without radicular symptoms. Wilson et al. (129) recently reported a series of 100 patients who underwent 235 CESIs. Patients in this study had no previous cervical spine surgery. Complications consisted of a dural puncture rate of 1 out of 50 patients. These investigators found that CESI was most efficacious in patients with radicular pain and signs. CESI supports the pathophysiology of root inflammation as a source of radicular pain.

Pain treatment centers may play a significant role in the non-operative management of patients particularly those with symptoms of long duration. In addition to traditional treatment modalities including therapeutic injections many centers use specialized techniques including behavioral modification, biofeedback, acupuncture, and acupressure in the management of such patients. Patients being treated long term with chronic pain should be evaluated periodically to verify the underlying diagnosis and to rule out occult neurological progression.

Chemonucleolysis has been reported as a treatment option for a herniated cervical disc (100). This treatment, however, is extremely controversial and certainly the experience in the lumbar spine has been associated with significant neurological risk including transverse myelopathy. A recent review of 38 patients undergoing cervical chemonucleolysis reported good to excellent results in 83% of the cases (100). However, the group of patients that respond best to this type of management are those who respond very effectively to standard treatment modalities, i.e., patients with radicular signs and symptoms who have failed conservative treatment and have positive neuroradiologic studies that correspond to the clinical signs and symptoms. Contraindications to this procedure include the previous use of chymopapain, cord involvement, cervical spine instability, and isolated neck pain (100). Because of the relative lack of well controlled studies one must view this treatment modality for cervical spondylosis with significant skepticism at the present time.

Cervical discography may play a role in the management of patients with cervical spondylosis. In general discography is reserved for those cases in which the diagnosis cannot be established by more traditional methods (48). Indeed the cervical discogram should be considered last as a diagnostic technique following myelography, CT scan, and/or MRI (23). Diagnostic cervical disc injection may be used to determine symptomatic levels in patients with internal disc derangement. Cervical arthrodesis should only be considered when prolonged treatment fails. As previously mentioned, positive surgical results have been reported in approximately two-thirds of patients when the pain pattern is reproduced by the injection (126).

It is beyond the scope of this chapter to discuss the surgical management of patients with cervical spondylosis. However, it is important to understand the advantages and disadvantages of surgical intervention in order to put non-operative treatment in its proper perspective. There are two basic approaches to the cervical spine: anterior and posterior. Anterior procedures primarily include intervertebral disc excision with or without fusion and vertebrectomy. The major posterior procedures include laminectomy and laminaplasty. Patients with single level disease and radicular findings may respond quite adequately to anterior intervertebral disc excision. Such patients may also respond to a posterior laminotomy/laminectomy with excision of disc material and/or osteophytes encroaching upon the neuroforamen. The number of levels involved may be important in deciding the approach to a patient with cervical spondylotic myelopathy. In general, patients with less than 2 to 3 levels of involvement may be most judiciously managed by an anterior procedure. Patients with greater than 3 to 4 levels involved may be best managed by a posterior approach. Certainly there are many different ways to manage myelopathy secondary to cervical spondylosis. Often the procedure which the treating physician is most comfortable with produces the best result. However, it is very important to individualize the surgical treatment plan based on the individual characteristics of the patient as well as the neuroradiographic findings. Therefore, the spine surgeon should be skilled in multiple approaches. The following general principles apply. Patients with central cord compression may be most directly managed with an anterior approach. The most direct approach to a specific anatomic lesion is often the most efficacious. Cervical kyphosis may be a contraindication to posterior procedures particularly laminectomy since adequate decompression may not be obtained and the cord is not allowed to migrate dorsally because of this sagittal deformity.

Cervical laminaplasty may play a significant role in the management of patients with cervical spondylosis. The Japanese have had a long and successful experience with the use of this procedure in patients with myelopathy secondary to ossification of the posterior longitudinal ligament as well as spondylosis (54,56,63). Laminaplasty has the advantages of maintaining the osseous protection of the spinal cord as well as potentially retaining stability (63). The development of a late swan-neck deformity has been a concern in patients undergoing multi-level laminectomies (28). This may be a particular problem in younger patients with more mobile spines. This is less of a concern in older patients with a relatively immobile spine.

In summary, many patients with cervical spondylosis can be effectively managed non-operatively and in most cases surgical intervention is not considered until the patient has undergone an adequate trial of non-operative management. Certainly the duration as well as severity of neurological signs and symptoms are important considerations in this regard. Accurate diagnosis and careful patient selection are essential to the successful management of this condition.

ACKNOWLEDGMENT

The author wishes to acknowledge the assistance of William A. Roberts, M.D., who provided significant input for the section on differential diagnosis.

REFERENCES

1. Aboulker J, Metzger J, David M, Engel P, Balliret J (1965): Les myelopathies cervicals d'origine rachidienne. *Neurochirurgie* 11:87–198.
2. Angelini L, Broggi G, Nardocci N, Savoiardo M (1982): Subacute

cervical myelopathy in a child with cerebral palsy. Secondary to torsion dystonia? *Childs Brain* 9:354–357.

3. Austin GM (1960): The significance and nature of pain in tumors of the spinal cord. *Surg Forum* 10:782–785.

4. Badami JP, Norman D, Barbaro NM, Cann CE, Weinstein PR, Sobel DF (1985): Metrizamide CT myelography in cervical myelopathy and radiculopathy: correlation with conventional myelography and surgical findings. *AJR* 144:675–680.

5. Ball J, Sharp J (1971): Rheumatoid arthritis of the cervical spine. In: Hill AGS, ed. *Modern trends in rheumatology, vol 2.* London: Butterworth, p. 117.

6. Barnes MP, Saunders M (1984): The effect of cervical mobility on the natural history of cervical spondylotic myelopathy. *J Neurol Neurosurg Psychiatry* 47:17–20.

7. Batzdorf U, Batzdorff A (1988): Analysis of cervical spine curvature in patients with cervical spondylosis. *Neurosurgery* 22:827–836.

8. Beatty RM, Fowler FD, Hanson EJ Jr (1987): The abducted arm as a sign of ruptured cervical disc. *Neurosurgery* 21:731–732.

9. Bertalanffy H, Eggert HR (1988): Clinical long-term results of anterior discectomy without fusion for treatment of cervical radiculopathy and myelopathy. A follow-up of 164 cases. *Acta Neurochir (Wien)* 90:127–135.

10. Bohlman HH, Sachs BL, Carter JR, Riley L, Robinson RA (1986): Primary neoplasms of the cervical spine. *J Bone Joint Surg [Am]* 68:483–494.

11. Bohlman HH, Emery SE (1988): The pathophysiology of cervical spondylosis and myelopathy. *Spine* 13(7):843–846.

12. Boni M, Denaro V (1982): The cervical stenosis syndrome with a review of 83 patients treated by operation. *Int Orthop* 6:185–195.

13. Bradshaw P (1957): Some aspects of cervical spondylosis. *Q J Med* 26:177–208.

14. Breig A, Turnbull I, Hassler O (1966): Effects of mechanical stresses on the spinal cord in cervical spondylosis: a study on fresh cadaver material. *J Neurosurg* 25:45–56.

15. Burrows EH (1963): The sagittal diameter of the spinal canal in cervical spondylosis. *Clin Radiol* 14:77–86.

16. Buszek MC, Szymke TE, Honet JC, Raikes JA, Gass HH, Leuchter W, Bendix SA (1983): Hemidiaphragmatic paralysis: an unusual complication of cervical spondylosis. *Arch Phys Med Rehabil* 64:601–603.

17. Campbell AM, Phillips DG (1960): Cervical disk lesions with neurological disorder. Differential diagnosis, treatment, and prognosis. *Br Med J* 2:481–485.

18. Clark CR (1984): Cervical spine involvement in rheumatoid arthritis. A primer for the practitioner. *Iowa Med* 74:57–62.

19. Clark CR (1987): Surgical treatment of bone destruction in the cervical spine. *Sem Orthop* 2(2):84–93.

20. Clark CR (1988): Cervical spondylotic myelopathy: history and physical findings. *Spine* 13(7):847–849.

21. Clark CR, Goetz DD, Menezes AH (1989): Arthrodesis of the cervical spine in rheumatoid arthritis. *J Bone Joint Surg [Am]* 71:381–392.

22. Clark CR (1989): Indications and surgical management of cervical myelopathy. *Sem Spine Surg* 1(4):254–261.

23. Clark CR (in press): The cervical spine. Pediatric and reconstructive aspects. In: *Orthopaedic knowledge update, 3rd ed.* Pos R, ed. Park Ridge: American Academy of Orthopaedic Surgeons.

24. Clark CR (in press): Rheumatoid arthritis. Surgical considerations. In: Rothman RH, Simeone FA, eds. *The spine, 3rd ed.* Philadelphia: W. B. Saunders.

25. Coin CG, Coin JT (1981): Computed tomography of cervical disc disease. Technical consideration with representative case reports. *J Comput Assist Tomogr* 5:275–280.

26. Conlon PW, Isdale IC, Rose BS (1966): Rheumatoid arthritis of the cervical spine. An analysis of 333 cases. *Ann Rheumat Dis* 25:120–126.

27. Crandall PH, Batzdorf U (1966): Cervical spondylotic myelopathy. *J Neurosurg* 25:57–66.

28. Crandall PH, Gregorius FK (1977): Long-term follow-up of surgical treatment of cervical spondylotic myelopathy. *Spine* 2:139–146.

29. Daniels DL, Grogan JP, Johansen JG, Meyer GA, Williams AL, Haughton VM (1984): Cervical radiculopathy. Computed tomography and myelography compared. *Radiology* 151:109–113.

30. Daskalakis MK (1983): Thoracic outlet compression syndrome: current concepts and surgical experience. *Int Surg* 68:337–344.

31. Dillin L, Hoaglund FT, Scheck M (1985): Brachial neuritis. *J Bone Joint Surg [Am]* 67(6):878–883.

32. Di Lorenzo N, Fortuna A (1987): High cervical (C2-C3) spondylogenetic myelopathy treated by transoral approach. Case Report. *J Neurosurg Sci* 31:71–74.

33. Dirheimer Y (1977): *The craniovertebral region in chronic inflammatory rheumatic diseases.* Berlin: Springer-Verlag.

34. Dobson J (1951): Tuberculosis of the spine. An analysis of the results of conservative treatment and of the factors influencing the prognosis. *J Bone Joint Surg [Br]* 33:517–531.

35. Dublin AB, McGahan JP, Reid MH (1983): The value of computed tomographic metrizamide myelography in the neuroradiological evaluation of the spine. *Radiology* 146:79–86.

36. [Editorial] (1984): Management of cervical spondylotic myelopathy. *Lancet* 1(8385):1058.

37. Edwards WC, La Rocca H (1983): The developmental segmental sagittal diameter of the cervical spinal canal in patients with cervical spondylosis. *Spine* 8:20–27.

38. Edwards WC, La Rocca H (1985): The developmental segmental sagittal diameter in combined cervical and lumbar spondylosis. *Spine* 10:42–49.

39. Ehni G (1982): Extradural spinal cord and nerve root compression form benign lesions of the cervical area. In: Youmans JR, ed. *Neurological Surgery, vol. 4.* Philadelphia: W. B. Saunders, pp. 2574–2612.

40. Epstein JA, Janin Y, Carras R, Lavine LS (1982): A comparative study of the treatment of cervical spondylotic myeloradiculopathy. Experience with 50 cases treated by means of extensive laminectomy, foraminotomy, and excision of osteophytes during the past 10 years. *Acta Neurochir (Wien)* 61:89–104.

41. Epstein JA (1985): Management of cervical spinal stenosis, spondylosis and myeloradiculopathy. In: Tindall GT, ed. *Contemporary Neurosurgery,* vol. 7. Baltimore: Williams and Wilkins, pp. 1–6.

42. Epstein NE, Epstein JA, Carras R, Murthy VS, Hyman RA (1984): Coexisting cervical and lumbar spinal stenosis. Diagnosis and management. *Neurosurgery* 15:489–496.

43. Epstein NE, Hyman RA, Epstein JA, Rosenthal AD (1988): Dynamic MRI scanning of the cervical spine. *Spine* 13:937–938.

44. Fielding JW, Cochran GvanB, Lawsing JF 3rd, Holh M (1974): Tears of the transverse ligament of the atlas. A clinical and biomechanical study. *J Bone Joint Surg [Am]* 56:1683–1691.

45. Forsythe M, Rothman RH (1978): New concepts in the diagnosis and treatment of infections of the cervical spine. *Orthop Clin North Am* 9:1039–1051.

46. Garcia A Jr, Grantham SA (1960): Hematogenous pyogenic vertebral osteomyelitis. *J Bone Joint Surg [Am]* 42:429–436.

47. Good DC, Couch JR, Wacaser L (1984): Numb, clumsy hands and high cervical spondylosis. *Surg Neurol* 22:285–291.

48. Gore DR, Sepic SB (1984): Anterior cervical fusion for degenerated or protruded discs. A review of one hundred forty-six patients. *Spine* 9:667–671.

49. Gore DR, Sepic SB, Gardner GM, Murray MP (1987): Neck pain. A long-term follow-up of 205 patients. *Spine* 12:1–5.

50. Gregorius FK, Estrin T, Crandall PH (1976): Cervical spondylotic radiculopathy and myelopathy. A long-term follow-up study. *Arch Neurol* 33:618–625.

51. Harrington KD (1986): Metastatic disease of the spine. *J Bone Joint Surg [Am]* 68:1110–1115.

52. Hawkins RJ (1985): Cervical spine and the shoulder. *Instructional Course Lectures* 34:191–195.

53. Hensinger RN (1984): Cervical spine. Pediatric. In: Asher MA, ed. *Orthop knowledge update,* Edition 1. Park Ridge: American Academy of Orthopaedic Surgery, p. 191.

54. Herkowitz HN (1989): The surgical management of cervical spondylotic radiculopathy and myelopathy. *Clin Orthop* 239:94–108.

55. Hirabayashi K, Miyakawa J, Satomi K, Maruyama T, Wakano K (1981): Operative results and postoperative progression of ossification among patients with ossification of cervical posterior longitudinal ligament. *Spine* 6(4):354–364.

56. Hirabayashi K, Satomi K (1988): Operative procedure and results of expensive open-door laminoplasty. *Spine* 13:870–876.

57. Hirano H, Suzuki H, Sakakibara T, Higuchi Y, Inove K, Suzuki Y (1982): Dysphagia due to hypertrophic cervical osteophytes. *Clin Orthop* 167:168–172.

58. Holzman RS, Bishko F (1971): Osteomyelitis in heroin addicts. *Ann Intern Med* 75:693–696.

59. Hoff JT, Wilson CB (1977): The pathophysiology of cervical spondylotic radiculopathy and myelopathy. *Clin Neurosurg* 24:474–487.

60. Hsu LCS, Yau ACMC (1983): Infections: tuberculosis. In: Bailey RW, ed. *The cervical spine, ed 1.* Philadelphia: J. B. Lippincott, pp. 336–355.

61. Hukuda S, Mochizuki T, Okata M, Shichikawa K, Shimomura Y (1985): Operations for cervical spondylotic myelopathy. A comparison of the results of anterior and posterior procedures. *J Bone Joint Surg* [Br] 67:609–615.

62. Kadoya S, Nakamura T, Kwak R, Hirose G (1985): Anterior osteophytectomy for cervical spondylotic myelopathy in developmentally narrow canal. *J Neurosurg* 63:845–850.

63. Kimura I, Oh-Hama M, Shingu H (1984): Cervical myelopathy treated by canal-expansive laminaplasty. Computed tomographic and myelographic findings. *J Bone Joint Surg* [Am] 66:914–920.

64. Lambert JR, Tepperman PS, Jimenez J, Newman A (1981): Cervical spine disease and dysphagia. Four new cases and a review of the literature. *Am J Gastroenterol* 76:35–40.

65. Landman JA, Hoffman JC Jr, Braun IF, Barrow DL (1984): Value of computed tomographic myelography in the recognition of cervical herniated disk. *AJNR* 5:391–394.

66. Lankford LL, Thompson JE (1977): Reflex sympathetic dystrophy, upper and lower extremity: Diagnosis and management. *Instructional Course Lectures* 26:163–178.

67. Lankford LL (1983): Reflex sympathetic dystrophy. In: Evarts CM, ed. *Surgery of the Musculoskeletal System.* New York: Churchill Livingstone, 1:145–201.

68. Leblhuber F, Reisecker F, Boehm-Jurkovic H, Witzmann A, Diesenhammer E (1988): Diagnostic value of different electrophysiologic tests in cervical disk prolapse. *Neurology* 38:1879–1881.

69. Lees F, Turner JW (1963): Natural history and prognosis of cervical spondylosis. *Br Med J* 2:1607–1610.

70. Leonard A, Comty CM, Shapiro FL, et al. (1973): Osteomyelitis in hemodialysis patients. *Ann Intern Med* 78:651–658.

71. Lipson SJ (1984): Rheumatoid arthritis of the cervical spine. *Clin Orthop* (182):143–149.

72. Long DM (1983): Cervical cord tumors. In: Bailey RW, ed. *The cervical spine, ed. 1.* Philadelphia: J. B. Lippincott, pp. 323–335.

73. Lunsford LD, Bissonette DJ, Zorub DS (1980): Anterior surgery for cervical disc disease. Part 2: Treatment of cervical spondylotic myelopathy in 32 cases. *J Neurosurg* 53:12–19.

74. MacFadyen DJ (1984): Posterior column dysfunction in cervical spondylotic myelopathy. *Can J Neurol Sci* 11:365–370.

75. Macnab I (1975): Cervical spondylosis. *Clin Orthop* 109:69–77.

76. Mackinnon SE, Holder LE (1984): The use of three-phase radionuclide bone scanning in the diagnosis of reflex sympathetic dystrophy. *J Hand Surg* [Am] 9:556–563.

77. Martel W (1961): The occipito-atlanto-axial joints in rheumatoid arthritis and ankylosing spondylitis. *Am J Roentgenol* 86:223–240.

78. Martin NS (1970): Tuberculosis of the spine: a study of the results of treatment during the last twenty-five years. *J Bone Joint Surg* [Br] 52:613–628.

79. Masaryk TJ, Modic MT, Geisinger MA, Standefer J, Hardy RW, Boumphrey F, Duchesneau PM (1986): Cervical myelopathy: a comparison of magnetic resonance and myelography. *J Comput Assist Tomogr* 10:184–194.

80. Mathews JA (1969): Atlanto-axial subluxation in rheumatoid arthritis. *Ann Rheum Dis* 28:260–266.

81. Mayfield FH (1979): Cervical spondylotic radiculopathy and myelopathy. *Adv Neurol* 22:307–321.

82. McAfee PC, Regan JJ, Bohlman HH (1987): Cervical cord compression from ossification of the posterior longitudinal ligament in non-orientals. *J Bone Joint Surg* [Br] 69:569–575.

83. McFarlin DE, McFarland HF (1982): Multiple sclerosis (second of two parts). *N Engl J Med* 307(20):1246–1251.

84. McLaughlin HL (1962): Rupture of the rotator cuff. *J Bone Joint Surg* [Am] 44:979–983.

85. Meikle JA, Wilkinson M: Rheumatoid involvement of the cervical spine. *Ann Rheum Dis* 30:154–161.

86. Modic MT, Ross JS, Masaryk TJ (1989): Imaging of degenerative disease of the cervical spine. *Clin Orthop* 239:109–120.

87. Nakagawa H, Okumura T, Sugiyama T, Iwata K (1983): Discrepancy between metrizamide CT and myelography in diagnosis of cervical disk protrusions. *AJNR* 4:604–606.

88. Neer CS 2nd (1983): Impingement lesions. *Clin Orthop* 173:70–77.

89. Northfield DW (1955): Diagnosis and treatment of myelopathy due to cervical spondylosis. *Br Med J* 2:1474–1477.

90. Nurick S (1972): The pathogenesis of the spinal cord disorder associated with cervical spondylosis. *Brain* 95:87–100.

91. Nurick S (1972): The natural history and the results of surgical treatment of the spinal cord disorder associated with cervical spondylosis. *Brain* 95:101–108.

92. Panjabi M, and White A 3rd (1988): Biomechanics of nonacute cervical spinal cord trauma. *Spine* 13(7):838–842.

93. Parke WW (1988): Correlative anatomy of cervical spondylotic myelopathy. *Spine* 13(7):831–837.

94. Paty DW, Poser C (1984): Clinical symptoms and signs of multiple sclerosis. In: Poser CM, ed. *The diagnosis of multiple sclerosis.* New York: Thieme-Stratton, pp. 27–43.

95. Paulson DL (1975): Carcinomas in the superior pulmonary sulcus. *J Thorac Cardiovasc Surg* 70:1095–1104.

96. Payne EE (1959): The cervical spine and spondylosis. *Neurochirurgia* 1:178–196.

97. Pellicci PM, Ranawat CS, Tsairis P, Bryan WJ: A prospective study of the progression of rheumatoid arthritis of the cervical spine. *J Bone Joint Surg* [Am] 63:342–350.

98. Perlik SJ, Fisher MA (1987): Somatosensory evoked response evaluation of cervical spondylotic myelopathy. *Muscle Nerve* 10:481–489.

99. Rasker JJ, Cosh JA (1978): Radiological study of cervical spine and hand in patients with rheumatoid arthritis of 15 years' duration: an assessment of the effects of corticosteroid treatment. *Ann Rheum Dis* 37:529–535.

100. Richaud J, Lazorthes Y, Verdie JC, Bonafe A (1988): Chemonucleolysis for herniated cervical disc. *Acta Neurochir (Wien)* 91:116–119.

101. Roberts AH (1966): Myelopathy due to cervical spondylosis treated by collar immobilization. *Neurology* 16:951–954.

102. Robinson RA, Afeiche N, Dunn EJ, Northrop BE (1977): Cervical spondylotic myelopathy: etiology and treatment concepts. *Spine* 2:89.

103. Roos DB (1976): Congenital anomalies associated with thoracic outlet syndrome. Anatomy, symptoms, diagnosis and treatment. *Am J Surg* 132:771–778.

104. Roos DB (1982): The place for scalenectomy and first-rib resection in thoracic outlet syndrome. *Surgery* 92:1077–1085.

105. Schlesinger EB, Antunes JL, Michelsen WJ, Louis KM (1981): Hydromyelia: clinical presentation and comparison of modalities of treatment. *Neurosurgery* 9:356–365.

106. Schmorl G, Junghann S (1932): Die gesunde and kranke wirbel saule in Rontgenbild. Leipzig.

107. Scotti G, Scialfa G, Pieralli S, Boccardi E, Valsecchi F, Tonon C (1983): Myelopathy and radiculopathy due to cervical spondylosis. Myelographic-CT correlations. *AJNR* 4:601–603.

108. Scoville WB (1961): Cervical spondylosis treated by bilateral facetectomy and laminectomy. *J Neurosurg* 18:423–428.

109. Sharp J, Purser DW, Lawrence JS (1958): Rheumatoid arthritis of the cervical spine in the adult. *Ann Rheum Dis* 17:303–313.

110. Sharp J, Purser DW (1961): Spontaneous atlanto-axial dislocation in ankylosing spondylitis and rheumatoid arthritis. *Ann Rheum Dis* 20:47–77.

111. Shaw RR (1984): Pancoast's tumor. *Ann Thor Surg* 37(4):343–345.

112. Simeone FA, Rothman RH (1982): Cervical disc disease. In: Rothman RH, Simeone FA, eds. *The spine.* Philadelphia: W. B. Saunders, pp. 440–476.

113. Stevens JC, Cartlidge NE, Saunders M, Appleby A, Hall M, Shaw DA (1971): Atlanto-axial subluxation and cervical myelopathy in rheumatoid arthritis. *Q J Med* 40:391–408.

114. Stone DB, Bonfiglio M (1963): Pyogenic vertebral osteomyelitis.

A diagnostic pitfall for the internist. *Arch Intern Med* 112:491–500.

115. Torg JS, Pavlov H, Genuario SE, Sennett B, Wisneski RJ, Robie BH, Jahre C (1986): Neurapraxia of the cervical spinal cord with transient quadriplegia. *J Bone Joint Surg* [Am] 68:1354–1370.
116. Torg JS (1989): Pavlov's ratio: determining cervical spinal stenosis on routine lateral roentgenograms. *Contemp Orthop* 18(2):153–160.
117. Tsairis P, Dyck PJ, Mulder DW (1972): Natural history of brachial plexus neuropathy. *Arch Neurol* 27:109–117.
118. Uhthoff HK, Sarkar K, Gomez J (1977): Calcifying tendinitis: a new concept of its pathophysiology. In: *Abstracts XV. Int Congress Rheum,* p. 106.
119. Upton AR, McComas AJ (1973): The double crush in nerve entrapment syndromes. *Lancet* 2:359–362.
120. Veidlinger OF, Colwill JC, Smyth HS, Turner D (1981): Cervical myelopathy and its relationship to cervical stenosis. *Spine* 6:550–552.
121. Verbiest H (1973): The management of cervical spondylosis. *Clin Neurosurg* 20:262–294.
122. Weidner A, Immenkamp M (1981): The operative management of extradural tumors of the cervical spine. *Orthop Trans* 5:116.
123. Weinstein JN, McLain RF (1987): Primary tumors of the spine. *Spine* 12(9):843–851.
124. White AA 3rd, Panjabi MM (1988): Biomechanical considerations in the surgical management of cervical spondylotic myelopathy. *Spine* 13(7):856–860.
125. Whitecloud TS (1983): Management of radiculopathy and myelopathy by the anterior approach. In: Bailey R, ed. *The cervical spine.* Philadelphia: J. B. Lippincott, pp. 411–424.
126. Whitecloud TS 3rd, Seago RA (1987): Cervical discogenic syndrome: results of operative intervention in patients with positive discography. *Spine* 12:313–316.
127. Wilberger JE Jr, Chedid MK (1988): Acute cervical spondylotic myelopathy. *Neurosurgery* 22:145–146.
128. Williams B (1979): Orthopaedic features in the presentation of syringomyelia. *J Bone Joint Surg* [Br] 61:314–323.
129. Wilson SP, Iacobo C, Rocco AG, Ferrante FM, Lipson SJ (1989): Cervical epidural steroid injection (CESI): Clinical classification as a predictor of therapeutic outcome. Read before the annual meeting of the Cervical Spine Research Society, New Orleans.
130. Wolf BS, Khilnani M, Malis LI (1956): The sagittal diameter of the bony cervical spinal canal and its significance in cervical spondylosis. *J Mt Sinai Hosp* 23:283–292.

The Adult Spine: Principles and Practice,
J. W. Frymoyer, Editor-in-Chief.
Raven Press, Ltd., New York © 1991.

CHAPTER 56

Cervical Spondylosis

The Anterior Approach

Thomas S. Whitecloud III

Degenerative disease of the cervical spine can produce a variety of clinical signs and symptoms, most of which are amenable to non-operative management. There are instances, however, when pain or neurological dysfunction is best managed by operative intervention. Depending on where pressure is exerted on neural structures, radiculopathy, myelopathy, or a combination of both may be produced (103). These symptoms may not be produced by the same etiological factors, although the resultant neurological lesion is the same. A soft disc herniation can produce an acute medullary or radicular symptom complex; progressive disc deterioration without a frank herniation may lead to the formation of posterior and posterolateral osteophytes with resultant similar compression on neurological structures. Disc degeneration without any frank neurological deficits may result in a condition known as a discogenic syndrome, which is characterized by chronic neck, shoulder, and interscapular pain and is frequently associated with occipital headaches (28,112,147). Failure of non-operative management for any of these symptom complexes requires the treating physician to consider operative intervention. It is now recognized that early surgical intervention, especially in cases of cervical spondylotic myelopathy, will

generally result in a better clinical outcome (5,6,10,48, 55,62,70,73,90,100,108,150).

Before the early 1950s, the routine surgical approach for symptoms produced by cervical spondylosis was posterior. The primary problem with this approach is the technical difficulty encountered in attempting to expose and remove compressive structures that lie primarily anterior to the spinal cord and nerve roots. In 1928, Stooky noted difficulty in removing "chondromas" by the posterior transdural route (126). The need for easier access to anterior compressive structures led to development of the anterior surgical approach to the cervical spine.

This approach was developed and popularized in the early 1950s. Bailey and Badgley performed an anterior cervical stabilization procedure in 1952 for a patient suffering from a lytic lesion of the fourth and fifth cervical vertebrae. The first published report of their technique of an onlay strut graft was in 1960 (7) (Fig. 1). It was recommended for use in destructive lesions of the vertebral column and in fracture dislocations. In 1955, Robinson and Smith described an operative technique for stabilizing a pathological cervical segment utilizing a horseshoe-shaped graft (113) (Fig. 2). Cloward, with no knowledge of the work done by others, first published his technique of anterior disc excision and direct removal of compressive structures in 1958 (27) (Fig. 3). Dereymaeker, in 1956, had developed a technique similar to that of Smith and Robinson (42). Interestingly, these various tech-

T. S. Whitecloud III, M.D.: Professor and Acting Chairman, Department of Orthopaedic Surgery, Tulane University School of Medicine, New Orleans, Louisiana, 70112.

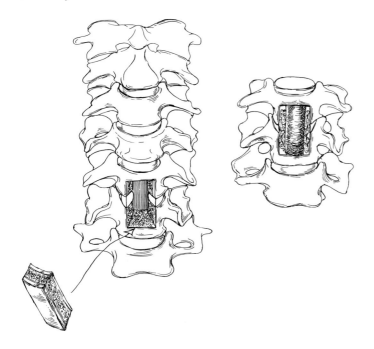

FIG. 1. A Bailey-Badgley type arthrodesis in which only a portion of the disc is removed and the posterior disc space is filled with cancellous bone and on-lay graft inserted. No attempt is made to remove compressive structures.

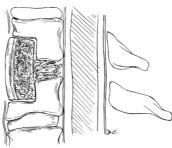

niques resulted in good or excellent results in the majority of cases.

The primary difference between the Cloward procedure and that of Robinson and Smith is not the configuration of graft constructs. The Cloward technique emphasizes direct visualization and removal of compressive structures (27,29,30), whereas Robinson and Smith felt that the removal of these offending structures was not necessary, and that posterior and posterolateral osteophytes will be resorbed once stabilization has been achieved (113,114).

Numerous refinements have been made in the anterior approach to the cervical spine for the treatment of cervical radiculopathy, myelopathy, or myeloradiculopathy. There are variations in configurations of bone graft (9,17,32,54,121), as well as variations in the source of graft material (21,31,35,64,119,120,129). Utilization of operative magnification allows better visualization of neural structures so compressive lesions can be easily seen and removed (8,16,67,74,78,83,86,117,123).

SURGICAL TECHNIQUE

The anterior approach to the cervical spine is relatively safe, technically easy, and relatively bloodless, and utilizes natural anatomical planes. The approach is essentially the same for any type of operative procedure to be performed on the anterior cervical spine. Anatomic details of the surgical approach have been well described (122).

Positioning of the patient for the surgical approach is critical. The patient is supine on the operating table with a head halter or skeletal traction in place. Traction helps to stabilize the spine in a neutral position. Distraction of the disc space can be obtained by adding more weight at the time of graft insertion, or a vertebral body spreader may be inserted. It is not necessary to elevate one side of the pelvis to harvest an iliac crest graft if one is to be used. Operative draping must be done so the cervical spine can be easily evaluated radiographically.

Although anatomical landmarks are present that will

help guide the surgeon to the pathologic interspace, a lateral roentgenogram taken prior to making the skin incision can help assure an accurate approach to the appropriate level. The incision can then be placed in relationship to the shoulders as they appear on the roentgenogram. The approach to the cervical spine can be made from either the right or the left side; most right-handed surgeons prefer to work from the right side. Generally, only one or two disc levels will be removed at the time of operative procedure. These can be quite adequately exposed by a transverse skin incision. However, if three or more levels are to undergo excision, it is easier to place the skin incision obliquely along the border of the sternocleidomastoid. Harvesting of the bone graft material is best done prior to making the neck incision.

Once the anterior aspect of the cervical spine has been exposed, it is mandatory to obtain a roentgenogram identifying the proper disc level. Proper illumination is necessary at the time of disc removal and can be obtained from a fiber-optic light source attached to a retractor, or utilization of an operating microscope. Magnifi-

cation loops and/or an operating microscope allows better visualization for removal of compressive structures, if this is the desire of the surgeon.

The anterior approach to the cervical spine has a low morbidity. Complications are rare but can be devastating. They can be minimized by a thorough anatomical knowledge of the area.

GRAFT CONFIGURATIONS FOR ANTERIOR CERVICAL FUSIONS

The pioneers of the anterior approach to the cervical spine for the treatment of a variety of pathological conditions are considered to be Bailey and Badgley, Robinson and Smith, and Cloward (7,27,113). Although their grafts are of different configurations, all these authors believe that stabilization following disc excision is necessary to achieve the best possible clinical result. As stated, Cloward emphasized the direct visualization and removal of compressive structures at the time of surgical

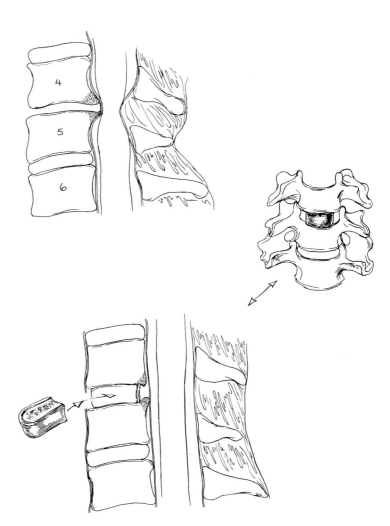

FIG. 2. An anterior disc excision followed by insertion of a cortical cancellous horseshoe-shaped Robinson-Smith bone graft. No attempt is made to remove posterior or posterolateral compressive structures. The cortical portion of the graft is inserted anteriorly in the original description of this procedure.

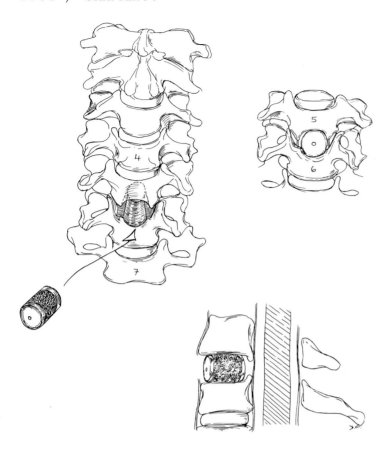

FIG. 3. The Cloward technique of insertion of a dowel of bone into the prepared disc space and vertebral bodies. Neural structures are decompressed directly posteriorly to the posterior longitudinal ligament which may be removed at the discretion of the surgeon. With this graft configuration, care must be taken to insert the bone graft so that both cortical ends of the graft are within the disc space, otherwise there is a tendency for graft collapse or extrusion.

intervention. Robinson and Smith did not recommend removal of compressive structures; but if desired, it is possible to remove compressive structures with the Robinson-Smith technique, especially with utilization of the operating microscope. The original technique of Bailey-Badgley simply stabilizes the involved segment and does not require complete disc removal. Biomechanically, White has shown that the horseshoe-shaped graft of Robinson-Smith resists compression forces better than the other graft configurations (141).

The individual surgeon must decide whether or not direct removal of compressive structures enhances the overall clinical result. However, it does appear that the risk of spinal cord injury at the time of surgery increases if there is a direct attempt to remove compressive structures or resect the posterior longitudinal ligament (8,15,57,87,98,112,128,149).

Robinson-Smith were the first to describe a technique of anterior cervical fusion done for symptoms of cervical disc degeneration (113). They postulated that disc degeneration led to osteophyte formation, disc narrowing, subluxation, instability of one cervical vertebra on another, or disc protrusion. Their technique of interbody fusion restores disc height and, by stopping excessive motion, theoretically allows resorption of posterior and posterolateral osteophytes (Fig. 4). Their method of graft

insertion consists of removing the pathological disc or discs at the appropriate interspace. Cartilaginous end plates and subchondral bone at the top and bottom of the disc space to be fused are also removed. (Subsequently, the authors recommended that the subchondral bone be left in place.) No attempt is made to remove any compressive structures. The prepared disc space is then measured, and a horseshoe-shaped graft obtained from the iliac crest is inserted and countersunk. The graft is inserted so that its cancellous portion is directed posteriorly.

Technical difficulties, such as collapse, extrusion, or non-union (5,34,40,51,110,114,142,148), which occurred on occasion with this type of graft, led to a modification described by Bloom and Raney (13). The graft is prepared in a similar fashion, but the cortical portion is inserted directly posteriorly (Fig. 5). This assures placement of the maximum amount of cortical bone within the disc space, and allows better maintenance of disc height. Whitecloud has reported a clinical series utilizing this modification that has a lower pseudarthrosis rate than found in series in which the original technique is used (145) (Fig. 6).

Cloward's technique of interbody fusion consists of drilling a round hole in the region of the intervertebral disc into which is inserted a pre-fit dowel of bone (27).

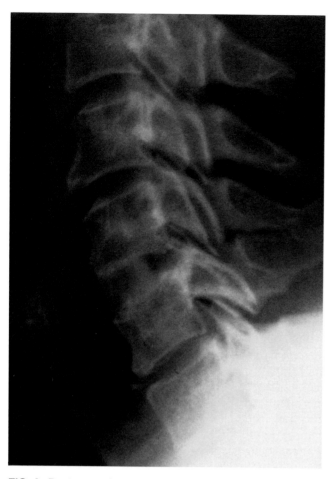

FIG. 4. Post-operative roentgenogram following anterior disc excision and fusion at C5-C6. No attempt was made to remove the posterior or posterolateral osteophytes. In this instance, the Robinson-Smith graft has been reversed. The patient had an excellent clinical result.

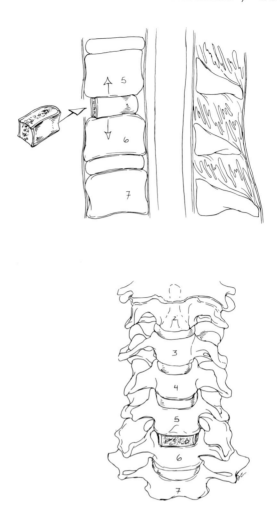

FIG. 5. A variation of the Robinson-Smith graft technique in which the graft is reversed so the cortical portion is posterior. This insures placement of a maximum amount of cortical bone within the disc space to resist compressive forces and extrusion. The graft does not have to be inserted in line with the posterior aspect of the vertebral bodies. The arthrodesis rate utilizing this technique is somewhat higher than that reported in the literature for the original description of bone graft insertion.

He modified instrumentation previously designed for posterior lumbar interbody fusion. A drill is used with a guard that permits drilling of the intervertebral disc space and adjacent vertebra to any desired depth. The drill and guard are removed several times in order to check their location. Drilling is continued downward until the bone at the bottom of the hole is entirely cortical in nature. This remaining cortical bone is then removed with curettes and rongeurs to expose the posterior longitudinal ligament. With care, the direct removal of posterior and posterolateral osteophytes or a soft disc is then possible. Once decompression has been carried out, a pre-cut dowel of bone obtained from the iliac crest is then tapped into place. It should be slightly shorter than the depth of the drill hole. The dowel of bone is cancellous in its mid-portion with cortical bone at both ends. Cloward recommends the use of allograft where possible (31). One of the difficulties with utilization of a dowel of bone is that care must be taken to place it exactly in the prepared hole, otherwise there is a tendency

for graft extrusion or collapse. If this occurs, a kyphotic deformity may develop (84). Because of this, Cloward subsequently modified multiple-level fusions so that a Robinson-Smith type of graft may be inserted at one disc space with a dowel of bone at an adjacent space (32). He also uses large blocks of bone when one or more vertebral bodies needs to be replaced.

The original technique of Bailey and Badgley requires the preparation of a trough in the anterior aspect of the vertebral body approximately one-half inch in width and three-sixteenths of an inch in depth (7). The trough is cut into the full vertical height of the vertebra, and the discs are cleaned with a rongeur to a depth of approximately one-half inch. The cartilaginous end plates of the inferior

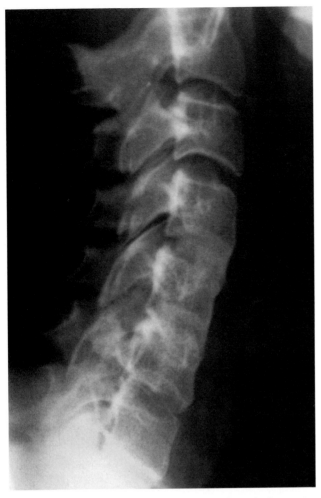

FIG. 6. Lateral roentgenogram of two-level cervical spondylosis treated by modified Robinson-Smith technique.

and superior aspects of the vertebral bodies to be fused are removed. A cortical cancellous graft from the iliac crest is shaped to fit into the prepared trough. Chips of cancellous bone are packed into the cleaned disc spaces and the cortical cancellous graft is morticed into the trough. If possible, sutures placed through the pre-vertebral fascia are tied over the graft, thus helping to maintain it in its correct position.

Besides these original three techniques regarding graft constructs, other graft configurations have been developed. They include the keystone graft of Simmons, and subsequent modification by Gore (54,121). With the advent of subtotal vertebrectomy for thorough removal of all compressive structures that may be contributing to compression of the spinal cord in patients with cervical spondylotic myelopathy, other surgeons have developed and described different graft configurations and techniques for insertion that will span multiple cervical segments (9,14,17,124,153). These grafts are either cortical cancellous bone obtained from the iliac crest or cortical bone generally obtained from the fibula.

There have been numerous reports in the literature reporting on the clinical results and rate of fusion in patients undergoing anterior disc excision and interbody fusion. As would be expected, the pseudarthrosis rates vary (5,30,34,40,55,114,121,127,142,148). There is no doubt that there is increased risk of pseudarthrosis if more than one level is fused (34,142). This is not true, however, if one long piece of cortical cancellous graft or cortical bone is used to span multiple segments (9,17,153). The presence of a pseudarthrosis does not necessarily compromise the clinical result (40), although it is the goal of the surgeon to stabilize the involved pathological spinal segment.

RESULTS OF ANTERIOR DISC EXCISION AND FUSION

Because of different pre-operative criteria and length of follow-up, it is not possible to critically compare the numerous reports that have appeared in the literature describing the clinical results of anterior disc excision and interbody fusion (25,34,40,43,55,58,80,110,114, 121,127,142,148). Table 1 is a list of selected series from the literature that have utilized Odom's criteria or a modification thereof for evaluation of their post-operative clinical results (102). His criteria are listed in Table 2. Patients in the excellent, good, or fair category have benefited from surgical intervention. In the series presented in Table 1, Stuck, Dohn, and Chirls utilized a Cloward technique, whereas the Robinson-Smith technique was utilized by all the other authors except for Simmons and Gore, who reported on their keystone type of arthrodesis.

Another large series, which cannot be listed in Table 1 because results are not reported by Odom's criteria, is that of Mosdal (96). In 1984 he reported on the results of 740 patients undergoing anterior disc excision with in-

TABLE 1. *Clinical results of anterior disc excision and fusion*

Reference	No. cases	Good, excellent	Fair	Poor
Robinson (114)	55	73%	22%	5%
Stuck (127)	151	73	21	6
Connolly (34)	63	54	24	22
Dohn (43)	210	51	29	20
Williams (148)	60	63	15	22
Riley (110)	93	71	18	10
Simmons (121)	68	81	15	4
Jacobs (80)	62	82	13	5
DePalma (40)	229	63	29	8
White (142)	65	67	22	11
Green (58)	33	97	1	0
Chirls (25)	467	92	6	2
Gore (55)	133	96	2	2
	1,689	74%	16.69%	9%

TABLE 2. *Odom's criteria*

Excellent:	All pre-operative symptoms relieved; abnormal findings improved
Good:	Minimal persistence of pre-operative symptoms; abnormal findings unchanged or improved
Fair:	Definite relief of some pre-operative symptoms; other symptoms unchanged or slightly improved
Poor:	Symptoms and signs unchanged or exacerbated

terbody fusion by the Cloward technique. For those patients having primarily radicular symptoms, 19% were totally pain-free and 62% had partial relief of their pre-operative symptoms. These would correspond to good or excellent results if they had been judged by Odom's criteria. Eighty-three percent of these patients had heterologous graft material utilized (Kiel surgibone). Kyphotic angulation was noted in 12% of patients and found to be more prevalent when more than one level was fused. This did not seem to compromise the surgical result.

It has been noted by several authors that results of surgery on patients involved in litigation are not statistically different from those on patients who are not in a litigious situation (142,147). Furthermore, the series of White pointed out that there is no difference in results in patients with an abnormal psychological profile (142).

There is no question that the best surgical results can be anticipated from those patients who present with a monoradiculopathy and a duration of symptoms of less than one year (5,6,48,55,73). Multilevel disease requiring surgery at more than one level usually does not provide an excellent result, especially as regards the relief of neck pain. It must be remembered that cervical disc degeneration is a progressive disease, and a recurrence or progression of symptoms should not be unanticipated (23). The large series of Mosdal, in which follow-up up to 13 years has been possible, shows a deterioration of his 81% good or excellent results to 71% on longer follow-up (96).

The series presented here did not directly address the question of cervical spondylotic myelopathy. Several of the authors included a few patients in this diagnostic category and generally found the results much poorer than those patients with radiculopathy only (43,96,142). Again, it must be emphasized that early surgical intervention will allow the best results from anterior surgery for cervical spondylotic myelopathy (12,48,70,90,150).

Without question, anterior disc excision followed by stabilization with any variety of graft configuration should result in satisfaction of both patient and surgeon most of the time. Literature review indicates that approximately 90% of patients undergoing this procedure derive benefit from it, and 70% can be anticipated to have a good or excellent result. It is not possible to ascertain whether or not compressive structures should be removed at the time of disc excision, since comparable

results are found in those patients in which the diseased cervical segment is simply immobilized by fusion. Each individual surgeon must decide whether or not direct neural decompression provides more benefit to each individual patient.

ANTERIOR DISC EXCISION WITHOUT FUSION

In addition to the controversy that has developed between surgeons who favor direct removal of compressive structures and those who favor simple stabilization of the involved segment following disc removal, another has developed between surgeons who do not insert a graft following disc removal and those who do (Fig. 7). Clinical results of those who recommend fusion and those who do not are very similar, i.e., 90% of patients undergoing disc excision without fusion will derive benefit from the procedure (8,10,12,16,39,44,52,61,67,72, 74,78,83,86,94,98,111,115,136,149).

In 1960, Dr. Carl Hirsch first described the partial ante-

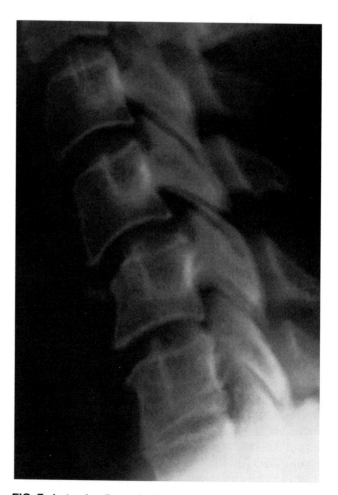

FIG. 7. Lateral radiograph of a patient following anterior disc excision without fusion at C6-C7. Spontaneous arthrodesis has occurred. The patient has had an excellent result for surgery performed for soft disc herniation with radiculopathy.

rior excision of a cervical disc without an accompanying interbody fusion (72). His operative technique consisted of incising the anterior annulus and curetting the disc. No attempt was made to remove the cartilaginous end plates, posterior annulus, osteophytes, or posterior longitudinal ligament. Twenty-nine of thirty-five patients (83%) undergoing this procedure had a good or excellent clinical result. All patients achieved a fibrous or bony union at the area of disc excision. Subsequent series demonstrated a bony union in 70% to 100% of cases (8, 10,12,16,39,44,52,61,67,72,74,78,83,86,94,98,111,115, 136,149). Hirsch was unable to explain why this procedure would eliminate the patients' symptoms. In 1964 and 1966, respectively, Boldey and Susen reported their series of simple anterior cervical disc excision without fusion and had results similar to Hirsch's. Again, their described surgical procedure consisted of only simple disc excision.

Murphy and Gado reported on a similar operation in a group of 26 patients undergoing anterior disc excision for a lateral cervical disc syndrome (98). Twenty-four of their patients, or 92%, had a good clinical result. Follow-up radiographic evaluation in 20 patients showed an instance of fusion of 72% when discectomy was performed at a single level. Even in those patients that did not have a complete fusion, dynamic roentgenograms demonstrated stability at the operative site. Interestingly, half their patients demonstrated some degree of resorption of posterior and posterolateral osteophytes at 12 months. This compares favorably with reported series of anterior cervical discectomy with interbody fusion, in which approximately half the patients studied demonstrated posterior osteophyte remodeling (55,114).

Although these surgical results were satisfactory, subsequent reported series emphasize a much more radical decompression of neural structures (10,12,16,44,74, 78,86,90,93,94,136). Most authors who prefer an anterior disc excision without fusion feel that the primary goal in obtaining relief of clinical symptoms is the removal of compressive structures in order to relieve the pressure on the cervical nerve root and/or the spinal cord (44,78,91,94,98,111,136). Numerous series emphasize the importance of removing posterior and posterolateral osteophytes in association with bilateral foraminotomies to prevent root compression by narrowing of intervertebral space, which occurs after radical discectomy (10,12, 16,44,46,74,78,86,90,94,98,111,136). A controversy exists regarding resection of the posterior longitudinal ligament. Some authors find that it is unnecessary and dangerous to resect the ligament (8,57,98,111,112,149), while others feel that it is an essential part of the procedure to visualize the roots and dura to be sure the decompression is adequate (10,12,67,78,86,94,123,136,139).

Utilization of the operating microscope has made the radical decompression procedures, which now seem to be favored, technically feasible. One of the first reported

series of a more radical excision was by Robertson in 1973 (111). He compared 53 patients that had undergone anterior disc excision and fusion with 40 patients that had not. He could find no difference in the clinical results, but felt that since a simple discectomy avoided the morbidity of bone grafting, he preferred this technique. He recommended thorough curettement of all disc material, including the cartilaginous end plates. The operating microscope was used to allow inspection for a hole in the posterior annulus through which a disc fragment could have migrated, and also for removal of posterior annulus and posterior longitudinal ligament if necessary. Clinically, 16 patients with radiculopathy had an excellent result, and 80% of the patients with a painful disc syndrome were markedly improved. A slightly different technique utilizing the operating microscope was reported by Hankinson and Wilson in 1975; it emphasized preserving columns of disc material on both sides of the disc space, recommending a central opening of no more than 10 mm (67). Using the operating microscope and an air drill with an angled adaptor, a portion of the superior intervertebral body is removed, thus allowing more vertical exposure in the central portion of the disc. Posterior and posterolateral osteophytes are then removed under direct vision. If possible, the posterior longitudinal ligament is generally opened. This series reported on the clinical results in 51 patients. In 26 of these, disc removal was performed at multiple levels, and three had four discs removed at the time of surgery. Instability did not develop in any of these patients, possibly due to the preservation of lateral column disc material and the minimal removal of anterior bone. Their results were similar to those of others, with 84% of their patients showing good or excellent results.

A more radical surgical procedure was described by Martins in 1976. His operative technique consisted of radical discectomy with foraminotomy (94). The entire disc is removed along with cartilaginous end plates. In addition, the posterior aspect of the superior and inferior vertebral bodies is removed to facilitate exposure of the posterior longitudinal ligament. The ligament is excised and removed along with any posterior osteophytes. At the end of the procedure the dura and nerve roots are checked visually to be certain they are free of any encroachment. Ninety-two percent of the patients undergoing surgery fell in the good or excellent category. This series of patients was compared to another group who underwent Cloward interbody fusion. The results were similar, with both groups having 92% good or excellent results. Comparing these results, Martins raised the question why a fusion should even be done.

Dunsker also had a small series in which two similar groups of patients either were fused or underwent a radical disc excision without fusion (44). He felt that grafting should be considered if a large amount of bone was removed from the posterior aspect of the vertebral bodies in order to visualize and decompress the neural structures. Again, the results in these patients undergoing either a radical disc excision or excision and fusion were quite similar, most falling in the good or excellent category. Martins also recommended grafting with the dowel technique in cases of advanced spondylosis requiring surgery at multiple levels (94).

Several large series have appeared in the literature that emphasize the value of radical disc excision and removal of all compressive structures in order to relieve pressure on the cervical nerve roots and/or the spinal cord (10,12,16,44,74,78,86,90,93,94,98,111,136). Utilization of the operating microscope allows relatively safe neural decompression. A detailed description of the generally accepted technique with utilization of the microscope is given by Seeger (117).

Bertalanffy and Eggert performed anterior microsurgical discectomy at one or more cervical segments without interbody fusion in 251 cases between 1976 and 1983 (12). They were able to follow 164 cases between one and eight years. Diagnostic categories included 109 patients with radiculopathy and 55 patients with myelopathy. As expected, the best results were found in patients with radicular symptoms; 82% had good or excellent long-term results. Fifty-five percent of those patients with myelopathy had good or excellent long-term benefit from surgery. These authors felt that their results clearly demonstrated that anterior cervical disc excision is an effective treatment of cervical myelopathy. This stands in contrast with other reports (92,96,100,101,150).

Another series by Lesoin et al. analyzed the results of 1,000 surgical procedures done for radicular myelopathy over a 20-year period (90). Eight hundred cases were performed anteriorly and 200 posteriorly. They were able to analyze the surgical results in 700 of these patients, and although the specific numbers treated by the various techniques are not possible to ascertain, they felt that 66% of the patients achieved excellent or good results. This large series allowed these authors to state that they prefer the radical discectomy to discectomy followed by a Cloward bone graft.

It is obvious from the literature reviewed that radical decompression anteriorly without bone grafting is an accepted modality for the treatment of cervical radiculopathy, myelopathy, or myeloradiculopathy. Certainly, complications related to bone grafting are completely avoided. However, there are some risks inherent to the procedure itself. They will be discussed later in this chapter.

Critical evaluation of the series available in the literature reveals that the results of disc excision without fusion are comparable to those in which an interbody fusion is performed. Obviously, the elimination of the donor site from the operative procedure decreases operative morbidity. Although generally minor in nature, complications from the donor site have been reported to occur in approximately 20% of patients undergoing autologous grafting (143). Lunsford compared a series of 334 patients in which some had undergone fusion and some had not, and stated that the post-operative complications were much more frequent and hospital stays longer in those patients undergoing fusion (91).

ANTERIOR SURGERY FOR CERVICAL SPONDYLOTIC MYELOPATHY

The most serious consequence of degenerative disease of the cervical spine is cervical spondylotic myelopathy (Fig. 8). This condition is obviously different from cervical spondylosis causing a radiculopathy. Myelopathy is due to direct compression on the spinal cord itself as opposed to nerve root compression only. It is the most common disease of the spinal cord developing during and after middle age (18,37), but must be differentiated from other diseases affecting the spinal cord such as amyotrophic lateral sclerosis or multiple sclerosis (24,47).

The pathophysiology of cervical spondylotic myelopathy is due to factors causing a reduction in the volume of the spinal canal (104,130,131). These can be both static and dynamic mechanical factors, and are frequently associated with vascular compromise (132). Anatomical factors that lead to reduction in the volume of the spinal canal include hypertrophy of the posterior arch, thickening of the ligamentum flavum, dural hypertrophy, tethering of the spinal cord by dentate ligaments, foraminal osteophytes compressing radicular vessels, anterior osteophytes compressing the spinal cord, ossification of the posterior longitudinal ligaments, and ossified ligamentum flavum (1,2,3,26,45,50,88,99,101,104,105, 106,125,130,131,132,138). Experimental studies have indicated that both compression and ischemia contribute to myelopathy (53,60,77,151). These are additive factors producing more symptoms in combination than when acting singularly (53). Dynamic compression, which has been described by Penning, Guidetti, and others, further reduces the functional diameter of the osseous canal (1,62,107,131). This occurs with motion, since flexion stretches the cord across ventral spurs, and extension may cause retrolisthesis of a vertebral body or inbuckling of the ligamentum flavum (20,109).

The clinical presentation of this disease is highly variable. The most common presenting symptoms are upper extremity weakness associated with a gait disturbance. Other findings can include spasticity, muscle atrophy, intrinsic bladder dystrophy, and, on occasion, radicular pain. In the most severe cases, posterior column dysfunction is noted. This is an ominous prognostic sign that indicates permanent spinal cord damage and is a poor prognostic sign as regards a patient's response to surgical intervention (15).

A

B

C

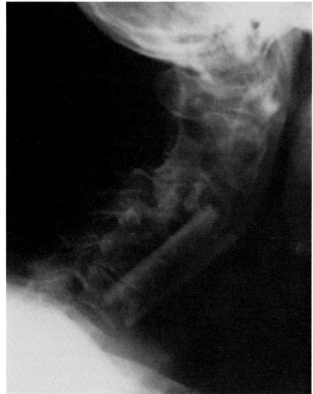

FIG. 8. Radiograph **(A)** and MRI **(B)** of a patient with severe cervical spondylosis with a secondary kyphotic deformity and herniation of the C3-C4 cervical disc. Patient manifested signs and symptoms of cervical spondylotic myelopathy. **C:** Surgery consisted of subtotal vertebrectomy of C4 and excision of herniated cervical disc at C3-C4 and anterior stabilization with a fibular allograft from C3-C7.

The natural history of cervical spondylotic myelopathy is one of intermittent progression with long periods in which the disease is static, followed by periods of exacerbation (47). Only a small group of patients will ever show a rapidly deteriorating disability. Few deaths are directly attributed to cervical spondylotic myelopathy (59). The episodic nature of this disease process has been documented by Lees and Turner and also Clark and Robinson (26,89). These authors felt that there was no prognostic sign that would identify those patients who would deteriorate rapidly.

Lees and Turner also pointed out that the long-term follow-up results of posterior surgery for cervical spondylotic myelopathy showed no significant difference between those treated operatively and those treated non-operatively (89). Delayed loss of neurological function following laminectomy as well as the hazards of perioperative neurological deficit are well recognized and estimated to occur from 19% to 53% of the time (19,26,37,59,63,108,135).

These relatively poor results from posterior procedures led to the utilization of the anterior approach for operative intervention in patients suffering from this disease process (9,15,17,33,34,37,38,41,43,62,65,66,68,79, 97,108,116,118,152,153,154). However, the type of anterior procedure to be performed on patients with cervical spondylotic myelopathy has not been delineated. Favorable surgical outcome has been reported in patients undergoing simple disc excision without fusion (4,10,12, 44,61,78,81,90,93,103) and also in patients undergoing disc excision plus radical decompression followed by stabilization procedures (9,17,33,34,37,38,41,43,62,65,66, 68,79,97,108,116,118,152,153,154). It has been noted that early operative intervention will provide the best clinical results (5,6,10,12,48,55,62,70,73,90,108,150).

Some of the early series reporting on clinical results of anterior disc excision and fusion included patients that had cervical spondylotic myelopathy. In Dohn's large series, 39 of his 210 patients were in this diagnostic category (43). Overall, he noted that the results are poorest in this group of patients. White also reported an overall poor result in patients with this disease process (142). In Connolly's series, two thirds of his patients with this diagnosis had good or excellent results from anterior disc excision and stabilization (34). Aronson's series had three patients with cervical spondylotic myelopathy from soft disc herniations, and all were treated successfully by the anterior approach (5,6). He found that the duration of symptoms in these patients with soft disc herniations was short and represented a disease process somewhat different from that of patients with longstanding deficits.

One of the earliest reports dealing only with the results of anterior disc excision and fusion for cervical spondylotic myelopathy was published in 1966 by Crandall and Batzdorf (37). They had 21 patients treated by the Cloward technique, and noted a 71% improvement following surgery. In 1969, Guidetti and Fortuna reported that of 45 patients undergoing a similar operative procedure, 82% had results in the very good, good, or fair category (62). They did note that two patients were made worse by surgery, and one continued to deteriorate following surgery. Phillips reported a 74% improvement rate following Cloward procedures performed in 65 patients (108). He felt that the results of anterior surgery were markedly superior to those of laminectomy or conservative management.

Crandall and Gregorius compared the results of laminectomy to those of anterior decompression followed by a Cloward fusion in 33 patients (38). Twelve of the 18 patients undergoing laminectomy deteriorated, while only 5 of the 15 patients lost function following decompression and fusion. In 1977, Bohlman reported on 17 patients requiring ambulatory aids prior to surgery who were treated by simple stabilization of the involved segment (15). Fifteen patients became independent ambulators after surgery.

Although simple stabilization of the pathological segment was shown by Bohlman to be beneficial, most series now recommend both decompression and stabilization of the involved spinal segments. This may be done at the disc level only (34,37,38,41,43,62,65,66,68,79, 97,108,116,118,152,153,154) or in combination with a partial vertebrectomy (9,17,65,66,68,152).

Another series with long-term follow-up was reported by Irvine in 1987 (79). Forty-six patients were evaluated at a mean of 10 years post-surgery, and it was found that 36 patients (78%) remained improved, 6 remained unchanged (13%), and 4 (9%) showed progression of the disease. It should be noted that these patients underwent surgery only at one or two levels.

One of the few series in which the Smith-Robinson technique was utilized exclusively was published by Zhang in 1983 (154). A total of 121 patients were presented; the average number of discs removed and fused per patient was 2.9. He reported a 91% improvement following surgery and a 73% instance of patients being able to return to their former activities.

Another series reporting the results of patients undergoing decompression and Cloward fusion for one- or two-level disease has been published by Moussa (97). In 125 patients, 70% were improved by surgery, and 30% were able to return to their former employment. The average follow-up was 2.3 years.

Surgery in the before-mentioned series was for disease at one or two levels. Utilization of the Cloward or the Smith-Robinson technique is difficult over multiple segments, and the pseudarthrosis rate is higher. For this reason, various techniques of partial vertebrectomy with decompression followed by stabilization with a variety of

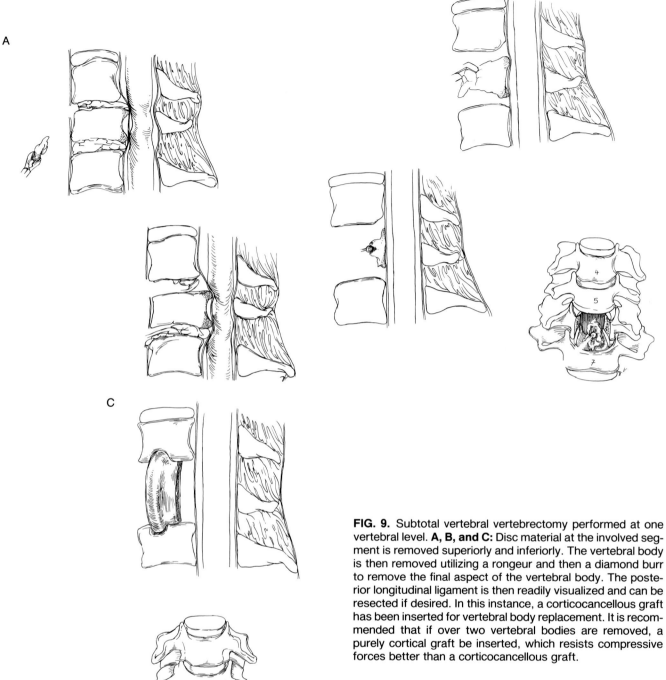

FIG. 9. Subtotal vertebral vertebrectomy performed at one vertebral level. **A, B, and C:** Disc material at the involved segment is removed superiorly and inferiorly. The vertebral body is then removed utilizing a rongeur and then a diamond burr to remove the final aspect of the vertebral body. The posterior longitudinal ligament is then readily visualized and can be resected if desired. In this instance, a corticocancellous graft has been inserted for vertebral body replacement. It is recommended that if over two vertebral bodies are removed, a purely cortical graft be inserted, which resists compressive forces better than a corticocancellous graft.

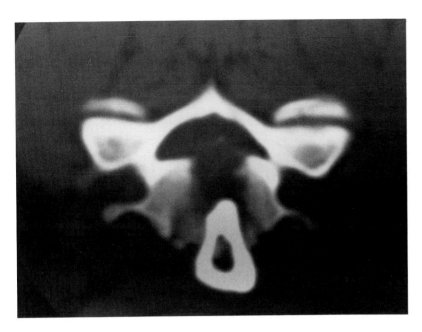

FIG. 10. Post-operative CT scan of partial vertebrectomy done for removal of compressive structures causing cervical spondylotic myelopathy.

graft configurations have been described (9,17,65,66, 68,152) (Fig. 9). Techniques for vertebral body resection and decompression were initially described for the treatment of trauma (14,124).

All the techniques developed for grafting following vertebral body resection have in common the utilization of purely cortical or cortical cancellous bone, which is fashioned in such a way as to be locked into the vertebral bodies above and below the area of resection. The purely cortical bone used for graft material is usually obtained from the fibula or tibia, whereas the cortical cancellous graft material is generally obtained from the iliac crest. The reported rate of fusion for these different varieties of grafts, which are usually inserted over at least two disc spaces, approaches 100% (9,17).

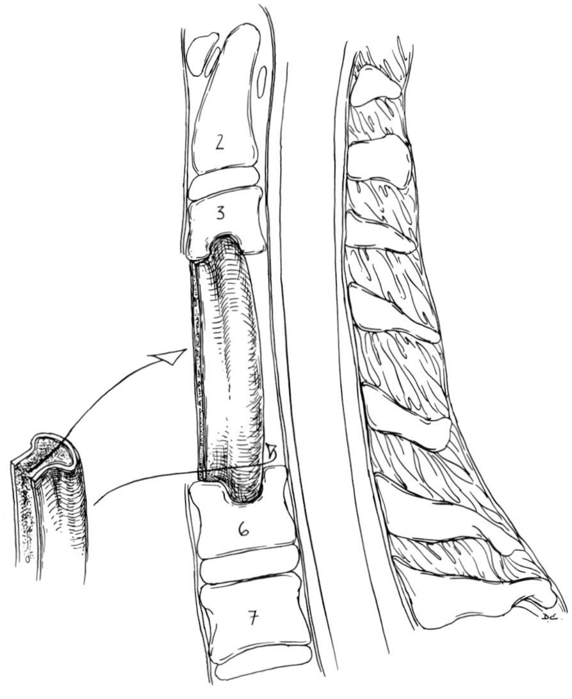

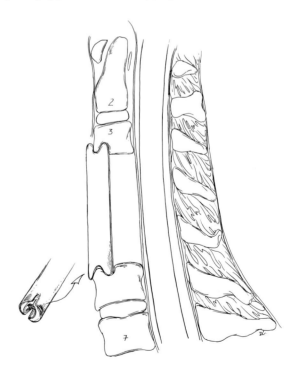

FIG. 12. Cortical graft obtained from the fibula and inserted so that it is notched into place. This graft is inserted with traction applied to the cervical spine. The neck does not have to be extended for insertion. This graft configuration helps prevent migration of the graft posteriorly into the area of the neural canal either at time of insertion or in the post-operative period.

FIG. 11. Corticocancellous graft locked into place following two-level vertebral body resection.

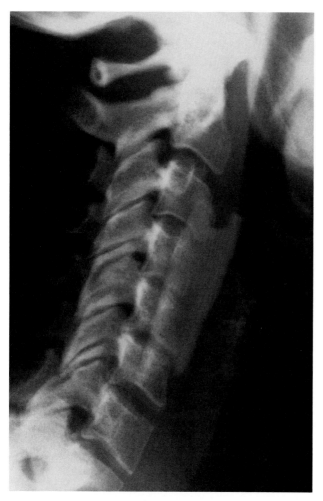

FIG. 13. Lateral radiograph of a three-level fusion done with fibula allograft. Three months have transpired since surgery.

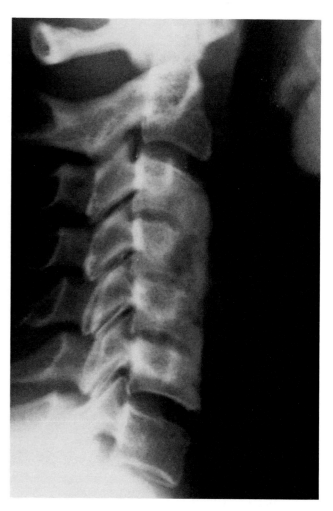

FIG. 14. Roentgenogram of cervical spine fused utilizing allograft four years following surgery.

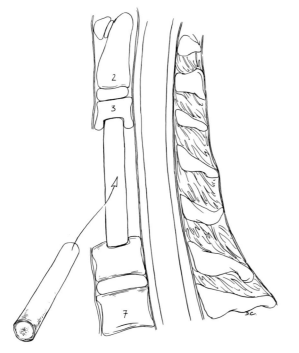

FIG. 15. Entire piece of fibula may be inserted following multiple level, subtotal vertebrectomies. In order for this graft to be inserted, the neck must be extended. This cannot be done safely unless any compressive structures have been totally removed. Care must be taken at the time of graft insertion not to impact the graft into the spinal canal.

Several series have been reported in which multilevel subtotal vertebrectomy with resection of all compressive structures has been performed. Senegas reported such a technique in 1975 (118) (Fig. 10). Boni reported on 39 cases in which the central portion of three or more vertebral bodies was removed followed by stabilization with a cortical cancellous graft (17). Fifty-three percent of patients were reported as having good results, with moderate improvement shown in 39%. Boni initially removed the disc and the portion of the vertebral body utilizing a Cloward drill (Fig. 11). Graft material was obtained from the iliac crest. Sakou reported on a similar procedure in 22 patients suffering from ossification of the posterior longitudinal ligament. Results were considered excellent in 2, good in 16, and fair in 4 (116). Hanai reported on a series of 15 patients undergoing subtotal vertebrectomy and fusion using iliac crest graft (65). This series again was in patients with ossification of the posterior longitudinal ligament.

A somewhat different method of vertebral body resection and grafting has been reported by Bernard and Whitecloud (9) (Fig. 12). In their operative technique, discs in the involved area are removed first, as would be done in performing a Smith-Robinson procedure. The intervening vertebral bodies are then removed utilizing a dental burr and rongeurs. The mid-portion of the vertebral body is removed down to the posterior longitudinal ligament. Compressive structures in the region of the disc itself are then removed using curettes and rongeurs. Decompression is thus carried out from a region of minimal compression toward the region of maximum compression. Following decompression the superior and inferior vertebral bodies are undercut in such a way as to retain the anterior portion of the vertebra (Fig. 13). The posterior extension of a previously notched fibula can then be locked into place. In the initial reported series of 21 patients, 19 benefited from surgical intervention. Autologous fibula was used in this series, but subsequently has been changed to fibular allograft (Fig. 14). With either type of graft, fusion rate approaches 100%.

Zdeblick and Bohlman reported on 8 patients with cervical spondylotic myelopathy treated with a similar procedure, but varied the method of insertion of the graft (153) (Fig. 15).

Yonenobu compared three surgical procedures for multisegment cervical spondylotic myelopathy in 95 patients (152). Of the 21 patients undergoing subtotal vertebrectomy and fusion, he felt that the results were superior to the other techniques of laminectomy and anterior fusion alone. He did state that if there is involvement of over four segments, a posterior procedure should be carried out.

Not all reports of anterior decompression and stabilization have been optimistic. Galera noted only a 39% improvement in 33 patients undergoing a Cloward procedure (51). He felt that there was a definite tendency toward deterioration with prolonged follow-up. Likewise, Lunsford noted only 50% improvement in patients who had undergone anterior cervical surgery that were followed for one to seven years (92). Fifty percent of the patients were not improved or deteriorated despite operative intervention. In his series, various types of anterior procedures were performed, none showing any better results than another. He did not feel that surgical intervention results were any better than non-operative management.

Some have been managed successfully by disc excision alone. Bertalanffy and Eggert performed radical disc excision in 105 patients having medullary or radiculomyelopathy signs and symptoms (12). The best results in this group of patients were in those that had a soft disc herniation causing medullary symptoms. Overall, 55% of patients with myelopathy had an excellent or good long-term result. Bollati performed a similar radical decompression in 10 patients having myelopathy and reported that 8 were in the excellent or good category (16). In Wilson's series, 9 patients with myelopathy had 1 excellent, 5 good, 2 satisfactory, and 1 poor result (149).

It is quite difficult to directly compare the various series that appear in the literature regarding results of anterior cervical surgery for cervical spondylotic myelopathy. Most results are evaluated according to Nurick's six grades of disability, which are based on the degree of difficulty in walking (100). Despite the numerous series that indicate anterior surgery should be of benefit to the patient, in approximately 70% to 80% of cases, there are still no clear-cut criteria as to when or how surgery should be performed. A short duration of symptoms prior to operative intervention does appear to have a better chance of a favorable surgical result.

Just as there is no clear-cut indication when surgery should be recommended for patients with this disease process, it is also not possible to determine whether the anterior approach is better than the posterior one (144). Quite favorable results have been reported by the different varieties of laminoplasties developed primarily for the treatment of ossification of the posterior longitudinal ligament (71,76,85,137). The answer to when or how to operate for cervical spondylotic myelopathy cannot be obtained until controlled prospective series have been initiated and completed.

COMPLICATIONS OF ANTERIOR CERVICAL SURGERY

The anterior approach to the cervical spine is relatively easy and makes use of natural anatomical planes. The results of surgery are generally satisfactory to both the patient and the surgeon in approximately 90% of procedures being performed. This is true whether or not an interbody fusion is done. As with any surgical procedure, there are inherent risks related to the surgical approach. This is due to the diversity of anatomical structures encountered as the anterior portion of the cervical spine is exposed. Once exposure has been achieved, disc excision, with or without removal of compressive structures, has a potential for injury to the spinal cord or cervical nerve roots (11,49,56,87,128). If the pathological segment is stabilized following disc removal, bone graft and donor site problems can be encountered (7,29,34,40,110,114,134,143). The spinal surgeon must be aware of these potential complications, their incidence according to the literature, and how to prevent them. Only then can the surgeon intelligently discuss the risks and benefits of a surgical procedure, which, in most cases, is elective in nature.

In the surgical exposure to the anterior cervical spine, there are a number of soft tissue structures that must be recognized, avoided, and/or retracted. Virtually any of the anatomical structures encountered are susceptible to injury, and such injuries have been reported.

Necessity of retraction of the pharynx, trachea, and esophagus across the midline for disc exposure render these structures susceptible to injury. In most circumstances, injury is caused by penetration by the sharp blades of a retractor (29,133). These structures should be carefully retracted, and if self-retaining retractors are utilized, their blades should be carefully placed under the edge of the longus colli muscles. Retractor blades should not be sharp. Prolonged retraction against the in situ tracheal tube can lead to the common complication of temporary dysphasia and hoarseness (95,140). This can be eliminated by not applying constant pressure against the trachea and by using detramexazone in the perioperative period (143).

Vocal cord paralysis can occur with injury to the recurrent laryngeal or vagus nerve (22,69). It is unlikely that these structures are divided directly during the exposure; more than likely it is again caused by prolonged pressure against the trachea. Fortunately, most of these injuries are transient in nature. Heeneman reported on 85 cases evaluated following anterior cervical surgery, and found 11% had post-operative voice changes with three permanent vocal cord paralysis (69). Anatomically, the recurrent laryngeal nerve is less likely to be injured when approached from the left side of the neck because of its longer course and more protective position in the trachea-esophageal groove (122).

Another potential complication that can occur as the disc and vertebral bodies are approached is an injury to the sympathetic chain (133,134). This can be avoided if care is taken not to dissect lateral to the longus colli muscles, and to avoid improper retractor placement. Most of these injuries are transient in nature and of little clinical consequence.

Vascular injuries to the carotid artery or jugular vein are fortunately rare, but have been reported (90,108).

Again, the most common cause of injury would be secondary to penetration by a sharp retractor. Prolonged, forceful retraction against the carotid artery can lead to cerebral ischemia.

Direct injury to the vertebral artery is, again, a rare complication and almost invariably occurs from direct injury by an instrument (36). Direct exposure is necessary at the foramen transversarium in order to control the resultant hemorrhage.

Utilization of a drain inserted down to the anterior portion of the cervical spine generally prevents accumulation of a post-operative hematoma (143). This is, however, a potentially serious problem if unrecognized in the early post-operative course. Tew and Mayfield have recommended that a cervical collar not be applied in the operating room so that the post-operative dressing can be inspected easily (134). This recommendation was made after one of their patients had a respiratory arrest due to tracheal compression secondary to hematoma accumulation.

Fortunately, the instance of post-operative wound infection of the cervical spine is less than 1% (133). This is probably due to the vascularity of the area. There is an increased risk of infection at the donor site if a graft has been harvested. Proper draping of the donor site, proper placement of the incision, utilization of a drain, and obtaining the graft and closing the wound prior to beginning the approach to the cervical spine can decrease this problem (143).

Many surgeons who prefer anterior disc excision without fusion have been swayed to this technique by complications occurring at the donor site and with the grafts themselves once inserted (7,29,34,110,114,134,143). The utilization of any type of graft configuration can result in partial graft extrusion, frank dislodgement, or graft collapse. Partial graft extrusion is of little consequence and usually does not require any treatment. Complete graft extrusion, however, especially when multilevels have been stabilized, obviously requires replacement of the graft (146). Another potential complication encountered with utilization of grafts at individual interspaces is the occurrence of avascular necrosis of the remaining vertebral body (96). This is more prone to occur utilizing the Cloward technique at two adjacent levels. Cloward has reported on alternating graft configuration at adjacent levels to help avoid this problem (32). When avascular necrosis or graft collapse occurs, an anterior kyphotic deformity may result (75,84). This, again, can be avoided by utilization of a cortical strut graft over multiple levels, or by alternating the type of grafts inserted. The pseudarthrosis rate utilizing different varieties of graft techniques varies from zero to as high as 26% (5,34,40,55,110,114,121,127,142,148).

The donor site is a source of a number of complications. These are generally minor in nature and can consist of persistent drainage, hematoma formation, superficial or deep wound infection (which has been previously addressed), a hernia through the area of bone removal, or an injury to the lateral femoral nerve. A review of 1,244 cases from various series reported a complication rate of 20% at the donor site, whereas there was only a 0.2% complication rate occurring from the neck incision (143).

Utilization of other materials to obtain fusion obviously eliminates donor site problems. Reports have appeared in the literature on utilization of Kiel bone grafts, allografts, hydroxylapatite, or polymethylmethacrylate (31,35,64,119).

Proponents of disc excision without fusion have obviously eliminated donor site and graft complications. There are, however, definite complications that can occur when disc excision alone is performed. One major problem is a transient exacerbation of cervical pain following disc removal. Most series report a 15% to 20% incidence (11,61,74). One series had a 60% occurrence, and the author elected to abandon the procedure (82). Wilson and Campbell consider post-operative neck pain as directly proportionate to the extent of vertebra spreading at the time of disc removal (149).

Another reported complication of this procedure is a radiculopathy occurring on the opposite extremity from what was present pre-operatively. It is felt to be due to inadequate anterior foraminotomy being performed bilaterally (11,52,67,78,91). Several series report an increased angular deformity occurring at the site of disc excision (11,98,134). This is generally of no consequence, but on occasion, is significant enough to require bone grafting (11,98). This is more likely to occur when multiple levels are operated on, especially if radical disc excision is carried out (11,134).

Although there are successful reports of treating myelopathy with anterior disc excision alone, several reports indicate a definite increased risk of worsening of symptoms (11,52), especially in elderly patients with multilevel disease or in patients with congenital stenosis.

By far the most devastating complication of anterior cervical surgery is injury to the spinal cord or nerve root. The exact incidence of this serious complication is not known; there are, however, a few mentioned in most large series. Flynn has published the most ambitious attempt to determine the magnitude of neurological problems following anterior cervical surgery (49). Members of the American Association of Neurological Surgeons were polled, and 52% responded. An analysis of the responses shows a 0.38% incidence of neurological complications. A radiculopathy was reported in 158 cases, and a myelopathy in 129. There were 70 cases in which a myelopathy resulted in which detailed evaluation could be made. Fifty-three of these were immediate and 17 were delayed. Surgical re-exploration did not make much difference in recovery.

There remains speculation as to what causes cord injury at the time of surgical procedure. Some undoubtedly are due to intra-operative trauma caused by actual impaction of the bone graft (108) or the utilization of instrumentation within the spinal canal (29,87). A post-operative epidural hematoma has been implicated in other cases (128,139). The vascular supply of the cord can be damaged at the time of surgery (87).

It must be remembered that mechanical factors such as manipulation of the neck during intubation or hyperextension of the neck in an anesthetized patient can cause inbuckling of the ligamentum flavum and annulus fibrosus and thus cause a cord injury (20,46,128). Some authors have recommended testing the tolerance of neck motion before surgery, and making certain it is not exceeded during the intubation procedure (128,133).

Radical neural decompression with removal of all compressive structures and the posterior longitudinal ligament remains controversial. There have been reported cases of the extensive dissection required for removal of these structures resulting in an increased instance of epidural bleeding (139). It is apparent that adequate visualization using accessory illuminative sources and operative magnification are necessary for safe removal of compressive structures. Also, epidural bleeding must be thoroughly controlled. A bone graft of any configuration must be properly shaped and inserted without excessive force. Obviously, care must be taken not to impact the bone graft into the neural canal.

The Cervical Spine Research Society has obtained further information regarding the incidence of complications in cervical spine surgery (56). This organization is composed primarily of both orthopedists and neurosurgeons. Five years' experience of this group has been obtained and published. In 3,894 reported anterior procedures, the instance of neurological complication has ranged from a low of 0.265% in 1983 and 1984 to a high of 0.91% in the period between 1985 and 1986. These large retrospective series indicate that the risk of spinal cord injury in anterior cervical surgery is probably less than 1%.

Sugar has made several recommendations regarding what to do if an increased neurological deficit is noted post-operatively (128). Certainly, each case must be treated individually, but general guidelines are useful. Make certain that the blood pressure is maintained at proper levels. Although there is no evidence of the benefit of the administration of corticosteroids in a traumatic injury to the spinal cord in humans, they may be of some benefit if given immediately following recognition of a profound neurological dysfunction. A lateral roentgenogram of the neck should be made in order to carefully visualize placement of the graft. An anesthetist should be notified that surgery may have to be performed as soon as possible, especially if the graft is obviously within the canal. This could be done under local anesthesia to avoid manipulation of the already compromised cord.

If there is no evidence of direct compression of the cord by the bone graft, diagnostic studies such as a myelogram, CT, or MRI can be obtained to look for a compressive lesion. Further anterior or posterior decompression can be considered. Consultation should be sought. It must be remembered that an etiological factor for deterioration in neurological function following anterior surgery is often not found, and the cause never known.

Although their occurrence is rare, a number of serious complications can result from anterior cervical spine surgery. Since this operative procedure is relatively easy, there is a tendency to underestimate the seriousness of these potential problems. The spinal surgeon must know how to intelligently discuss these potential problems with the patient prior to embarking on any type of anterior cervical procedure. Certainly, the surgeon also must know how to deal with them if any are encountered.

ACKNOWLEDGMENTS

I wish to acknowledge Ms. Judi Clay and Mr. Jacques Whitecloud for their help in preparing this manuscript.

REFERENCES

1. Adams CBT, Logue V (1971): Studies in cervical spondylotic myelopathy: I. Movement of the cervical roots, dura and cord, and their relation to the course of the extrathecal roots. *Brain* 94:557–568.
2. Adams CBT, Logue V (1971): Studies in cervical spondylotic myelopathy: II. The movement and contour of the spine in relation to the neural complications of cervical spondylosis. *Brain* 94:569–586.
3. Adams CBT, Logue V (1971): Studies in cervical spondylotic myelopathy: III. Some functional effects of operations for cervical spondylotic myelopathy. *Brain* 94:587–594.
4. Arnasson O, Carlsson CA, Pellettieri L (1987): Surgical and conservative treatment of cervical spondylotic radiculopathy and myelopathy. *Acta Neurochir* (Wien) 84:48–53.
5. Aronson N, Filtzer DL, Bagan M (1968): Anterior cervical fusion by the Smith-Robinson approach. *J Neurosurg* 29:397–404.
6. Aronson NI (1973): The management of soft cervical disc protrusions using the Smith-Robinson approach. *Clin Neurosurg* 20:253–258.
7. Bailey RW, Badgley CE (1960): Stabilization of the cervical spine by anterior fusion. *J Bone Joint Surg* [Am] 42(4):565–594.
8. Benini A, Krayenbuhl H, Bruderl R (1982): Anterior cervical discectomy without fusion. Microsurgical technique. *Acta Neurochir* (Wien) 61:105–110.
9. Bernard TN Jr, Whitecloud TS III (1987): Cervical spondylotic myelopathy and myeloradiculopathy: Anterior decompression and stabilization with autogenous fibula strut graft. *Clin Orthop* (221):149–160.
10. Bertalanffy H, Eggert H-R (1988): Clinical long-term results of anterior discectomy without fusion for treatment of cervical radiculopathy and myelopathy: A follow-up of 164 cases. *Acta Neurochir* (Wien) 90:127–135.
11. Bertalanffy H, Eggert H-R (1989): Complications of anterior cervical discectomy without fusion in 450 consecutive patients. *Acta Neurochir* (Wien) 99:41–50.
12. Bertalanffy H, Eggert H-R (1990): Anterior discectomy without fusion for treatment of cervical degenerative disc disease. Twelve years' experience based on 450 consecutive cases. In: Louis R, Weidner A, eds. *Cervical spine II. Marseille 1988.* New York: Springer-Verlag, pp. 208–215.
13. Bloom MH, Raney FL: Anterior invertebral fusion of the cervical spine: A technical note. *J Bone Joint Surg* [Am] 63(5):842.
14. Bohlman HH (1972): Pathology and current treatment for cervical spine injuries. *AAOS Instructional Course Lectures, vol 21.* St. Louis: C V Mosby, pp. 108–115.
15. Bohlman HH (1977): Cervical spondylosis with moderate to severe myelopathy: A report of 17 cases treated by Robinson anterior cervical discectomy and fusion. *Spine* 2(2):151–162.
16. Bollati A, Galli G, Gandolfini M, Marini G, Gatta G (1983): Microsurgical anterior cervical disk removal without interbody fusion. *Surg Neurol* 19:329–333.
17. Boni M, Cherubino P, Benazzo F (1984): Multiple subtotal somatectomy: Technique and evaluation of a series of thirty-nine cases. *Spine* 9(4):358–362.
18. Brain R (1954): Spondylosis: The known and the unknown. *Lancet* 1:687–693.
19. Brain WR, Northfield D, Wilkerson M (1952): The neurological manifestations of cervical spondylosis. *Brain* 75:187–225.
20. Breig A, Turnbull I, Hassler O (1966): Effects of mechanical stresses on the spinal cord in cervical spondylosis. *J Neurosurg* 25:45–56.
21. Brown MD, Malinin TI, Davis PB (1976): A roentgenographic evaluation of frozen allografts versus autografts in anterior cervical spine fusions. *Clin Orthop* (119):231–236.
22. Bulgar RF, Rejowski JE, Beatty RA (1985): Vocal cord paralysis associated with anterior cervical fusion: Considerations for prevention and treatment. *J Neurosurg* 62:657–661.
23. Busch G (1978): Anterior fusion for cervical spondylosis. *J Neurol* 219:117–126.
24. Campbell A, Phillips D (1960): Cervical disc lesion with neurological disorder. Differential diagnosis, treatment, and progression. *Br Med J* 2:481–485.
25. Chirls M (1978): Retrospective study of cervical spondylosis treated by anterior interbody fusion (in 505 patients performed by the Cloward technique). *Bull Hosp Joint Dis* 39:74–82.
26. Clark E, Robinson PK (1956): Cervical myelopathy: A complication of cervical spondylosis. *Brain* 79:483–510.
27. Cloward RB (1958): The anterior approach for removal of ruptured cervical disks. *J Neurosurg* 15:602–617.
28. Cloward RB (1959): Cervical discography contribution to the etiology and mechanism of neck, shoulder and arm pain. *Ann Surg* 150(6):1052.
29. Cloward RB (1962): New method of diagnosis and treatment of cervical disc disease. *Clin Neurosurg* 8:93–132.
30. Cloward RB (1963): Lesions of the intervertebral disks and their treatment by interbody fusion methods. *Clin Orthop* (27):51–77.
31. Cloward RB (1980): Gas-sterilized cadaver bone grafts for spinal fusion operations: A simplified bone bank. *Spine* 5(1):4–10.
32. Cloward RB (1988): The anterior surgical approach to the cervical spine: The Cloward procedure: Past, present and future. *Spine* 13(7):823–827.
33. Concha S, McQueen J (1977): Anterior cervical fusions for spondylotic myelopathy: A preliminary report. *Spine* 2(2):147–150.
34. Connolly ES, Seymore RJ, Adams JE (1965): Clinical evaluation of anterior cervical fusion for degenerative cervical disc. *J Neurosurg* 23:431–437.
35. Cook SD, Whitecloud TS, Reynolds MC, Harding AF, Routman AS, Kay JF, Jarcho M (1987): Hydroxylapatite graft materials for cervical spine fusions. In: Kehr P, Weidner A, eds. *Cervical spine I. Strasbourg 1985.* New York: Springer-Verlag, pp. 257–262.
36. Cosgrove GR, Theron J (1987): Vertebral arteriovenous fistula following anterior cervical spine surgery. Report of two cases. *J Neurosurg* 66:297–299.
37. Crandall PH, Batzdorf U (1966): Cervical spondylotic myelopathy. *J Neurosurg* 25:57–66.
38. Crandall PH, Gregorius FK (1977): Long-term follow-up of surgical treatment of cervical spondylotic myelopathy. *Spine* 2(2):139–146.
39. Cuatico W (1981): Anterior cervical discectomy without interbody fusion: An analysis of 81 cases. *Acta Neurochir* (Wien) 57:269–274.
40. DePalma AF, Rothman RH, Lewinneck RE, Canale S (1972): Anterior interbody fusion for severe cervical disc degeneration. *Surg Gynecol Obstet* 134:755–758.

41. Dereymaeker A, Ghosez J-P, Henkes R (1963): Le traitement chirurgical de la discopathie cervicale. Resultats compares de l'abord posterieur (laminectomie) et de l'abord ventral (fusion corporeale) dans une cinquantaine de cas personels. *Neurochir* 9:13–20.

42. Dereymaeker A, Mulier J (1956): Nouvelle cure neurochirurgicale des discopathies cervicoles. *Neurochirurgie* 2:233–234.

43. Dohn DF (1966): Anterior interbody fusion for treatment of cervical disk condition. *JAMA* 197(11):897–900.

44. Dunsker SB (1977): Anterior cervical discectomy with and without fusion. *Clin Neurosurg* 24:516–521.

45. Epstein J, Carras R, Epstein B, Levine L (1970): Myelopathy in cervical spondylosis with vertebral subluxation and hyperlordosis. *J Neurosurg* 32:421–426.

46. Epstein JA, Carras R, Lavine LS, Epstein BS (1969): The importance of removing osteophytes as part of the surgical treatment of myeloradiculopathy in cervical spondylosis. *J Neurosurg* 30:219–226.

47. Epstein JA, Janin Y, Carras R, Levine LS (1982): A comparative study of the treatment of cervical spondylotic myeloradiculopathy: Experience with 50 cases treated by means of extensive laminectomy, foraminotomy, and excision of osteophytes during the past 10 years. *Acta Neurochir* (Wien) 61:89–104.

48. Eriksen EF, Buhl M, Fode K, et al. (1984): Treatment of cervical disc disease using Cloward's technique. The prognostic value of clinical preoperative data in 1,106 patients. *Acta Neurochir* (Wien) 70:181–197.

49. Flynn TB (1982): Neurologic complications of anterior cervical fusion. *Spine* 7(6):536–539.

50. Frykholm R (1951): Cervical nerve root compression resulting from the disk degeneration and nerve root sleeve fibrosis: A clinical investigation. *Acta Chir Scan* (Suppl) 160:1–149.

51. Galera GR, Tovi D (1968): Anterior disc excision with interbody fusion in cervical spondylotic myelopathy and rhizopathy. *J Neurosurg* 28:305–310.

52. Giombini S, Solero CL (1980): Consideration on 100 anterior cervical discectomies without fusion. In: Grote W, Brock M, Clar HE, Klinger M, Nau HE, eds. *Advances in neurosurgery, vol 8.* Berlin, Heidelberg, New York: Springer-Verlag, pp. 302–307.

53. Gooding MR, Wilson CB, Hoff JT (1975): Experimental cervical myelopathy: Effects of ischemia and compression of the canine cervical spinal cord. *J Neurosurg* 43:9–17.

54. Gore DR (1984): Technique of cervical interbody fusion. *Clin Orthop* (188):191–195.

55. Gore DR, Sepic SB (1984): Anterior cervical fusion for degenerated or protruded discs: A review of one hundred forty-six patients. *Spine* 9(7):667–671.

56. Graham J (1989): Complication of cervical spine surgery. In: *The cervical spine, 2nd ed.* The Cervical Spine Research Society. Philadelphia: J.B. Lippincott, pp. 831–837.

57. Granata F, Taglialatela G, Graziussi G, Avella F (1981): Management of cervical disc protrusions by anterior discectomy without fusion. *J Neurosurg Sci* 25:231–234.

58. Green PWB (1977): Anterior cervical fusion: A review of thirty-three patients with cervical disc degeneration. *J Bone Joint Surg* [Br] 59(2):236–240.

59. Gregorius F, Estrin T, Crandall P (1976): Cervical spondylotic radiculopathy and myelopathy. A long-term follow-up study. *Arch Neurol* 33:618–625.

60. Griffiths IR (1972): Some aspects of the pathology and pathogenesis of the myelopathy caused by disc protrusions in the dog. *J Neurol Neurosurg Psychiatr* 35:403–413.

61. Guarnaschelli JJ, Dzenitis AJ (1982): Anterior cervical discectomy without fusion: comparison study and follow-up. In: Brock M, ed. *Modern neurosurgery I.* New York: Springer-Verlag, pp. 284–291.

62. Guidetti B, Fortuna A (1969): Long-term results of surgical treatment of myelopathy due to cervical spondylosis. *J Neurosurg* 30:714–721.

63. Haft H, Shenkin HA (1963): Surgical end results of cervical ridge and disk problems. *JAMA* 186(4):312–315.

64. Hamby WB, Glaser HT (1959): Replacement of spinal intervertebral discs with locally polymerizing methylmethacrylate. Experimental study of effects upon tissue and report of a small clinical series. *J Neurosurg* 16:311–313.

65. Hanai K, Fujiyoshi F, Kamei K (1986): Subtotal vertebrectomy and spinal fusion for cervical spondylotic myelopathy. *Spine* 11(4):310–315.

66. Hanai K, Inouye Y, Kawai K, Tago K, Itoh Y (1982): Anterior decompression for myelopathy resulting from ossification of the posterior longitudinal ligament. *J Bone Joint Surg* [Br] 64(5): 561–564.

67. Hankinson HL, Wilson CB (1975): Use of the operating microscope in anterior cervical discectomy with fusion. *J Neurosurg* 43:452–456.

68. Harsh GR IV, Sypert GW, Weinstein PR, Ross DA, Wilson CB (1987): Cervical spine stenosis secondary to ossification of the posterior longitudinal ligament. *J Neurosurg* 67:349–357.

69. Heeneman H (1973): Vocal cord paralysis following approaches to anterior cervical spine. *Laryngoscope* 83:17–21.

70. Hicks D, Whitecloud T, LaRocca SH (1980): Cervical spondylotic myelopathy: Results of anterior decompression and stabilization. *Orthop Trans* 4:44.

71. Hirabayashi K, Watanabe K, Wakano K, Suzuki N, Satomi K, Ishii Y (1983): Expansive open-door laminoplasty for cervical spinal stenotic myelopathy. *Spine* 8(7):693–699.

72. Hirsch C (1960): Cervical disc rupture: Diagnosis and therapy. *Acta Orthop Scand* 30:172–186.

73. Hirsch C, Wickbon I, Lidstrom A, et al. (1964): Cervical disc resection. A follow-up of myelographic and surgical procedure. *J Bone Joint Surg* [Am] 46(8):1811–1821.

74. Hoff JT, Wilson CB (1979): Microsurgical approach to the anterior cervical spine and spinal cord. *Clin Neurosurg* 26:513–528.

75. Horwitz NH, Rizzoli HV (1967): *Postoperative complications in neurosurgical practice; recognition, prevention, and management.* Baltimore: Williams and Wilkins Co.

76. Hukuda S, Mochizuki T, Ogata M, Shichikawa K, Shimomura Y (1985): Operations for cervical spondylotic myelopathy. *J Bone Joint Surg* [Br] 67(4):609–615.

77. Hukuda S, Wilson C (1972): Experimental cervical myelopathy: Effects of compression and ischemia on the canine cervical cord. *J Neurosurg* 37:631–652.

78. Husag L, Probst C (1984): Microsurgical anterior approach to cervical discs. Review of 60 consecutive cases of discectomy without fusion. *Acta Neurochir* (Wien) 73:229–242.

79. Irvine GB, Strachan WE (1987): The long-term results of localised anterior cervical decompression and fusion in spondylotic myelopathy. *Paraplegia* 25:18–22.

80. Jacobs B, Krueger EG, Leivy DM (1970): Cervical spondylosis with radiculopathy: Results of anterior diskectomy and interbody fusion. *JAMA* 211(13):2135–2140.

81. Jomin M, Lesoin F, Lozes G, Thomas CE III, Rousseaux M, Clarisse J (1986): Herniated cervical discs. Analysis of a series of 230 cases. *Acta Neurochir* (Wien) 79:107–113.

82. Kadoya S, Kwak R, Hirose G, Yamamoto T (1982): Cervical spondylotic myelopathy treated by a microsurgical anterior approach with or without interbody fusion. In: Brock M, ed. *Modern neurosurgery I.* Berlin, Heidelberg: Springer-Verlag, pp. 292–297.

83. Kadoya S, Nakamura T, Kwak R (1984): A microsurgical anterior osteophytectomy for cervical spondylotic myelopathy. *Spine* 9(4):437–441.

84. Keblish PA, Keggi KJ (1967): Mechanical problems of the dowel graft in anterior cervical fusion. *J Bone Joint Surg* [Am] 49(1):198–199.

85. Kimura I, Oh-Hama M, Shingu Y (1984): Cervical myelopathy treated by canal-expansive laminaplasty. *J Bone Joint Surg* [Am] 66(6):914–920.

86. Kosary IZ, Braham H, Shacked I, Shacked R (1976): Microsurgery in anterior approach to cervical discs. *Surg Neurol* 6:275–277.

87. Kraus DR, Stauffer ES (1975): Spinal cord injury as a complication of elective anterior cervical fusion. *Clin Orthop* (112):130–141.

88. Kubota M, Babe I, Sumida T (1981): Myelopathy due to ossification of the ligamentum flavum of the cervical spine: A report of two cases. *Spine* 6(6):553–559.

89. Lees F, Turner JWA (1963): Natural history and prognosis of cervical spondylosis. *Br Med J* 2:1607–1610.

90. Lesoin F, Bouasakao N, Clarisse J, Rousseaux M, Jomin M (1985): Results of surgical treatment of radiculomyelopathy caused by cervical arthrosis based on 1,000 operations. *Surg Neurol* 23:350–355.

91. Lunsford LD, Bissonette DJ, Jannetta PJ, Sheptak PE, Zorub DS (1980): Anterior surgery for cervical disc disease. Part 1: Treatment of lateral cervical disc herniation in 253 cases. *J Neurosurg* 53:1–11.

92. Lunsford LD, Bissonette DJ, Zorub DS (1980): Anterior surgery for cervical disk disease: Treatment of cervical spondylotic myelopathy in thirty-two cases. *J Neurosurg* 53:12–19.

93. Mann KS, Khosla VK, Gulati DR (1984): Cervical spondylotic myelopathy treated by single-stage multilevel anterior decompression: A prospective study. *J Neurosurg* 60:81–87.

94. Martins AN (1976): Anterior cervical discectomy with and without interbody bone graft. *J Neurosurg* 44:290–295.

95. Mayfield F (1966): Cervical spondylosis: a comparison of the anterior and posterior approaches. *Clin Neurosurg* 13:181–188.

96. Mosdal C (1984): Cervical osteochondrosis and disc herniation. Eighteen years' use of interbody fusion by Cloward's technique in 755 cases. *Acta Neurochir* (Wien) 70:207–255.

97. Moussa AH, Nitta M, Symon L (1983): The results of anterior cervical fusion in cervical spondylosis: Review of 125 cases. *Acta Neurochir* (Wien) 68:277–288.

98. Murphy MG, Gado M (1972): Anterior cervical discectomy without interbody bone graft. *J Neurosurg* 37:71–74.

99. Nugent GR (1959): Clinicopathologic correlations in cervical spondylosis. *Neurology* 9:273–281.

100. Nurick S (1972): The natural history and the results of surgical treatment of the spinal cord disorder associated with cervical spondylosis. *Brain* 95:101–108.

101. Nurick S (1972): The pathogenesis of the spinal cord disorder associated with cervical spondylosis. *Brain* 95:87–100.

102. Odom GL, Finney W, Woodhall B (1958): Cervical disk lesions. *JAMA* 166(1):23–28.

103. O'Laire SA, Thomas DGT (1983): Spinal cord compression due to prolapse of cervical intervertebral disc (herniation of nucleus pulposus): Treatment in 26 cases by discectomy without interbody bone graft. *J Neurosurg* 59:847–853.

104. Olsson SE (1958): The dynamic factor in spinal cord compression: A study on dogs with special reference to cervical disc protrusion. *J Neurosurg* 15:308–321.

105. Ono K, Ota H, Tada K, Hamada H, Takaoka K (1977): Ossified posterior longitudinal ligament. *Spine* 2(2):126–138.

106. Payne EE, Spillane JD (1957): The cervical spine. An anatomico-pathological study of 70 specimens (using a special technique) with particular reference to the problem of cervical spondylosis. *Brain* 80:571–576.

107. Penning L, Van der Zwaag P (1966): Biomechanical aspects of spondylotic myelopathy. *Acta Radiol* (Diagn) 5:1090–1103.

108. Phillips DG (1973): Surgical treatment of myelopathy with cervical spondylosis. *J Neurol Neurosurg Psychiatr* 36:879–884.

109. Reid JD (1960): Effects of flexion-extension movements of the head and spine upon the spinal cord and nerve roots. *J Neurol Neurosurg Psychiatr* 23:214–221.

110. Riley LH Jr, Robinson RA, Johnson KA, et al. (1969): The results of anterior interbody fusion of the cervical spine: Review of ninety-three consecutive cases. *J Neurosurg* 30:127–133.

111. Robertson JT (1973): Anterior removal of cervical disc without fusion. *Clin Neurosurg* 20:259–261.

112. Robertson JT (1978): Anterior operations for herniated cervical disc and for myelopathy. *Clin Neurosurg* 25:245–250.

113. Robinson RA, Smith GW (1955): Anterolateral cervical disc removal and interbody fusion for cervical disc syndrome. *Bull of the Johns Hopkins Hosp* 96:223–224.

114. Robinson RA, Walker AE, Ferlic DC, et al. (1962): The results of an anterior interbody fusion of the cervical spine. *J Bone Joint Surg* [Am] 44(8):1579–1586.

115. Rosenorn J, Hansen EB, Rosenorn M-A (1983): Anterior cervical discectomy with and without fusion: A prospective study. *J Neurosurg* 59:252–255.

116. Sakou T, Miyazaki A, Tomimura K, Maehara T, Frost HM (1979): Ossification of the posterior longitudinal ligament of the cervical spine: Subtotal vertebrectomy as a treatment. *Clin Orthop* 140:58–65.

117. Seeger W (1982): *Microsurgery of the spinal cord and surrounding structures.* New York: Springer-Verlag.

118. Senegas J, Guerin J (1975): Technique de decompression medullaire anterieure daus les stenoses Canalaires estendues. *Rev Chir Orthop* 61:219–223.

119. Senter HJ, Kortyna R, Kemp WR (1989): Anterior cervical fusion with hydroxylapatite fusion. *Neurosurgery* 25(1):39–43.

120. Shima T, Keller JT, Alvirn MM, Mayfield FH, Dunsker SB (1979): Anterior cervical discectomy and interbody fusion: An experimental study using a synthetic tricalcium phosphate. *J Neurosurg* 51:533–538.

121. Simmons EH, Bhalla SK (1969): Anterior cervical discectomy and fusion: A clinical and biomechanical study with eight year follow-up. *J Bone Joint Surg* [Br] 51(2):225–237.

122. Southwick WO, Robinson RA (1957): Surgical approaches to the vertebral bodies in the cervical and lumbar regions. *J Bone Joint Surg* [Am] 39(3):631–644.

123. Spetzler RF, Roski RA, Selman WR (1982): The microscope in anterior cervical spine surgery. *Clin Orthop* (168):17–23.

124. Stauffer ES, Kaufer H (1975): Fractures and dislocations of the spine. In: Rockwood CA, Green DP, eds. *Fractures.* Philadelphia: J.B. Lippincott, pp. 851–853.

125. Stoltmann H, Blackwood W (1964): The rule of the ligamenta flava in the pathogenesis of myelopathy in cervical spondylosis. *Brain* 87:45–50.

126. Stookey B (1928): Compression of the spinal cord due to ventral extradural cervical chondromas: Diagnosis and surgical treatment. *Arch Neurol Psychiatry* 20:275–291.

127. Stuck RM (1963): Anterior cervical disc excision and fusion: Report of two hundred consecutive cases. *Rocky M Med J* 60:25–30.

128. Sugar O (1981): Spinal cord malfunction after anterior cervical discectomy. *Surg Neurology* 15:4–8.

129. Taheri ZE, Gueramy M (1972): Experience with calf bone in cervical interbody spinal fusion. *J Neurosurg* 36:67–71.

130. Tarlov IM, Klinger H (1954): Spinal cord compression studies: II. Time limits for recovery after acute compression in dogs. *Arch Neurol Psychiatry* 71:271–290.

131. Tarlov IM, Klinger H, Vitale S (1953): Spinal cord compression studies: I. Experimental techniques to produce acute and gradual compression. *Arch Neurol Psychiatry* 70:813–819.

132. Taylor AR (1953): Mechanism and treatment of spinal-cord disorders associated with cervical spondylosis. *Lancet* 1:717–723.

133. Tew JM Jr, Mayfield FH (1975): Complications of surgery of the anterior cervical spine. *Clin Neurol* 23:424–434.

134. Tew JM, Mayfield FH (1981): Surgery of the anterior cervical spine: Prevention of complications. In: Dunsker SB, ed. *Cervical spondylosis.* New York: Raven Press, pp. 191–208.

135. Tezuka A, Yamada K, Ikata T (1976): Surgical results of cervical spondylotic radiculo-myelopathy observed more than five years. *Tokushima J Exp Med* 23:9–18.

136. Tribolet N de, Zander E (1981): Anterior discectomy without fusion for the treatment of ruptured cervical discs. *J Neurosurg Sci* 25:217–22.

137. Tsuji H (1982): Laminoplasty for patients with compressive myelopathy due to so-called spinal canal stenosis in cervical and thoracic regions. *Spine* 7(1):28–34.

138. Tsuyama N (1981): The ossification of the posterior longitudinal ligament of the spine (OPLL). *J of the Japanese Orthop Assoc* 55:425–440.

139. U HS, Wilson CB (1978): Postoperative epidural hematoma as a complication of anterior cervical discectomy. *J Neurosurg* 49:288–291.

140. Verbiest H, Paz Y, Geuse HD (1966): Anterolateral surgery for cervical spondylosis in cases of myelopathy or nerve root compression. *J Neurosurg* 25:611–622.

141. White AA III, Hirsch C (1971): An experimental study of the immediate load bearing capacity of some commonly used iliac grafts. *Acta Orthop Scand* 42:482–490.

142. White AA III, Southwick WO, DePonte RJ, Gainor SW, Hardy R (1973): Relief of pain by anterior cervical spine fusion for spondylosis: A report of sixty-five cases. *J Bone Joint Surg* [Am] 55(3):525–534.

143. Whitecloud TS III (1978): Complication of anterior cervical fusion. In: American Academy of Orthopaedic Surgeons: *Instructional Course Lectures, vol 27.* St. Louis: CV Mosby, pp. 223–227.
144. Whitecloud TS III (1988): Anterior surgery for cervical spondylotic myelopathy: Smith-Robinson, Cloward and vertebrectomy. *Spine* 13(7):861–863.
145. Whitecloud TS III, Geibel PT, Olive PM, Levet B (submitted for publication): Anterior cervical fusion using a reversed Robinson-Smith graft.
146. Whitecloud TS III, LaRocca SH (1976): Fibular strut graft in reconstructive surgery of the cervical spine. *Spine* 1(1):33–43.
147. Whitecloud TS III, Seago RA (1987): Cervical discogenic syndrome: Results of operative intervention in patients with positive discography. *Spine* 12:313–315.
148. Williams JL, Allen MD Jr, Harkess JW (1968): Late results of cervical discectomy and interbody fusion: Some factors influencing the results. *J Bone Joint Surg* [Am] 50:277–286.
149. Wilson DH, Campbell DD (1977): Anterior cervical discectomy without bone graft: Report of seventy-one cases. *J Neurosurg* 47:551–555.
150. Wohlert L, Buhl M, Eriksen EF, et al. (1984): Treatment of cervical disc disease using Cloward's technique III. Evaluation of cervical spondylotic myelopathy in 138 cases. *Acta Neurochir* (Wien) 71:121–131.
151. Wolf BS, Khilnani M, Malis L (1956): The sagittal diameter of the bony cervical spinal canal and its significance in cervical spondylosis. *J of Mt Sinai Hosp* 23:283–292.
152. Yonenobu K, Fuji T, Ono K, Okada K, Yamamoto T, Harada N (1985): Choice of surgical treatment for multisegmental cervical spondylotic myelopathy. *Spine* 10(8):710–716.
153. Zdeblick TA, Bohlman HH (1989): Myelopathy, cervical kyphosis and treatment by anterior carpectomy and strut grafting. *J Bone Joint Surg* [Am] 71(2):170–182.
154. Zhang ZH, Yin H, Yang K, Zhang T, Dong F, Dang G, Lou SQ, Cai Q (1983): Anterior intervertebral disc excision and bone grafting in cervical spondylotic myelopathy. *Spine* 8(1):16–19.

The Adult Spine: Principles and Practice,
J. W. Frymoyer, Editor-in-Chief.
Raven Press, Ltd., New York © 1991.

CHAPTER 57

Cervical Radiculopathies and Myelopathies

Posterior Approaches

Thomas B. Ducker

When spinal surgery developed at the turn of the century, the neurologist made an anatomical diagnosis and then advised the surgeon (who carried the title of Mister, not Doctor) on where to cut to correct the problem. A midline incision over the spinous process was made and multiple segments were exposed until the pathology was found. In the early 1920s, the conditions of nerve root pain (sciatica) and myelopathy became better appreciated and separated. Specific root syndromes were identified in the 1940s, and in the 1950s the posterior decompression keyhole surgical procedure to remove a lateral ruptured cervical intervertebral disc and/or osteophytes was described (59,62,63). By the 1960s, neurosurgeons and orthopedists began treating the various root syndromes resulting from a single disc rupture (45). Myelopathies due to cervical spondylytic stenosis, either acquired or congenital, were also well described (6), and their surgical care by a posterior approach became well defined (1,11,18,42).

With the advent and utilization of anterior approaches to the cervical spine in the 1950s, the debate on the appropriate approach to these conditions was initiated (10,42,61). The debate continues concerning the posterior procedure versus the anterior procedure.

In this chapter, I take the position that posterior procedures for the many problems of cervical spondylosis are not only acceptable but may be more desirable in many cases. However, the physician who utilizes a posterior exposure to the exclusion of an anterior procedure and vice versa is not providing the patient with the best possible care since each situation needs to be individualized. In this context, the posterior approach has certain advantages over anterior procedures. In the exposure, the midline structures and muscles can be safely divided without danger to any major vessels, the esophagus, trachea, or major nerves. If the muscles are sewn back tightly in multiple layers, the cosmetic result is quite acceptable. In general, the posterior exposure carries a low potential for instability or malalignment, providing care is taken to preserve the integrity of the facet joints and capsules. Multilevel disease can easily be decompressed from the posterior approach and there is good visualization of the dura and full appreciation of the decompres-

T. B. Ducker, M.D.: Department of Neurological Surgery, The Johns Hopkins University School of Medicine, Baltimore, Maryland 21205.

sion. Furthermore, the entire length of the cervical spine can be treated because one has good access to the very high lesions around C1, C2, and C3 and to the very low pathology around C7 and T1. Finally, if there are any questions which require visualization of the spinal cord over several segments, this is by far more easily accomplished with posterior exposure.

However, the posterior exposure is not ideal in all cases. When there is clearcut pathology at one or two disc levels anteriorly and/or single focal instability at only one space, the anterior procedure can be safely and quickly carried out with minimal morbidity and mortality. When pre-operative diagnostic images reveal the major pathology is anterior, posterior operations are not noted for excellent results. In particular, when anterior compression is combined with a cervical kyphos, anterior decompression and fusion are preferred.

Lengthy laminectomies in children can result in instability and kyphotic deformities as well. It is obvious that understanding the patient's complaints and analysis of imaging studies will lead to proper selection of the procedure for each individual patient.

CLINICAL ASSESSMENT

Before a patient is treated surgically for a radiculopathy or myelopathy, repeated evaluations should be done with efforts to treat the problem medically if possible. The interval between visits varies widely. If the patient has an acute problem with severe pain requiring narcotics or is demonstrating progressive serious neurologic loss, then evaluation may need to be carried out as often as daily and definitive diagnostic studies completed so the treatment can be done. If the problem is chronic and/or that of recurring pain and only mild weakness, then the visits can be every week or month, until a full appreciation of the neurologic syndrome is possible. Making a neurologic diagnosis is essential in treating radiculopathies and myelopathies. Although certain axial spinal cervical pain syndromes with referred discomforts can, on occasion, be successfully treated with an anterior cervical fusion, that is rarely the case posteriorly. With posterior operations, the compressed nerve roots and/or cord need to be specifically identified. With the clinical identification of the single diseased root or roots, the confirmation of the problem must then be done by neuroradiological studies.

In all patients, plain cervical spine x-rays are needed, often with flexion and extension to evaluate stability. The next diagnostic study need not entail any injections. Generally speaking, the more bony abnormalities the patient has on plain x-rays, the more likely it is that a CT scan will provide the definitive diagnosis. The CT is an excellent study in most older patients. If the plain x-rays are basically normal and show little bony pathology,

then attention is directed to a soft tissue lesion. In this case the MRI is clearly superior. If the first CT or MRI fails to give a diagnosis and a neurologic syndrome is still strongly suspected, then use of the other study may provide the diagnosis. Unfortunately, there are those patients who will have an osteophyte at one level and a soft disc herniation at the next level, and the MRI and CT scan may be necessary to fully appreciate the pathologic abnormality. If the diagnosis has not been achieved by plain x-ray, CT, and MRI, then invasive diagnostic studies are needed. Depending on the index of suspicions and the seriousness of pathology, one can choose an enhanced CT scan, commonly referred to as a myelographic CT, or a full column myelogram followed by selected CT images at levels of involvement. At the same time, the cerebral spinal fluid should be fully evaluated. Finally, there are those patients in which the clinical symptoms and signs are confusing. In these patients intracranial pathology needs to be excluded by a brain MRI. Also the treating surgeon must remember that some patients will have two pathological processes, such as a myelopathy accompanied by intracranial lesions of multiple sclerosis (MS). Accurate diagnosis is possible only with the newer diagnostic techniques.

Concurrent disease influences the outcome of care of the patient with myelopathies and radiculopathies. Obviously, the metabolic disease that has the most adverse influence is diabetes. Particularly in the older patient vascular, heart, and pulmonary disease may preclude operative treatment. Finally, neurologic disorders (such as MS, amyotrophic lateral sclerosis), always make diagnosis challenging when considering operative intervention. Each spinal surgeon has his own rare case wherein standard surgery failed to relieve the patient of his problem and the extremely rare diagnosis is made at a later date. One such example is a patient succumbing to Shy-Drager syndrome, severe dysautonomia, and concurrent myelopathy.

With repeated assessments of any patient's disease, the appropriate neurologic syndrome should be identified and these are well described in Chapters 30 and 49.

INFORMED CONSENT AND ANTICIPATED RESULTS

The natural history of untreated radiculopathies and myelopathies is quite different. Radiculopathies, even when severe, tend to improve even though there may be persistent weakness and often persistent pain. A truly devastating outcome from an untreated radiculopathy is quite rare. Therefore, proceeding with surgical treatment often deals more with the quality of the patient's life than with any other single factor. With radiculopathies, the persistence of pain and/or weakness which interferes with one's activities in spite of adequate treatment with anti-inflammatory drugs and other medical regimes, is a common justification for operative intervention.

The natural history of untreated myelopathies is entirely a different matter. Clearly two-thirds of those patients will have a progressive myelopathy, numbness and clumsiness of the hands, weakness in the legs, and may over a period of years become confined to wheelchair and/or a bed. When operative intervention is delayed until the late stages of the disease irreversible damage has been done to the cord and a good recovery is not possible. Myelopathy complicated by the ossification of the posterior longitudinal ligament is a disorder common in the Orient and rare in the Americas or Europe. It carries with it the same ominous signs that myelopathy does in general. The description of end-stage myelopathy with scarring and gliosis in the cord is well documented.

In giving a patient informed consent and anticipated results when operative intervention is being planned, there are both general statements about operative care as well as specific statements about the patient's disorder which are necessary. General broad statements dealing with anesthesias and drug reactions are appropriate, but admittedly these complications are rare. A general statement about infection must be included. The infection rate in spinal procedures typically is 1% to 2% and appears to be even less when 24 hours of antibiotic coverage is provided (12,30,31,56,57,60). While the consequences of infection need to be outlined, a reassuring statement to the effect that most of these are treated successfully with antibiotics can be added. Thrombophlebitis in the lower extremities or thrombophlebotic phenomenon still occurs and seems to be more common in the older patient, especially when the operation is of long duration. Again, this seems to affect only 1 patient per 100. The advent of the intermittent pressure device or sequential compression devices on the lower extremities during operative care and immediately in the recovery room has lowered the incidence of lower extremity venous problems substantially in our practice. Post-operative urinary tract infections still occur, and if the male has pre-existing prostatism or the female has a history of recurrent urinary tract infection, it is obviously a greater risk.

Specific problems related to the spinal surgery itself have to do with instability of the spine, damage to the spinal nerve roots, or injury to the spinal cord. Treating radiculopathies, with removal of cervical herniated discs, decompressing cervical foraminal stenosis, or reduction of a very specific osteophytic spur may lead to adverse changes in neurological function in the specific nerve root in 2% to 3% of cases. In treating radiculopathies, damage to the spinal cord is rare, but does occur in 1 out of 200–300 cases. Another disease, such as longstanding juvenile diabetes, does change the risks. Such patients may have diabetic end-artery disease and manip-

ulation of the root can lead to a central ischemic episode in the spinal cord itself. Spinal instability after laminoforaminotomies is extremely rare, providing careful attention is paid to the facets.

In summary, 90% to 95% of patients undergoing posterior cervical surgery for radiculopathies have a satisfactory outcome (17,22,33,44,46,50,59,62,63). This figure clearly exceeds the number of good results achieved in lumbar disc surgery, and it exceeds the number of good results found in treating the serious myelopathies.

In comparison to the treatment of radiculopathies, carrying out operative decompressions for myelopathy is technically dangerous. If it were not for such a grave prognosis without operative decompression, surgeons would not be eager to do these procedures. In providing informed consent for these patients, the overwhelming evidence indicates that two-thirds of the patients continue to deteriorate if not decompressed (5,6,39,49,55). However, a well executed decompressive laminectomy with limited foraminotomies as needed will lead to some or complete improvement in the patient's clinical condition in over 70% of patients (2,8,16,20,43). How aggressive the surgeon is in removing osteophytes in and around the foramen depends on preference and skills, but certainly the experience reported by Epstein indicates that foraminotomy may further enhance recovery after the surgical procedure (20). Carrying out laminectomies with dura grafts and with/without sectioning of the dentate ligaments does not increase the patient's chances of a good result (2,11,26,28,29,43,50,52,66). For practical purposes, the major goal is to perform an adequate posterior decompressive laminectomy and this is usually all that is required (8,11,16,17,23).

COMPARISON OF SURGICAL RESULTS AFTER ANTERIOR AND POSTERIOR DECOMPRESSION

In Table 1, the posterior approach and anterior approach are compared by adding together several large series. In many of these series, the patients treated with

TABLE 1. *Comparing anterior and posterior decompressive procedures in cervical myelopathy patients. Numbers reflect summations of several large series*

Approach	Patients	Improved	Unimproved
Anterior	434	73%	27%
Posterior	685	71%	29%

References for this table are available in the articles by Epstein (16) and Carol and Ducker (8). Additional references concerning the anterior approach are in Chapter 56 by Whitecloud (this volume) and in references 27, 43, 67, 68, and 69.

There is no randomized comparative series. In most comparative evaluations, the patients having the posterior decompressive procedures were older, had disease at many levels, and presented with worse neurologic deficits (8).

posterior procedures were older and had a more severe cord deficit (8,17). Yet, the results of treatment are comparable. These data support both anterior and posterior operative approaches, but also indirectly support the concept that individualizing each case to pick the most appropriate decompressive procedure is the responsibility of the attending surgeon (6,8,11,17,22,28,42,53, 67,69). However, it also has to be recognized that not all patients do well.

Clearly, older patients who have severe myelopathy, where they are unable to ambulate, run a risk of dying from the procedure. As previously noted, these patients are more prone to cardiovascular and thromboembolic complications. The percent of patients actually worse following a decompressive laminectomy varies from 3% to 10%, and in my experience, it is 4% to 5% (8).

KYPHOSIS

Great care should be taken to evaluate the contour of the cervical spine pre-operatively. With a lordotic or straight curve and myelopathy, a laminectomy over several segments can allow the cord to migrate posteriorly, relieving even anterior impingement. However, with a kyphotic curve and myelopathy, the spinal cord is placed under tension over the angular deformity. Laminectomy will then be less effective in relieving cord impingement, and may in fact serve to destabilize the spine, and increase the kyphosis (4,8,27,28,42,67,69). In those situations where myelopathy and cervical kyphosis co-exist anterior decompression and fusion are recommended. These problems are discussed in Chapters 56 and 58.

OSSIFICATION OF POSTERIOR LONGITUDINAL LIGAMENTS

Myelopathy associated with ossification of the posterior longitudinal ligament (OPLL) is even a more serious problem (13). Ossification of the posterior longitudinal ligament can take on many configurations with protrusions into the canal, being square-shaped, mushroom-formed, or Hill types (Fig. 15) (3,13,25,35,37,47,48). When bony compression impinges on the anterior spinal artery complex, pathology is associated with ischemic phenomenon in the spinal cord. Surgical results for OPLL diseases do not have the 70% good results for myelopathy associated with degeneration; even the Japanese can only improve 60% of these patients (34,35,38). OPLL continues in its growth and impingement upon the spinal cord even after operative intervention. This progressive pathology is seen in anywhere from 25% to 80% of the patients who have had operative decompression (37). There is some evidence that fusion or various laminoplasties, as opposed to a standard decompressive laminectomy, retard the transverse and longitudinal

growth of the OPLL. Our standard decompressive procedure is less commonly carried out on this particular subgroup of patients. It is in this same subgroup of patients that the chances of being neurologically worse after the decompression is higher, and exceeds 10%. Of course, all other risk factors are still present, particularly in older patients.

ANESTHESIA: POSITIONING AND MONITORING

The positioning of the patient clearly is the physician's and anesthesiologist's preference. There are advantages and disadvantages to either prone or sitting positions. The prone position may cause more engorgement of the adjacent veins and subsequent tissue which, in turn, can hinder good visualization of the pathology and compromise the decompression. While the sitting position leads to less engorgement of the venous structures, and to drainage of the fluids and blood away from the surgical area, there is the never ending risk of air emboli and cardiovascular instability. Unfortunately, if an adverse problem develops with either position, there are self styled experts who travel for plaintiff's attorneys around the country to say that that particular physician or anesthesiologist made the wrong choice. The fact is that either the prone or sitting position are acceptable for the treatment of radiculopathies and myelopathies.

For a variety of reasons, many surgeons tend to use the sitting position for the radicular nerve root decompressions, and the prone position for the myelopathy. In treating radiculopathies, the bony resection is unilateral and usually quite limited, and the operation is swiftly carried out. It is in those positions in which we consistently work in front of the nerve root to remove a herniated disc and/or osteophyte. Good visualization of the nerve root without engorgement of fluid, blood, etc., is important. In my own personal experience of nearly 500 cases, I have not seen serious air embolic phenomenon leading to any cardiovascular instability or change in the end tidal PCO_2. While the Doppler has heard air on a few occasions, this has never been a major problem. Our experience parallels Henderson et al. (33).

For myelopathy, the prone position is more commonly used. But Epstein's experience (18,20) clearly shows that a patient properly positioned and properly hydrated can have these procedures carried out in the sitting position as well. If the patient has a severe myelopathy, which leads to alterations in sympathetic tone, and causes low blood pressure and perfusion compromise to the cord itself, utilizing the prone position may be safer. At the present time both the prone and sitting positions are acceptable in operative care of these patients. A more complete analysis of over 500 cases by Matjasko et al. is available for review (41).

Holding the patient's head during operative intervention on the cervical spine is usually done by the three pin holders of the Mayfield frame. In some of the patients who have severe myelopathies, traction can afford them some minor relief even before operative intervention is carried out. In those patients who have had an acute traumatic event the utilization of traction in the hospital bed with the head and shoulders elevated 10–20 degrees helps. The 15–20 pounds of traction helps many by simply opening up the joints, taking the pressure off of the collapsing ligaments. In patients with significant myelopathy, it is recommended to use skeletal tong traction with 15–20 pounds during the operation (8). The traction can be done with an operative wedge frame or an operative Stryker frame. Or, it can be carried out with standard operating room equipment with horseshoe head apparatus and a traction attachment. Also, the tongs in the skull certainly make it easier to turn the patient from supine to prone without any unusual positioning. Traction most commonly is used in selected cases of myelopathies undergoing decompressing.

Intubation techniques are dependent on the patient's diagnosis. If this patient has a supple neck and radiculopathy, a standard intubation technique is safe. When the endotracheal tube is in position, primary extension is at the occipital C1–C2 area, with flexion occurring in the lower cervical areas, where the pathology commonly occurs. In patients with early myelopathy, who have a good range of motion of the neck, a transient extension to place the endotracheal tube rarely causes any problem. However, there are those patients who have severe myelopathies and who have severe stenosis involving C3–C4 or higher. It is in these patients that most anesthesiologists and surgeons prefer an awake fiberoptic assisted intubation under local anesthesia. It is also these patients who are more likely to be operated on in a Stryker frame and with traction. Once the patient is properly intubated, he can be placed under general anesthesia, maintained or placed in traction, and turned safely without significant risks. In some instances, patient positioning is best done prior to administration of general anesthesia, after awake intubation.

Intravascular volume controlled by peripheral and central venous lines is assessed on an individual basis. If the sitting position is used, it is wise to keep the patient well-hydrated unless there is a specific cardiovascular contraindication. Certain centers have advocated placing a central line in all these patients. One of the goals of having a central cardiac line is to remove air from the right side of the heart if air embolism should occur. In my personal experience, I have been unimpressed with the ability to remove air through these lines. In fact, suctioning on a central cardiac line may further compromise cardiac output. Using the central line as a measure of central blood volume is of more value (19,41), and in the unstable patient is justified. With limited laminofor-

aminotomies for a root decompression, maintaining good hydration, Doppler monitoring to listen for air, and careful monitoring of vital signs and end tidal PCO_2 are all that is required. End tidal PCO_2 monitoring will also alert the anesthesiologist to kinks in the endotracheal tube. Placing a central line in all of these patients is simply not needed and may even lead to complications (33). In my experience treating radiculopathies with one or two space laminoforaminotomies, we have had more difficulty with pneumothoraxes from line placement (3 patients) than serious air embolic phenomenon (0 patients). It is true that the Doppler will suggest some air in roughly 3% of these patients, but the vital signs, end tidal PCO_2, etc., do not change and the volume of air must be very small (41). Consequently, a central venous or pulmonary wedge pressure line in a simple unilateral laminoforaminotomy are being placed in less than half of my patients and the decision is the preference of the anesthesiologist.

However, if the patient to be treated has a myelopathy, especially the elderly patient who may be on anti-hypertensive medications, monitoring to include central venous pressure and/or pulmonary arterial wedge pressures may be needed. Central lines may be needed in the patient who is prone. This particular group of patients has an abnormal sympathetic nervous system due to compression of the cervical spinal cord. The central fibers on the reticulospinal system are damaged along with all of the other motor and sensory fibers. With an unstable sympathetic system, and if there is an unstable cardiac condition, these patients may be more difficult to manage in either position. If one elects to do the sitting position in this particular group of patients, proper hydration and monitoring are absolutely required (41). Furthermore, in these patients treated in the sitting position, the importance of Doppler monitoring cannot be overemphasized. When air is heard, even though it may not alter the vascular dynamics, the source of the air should be searched for and the vessel coagulated with a bipolar cautery. If it is not readily accessible, temporarily packing the wound with wet sponge for a minute or two will often stop this air influx permanently. Doppler monitoring should be utilized by the surgeon as a warning to find the source of any open vessel. Once the air is heard, the next important monitor is the end tidal PCO_2. If there is significant air, the end tidal PCO_2 will fall and blood pressure and cardiac output may be diminished. The wound must be packed with wet sponges if this event occurs, until hemodynamic stability is regained.

EVOKED POTENTIALS

Evoked potential monitoring of the spinal cord during operations for myelopathy is now commonplace and there are numerous articles as well as books on the subject matter (14). Evoked potential monitoring is not needed for treating radiculopathies, but it is helpful in certain patients with myelopathies. By utilizing certain anesthetic agents, an evoked potential which is not present on routine study can be augmented so that recordings can be made throughout the surgical procedure (4). Most evoked potential monitoring measures the sensory systems through the posterior columns. With posterior cervical operations and decompression, this is a valuable tool. However, there are limitations. Certain anesthetics depress the response making it difficult to interpret. Also, the patients with severe myelopathy may not have any evoked potentials pre-operatively and trying to record them intra-operatively is impossible. Information from evoked potentials alters the care in only 3% of patients (9). Commonly, the position of the patient can be changed because of evoked potentials. We have found that having the patient in a neutral, slightly flexed position the potentials are the strongest. Hyper-flexion or hyper-extension is detrimental to the evoked potentials and obviously detrimental to the cord. Hypotension is definitely detrimental to the evoked potentials. Any pressure applied to the spinal cord during the surgical procedure will alter the potential (9).

INTRA-OPERATIVE RADIOGRAPHY

No matter how trivial it may seem, a single localizing intra-operative x-ray should be utilized in all cases. This film helps the surgeon to confine his dissection to the pathological area. It also is a means of defense to mitigate against our litigious society that may accuse the surgeon of not carrying out the procedure properly. It helps eliminate exploring a nerve root that does not require inspection.

ANTIBIOTICS AND STEROIDS

Use of peri-operative antibiotics and steroids is still somewhat debated. My own early research showed that steroids given before injury to the spinal cord were more helpful than giving them afterwards (15). There is a definite place for this medication, even though it is limited (7,8,32). It is common for surgeons to give the patient 4 to 6 mg of dexamethasone or equivalent dose in methylprednisolone two hours before the procedure, intra-operatively, and three doses every six hours after the surgical procedure. Twenty-four hour coverage is all that is needed. Utilizing the medication for longer periods, while advocated by some, seems unnecessary (8,17). Conversely, the short time use of steroids appears beneficial experimentally and clinically (7,32).

Peri-operative antibiotics do appear to be beneficial (12,30,31,40,56,57,60,64). A voluminous literature has been reviewed by Haines and summarizes the more than 100 articles on this subject and concluded an antibiotic should be given in the peri-operative period (30). The major intra-operative infection organism is usually a *Staphylococcus*. Consequently, a newer penicillin or one of the cephlosporins is most acceptable. If the patient is truly allergic to penicillin, then either no drug or an entirely different family of medications such as vancomycin would be needed. Having the steroid given before the antibiotic and having both given pre-operatively allows recognition of an allergic reaction prior to surgery. If one occurs, no further antibiotics are given.

OPERATIVE TECHNIQUE

Laminotomy and Laminoforaminotomy

Exposure of the lamina and the foramen to decompress the nerve root for a radiculopathy can be either from a straight posterior incision or a posterior lateral incision. The former is the traditional approach (17,22,33,46,53,59,63) while the latter has been developed more recently and is quite effective (Fig. 1) (44). The pure posterior approach takes down the muscle attachments off the midline and the spinous processes in order to expose the lamina and facets. The posterolateral approach is more of a muscle splitting procedure, but again, the muscles are taken off of part of the lamina and facet area. The older posterior procedure was developed, in part, in the 1940s and clearly described in the 1950s (50,59,62,63). The "keyhole" foraminotomy became common use in the 1950s and early 1960s (21,46,58). The incision has to be long enough so that instruments can be placed in the operative hole without obliterating the surgeon's view. With good exposure of the lamina and two-thirds of the facet, a single bladed retractor is all that is required to hold the muscles laterally. While we have had special instruments made for this common procedure, there are commercially available retractors to accomplish the same task. If the neck is hyperflexed, the muscles and adjacent tendons are extremely tight making it difficult to achieve retraction of the muscles laterally. If the neck is only slightly flexed, then the retraction is easily achieved without a great deal of strain on the tissues. If the neck is extended, then it is harder to get in the interlamina space to accomplish the exposure for decompression. Neck position is a factor in both the sitting or prone position of the patient.

A localizing x-ray is commonly employed at the dissecting stage of exposure. By placing an instrument such as a small dissector probe into the apophyseal joint at the level which has been exposed, the intra-operative film will confirm that one is indeed operating at the right interlamina space. The marker will point slightly to the vertebral body above the joint space itself. Others prefer to mark a spinous process or an intraspinous process

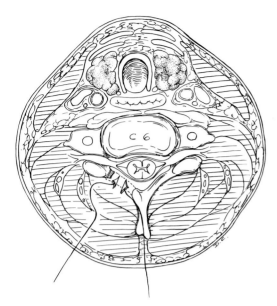

FIG. 1. The most common approach posteriorly to the cervical spine for radiculopathy is midline posterior, but the posterolateral approach is equally acceptable. Both approaches to the nerve root allow adequate views of any pathology.

area for the film. All of these techniques are acceptable, and do provide intra-operative confirmation at the time of initial exposure so that the bony removal will be at the correct level. The incisions are not long and the exposures are limited; so it is difficult to count, with certainty, the various spinous processes to be confident of proper exposure without an intra-operative film. Studying both the lateral and AP plain x-rays, with identification of the last bifid spine, whether this be either C5 or C6, aids in creating the proper limited exposure. If one is using a straight posterior exposure, one side of a bifid spine may be excised without any loss of mobility or stability, in order to achieve a better visualization of the lamina and facet areas. Removing that small part of the spinous process may also facilitate placing the retractors to hold the muscle laterally.

Bony removal is initiated in the intervertebral joint area. This can be safely done without introducing any instruments into the canal or on the nerve root. The same bone can be taken away quickly with a high speed drill. Either the drill or rongeur forceps can be utilized to reduce the bulk of the bone superiorly even in the facet area. In patients who have a lateral disc rupture without canal stenosis, utilization of small rongeurs and the very small angled Kerrison's punches can be safely done. However, in patients who have any canal compromise and severe bony stenosis, high speed drills work better in thinning the bone down. In either case, the roof of the foramen or spinal root canal can be further decompressed with angled 2.0 and 3.0 curettes. This can be carried out with undercutting one-third or one-half of the facet area and the joint (Fig. 2). The majority of the

posterior apophyseal joint is maintained, and later spinal instability is rarely a problem (53,54,70). Spinal instability does not occur when surgery is performed posteriorly for radiculopathy. When focal instability develops at one level, it is usually associated with neurofibroma tumor surgery where much of the facet anatomy has been previously destroyed and there are further changes with the operative exposure in order to rid the patient of the tumor.

If the bony removal is carried out properly, the lateral aspects of the dura sac can readily be visualized by removing only the lateral one-third of the remaining ligamentum flavum and soft tissues. The nerve root as it exits from the dura sac should be visualized above and below, although most of the visualization is clearly inferiorly. The anatomy is usually clearly identified by gently sweeping away any remaining small epidural fat present, bipolar coagulation of any obvious veins, and by removing fibrous tissue over the posterior aspect of the nerve root itself (Figs. 4 and 5).

In by far the majority of clinical situations (90%), the decompression of a cervical nerve root and the dura sac can be accomplished through this limited exposure. By taking a small dissector, the plane between the nerve root and the dura sac can be developed well up into the axilla of that junction of the dura (Fig. 6). The nerve root can be gently mobilized superiorly and then be retracted without fear of significant damage, especially when the foraminotomy has been carried out so that the nerve root is free (Fig. 7). Again, any veins which are a problem can be bipolar coagulated at that time, or a small micropledget or a cutdown pledget may be placed inferiorly if there is any oozing. Hemostatic cellulose material is rarely needed, but can be placed epidural and laterally if required.

By holding the nerve root axilla superiorly, a small microblunt nerve hook may then be passed beneath the nerve root and the dura and with a 360 degree sweeping motion, removal of any herniated disc fragments that have traversed the posterior longitudinal ligament can be safely done. The various size 90 degree nerve root hooks recommended are both 2 mm and 3 mm and on very rare occasions a 4 mm. If the posterior longitudinal ligament is deformed over a disc or spur, this will be apparent at this stage of the operation and the actual pathology can be appreciated with the smaller and shorter nerve hook. To remove a disc fragment which is still beneath the ligament and/or to reduce an osteophyte in the same area, the posterior lateral aspect of the posterior and longitudinal ligament needs to be incised. This is done with a pointed no. 11 knife, while one hand carefully holds the nerve root superiorly and the dura sac slightly medially. The cut into the posterior longitudinal ligament should extend directly behind the small dissector which is holding the nerve root superiorly and slightly medially, and the cut into that posterior longitudinal liga-

Text continues on page 1198.

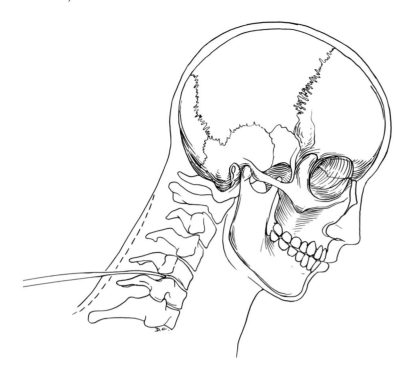

FIG. 2. In cervical hemilaminectomy for herniated disc, the incisions now are shorter. It may not be possible to identify the vertebral level with certainty. An intra-operative localizing film is necessary. Placing a probe at the laminoforaminotomy site or in the facet joint makes the level decompression identification absolutely accurate.

FIG. 3. The "keyhole" laminoforaminotomies for 3 decades have provided good exposure to the nerve root and the lateral dura. Only a very small portion of the ligamentum flavum needs to be removed. Occasionally, epidural veins posteriorly will need to be coagulated. Or tiny cotton pledgets can be placed laterally to compress the epidural veins. The dura covering the spinal cord is not retracted for this laterally extruded disc.

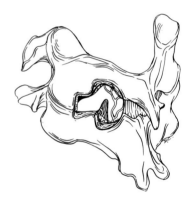

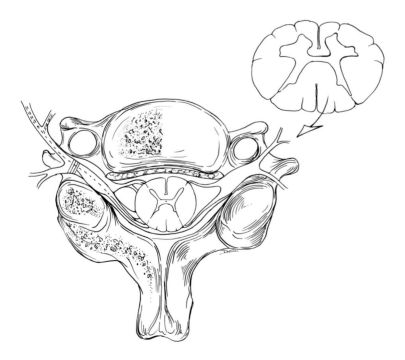

FIG. 4. The normal cross section anatomy at C5-C6 illustrates the relation of the roots to the spinal cord itself. Gentle retraction of the roots in the axilla of the dura sleeve results in very little pressure on the cord.

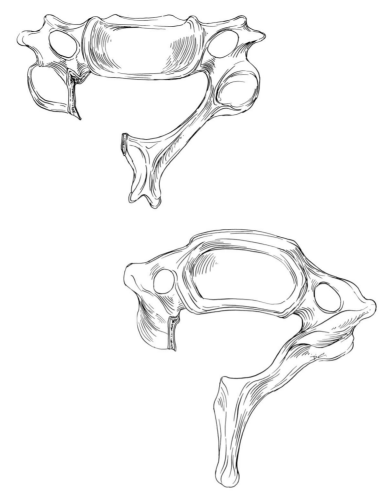

FIG. 5. In removing the bone posteriorly for radiculopathy, only one third of the facet itself needs to be removed and that will not cause any instability.

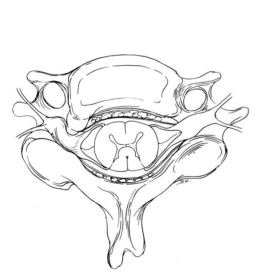

FIG. 6. Soft disc herniation in radiculopathy is lateral and beneath the nerve root. In some cases it can be pulled from beneath the nerve root and in others it remains beneath a thinned layer of posterior longitudinal ligament.

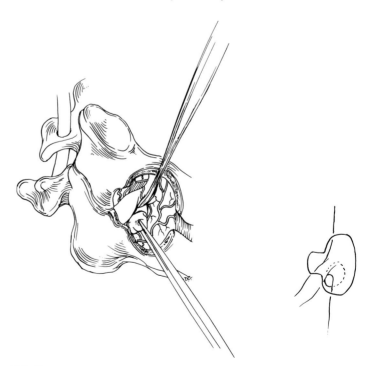

FIG. 7. In nearly all cases, the nerve root can be lifted safely. A micro nerve hook will mobilize the disc. Long, small toothed forceps can then remove a free fragment of disc.

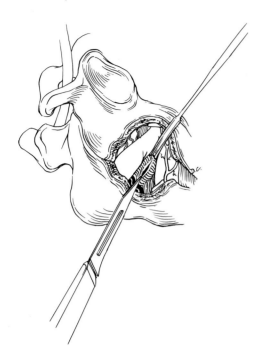

FIG. 8. In some cases the disc herniation is beneath the posterior longitudinal ligament. In those cases the ligament needs to be cut open. The incision is down and lateral—away from the cord and roots.

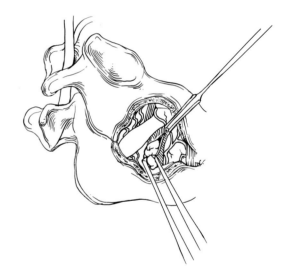

FIG. 9. Once there is an opening in the posterior longitudinal ligament, the micro nerve hook can free the herniated fragments. Then, the herniated disc can be removed with the forceps.

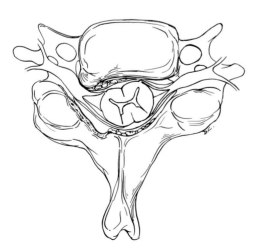

FIG. 10. Diffuse foraminal stenosis will respond to posterior decompression. In the drawing, the bone posterior to the root has been removed. In many cases, the foraminotomy is all that is required. But in some cases the osteophyte from the uncinate process distorts the nerve root.

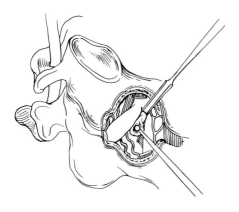

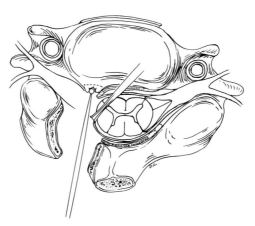

FIG. 11. When there is focal distortion of the nerve root due to osteo-phyte, removal of that bony prominence assures decompression. The posterior longitudinal ligament in front of the root needs to be bipolar coagulated and incised. Either a small reverse curette or a 2 mm diamond burr is needed to remove that bone.

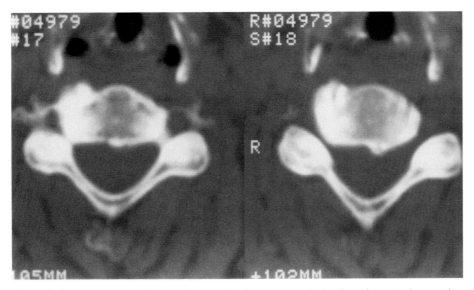

FIG. 12. A high quality plain CT often will confirm the level of diffuse foraminal stenosis. In a few cases, the stenosis will be at two levels. Posterior laminoforaminotomies are quick, safe, and effective in these cases.

ment should be made inferiorly and laterally (Fig. 8). In this fashion, the movement of the knife is always away from the spinal cord and the nerve root sleeve itself. If there is any bleeding at this time, bipolar coagulation can be utilized. If a soft disc is the diagnosis as proven by the pre-operative study (such as MRI), then the right angle small nerve hooks or dissectors can again be introduced and with a sweeping motion the herniated disc fragment will commonly present itself. Removing the disc fragment is easily done with toothed forceps (Fig. 9). Rarely are larger pituitary forceps needed. For herniated disc fragments, it is important to try to mobilize them so that they present away from the spinal cord and nerve root into the small opening made in the posterior and longitudinal ligament. By repeated sweeping motions, the sizeable disc fragments can be removed. One must remember that a large cervical disc would be very small for the lumbar area. Rarely, if ever, is a single huge disc fragment removed. In the two cases in which this was done by the author, it was regretted, for in one case it was definitely associated with a transient worsening of a patient's neurologic signs and symptoms, and in the other case, a central cord symptom developed. Fortunately, these both entirely cleared.

If on opening the posterior longitudinal ligament, the problem beneath the nerve root is an obvious osteophyte (Fig. 10), then this can easily be reduced with a small reversed angled curette, utilizing a motion which again is both inferiorly and slightly laterally coming away from the cord and root. These techniques have been available since the 1960s (Fig. 11) (17,19,46). If there is not a single bony spur or hump, then a carefully executed laminoforaminotomy with decompression posteriorly will achieve relief of the patient's symptoms. This type of bony stenosis can be identified on pre-operative CT scan and is often a reflection of facet hypertrophy more than any anterior spurring (Fig. 12). It is also in this group of patients that the clinical syndrome between two adjacent roots makes it difficult to identify a single root as the cause of the patient's symptoms. Consequently, it is in this group of patients that a level two foraminotomy is carried out to relieve the patients of the diffuse symptoms in the upper extremity which could be either a C6 or C7 root syndrome. In these cases, the pain extends down into the arm, is often worse with traction, is unrelenting, and present for a long period of time. There is some triceps weakness and the sensory loss is more diffuse, and rarely dermatomal. When the patient has this diffuse foraminal or nerve root canal stenosis due to facet disease wherein the apophyseal joint needs to be undercut some 50%, the straight posterior approach is better because 60% of the posterior aspect of that joint can be maintained in the surgical procedure. If one is removing a simple lateral disc herniation or a very focal osteophytic posterior spurring coming off aspects of the

uncovertebral joint, then the posterior lateral approach is equally good and, on occasion, superior.

Control of bleeding is often easily achieved with bipolar coagulation or temporary placement of micropaddies. If that fails, using hemostatic cellulose agents with small pledgets will achieve the hemostasis needed. Placing large pledgets is contraindicated. If one simply waits with a small pledget, the bleeding will stop. If there is a minor ooze at the end of the procedure, a small drain may be placed and can be removed in 12 to 24 hours. Post-operative hematomas for the laminotomies and the laminoforaminotomies are extremely rare.

Closure of even the simpler laminoforaminotomies needs to be carefully done. If one chooses posterolateral exposure, the incision is more muscle splitting and simply by removing the retractors, the wound almost appears to be closed on its own. Only the outer two layers of fascia need to be closed with single 0 polyglactin, a subcutaneous layer can be closed with 3-0 polyglactin, and the skin may be closed with either a small subcuticular nylon or staples. Patients prefer the former for comfort and cosmetic reasons. If one chooses to do the straight posterior exposure, then four layers of polyglactin suture are needed. The deep muscles next to the spinous processes should be closed. Then the heavy fascial layer needs to be closed in almost two layers getting the inferior aspect, and then the superior aspect with a different row of sutures. The second fascial layer includes much of the ligamentum nuchal layer, especially in the inferior aspect of the cervical area. Even the deep subcutaneous tissue should be closed with inverted polyglactin to prevent spreading of the wound. The subcutaneous layer can then be closed with 3-0 polyglactin and the skin closed with either a small subcuticular nylon, a nonlocking running nylon, or staples. All of these lead to good cosmetic results. The most important aspect of closure of posterior cervical wounds is to prevent any separation of the muscles which can lead to indentation and/or a cavitation which is quite unsightly.

What are the surgeon's responsibilities if the patient, immediately after the operative procedure, is worse neurologically, either at the root or cord level? Obviously, appreciation of this problem should be in the recovery room. It behooves the surgeon never to leave the hospital until he is quite certain that the patient's arms and legs are functioning as well as they did pre-operatively. If there is any problem, an immediate lateral cervical spine x-ray is indicated to check for alignment. After that, the patient needs a contrast diagnostic study. In the past, a full myelogram was utilized. More recently, an intrathecal enhanced CT scan with good visualization of the operative area will suffice and will rule out any retained disc fragments or hematoma.

If the myelogram and CT scan show no compression at the operative area, then the patient should be treated as if there was a vascular spinal cord injury which includes maintenance of good blood volume, adequate profusion pressure, and maintenance of normal blood pressure, as described in Chapters 51 and 59. If there is any suspicion of spinal instability, either traction or a firm cervical collar should be applied.

If there is any contrast blockage or compression documented on the CT diagnostic study such as hematoma, then the patient should be taken back to the operating room within a few hours and have a wider decompressive laminectomy, and removal of any residual pathology. The wound should be closed meticulously, and a small suction drainage catheter should be placed at the base of the wound to prevent reoccurrence of the same problem.

In the closure after a cervical laminectomy or in the closure of some complicated laminotomy, utilization of a small suction catheter at the base of the wound is recommended. If the surgery went well, but there is only a minor ooze, such catheters can be removed in 24 hours. If there is any persistent drainage, removal of such catheters after 48 hours is equally acceptable.

Post-Operative Care

The post-operative care of a patient having a laminotomy for pathology on a nerve root should include encouragement of the patient to be up and active as soon as possible including bathroom privileges the day of the operation. For comfort, a soft cervical collar can be utilized; however, the majority of patients prefer to have no collar. For the first 18 to 24 hours after the procedure, antibiotic and steroid coverage can, respectively, reduce the incidence of wound infection and reduce the incidence of nerve root swelling and pain. If steroids are used for 24 hours, it is wise to warn patients that at 48 hours after surgery they will be considerably stiffer than they were the day immediately after the operation. By 48 hours, all drains, medicines such as IV fluids, steroids, antibiotics, should be stopped and patients should be fully ambulatory so that they can be sent home then or within 72 hours. The skin closure, be it a 4.0 or 5.0 nylon suture or staples, should be removed 7 to 10 days after the procedure. The better the closure of the subcutaneous layer is, the less there will be separation of the skin itself. Patients need to be encouraged to maintain good posture in holding their head erect. I discourage neck motion in the early post-operative period because that leads to fibrosis and tearing on the deep fascial suture line. In the neck, exercises are not needed at any time to increase muscle strength, range of motion, etc. It is more important to constantly emphasize that the patient have good posture, and maintain proper curvature of the spine. I also instruct the patients not to read or study in a position where there is marked flexion of the neck.

Commonly, patients having a 1 or 2 nerve root decompression on one side are back to work within 2 to 3 weeks. Few patients are unable to work more than one month. Heavy laborers may miss 6 weeks of work, because the large muscles attaching to the scapula and the upper part of the shoulder girdle posteriorly need to be well healed before one can do extremely heavy shoveling, pulling, etc. Even those patients returning to professional contact sports have resumed all of their activities by the end of 8 weeks. Spinal instability, as previously mentioned, is such a rare problem follow-up x-rays are probably not needed.

Laminectomy for Myelopathy

A standard decompressive laminectomy in the cervical area over several segments now can be safely carried out in the majority of patients. The reported serious neurologic deterioration with such procedures is now in the range of 2% or less (8), although there are reports of a higher incidence (27,49). The problem is almost always in the patient who already has a severe neurologic myelopathy, accompanying cardiovascular disease, and not infrequently has a poor nutritional status. In that subgroup of patients, the risks are considerable, but there is really no other alternative therapy.

The exposure for cervical decompressive laminectomy has to be sufficient for one to work with good visualization. This is certainly not microscopic surgery. The skin should be marked before draping, for the midline may be elusive once all the drapes are placed. For most cervical decompressive laminectomies for spinal stenosis, the spinous process in the lamina from C3 through C7 inclusive must be removed. For this, the incision has to begin over the C2 spinous process and extend over the C7 spinous process.

Once the skin is incised, skin bleeders can be controlled using cautery. The utilization of Dandy snaps is now not common. The muscle dissection is in the midline utilizing self-retaining retractors to pull the tissues laterally to reduce the cautery dissection. If one uses self-retaining retractors, constantly moving them deeper and deeper, the amount of tissue which is cauterized or burned is kept to a minimum. Bleeders are quickly identified. Dissection can be carried out in the midline more accurately right down to the spinous processes on the back of C2 so that one can feel the bifid spines of C3, C4, and C5, and then the more straight nonbifid spines of either C6 or C7. The C6 spinous process may or may not be bifid. With good identification of the spinous processes, the muscles can be detached around the end of the spinous processes. If the bifid parts are in the way of good exposure of the lamina, they can be removed at this initial exposure. The muscles arising from the superior aspect of C2 should be kept intact if at all possible if C2 is not to be removed, because the major extensors of the neck insert here. Once the muscles are detached from the ends of the spinous process, the muscles can easily be stripped subperiosteal from the lamina. Operative exposure is aided by turning the cautery down to a lower electrical intensity when placing the retractors deeper and deeper. The retractors can then be placed well down the lateral to the C7 lamina and well lateral to the C3 and C4 lamina with retraction in between if necessary. Throughout this part of the exposure, the blood loss needs to be only 50 to 75 cc. With good visualization of all of the spinous processes, the lamina, and at least half of the facet area, the full laminectomy can begin. This is done by removing the spinous processes, and this is typically done from caudal to cephalad. After the lamina are off, one can judge the position of the hidden spinal canal more accurately.

Removing the lamina is done either with large bony rongeur forceps or with a high speed drill. If bony rongeurs are utilized, these have to be kept parallel to the spinal canal and at no time should the lip of the instrument enter into the canal. Standard Kerrison punches should not be used in the initial part of the laminectomy. The spinal canal is often compromised in these cases; we have observed diameters down to 5 mm. The tighter the stenosis, obviously, the more caution is used in removing the bone. Placing a 3 mm Kerrison punch beneath the lamina obviously can compromise the canal very severely. Any canal below 14 mm in AP central diameter increases the potential risk of damaging the cord during placement of the punch.

The basic anatomical numbers to remember at this stage of the operation are the following: (a) AP diameter of the spinal cord in the cervical area is roughly 8 mm; (b) longitudinal diameter is more, in the range of 11 to 11.5 mm; (c) around the spinal cord, there is commonly at least 1 mm of spinal fluid and an additional 1 mm of dura. Therefore, the AP diameter of the spinal canal should allow for 8 mm of spinal cord, 1 mm on either side of cerebral spinal fluid for a total of 2 mm, plus 1 mm of dura on either side for a total of 2 mm which adds up to 12 to 13 mm. Any space smaller than that has the potential of compressing and altering the dynamics, the cord, and the surrounding structures. Introducing into a stenotic canal an instrument with a footplate of 3 to 4 mm can only lead to disastrous sequelae.

If bony rongeurs are used for the majority of the lamina, this is done from inferiorly to superiorly. The inferior lip of the lamina protrudes and will provide a purchase point from which to initiate the majority of the laminectomy. By using a very small angled curette, the superior lip of the same lamina can be identified. Then the rongeur can be placed exactly perpendicular to the spinal cord so that the lips of the rongeur are biting parallel to the canal and the bone can safely be removed over the midline and partly laterally. This decompression can

be done for C7, C6, C5, C4, and even C3 (Figs. 13 and 14). But the C3 lamina will be more difficult to remove. Sometimes a thinner Lexell is required at that time.

An equally good and effective way of doing the laminectomy is to use a high speed air drill. Whether one uses a very rapid Midas Rex drill or the more standard Hall drill, is a matter of equipment and preference in the operating room. Typically, a 4 or 5 mm burr or round pineapple burr will give a wide enough trough in order to safely carry out the bony removal. The bony removal will be two parallel strips at the lamina-facet junction. With skill and time, one can feel the actual bone disappear so that there is not a risk of drilling down into the dura and other soft tissues. If there is any question, a small angled curette can often break through the small filament of bone that is left behind. This trough can extend over all of the lamina which are to be removed. Then the entire lamina structure, including the ligamentum flavum, can be lifted from interior to superior and cut away and removed as a whole unit.

If Kerrison punches are to be used, it is only at the end of the procedure. At that time, the lateral aspect of the canal can be further opened laterally with angled punches of 1, 1.5, and even 2 mm (Fig. 13). At the same time, if a particular root is clinically involved, the foraminotomy can be done with this exposure. If one needs to take out a particular osteophyte, the same foraminotomy which was described earlier for a root decompression can be added to the laminectomy.

The need to remove C2 is rare, but there are certainly some cases where it is needed. Those patients who have severe long standing congenital stenosis complicated by superimposed cervical osteoarthritic spondylytic stenosis are the most likely candidates for C2 removal. The principles of removing that spinous process and the lamina are exactly the same as for other lower levels. Even more rare is the need to remove the ring of C1 with the exception of complex congenital stenosis such as seen in achondroplastic dwarfs.

The dura need not be opened for the majority of decompressions for cervical spondylytic stenosis with myelopathy (Fig. 14). The data indicates that opening the dura even with grafts does not substantially improve the final results of the decompressive procedure (11,52,66). Adding dentate sectioning to the procedure with or without dura grafts also does not necessarily improve the results (26,28,29,50,51,66). Therefore, opening the dura and sectioning the dentate ligaments is rarely if ever done for cervical spondylytic stenosis with myelopathy. If the laminectomy is properly carried out and the entire dura sac balloons back into the decompressive area, then the dentate attachments themselves migrate posteriorly and the entire spinal cord is away from the anterior osteophytes. Only in those patients who have a significant kyphosis of the cervical spine, with significant ridging, will the spinal cord still ride next to the diseased bone. It

A

B

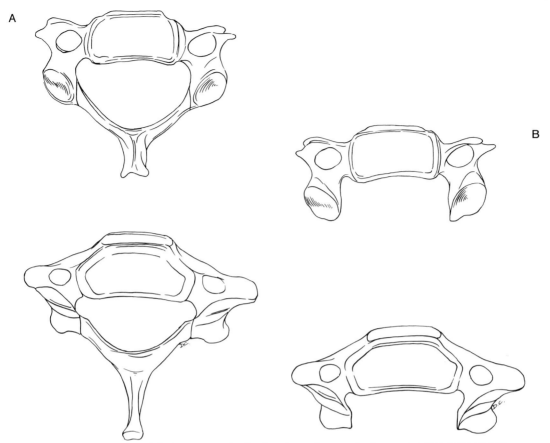

FIG. 13. A and B: A full decompressive laminectomy for acquired or congenital stenosis can be done from C3 to C7 inclusive without significant damage to the apophyseal facet joints. But the anatomy does differ slightly with each level.

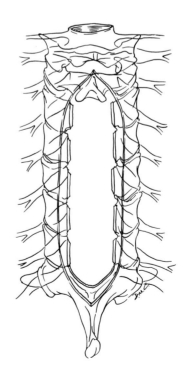

FIG. 14. Full laminectomies are done without placing any instruments beneath the lamina itself. Only after the vast majority of the decompression is accomplished can the smaller Kerrison be used next to the lateral mass and apophyseal facet joint. In spondylytic stenosis, the dura need not be opened.

is in these patients that the results of the decompressive laminectomy are not favorable (4,38) and the importance of appreciating this particular problem is the subject of Chapter 58. These complex cervical myelopathies are a special group to themselves and require special treatment which may include not only laminectomies, but anterior decompressions as well and even staged procedures.

As pointed out by Epstein, some bony spurs and osteophytes need to be excised in selected patients. By carrying out that procedure, the number of patients who improve may exceed the usual reported 70% success rate and climb to over 80% (16,18,42). Removing the osteophytes is identical to that described in the laminotomies for radiculopathies. Working in the axilla of the nerve root and at the level involved, reversed angled curettes and a high speed drill with a burr of 2 mm can often take down the offending bone without further compromising the stability of the spine and/or the spinal cord. Admittedly, if anterior osteophyte removal is a major part of the planned operative care, then placing the patient in a sitting position is easier on the surgeon in order to prevent venous engorgement and pooling of blood in the area of the pathology. If the osteophytes are huge ridges completely across the spinal axis, then their removal is not as important as a well executed laminectomy.

Bleeding, for the most part, with decompressive laminectomies can be successfully handled with bipolar coagulation. Unipolar coagulation is not to be utilized near the dura. Gentle retraction and bipolar coagulation can often stop any epidural veins. Very small pledgets of oxidized cellulose or microfibulary collagen, held in place with very small paddies, usually will stop all of the bleeding. The newer microfibulary collagen (Avitene) is very effective even though it is more expensive. If there is a small continuous ooze from the epidural space, bone, or even muscle, then use of suction drainage post-operatively with the various devices now available on the market is wise.

Closure of these wounds is identical with that described for laminoforaminotomies.

The post-operative medicines are similar to those used in foraminotomies. As noted, prophylactic antibiotics for 24 to 48 hours will reduce the incidence of wound infection from 1% and 2% (64) to less than 1%.

Pain medications for these patients should include narcotics at fairly low doses given very often. Giving the patient medicine every 2 to 3 hours at a low dose is more effective than giving a large dose with a longer interval of time between doses. In addition, the new patient control devices for IV narcotics for the first 24 to 48 hours are equally effective. Their pain medication may include an injection at night time, while they are on the oral synthetic codeine combination drugs with Tylenol by the second night of their surgical procedure. Bracing and collars are only rarely utilized. However, if a fusion is

required with the laminectomy, obviously, the patient will have to be immobilized. Finally, when patients are out of the recovery area, placing them in a slight jack-knife position with the head of the bed up some 20° will promote venous drainage from the operative area and may minimize some of the swelling. For those patients who do not have a significant myelopathy and who do not require canes or crutches for ambulation, discharge on the fourth or fifth day is common. In those patients with a marked gait disturbance, up to a week of hospitalization is required. Many of these patients also require physical therapy in order to improve their strength and ambulation. Those patients who have severe neurologic deficit, with a very spastic myelopathy, may require transfer to a rehabilitation center.

Central Soft Disc Herniation

Soft central disc herniations should not be removed posteriorly. Now that we have modern CT scans and MRIs, these problems can be identified prior to operative intervention. In the past, before diagnostic studies could completely outline the pathology, the disc was mobilized and removed. In two-thirds of such cases, the patients had a satisfactory outcome; however, removing a soft disc posteriorly when it is placed central and anterior can be associated with a transient neurologic deterioration (27). Now that surgical procedures have been developed for removing soft discs anteriorly with a cervical discectomy, decompression, and fusion, it is the recommended surgical approach (10,42,61,69). This is true even if it means closing a patient posteriorly, turning him over, and proceeding with the anterior decompression, when a soft central disc is identified during posterior decompression.

Laminoplasty

Laminoplasty has been found to be of benefit in those patients with ossification of the posterior and longitudinal ligaments (OPLL) (Fig. 15) (3). It is our Japanese colleagues who have championed this procedure (34,35,37,38,47,48,51,65). In the Japanese Public Health study (37), longitudinal and transverse growth of OPLL in asymptomatic patients was found to be 24% and 11% respectively over 5 years. This means that nearly one-quarter of the patients in a 5 year period by the natural history of the disease have longitudinal extension of the OPLL. Once a laminectomy is done, this longitudinal extension may increase to 85% to 90% of patients (35). If laminectomy is converted back to a laminoplasty so that there are some posterior elements, this extension is reduced to 34%. If one achieves a solid spinal fusion anteriorly, it is further reduced to 20%, or approximately equal to the natural history of the disease

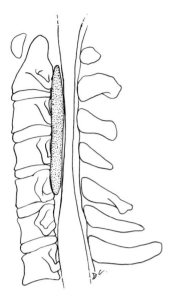

FIG. 15. In many cases of OPLL, the pathology is as high as C2 and, therefore, the decompression needs to include even C1.

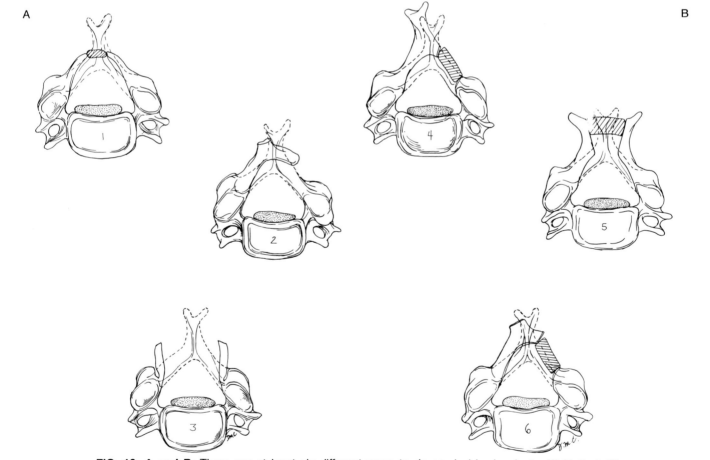

FIG. 16. A and B: There are at least six different ways to do cervical laminoplasty: (1) Hattori, (2) Hirabayashi, (3) Iwaski, (4) Itoh and Matsuzaki, (5) Kurokawa, and (6) Ducker. Hirabayashi's review (ref. 35) provides the data for this operation, which occurs considerably more often in Japan.

if left untreated. It is this kind of data that has led to the laminoplasty, especially in the patient who is young and has OPLL.

There are five common ways to carry out laminoplasty (Fig. 16) (35). Two of the five techniques require bone grafts. Currently, it is difficult to say which is the most effective technique. My own experience is limited, but I have found the open door hemi-lateral technique utilizing a bone graft to be effective (Fig. 16). In about one-half of these cases, the spinous process itself has been utilized as the bone graft to fill in the lamina on the side where the opening is achieved. In other cases, the graft has been taken from the ilium. Bank bone can also be safely used.

To carry out a laminoplasty, a high speed drill is essential. The basic exposure is the same as the laminectomy with a fusion. With good visualization of the lamina and spinous process, the spinous process is cut away with one bone cut so that it can be used as a bone graft. Then the high speed drill is used to thin the bone down to a single cortical layer posterolateral to the spinal cord on both sides. On the side to be opened, a very small angled curette can be used to crack through the remaining thin bone. The bone can then be opened gently. A small hole can be made into the lamina with the 1 mm drill. Then, 2.0 nylon suture can be passed through the hole and to the graft affixing the graft to the lateral aspect of inner-facet area (Fig. 16F). We do not use wire for bone fixation in those cases. The grafts are commonly incorporated quickly. The closure of the wound is slightly different than the standard laminectomy. The muscles next to the laminoplasty are not closed. Instead of the four-layer closure, a three-layer on the fascia is all that is required. The placement of a small suction drainage should be on the bony side away from the graft.

The results in stopping the progression of myelopathy in OPLL are not as good as the improved success rate after treating degenerative cervical spondylytic stenotic myelopathy. Instead of 70% of the patients being improved, the good results are in the range of 60% (34,36,37). Practically speaking, half of the patients should remain improved over an extended period. Older patients, patients with superimposed trauma, and patients who have a kyphotic spinal curvature do poorly. Unfortunately, there are no other alternatives in treatment that offer better results. The anterior procedure has major limitations in this disease.

Posterior Cervical Fusion for Degenerative Disease

Posterior spinal fusion for those patients who have recurrent osteophytes and/or a failed anterior cervical discectomy and fusion with continued pain and deformity is an appropriate operative procedure. If a radiculopathy is the major symptom, then the standard laminoforaminotomy as previously described is chosen.

Failed Anterior Cervical Fusion

Between 4% and 12% of anterior cervical fusions will progress to a non-union. Approximately half of these patients remain symptomatic with neck and arm pain. With myelopathy and continued canal compromise, repeat anterior decompression and fusion can be successful. This requires a partial or hemi-corpectomy above and below the disc space to safely remove the posterior osteophyte ridge. A tall tri-cortical bone graft can then be used (70).

In a non-union of an anterior cervical fusion where neck and arm pain or neck pain alone persists, we prefer a posterior approach. As previously described, a keyhole foraminotomy is performed for decompression of the symptomatic nerve root. This is followed by a posterior interspinous process wiring and bone grafting at the non-union level. With a solid posterior fusion the anterior non-union often will also consolidate (24).

REFERENCES

1. Aboulker J, Metzger J, David M, Engel P, Ballivet J (1965): Les myelopathies cervicales d'origine rachidienne. *Neurochirurgie* 11:87.
2. Allen KL (1968): Cervical spondylosis with accompanying myelopathy: Its alleviation by removal of the bony spur. *S Afr J Surg* 6:5.
3. Bakay L, Cares HL, Smith RJ (1970): Ossification in the region of the posterior longitudinal ligament as a cause of cervical myelopathy. *J Neurol Neurosurg Psychiatr* 33:263.
4. Batzdorf U, Batzdorff A (1988): Analysis of cervical spine curvature in patients with cervical spondylosis. *Neurosurg* 5:827–836.
5. Bradshaw P (1957): Some aspects of cervical spondylosis. *Q J Med* 26:177.
6. Brain WR, Wilkinson JL (1967): *Cervical spondylosis and other disorders of the spine.* Philadelphia: W.B. Saunders.
7. Braughler JM, Hall ED (1985): Current application of "high-dose" steroid therapy for CNS injury. *J Neurosurg* 62:806–810.
8. Carol MP, Ducker TB (1988): Cervical spondylytic myelopathies: surgical treatment. *J Spinal Disorders* 1:59–65.
9. Cassidy J, Ducker TB (1990): Clinical correlations of intraoperative evoked potential monitoring in spinal cord disorders. In: *Spinal cord monitoring and electrodiagnosis.* Heidelberg: Springer Verlag.
10. Cloward RB (1952): Treatment of ruptured intervertebral discs: observations on their formation and treatment. *Am J Surg* 84:151.
11. Crandall PH, Barzdorf I (1966): Cervical spondylotic myelopathy. *J Neurosurg* 25:57.
12. Dempsey R, Rapp RP, Young B, et al (1988): Prophylactic parenteral antibiotics in clean neurosurgical procedures: a review. *J Neurosurg* 69:52–57.
13. Dietemann JL, Dirheimer Y, et al (1985): Ossification of the posterior longitudinal ligament (Japanese disease): a radiological study in 12 cases. *J Neuroradiol* 12:212.
14. Ducker TB, Brown RH (1988): *Neurophysiology and standards of spinal cord monitoring.* New York: Springer Verlag.
15. Ducker TB, Hamit HF (1969): Experimental treatments of acute spinal cord injury. *J Neurosurg* 6:693–697.
16. Epstein JE, Carras R, Lavine LS, Epstein BS (1969): The importance of removing osteophytes as part of the surgical treatment of myeloradiculopathy in cervical spondylosis. *J Neurosurg* 30:219.
17. Epstein JA, Epstein NE (1989): The surgical management of cervical spinal stenosis, spondylosis, and myeloradiculopathy by means of the posterior approach. In: Sherk HH, et al., eds. *The cervical spine, 2nd ed.* Philadelphia: JB Lippincott Company, pp. 625–643.
18. Epstein JA, Epstein BS, Lavine LS (1963): Cervical spondylotic myelopathy: the syndrome of the narrowed canal treated by lami-

nectomy, foraminotomy, and the removal of osteophytes. *Arch Neurol* 8:307.

19. Epstein JA, Epstein BS, Lavine LS, et al. (1978): Clinical monoradiculopathy caused by arthrotic hypertrophy. *J Neurosurg* 49:387.

20. Epstein JA, Janin Y, Carras R, Lavine LS (1982): A comparative study of the treatment of cervical spondylotic myeloradiculopathy: experience with 50 cases treated by means of extensive laminectomy, foraminotomy and excision of osteophytes during the past 10 years. *Acta Neurochir (Wein)* 61:89–104.

21. Epstein JA, Lavine LS, Aronson HA, et al (1965): Cervical spondylotic radiculopathy. *Clin Orthop* 40:113–122.

22. Fager CA (1976): Management of cervical disc lesions and spondylosis by posterior approaches. *Clin Neurosurg* 24:488.

23. Fager CAL (1973): Results of adequate posterior decompression in the relief of spondylotic cervical myelopathy. *J Neurosurg* 38:684.

24. Farey I, McAfee P (in press): Posterior foraminotomies: Stabilization and fusion for failed anterior cervical fusions.

25. Firooznia H, Rafii M, et al (1984): Computed tomography of calcification and ossification of posterior longitudinal ligament of the spine. *J Comput Assist Tomogr* 8:317.

26. Gorter K (1976): Influence of laminectomy on the course of cervical myelopathy. *Acta Neurochir (Wein)* 33:265.

27. Gregorius FK, Estrin T, Crandall PR (1976): Cervical spondylotic radiculopathy and myelopathy. A long term follow-up study. *Arch Neurol* 33:618–625.

28. Guidetti B, Fortuna A (1969): Long term results of surgical treatment of myelopathy due to cervical spondylosis. *J Neurosurg* 30:714–721.

29. Haft H, Shenkin HA (1963): Surgical end results of cervical ridge and disc problems. *JAMA* 186:312.

30. Haines SF (1980): Systemic antibiotic prophylaxis in neurological surgery. *Neurosurg* 6:355–361.

31. Haines SJ (1985): Prophylactic antibiotics. In: Wilkins RH, Rengachary SS, eds. *Neurosurgery* vol. 1. New York: McGraw-Hill, pp. 448–452.

32. Hall ED, Wolf MS, Braughler MJ (1984): Effects of a single large dose of methylprednisolone sodium succinate on experimental post-traumatic spinal cord ischemia. *J Neurosurg* 61:124–130.

33. Henderson CA (1983): Posterolateral foraminotomy as exclusive operative technique for cervical radiculopathy: a review of 846 consecutively operated cases. *Neurosurg* 13:504–512.

34. Hirabayashi K, Miyakawa J, Satomi K, et al (1981): Operative results and postoperative progression of ossification among patients with cervical posterior longitudinal ligament. *Spine* 6:354–364.

35. Hirabayashi K, Satomi K, Sasaki T (1989): Ossification of the posterior longitudinal ligament in the cervical spine. In: Sherk HH, et al., eds. *The cervical spine, 2nd ed.* Philadelphia: JB Lippincott Company, pp. 678–691.

36. Hirabayashi K, Watanabe K, Wakano K, et al (1983): Expansive open-door laminoplasty for cervical spinal stenotic myelopathy. *Spine* 8:693.

37. Japanese Ministry of Public Health and Welfare (1981–1985): Investigation committee reports on OPLL. Tokyo.

38. Kojima T, et al. (1989): Anterior cervical vertebrectomy and interbody fusion for multi-level spondylosis and ossification of the posterior longitudinal ligament. *Neurosurg* 6:864–872.

39. Lees F, Aldren Turner JS (1963): Natural history and prognosis of cervical spondylosis. *Br Med J* [Clin Res] 2:1607–1610.

40. Malis LI (1979): Prevention of neurosurgical infection by intraoperative antibiotics. *Neurosurg* 5:339–343.

41. Matjasko J, Petrozza P, Cohen M, Steinberg P (1985): Anesthesia and surgery in the seated position: Analysis of 554 cases. *Neurosurg* 17:695.

42. Mayfield FH (1965): Cervical spondylosis: A comparison of the anterior and posterior approaches. *Clin Neurosurg* 13:181.

43. McPherson RW, Ducker TB (1988): Augmentation of somatosensory evoked potential waves in patients with cervical spinal stenosis. In: Ducker TB, Brown RH, eds. *Neurophysiology and standards of spinal cord monitoring.* New York: Springer-Verlag, pp. 168–176.

44. Miller C, Hunt W (1985): Neurosurgical correlation in acute cervical monoradicular syndrome: treatment by muscle splitting approach. *J Neurosurg.*

45. Mollman HD, Haines SJ (1986): Risk factors for postoperative neurosurgical wound infection. A case-control study. *J Neurosurg* 64:902–906.

46. Murphey F, Simmons J (1966): Ruptured cervical discs. *Am J Surg* 32:83–88.

47. Nagashima C (1972): Cervical myelopathy due to ossification of the posterior longitudinal ligament. *J Neurosurg* 37:653–660.

48. Nakanishi T, Mannen T, Toyokura Y, et al (1974): Symptomatic ossification of the cervical spine. *Neurology* 24:1139–1140.

49. Nurick S (1972): The natural history and the results of surgical treatment of the spinal cord disorder associated with cervical spondylosis. *Brain* 9S:101.

50. Odom GL, Finney W, Woodhall B (1958): Cervical disk lesions. *JAMA* 166:23–28.

51. Ono K, Ota H, Tada K, Yamamoto T (1977): Cervical myelopathy secondary to multiple spondylotic protrusions. *Spine* 2:218.

52. Piepgras DG (1977): Posterior decompression for myelopathy due to cervical spondylosis: laminectomy alone vs laminectomy with dentate ligament section. *Clin Neurosurg* 24:508–515.

53. Raynor RB (1983): Anterior or posterior approach to the cervical spine: An anatomical and radiographic evaluation and comparison. *Neurosurg* 12:7.

54. Raynor RB, Pugh J, Shapiro I (1985): Cervical facetectomy and its effect on spine strength. *J Neurosurg* 63:278–282.

55. Roberts AH (1966): Myelopathy due to cervical spondylosis treated by collar immobilization. *Neurology* 16:951–954.

56. Savitz MH, Katz SS (1981): Rationale for prophylactic antibiotics in neurosurgery. *Neurosurg* 9:142–144.

57. Savitz MH, Katz SS (1986): Prevention of primary wound infection in neurosurgical patients: A 10-year study. *Neurosurg* 18:685–688.

58. Scoville WB (1961): Cervical spondylosis treated by bilateral facetectomy and laminectomy. *J Neurosurg* 18:423–428.

59. Scoville WB, Whitcomb BB, McLaurin RL (1951): The cervical ruptured disc: report of 115 operative cases. *Trans Am Neurol Assoc* 76:222–224.

60. Shapiro M, Wald U, Simchen E, et al. (1986): Randomized clinical trial of intra-operative antimicrobial prophylaxis of infection after neurosurgical procedures. *J Hosp Infect* 8:283–295.

61. Smith GW, Robinson RA (1955): Anterior lateral cervical disc removal and interbody fusion for cervical disc syndrome. *Bull Johns Hopkins Hosp* 96:223.

62. Spurling RG, Scoville WB (1955): Lateral rupture of the cervical intervertebral discs: a common cause of shoulder and arm pain. *Surg Gynecol Obstet* 78:350.

63. Spurling RB, Segerberg LH (1953): Lateral intervertebral disc lesions in the lower cervical region. *JAMA* 151:354.

64. Tenney JH, Valahov D, Salcman M, Ducker TB (1985): Wide variation in risk of wound infection following clean neurosurgery: implications for perioperative antibiotic prophylaxis. *J Neurosurg* 62:243–247.

65. Tsuji H (1982): Laminoplasty for patients with compressive myelopathy due to so-called spinal canal stenosis in cervical and thoracic regions. *Spine* 7:28–34.

66. Thomalski G, Wilk von K, Lammert E (1972): Zur chirurgischen behandlung der cervicales myelopathie. *Nervenarzt* 43:520–524.

67. Veidlinger OF, Coleill JC, Smyth HS, Turner D (1981): Cervical myelopathy and its relationship to cervical stenosis. *Spine* 6:550–552.

68. Verbiest H (1973): The management of cervical spondylosis. *Clin Neurosurg* 20:262.

69. Verbiest H, Paz Y, Geuse HD (1966): Anterolateral surgery for cervical spondylosis in cases of myelopathy or nerve root compression. *J Neurosurg* 25:611.

70. Zdeblick T, Bohlman HH (in press): *Failed anterior cervical discectomy.*

71. Zdeblick T, Zou D, Warden KE (in press): Cervical stability following foraminotomy: A biomechanical in-vitro analysis.

The Adult Spine: Principles and Practice,
J. W. Frymoyer, Editor-in-Chief.
Raven Press, Ltd., New York © 1991.

CHAPTER 58

Complex Cervical Myelopathies

Ulrich Batzdorf

Cervical spondylotic myelopathy is defined as a neurologic disorder generally manifested in its severe (complex) form by a spastic gait, sometimes spastic hands with atrophy and sensory impairment, sphincter disturbances, and related underlying spondylosis of the cervical spine. These symptoms may exist in every different combination and proportion. Although there is often some degree of associated neck stiffness, severe neck pain is not usually part of the syndrome.

PATHOPHYSIOLOGY

Two major schools of thought exist with respect to the basic mechanisms responsible for the myelopathic clinical features and the often profound changes seen in autopsy specimens of the cervical cord.

Mechanical

The classical concept is that spondylotic myelopathy is the result of spinal cord *compression,* focal or extend-

ing over several segments, with osteophytes or a combination of osteophytes and degenerated disc constituting the compressive material (15). The varying mechanisms by which osteophyte growth or disc degeneration might be produced are discussed below in the section on etiologies. Even this very elementary concept must, however, be qualified. While it is inherent in the postulated mechanism that the osteophyte or degenerated disc is hard, it is also known that the spinal cord can tolerate quite extensive compression by osteophyte or disc, as judged by magnetic resonance (MR) scans for example, without any clinical manifestations of myelopathy (24).

The development of significant myelopathy seems to depend on the interaction of three factors: (a) degree of cord compression; (b) the period of time (i.e., rate) over which these compressive changes have taken place; and (c) the constancy or intermittency of the compressive force. Thus, the spinal cord notoriously will tolerate extensive compression if the narrowing of the canal develops very slowly, that is, over a period of many years. Relatively constant compression also seems to be better tolerated by the spinal cord than frequent repetitive compressive forces, such as might be seen in the patient with a hypermobile spine segment. Intermittent subluxation at a motion segment, or several adjacent motion

U. Batzdorf, M.D.: Professor of Surgery/Neurosurgery, University of California, Los Angeles, School of Medicine, Los Angeles, California 90024.

segments, as is sometimes seen, seems to resemble repeated episodes of sub-acute trauma rather than chronic compression. However, as discussed below, once the spinal cord is compressed, though asymptomatically, it sometimes takes very little additional compression (such as might result from a seemingly trivial fall) to produce sudden and severe neurologic deterioration. Changes in viscoelastic properties of the degenerated cord may also play a role (21).

Vascular

A vascular mechanism for the development of spinal cord changes and the associated myelopathic symptoms and signs has been postulated for many years (23). The close resemblance of the clinical syndrome of anterior spinal artery occlusion to that seen in many patients with severe cervical myelopathy led to the belief that the rough anterior osteophytes rub against the spinal cord and produce focal areas of ischemia or hypoperfusion. Some have also shown that fibrosis of the root sleeve due to foraminal compression can involve the delicate accompanying radicular vessels which contribute to spinal cord perfusion.

The strongest argument against the vascular theory has always been the slow clinical progression in most instances of myelopathy due to spondylosis, whereas a vascular occlusive mechanism would be expected to present more abruptly.

Combination of Mechanical and Vascular

The possibility that mechanical and vascular factors may work in combination to produce myelopathic changes must be considered. A compressed cord will tolerate diminished perfusion poorly; a marginally vascularized cord will tolerate compression equally poorly. One must further consider the added injury to the cord which might come about from temporarily reduced perfusion on a systemic basis, similar to that postulated in the secondary insult concept considered responsible for some of the more severe effects of a head injury (4).

ETIOLOGIES

A number of different etiologies of cervical myelopathy must be considered. All may cause cord injury by either compression, vascular changes, or a combination thereof, as discussed above and in Chapters 56 and 57.

Acute Disc Herniation

A significant disc herniation, particularly if central, can result in acute myelopathy.

Spondylosis

Typically, spondylosis consists of protrusion of the annulus fibrosus due to intrinsic degenerative changes of the intervertebral disc, which involve loss of water and changes in collagen, resulting in loss of disc height with some spreading effect, i.e., increase in disc diameter. Not infrequently, this process occurs at several levels simultaneously.

While normal aging processes result in these changes in many patients, chronic repetitive disc trauma such as produced by certain occupations (for example, hod carriers) or even a single episode of severe disc injury, can accelerate these degenerative changes. Ligamentous changes following a spine injury conceivably could also favor the late development of disc and intervertebral joint degeneration.

A sequence of related changes may follow degenerative disc pathology (7):

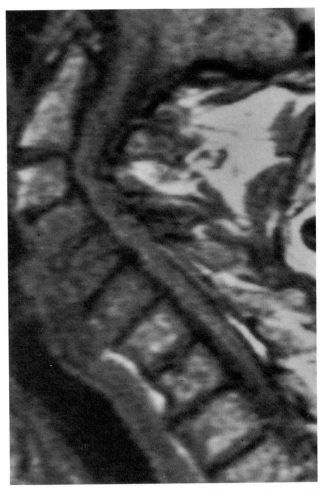

FIG. 1. Magnetic resonance scan of a 79-year-old man with hyperlordotic deformity resulting in cord compression at the C3 and C4 levels. Patient was treated with a C1 to C5 laminectomy.

1. bony overgrowth at the annulus margin to form an osteophytic ridge;
2. facet joint stress leading to joint narrowing, cartilage degeneration, and osteoarthritic spurs originating from the joint margin;
3. hypermobility of the spine or segments thereof, including subluxation of vertebrae with secondary stretching of the supporting ligaments of the spine (6,8);
4. loss of disc height leading to telescoping of the cervical spine with shingling of cervical vertebrae and con-

traction of the ligamentum flavum which, in its contracted state, is thicker;
5. spontaneous fusion due to bridging osteophytes.

Loss in Height of Vertebrae and Postural Changes

Vertebral compression may occur as an aftermath to the vertical component of spine trauma, or as a consequence of osteoporosis, or from other less clearly understood mechanisms such as impairment of bone vascularity.

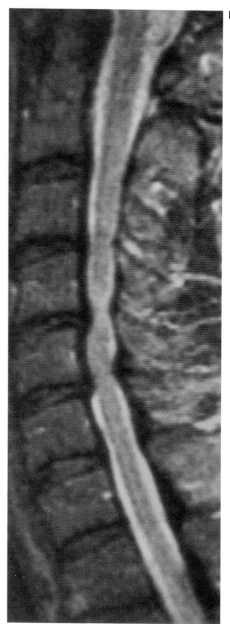

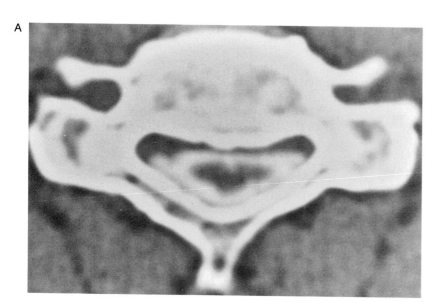

FIG. 2. Computed tomographic scan of the cervical spine in a 58-year-old patient following intrathecal injection of Omnipaque. **A:** The spinal canal is very narrow in the anterior-posterior dimension due to unusually short pedicles. **B:** Multiple levels of cord compression are evident in the sagittal scan of the same patient. Even small disc protrusions or osteophytes like these can cause myelopathy in a patient with a congenitally narrow canal; treated by laminectomy.

When these forces are applied in an uneven manner, they will result in a change in the shape of the vertebral body. Most commonly this is in the form of wedging, the result of the anterior vertebral body being compressed more than the posterior margin. This may then result in an alteration of the curvature of the spine from its lordotic curve. Secondary ligamentous stretching may then occur and ultimately a combination of soft tissue, bony, and cartilaginous changes may make the deformity irreversible.

Postural changes of the cervical spine probably can also result from primary ligamentous problems, i.e., ligamentous weakness or stretching, such as might occur following a flexion injury (8). Finally, severe kyphotic deformities of the upper thoracic spine, such as are sometimes seen in the elderly, may generate a compensatory lordotic deformity of the cervical area as a result of the patient's need to look forward (Fig. 1).

Degenerative Changes Superimposed on Previous Acute Trauma

As noted above, the normal processes of aging of the intervertebral disc may be given a premature start or accelerated by the internal disruption of a disc following an acute injury.

Degenerative Changes Superimposed on Congenital Abnormalities of the Cervical Spine

Three categories are important. They are (a) the congenitally narrow spinal canal (Fig. 2); (b) Klippel-Feil deformities; and (c) cranio-cervical junction abnormalities. These entities are discussed in Chapters 48, 49, 56, and 57. While Klippel-Feil and cranio-cervical junction abnormalities tend to be immediately recognizable on plain radiographs, the congenitally narrow canal may be less obvious. Complete overlapping of the facet joints on the laminae in a lateral cervical radiograph is strongly suggestive of a congenitally narrow canal. A thin-slice CT scan in the axial projection would provide the best confirmation of short pedicles.

The significance of a congenitally narrow canal in the context of cervical myelopathy is that a relatively small osteophyte or disc protrusion can result in spinal cord compression and myelopathy when the "tolerance" for the cord is marginal at the outset. This is exemplified to the extreme in achondroplastics.

Klippel-Feil deformities, characterized by block vertebrae, may show evidence of accelerated degenerative change at the first mobile segment above and below the block vertebra; presumably motion, which is normally distributed over many segments, is greater at the remaining mobile segment when a block vertebra is present. Cranio-cervical junction abnormalities can cause my-

elopathy by a number of different mechanisms, including displacement of the cord by a non-united odontoid, basilar invagination, and congenital anomalies of the atlanto-axial joint (16).

Idiopathic Ossification of the Posterior Longitudinal Ligament

The etiology of this condition is poorly understood. Calcified thickening of the posterior longitudinal ligament may be focal or spread over several spinal segments. Incorporation of the dura into the calcified or ossified ligament has been described and obviously creates management problems.

CLINICAL DIAGNOSIS

Symptoms

In a comprehensive analysis (9), gait abnormalities, together with lower extremity weakness, sensory symptoms, and sphincter disturbances were noted in over 60% of patients with cervical myelopathy (Table 1). Signs on examination (Table 2) reflected a similar pattern, with upper and lower extremity spasticity and lower extremity weakness being most common. Upper extremity weakness was almost as common, with atrophy present in the proximal or distal portion of the limb in many patients.

Differential Diagnosis

The differential diagnosis should include a consideration of vascular malformations of the cord, syringomyelia, and cord tumors. These conditions should be readily differentiated by magnetic resonance imaging. More difficult might be the differential diagnosis of amyotrophic lateral sclerosis, particularly in the elderly patient who also has some spondylotic changes of the cervical spine. The major point in the differential diagnosis of this condition, as well as multiple sclerosis, is the presence of findings, clinical or by imaging, above the spinal level. Sub-acute combined degeneration and even early stages of extrapyramidal disorder may mimic cervical spondylotic myelopathy.

Confirmatory Tests

The diagnosis of cervical spondylotic myelopathy is today often made by an initial magnetic resonance scan, the appeal of this study being its non-invasive nature, its capacity to generate both sagittal and axial images, and the ability to exclude almost immediately several other conditions such as syringomyelia. This diagnostic tech-

TABLE 1. *Symptoms at admission in radiculopathy and myelopathy groups, including all symptoms in all patients*

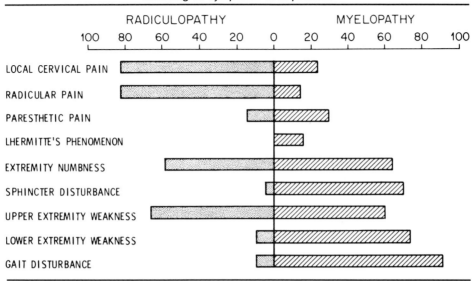

With permission from ref. 9.

nique does, however, have some limitations quite aside from those relating to the technical features of the particular scanner. MR scans are, for the most part, static and do not reflect abnormalities that may be seen in positions of flexion or extension, but occasionally such studies can be requested. Gliosis due to chronic cord compression is sometimes recognizable on MR scans and may correlate with a fixed myelopathic picture (22). Actual cord compression is best recognized in the sagittal MR image. MR scans are, however, not ideal for visualization of bony abnormalities, and such features as congenital narrowing of the canal may not be immediately

apparent. For this reason, it is best to obtain plain films of the cervical spine, as well as flexion and extension views (19). The latter are particularly helpful in assessing abnormal motion of the cervical spine.

Computed tomography (CT) scans, especially when obtained in conjunction with a myelogram using water soluble contrast material, provide an excellent means of assessing the patient with spondylotic myelopathy. CT scans show bony abnormalities very clearly, and with contrast will demonstrate deformation or compression of the cord, especially on axial views. The same limitations of a static examination do, however, apply. When

TABLE 2. *Physical findings at admission in radiculopathy and myelopathy groups, including all signs in all patients*

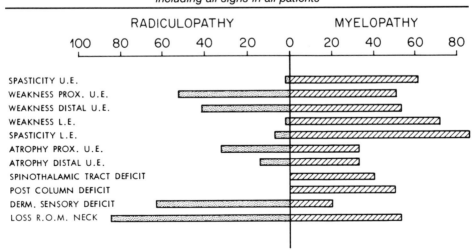

With permission from ref. 9.
UE: upper extremity; PROX: proximal part; LE: lower extremity; DERM: dermatoma; ROM: range of motion.

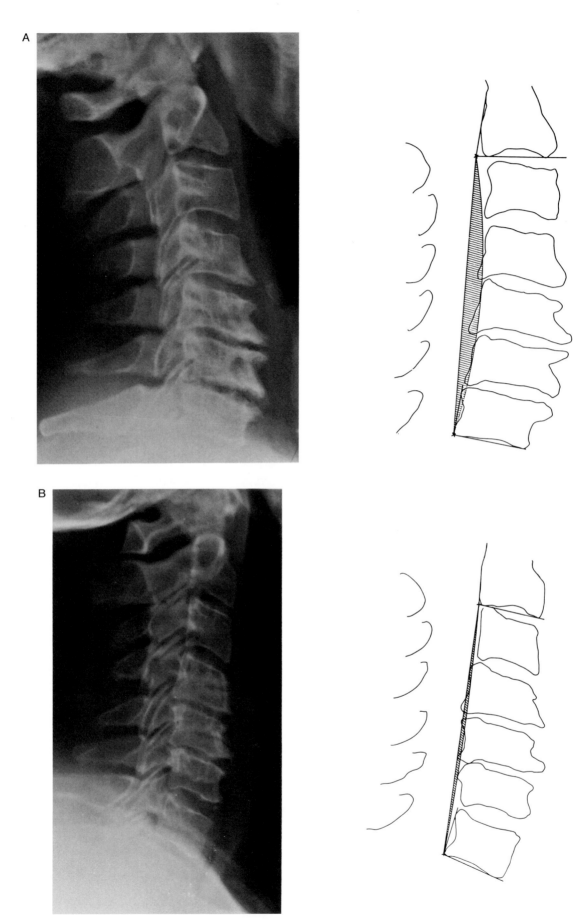

FIG. 3. Spondylosis may give rise to varying deformities of the spine, often in conjunction with narrowing of the spinal canal. **A:** Normal cervical curvature. **B:** Straightened cervical spine.

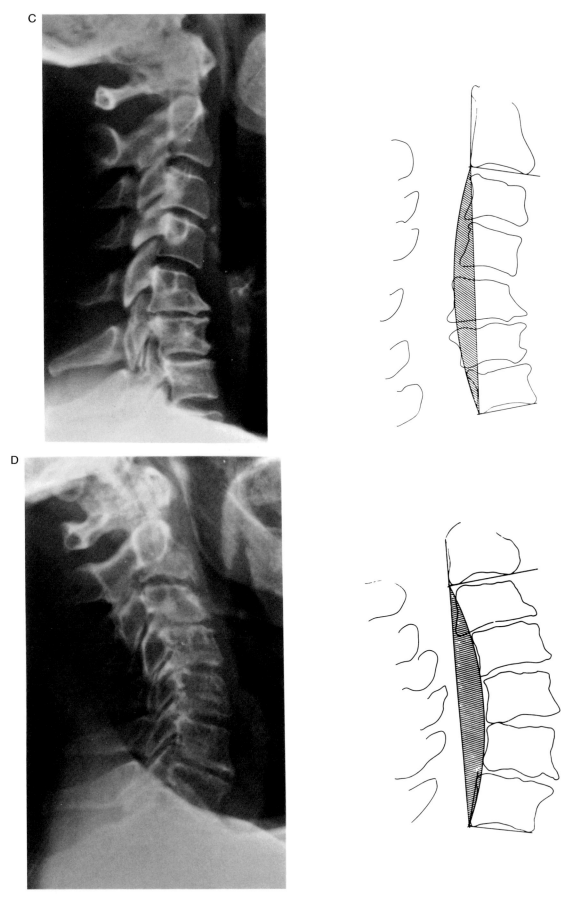

FIG. 3 *Continued.* **C:** Kyphotic spine. **D:** Hyperlordotic spine. The shaded area represents the area under the arc, constructed from C2 to C7, and quantifies the degree of deformity (with permission from ref. 1).

performed with intrathecal contrast, this study is invasive, although very few complications have been encountered with currently used contrast agents.

PRINCIPLES OF TREATMENT

Non-Surgical Treatment

Medical therapy can be instituted to help relieve some symptoms of cervical myelopathy, notably spasticity. Carefully titrated doses of Baclofen seem to be effective for some patients. Sometimes spasticity may generate pain in spastic muscle groups and medical therapy in conjunction with physical medicine may be very helpful.

In patients in whom hypermobility of the cervical spine can be demonstrated (see above), external stabilization will help to protect the cord from additional trauma. Only rarely would such immobilization be expected to achieve any clinical improvement, but it may be a useful interim measure while plans for definitive therapy await completion.

Surgical Considerations

The pre-operative evaluation of patients with complex spondylotic cervical myelopathy should take the following into consideration:

1. hypermobility or instability of the cervical spine;
2. abnormal curvature of the cervical spine;
3. number of vertebral levels involved in the spondylotic process;
4. presence of congenital canal narrowing or other congenital anomalies;
5. evaluation of relative degrees of anterior spinal pathology (e.g., osteophytes, discs) versus posterior spinal pathology (e.g., ligamentous hypertrophy, shingling).

In addition, the patient's general condition should be taken into account, particularly the presence of osteopenia if some form of arthrodesis is under consideration as part of the surgical management.

Hypermobility or Instability

Subluxation of the cervical spine at one or more segments, in the presence of myelopathy, requires that stabilization be part of the operative management. Hypermobility implies disc degeneration and ligamentous stretching, including the capsular ligaments of the intervertebral joints. In the author's experience, stabilization and anterior decompression is best performed by an anterior cervical disc excision and interbody fusion. External immobilization is essential post-operatively until complete fusion has been achieved, as evidenced by serial cervical spine radiographs. Both the Cloward dowel construct (3) and the tricortical wafer-type bone graft (20), as discussed in Chapters 56 and 57, are acceptable techniques for achieving stability in these cases.

Vertebrectomy, as opposed to multiple level osteophyte or disc removal, with fusion, has also been advocated (13). However, some surgeons achieve decompression and stabilization by a posterior approach, as is discussed in Chapter 59. In severe cases of subluxation and instability, it may be necessary to apply pre-operative traction and halo immobilization.

Abnormal Curvature

Kyphosis, straightening, and hyperlordosis of the cervical spine may all be seen in conjunction with spondylotic myelopathy, while in other patients the normal curvature is preserved (1) (Fig. 3). These alterations in curvature must be taken into consideration during preoperative surgical planning.

When the cervical spine is straightened or kyphotic, anterior osteophyte removal and decompression of the cord is indicated; laminectomy cannot be expected to accomplish adequate canal decompression of a kyphotic spine. When the spine is straightened but not angulated, laminectomy may be considered, particularly if the consideration of spine geometry includes removal of the C2 and C1 laminae, as well as the mid- and lower cervical vertebrae (extended laminectomy). A post-operative MR scan should be obtained and any osteophytes still compromising the cord should be removed by the anterior approach as a staged, secondary procedure (2) (Fig. 4).

In the patient with a normally preserved lordosis, anterior osteophyte removal with interbody fusion or posterior laminectomy can be considered. In general, if three or more vertebral levels are involved, this author prefers laminectomy to multiple arthrodeses, because of the somewhat greater risk of non-union and the more significant reduction in spine mobility when fusion occurs. Multiple level vertebrectomies with fusion have, however, been performed (13). The same option mentioned above, of dealing with a remaining compressive osteophyte by the anterior approach if this is indicated on the basis of a post-operative MR scan, should be considered. The resulting decrease in mobility would probably still be less than with a multiple-level arthrodesis. When one or two levels of anterior compression are the basis of the patient's myelopathy, the anterior approach of osteophyte and disc removal with arthrodesis is the preferred approach.

Decompressive laminectomy covering multiple levels is also the indicated procedure for patients with myelopathy and a congenitally narrow spinal canal. In patients in whom the normal lordotic cervical curvature is preserved, cord disengagement from the osteophytes can usually be achieved without removing the C1 and C2 laminae. The normally wider canal diameter at these two

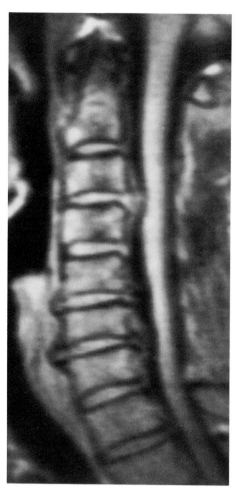

FIG. 4. Magnetic resonance scan of a 48-year-old patient who underwent a C2-C7 laminectomy. The scan shows that the cervical spine is straightened and the cord is not disengaged from a large osteophyte at C3-C4. Some cord atrophy is also evident.

levels is a well recognized anatomical feature. Section of the dentate ligament (12) and dural grafting (5) are no longer carried out by this author as part of a standard decompressive laminectomy.

Hyperlordosis of the spine may pose a difficult management problem. A laminectomy covering many levels, even the commonly performed C3 to C7 laminectomy covering the most frequently involved levels, may result in such extensive posterior migration of the cord that excessive angulation or tension can be applied to several nerve roots. The accompanying radicular vessels may also be compromised. An anterior procedure will often do little to eliminate the factors causing cord compression in such patients. A judiciously planned, limited laminectomy, with geometrical considerations in mind, is the preferred approach.

"S" Curves

Kyphosis and hyperlordosis may coexist and this gives rise to an S-shaped deformity of the spine, causing greater instability and management problems. Both "S-

type" deformities and "reversed S-type" deformities have been described in patients following cervical laminectomy (11). The "S-type" has a kyphosis in the lower cervical level and increased lordosis in the upper cervical region; the "reversed S-type" has an increased lordosis in the lower cervical segment, and kyphosis in the upper cervical area, the more typical "swan" deformity. Such deformities can also exist pre-operatively as a result of the multifactorial degenerative changes of spondylosis (Fig. 5). These patients may require both anterior decompression (for the kyphotic deformity) and posterior decompression (at the hyperlordotic levels) at one operation. The potential role of upper cervical muscle and ligamentous injury at the time of surgery is cited as playing a role in the post-operative deformities. It is tempting to speculate that ligamentous injuries may set the stage for such deformities occurring spontaneously in the course of spondylosis (8).

The foregoing should make it clear that detailed decision making is necessary pre-operatively, based on considerations particular to the patient, rather than on a pre-existing formula. The potential delayed hazards of laminectomy, particularly if the facet joints are injured, have been analyzed in detail and are discussed below (11).

Congenital Canal Narrowing and Other Anomalies

Laminectomy has already been mentioned as the preferred technique for decompressing the cord in the patient with a congenitally narrow canal. Klippel-Feil deformities tend to be associated with degenerative disc changes at the first mobile segment above and below the block vertebra. Anterior osteophyte and disc excision with arthrodesis is generally the preferred surgical approach, but in specific limited situations laminectomy may be preferable. Cranio-cervical junction abnormalities may be very complex. If there is evidence of odontoid impingement on the spinal cord which cannot be relieved by realignment in gradual traction, odontoid resection must be considered (17). When the cord compression can be relieved with realignment, posterior fusion should be performed. This would usually be limited to a C1-C2 arthrodesis, although occasionally the occiput must be included in the fusion. High cervical laminectomy and foramen magnum decompression may be indicated in certain specific instances of high cervical cord compression.

Ossification of the Posterior Longitudinal Ligament (OPLL)

OPLL can result in severe myelopathy (Fig. 6). Recent experience (10,13) has favored extensive anterior resections at multiple levels, stabilization being accomplished by fibular strut graft or iliac crest. Depending on the particular spine alignment, some patients with OPLL may also be managed by laminectomy, with or without

A

B

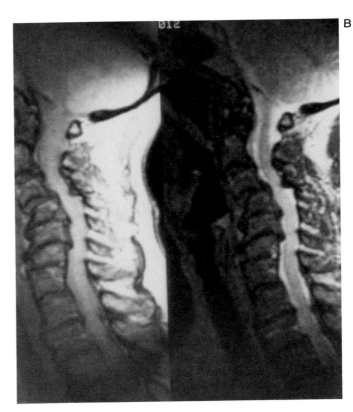

FIG. 5. Radiograph (**A**) and magnetic resonance scan (**B**) of a male patient with a kyphotic deformity at C4-C6 and hyperlordosis of C2-C4 with instability at the C2-C3 and C3-C4 levels, an ''S-type'' deformity. He was managed by upper cervical laminectomy and anterior decompression and fusion below (with permission from Dr. Thomas B. Ducker).

fusion, or by laminoplasty. The laminoplasty techniques are described in Chapter 57.

Delayed Sequelae of Surgical Management

Late changes, not properly called complications, may develop after either anterior or posterior cervical procedures for myelopathy, and such changes may result in secondary deterioration of the patient's condition. Secondary deformity of the cervical spine after extensive laminectomy has been well described and was studied extensively (11). Concerns over spinal instability, delayed deformities, dural compression by epidural scar formation and lack of bony protection of the cervical cord led to the development of a modified laminectomy technique (18). Suspension laminotomy, a form of laminoplasty described by Ohmori et al. (18) preserves the posterior arches as one unit by using an air drill to divide the laminae on each side. The resulting laminar flap is then suspended from the preserved nuchal and supraspinous ligaments and anchored to several of the facets. Bone grafts may be interposed to maintain the position of the laminar flap. A lower incidence of spinal deformity and dural constriction is reported for this procedure (11) compared to conventional laminectomy. This

author has had no personal experience with the technique. The importance of preserving the integrity of the facet joints in performing a laminectomy is well recognized. The development of a laminectomy membrane has also been described extensively (14), although its role in producing recurrent cervical cord compression is not clear.

Late changes may also follow anterior cervical disc excision and interbody fusion. The technical problems of early graft absorption and non-union are well recognized. The use of properly prepared bank bone in place of autologous bone is particularly justified in the osteopenic patient. Excessive late bone formation at the site of an anterior interbody fusion (autologous bone graft), can result in recurrent cord compression. Such problems should be helped by laminectomy.

Anterior versus Posterior Surgical Approach: An Epilogue

The details of surgical decompressive procedures by the anterior and posterior approaches are covered in Chapters 56 and 57. Each has its advocates. Careful preoperative analysis is essential, and the special considerations that affect decision making have been detailed in this chapter. It is of greatest importance that the surgeon

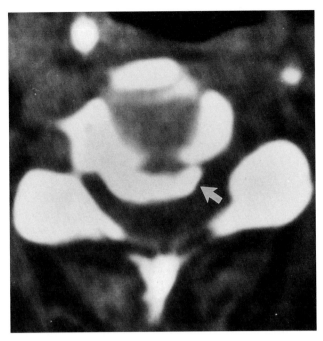

FIG. 6. Computed tomographic scan of a 63-year-old patient with OPLL. The densely calcified ligament (arrow) occupies more than a third of the anterior-posterior dimension of the spinal canal.

be prepared to employ either approach, or a combination of staged procedures, in the management of any patient with spondylotic myelopathy.

REFERENCES

1. Batzdorf U, Batzdorff A (1988): Analysis of cervical spine curvature in patients with cervical spondylosis. *Neurosurgery* 22:827–836.
2. Batzdorf U, Flannigan B (1991): Evaluation of the efficacy of surgical decompressive procedures for cervical spondylotic myelopathy: A study utilizing magnetic resonance imaging. *Spine.*
3. Cloward RB (1958): The anterior approach for removal of ruptured cervical disks. *J Neurosurg* 15:602–617.
4. Cooper PR (1985): Delayed brain injury: Secondary insults. In: *Central nervous system trauma status report* (1985). DP Becker, JT Povlishock, eds. Bethesda: National Institutes of Health, pp. 217–228.
5. Crandall PH, Batzdorf U (1966): Cervical spondylotic myelopathy. *J Neurosurg* 25:57–66.
6. Epstein JA, Carras R, Epstein BS, et al (1970): Myelopathy in cervical spondylosis with vertebral subluxation and hyperlordosis. *J Neurosurg* 32:421–426.
7. Epstein JA, Davidoff LM (1951): Chronic hypertrophic spondylosis of the cervical spine with compression of the spinal cord and nerve roots. *Surg Gynecol Obstet* 93:27–38.
8. Green JD, Harle TS, Harris JH Jr (1981): Anterior subluxation of the cervical spine: Hyperflexion sprain. *AJNR* 2:243–250.
9. Gregorius FK, Estrin T, Crandall PH (1976): Cervical spondylotic radiculopathy and myelopathy. *Arch Neurol* 33:618–625.
10. Harsh GR 4th, Sypert GW, Weinstein PR, et al (1987): Cervical spine stenosis secondary to ossification of the posterior longitudinal ligament. *J Neurosurg* 67:349–357.
11. Ishida Y, Suzuki K, Ohmori K, et al (1989): Critical analysis of extensive cervical laminectomy. *Neurosurgery* 24:215–222.
12. Kahn EA (1947): The role of the dentate ligaments in spinal cord compression and the syndrome of lateral sclerosis. *J Neurosurg* 4:191–199.
13. Kojima T, Waga S, Kubo Y, et al (1989): Anterior cervical vertebrectomy and interbody fusion for multi-level spondylosis and ossification of the posterior longitudinal ligament. *Neurosurgery* 24:864–872.
14. LaRocca H, Macnab I (1974): The laminectomy membrane: Studies in its evolution, characteristics, effects and prophylaxis in dogs. *J Bone Joint Surg* [Br] 56:545–550.
15. Mair WGP, Druckman R (1953): The pathology of spinal cord lesions and their relation to the clinical features in protrusion of cervical intervertebral discs. *Brain* 76:70–91.
16. McRae DL (1960): The significance of abnormalities of the cervical spine. *Am J Roentgenol Radium Ther* 84:3–25.
17. Menezes AH, VanGilder JC, Graf CJ et al (1980): Craniocervical abnormalities: A comprehensive surgical approach. *J Neurosurg* 53:444–455.
18. Ohmori K, Ishida Y, Suzuki K (1987): Suspension laminotomy: A new surgical technique for compression myelopathy. *Neurosurgery* 21:950–957.
19. Payne EE, Spillane JD (1957): The cervical spine: An anatomico-pathological study of 70 specimens (using a special technique) with particular reference to the problem of cervical spondylosis. *Brain* 80:571–596.
20. Robinson RA, Smith GW (1955): Antero-lateral cervical disc removal and interbody fusion for cervical disc syndrome. *Bull Johns Hopkins Hosp* 96:223–224.
21. Stevens JM, O'Driscoll DM, Yu YL, et al (1987): Some dynamic factors in compressive deformity of the cervical spinal cord. *Neuroradiol* 29:136–142.
22. Takahashi M, Sakamoto Y, Miyawaki M, et al (1987): Increased MR signal intensity secondary to chronic cervical cord compression. *Neuroradiol* 29:550–556.
23. Taylor AR (1964): Vascular factors in the myelopathy associated with cervical spondylosis. *Neurology* 14:62–68.
24. Teresi LM, Lufkin RB, Reicher MA, et al (1987): Asymptomatic degenerative disk disease and spondylosis of the cervical spine: MR imaging. *Radiology* 164:83–88.

The Adult Spine: Principles and Practice,
J. W. Frymoyer, Editor-in-Chief.
Raven Press, Ltd., New York © 1991.

CHAPTER 59

Post-Laminectomy Instability of the Cervical Spine

Etiology and Stabilization Technique

John G. Heller and Thomas S. Whitecloud III

The posterior approach provides convenient, extensile, and appropriate access for certain disorders of the cervical spine and spinal cord. However, adequate exposure requires detachment of various muscle groups and ligaments, as well as violation of the posterior column, which has implications for spinal stability. In this chapter, we describe the variables influencing cervical stability and some of the methods for managing instabilities.

The posterior column is defined as the osteoligamentous complex dorsal to the posterior longitudinal ligament (94). This complex includes the laminae, facet joints, and spinous processes, as well as the supraspinous and interspinous ligaments, ligamentum flavum, and facet capsules. In vitro biomechanical testing has demonstrated the importance of these structures to cervical stability (47,62,94,95). In vertical compression, the anterior column transmits only 36% of the applied load, while each pillar of facets transmits 32% of the total applied load (61).

Flexion and extension testing has further defined the role of posterior elements. At least one of the elements that make up the posterior column must be intact, in addition to all of the anterior column, in order to maintain stability (94).

Considerable controversy exists over the relative incidence of instability following posterior approaches to the cervical spine (Fig. 1). A review of the literature of the last four decades makes it apparent that the controversy has arisen from heterogeneity in patient populations, pathological processes, and surgical procedures. An all-encompassing reference to post-laminectomy instability is fruitless. The importance of age, pre-operative cervical alignment, disease type, number and location of laminae excised, and degree of facet violation must be specified (51).

The occurrence of post-laminectomy deformity in children is well recognized, with the highest incidence occurring in the cervical spine (2,6,16,53,89,99,100). In reviewing 132 children who underwent cervical laminectomy, Bell et al. found a 38% incidence of kyphosis and a 15% incidence of hyperlordosis (6). When laminectomy was combined with suboccipital decompression, Aronson et al. found instability in 95% of operated children (2). Yasuoka et al. noted that post-operative kyphosis will develop in children without pre-existing deformity or facet violation. They felt that the evolution of kyphosis and vertebral wedging was a reflection of altered static and dynamic stabilization amplified through their influence on spinal growth and development (99,100). As an alternative approach, Raimondi and co-workers have

J. G. Heller, M.D.: Assistant Professor, Department of Orthopaedic Surgery, Emory University School of Medicine, Atlanta, Georgia, 30322.
T. S. Whitecloud III, M.D.: Professor and Acting Chairman, Department of Orthopaedic Surgery, Tulane University School of Medicine, New Orleans, Louisiana, 70112.

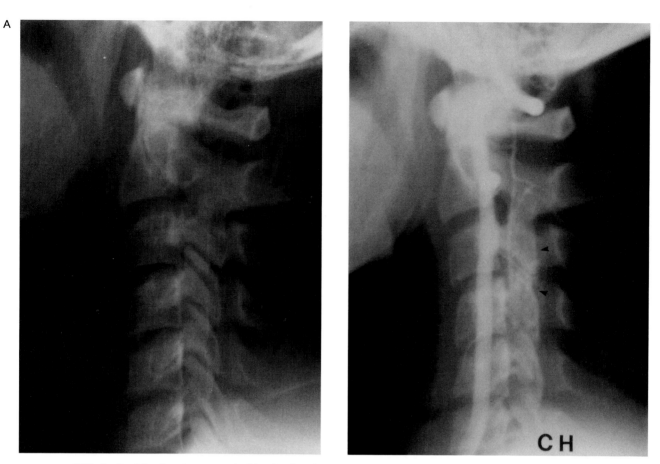

FIG. 1. Post-laminectomy cervical kyphosis with myelopathy. **A:** Pre-operative lateral cervical radiograph. **B:** Vertebral angiogram demonstrating a spinal cord arteriovenous malformation.

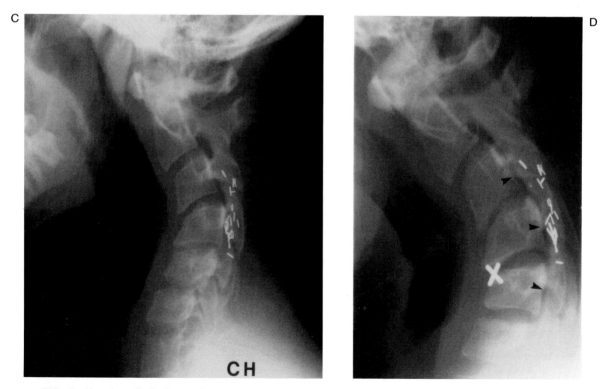

FIG. 1. *(Continued)* **C:** Cervical kyphosis acquired after laminectomies of C3, C4, and C5. **D:** Lateral view from a cervical myelogram demonstrating tethering of the cervical spinal cord across the kyphotic segment (arrowheads). (Figs. 1E–1F follow.)

E

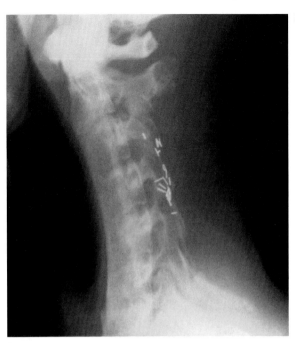

F

FIG. 1. *(Continued)* **E:** Metrizamide enhanced CT scan revealing the flattened, atrophic spinal cord (arrowheads). **F:** Lateral radiograph with solid arthrodesis two years after anterior decompression, reduction, and fibula strut grafting. The patient showed significant though incomplete neurologic recovery (photographs courtesy Dr. Henry H. Bohlman).

performed multilevel en bloc excision of laminae with reconstruction of the posterior arch, thereby avoiding the risk of kyphosis and the need for fusion (67).

Fortunately, in adults with normal cervical alignment and no pre-operative instability, laminar excision alone usually is not associated with a significant incidence of post-operative instability or kyphosis (3). However, the presence of pre-operative deformity or instability will create later deformity or instability (50,57,80). Because of disproportionately poor results from laminectomies in patients with spondylotic myelopathy and cervical malalignment, Miyazaki et al. began to include posterolateral fusion in all such cases. Their recent work substantiates the improved results obtained by this approach and emphasizes the tendency for malalignment to progress if fusion is not performed. In spite of attempted fusion, 50% of their patients developed either new deformity or worsening of pre-existing malalignment (58). These results are all the more compelling, since their operative technique is a laminoplasty variant in which the majority of the ligamentum flavum is preserved and no facetectomy is performed.

The contribution of facetectomy to post-operative instability cannot be overemphasized (55). Although Scoville stated that partial or complete facetectomy engendered no risk of instability (78), it is now clear that such is not the case. Fager often performed laminectomy from C1 to T1 without significant post-operative instability; however, he carefully distinguished between laminec-

tomy alone and laminectomy done in combination with facetectomy (29,30).

In a recent symposium, Epstein underscored the importance of the facet's contribution to stability as he emphasized that not more than one quarter to one third of the facet should be removed in foraminal decompression (28).

Laboratory data support these clinical deductions. Munechika demonstrated the relative contribution of facets and laminae to spinal stability in monkeys. Laminectomy alone was not associated with deformity when fewer than five laminae were removed; however, a gibbus developed when laminectomy was combined with resection of even one facet joint (59).

Raynor has shown that bilateral facetectomy of greater than 50% significantly reduces resistance to loads in shear (70). He has further demonstrated alterations in coupled cervical motions secondary to facetectomy that might predispose motion segments to injury or degeneration (69). White et al. demonstrated with flexion loads that clinical instability in horizontal translation is significantly greater following facetectomy (94).

Cusick et al. examined the influence of complete facetectomy on cervical stability in compression-flexion loading (22). They noted a 32% and 53% reduction in strength with unilateral and bilateral facetectomies, respectively.

Zdeblick et al. recently studied the effect of progressive facetectomy on cervical stability. This work is particu-

A

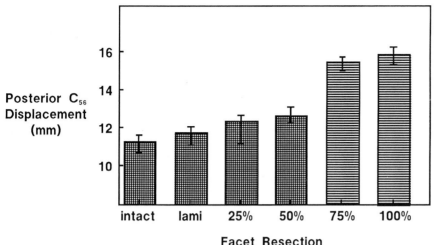

Flexion

Posterior C_{56} Displacement (mm)

Facet Resection

B

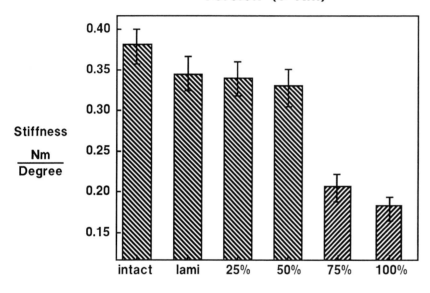

Torsion (5 Nm)

Stiffness

$$\frac{Nm}{Degree}$$

FIG. 2. The effect of progressive facetectomy on cervical spine stability. **A:** In flexion testing, a significant increase in posterior displacement occurs when more than 50% facetectomy is performed. **B:** Likewise, torsion stiffness decreases significantly with more than 50% facetectomy (courtesy Dr. Thomas A. Zdeblick).

larly important in that human specimens were tested in axial load, flexion, extension, and torque. Each test was repeated for the intact specimen as well as 25%, 50%, 75%, and complete C5-C6 bilateral facetectomy. Facetectomy of greater than 50% caused a statistically significant loss of stability in flexion and torsion (102) (Fig. 2).

It has been assumed that the cervical muscle groups contribute little to clinical stability (94). Perry and Nickel demonstrated that severe paracervical muscle paralysis did not lead to significant instability, as long as the bony and ligamentous structures remain intact (63). However, Nolan and Sherk have questioned the validity of these observations. Based on their cadaver dissections and biomechanical modeling, they believe that the semispinalis cervicis and semispinalis capitis groups are primarily responsible for head and neck extension. Be-

cause of this presumed role in dynamic stabilization of the head and neck, they recommend preserving the insertion of these muscle groups into the arch of C2 and the occiput whenever possible (60). Epstein advocates similar restraint in posterior cervical exposures (28).

Clinical evidence in support of these conclusions is available. Simmons and Bradley reported six cases of neuromyopathic flexion deformities of the cervical spine (82). Similar deformities may occur with myasthenia gravis, Parkinsonism, and post-irradiation myofibrosis (8,31).

In summary, there are many determinants of clinical stability that must be kept in mind during posterior cervical surgery. The extent of soft tissue stripping is now presumed to have potential influence on post-operative stability. Clinical and laboratory data clearly demonstrate the adverse consequences of excessive facet resection. Pre-existing segmental instability or deformity amplify any adverse influence of laminectomy and/or facetectomy in the adult. Children represent a distinct high-risk population because of their remaining growth potential and relative ligamentous laxity. The addition of stabilization procedures at the time of posterior cervical surgery is based on a thorough understanding of these variables.

Based on these considerations, cervical stabilization techniques may be adapted to virtually any clinical circumstance ranging from the occiput to the cervicothoracic junction.

SUBAXIAL CERVICAL FUSION TECHNIQUES

Subaxial Cervical Fusion

For most posterior cervical procedures in which fusion is anticipated, the patient should be positioned prone or in some amount of reverse Trendelenberg position. The sitting position does not allow intra-operative access to the iliac crests for bone graft harvest. The head/neck complex is held in appropriate alignment by Mayfield cranial calipers, a halo ring, or Gardner-Wells tongs in association with a horseshoe headrest.

If a halo vest will be used post-operatively, the ring should be applied before positioning the patient, since this gives optimal control of the head and neck and minimizes post-operative manipulation. Halo fixation can be used in virtually any patient (35). Through careful attention to detail, complications of halo fixation can be avoided (10,33,35,38). In the child, prior to closure of the cranial sutures, pin placement is guided by a CT scan, which documents the position of the sutures. A custom ring with 8 to 12 pins is used; the pins are torqued only 2 to 4 inch pounds (35). The halo also may be used in the elderly and for rheumatoids. In those patients, custom molded vests may help reduce problems with fitting and skin complications.

With the patient appropriately positioned, a lateral radiograph is taken to confirm proper positioning. Generous fields should be prepped for both the primary surgical site and the intended graft donor site. The surgeon must anticipate the need to significantly extend the exposure, if required by intra-operative findings. Both iliac crests should be prepped for access in case of inadequate graft from one side or graft fracture.

The least complicated subaxial fusion technique is illustrated in Figure 3. The principles of an on-lay fusion are critical in that they are the cornerstone on which all other techniques build. Without meticulous attention to detail, results will be compromised. The levels to be fused are determined by the variables discussed above.

Meticulous subperiosteal exposure is carried laterally

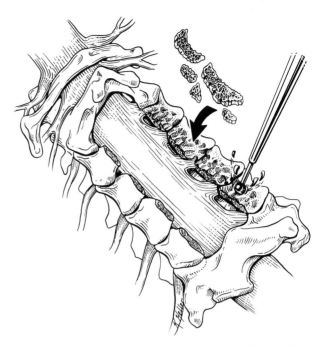

FIG. 3. On-lay fusion technique from C3 to C6. The facet capsules at C2-C3 and C6-C7 must be left intact. A high speed burr is used to decorticate the lateral masses. Cancellous autograph is then placed over the decorticated surfaces. Care is taken during closure to avoid graft displacement medially.

to the edge of the lateral masses, but only over the levels of intended fusion. The facet capsules of unfused segments must not be disturbed. Decortication of the exposed bone surfaces is performed with a high-speed burr. Cancellous and corticocancellous strips of iliac autograft are then placed over the decorticated surfaces. Care should be taken not to displace the grafts when closing the wound. Both the cervical and iliac wounds are drained appropriately. A halo is recommended post-operatively in most circumstances because the technique does not provide immediate stability. To overcome this deficiency, Southwick introduced segmental fixation by facet wires (14,39,72) (Fig. 4). With a Freer elevator passed into the facet joint, a 2 mm to 3 mm burr is used to drill a hole in the center of each inferior articular process of the levels to be fused (Fig. 4B). A transspinous burr hole is made at the subjacent intact posterior arch, as this level must be included in the fusion (14). All surfaces are then decorticated prior to passing the wires. Wire passage is facilitated by the use of an angled dural guide (Fig. 4C). Figure 4A demonstrates the construct utilizing a rib graft. Southwick preferred iliac crest to rib (14), but secured his grafts, as seen in Figure 4A. Figure 4D illustrates a modified iliac technique, which may increase the strength of the construct. Cancellous graft chips are then placed laterally between the strut grafts and the cervical musculature.

The strength of the Southwick technique, and indeed

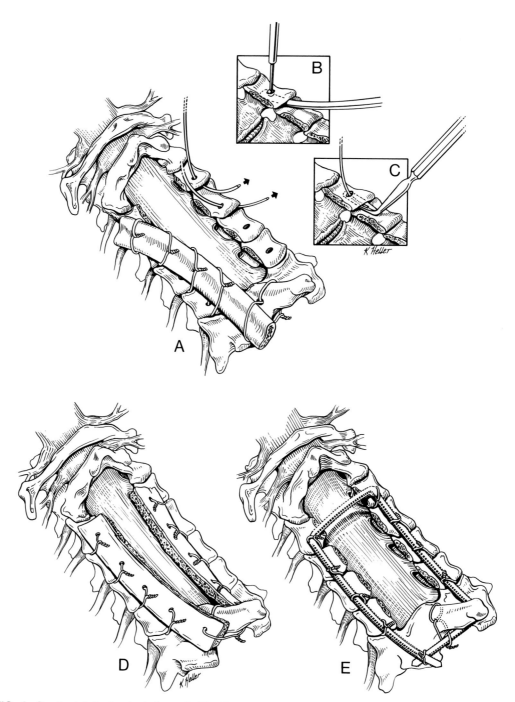

FIG. 4. Southwick fusion technique. **A:** The facet wiring construct illustrated with a rib graft. Note that the subjacent intact level is included in the fusion. **B:** A high speed burr is used to drill a hole in each lateral mass. The Freer elevator defines the depth and orientation of each hole and protects against over-drilling. **C:** Passage of each wire is facilitated by an angled dural guide. **D:** A variation of Southwick's original construct in which the wires are passed through drill holes in an iliac strut graft rather than around it. Supplemental cancellous graft is added lateral to each strut. **E:** Metallic implants may be used to enhance segmental stability, especially when bone grafts are mechanically deficient or in the event of malignancy. In this case, a threaded Steinman pin has been fashioned into a contoured rectangular implant. (Figs. 4F–4J follow.)

F

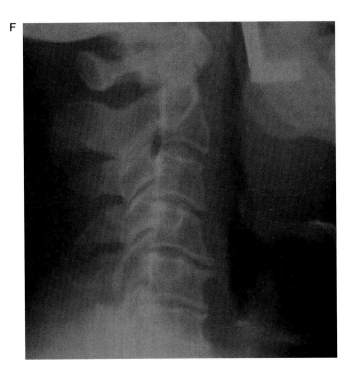

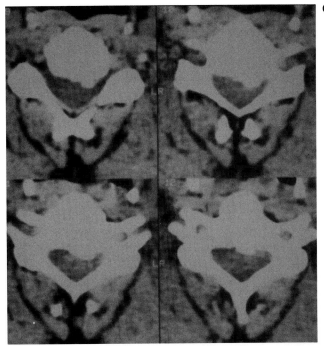

G

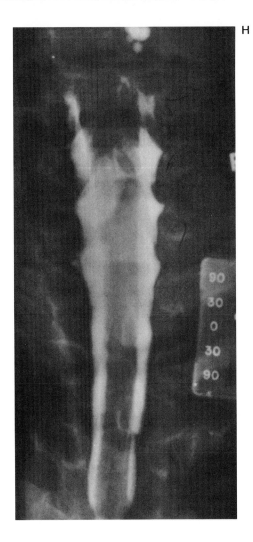

H

FIG. 4. *(Continued)* **F:** Lateral cervical spine x-ray in a 52-year-old man showing marked degenerative changes and very early kyphotic reversal of the normal spinal curvature. **G:** Axial cuts in the CT scan at several levels show diffuse spinal stenosis with multiple osteophytic ridging. **H:** Myelogram in the same patient demonstrates spinal cord compression and blockage from C5-C6 up to C3-C4, with three levels involved and the osteophytes extending not only behind the discs, but behind the vertebral bodies as well. (Figs. 4I–4J follow.)

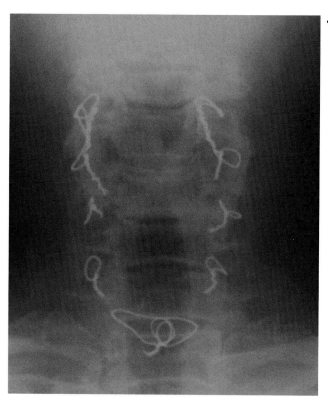

FIG. 4. *(Continued)* **I:** Post-operative film of the same patient after decompressive cervical laminectomy. In addition, posterolateral facet wiring fusion was done in order to immobilize the spine completely, stop the arthritic changes, and prevent further kyphotic deformity. **J:** AP spine x-ray of the same patient shows the wire placement (see Figs. 4B–4C). The patient has a long, segmental decompression as well as a stable fusion. The patient did extremely well with complete clearing of his myelopathy and radiculopathy complaints.

its weakness, has always been the quality of the host bone, both in the graft and at the wire-facet interface (39). Proper positioning of the drill hole will maximize the latter. Graft strength may be poor in the elderly and in patients with connective tissue disease, steroid use, or long-standing spinal cord injuries. In such instances, acute stability may be enhanced by segmental fixation to a contoured rectangle fashioned from a threaded Steinmann pin or stainless steel rod (34) (Fig. 4E). A Luque rectangle or bone graft is then applied to all exposed decorticated surfaces, as in the on-lay grafting procedure. Alternatively, if one wishes to avoid metallic implants, allograft iliac struts can be used in association with autogenous cancellous bone. In any of the above constructs, post-operative immobilization is recommended (14).

As an alternative to wiring, posterior cervical fixation with lateral mass screws and plates was introduced by Roy-Camille and Saillant (76). Although these techniques have not been widely accepted in this country, early reports have been encouraging (26,41,77).

A variety of screw insertion techniques have been proposed. Each shares the goal of obtaining screw purchase in the lateral articular mass. Biomechanical studies have documented the efficacy of these constructs compared to standard wiring techniques (88,91). Furthermore, in most testing modes, posterior plates are superior to anterior plates in stabilizing cervical motion segments (88,91).

In the presence of intact posterior arches and spinous processes, wiring techniques are simple, cost-effective, and mechanically sound (22,75,85,88,91). However, when the posterior arches are surgically removed or fractured, the wiring techniques may be less applicable, and the plating technique allows for fusion of only the destabilized or injured segments. Transspinous wiring also generally requires extension to one level above and one level below the involved segments (85). Southwick recommends including the first intact level below in his facet wiring technique (14).

If posterior plating is biomechanically equivalent to the best-known wiring techniques and is able to spare additional fusion levels, why has it been slow to gain popularity? The procedure is technically demanding, with some theoretically greater risks. In an attempt to define these risks, Heller and associates performed a cadaveric study to compare the two principal styles of screw insertion (45). Figure 5 illustrates the differences between the Roy-Camille and Magerl screw techniques.

Each method seeks to avoid the central zone ventral to the articular mass through which the exiting nerve root traverses.

We found that neither the spinal cord nor the vertebral arteries were injured or placed "at risk" for injury with either method. There was no statistically significant difference in the actual occurrence of nerve root injury between the Roy-Camille and Magerl techniques (2% and 6%, respectively) (Fig. 6A). However, the trajectory of a given screw placed a nerve root "at risk" for injury in 33% of the Magerl screws, but only 6% of the Roy-Camille screws. In such a circumstance, injury could have occurred with insertion of too long a screw or past-point-

ing with a drill. Thirty-four percent of Roy-Camille screws violated their associated facet joint, whereas no Magerl screw did so (Fig. 6B). This poses a problem at the caudal end of a fusion segment where the facet is to be preserved. Finally, the study demonstrated a learning curve in that the accuracy of insertion tended to improve with increasing operator experience and familiarity with cervical anatomy.

Figure 7 illustrates the use of three-hole Roy-Camille plates after laminectomies of C4 through C6. This procedure is adaptable for fusions of one or more motion segments; however, contrary to Roy-Camille, we recommend the routine use of bone graft.

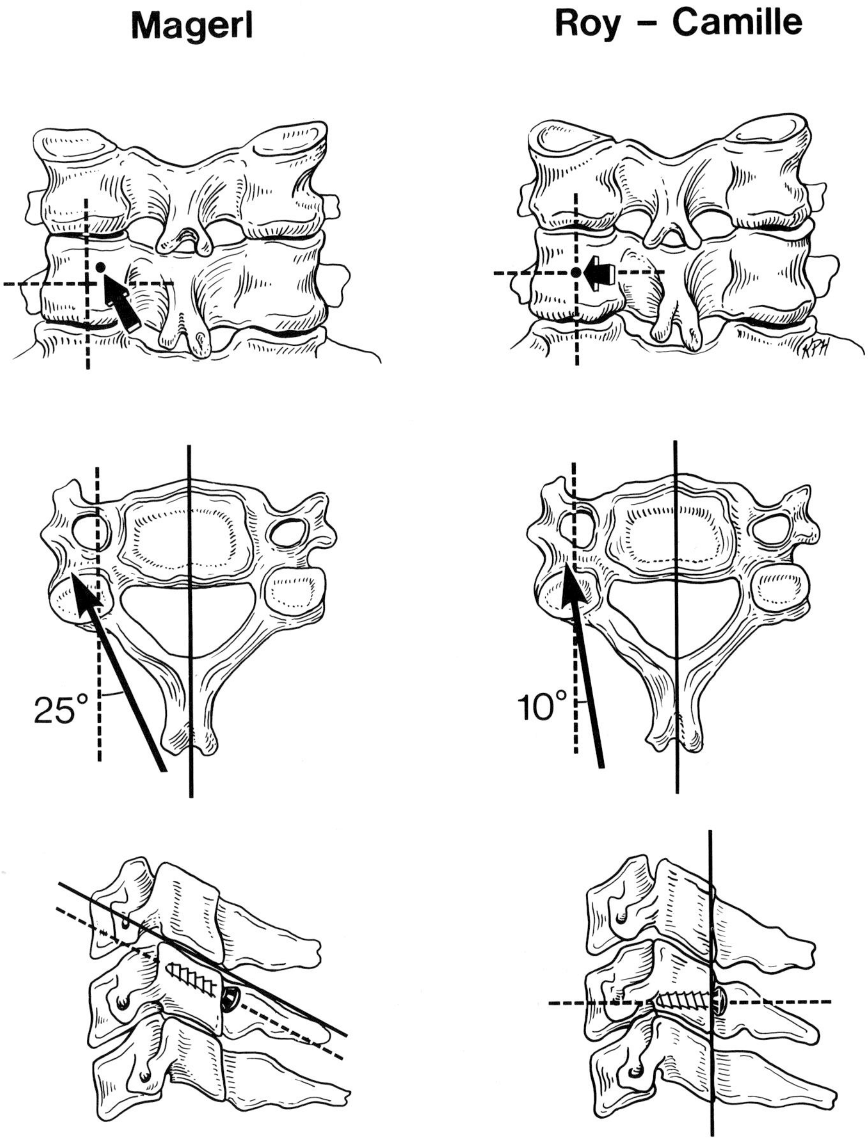

Magerl   Roy – Camille

FIG. 5. Comparison of the Magerl and Roy-Camille techniques for lateral mass screw insertion: Magerl's starting point is 2–3 mm medial and cephalad to the intersection of lines bisecting the exposed lateral mass. Roy-Camille's starting point is at the intersection of these lines. Magerl then angles the drill 25° laterally and parallel to the surface of the superior articular process. Roy-Camille screws are angled 10° laterally and perpendicular to the posterior vertebral cortex.

A

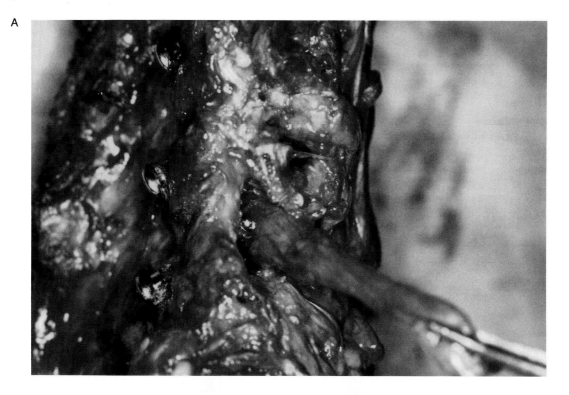

B

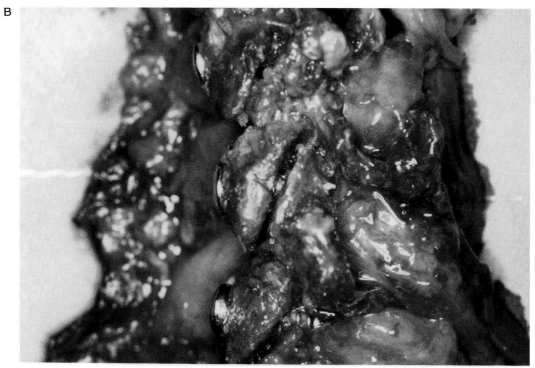

FIG. 6. Gross anatomic specimen showing **(A)** a Magerl screw tip against a cervical root, and **(B)** facet joint violation with a Roy-Camille screw.

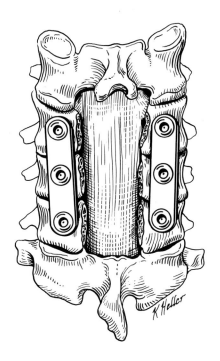
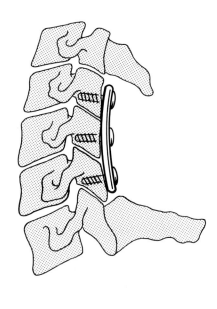

FIG. 7. Roy-Camille plates used for stabilization and fusion from C4 to C6 after laminectomy. Decortication and bone grafting are recommended.

A variety of other techniques are available. Figure 8 demonstrates the use of Magerl's hook plate. When the interspinous bone block is properly seated, this technique is biomechanically equivalent to other posterior cervical plates (88,91). However, this technique has a relative disadvantage; each plate must grasp a portion of an intact lamina at the caudal end of the fusion. Further-more, it is generally limited to one or two motion segments.

The Halifax clamp is another alternative (46), but it requires intact lamina above and below the laminectomy level (Fig. 9). Again, supplemental cancellous graft should be placed over the exposed decorticated surfaces of the lateral masses.

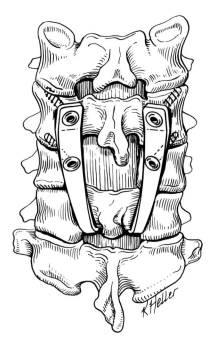
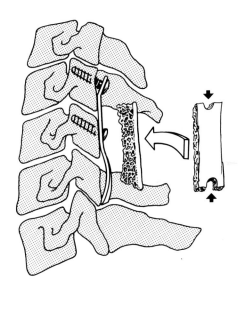

FIG. 8. Magerl's hook plate used for stabilization and fusion from C4 to C6 after C5 laminectomy. A corticocancellous bone block is contoured and fitted into notches in the spinous processes of C4 and C6. The graft blocks overreduction of the facets and increases the construct's stiffness. Cancellous graft is added lateral to the plates.

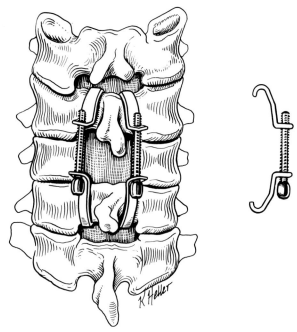

FIG. 9. Halifax clamps used from C4 to C6 after C5 laminectomy. An interspinous bone block may be added to strengthen the construct (see Fig. 8). Decortication and grafting over the lateral masses are required.

The key to safe insertion of either the Roy-Camille or Magerl screw is possessing a thorough grasp of cervical anatomy and osteology (45). The surgeon should be wary of how posterior landmarks are distorted by degenerative disease. Osteophytes should be excised to reveal the true boundaries of the lateral masses. An image intensifier will increase the margin of safety. Pointed, self-tapping screws may increase the risks of nerve root injury unnecessarily. Therefore, smooth-tipped 3.5 mm

cortical screws should be inserted after tapping the drill hole. Screw purchase should be bicortical (37); however, care must be taken not to penetrate beyond the ventral cortex of the lateral mass.

In circumstances in which the superior articular process of one level is deficient as a result of fracture or excision, other fusion methods can be adapted to maintain anatomic alignment. The use of a "tile plate" is illustrated in Figure 10B. This angled plate serves as a prosthetic replacement for the absent superior articular process (77). Alternatively, if a subjacent spinous process is present, one may use an oblique wiring technique to supplement the construct of choice (11,22,27,85) (Fig. 10A).

The type of brace to be used after cervical plating must be individualized. In general, these constructs provide immediate stiffness similar to the intact spine. Sutterlin et al. demonstrated that these constructs endure short-term fatigue testing. However, they rightfully observe that healing of a fusion occurs over months (88), and the properties of screw-plate constructs during such an interval cannot be determined from short-term biomechanical studies (98). In deciding about post-operative support, it is critical to remember that the quality and duration of fixation depends on the host's bone. Relatively deficient bone requires greater protection until there is radiographic evidence of healing.

Cervicocranial Fusion

Instability of the atlanto-occipital and atlanto-axial joints can present a difficult problem. With an intact C1 posterior arch, any of a number of techniques may be used to perform atlanto-axial (85) or occipitocervical fusion (93). When a laminectomy of C1 is required, possi-

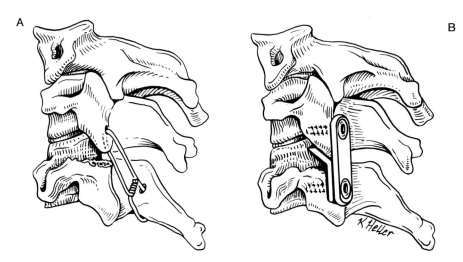

FIG. 10. Stabilization techniques in the presence of a fractured or resected superior articular process. Rotational and transnational stability can be increased by using **(A)** an oblique facet wiring technique or **(B)** a "tile plate" in conjunction with a screw-plate construct.

bly in combination with a suboccipital decompression, other techniques may be considered.

Atlanto-axial fusion may be performed with posterior transarticular screws, as described by Magerl (42,54) (Fig. 11). Although he has reported 51 consecutive cases without significant complications (42), Magerl cautions that this procedure is exacting. The entrance point and trajectory of the screws are critical and difficult to achieve. Deviation medially can injure the spinal cord, while lateral deviation threatens the vertebral artery. Failure to angle the screws sufficiently cephalad will compromise purchase in the C1 articular mass. Furthermore, examination of a large number of C2 specimens has demonstrated that the size and location of the vertebral arteries within the lateral masses of C2 are quite variable. On occasion, a vertebral artery and its associated venous plexus may fill an entire lateral mass (44).

Because of these potential problems, careful analysis of thin section CT scans with appropriate reformations should identify these high-risk variants. Furthermore, the screws should cross the posterior-most portion of the atlanto-axial joint such that it can just be seen traversing the articular space. Such a trajectory is difficult to achieve, but it ensures adequate purchase in C1 and minimizes the risk of vertebral artery injury. The authors are aware of one incident of vertebral artery laceration that was controlled by local measures, without adverse neurologic sequelae (1). Magerl does not recommend post-operative immobilization when this technique is used to augment a conventional fusion (42). In the absence of a C1 posterior arch, bracing and a halo are probably advisable.

Occipitocervical fusion can be made more difficult and less predictable after C1 laminectomy and/or suboccipital decompression. The diminished bone surface available for fusion is a theoretical concern. Again, standard techniques may be readily adapted to this situation. Figure 12 illustrates the technique of Wertheim and Bohlman (93) (see Chapter 52), except that the C1 sublaminar wire is conspicuously absent. A high-speed burr is used to create a trough on either side of the inion process. The troughs are then connected by undermining the outer cortex with a burr and angled curettes. Care should be taken to preserve the full thickness of the cortical bone. Transspinous holes are prepared in C2 and as many other spinous processes as deemed appropriate. Either 18- or 20-gauge wires are then passed twice through each hole to increase their pull-out strength (84).

The hazards of passing transspinous wires are well defined (19). Care should be taken in choosing the location of the burr holes and in the passage of the wires. Bone grafts are harvested from the outer table of the iliac crest. Two stout corticocancellous struts are required in addition to a generous amount of cancellous bone. If the patient's iliac bone is unsuitably weak, consideration

should be given to using allograft iliac struts supplemented by cancellous autograft. The cancellous bone is used to fill the voids ventral to the strut grafts. In these instances, halo immobilization is required for three to six months.

As an alternative, internal fixation may be added to the standard occipitocervical fusion to avoid halo immobilization (48). Figure 13 illustrates the use of a contoured threaded Steinmann pin to provide additional stability. Alternatively, Roy-Camille occipitocervical plates (Fig. 14) may be used for rigid internal fixation (77). Whether these constructs obviate the need for external support is uncertain. Both biomechanical data and adequate clinical reports are wanting. Bone grafting in the latter two constructs is similar to that seen in Figure 12.

Methylmethacrylate

The indications for methylmethacrylate stabilization techniques in the cervical spine are well defined (24,56). Such constructs are to be used for instability secondary to malignancy when life expectancy is less than one year. Methylmethacrylate serves well as an anterior load-bearing column, but posterior arthrodesis is frequently recommended for additional stability and durability (24,56).

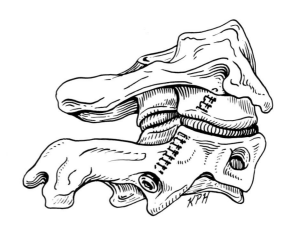

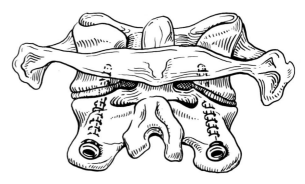

FIG. 11. Magerl's C1-C2 transarticular screw technique.

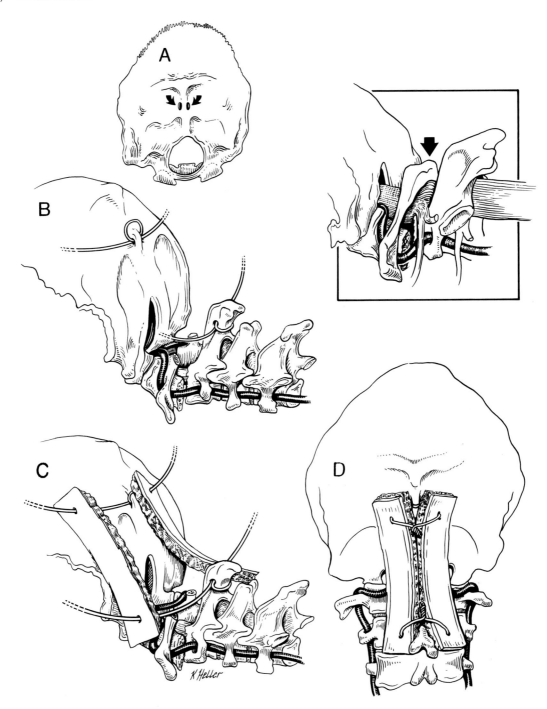

FIG. 12. Occipitocervical fusion technique to stabilize the cervicocranium after C1 laminectomy and/or suboccipital decompression. Exemplified is cord compression due to irreducible atlanto-axial subluxation requiring C1 laminectomy (inset). **A:** Burr holes on either side of the inion process are connected to provide purchase of the skull by wire. **B:** Transspinous drill holes are made at the appropriate levels. Double looped wires are then passed at each level. **C:** The exposed bone surfaces are decorticated before wiring contoured iliac struts in place. Cancellous graft is used to fill any voids between the struts and the underlying recipient surfaces. **D:** Posterior view of an occiput to C2 construct.

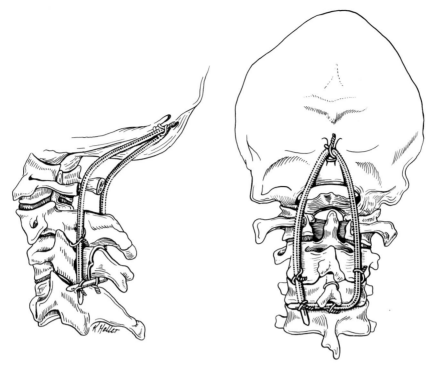

FIG. 13. A contoured threaded Steinman pin can be wired in place to impart greater immediate stability when autogenous struts are mechanically inadequate. Bone grafting is still performed as in Figure 12.

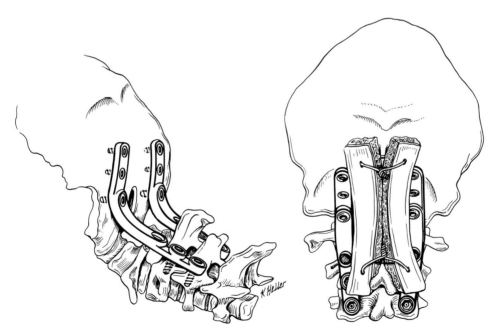

FIG. 14. Roy-Camille occipitocervical plates for rigid internal fixation. Bone grafting is performed as in Figure 12.

The use of methylmethacrylate posteriorly is limited, if not contraindicated, by its mechanical and biological properties. A sound posterior construct should provide immediate and sustained stability until arthrodesis occurs but should not limit access to decorticated surfaces. The rate of operative complications, such as infection and wound dehiscence, should not be increased unless the anticipated benefits clearly outweigh such additional risk.

The mechanical deficiencies of posterior methacrylate techniques are emphasized in the laminectomized spine. Methylmethacrylate does not cause fusion to occur; it is a grouting material. It cannot adhere to bone primarily, but rather holds a vertebra by either encasing a bony prominence (e.g., spinous process) or incorporating some other material anchored into bone (e.g., wires or screws). After laminectomy, as with the other internal fixation techniques discussed above, the bone-implant interface will be the weak link. Whitehill and Barry demonstrated failure of methylmethacrylate constructs at the bone-wire interface in their dog model (98). Furthermore, although immediate stability is achieved with such constructs, it is not superior to other conventional posterior wiring or plating techniques. The stability achieved also tends to deteriorate within the first post-operative month, while that of bone constructs improves steadily with time (98).

Segmental facet wiring to methylmethacrylate tends to retard access of bone graft to the recipient bed, theoretically increasing the risk of non-union.

Posterior methylmethacrylate struts require the material to function in modes for which it is least suited. The polymer resists compression well; however, it is brittle and resists bending and tension poorly. These deficiencies are exaggerated by the voids and surface irregularities that occur when the material is used in the clinical setting.

Finally, methylmethacrylate has been shown to have adverse biological effects. It retards local immune response (64,65) and is associated with a higher infection rate than other implant materials (66). In total joint replacement, the cement may be associated with a synovial-like membrane sometimes associated with osteolysis and implant failure.

McAfee et al. have reported a large series of clinical failures with methylmethacrylate (56). Nineteen of their 24 cases represented a failure of posterior constructs; 6 of these 19 cases were infected, either early or late. Failure of fixation typically occurred at the bone-implant interface, as predicted by Whitehall and Barry's work (98). Worsening of neurologic function frequently accompanied such failures (56).

Branch et al. recently reported a series of traumatic instabilities treated with posterior methacrylate-wire fixation, claiming a 97% success rate (11). This technique was applied without bone grafting and typically included

two levels above and two levels below the injured motion segment. Close inspection of the data reported for the 45 patients followed more than one year provides a different outlook on this procedure. Four patients required a second operation, three for loss of fixation and one for progressive kyphosis. Fifteen patients had radiographic non-unions demonstrated by pinhole erosions and broken wires. From this more critical perspective, the failure rate approaches 42%.

These considerations lead to the conclusion that methylmethacrylate fusion is a misnomer. This material is one among numerous choices of temporary internal splints. The ultimate clinical success of any stabilization construct hinges on eventual and timely arthrodesis. Methylmethacrylate has many mechanical and biological disadvantages compared to the other posterior techniques described in this chapter; laboratory and clinical experience suggests that it should be used only for short-term anterior reconstruction supplemented with posterior fusion. Methylmethacrylate cannot be recommended for posterior stabilization of the cervical spine, especially after laminectomy.

ALTERNATIVES TO THE POSTERIOR APPROACH

Thus far, this chapter has dealt with the various modalities available to stabilize the cervical spine following laminectomy. Fortunately, it is uncommon for adults to develop a post-operative cervical kyphosis (29,49,74,78). If the pathological process that requires decompression does not necessitate facetectomies, there is little likelihood that a kyphotic deformity will result. However, if facetectomy is required, a prophylactic fusion done at the time of decompression is much more easily accomplished at the time of the laminectomy. Although all the previously described posterior procedures can be done after a kyphosis has developed, it is certainly technically easier to have obtained stabilization initially. The optimal surgical procedures for a kyphotic deformity are those that prevent the kyphosis from developing.

Another alternative to posterior procedures for a post-laminectomy kyphotic deformity is to achieve stability and arthrodesis via the anterior route (4,17,81,83). Anterior stabilizing procedures are obviously technically easier, since the surgery is being performed in an area that has not been subjected to an operation. Another distinct advantage to anterior surgery in the presence of a kyphotic deformity is that the grafts are in compression and thus not subjected to tensile forces.

As already emphasized, it is generally mandatory to apply pre-operative skeletal traction utilizing a halo device or skull tongs whenever a significant cervical kyphotic deformity is going to be stabilized. Some deformities are relatively rigid, and little reversal of the kyphosis is demonstrated with pre-operative traction. A fusion in situ may be performed or selective osteotomies can be done at the time of graft insertion to improve the deformity. Any improvement in the kyphotic deformity prior to surgery makes the procedure technically easier.

Chapter 56 describes the numerous techniques for stabilizing the spine anteriorly. However, anterior interbody fusion techniques were developed for management of one- or two-level disease secondary to spondylitic changes (3,20,23,40,71,73,74,92,96). The most common of these techniques, the Robinson-Smith or Cloward, provides no immediate spinal stability (17,71). Stauffer and Kelly have noted loss of stability when anterior interbody fusion is utilized in the treatment of certain types of fracture dislocations (86). This situation can be considered analogous to the laminectomized cervical spine that has obviously lost posterior stability. Interbody fusion techniques at more than one level also have an increased risk of extrusion or non-union (17,18,20,96). Therefore, it is not recommended that interbody fusion techniques be performed in the face of a laminectomized spine when more than two motion segments require stabilization (Fig. 15).

The technique of Bailey and Badgley theoretically would offer more strength and would be able to span multiple motion segments (4). However, it has been shown that corticocancellous graft materials do not have enough inherent strength to resist fracturing when more than two levels are spanned. This has led to the development of the various surgical techniques in which purely cortical bone, generally obtained from the fibula, is utilized to span multiple motion segments and resist compressive forces without fracturing (7,97). Stauffer initially described utilization of the fibula for graft material for stabilization following fractures (86). Subsequently, Whitecloud and LaRocca utilized fibula following anterior decompression after multiple cervical segments had been decompressed to provide relief of the symptoms of cervical myelopathy (97). These and other authors have reported a high rate of union utilizing fibula as graft material, with essentially no incidence of graft failure. Successful fusion has been achieved over as many as five cervical segments, and the extent of the fusion that can be done is limited only by the fact that the fibula is a straight piece of bone and the cervical spine has a normal kyphosis beginning at the cervicothoracic junction.

The surgical technique for multilevel cervical stabilization is described in detail in Chapter 56. Briefly, in the face of a kyphotic deformity, skeletal traction is applied prior to and during the operative procedure. Individuals with significantly long-standing kyphotic deformities will develop varying amounts of scar tissue at the apex of the deformity, which will require removal for adequate visualization. If the deformity is fixed in an acceptable position, no attempt should necessarily be made to achieve correction by vertebrectomy. However, if there are signs of continued neural compression because of the kyphotic deformity, the source of compression should be removed at the time of surgical stabilization. Once the levels to be stabilized have been correctly identified by intra-operative roentgenogram, the discs of involved segments to be fused are removed. Once this has been done, a trough is prepared in the anterior aspect of vertebral bodies utilizing rongeurs and a dental burr. A trough is thus created whose depth will allow the insertion of the bone graft. If decompression of neural structures is not required, the posterior cortex of the vertebral body is left intact. Once the trough has been prepared, holes are cut at the superior and inferior end of the trough. The size of the holes will depend on the method of insertion of the graft. Either iliac or fibula graft may be utilized, but it is recommended that purely cortical bone be used for more extensive procedures. It has now been demonstrated that the allograft can be used successfully in the cervical spine (43). This has allowed a variation in the technique of graft insertion. Because allograft fibula obviously comes in different sizes, the trough can be prepared so that the graft can be wedged in along the sides of the vertebrae, not only superiorly and inferiorly. Once the superior and inferior vertebrae have been prepared to receive the graft, more traction is applied to the cervical spine and the graft, which has been fashioned to the correct length, is inserted.

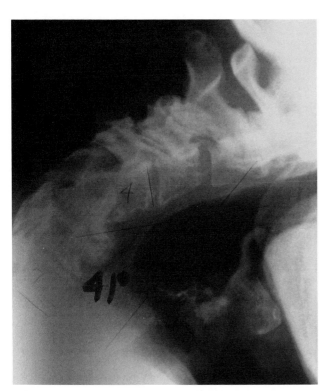

FIG. 15. Lateral radiograph of a patient who developed a kyphotic deformity following a laminectomy. An attempt at stabilization by a two-level arthrodesis at C4-C5 and C5-C6 has failed due to graft collapse.

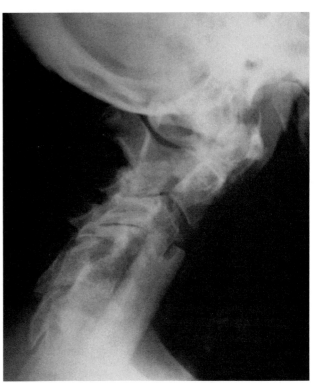

FIG. 16. The same patient as in Figure 15. **A:** Traction has been applied prior to anterior stabilization. **B:** A notched fibular graft has been inserted with spinal alignment maintained. This patient utilized only a Philadelphia collar post-operatively.

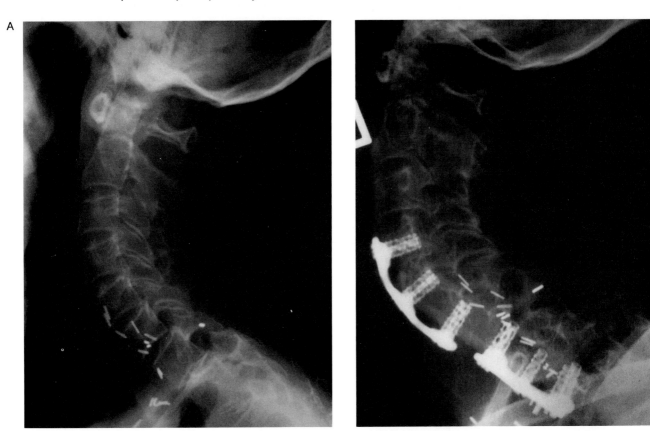

FIG. 17. Kyphotic deformity **(A)** developing following extensive posterior decompression. In this instance **(B)**, anterior stabilization has been achieved by utilization of a cortical graft, and the hollow titanium screws developed by Mosher. Note that the screws do not need to penetrate the posterior cortex of the vertebral bodies.

A

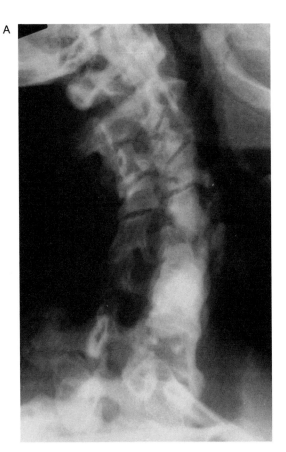

B

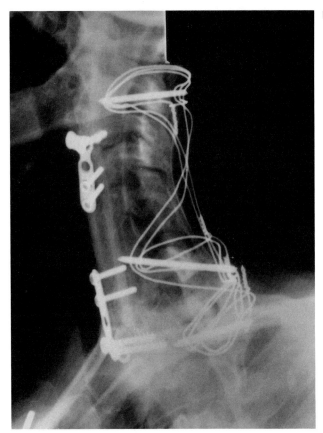

FIG. 18. Pre- and post-operative radiographs **(A)** of a patient's cervical spine destabilized because of the necessity for adequate tumor removal. In this case **(B)**, a posterior Dewar compression arthrodesis has been combined with an anterior cortical graft from the fibula which, in turn, has been stabilized by an anterior plating system.

There are two methods of inserting fibula when utilized to span multiple segments. One is to prepare an undercut area in the superior and inferior vertebrae and insert the entire fibula so that it lies within the prepared trough (101). One problem with this technique is that the spine must be extended to some degree to insert the graft properly, and since the graft must be driven into place, there is a chance that it may inadvertently enter the neural canal if the posterior portion of the vertebral body has been removed during decompression. Another technique reported by Whitecloud and LaRocca is utilization of a notched fibula (97) (Figs. 16A and 16B). With the notched fibula, only its widest portion is inserted within the trough, and the way the graft is fashioned prevents it from being inadvertently inserted into the neural canal at the time of insertion.

There have been numerous other techniques described for the insertion of corticocancellous grafts obtained from the ilium to span multiple segments (4,9). As stated, it is not felt that these constructs are strong enough to resist compressive forces if more than two motion segments are stabilized.

A variety of spinal implants have been designed for utilization on the anterior aspect of the cervical spine.

All these various plating systems have in common two rows of vertical screw holes like the H-plate developed by ASIF for anterior cervical plating (12,21,36,52). The systems developed by Senegas, Strehli, Fuentes, and Caspar share this design (15,32,79,87). All these systems require penetration of the posterior cortex of the vertebral body for maximal security and are obviously somewhat technically difficult to insert. There has been one system developed by Mosher utilizing hollow titanium screws that does not require the penetration of the posterior cortex of the vertebral body (Figs. 17A and 17B). All these systems can be used to span multiple vertebral levels to provide some stability while arthrodesis is occurring. As with posterior constructs, these systems have all been used to a much greater extent in Europe.

Biomechanical studies have demonstrated that the anterior plating systems are not as inherently stable as the various posterior constructs that have been devised (90). The highest degree of stability is achieved with both an anterior and posterior stabilizing device (Figs. 18A and 18B).

Currently, the criteria for utilization of anterior spinal plating devices are being developed. In most instances, the utilization of cortical bone provides enough inherent stability so that internal fixation devices are not necessary. Certainly it is still possible to utilize halo stabilization in cases in which the stability of the cortical construct is suspect.

Post-laminectomy instability of the cervical spine may be managed either anteriorly or posteriorly. The variety of posterior procedures that have been described in this chapter are best performed at the time of the original decompressive procedure. Thus the development of a kyphotic deformity is prevented. Generally, it is technically easier to achieve anterior stabilization and arthrodesis if a post-laminectomy kyphosis develops.

REFERENCES

1. Anderson PA: Personal communication.
2. Aronson DD, Kahn RJ, Canady A (1989): Cervical spine instability following suboccipital decompression and cervical laminectomy for Arnold-Chiari syndrome (abs). Presented at 56th Annual Meeting of the American Academy of Orthopaedic Surgeons, Las Vegas.
3. Aronson N, Filtzer DK, Bagan M (1968): Anterior cervical fusion by the Smith-Robinson approach. *J Neurosurg* 29:397–404.
4. Bailey RW, Badgley CE (1960): Stabilization of the cervical spine by anterior fusion. *J Bone Joint Surg* [Am] 42:565–594.
5. Batzdorf U, Batzdorf A (1988): Analysis of cervical spine curvature in patients with cervical spondylosis. *Neurosurgery* 22:827–836.
6. Bell DF, Walker JL, O'Connor G (1989): Spinal deformity following multiple level cervical laminectomy in children (abs). Presented at the 56th Annual Meeting of the American Academy of Orthopaedic Surgeons, Las Vegas.
7. Bernard TN, Whitecloud TS (1987): Cervical spondylotic myelopathy and myeloradiculopathy: Anterior decompression and stabilization with autogenous fibula strut graft. *Clin Orthop* 221:149–160.
8. Bohlman HH: Personal communication.
9. Boni M, Cherubino P, Benazzo F (1984): Multiple subtotal somatectomy: Technique and evaluation of a series of thirty-nine cases. *Spine* 9:358–362.
10. Botte MJ, Byrne TP, Garfin SR (1987): Application of the halo device for immobilization of the cervical spine utilizing an increased torque pressure. *J Bone Joint Surg* [Am] 69:750–752.
11. Branch CL Jr, Kelly DL Jr, Davis CH Jr, McWhorter JM (1989): Fixation of fractures of the lower cervical spine using methylmethacrylate and wire: Technique and results in 99 patients. *Neurosurgery* 25:503–512.
12. Brenner A, Roosen K, Wissing HJ, Grote W, Schmitt-Neuerburg KP (1986): Osteosynthesis with AO plates in the cervical and lumbal regions of the vertebral column in cases of spinal metastases. In: Wenker H et al., eds. *Advances in neurosurgery, vol 14.* New York: Springer-Verlag, p. 133.
13. Cahill RA, Bellegarrigue R, Ducker TB (1983): Bilateral facet to spinous process fusion: A new technique for posterior spinal fusion after trauma. *Neurosurgery* 13:1–4.
14. Callahan RA, Johnson RM, Margolis RN, Keggi KJ, Albright JA, Southwick WO (1977): Cervical facet fusion for control of instability following laminectomy. *J Bone Joint Surg* [Am] 59:991–1002.
15. Caspar, W (1987): Anterior stabilization with the trapezial osteosynthetic plate technique in cervical spine injuries. In: Kehr P, Weidner A, eds. *Cervical spine I,* Wien, New York: Springer-Verlag, pp. 198–204.
16. Cattell HS, Clark GL Jr (1977): Cervical kyphosis and instability following multiple laminectomies in children. *J Bone Joint Surg* [Am] 59:991–1002.
17. Cloward RB (1958): The anterior approach for removal of ruptured cervical discs. *J Neurosurg* 15:602–617.
18. Cloward RB (1961): Treatment of acute fractures and fracture dislocations of the cervical spine by vertebral-body fusion. A report of eleven cases. *J Neurosurg* 18:201–209.
19. Coe JD, Simpson MB (1989): Potential neurological hazards with interspinous wiring in the cervical spine (abs). Presented at the 17th Annual Meeting of the Cervical Spine Research Society, New Orleans.
20. Connolly E, Seymour R, Adams J (1965): Clinical evaluation of anterior cervical fusions for degenerative cervical disc disease. *J Neurosurg* 23:431–437.
21. Correia Martins MA (1987): Anterior cervical fusion—indications and results. In: Kehr P, Weidner A, eds. *Cervical spine I.* Wien-New York: Springer-Verlag, p. 205.
22. Cusick JF, Yoganandan N, Pintar F, Myklebust J, Hussain H (1988): Biomechanics of cervical spine facetectomy and fixation techniques. *Spine* 13:808–812.
23. Depalma AF, Rothman RH, Levinneck RE, et al (1972): Anterior interbody fusion for severe cervical disc degeneration. *Surg Gynecol Obstet* 134:755–758.
24. Dunn EJ (1977): The role of methylmethacrylate in the stabilization and replacement of tumors of the cervical spine: A project of the Cervical Spine Research Society. *Spine* 2:15–24.
25. Dunsker SB (1976): Summary of panel on management of myelopathy and radiculopathy of cervical spondylosis. *Clin Neurosurg* 24:522–526.
26. Ebraheim NA, An HS, Jackson WT, Brown JA (1989): Internal fixation of the unstable cervical spine using posterior Roy-Camille plate: Preliminary report. *J Orthopaedic Trauma* 3:23–28.
27. Edwards EC, Matz SO, Levins AM (1985): The oblique wiring technique for rotational injuries of the cervical spine. *Trans Orthop* 9:142.
28. Epstein JA (1988): The surgical management of cervical spinal stenosis, spondylosis and myeloradiculopathy by means of the posterior approach. *Spine* 13:864–869.
29. Fager CA (1973): Results of adequate posterior decompression in the relief of spondylotic cervical myelopathy. *J Neurosurg* 38:684–692.
30. Fager CA (1977): Management of cervical disc lesions and spondylosis by posterior approaches. *Clin Neurosurg* 24:488–507.
31. Fielding JW, quoted in Simmons EH, Bradley DD (1988): Neuro-myopathic flexion deformities of the cervical spine. *Spine* 13:760.
32. Fuentes JM (1984): Description d'une plaque d'osteosynthese cervicale anterieure. *Neurochirurgie* 30(5):351–353.
33. Garfin SR, Botte MJ, Waters RL, et al (1986): Complications in the use of the halo fixation device. *J Bone Joint Surg* [Am] 68:320–325.
34. Garfin SR, Moore MR, Marshall LF (1988): A modified technique for cervical facet fusion. *Clin Orthop Rel Res* (230):149–153.
35. Garfin SR, Mubarak SJ, Camp JF, Wenger DR (1988): Halo application in the child under two (abs). Presented at the 16th Annual Meeting of the Cervical Spine Research Society, Key Biscayne.
36. Gassmann J, Seligson D (1983): The anterior cervical plate. *Spine* 8:700.
37. Gill K, Paschal S, Corin J, Ashman R, Bucholz RW (1988): Posterior plating of the cervical spine: A biomechanical comparison of different posterior fusion techniques. *Spine* 13:813–816.
38. Glaser MA, Whitehill R, Stamp WG, Jane JA (1986): Complications associated with the halo-vest. *J Neurosurg* 65:762–769.
39. Goel VK, Clark CR, Harris KG, Kim YE, Schulte MR (1989): Evaluation of effectiveness of a facet wiring technique: An in vitro biomechanical investigation. *Annals of Biomed Engineering* 17:115–126.
40. Gore DR, Sepic SB (1984): Anterior cervical fusion for degenerated or protruded discs: A review of one hundred forty-six patients. *Spine* 9:667–671.
41. Grady SM, Anderson PA, Henley MB (1990): Posterior cervical fusion using A.O. reconstruction plates and iliac bone graft (abs). Presented at the 57th Annual Meeting of the American Academy of Orthopaedic Surgeons, New Orleans.
42. Greenfield GQ Jr, Jeanerette B, Magerl F (1989): Transarticular screw fixation for atlanto-axial instability (abs). Presented at the

56th Annual Meeting of the American Academy of Orthopaedic Surgeons, Las Vegas.

43. Hanley EN, Harvell JC, Shapiro DE, Kraus DR (1989): Use of allograft bone in cervical spine surgery. *Seminars in spine surgery* 1(4):262–270.

44. Heller JG: Unpublished data.

45. Heller JG, Carlson GD, Abitbol J-J, Garfin SR (1989): Anatomical comparison of the Roy-Camille and Magerl techniques for screw fixation of the lower cervical spine (abs). Presented at the 17th Annual Meeting of the Cervical Spine Research Society, New Orleans.

46. Holness RO, Huestis WS, Howes WJ, Langille RA (1984): Posterior stabilization with an interlaminar clamp in cervical injuries: Technical note and review of the long term experience with the method. *Neurosurg* 14:318–322.

47. Huelke DF, Nusholtz GS (1986): Cervical spine biomechanics: A review of the literature. *J Orthop Res* 4:232–245.

48. Itoh T, Tsuji H, Katoh Y, et al (1988): Occipito-cervical fusion reinforced by Luque's segmental spinal instrumentation for rheumatoid diseases. *Spine* 13:1234–1238.

49. Jenkins DHR (1973): Extensive cervical laminectomy: Long term results. *Br J Surg* 60:852–854.

50. Kamioka Y, Yamamoto H, Tani T, Ishida K, Sawamoto T (1989): Postoperative instability of cervical OPLL and cervical radiculomyelopathy. *Spine* 14:1177–1183.

51. Katsumi Y, Honma T, Nakamura T (1989): Analysis of cervical instability resulting from laminectomies for removal of spinal cord tumor. *Spine* 14:1172–1176.

52. Knoringer P (1986): Osteosynthesis in patients with malignant tumors of the cervical vertebral column: Indications, technique, and results. In: Wenker H et al., eds. *Neurosurgery, vol 14.* New York: Springer-Verlag, p. 125.

53. Lonstein JE (1977): Post-laminectomy kyphosis. *Clin Orthop Rel Res* (128):93–100.

54. Magerl F, Seemann P (1985): Stable posterior fusion of the atlas and axis by transarticular screw fixation. In: Kehr P, Weidner A, eds. *Cervical spine I.* Strassburg, Wien, New York: Springer-Verlag.

55. Mayfield FH (1965): Cervical spondylosis: A comparison of the anterior and posterior approaches. *Clin Neurosurg* 13:181–188.

56. McAfee PC, Bohlman HH, Ducker T, Eismont FJ (1986): Failure of stabilization of the spine with methylmethacrylate: A retrospective analysis of twenty-four cases. *J Bone Joint Surg* [Am] 68:1145–1157.

57. Mikawa Y, Shikata J, Tamamuro T (1987): Spinal deformity and instability after multilevel cervical laminectomy. *Spine* 12:6–11.

58. Miyazaki K, Tada K, Matsuda Y, Okuno M, Yasuda T, Murakami H (1989): Posterior extensive simultaneous multisegment decompression with posterolateral fusion for cervical instability and kyphotic and/or S-shaped deformities. *Spine* 14:1160–1170.

59. Munechika Y (1973): Influence of laminectomy on the stability of the spine: An experimental study with special reference to the extent of laminectomy and the resection of the intervertebral joint. *J Jap Orthop Assn* 47:111–125.

60. Nolan JP Jr, Sherk HH (1988): Biomechanical evaluation of the extensor musculature of the cervical spine. *Spine* 13:9–11.

61. Pal GP, Sherk HH (1988): The vertical stability of the cervical spine. *Spine* 13:447–449.

62. Panjabi MM, Summer DJ, Pelker RR, Videman T, Friedlaender GE (1986): Three-dimensional load-displacement curves due to forces on the cervical spine. *J Orthop Res* 4:151–152.

63. Perry J, Nickel VL (1959): Total cervical spine fusion for neck paralysis. *J Bone Joint Surg* [Am] 41:37–60.

64. Petty W (1978): The effect of methylmethacrylate on bacterial phagocytosis and killing by human polymorphonuclear leukocytes. *J Bone Joint Surg* [Am] 60:752–757.

65. Petty W (1978): The effect of methylmethacrylate on chemotaxis of polymorphonuclear leukocytes. *J Bone Joint Surg* [Am] 60:492–498.

66. Petty W, Spanier W, Shuster JJ, Silverthorne C (1985): The influence of skeletal implants on incidence of infection. *J Bone Joint Surg* [Am] 67:1236–1244.

67. Raimondi AJ, Gutierrez FA, DiRocco C (1976): Laminotomy and total reconstruction of the posterior spinal arch for spinal canal surgery in childhood. *J Neurosurg* 45:555–560.

68. Raynor RB (1983): Anterior or posterior approach to the cervical spine: An anatomical and radiographic evaluation and comparison. *Neurosurgery* 12:7–13.

69. Raynor RB, Moskovich T, Zidel P, Pugh J (1987): Alterations in primary and coupled neck motions after facetectomy. *Neurosurgery* 21:681–687.

70. Raynor RB, Pugh J, Shapiro I (1985): Cervical facetectomy and its effect on spine strength. *J Neurosurg* 63:278–282.

71. Robinson RA, Smith GW (1955): Anterolateral cervical disc removal and interbody fusion for cervical disc syndrome. *Bull of the Johns Hopkins Hosp* 96:223–224.

72. Robinson RA, Southwick WO (1960): Indications and techniques for early stabilization of the neck in some fracture dislocations of the cervical spine. *South Med J* 53:565–579.

73. Robinson RA, Walker AE, Ferlic DC, et al (1962): The results of an anterior interbody fusion of the cervical spine. *J Bone Joint Surg* [Am] 44:1569–1587.

74. Rogers L (1961): The surgical treatment of cervical spondylotic myelopathy: Mobilization of the complete cervical cord into an enlarged canal. *J Bone Joint Surg* [Br] 43:3–6.

75. Rogers WA (1957): Fractures and dislocations of the cervical spine. *J Bone Joint Surg* [Am] 39:341–376.

76. Roy-Camille R, Saillant G (1972): Chirurgie du rachis cervical. *Nouv Presse Med* 1:2707–2709.

77. Roy-Camille R, Saillant G, Mazel C (1989): Internal fixation of the unstable cervical spine by a posterior osteosynthesis with plates and screws. In: Sherk HH, Dunn EJ, Eismont FJ, et al., eds. *The cervical spine, 2nd ed.* Philadelphia: J.B. Lippincott, pp. 390–403.

78. Scoville WB (1961): Cervical spondylosis treated by bilateral facetectomy and laminectomy. *J Neurosurg* 18:423–428.

79. Senegas J, Gauzere JM (1977): Traitment des lesions cervicales par voie anterieure. *Rev Chir Orthoped* 63:466.

80. Sim FH, Svien HJ, Bickel WH, Janes JM (1974): Swan-neck deformity following extensive cervical laminectomy: A review of twenty-one cases. *J Bone Joint Surg* [Am] 56:564–580.

81. Simmons EH, Bhalla SK (1969): Anterior cervical discectomy and fusion: A clinical and biomechanical study with eight year follow-up. *J Bone Joint Surg* [Br] 51:225–237.

82. Simmons EH, Bradley DD (1988): Neuro-myopathic flexion deformities of the cervical spine. *Spine* 13:756–762.

83. Smith GW, Robinson RA (1958): The treatment of certain cervical spine disorders by anterior removal of intervertebral disc and interbody fusion. *J Bone Joint Surg* [Am] 40:607–624.

84. Stambrough JL, Jauch EC, Norrgran CL (1989): Posterior spinous process wiring in the cervical spine (abs). Presented at the 17th Annual Meeting of the Cervical Spine Research Society, New Orleans.

85. Stauffer ES (1988): Wiring techniques of the posterior cervical spine for the treatment of trauma. *Orthopedics* 11:1543–1548.

86. Stauffer ES, Kelly EG (1977): Fracture-dislocations of the cervical spine. Instability and recurrent deformity following treatment by anterior interbody fusion. *J Bone Joint Surg* [Am] 59:45–48.

87. Strehli R (1987): Double hole plate fixation of the lower cervical spine. In: Kehr P, Weidner A, eds. *Cervical spine I.* Wien, New York: Springer-Verlag, pp. 175–179.

88. Sutterlin CE 3rd, McAfee PC, Warden KE, Rey RM Jr, Farey ID (1988): A biomechanical evaluation of cervical spinal stabilization methods in a bovine model: Static and cyclical loading. *Spine* 13:795–802.

89. Taddonio RF Jr, King AG (1982): Atlantoaxial rotatory fixation after decompressive laminectomy: A case report. *Spine* 7:540–544.

90. Ulrich C, Worsdorfer O, Claes L, Magerl F (1987): Comparative stability of anterior or posterior cervical spine fixation in vitro investigation. In: Kehr P, Weidner A, eds. *Cervical spine I.* Wien, New York: Springer-Verlag, p. 65.

91. Ulrich C, Worsdorfer O, Claes L, Magerl F (1987): Comparative study of the stability of anterior and posterior cervical spine fixation procedures. *Arch Orthopaedic Trauma Surg* 106:226–231.

92. Verbiest H (1973): The management of cervical spondylosis. *Clin Neurosurg* 20:262–294.

93. Wertheim SB, Bohlman HH (1987): Occipitocervical fusion: Indications, technique and long-term results in thirteen patients. *J Bone Joint Surg* [Am] 69:833–836.

94. White AA, Johnson RM, Panjabi MM, Southwick WO (1975): Biomechanical analysis of clinical stability in the cervical spine. *Clin Orthop Rel Res* 109:85–96.

95. White AA 3rd, Panjabi MM (1988): Biomechanical considerations in the surgical management of cervical spondylotic myelopathy. *Spine* 13:856–860.

96. White AA III, Southwick WO, DePonte RJ, et al (1973): Relief of pain by anterior cervical spine fusion for spondylosis: A report of sixty-five cases. *J Bone Joint Surg* [Am] 55:525–534.

97. Whitecloud TS, LaRocca H (1976): Fibular strut graft in reconstructive surgery of the cervical spine. *Spine* 1:33–43.

98. Whitehill R, Barry JC (1985): The evolution of stability in cervical spinal constructs using either autogenous bone graft or methylmethacrylate cement: A follow-up report on a canine *in vivo* model. *Spine* 10:32–41.

99. Yasouka S, Peterson HA, Laws ER, MacCarty CS (1981): Pathogenesis and prophylaxis of postlaminectomy deformity of the spine after multiple level laminectomy: Difference between children and adults. *Neurosurgery* 9:145–152.

100. Yasouka S, Peterson HA, MacCarty CS (1982): Incidence of spinal column deformity after multilevel laminectomy in children and adults. *J Neurosurg* 57:441–445.

101. Zdeblick TA, Bohlman HH (1989): Myelopathy, cervical kyphosis and treatment by anterior carpectomy and strut grafting. *J Bone Joint Surg* [Am] 71:170–182.

102. Zdeblick TA, Zou D, Warden KE (1989): Cervical stability following foraminotomy: A biomechanical *in vitro* analysis (abs). Presented at the 17th Annual Meeting of the Cervical Spine Research Society, New Orleans.

PART V

Thoracic and Thoracolumbar Spine

The Adult Spine: Principles and Practice,
J. W. Frymoyer, Editor-in-Chief.
Raven Press, Ltd., New York © 1991.

CHAPTER 60

Surgical Approaches to the Thoracic and Thoracolumbar Spine

John P. Kostuik

The selection of approach to the thoracic and thoracolumbar spine is determined by the aim of the operative procedure and the location of the vertebral elements to be accessed. Three general methods are available:

1. *Transthoracic:* The transthoracic approach may be transpleural or retropleural. Both allow good access to the vertebral body, including the pedicle nearest to the operator, but access is poor to the opposite vertebral pedicle (Fig. 1).
2. *Posterior:* These approaches are used to access the vertebral arch and are most appropriate for laminectomies and posterior or posterolateral fusions. However, it may be possible to visualize the lateral or even anterior part of the spine in scoliotic deformities, depending on the degree of rotation.
3. *Posterolateral:* These include costotransversectomy

or an extensile posterior approach, which can be made bilaterally or unilaterally.

If the pathology involves the cervical as well as the thoracic spine, four basic strategies are available: (a) posterior approaches, (b) approaches anterior to the sternomastoid, (c) cervicosternotomy, and (d) transpleural axillary thoracotomy.

Approaches to the thoracolumbar spine include posterior and anterolateral approaches. The posterior approaches are simple and well known, and are usually indicated for procedures such as laminectomies and posterior or posterolateral fusions. Anterolateral approaches may be retroperitoneal, transpleural retroperitoneal, or transpleural transdiaphragmatic retroperitoneal. The last approach is the most extensive.

Thoracolumbar approaches may, of course, be extended to involve the entire lumbar spine. Indeed, the entire thoracolumbar spine can be accessed through a thoracoabdominal approach.

In addition to the cervical-thoracic, thoracic, thoracolumbar, or lumbar approach, approaches may be performed in combination, such as a combined posterior and anterior, or anterolateral approach. These proce-

J. P. Kostuik, M.D., F.R.C.S.(C): Professor of Orthopaedics, University of Toronto, Toronto, Ontario; Director, Spinal Surgery; Director, Biomechanics Laboratory, The Toronto Hospital, Toronto, Ontario, M5G 2C4.

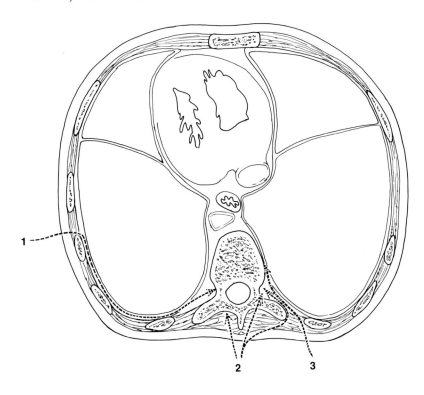

FIG. 1. Possible approaches to the thoracic spine. 1: Transthoracic. 2: Posterior or extended posterior. 3: Posterolateral (costotransversectomy).

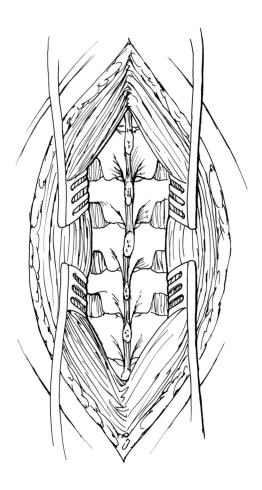

FIG. 2. Exposure is extended laterally to include the transverse processes.

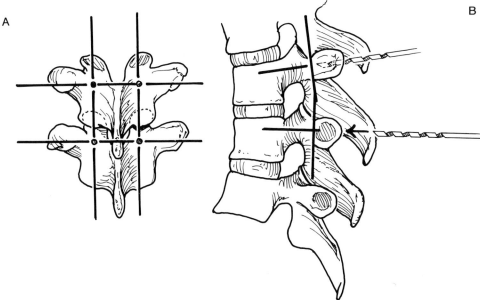

FIG. 3. Localization of the pedicular holes in the thoracic spine. **A:** Posterior view. **B:** Lateral view.

dures are usually reserved for patients requiring an osteotomy or for primary malignant tumors.

POSTERIOR APPROACHES TO THE CERVICAL-THORACIC, THORACIC, AND THORACOLUMBAR SPINE

The indications for posterior approaches are laminectomy and fusions, with or without instrumentation. These incisions are straightforward, because of the superficial presentation of the spinous processes. The patient is placed in the prone position usually on a frame, which allows the abdomen and thorax to be free from pressure. The anterosuperior aspect of the iliac crest is carefully protected, since the lateral cutaneous nerve of the thigh is vulnerable and neuralgia resulting in parasthetica may be a problem post-operatively. Fortunately, this complication is usually transitory in nature. The positioning of the head is determined by the anesthetist, but usually a headrest is preferred.

Prior to the injection of hypotensive agents, I prefer to score the skin with a scalpel. Then I infiltrate the skin and underlying musculature with a weak solution comprising 1 cc of 1/1,000 adrenaline and 500 cc of normal saline. If the patient is under the age of 50, hypotensive anesthesia, which maintains upper systolic blood pressure between 80 and 90 mmHg, is used as another means to control bleeding, provided there are no medical contraindications. The fascia typically is incised in line with

the skin incision, and the spinous processes and lamina exposed by subperiosteal dissection.

In contrast to the lumbar spine, the lamina of the thoracic spine run obliquely. When using the periosteal elevator to remove soft tissues, this anatomic perspective must be kept in mind in order to decrease bleeding (Fig. 2). Care must be taken to cauterize the small artery that appears between the transverse processes as the soft tissues are dissected from these structures.

Instrumentation is common as part of the posterior surgery. The pedicle has received increasing attention with the growing popularity of pedicle screw fixation. Pre-operative radiographs, including computerized axial scans, provide information regarding pedicle orientation. Anatomical variations of thoracic pedicles are minor when compared to the diversities encountered in the lumbar spine. The structure is ideally located in the upper corner of the outer inferior quadrant to two bisecting lines (Figs. 3A and 3B). These lines run from the midpoint of the transverse process horizontally and are intersected by a vertical line that passes through the center of the facet joints. A drill or awl may be inserted at this point.

The drill point or awl must be angled no more than five degrees medially, while angulation in the sagittal plane depends on an analysis of the lateral radiograph. Also, the pedicle is closer to the superior aspect of the vertebral body in the thoracic spine, in comparison to the thoracolumbar spine. It is useful to obtain a lateral radiograph on the operating table, since the sagittal angle may change when the patient is positioned supine.

Extended Posterior Approach

This approach is used primarily for tumors. It gives access to the entire spine, including the contents of the spinal canal; allows for the combined exposure of both the posterior and anterior structures of the spine; and may be unilateral or bilateral. Total vertebrectomies can be performed in the thoracic spine with one procedure. Because the approach is so extensive, the risk of neurological damage is high from direct damage to neurostructures or interruption of the blood supply in the watershed area of the thoracic spine (Fig. 4).

The patient is placed in the prone position on a frame to prevent compression of the thoracic and abdominal contents. A midline posterior incision is used to permit complete visualization of the posterior vertebral arch and the posterior aspect of the ribs for at least 5 cm. The incision must be three to four levels proximal and distal to the area of resection in order to allow sufficient retraction. In some cases, exposure is facilitated by dividing the paravertebral muscles transversely.

A complete laminectomy of the desired number of vertebral levels is performed (Figs. 5, 6A, and 6B), thus permitting the spinal canal and its contents to be visualized. The ribs are divided 3 cm lateral to the costotransverse joints. The neurovascular pedicles may or may not be ligated. Usually, a minimum of three levels is necessary. The posterior mediastinum can then be entered. Ideally, resection of the ribs is done extrapleurally, but in most adults the pleura is very thin and tenuous. It is common for an intrapleural approach to result in a pneumothorax necessitating insertion of a chest tube at the completion of the procedure. The articular processes and the pedicles are resected. The posterior mediastinal structures are swept away from the vertebral body, preferably by hand with the use of swabs (Figs. 7A and 7B). Mobilizing the vascular structures requires the segmental vessels to be ligated. A malleable retractor is inserted

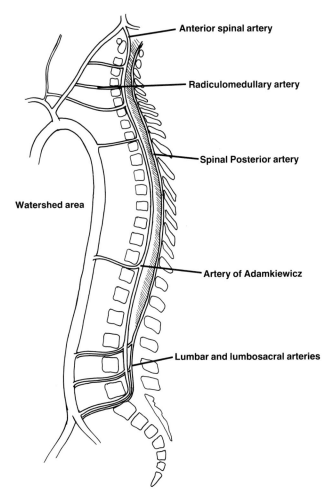

FIG. 4. Blood supply to the spinal cord.

to protect and displace the anterior structures (Fig. 8). The vertebral bodies are excised, generally through the disc space above and below the pathology. Less blood loss usually occurs with this procedure, but the length of resection is greater. Alternatively, vertebral bodies may be sectioned with a Gigli saw, starting anteriorly and ex-

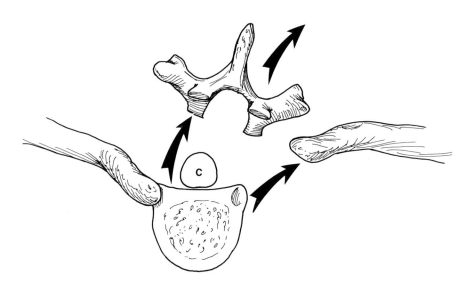

FIG. 5. Bilateral laminectomy and resection of transverse processes, pedicles, and one rib (C, spinal cord).

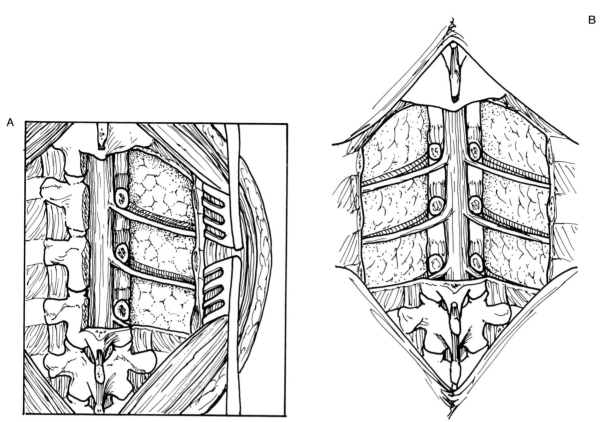

FIG. 6. A: Resection of three ribs allows the posterior mediastinum to be approached. **B:** Completion of laminectomy, bilateral costotransversectomy, and pedicular resection.

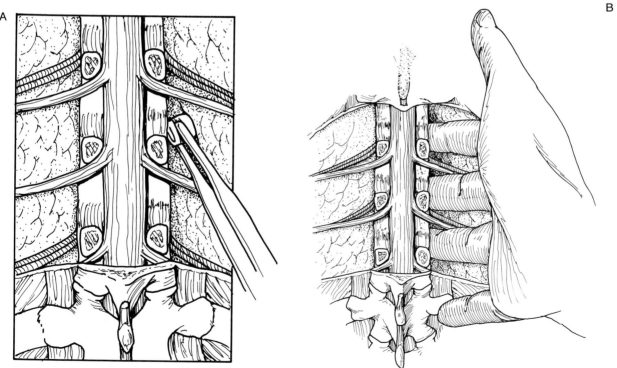

FIG. 7. A: The posterior mediastinum is separated from the vertebral body with a swab mounted on a forceps and then with fingers. **B:** Anterior pleural dissection on either side of the vertebral bodies is carried out using fingers (1-2).

tending through vertebral bodies, from anterior to posterior, through the anterior two thirds of the vertebral body. The osteotomy is then completed in the remaining posterior one third of the vertebral body from either side with a thin osteotome. The posterior longitudinal ligament is then easily cut with a knife (Figs. 9A, 9B, and 10).

Prior to this anterior resection, the posterior part of the spine should be stabilized. Otherwise, the spine is temporarily completely destabilized and at even greater risk of neurological compromise (Fig. 11). Following resection of the vertebral bodies, posterior stabilization and grafting can be added. The extended posterior approach is often long, laborious, and tedious, and must be done with great care (Fig. 12).

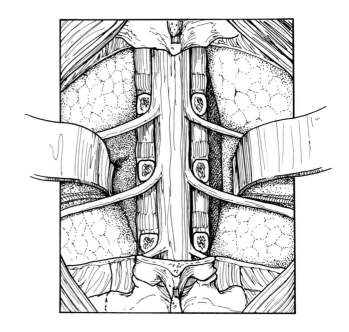

FIG. 8. The pleura and lungs are retracted anteriorly with malleable retractors.

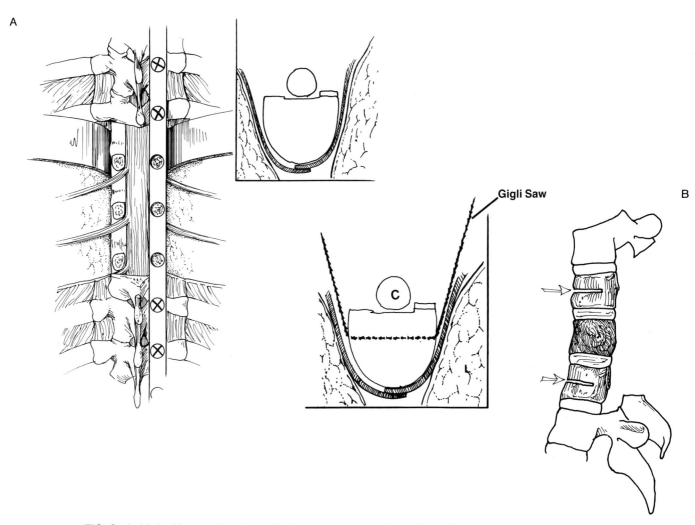

FIG. 9. A: Malleable retractors to protect posterior mediastinum. **B:** Partial anterior vertebral body section with Gigli saw (C, cord).

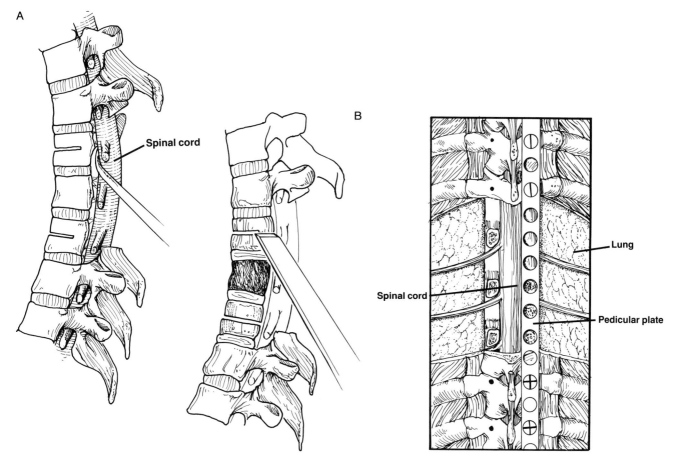

FIG. 10. A: The dura is dissected from posterior vertebral body. **B:** Transverse posterior vertebral body wall osteotomy using fine osteotomies is done to join the Gigli saw vertebral section.

FIG. 11. Provisional pedicular plate stabilization.

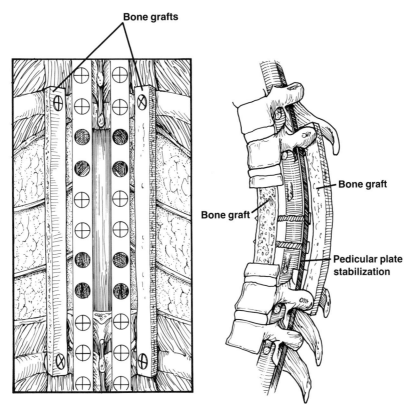

FIG. 12. Posterior stabilization, anterior reconstruction, and lateral grafts.

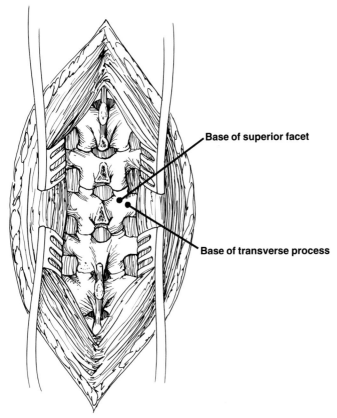

FIG. 13. Point of entry into the pedicle at the lumbar level.

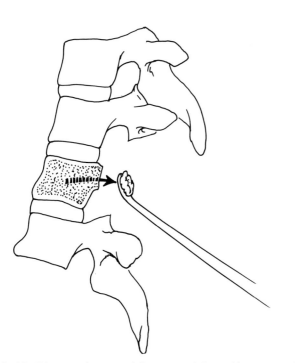

FIG. 14. Biopsy using a straight curette followed by a curved curette. This vertebral body may be evacuated producing an "eggshell" as described by Heinig.

Eggshell Procedure

Heinig has described an alternative extended posterior approach for the treatment of sharp angular kyphotic or kyphoscoliotic deformities that may be performed at one or more levels (personal communication) (see Chapter 88). This technique is termed the "eggshell procedure." The posterior incision is the same as described for the standard posterior approach to the thoracic spine. The ribs do not need to be exposed. After exposure of the posterior arch, the spinous processes in the area are removed. The laminae are thinned down, or may be removed. The pedicle is located bilaterally at the levels of interest and evacuated with the aid of small curettes. Angled curettes are used to remove the cancellous bone of the vertebral body to the limits of the anterior and posterior cortex of the vertebral body (Figs. 13 and 14). Following this maneuver, the posterior shell of the vertebral body is removed together with the pedicles if necessary. Posterior laminar elements are thinned out but may be preserved to protect the contents of the dural sac. After removal of the posterior aspect of the vertebral body, the spine is malleable, and correction of the deformity may be carried out with the various forms of instrumentation.

POSTEROLATERAL APPROACHES

Costotransversectomy

The costotransversectomy provides access to the lateral aspect of the vertebral bodies and to the posterior elements. If the approach is extended, the anterior part of the vertebral bodies can also be accessed. It is particularly valuable in the upper thoracic spine, where access to the vertebral bodies may be difficult by a more conventional anterior approach. Traditionally, the costotransversectomy has been used for evacuation of tuberculous abscesses of the thoracic spine. Usually, the approach is extrapleural, but it need not be.

The patient is placed in a lateral position with an axillary roll padding the contralateral side to avoid compression of the neurovascular structures. The rib to be excised is determined by the pathology. Proximal to T7, the incision is made posteriorly in a straight line midway between the vertebral border of the scapula and the spinous processes. This selection of incision depends to some degree on the extent of exposure to the posterior elements required. As an alternative, the skin incision may be made in line directly over the spinous processes. When this incision is done, the paravertebral muscles need to be divided horizontally. In the upper thoracic spine, tumor resections may require mobilization of the entire scapula. This maneuver will allow a complete approach to the cervical thoracic spine.

Between T7 and T10, the longitudinal part of the incision usually lies at the lateral quarter of the vertebral

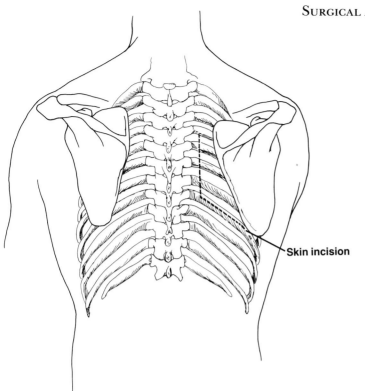

FIG. 15. Position of the patient and skin incision.

Skin incision

muscles. The distal limb of the incision is slightly oblique and follows the rib to be approached (Fig. 15).

During mobilization of the scapula for more proximal lesions of the thoracic spine, the trapezius and rhomboid muscles are divided. The lateral border of the trapezius and the medial border of the latissimus dorsi are also cut. The ribs then come into view. The paravertebral muscles are lifted and retracted to expose the costotransverse joints and transverse processes; alternatively, these muscles may be divided. The approach may be extrapleural, dividing the periosteum of the rib longitudinally, or an intrapleural violation may occur. The rib is cut at a distance of approximately 8 cm from the costotransverse joint to permit easy access. The ligaments of the costotransverse joint are then released. The pleura is usually protected anteriorly prior to cutting the rib. The anterior ligaments of the costovertebral joint are cut and the rib is removed completely. Alternatively, the rib may be released at its neck rather than through its ligamentous attachments (Figs. 16 and 17), followed by removal of the stump of the main rib. The approach may be enlarged by removing adjacent ribs. Intercostal vascular pedicles may be ligated if necessary, but should be preserved if possible (Fig. 18). Access to the intervertebral foramina is facilitated by removal of the transverse process. The pleura and lung should be protected by use of malleable retractors (Fig. 19). The posterior mediastinum is opened and the lateral surface of the vertebral bodies is exposed. The approach on the vertebral bodies may be extended above and below. A one- or two-rib costotransversectomy permits two and sometimes three vertebrae to be accessed (Fig. 20). Greater exposure may be obtained by resection of more of the chest wall, particularly for the resection of larger tumors.

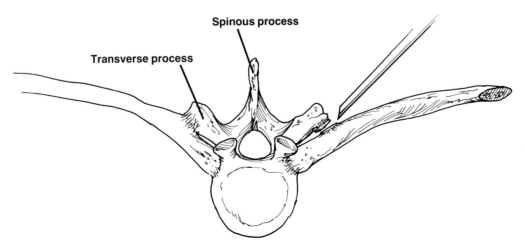

Spinous process

Transverse process

FIG. 16. Division of the posterior costotransverse ligaments is made under direct vision.

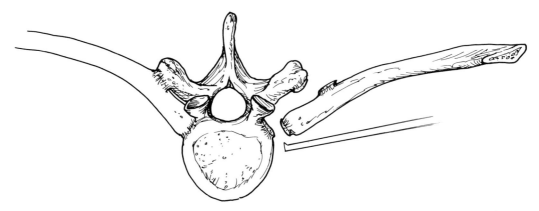

FIG. 17. The anterior costotransverse ligament is shown divided.

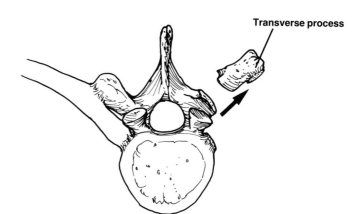

FIG. 18. Division of the transverse process is not usually done.

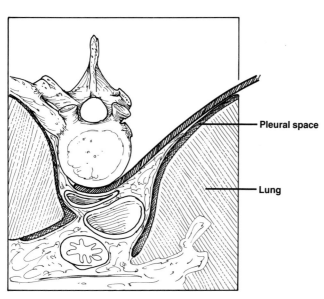

FIG. 19. The pleura and lung are retracted.

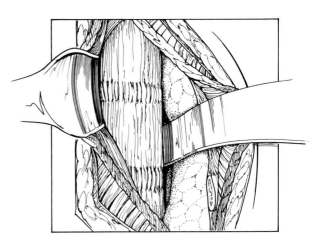

FIG. 20. Access to the lateral aspect of one, two, or three vertebral bodies is possible.

ANTERIOR APPROACHES TO THE THORACIC AND THORACOLUMBAR SPINE

Via the Sternomastoid

The first thoracic vertebra and the T1-T2 disc can be reached through a standard anterior approach to the cervical spine (see Chapter 47). Resection of the body of T2 or correction of deformity to the T1-T2 level is, however, difficult (Fig. 21). The T1-T2 levels can also be reached through an upper thoracic thoracotomy, particularly through the third rib.

In the anterior sternomastoid approach, hyperextension of the neck, if not contraindicated, aids in the exposure. Intra-operative radiographic confirmation is difficult to obtain, and it may be necessary to apply traction to the shoulders in order to obtain satisfactory views.

The approach is through a vertical incision anterior to the medial border of the sternomastoid muscle, which, if possible, is made from the left side in order to prevent damage to recurrent laryngeal nerves. The omohyoid and inferior thyroid vascular pedicle are divided. Exposure may be difficult and significant retraction necessary. Danger to the great vessels, particularly the innominate artery and especially the vein, must be considered.

Cervical Sternotomy

The lower cervical and upper three thoracic vertebrae levels may be accessed through a cervical sternotomy. Again, it is preferable to use the left side to avoid damage to recurrent laryngeal nerves. The head is, therefore, rotated to the right.

A vertical incision is made (Fig. 22) anterior to the sternomastoid, then distally towards the jugular notch and the xiphoid-sternum. The brachiocephalic vein at the upper border of the manubrium sterni is ligated. The innominate veins can be well visualized. The sternum is divided by an oscillating saw, usually proximal to distal along its entire length. The sternum is retracted after coating the bone edges with wax to decrease bleeding. The pericardium and costomediastinal pleural recesses are separated. The esophagus and trachea are retracted anteriorly to the right, and the common carotid artery posteriorly to the left. The best exposure may be obtained by ligation of the left brachiocephalic vein. Care must be taken to avoid vascular damage (Fig. 23). Mobilization of the esophagus and trachea with displacement to the right will allow exposure of the thoracic spine to the third thoracic level.

Partial division of the sternum can achieve the same exposure. In this case, the sternum is longitudinally osteotomized to the third or fourth intercostal level, where it is divided transversely. This approach is rarely used, but may assist in tumor excision at the cervicothoracic junction or correction of deformity at this level. Again,

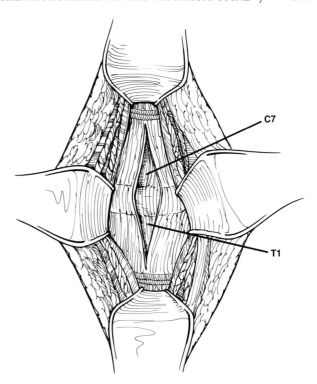

FIG. 21. Cervicothoracic lordosis limits access distal to T1. Exposure of T1 is relatively easy though the wound is deep.

dangers lie in possible damage to the vascular structures, particularly the innominate vein.

A disadvantage of both these techniques is that sternotomy carries a relatively high risk for infection or dehiscence.

An anterior approach to the upper thoracic spine in which the medial portion of one clavicle and part of the manubrium sterni are excised has also been described. A left-sided approach is preferred in order to decrease the risk of damage to the recurrent laryngeal nerves.

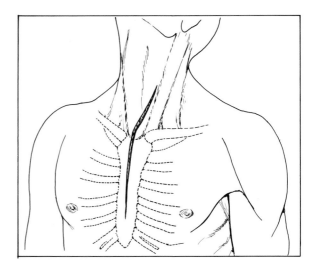

FIG. 22. Cervical sternotomy. The approach is anterior to the sternomastoid and is extended distally by a vertical midline sternal incision.

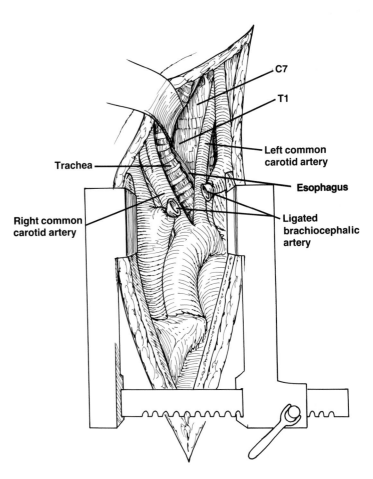

FIG. 23. The left common carotid lies laterally. The trachea and esophagus are identified with the finger and are retracted medially and anteriorly to expose the spine. The arch of the aorta and the left brachiocephalic (innominate) vein are in the lower part of the wound. Ligation of the brachiocephalic vein increases exposure but is not essential. A thorough knowledge of the vasculature is important.

Transpleural Axillary Thoracotomy

This approach has been used for resection of cervical ribs in thoracic outlet syndromes. It may be used for unusual conditions affecting the cervical-thoracic or upper thoracic spine. However, the exposure is difficult because of the depth of the wound.

When this approach is used to access the spine, it is preferable for patients to lie on the left side, where the aorta and thoracic duct are more prominent. The shoulder is in full abduction and is positioned in external rotation with the patient's hand behind the neck; this position opens the axilla. The upper extremity on the side to be operated on must be prepared and be mobile. The incision is carried from behind downward and forward along the intercostal space, usually the third space. The incision averages about 15 cm in length and lies between the latissimus dorsi posteriorly and pectoralis major anteriorly. It may be extended into the submammary crease. In retracting the latissimus dorsi, care must be taken to avoid injury to the long thoracic nerve of Bell and the nerves of the latissimus dorsi. For greater exposure, the inferior portion of the pectoralis major may be released (Fig. 24). The chest may be opened along the upper border of the fourth rib. If the pleura is opened and the chest entered, the apex of the lung is retracted distally to reveal the costovertebral region. The mediastinal pleura is then divided and the intercostal vessel and

esophagus retracted anteriorly. Closure is achieved by approximation of the ribs.

TRANSTHORACIC APPROACHES

The thoracic spine from T2 to T12 may be exposed through a transthoracic approach. These approaches are used for a variety of reasons such as biopsy, anterior spinal cord decompression and instrumentation, spinal osteotomy, correction of kyphosis, correction of scoliosis, vertebral body resection and reconstruction for tumor or infection, and anterior interbody fusion. The approaches are simple; however, for the uninitiated, the assistance of an experienced cardiovascular or thoracic surgeon may be necessary.

Many surgeons prefer a retropleural rather than a transpleural approach, but I have found that in adults, the pleura frequently becomes torn. Nor do I feel that a transpleural approach is more traumatic or requires more post-operative care.

Transpleural Approach

I prefer to approach the patient from the left side. Release of segmental vessels at the midpoint of the vertebral body allows the great vessels (aorta, inferior vena cava, azygos system) to fall away from the spine. The aorta

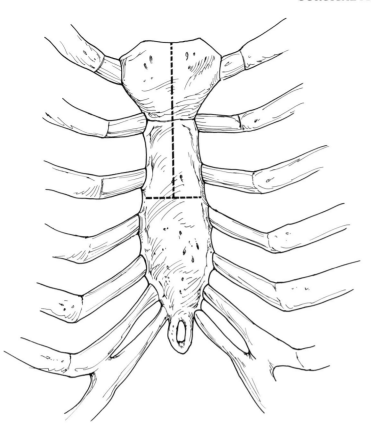

FIG. 24. A variation of vertical division of the sternum is possible. The sternal division stops at the level of the third or fourth intercostal space where the sternum is divided transversely.

protects the more fragile venous structures. Some surgeons prefer to approach the thoracic and lumbar spine from the right-hand side, unless pathology dictates otherwise, especially when internal fixation devices are to be used (Fig. 25). They feel that the proximity of internal fixation devices to arterial structures may result in traumatic aneurysms. Indeed, the Dunn device on the left-hand side did cause aneurysms in a number of cases, although none in its inventor's hands (see Chapters 61 and 93). In over 500 cases of anterior instrumentation of the spine, I have not encountered this complication from an internal fixation device inserted from the left side. Release of two segmental vessels proximally and, if possible, distal to the site of insertion of the internal fixation devices allows the great vessels to fall away to the opposite side. However, care must be taken not to place internal fixation devices directly anterior. Whenever possible, an anterolateral placement of internal fixation devices is preferred. As part of this procedure, venules and arterioles may be cauterized and intermediate vessels clipped, while larger vessels are preferably tied off, since the release of a clip may result in significant blood loss.

The patient is placed on his side. Ideally, he is positioned over a break in the table to allow the table position to be manipulated if necessary to improve exposure or correct deformity. An axillary roll is used to prevent damage on the down side. The upper extremity on the side of the surgical approach may be draped free or out of the field (Fig. 26). Selective bronchial intubation may

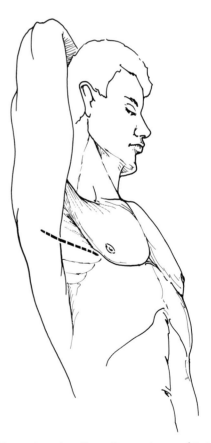

FIG. 25. Transpleural axillary thoracotomy. An approach from the right is preferable. The shoulder is in full abduction with the patient's hand behind the head and neck. The incision is oblique from behind downward and forward along the third intercostal space over a length of 15 cm.

allow for collapse of the lung on the ipsilateral side, permitting a clearer field (Fig. 27).

The level of the incision depends on the vertebra to be reached. Ideally, the incision should be two ribs above the vertebral lesion, but this depends to some degree on the obliquity of the ribs. The incision usually runs from the lateral border of the vertebral muscles to as far anterior as necessary. The muscles are divided, preferably with cutting diathermy. The rib is removed, usually subperiosteally, and saved for grafting (Fig. 28). Thoracotomy may be done without rib resection, but excision of the ribs gives better exposure. The latissimus dorsi and the lateral part of the trapezius muscle or the rhomboids in the upper approach may be divided, but it is rarely necessary to cut the rhomboids.

I have been able to expose entire thoracic spines from T1 down to the diaphragm through the fifth rib if necessary. This is relatively easily achieved in short patients. In taller patients, exposure of the entire thoracic spine may require two incisions, one through the fourth rib and one through the eleventh rib. With the lung selectively deflated, exposure of the spine is easy. If the lung remains inflated, it may need to be retracted out of the field.

The mediastinal pleura is excised, exposing the intercostal vessels, which are usually easily visualized, depending on the amount of fat present (Fig. 29). The intercostal vessels should be ligated or clipped in the midpoint of the spine (Fig. 30). Large veins are preferably ligated, or locking clips may be applied. The vertebral bodies are exposed either subperiosteally or extraperiosteally. The periosteum becomes adherent to the annulus of the disc at each disc level and results in more difficult exposure. Subperiosteal dissection will result in greater earlier blood loss, but may be preferable at the time of closure (Fig. 31). The neurovascular intercostal bundle is vulnerable and is often coagulated.

At the time of closure, the mediastinal pleura is

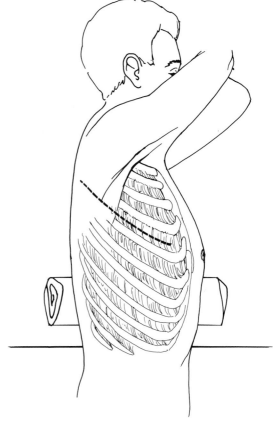

FIG. 26. Rib incision is usually two levels proximal to the vertebral body to be approached.

usually left open, as it is thin and often difficult to approximate, but this is not usually an important concern (Figs. 32 and 33). A large chest tube is necessary to evacuate the post-operative accumulations of fluid. It is not necessary to have an airtight pleural closure in a transpleural approach, as the muscles become rapidly repleuralized.

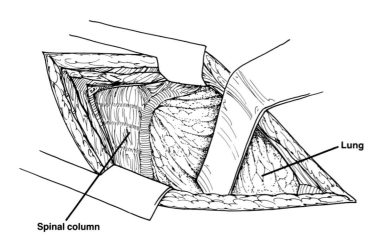

FIG. 27. The retracted lung allows visualization of the spine. It is helpful if the anesthesiologist collapses the ipsilateral lung.

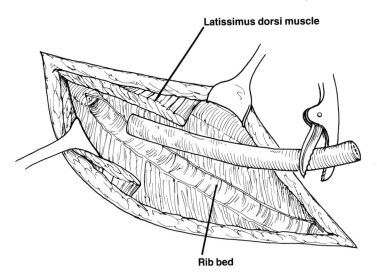

FIG. 28. Resection of the rib is helpful in adults with a rigid thorax.

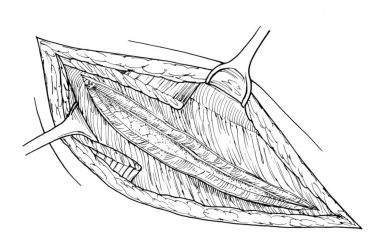

FIG. 29. The pleura is opened in the bed of the rib.

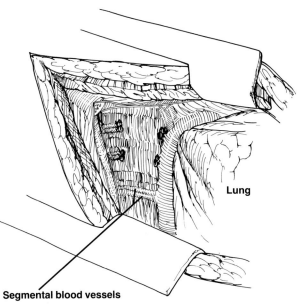

FIG. 30. The segmental vessels are ligated in the midline. The pleural foramina must be avoided in order not to interfere with the blood supply to the spinal cord.

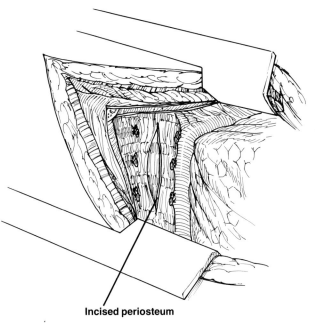

FIG. 31. The periosteum may be incised with cutting diathermy after ligation of the vascular pedicles (subperiosteal dissection).

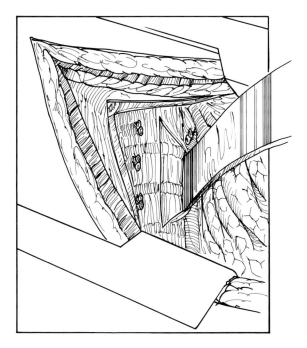

FIG. 32. A malleable retractor is placed on the opposite side of the vertebral body to protect structures on that side from damage.

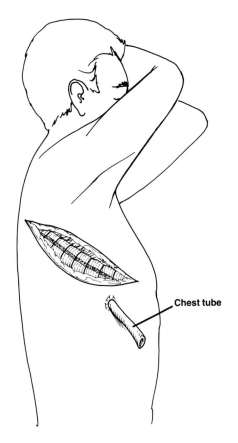

Chest tube

FIG. 33. Closure is obtained by bringing the adjacent ribs together with sutures. Drainage of the thoracic cavity is essential. The chest tube emerges in line with the mid-axillary line.

Retropleural Approach

This approach is similar to the transpleural approach and is generally performed one rib proximal to the involved vertebra. The rib is exposed subperiosteally and resected. The parietal pleura is then separated from the rib and muscle layers with fingers or swabs (Figs. 34 and 35). This is best started posteriorly at the posterior mediastinum. Resection of the head and neck of rib helps at this point. At the lateral part of the thoracic wall the pleura is more adherent. If the pleura is torn a transpleural approach may be made, or the pleura can be closed and an extrapleural dissection continued. It is not necessary to open the parietal pleura as the vertebral bodies are approached. The intercostal vessels in the plane of dissection can be ligated easily. An intercostal nerve often serves as a guide to the intravertebral foramina. However, care must be taken to avoid coagulation of these vessels near any of the foramina so as not to damage the blood supply to the spinal cord, particularly in the watershed area.

When a more limited access to the spine is desired, e.g., thoracic disc, the rib excised is dictated by the pathology. The rib that lies directly horizontal to the vertebral level at the mid auxiliary line of the anteroposterior chest x-ray is usually chosen. The rib removed must be proximal to the lesion and provide adequate exposure while working down on the lesion. For example, the eighth rib is resected for a T7-T8 disc. In the thoracic spine, the disc is the most prominent anterior structure. It is soft and white and relatively avascular and provides a safe area for dissection. The intercostal vessels cross the mid portion of each vertebral body. Because the disc is raised, the intercostal vessels at each level are easily delineated. If the segmental vessels are cut in the midline over the vertebral body, damage to the spinal cord blood supply will not be a problem. Coagulation in the intervertebral foramina must be avoided. The thoracic duct usually passes from right to left in the T4-T5 area. The sympathetic chain should be preserved, but interruption is not of major consequence, except in the upper thoracic spine, where disruption may result in a Horner's syndrome. Resection of the rib may be necessary to gain access to the posterior disc in the spinal canal in decompressive procedures. For greater exposure of a vertebral body, the discs above and below are resected, allowing for identification of the posterior vertebral body wall and the canal.

ANTEROLATERAL APPROACHES TO THE THORACOLUMBAR SPINE

Two anterolateral approaches are available, and the choice depends on the required exposure (Fig. 36). Generally, a transpleural retroperitoneal approach will allow for full access at all levels. In this approach, I prefer to

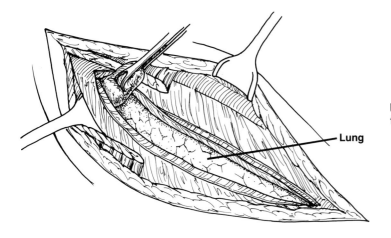

FIG. 34. Separation of the parietal pleura begins in the posterior mediastinum.

Lung

incise and detach the diaphragm from the chest wall.

A retropleural retroperitoneal approach gives limited access to only the lower thoracic spine from T10 distally, and exposure to the sacrum may be difficult. Some surgeons prefer a transpleural retroperitoneal approach in which the diaphragm is incised but not detached. However, I use the more extensive transpleural diaphragmatic retroperitoneal approach in almost all cases.

For all three approaches—retropleural retroperitoneal, transpleural retroperitoneal, and the extended anterior transpleural transdiaphragmatic retroperitoneal—the patient is usually positioned on the lateral side with an axillary roll under the contralateral axilla to avoid neurovascular compression of the contralateral upper extremity. I prefer to have the patient rolled slightly posteriorly at about 60 to 70 degrees. If radiographs are to be taken during the procedure, an adjustable radiolucent table is necessary.

As an alternative position, the patient may be placed directly lateral. This is necessary if the spine will also be approached posteriorly, or if a corrective procedure, such as an osteotomy, is planned.

FIG. 35. The pleura is gradually pushed away.

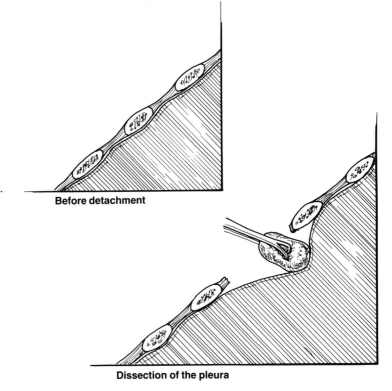

Before detachment

Dissection of the pleura

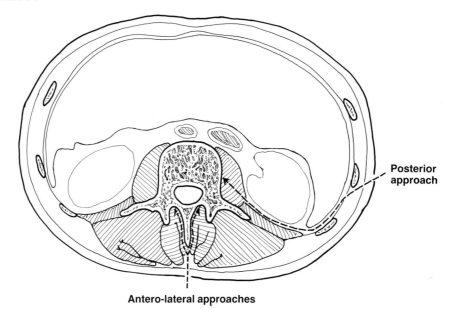

FIG. 36. Anterolateral approaches to the thoracolumbar spine, whether retropleural and retroperitoneal or transpleural, transdiaphragmatic, and retroperitoneal, give access to the vertebral bodies. An anterolateral approach gives exposure to T11, T12, and L1 and is not extensive. The classical posterior approach gives access to all vertebrae from T4 distally.

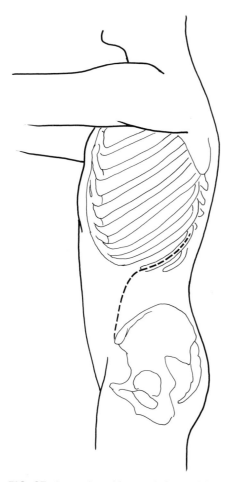

FIG. 37. Lateral position and skin incision.

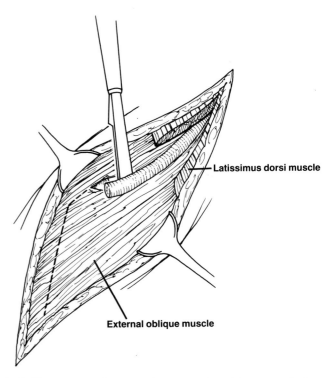

FIG. 38. Incision of the muscles, resection of the eleventh rib, and opening of the retroperitoneal space at the tip of the rib. If a more proximal rib is chosen, the distal ribs may have to be osteotomized in a transpleural, transdiaphragmatic, retroperitoneal approach.

Retropleural Retroperitoneal Approach

The incision is centered over the eleventh rib (Fig. 37). The twelfth rib may be resected or osteotomized. The incision extends from the lateral border of the paravertebral muscles, but generally aims anterior to the anterior/superior iliac spine, depending on the exposure required to the lumbar level. Musculature is preferably cut with cutting diathermy to decrease bleeding and improve hemostasis. The thoracic portion of the procedure is done first. The rib is located and the periosteum stripped. Care must be taken to remain extrapleural, which in older adults may be difficult. If the pleura is torn, it may be sewn or left open with subsequent insertion of a chest tube for drainage. The retroperitoneal space is entered by following the eleventh rib tip, which is usually detached and then split (Fig. 38). The diaphragm usually attaches to this cartilaginous tip. After osteotomy of the rib posteriorly, the approach passes anteriorly, dividing the musculature after stripping the periosteum from the ribs under the surface (Fig. 39).

Mobilization of the parietal pleura is preferably done

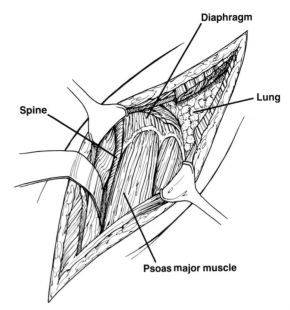

FIG. 39. Anatomical cross-section after removal of the peritoneum to show the relationship between lungs, diaphragm, crura, arcuate ligaments, and spine.

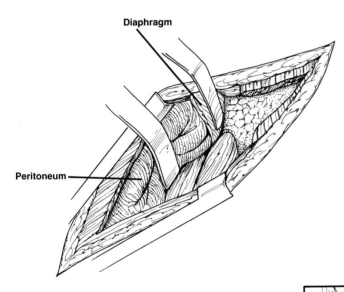

FIG. 40. Gradual mobilization of the peritoneal sac. The pleura above, the diaphragm centrally, and the peritoneum below are mobilized simultaneously en bloc.

FIG. 41. The release of the peripheral attachments of the diaphragm is achieved by manual traction and cutting diathermy.

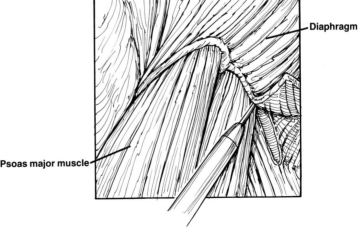

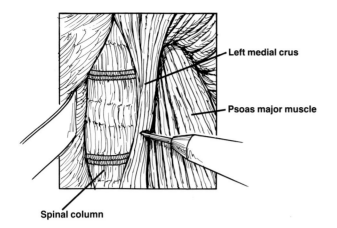

Left medial crus

Psoas major muscle

Spinal column

FIG. 42. Division of the fleshy body of the crus to permit its later reattachment. It should be tagged for reattachment.

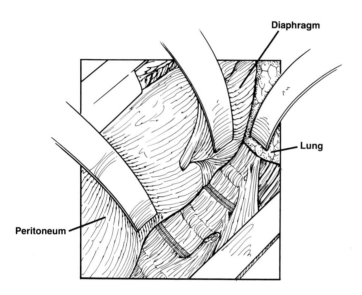

Diaphragm

Lung

Peritoneum

FIG. 43. The two viscera sacs and the diaphragm are retracted anteriorly to the spine and held by malleable retractors.

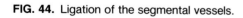

FIG. 44. Ligation of the segmental vessels.

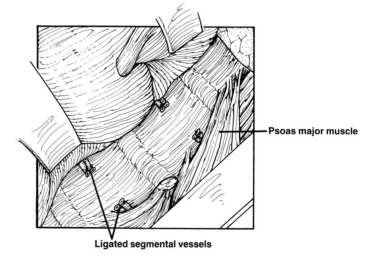

Psoas major muscle

Ligated segmental vessels

with blunt dissection using fingers or a sponge on a forcep. This begins anteriorly and progresses posteriorly. The pleura, diaphragm, and peritoneum are mobilized (Fig. 40). Following release of the diaphragm from the eleventh rib, mobilization continues posteriorly and through the twelfth rib and lateral arcuate ligament (Fig. 41). The medial attachment of the lateral arcuate ligament and the lateral attachment of the medial arcuate ligament are divided close to the tip of the transverse process of L1. Sufficient tissue must be left to reapproximate the diaphragm (Fig. 42).

The crus of the diaphragm is divided approximately 2 cm away from the vertebral body. Blood vessels in the midline may be ligated or clipped, but care must be taken to avoid coagulation near the foramina in order to prevent any damage to blood supply to the spinal cord. After division of the arcuate ligament, chest retractors are inserted. The viscera and diaphragm are retracted (Fig. 43). The parietal pleura is detached as far as T10. The pleura may be more adherent to the vertebral bodies in the area of the posterior mediastinum. The intercostal and lumbar vessels are ligated in the midline of the spine or close to the aorta as possible (Fig. 44). This maneuver allows the great vessels (aorta, inferior vena cava) to be displaced. With dissection, the pleura can be detached from the mediastinum to T10 (Fig. 45). It is preferable to mobilize the psoas to allow full exposure to the lumbar motion segments required. The psoas may be detached as far lateral as the pedicle. Care must be taken to avoid coagulation in the area of the intravertebral foramina.

Some authors prefer to incise the periosteum with cutting diathermy (Fig. 46) and subsequently expose the vertebral body with a periosteal elevator. I find that this method often results in excessive bleeding from the vertebral body.

A dissector may be inserted in the vertebral foramina

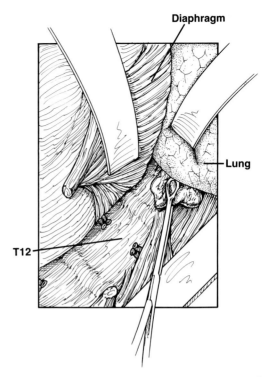

FIG. 45. Detachment of the mediastinal pleura can be extended proximally.

at the base of the pedicle if one wishes to gain access to the posterior vertebral wall (Fig. 47). I prefer to identify the root in the area of each foramina first. A preferable and, I believe, safer alternative is to approach the posterior wall of the vertebral body by excising the intervertebral disc. Dissection then may proceed proximally or distally. In the area of the thoracolumbar spine, the posterior longitudinal ligament is very thin and usually incised. Indeed, in burst fractures the posterior longitu-

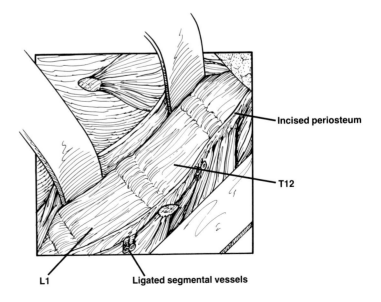

FIG. 46. After incision and elevation of the periosteum in a subperiosteal approach, malleable retractors are placed on the opposite side of the vertebral bodies protecting the viscera and great vessels.

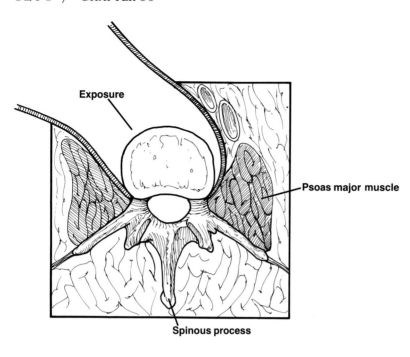

FIG. 47. A malleable retractor retracts and protects the opposite psoas and great vessels. The ipsilateral psoas is dissected off the vertebral body.

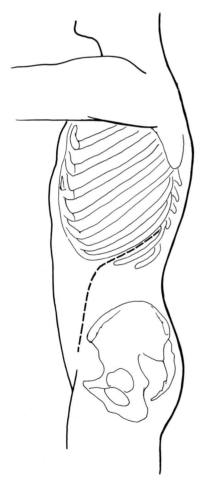

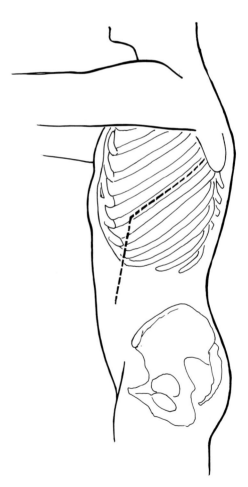

FIG. 48. Oblique incision of the intercostal space. It curves down onto the abdomen at the lateral border of the rectus abdominis to the level of the anterior superior iliac spine. The incision should be placed at least two levels proximal to the most proximal vertebral body chosen in the reconstructive process.

FIG. 49. Position of the patient and skin incision centered on the seventh rib giving access up to T7 and T8. Distal ribs are osteotomized.

dinal ligament may be torn.

The diaphragm at the closure is reattached by repairing the crus to the medial and lateral arcuate ligaments. The abdominal and chest walls are then closed in layers. The advantage of the retropleural retroperitoneal approach is that it is felt that post-operative care is easier. However, in my experience this has not necessarily been the case.

Transpleural Retroperitoneal Approach

In the transpleural retroperitoneal approach, considerable exposure is achieved by selective intubation of the lungs in order to allow collapse of the lung on the ipsilateral side. This is, however, not necessary—especially if exposure is at the lower part of the thoracic spine. Again, I prefer to do this exposure through the left side. The preferable rib to be excised is two levels proximal to the most proximal level of pathology to be dealt with. The incision begins posteriorly from the lateral border of the paravertebral muscles and continues on the length of the rib (Fig. 48). If there is a need to be proximal to the tenth or eleventh rib, I prefer to carry the incision anteriorly toward the costal margin and then osteotomize the distal

ribs (Fig. 49). The intercostal vessels require ligation in this more proximal approach in order to mobilize the chest wall. If the approach is through the tenth or eleventh rib, incision is carried to the mid axillary line by turning the incision distal towards the anterior/superior iliac crest and the lateral margin of the rectus abdominus.

In this approach I prefer to remove the rib and use it as graft, although occasionally the incision through the intercostal muscle may be carried out on the superior border of the rib. The rib is removed extraperiosteally and the pleura is opened. After careful division of the abdominal muscles the peritoneum is swept from under the transversalis muscle. The eleventh costal cartilage is divided at the junction of the retroperitoneal space and thoracotomy. Following this, the peritoneum and its contents are swept off the abdominal wall laterally and from the undersurface of the diaphragm. The diaphragm is then cut approximately 1 cm from the costal margin using cutting diathermy (Fig. 50). The vertebral bodies are approached as for the extrapleural extraperitoneal approach. Closure for the transpleural retroperitoneal transdiaphragmatic approach is performed in a standard manner with repair to the diaphragm. The retroperitoneal space is drained, as is the chest.

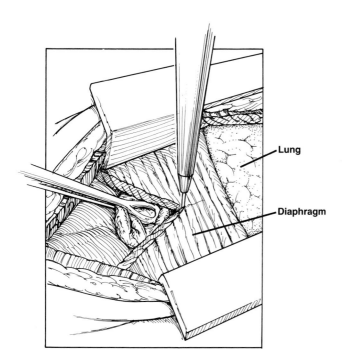

FIG. 50. Division of the periphery of the diaphragm under direct vision after retroperitoneal and transpleural exposure.

SUGGESTED READING

1. Bradford DS, Lonstein JE, Ogilvie JW, Winter RB (1987): *Moe's textbook of scoliosis and other spinal deformities, 2nd ed.* Philadelphia: W.B. Saunders, pp. 135–189.
2. Crenshaw AH (1987): *Campbell's operative orthopaedics, 7th ed.* St. Louis: Mosby, pp. 3091–3107.
3. Dwyer AF, Newton NC, Sherwood AA (1969): An anterior approach to scoliosis. *Clin Orthop* 62:192.
4. Freebody D, Bedall R, Taylor RD (1971): Anterior trauma transperitoneal lumbar fusion. *J Bone Joint Surg* [Br] 53:617–627.
5. Hall JE (1972): The anterior approach to spinal deformities. *Orthop Clin North Am* 3:81.
6. Harmon PH (1963): Anterior extraperitoneal lumbar disc excision and vertebral body fusion. *Clin Orthop* 16:169–198.
7. Hodgson AR et al. (1960): Anterior spinal fusion: The operative approach and pathological findings in 412 patients with Pott's disease of the spine. *Br J Surg* 58:172.
8. Hodgson AR, Yau AC (1964): Anterior approach to the spinal column. In: Appley, ed. *Recent advances in orthopaedics.* Baltimore: Williams and Wilkins, pp. 289–326.
9. Hoppenfeld S (1984): *Surgical exposures in orthopaedics.* Philadelphia: J.B. Lippincott, pp. 210–297.
10. Laurin CA, Riley LH, Roy-Camille R (1989): *Atlas of orthopaedic surgery, vol 1: General principles and spine.* Paris: Masson.
11. Riseborough EJ (1973): The anterior approach to the spine for the correction of deformity of the axial skeleton. *Clin Orthop* 93:207.
12. Watkins RG (1983): *Surgical approaches to the spine.* New York: Springer-Verlag.

Trauma of the Thoracolumbar Spine

The Adult Spine: Principles and Practice,
J. W. Frymoyer, Editor-in-Chief.
Raven Press, Ltd., New York © 1991.

CHAPTER 61

Thoracolumbar Spine Fracture

John P. Kostuik, Robert J. Huler, Stephen I. Esses, and E. Shannon Stauffer

Each year 162,000 Americans sustain a fracture of the vertebral column which leads to a physician visit or causes restriction of activity (87). The thoracolumbar spine is the predominant site for these injuries, and of these 4,700 result in paraplegia. Seventy-five percent occur in the age group 15 to 64, but the number of fractures occurring in elderly, osteoporotic females is probably significantly underestimated. Exclusive of osteoporosis, these injuries can be broadly categorized as follows: (a) stable fractures without neurologic injury, the majority of which go on uneventfully to healing and result in minimal long-term disability; (b) penetrating injuries, most commonly from gunshot wounds (see Chapter 40); (c) pathologic fractures associated with tumors and ankylosing spondylitis (see Chapters 36, 41, and 42); and (d)

high-energy trauma producing either stable or unstable injuries, with or without neurologic sequelae. It is this last group of patients who form the major focus for this chapter.

HISTORY

Although fractures of the thoracolumbar spine have been recognized for over 30 centuries, modern theories of reduction and stabilization can be traced to Lorenz Boehler (17) of Vienna, Austria, 60 years ago. He advocated postural reduction by hyperextending the spine and holding that position in an extension body cast. He also placed great emphasis on ambulation and rehabilitation exercises to strengthen the trunk muscle while fracture healing progressed. Before Boehler's publications, treatment had consisted of extended bed rest. If the patient had significant neurologic deficits, the usual outcome was death secondary to sepsis, pneumonia, or pressure sores. Indeed, prior to World War I, less than 10% of patients with neurologic injury survived.

Boehler's basic approach was furthered by two significant events during World War II, the availability of antibiotics and the establishment of specialized centers to provide comprehensive care for paralyzed soldiers and veterans. The National Spinal Injury Center was devel-

J. P. Kostuik, M.D., F.R.C.S.(C): Professor of Orthopaedics, University of Toronto; Director, Spinal Surgery; and Director, Biomechanics Laboratory, The Toronto Hospital, Toronto, Ontario, M5G 2C4.
R. J. Huler, M.D.: The Toronto Hospital, Toronto, Ontario, M5G 2C4.
S. I. Esses, M.D., F.R.C.S.: Assistant Professor, Department of Surgery, University of Toronto; Consultant, Dewar Spine Unit, The Toronto Hospital, Toronto, Ontario, M5G 2C4.
E. S. Stauffer, M.D., F.R.C.S.: Professor and Chairman, Division of Orthopaedics and Rehabilitation, Southern Illinois University School of Medicine, Springfield, Illinois, 62708.

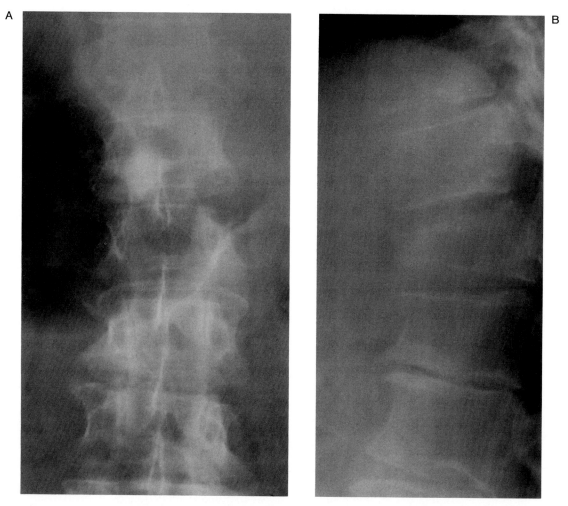

FIG. 1. A: Anteroposterior x-ray of a 56-year-old man demonstrating a burst fracture of T12 following a fall. **B:** Lateral x-ray reveals a fracture of T10 as well as the fracture of T12. (Figs. 1C-1D follow.)

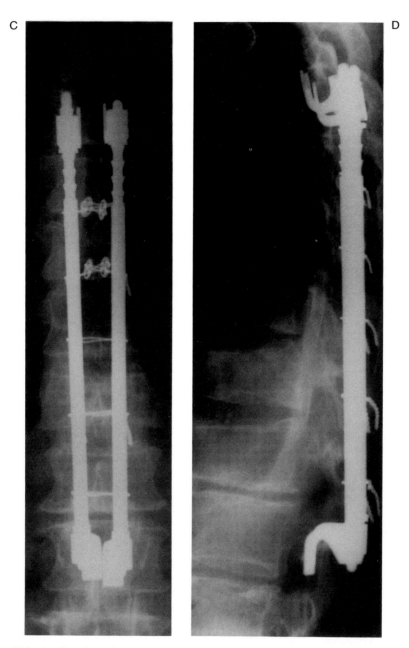

FIG. 1. *(Continued)* Post-operative x-rays **(C and D)** demonstrating dual Harrington rod system spanning T8-L2 with trans-spinous process wires through T11-T12 and L1 and Wisconsin button wires through T9 and T10.

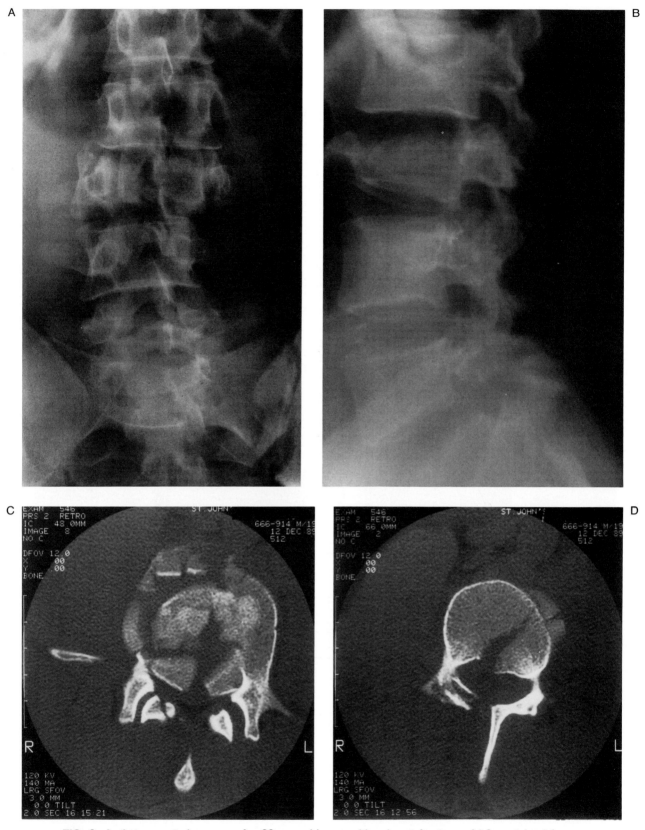

FIG. 2. A: Anteroposterior x-ray of a 20-year-old man with a burst fracture of L3 sustained from a 40-foot fall. **B:** Lateral x-ray shows a fracture of L2 posterior and middle columns as well as the burst fracture of L3. **C:** CT scan of L3. **D:** CT scan of L2. (Figs. 2E–2G follow.)

E

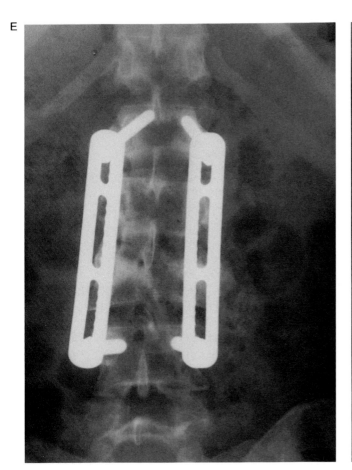

F

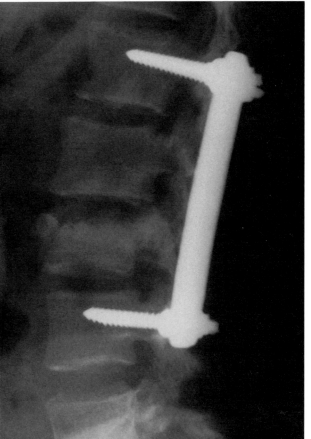

G

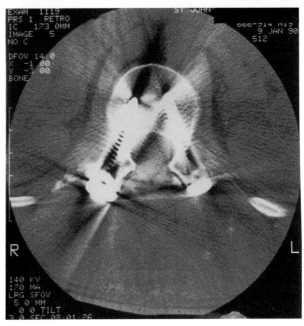

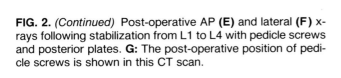

FIG. 2. *(Continued)* Post-operative AP **(E)** and lateral **(F)** x-rays following stabilization from L1 to L4 with pedicle screws and posterior plates. **G:** The post-operative position of pedicle screws is shown in this CT scan.

oped at Stokes Manville Hospital in England under the direction of Ludwig Guttman in anticipation of the casualties expected from the invasion of Europe by the allied forces. Soon thereafter, the United States Veterans Administration created several geographically dispersed centers for the care of paralyzed veterans. Both the English and American centers emphasized non-surgical care of the spinal fracture, strict nursing management to prevent complications, and comprehensive rehabilitation including exercise, vocational counseling, and community resettlement. Such centers have proven the value of aggressive, comprehensive care as measured by reduced societal costs, increased survival, and improved patient function.

After World War II, Guttman (91,93,94) continued to advocate postural reduction as the optimal treatment for thoracolumbar fractures. He rightfully emphasized the many complications of operative care which, at the time, was destabilizing laminectomy. Watson-Jones (212) further popularized extension cast management and early mobilization. Aggressive conservative management also was advocated by Bedbrook (10,11).

Despite the often favorable outcome of conservative management, dissatisfaction with non-operative care led Holdsworth (109,110) to advocate surgical stabilization with plates attached to the spinous processes. He thought such an approach prevented further neurologic damage, as well as allowed easier bed care by the nursing staff with less pain to the patients. However, 6 to 8 weeks of bed rest often were required because insufficient stability was provided by his surgical construct.

After achieving success with the management of scoliosis by distraction rods and laminar hooks, Harrington (57,102) extended his instrumentation to the treatment of spinal fractures and advocated a double-distraction rod technique to stabilize the fractured spine. His principles and techniques have been modified over the years but still serve as the standard method for surgical treatment of unstable fractures of the thoracolumbar spine (Fig. 1). In the past decade, newer methods of internal fixation have been developed, including pedicle fixation devices and anterior instrumentation.

Today, the management of spine fractures has some similarities and some significant differences compared to the management of long bone fractures. The shared principles are reduction, stabilization, promotion of fracture healing and joint motion, and early patient mobilization. The significant differences are that virtually all fractures of the spine involve multiple joints. Facet articular surfaces are fractured, facets are dislocated, and intervertebral discs are disrupted in many spinal fractures. Therefore, fracture healing alone is not sufficient for a full function restoration in some patients. Permanent stabilizing of disrupted joints, either by spontaneous interbody ankylosis, surgical fusion, or soft tissue healing, is the treatment goal. The ideal is to have the unstable fracture reduced to the anatomic position and the disrupted joints fused without involving normal joints above or below the injured segment. Sometimes this is not possible and several joints above and below have to be instrumented to achieve reduction and stabilization, as shown in Figure 1. However, newer instrumentation allows the surgeon to leave as many movable segments in the lumbar spine as possible (Fig. 2).

SPINAL STABILITY AND CLASSIFICATION OF SPINAL INJURIES

A useful classification of spinal fractures must be both simple and complete, reflect an understanding of the mechanisms of injury, correspond to the anatomic pathology, determine the treatment options, and be relevant to the prognosis. The criteria on which most classifications are based have been fracture stability and neurologic injury. However, there have been major difficulties in using only these two parameters. Stability represents a spectrum rather than an "all or none" phenomenon. In many instances it has not been possible to state that a spinal fracture was frankly unstable or stable (168,219,220). To further complicate classifications, the presence or absence of neurologic injury cannot, in and of itself, be used as a gauge of mechanical instability. There are many instances in which a stable fracture can be associated with neurologic injury, such as a nerve root injury after a transverse process fracture. Similarly, grossly unstable fractures may occur without neurologic deficits, particularly at the thoracolumbar junction and lumbar spine (187). Thus, the current classification schemes represent an evolution of thinking which has proceeded over many years.

Nicoll (157) proposed an anatomic classification and stressed the importance of distinguishing between stable and unstable injuries. He proposed that anterior and lateral wedge fractures were stable, and fracture subluxations and fracture dislocations were unstable. In his view, the major determinant of stability was the intraspinous ligaments. He further observed that laminar fractures above the level of L4 usually were stable, whereas those at L5 were often unstable. Although crude by today's standards, Nicoll's classification represented a significant advance and allowed early, aggressive mobilization of patients with stable injuries.

Holdsworth (109,110) departed from Nicoll by suggesting a mechanistic scheme for classification rather than one based on anatomy. He postulated multiple injury mechanisms including flexion, flexion and rotation, extension, or compression. As part of this classification, he stressed the importance of the entire posterior ligamentous complex consisting of intraspinous ligament, supraspinous ligament, and ligamentum flavum. Thus, he thought a flexion injury did not cause disruption of the posterior ligamentous complex and was stable. In comparison, a flexion-rotation injury caused disruption of these structures, rendering the spine unstable. Although extension forces could result in fractures of the posterior elements, the anterior spinal column remained intact, as did the ligamentous complex, and these also were classified as stable. However, Holdsworth recognized a frustrating dilemma in his assessment of compression injuries. Despite his classification of these injuries as stable, he acknowledged that major neurologic deficits and delayed recovery often occurred, suggesting mechanical insufficiency.

Bedbrook (9,10) recognized that often it was impossible to classify a fracture as stable or unstable, particularly in the acute phase after injury. He further demonstrated that disruption of the entire posterior ligamentous complex was not always synonymous with spinal instability. Additionally, he determined that instability could occur if the disc was disrupted and the anterior longitudinal ligaments stripped from the vertebral bodies. He stressed the need to recognize and document both the neural injury and the bony fracture pattern. His organized, comprehensive approach to the treatment of thoracolumbar injuries emphasized the importance of understanding the mechanisms by which trauma occurred, the neural pathology, and the associated bony and ligamentous injuries. The later developments in classification represent refinements of these concepts.

Whitesides (222) has characterized a stable spine as one that can withstand stress without progressive deformity or further neurologic damage. His approach is similar to that of White and Panjabi (219) who define clinical instability as "the loss of the ability of the spine under physiologic loads to maintain relationships between vertebrae in such a way that there is neither initial damage nor subsequent irritation to the spinal cord or nerve roots; and, in addition, there is no development of incapacitating deformity or pain due to structural changes."

These basic definitions have been furthered by biomechanical studies in the laboratory. For example, Posner et al. (168) tested functional spinal units in which individual components were sequentially transsected and the mechanical integrity of the segment was measured. These experiments were performed both from front to back and back to front, simulating flexion and extension injuries. In the flexion sequence, failure occurred when all the posterior components plus one anterior component had been destroyed. In the extension sequence, failure occurred when all of the anterior components plus two posterior components were disrupted. This basic work suggests that a simple two-column concept of the spine is inadequate to assess stability, and lends credence to a three-column conceptualization of the spine.

In addition to these basic studies to determine the anatomic determinants of stability, human cadaveric and calf spine models have been used to simulate the forces producing spinal destabilization, as well as the mechanical properties of surgical constructs (143,155,163,

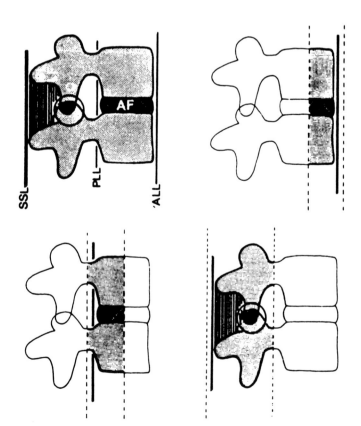

FIG. 3. Three columns of the spine (with permission from ref. 52).

204,205). Given the 6 degrees of freedom of the spine, these mechanisms include flexion, extension, axial compression, distraction, axial rotation, and shear (219). Anatomic studies and CT scans have further defined the three-column spine (52,140) which is conceptualized in Figure 3.

The anterior column is formed by the anterior one half of the vertebral body together with the anterior longitudinal ligament and anterior fibers of the annulus fibrosus. The middle column is formed by the posterior fibers of the annulus fibrosus together with the posterior wall of the vertebral body and posterior longitudinal ligaments. The posterior column is formed by the posterior ligamentous complex including the supraspinous and intraspinous ligaments, facet joint capsules, and ligamentum flavum, as well as the posterior bony arch.

Based on this anatomic description, Denis (52) identified four major types of spinal injuries: compression fractures, burst fractures, seatbelt injuries, and fracture-dislocations. He proposed that the key in distinguishing among these injuries is the middle column's mode of failure. In compression fractures the middle column is not injured and the fracture is stable. In burst fractures the middle column fails in compression and the injury is most likely unstable. In shearing injuries, such as seatbelt-related fractures, the middle column fails in distraction, whereas in fracture-dislocations the middle column fails in rotation or shear. These basic concepts form much of the basis for injury classification today.

In addition to the injury to individual motion segments, stability relates to anatomy of the thoracic, thoracolumbar, and lumbar spine, as well as to the presence or absence of neurologic injury.

Stability of Different Anatomic Areas

Fractures from T1 to T9 have inherently greater stability than fractures below this level due to the rib cage and sternum. However, if there are multiple rib fractures, the fracture is more likely to be unstable and to show significant displacement (189) (Table 1).

The thoracolumbar junction, T11, T12, and L1 are particularly vulnerable to instability. This area represents a transition from the relatively stable thoracic spine

TABLE 1. *Screening method to determine level of neurologic injury*

Level	Muscle power	Sensory	Reflexes
T2–T5	Upper extremity intact. Intercostals paralyzed. Breathing diaphragmatic.	T2 axialla lost T5 nipple line	None
T6–T9	Intact intercostals above level of involvement. Supraumbilical segments of rectus abdominus intact. Umbilicus moves cephalad with forced respiration.	T6 xiphoid T7 costal margins	Abdominals absent
T10	Infraumbilical segments of rectus abdominus intact. Umbilicus shifts caudad with forced respiration.	Umbilicus	
T12	Abdominal muscles intact.	Groin	Abdominals present
L1	No lower extremity.	Buttocks	Intact ankle jerk, knee jerk = upper motor neuron paralysis Cremasteric present
L2	Possible iliopsoas.	Anterior upper third of the thighs	Cremasteric absent
L3	Hip flexion sartorius and iliopsoas intact.	Anterior two thirds of the thighs	Knee jerk absent
L4	Hip flexion. Hip adduction. Intact sartorius permits some knee flexion.	Anterior thigh, medial leg	Knee jerk present
L5	Ankle dorsiflexion. Anterior tibial intact.	Medial ankle Dorsum of the foot, great toe absent	
S1	As above.	Plantar, lateral border of foot absent	
S2	Plantar flexion intact.	Peripheral sensation intact	Ankle jerk present
S3–S4	Cauda equina-type syndrome including potential loss of bladder and bowel control with sensory losses confined to the genitalia, perineum, anus, and posterior upper thigh. No peripheral motor loss.		

to the more mobile lumbar spine (219). This transition is also marked by a significant increase in the size of the disc space, a change from a kyphotic to a lordotic curve, and the reorientation of the facets from a frontal to a sagittal, more mobile plane (132). The thoracolumbar junction also marks the emergence of the nerve roots of the cauda equina. The cross-sectional area of the spinal cord relative to its bony confines is decreased. Vascularity is less precarious then in the "water shed" region of the thoracic spine (132,164). Therefore, injury at the thoracolumbar junction is often characterized by incomplete lesions of the conus medullaris or cauda equina, which have a greater potential for recovery (48,195,196) (Fig. 4). At this level there tends to be poor correlation between the degree of bony spinal canal compromise, as shown by CT scan, and the degree of neural injury (139,140). Therefore, it is proposed that most of the neurologic damage occurs at the time of injury or impact (26,48,51,100,139).

At this level there is also some controversy as to the importance of bony spinal canal compromise and the potential for neurologic deterioriation. Trafton and Boyce (207) felt there was a significant risk of neurologic deterioration if there was more than 50% canal compromise or an associated laminar fracture. In comparison, Weinstein demonstrated in a long-term follow-up study (215,216) that even greater than 50% compromise was compatible with a good, long-term outcome.

At the L2-L3 and L3-L4 levels fractures tend to have more inherent stability due to the size of the vertebral bodies and the surrounding musculature. Similarly, L4-L5 fractures are usually stable due to large vertebral bodies and the lordotic posture placing the vertebral bodies anterior to the weight-bearing line. Also, the cauda equina is less vulnerable to neurologic injury. Frequently fractures producing 60% to 80% canal compromise result in no neurologic injury, although this is not always the case (Fig. 5).

At L5-S1 the forces necessary for disruption are significant so these injuries may be less stable (Fig. 6). Moreover, associated pelvic trauma implies a mechanical history of high-energy injury and the potential for instability.

Clinical Classification

Magerl et al. (137) have recently proposed a classification of spinal fractures based on morphologic injury patterns. Three basic forces (compression, distraction, rotation) produce extreme main injury types. These have been applied to all levels of the spine and are divided into A, B, and C with subcategories (A1, A2, A3; B1, B2, B3; C1, C2, and C3), and with a further subdivision of 1, 2, and 3, based on severity. A, B, and C types, namely, compression, distraction, and rotation, can be interre-

lated. Type A are compression lesions (loss of vertebral body height). Type B are distractive (increased distance between posterior elements and B1 and B2 fractures, and between the anterior structures and B3 fractures). Type 3 are torsional injuries.

Type A fractures are further divided into body impaction A1, splitting A2, and burst A3.

Further subdivision into 1, 2, and 3 is given. For example, A1-1 is end plate impaction, A1-2 is wedge, and A1-3 is body collapse. Another example is A2-1 which is sagittal split fracture, with A being compression and 2 being splitting. A2-2 is a coronal split and A2-3 is a pincer type fracture. Another example is A3-1, which is A being compressive, 3 being burst, and 1 being incomplete (inferior, superior, or lateral). A3-2 is a burst split (sagittal split and burst of one half of the body). A3-3 is a complete burst fracture (both upper and lower halves. Category B and C fractures are similarly divided.

In Type C fractures there is anterior-posterior element destruction with torsion. These are the most unstable injuries and are a combination of types A and B with rotation.

A criticism of this all-inclusive classification is its length, which may prove to be cumbersome. It has, however, major advantages over other classifications in that it is descriptive and allows for ease of documentation and enhances a logical treatment plan.

Compression Fractures

Compression fractures result from an axial load combined with flexion or lateral bend (Fig. 7). They are the most common injury, comprising 89.1% of Denis's series (52), and have a predilection for the thoracolumbar junction. A variety of fracture patterns are identified: the most common involves the anterior one-half of the upper end plate; less common are isolated injuries of the inferior end plate or involvement of both end plates. If the injury mechanism involves lateral rather than forward flexion forces, lateral wedging is identified in the frontal plane (Fig. 8).

If the loss of vertebral body height is less than 50% or the angulatory deformity is less than 20 degrees, the fractures have been considered stable, although two of the authors (Kostuik and Esses) suggest 40% compression is a safer value.

As the degree of compression increases, particularly to 50%, it becomes absolutely essential to distinguish between a simple compression fracture and a burst fracture, which may be difficult with plain radiography. CT scanning is often necessary (140).

In those instances where compression injuries are contiguous, the angulatory and compression deformities are summated. Thus, if a patient has 30% compression and 15 degrees kyphosis at each level, the injury is appraised

Text continues on page 1286.

A

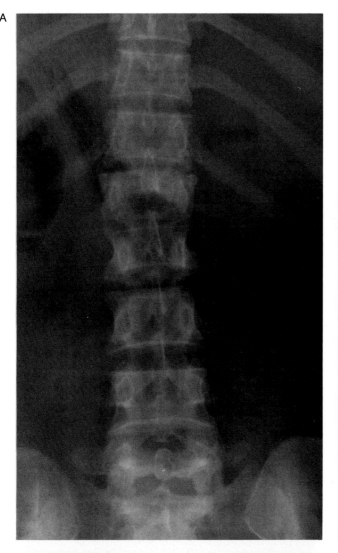

B

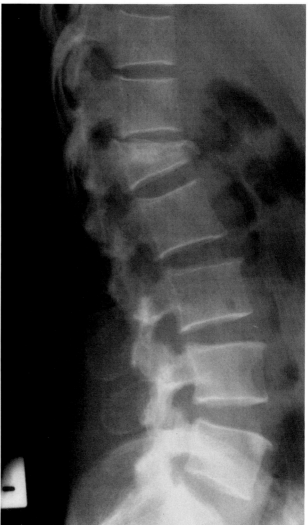

C

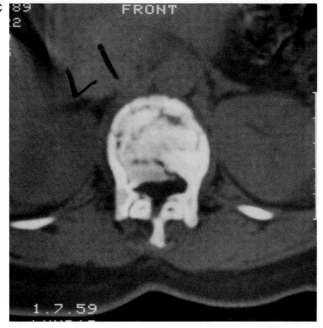

FIG. 4. A 22-year-old female student was involved in a motor vehicle accident. Examination was consistent with an incomplete neurologic injury, Frankel Grade B, with loss of bowel and bladder control. Radiographs **(A and B)** revealed an L1 burst fracture and thoracolumbar junctional kyphosis. CT scan **(C)** revealed 50% canal compromise at the level of the conus medullaris. (Figs. 4D–4E follow.)

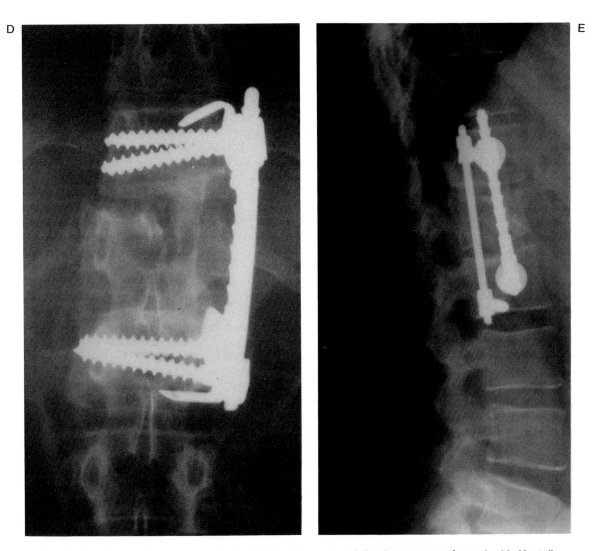

FIG. 4. *(Continued)* Urgent anterior decompression and stabilization were performed with Kostuik-Harrington instrumentation **(D and E)**. Seven months post injury the patient walks with a cane but requires intermittent self-catheterization.

A

B

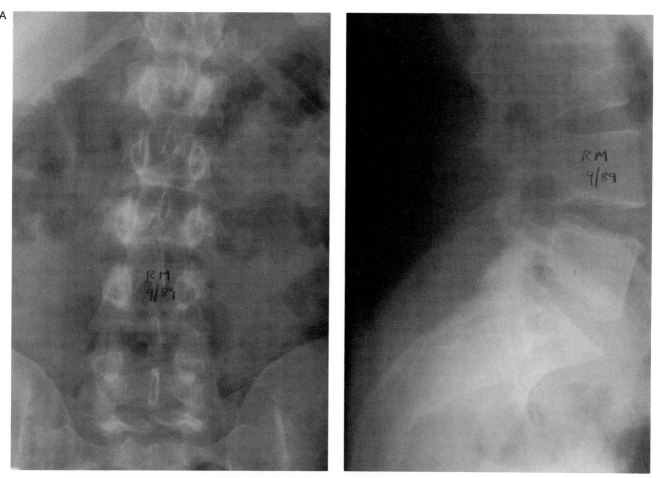

FIG. 5. A 26-year-old male was involved in a motor vehicle accident. Examination showed an incomplete neurologic injury Frankel Grade B, with loss of bowel and bladder control. Radiographs **(A and B)** demonstrated an L3 burst fracture. Note the subtle pedicular widening on the AP radiographic view.

C

D

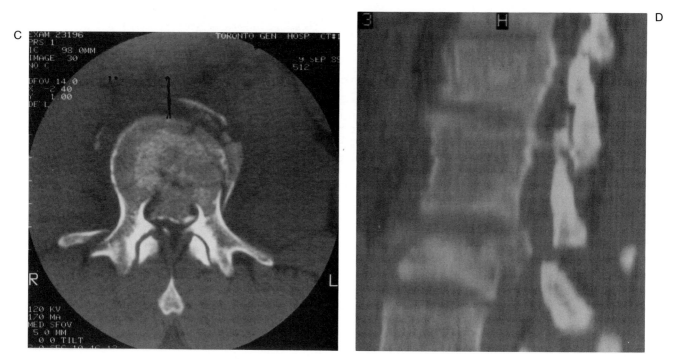

FIG. 5. *(Continued)* CT scan **(C and D)** with sagittal reconstruction revealed over 80% canal compromise. Note the characteristic retropulsion of the posterior superior endplate into the spinal canal. (Figs. 5E–5G follow.)

E

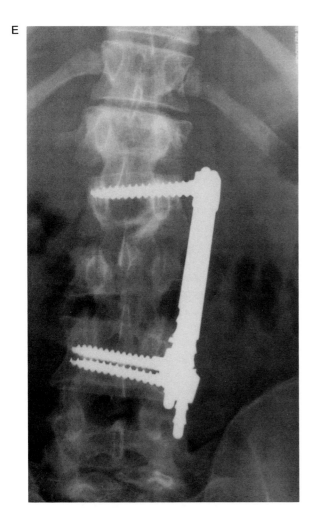

F

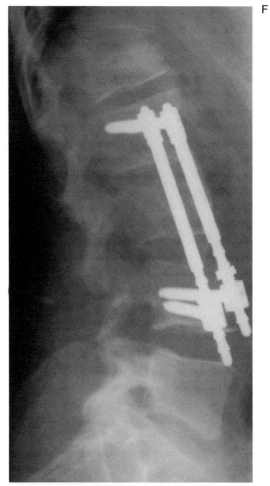

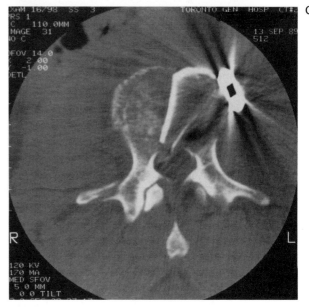

G

FIG. 5. *(Continued)* Urgent anterior decompression **(E and F)** using tricortical strut grafts and Kostuik-Harrington instrumentation was performed. The post-operative CT scan **(G)** was done at the same level as shown in Figure 2C (note the transverse process fracture) and demonstrates nearly complete restoration of canal. The patient recovered bowel and bladder control and was able to ambulate with a cane within 3 months of the injury.

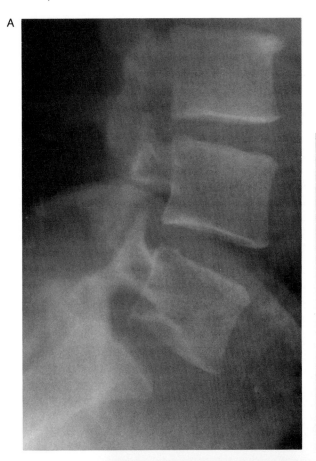

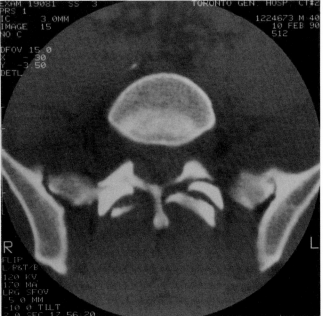

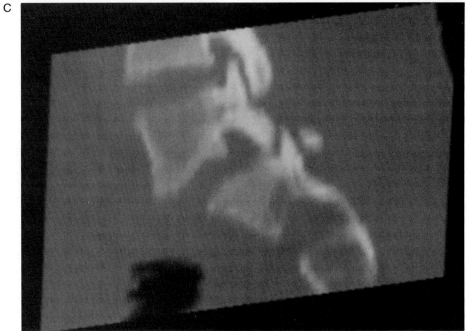

FIG. 6. A 34-year-old male construction worker was struck with a steel beam. Examination revealed skin abrasions, swelling over the low lumbar spine, and bilateral S1 radiculopathy. The lateral radiograph **(A)** revealed a lumbosacral spondylolisthesis. The CT scan **(B)** revealed fractures of the lumbosacral facet joints. Sagittal reconstructions from the CT scan **(C)** demonstrated "jumped" lumbosacral facets. Note that the superior sacral facet is displaced and *posterior* to the inferior facet of L5. (Figs. 6D–6E follow.)

D

E

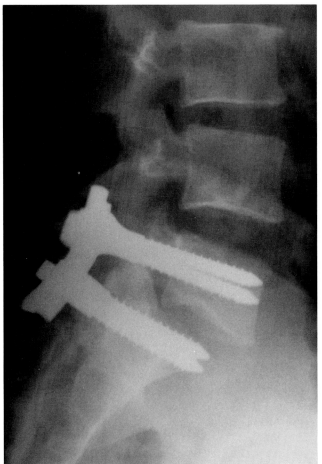

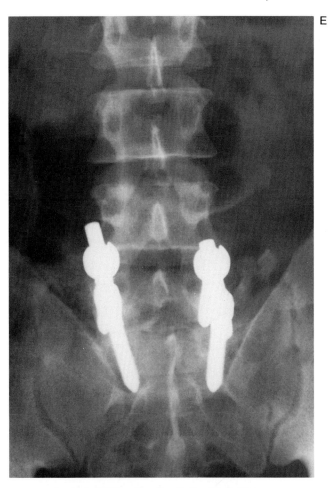

FIG. 6. *(Continued)* Following decompression of S1 nerve roots, and stabilization "in situ" with Cotrel-Dubousset instrumentation **(D and E),** the patient had return of plantar flexion strength within one month.

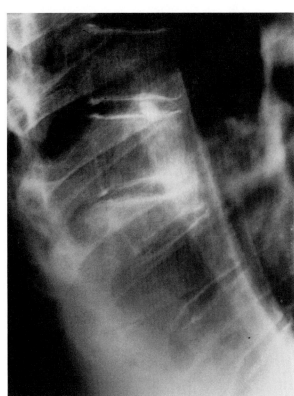

FIG. 7. A lateral radiograph of a typical wedge compression fracture.

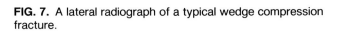

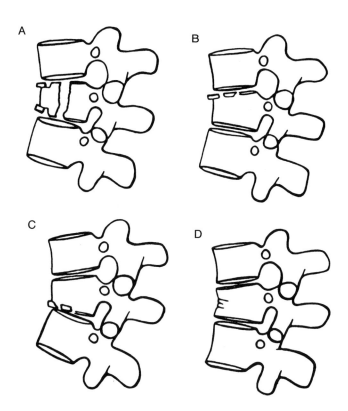

FIG. 8 (left). Wedge-compression fracture types (with permission from ref. 52).

FIG. 9 (below). A 19-year-old female student was involved in a motorcycle accident; she was neurologically intact. Radiographs **(A and B)** reveal L2 burst fracture and L3 compression fracture. Note the subtle vertical laminar fracture at L2.

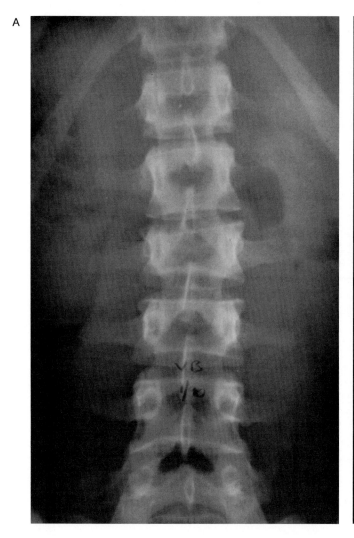

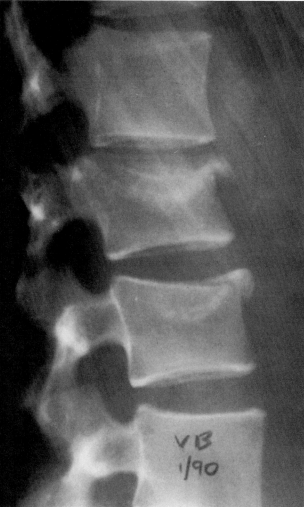

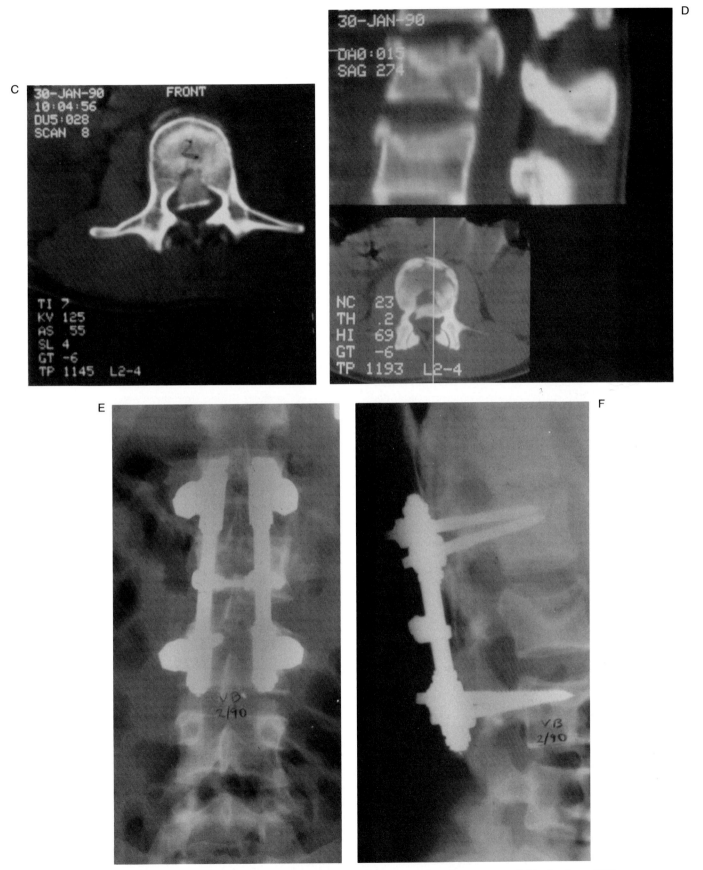

FIG. 9. *(Continued)* **C and D:** CT scan with sagittal reconstruction shows an unstable fracture, 60% canal compromise, and a typical pattern of retropulsion of posterior superior endplate into spinal canal. **E and F:** Reduction and stabilization with "Fixateur Interne."

as a total of 60% compression and 30 degrees kyphosis, and a more aggressive surgical correction may be warranted.

Burst Injuries

The essential feature of the burst injury is disruption of the middle column with varying degrees of retropulsion into the neural canal, best identified on CT scan (140) (Fig. 9). Involvement of the posterior elements is common. Of those with involvement, 50% have a bilateral posterior element injury, and 40% have unilateral injury. When the posterior elements are involved, neurologic injury is present in 50% of cases. In these instances it is important to recognize that the neural injury may be the result of neural element entrapment in laminal fractures. Dural laceration is to be anticipated (36,166). These patients may be improved by early laminectomy and stabilization. Five subtypes have been identified by Denis (52) based on which end plate is involved, whether both end plates are involved, and on the rotational or lateral flexion component (Fig. 10). These patterns may be relevant to neurologic recovery. Dall and Stauffer (48) reviewed recovery patterns in patients with burst fractures with over 30% canal compromise, and concluded those with superior body fractures and posterior ligamentous disruption with over 15 degrees of kyphos had a

better potential for recovery than those with burst fractures in the middle of the vertebral body.

Fracture Dislocations

These injuries are unstable because all three columns have failed. Multiple forces are involved including rotation, distraction, compression, and shear. Complete dislocation or subluxation may ensue, but some may reduce spontaneously. The magnitude of the injury may not be appreciated in the initial evaluation (49,76,105, 151,187,213). In general, these injuries are divided into flexion rotation, distraction (shear, flexion-distraction), and extension injuries (Fig. 11). Some have added a fourth category, the combined dislocation-burst injury (82).

Flexion Rotation Injuries

In this type, the posterior and middle columns fail by rotation and shear, and the anterior column fails under compression and rotation. In the thoracolumbar junction and lumbar spine, the orientation and size of the facets resist these forces, therefore complete dislocation is rare compared to the cervical spine. Disruption of the facets implies a grossly unstable injury.

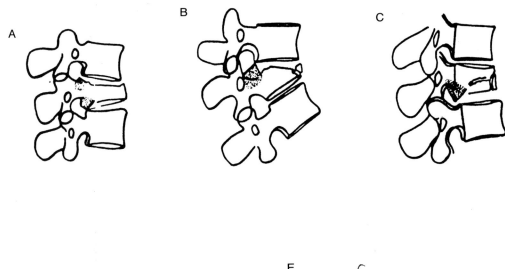

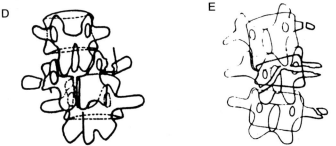

FIG. 10. Types of burst-fractures (with permission from ref. 52).

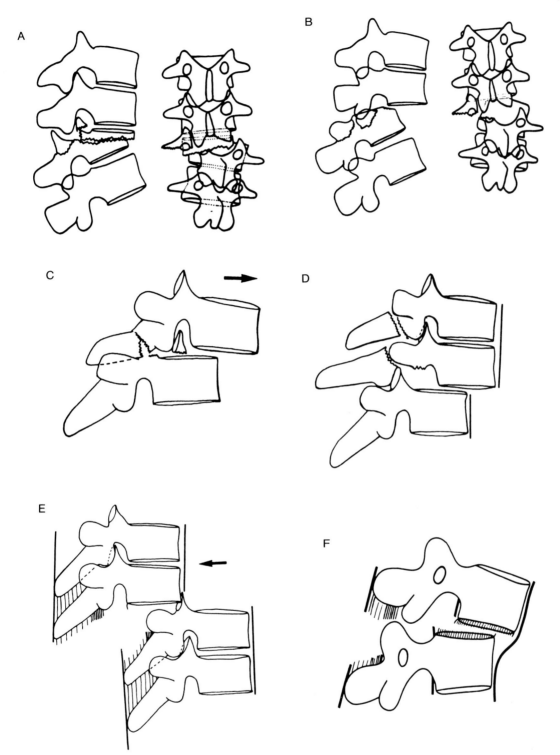

FIG. 11. Types of fracture dislocations (with permission from ref. 52).

Flexion-Distraction Injuries

Chance (38) first described this injury in 1948 as a fracture involving the upper half of the spinous process extending anteriorly through the pedicles, to emerge on the superior aspect of the vertebral body. Rennie and Mitchell (173) described two similar cases and concluded that the mechanism of injury was flexion and distraction. Smith and Kaufer (192) surmised the fracture was secondary to flexion around an anterior fulcrum, most commonly a seatbelt, a conclusion reached by others (8,31,32,39,111,190). Gertzbein and Court-Brown (79) felt the proposed mechanism did not explain adequately the compression or burst component sometimes seen in association with this injury. They concluded that the compression component occurs during the deceleration phase of the injury.

The stability depends on the magnitude of the forces, the intactness of the anterior longitudinal ligaments, and the pattern of structural involvement which may be purely ligamentous, purely osseous, or mixed osseo-ligamentous (79) (Fig. 12). Osseous injuries are compatible with bony union, whereas pure ligamentous and mixed lesions do not have this potential, resulting in a greater risk for long-term instability.

Extension Injuries

In extension injuries, the trunk or head is forced backward, applying tensile forces to the anterior longitudinal ligaments and anterior disc, and compression forces to the posterior elements. This may result in radiographic evidence of anterior vertebral body avulsion fracture, as well as fractures of the spinous processes, laminae, and occasionally the pedicles. These are usually stable.

Isolated Injuries of the Posterior Elements

Transverse Process Fractures. These injuries are the result of blunt trauma or violent contraction of the paraspinal musculature. When multiple fractures are present, or particularly when the L5 transverse process is fractured, there is a significant association with intra-ab-

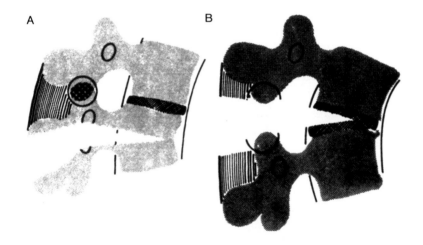

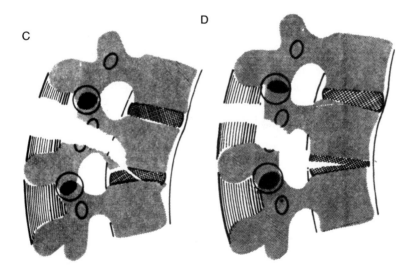

FIG. 12. Types of flexion distraction injuries (with permission from ref. 52).

dominal (renal) injuries and pelvic disruption (175,186). Occasionally neuropraxias results, most typically involving the L3 and L4 nerve roots.

Spinous Process Avulsions. Spinous process avulsions are fairly rare in the lumbar spine and are usually the result of direct trauma. Unless associated with a more complex pattern of involvement (e.g., flexion-distraction), these are considered stable injuries.

Isolated Facet Fractures. These are uncommon but may occur in patients with prior laminectomies, most commonly by a fatigue, rather than an acute, injury mechanism (see Chapter 89).

Traumatic Spondylolisthesis. True traumatic spondylolisthesis is rare compared to the far more common isthmic defect. Its description and treatment is to be found in Chapter 78 (see also Fig. 6).

APPROACH TO THE PATIENT WITH A THORACOLUMBAR SPINAL INJURY

The management of a patient with a spinal injury, with or without neurologic deficit, starts at the scene of the accident where attention to immobilization of the spine and prevention of further injury is paramount. Indeed, better training of paramedical personnel and greater attention to immobilization may account for the significant reduction in complete spinal cord injuries which has occurred over the past two decades (33). On arrival at the emergency room, the patient is left immobilized and a general physical examination is performed to evaluate for multiple potential associated injury to other organ systems or extremities (7,66,103,116, 167,189,193,194,199,200). Coordination of care by a trauma team leader is essential and the unusual priorities for emergent care are observed. Even if the injury appears to be limited to the spine, it is important to remember thoracolumbar fractures are commonly associated with abdominal trauma, including bowel, liver, spleen, and urologic injuries (103,192,193,200). This is particularly true when there is an associated neurologic deficit. Generally speaking, the most likely areas of visceral involvement correspond to the level of the spinal injury. For example, Woodring, Lee, and Jenkins (226) identified occult, unstable thoracic fractures in a few patients only after negative aortograms led to a search for other causes of the radiographic abnormalities. Although they emphasized that aortic rupture was the most common cause of mediastinal hemorrhage (18%), thoracic spinal fracture as the major causation was identified in 10% of these patients. Similarly, Harrington and Barker (103) reviewed 322 multiple injured patients with vertebral fractures. Intrathoracic lesions were commonly associated with thoracic fractures, while abdominal or urologic trauma occurred with lumbar injuries. Notably, pelvic and sacral fractures were associated with multi-or-

gan system injury because of the higher biomechanical forces involved. Bohlman (18) noted one third of thoracic spine fracture patients with paralysis had associated intrathoracic injury including hemopneumothorax, aortic tear, or ruptured diaphragm. Sternal fractures may occur as an indirect result of hyperflexion thoracic spinal fractures (72,116,189). The association of thoracic spinal fractures with mediastinal hemorrhage documented by chest radiographs is well described (50,54,200,225). Although radiographic evidence of mediastinal widening mandates thoracic aortography or CT scan, in many instances the study is negative and is ascribed to a "nonaortic" cause (225,226).

The issue of associated injury is particularly difficult when the patient presents with neurologic deficit. Soderstrom et al. (194) pointed out these problems and advocated immediate peritoneal lavage or minilaparatomy (Fig. 13). With this technique they were able to limit the number of interabdominal injuries which presented later, often compromising the patient's care. Similarly, seatbelt or "Chance" thoracolumbar fractures of the flexion-distraction type have a higher association with interabdominal trauma (8,32,39,58,111,119,178,190, 192,193,199,229).

Finally, at the same time one looks closely for associated injuries to other organ systems, the examiner should also be aware that beyond the obvious fracture, there is a 10% to 20% likelihood of other contiguous or somewhat more remote associated spinal fracture (12,35,100,124). Thus, it is recommended that complete radiologic evaluation of the entire spine be carried out, rather than focusing on the area of obvious deformity.

Once the initial patient assessment has taken place and the immediate life-threatening conditions are brought under control, greater attention can be focused on the spinal injury. A description of the accident alerts the examiner to potential injury types. Minimal trauma followed by significant pain is most likely to be associated with pathologic fractures, often from osteoporosis but also related to tumors. Falls from greater heights and motor vehicle accidents are associated with more serious and potentially unstable injuries. It is also important to understand the seatbelt system in place at the time of the automotive injury. The patient is carefully examined for chest and abdominal skin abrasions, gibbous deformity, and palpably displaced or separated spinous processes, all of which help to reconstruct the mechanism of injury (120).

A detailed neurologic evaluation is carried out with particular emphasis on the sensory level, if one is present, the sites and degree of muscle weakness, the presence or absence of peripheral reflexes, Babinski's sign, and the bulbocavernosus reflex. All of these are critical to establishing whether the associated neurologic injury is complete or incomplete, as well as forming a baseline for further observation. A spinal cord injury evaluation

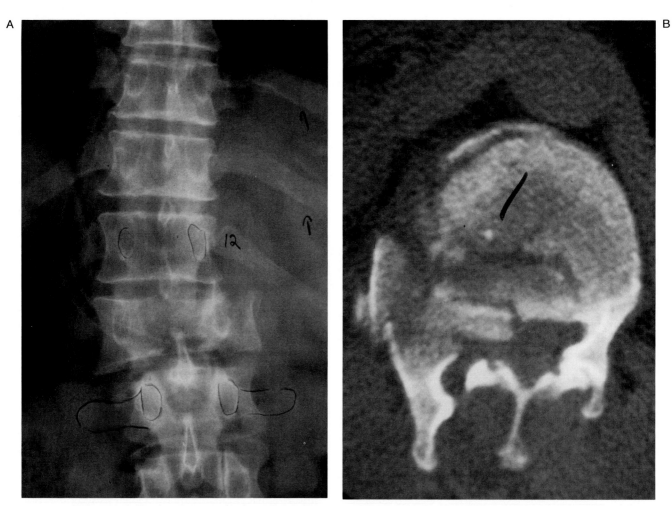

FIG. 13. A 52-year-old male fell from the roof of a house. Examination revealed complete motor and sensory deficit at the L1 level. Peritoneal lavage was positive for gross blood and laparotomy confirmed splenic rupture. **A:** Burst rotation injury at L1 with pedicular widening, vertical laminar fractures, and rib fractures. **B:** CT scan shows canal compromise mostly from posterior by anterior implosion of the posterior arch. (Figs. 13C–13D follow.)

C
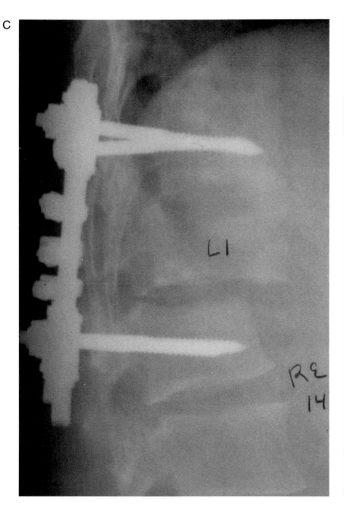

D
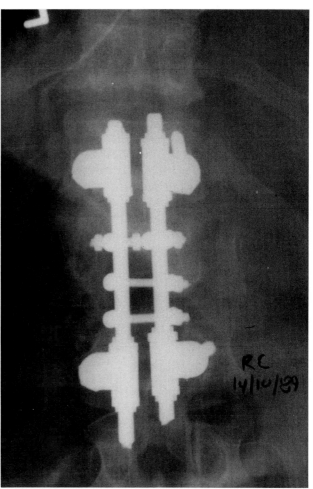

FIG. 13. *(Continued)* **C and D:** Posterior decompression and stabilization with "Fixateur Interne." Patient regained only minimal sensation and non-useful motor function (Frankel B) from this mixed conus medullaris/cauda equina injury.

form helps ensure that critical information is recorded (120). Table 1 outlines a clinically useful screening method to determine the level of neurologic injury.

In evaluating these patients, it is also critical to carefully examine the rectal sphincter tone, strength of sphincter contraction, and the bulbocavernosus reflex. The bulbocavernosus reflex involves the S2, S3, and S4 nerve roots and is a spinal cord-mediated reflex arc. In males, the bulbocavernosus reflex is tested by pulling on the Foley catheter or squeezing the glans penis while performing a rectal examination. Contraction of the striated muscle of the internal anal sphincter indicates an intact and functioning reflex arc. In females, tapping the clitoris initiates the same reflex arc. The presence or absence of this reflex carries great prognostic significance. Its absence documents the continuation of spinal shock or spinal injury at the level of the reflex arc itself. Rarely does spinal shock last in excess of 24 to 48 hours. Its return is used to document the termination of spinal shock. The

recovery of the bulbocavernosus reflex, in combination with the complete absence of distal motor or sensory function or perirectal sensation, describes a complete cord injury and significant neurologic function is unlikely ever to return. Incomplete cord injuries present when there is any distal sparing of motor or sensory function, and the presence of perirectal sensation. In the presence of an incomplete cord injury, the bulbocavernosus reflex is no longer prognostic for the return of function.

It is also extremely important to evaluate caudal control of urinary function. Unfortunately, most patients by necessity have an indwelling catheter placed in the emergency room and the ability to void cannot be established. However, before any surgical procedure is carried out, it is important to document intactness of bladder control. Stauffer (195) recommends cystometric examination, urodynamic flow studies, or sphincter electromyograms, particularly in the patient who appears otherwise neurologically intact but has an unstable spinal injury. Sometimes this ideal approach may not be possible in the multiply injured patient.

Neurologic Grading Scales

Once a complete neurologic evaluation has been carried out, this information should be compiled to document the grade of neurologic injury. A variety of neurologic injury rating scales have been developed, including the Frankel classification (73), the Sunnybrook cord injury scale (203), the spinal cord injury severity scale (23), and the motor index of Lucas and Ducker (133). All of these are designed to monitor the extent of the initial neurologic injury and its progression, as well as to provide a method for assessing treatment efficacy by different methods. The Frankel grading scale is shown in Table 2. Its advantage is that it is extremely well known and widely used. Its disadvantage is that it does not include complete assessment of rectal or bladder function, nor is it sensitive to significant neurologic improvement in those patients classified as grade D. An additional problem is that the lesion level is not indicated so that a paraplegic falls into the same category as a quadriplegic.

The Sunnybrook cord injury scale consists of 10 neurologic grades as seen in Table 3. This differs from the Frankel system since sensory loss can be classified as complete or incomplete. There is also a coding system to assess change in neurologic status. Unfortunately, motor grades 6 through 8 comprise a large and heterogeneous group. The differentiation between grades 3 through 5 and 6 through 8 correspond to Frankel grades C and D. Bladder and bowel function are not assessed. Although it represents some improvement over the Frankel system, it is not easy to commit to memory and, thus, has diminished bedside utility, particularly in acute management.

The motor index of Lucas and Ducker has been modified by the American Spinal Injury Association into a motor index score where 100 represents the perfect scale (Table 4). These scales are more precise and the score is calculated by summing separate measurements of the individual muscles with each individual measure, easily categorized by the usual 1 to 5 rating. Again, its deficiency is that bowel and bladder function are not evaluated.

The classification of Bracken et al. (24) has many of the features of the Sunnybrook cord injury system and,

like it, is difficult to memorize and apply at the bedside. It also makes no specific mention of bowel or bladder function.

Esses and Botsford (65) recently described a neurologic grading system attempting to overcome some of these deficits. It requires no special test other than those done in routine clinical neurologic examination. The scale includes assessment of motor and sensory function, rectal tone, and bladder control. Motor index is assessed by function. Using this system, a significant number of patients were noted to have had improvement with treatment which would have been overlooked using the Frankel classification.

Radiologic Evaluation

The initial assessment consists of anteroposterior (AP) and lateral radiographs of the spine. Unless the spinal injury is minor, the survey must include the entire spinal column. Five percent to 30% of these patients have multi-

TABLE 3. *Sunnybrook Cord Injury Scale (203)*

Grade	Description	Corresponding Frankel grade
1	Complete motor and sensory loss	A
2	Complete motor loss; incomplete sensory loss	B
3	Incomplete motor but unclear	C
4	Incomplete motor loss; incomplete sensory loss	
5	Incomplete motor but useless; normal sensory	C
6	Incomplete motor; complete sensory	D
7	Incomplete motor; incomplete sensory	D
8	Incomplete motor: normal sensory	D
9	Normal motor; incomplete sensory	D
10	Normal motor; normal sensory	E

TABLE 2. *Frankel classification (73)*

A. Complete neurologic injury
B. Incomplete: preserved sensation only
C. Incomplete: non-functional motor
D. Incomplete: functional motor
E. Complete recovery (may have abnormal reflexes)

TABLE 4. *Motor index score adapted for ASIA (133)*

Grade on right	Muscle	Grade on left
0–5	C5	0–5
0–5	C6	0–5
0–5	C7	0–5
0–5	C8	0–5
0–5	T1	0–5
0–5	L2	0–5
0–5	L3	0–5
0–5	L4	0–5
0–5	L5	0–5
0–5	S1	0–5
50		50
	Total score: 100	

ple rather than single-level injuries (5,7,12,35,97, 103,124,161). Generally, the first and most important radiographic view is the cross-table lateral, with the patient still immobilized. In 70% to 90% of cases, this single film will show the spinal injury (1,13,45,75). An anteroposterior radiograph is then taken which is of particular importance in identifying posterior element involvement (34). Watkins suggests that an organized sequence should be done by scrutinizing structures from posterior midline to anterior at each level, just as one would expose the posterior elements at the time of surgery (211). Subtle or significant widening of the distance between spinous processes may be the only clue to a flexion-distraction injury (Fig. 14). Vertical laminae fractures are common in burst injury, while horizontal laminae fractures may be present in slice injuries, seatbelt, Chance, or flexion-distraction injuries (Fig. 15). Subtle disruption of the superior and inferior articular facets denotes that significant ligamentous injury may have occurred (158). Fracture of the transverse process may be the only indicator of occult renal trauma (200). Widening of the intrapediculate distance indicates disruption of the posterior vertebral wall, seen most commonly in burst fractures (see Fig. 13A).

Usually these two radiographic views will identify most of the major pathology. However, oblique radiographs may be useful in defining facet fractures and injuries to the pars interarticularis. Sometimes the differentiation of acute traumatic lesions of the pars interarticularis from an old isthmic defect may ultimately require a bone scan.

Despite an organized approach to plain anteroposterior and lateral radiography, there are a number of pitfalls which may be encountered. Reid et al. evaluated 38 patients with "missed" or delayed diagnosis of spinal fracture (171). The most common predisposing factors were patient intoxication, multilevel spinal fractures, multiple trauma, or head injury.

There are also a number of specific pitfalls in diagnosis. For example, the pediatric population is at greater risk for spinal cord insult with the absence of apparent osseous injury (98,162). Pang and Pollack (162) coined the acronym SCIWORA, (Spinal Cord Injury Without Radiographic Abnormality) to describe this occurrence. It is proposed that the inherent ligamentous elasticity of the pediatric spine permits neurologic injury to occur without apparent osseous trauma. Therefore, a child with ongoing spinal pain or neurologic deficit often requires a more complete evaluation including CT scan and dynamic radiography.

A second group of patients are those with pre-existent diseases such as ankylosing spondylitis, diffuse idiopathic skeletal hyperostosis (DISH) (20–22,29,77,101, 112,153,174,208,214,229), and pre-existent spinal stenosis (69). Although spondylitis has been discussed in detail in Chapter 36, it is worth re-emphasizing certain im-

portant features. First, these fractures are often the result of minor trauma and a fracture is not suspected. Second, the fractures are not well visualized by routine radiography and the distorted anatomy and osteopenia further confounds the interpretation. Thus, all patients with ankylosing spondylitis complaining of acute back pain should be treated as fractures until proven otherwise (88,92,208). Evaluation often includes a necessary CT scan, bone scan, or magnetic resonance image to visualize the injury (174) (see Fig. 16).

Conventional Tomography

Despite the advent of CT scan, conventional tomography still may be useful in the evaluation of acute spinal trauma (13,15,104,169). The advantages are that plain tomography is more often available; the patient can be imaged in flexion and extension (45); and the technique may prove superior in the evaluation of axially oriented, thoracolumbar fractures including lap belt injuries, horizontal laminar fractures, and some facet injuries (see Fig. 15B). An important disadvantage is the requirement that the patient be positioned side lying, which may be risky for those with unstable fractures.

CT Scanning

In many hospitals the CT scan has virtually replaced conventional tomography (27). The distinctive advantages of CT scanning are its accurate reflection of the degree of bone and soft tissue injury in comparison to plain films (139); it requires less patient positioning, it is safer; and it has a lower radiation dose. As already noted, the disadvantage of axial CT is its inability to reflect the spinal canal and the degree of neural compromise, and to clearly delineate the posterior element involvement, particularly in burst fractures (89,122,139). Anatomic information gained from CT is largely responsible for the later development of clinically useful classifications for spinal fractures (5,52,139). The technique, as it is evolving, has the capacity for dynamic as well as static views (30).

In evaluating a CT scan, it is particularly important to pay attention to the facet joint relationships. Normally these structures are tightly opposed, symmetric, and paired. Separation or asymmetry of the facet joints is evidence of significant trauma. The term "naked facet" (158) is used to describe potential disruption of the facet joint (Fig. 17). In this situation, the inferior facet of the superior vertebra and the superior facet of the inferior vertebra are seen on different image cuts.

As already noted, the disadvantage of axial CT is its inability to detect subtle horizontally oriented fractures of the vertebral bodies, pedicles, or laminae, and minimal vertebral body compression fractures may not be

Text continues on page 1297.

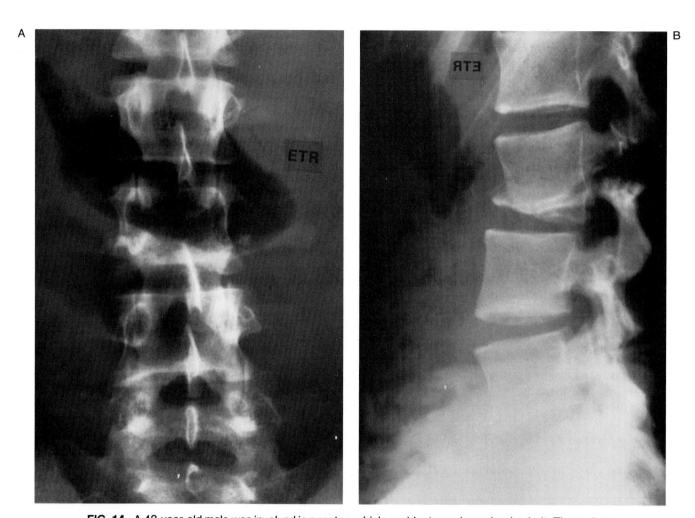

FIG. 14. A 42-year-old male was involved in a motor vehicle accident wearing only a lap belt. The patient was neurologically normal. Radiographs **(A and B)** demonstrated spinous process widening, horizontal laminar fractures, and a "Chance" type bony flexion distraction injury exiting anteriorly through L2-L3 disc space. (Figs. 14C–14E follow.)

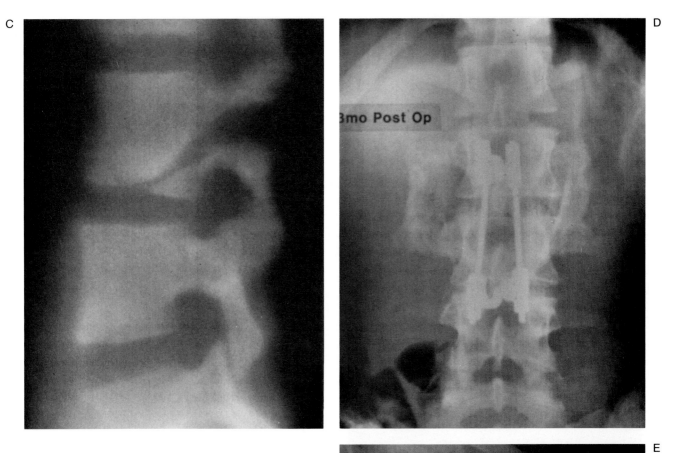

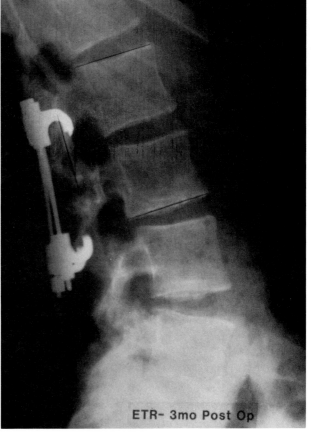

FIG. 14. *(Continued)* **C:** Tomograms demonstrated the course of the bony injury. **D and E:** Stabilization with a Harrington compression device was performed since the injury went through the disc space and was felt to have the potential for chronic instability.

A

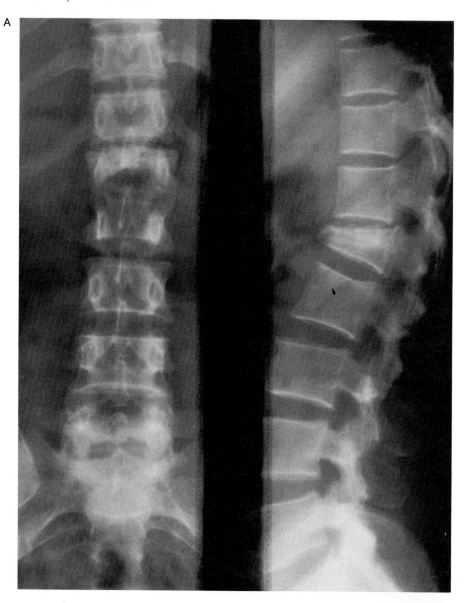

FIG. 15. A 34-year old female was involved in a motor vehicle accident wearing only a lap belt. She was neurologically normal. Radiographs **(A)** revealed spinous process widening between L1 and L2.

FIG. 15. *(Continued)* Tomograms **(B)** demonstrated facet subluxation and horizontal laminar fractures consistant with the mechanism of the lap belt injury.

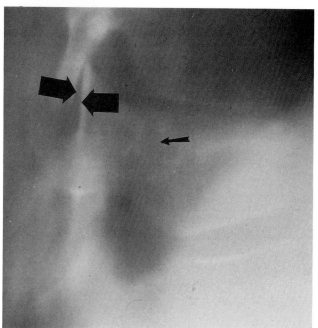

B

detected. Many of these problems can be overcome by accurate frontal and sagittal reformation (29,122,121).

An adjunct to CT scan may be myelography, often performed by lateral C1-C2 puncture with a few milliliters of metrizamide. This technique enhances the CT evaluation (41,46,47,121,122). Spinal cord hemorrhage or edema may be detected as a high density focus within the cord. Epidural hematomas or traumatic disc herniations may be seen as high density collections adjacent to the cord or cauda equina, with displacement accompanied by attenuation of the subarachnoid space (169). Lastly, three-dimensional reformations may be invaluable for pre-operative planning in complex injuries, as well as for understanding the various components of the injury (138) (Figs. 18A and 18B).

Magnetic Resonance Imaging

The authors view magnetic resonance imaging (MRI) as a complementary rather than a replacement study for CT scanning (13,45,104). CT scan continues to better define the osseous anatomy, while MRI can better demonstrate the status of the intervertebral disk, potential sites of ligamentous injury, epidural hematoma, and more precisely quantified spinal cord injury (14,37,84, 96,130,144,152,224). Kulkarni et al. (130) and others have correlated three patterns of MRI signal abnormalities with spinal cord injury patterns (16,22,152,206). Of prognostic significance are intradural traumatic lesions including cord edema, hemorrhage, and vascular infarction (226). Acute cord hemorrhage is noted as central hypointensity on T1-weighted images. Spinal cord edema and contusion have hyperintensity on T1-weighted images, as do areas of ligamentous and paravertebral edema and hemorrhage. A third mixed pattern most likely represents both edema and hemorrhage. In addition, cord transection, and later the formation of post-traumatic syrinx are well evaluated by MRI (see Chapter 53). The technique is particularly ideal in identifying and evaluating pathologic fracture caused by tumor or infection, as well as in evaluating perineural tissues, the spinal cord, nerve roots, and discs if the patient has a neurologic deficit unexplained by plain radiography or CT (152,169,226).

The indications for MRI therefore include spinal cord injury without obvious explanation, including fractures or fracture subluxations which are not of the magnitude sufficient to produce neural or clinical progression of a neural defect without an apparent explanation (Fig. 19). In the face of neurologic deficit and ostensibly normal radiographs, a variety of conditions can be considered. These include significant ligamentous injury, a spinal canal compromise through pre-existing degenerative or congenital stenosis, vascular insufficiency or tumor (Fig. 19) (69), and epidural hemorrhage which is a particular

risk in those taking anticoagulants (208) as well as those with known coagulopathy (4,20,169,183). MRI imaging is also particularly useful when traumatic disc herniations may accompany the injury. In Chance and slice fractures, MRI ideally should be performed before reductive manipulation is instituted (188).

Despite these obvious advantages, MRI has a number of significant disadvantages. It is not applicable to those who have cardiac pacemakers, ferromagnetic implants, or are claustrophobic (152). Most units have restricted emergency access and it is difficult to image a patient who requires mechanical ventilation. The development of MRI-compatible monitoring and life support systems are potential means to overcome these limitations (144,156).

Myelography

Today, myelography is rarely indicated for the acute evaluation of spinal trauma, particularly in units where the MRI is available (152). Historically, the indications have been the same as those for MRI (16,67). Its particular utility is the evaluation of nerve root avulsions or suspected dural tears (166). It still has utility when MRI is not available or cannot be performed due to the presence of metallic life support equipment or a cardiac pacemaker. A more detailed discussion of these issues and techniques of myelography is found in Chapter 19.

PATIENT MANAGEMENT

At the completion of the history, physical examination, plain radiography, and additional imaging studies if warranted, a definitive plan can be formulated for the patient's management. Obviously, the timing of management is first and foremost dependent on associated injury to other organ systems which may take precedence. The two most important determinants of management of the spine injury are stability and neurologic function, while the goals of management are: (a) to prevent further neurologic deterioration and to improve neurologic function if possible; (b) to stabilize the spine and prevent later deformity; and (c) to maximize early rehabilitation and prevent complications.

Influence of Neurologic Deficits on Management

If the patient has a normal neurologic examination and an injury with inherent stability, the preferred treatment has been non-surgical to allow the spine to heal without jeopardizing the spinal cord. The patient is kept on bed rest until the ilius resolves and there is no question of other injuries. If the injury is a minimal compression fracture (wedging less than 20–30 degrees), ambula-

Text continues on page 1304.

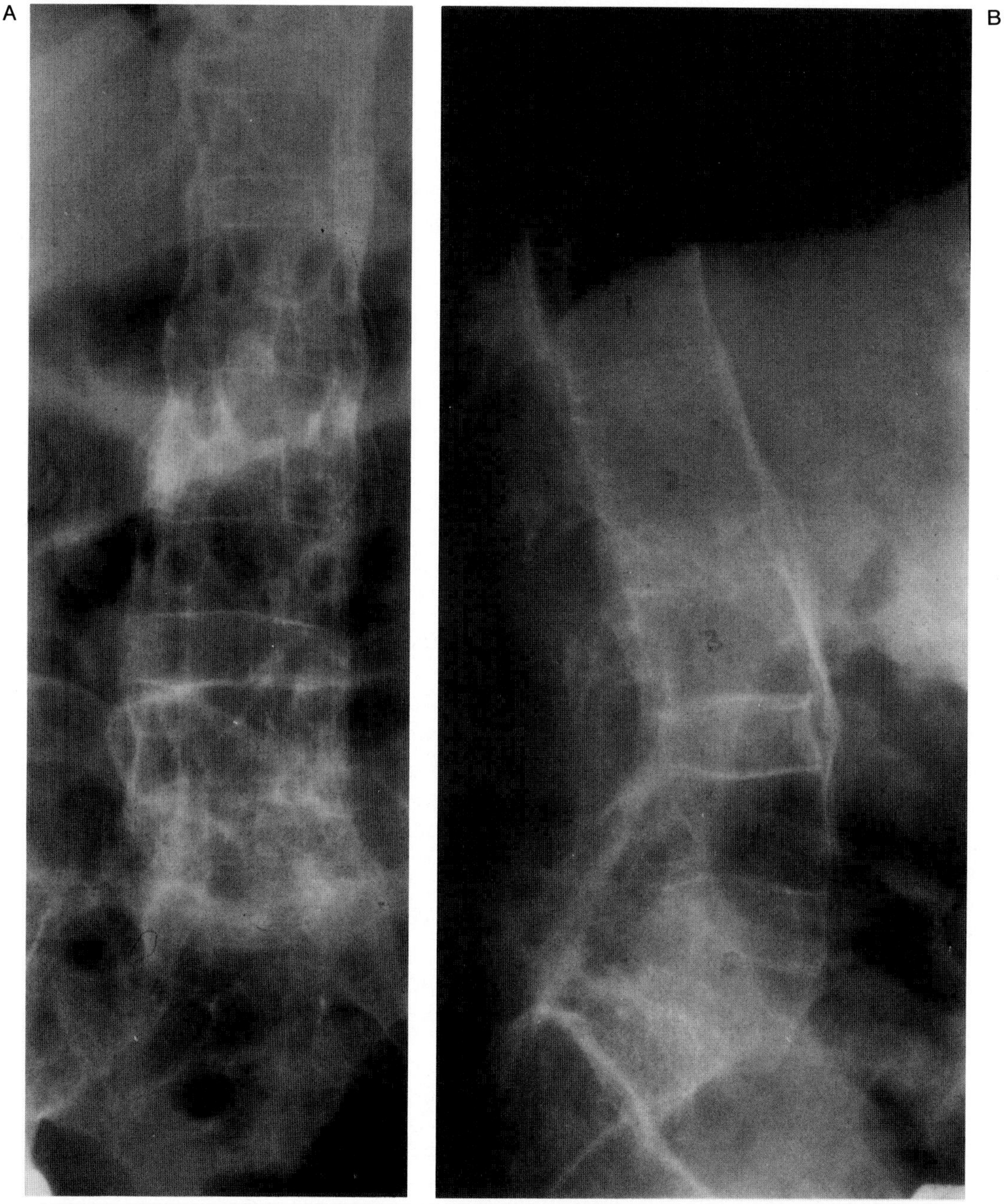

FIG. 16. A 50-year old male with known ankylosing spondylitis was unable to walk because of severe low back pain. In addition, osteomalacia was suspected on routine laboratory examination and confirmed through bone biopsy. A parathyroid adenoma was diagnosed. AP **(A)** and lateral **(B)** radiographs demonstrate severe osteopenia and an equivocal fracture at L5-S1 on the lateral view with loss of vertebral body height. (Figs. 16C–16D follow.)

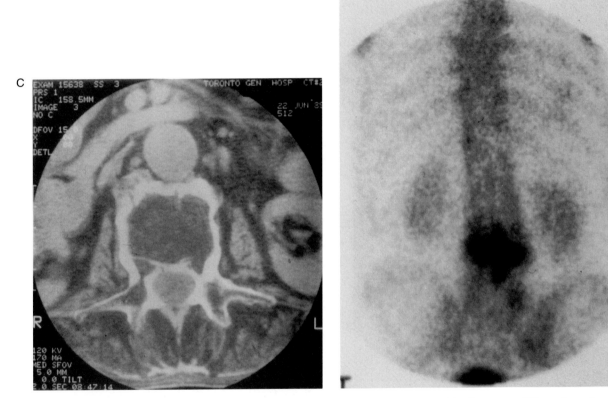

FIG. 16. *(Continued)* Thoracic CT scan **(C)** demonstrated severe osteopenia. Bone scan **(D)** confirmed a new stress fracture at L4.

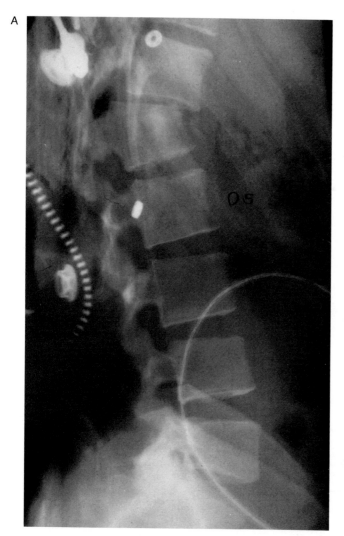

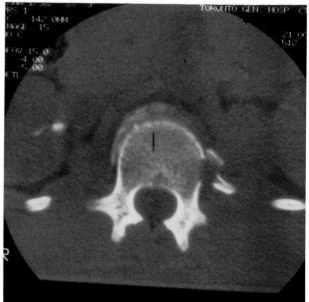

FIG. 17. A 34-year-old male jumped from a window. Examination revealed a Frankel Grade C injury with loss of bowel and bladder control. **A:** Fracture dislocation T12 on L1. **B:** CT demonstrated a "naked" superior facet of L1. Note that it no longer articulates with inferior facet of T12. (Figs. 17C–17D follow.)

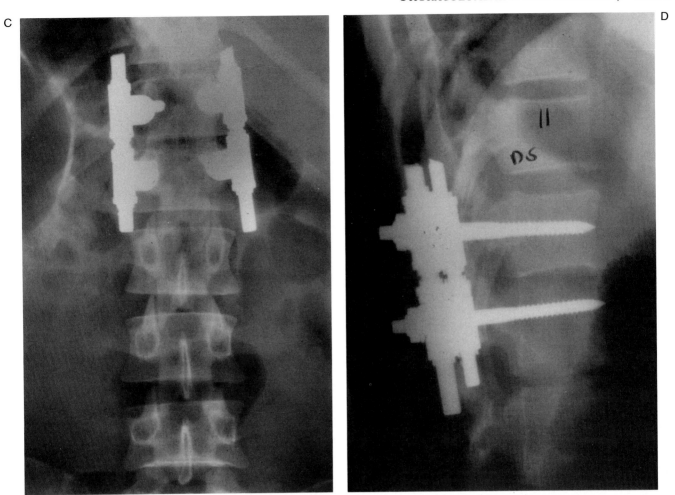

FIG. 17. *(Continued)* **C and D:** Reduction and demobilization was accomplished with the ''Fixateur Interne.''

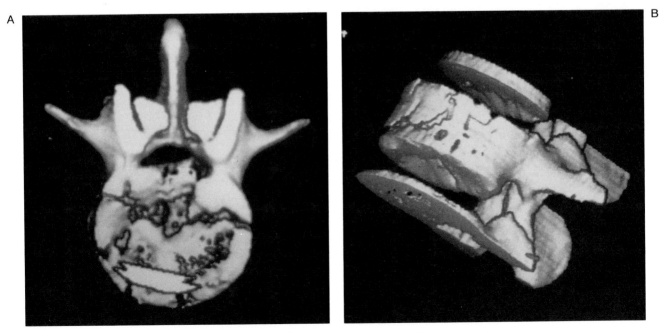

FIG. 18. Three-dimensional CT reconstructions **(A and B)** of a burst fracture.

A

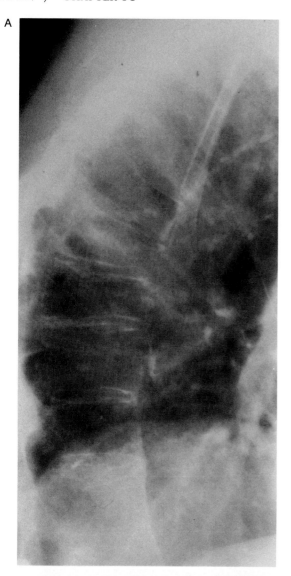

FIG. 19. A 62-year old male with known ankylosing spondylitis and rapidly progressive paraplegia after a trivial fall. An expanding epidural hematoma was suspected. Radiographs **(A)** revealed severe osteopenia.

B

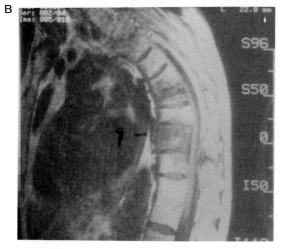
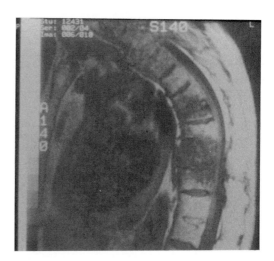

FIG. 19. *(Continued)* The MRI **(B)** was consistent with an infiltrative process at T9. (Figs. 19C–19D follow.)

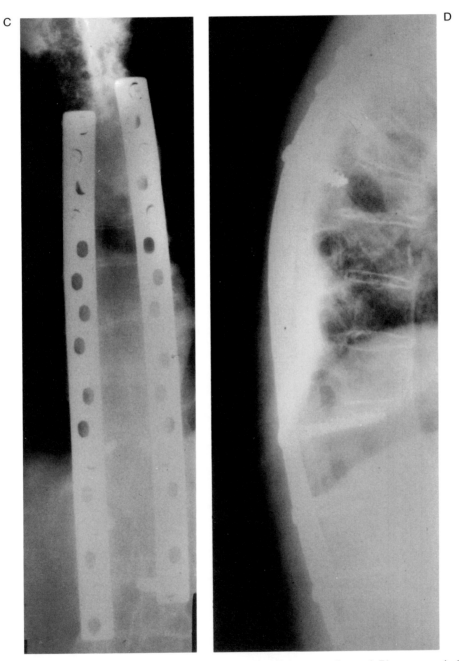

FIG. 19. (Continued) **C and D:** Decompression and stabilization was performed. Biopsy revealed a high grade sarcoma, likely from megavoltage radiation received for ankylosing spondylitis 30 years previously.

tory treatment without external supports may be considered. If there is a question of instability or pain management is a significant consideration, the patient initially is managed by bed rest and then placed in a body cast or thoraco-lumbar spinal orthosis (TLSO) and treated with bed rest at home or ambulation as tolerated (115) (Fig. 20). Assuming a compression fracture is at one level and has less than 20 degrees kyphos and less than 40% to 50% body compression, it usually will heal with no significant disability. If the spinal radiographs show any progressive deformity at follow-up evaluation, a posterior fusion can be performed as a delayed procedure. In general, advocates of this philosophy felt it was safer to perform a spinal fusion after the injury had obtained some stability of its own and the period of potential spinal cord edema had passed (21,23).

During the past decade there has been a shift, in general, toward a more aggressive approach in those patients who have suspected fracture patterns with the potential for instability. Denis et al. (53) felt that non-operative patients had more pain and 17% of his non-operatively treated patients later developed neurologic problems. He concluded that early surgical intervention resulted in less pain and more reliable return to work. His opinion was shared by Osebold et al. (160), who also advocated early instrumentation for potentially unstable injuries followed by aggressive rehabilitation. Jacobs et al. (113) likewise felt that mobilization was quicker and rehabilitation was more certain in patients treated operatively. They advocated longer posterior rodding incorporating three vertebrae above and three vertebrae below the area of spinal instability for better reduction, and because it was a stronger biomechanical construct. A study at Rancho Los Amigos Hospital by Gordon et al. (86) compared 45 patients with fractures of the thoracic spine treated non-operatively with 63 patients treated operatively. Their conclusions were that the operative patients had a shorter rehabilitation time and a shorter hospital-

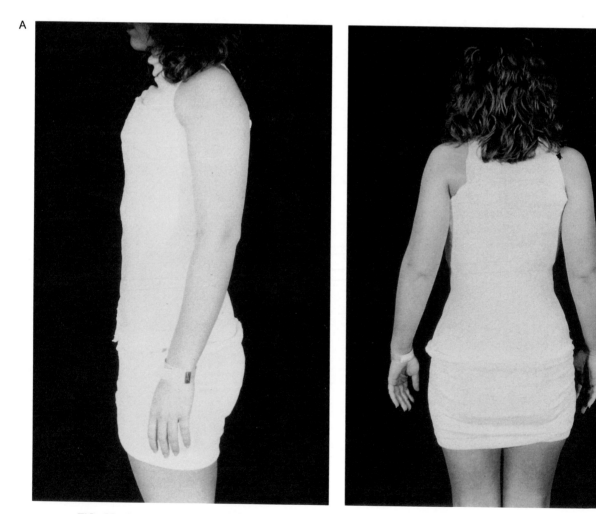

FIG. 20. Side **(A)** and back **(B)** views of body jacket applied for ambulatory treatment of moderately unstable fracture with no neurologic deficit.

ization, but that the surgical group also had a higher incidence of post-operative pain, pseudarthroses, and operative complications.

However, Krompinger et al. (129) in their follow-up evaluations felt that non-operative care was the best treatment for the neurologically intact. This position has also been supported by the long-term follow-up studies of burst fractures by Weinstein et al. (215,216).

Complete Neurologic Injuries

If a patient has a complete neurologic injury based on the criteria previously given, the major therapeutic consideration is what treatment method will facilitate the most rapid rehabilitation. In general, injuries located within the thoracic spine have inherent stability because of rib cage support and can be treated by TSLO and early mobilization as soon as the local injury pain subsides. At the thoracolumbar junction and below, the inherent instability of these anatomic regions makes it relatively more desirable to consider early operative intervention so that mobilization and rehabilitation can proceed rapidly.

Incomplete Neurologic Injuries

If the person has an incomplete neurologic lesion, one school of thought holds that it is important to manage this patient carefully for at least 24 hours to observe for improvement. Historically, log-rolling in bed or the Stryker frame have been used to control spinal stability. However, the degree of spinal immobilization produced by these methods is uncertain (145). A more secure method is the Rotokinetic bed (146). For many years the benefits of steroids, spinal cord cooling, and other therapeutic adjuncts have been debated (59). Recently it has been shown in a randomized, prospective study that methylprednisolone is effective when compared to a non-steroidal anti-inflammatory drug (24).

Based on the more conservative philosophy, surgical treatment is delayed to observe the patient's neurologic status. If improvement occurs over the first 24 to 48 hours and then plateaus, further imaging such as MRI is carried out to determine the possible benefits of surgical stabilization and/or decompression of offending bone fragment. If the patient shows a progressive worsening of a neurologic deficit, immediate surgery is indicated after appropriate imaging studies to explore the spinal canal. However, this approach is controversial. Two of the authors of this chapter (Kostuik and Esses) suggest that early decompression and stabilization may be more desirable and will produce a more certain outcome. If surgery is performed, there appears to be definite benefit to intra-operative monitoring of somatosensory-evoked potentials (147) (see Chapter 27). Today there is no clear-cut clinical investigation to document one or the other belief.

Treatment of Specific Fractures

Compression Fractures

These injuries are treated by short-term bed rest for pain control only. Depending on the degree of compression, the patient may be treated effectively by hyperextension exercises and the avoidance of compression overloads for a period of 12 weeks. For more significant compression, a hyperextension brace or TSLO may be advisable during that time interval, combined later with hyperextension exercises.

As the degree of compression increases, particularly beyond 40% to 50% compression or greater than 20 degrees angulation, the therapeutic options become more debatable. One of the authors (Stauffer) believes the appropriate treatment is initial bracing. If the follow-up evaluation 4 to 6 weeks following injury shows increasing kyphotic deformity or the patient's pain is not resolving, elective stabilization and fusion can then be done. The other authors (Kostuik, Esses) are more aggressive and recommend early stabilization and fusion. The rationale is that the deformity can be corrected by a posterior approach soon after injury, whereas an anterior approach is required when surgery is delayed. Moreover, they believe delay in surgical treatment serves to prolong the recovery and extends the disability period.

Burst Fractures

The management of burst fractures is based on the assessed stability and presence of a complete or incomplete neurologic injury. The conservative approach originated by Guttman (91) is still followed in many centers for patients who are neurologically intact. It consists of postural reduction followed by extension bracing or casts (148). One of the principle reasons for this philosophy was the failure of laminectomy to improve neurologic lesions, often accompanied by increased instability and deformity (10,73,93,150,178), a conclusion also derived from biomechanical analysis (204).

That conservative treatment can be effective for these fractures over the long-term has been established by Weinstein et al. in their study of patients with burst fracture and no neurologic involvements (215,216). At an average follow-up interval of 20 years, they demonstrated that 88% of the patients were working. Most had mild residual backache but none were taking narcotic medication. There was no long-term neurologic deterioration. The residual kyphos averaged 26.5 degrees, and there was no correlation between kyphotic deformity and pain. These results are comparable to those obtained by others (107,172). More intriguing was the demonstration that retropulsed fragments gradually resorbed (68). They speculated that bony remodeling was mediated by pulsations of the neural contents within the bony canal.

Others have questioned this conservative approach. The development of posterior stabilization devices by Harrington et al. (57,197,202) followed by modifications such as those introduced by Jacobs et al. (113) and the Edwards sleeve (62) allowed many to conclude that these fractures could be predictably stabilized. Reduction of the retropulsed fragments was also observed (25,57,228). The proposed mechanism was that the fragments remain attached to the posterior and/or anterior longitudinal ligaments. Early reduction was also promoted by an accumulated experience with later neurologic deterioration as the result of progressive kyphosis with tethering of the spinal cord and conus, and/or from spinal stenosis (see Chapter 62) (154).

If the operative approach is selected, a variety of strategies are available. The traditional posterior approach still favored by many surgeons is the Harrington distraction implant, or one of its modifications such as the Wisconsin (123), Jacob's hooks (114) or the Edwards sleeve (62) (see also Figs. 1A–1D). The underlying principle is three-point fixation which is enhanced by placing the rods at least two levels above and two levels below (the "rod long, fuse short" approach) (42). This principle is enhanced by the Edwards sleeve. Enhanced stabilization may also be promoted by the addition of sublaminar or spinous process wires. Although sublaminar wires give more rigid fixation, their passage in a neurologically compromised patient increases the risk of further injury (180,217) and, thus, are recommended only for patients with complete paraplegia.

The advantages of the Harrington system and its modifications are its widespread availability, surgeon familiarity, and relative ease of insertion. The disadvantages are the possibility that the device is insufficient to stabilize many burst fractures (78); the lack of predictable reduction or the inability to completely reduce the retropulsed fragments (19,28,55,118,125–128,141,149,165, 178,221,223); the necessity to incorporate normal levels with resultant secondary arthritic changes in the facet joints (117), a consideration of particular importance when only a few mobile lumbar segments remain (40); and the potential risk of producing a painful flat back deformity when the fixation extends into the mid or lower lumbar spine (106) (see Chapters 64 and 65). Early in the post-operative course, the hooks may dislodge with loss of correction. Over time the device may break or require removal (141). In these instances, one of the authors (Stauffer) has noted some correction loss, although the other authors have not.

Numerous alternatives have continued to evolve to supplant the basic Harrington instrumentation. The Luque system (134) has the advantage of greater stabilization of the rotational and translational components, but provides no distractive force and minimally resists axial compression. Additionally, there is an inherent danger in passing sublaminar wires, particularly in the face of recent spinal injury accompanied by spinal cord edema. Thus, these devices have found little place in the management of burst injuries, but still are useful in selected injuries accompanied by acute paraplegia.

Pedicle screw implants have the advantage of controlling the anterior column via a posterior approach, provide four-point fixation, and significantly reduce the number of levels that need to be incorporated in the construct, although there is considerable variation in the rigidity of fixation provided (6,90,95,142). The screws provide lever arms which facilitate reduction maneuvers and lordosis can be maintained. A large variety of possible implants are available which vary in their linkage systems, screw design, and flexibility of application, as described by Krag in Chapter 92 (2,3,43,56,64,131,135, 136,159,176,181,198). The disadvantages are the commercial unavailability of many of the devices and particularly the level of surgical skill necessary to avoid penetrating the pedicle with the potential risk of further neurologic damage.

The posterior approach remains the choice of most surgeons and is essential when laminal fractures with potential entrapment of neural elements are suspected. In these instances laminectomy is the method of choice (36). The posterolateral approach described by Flesch et al. (70) and others (74,210) is an alternative to decompression. Regardless of which means of decompression is employed, the benefit of ultrasonography in evaluating residual canal deformation has been shown (170).

Another school of thought has promoted the anterior approach in selected cases. This is particularly true when there is major canal involvement (60%–80%) by retropulsed fragments, irrespective of the patient's neurologic status. The rationale for this philosophy is that posterior approaches do not reliably reduce all fracture fragments, although some have argued that this can be done by a transpedicular approach, still utilizing posterior surgery.

The evolution of this approach can be traced to Royle (181), its popularization by Hodgson and Stock (108), and the development of anterior instruments used initially for the treatment of spinal deformities (61,99), the widespread experience in degenerative conditions (71,85,184,185), and the application of an anterior fixation device by Dunn (60) for the treatment of burst injuries. Although Dunn's device (Fig. 21) was withdrawn because of later vascular injuries, others applied their devices to the management of thoracolumbar fractures, most notably burst injuries (118,127,176,190,229), (personal communications: G. Armstrong, H. Yuan). The multiple devices are shown in Figures 22 through 27. These anterior distractive devices or fixation devices generally fall into the following categories: (a) plates; (b) external devices, that is, rods that lie outside the vertebral bodies; and (c) interbody devices. Distractive devices include the Kostuik-Harrington, Dunn, Slot, and Zielke devices, and the plates include the AO plate, the Arm-

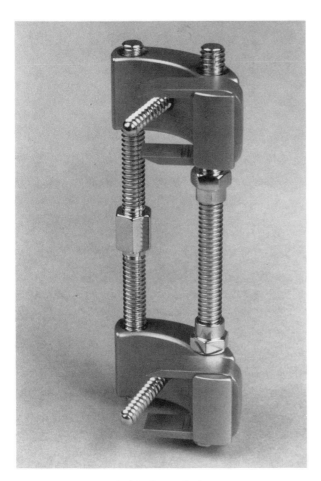

FIG. 21. Dunn device.

strong plate, and the I beam plate of Yuan. Interbody devices include the Rezinian device or temporary devices such as the Pinto distractor.

Plates provide fixation only, whereas most distractive devices are corrective as well. The rationale underlying these instruments is the inability of anterior grafts alone to withstand loads in the erect posture (218) or to provide adequate rotational control (see Chapter 93 for the historic details and evolution of these devices). The rates of non-unions, where no stabilizing devices are used, have ranged from 18% to 100% in the historic series, but on the average have been 10% to 20%. Another device with which two of the authors have had extensive experience is the Kostuik-Harrington device (Figs. 28A and 28B).

Two of the authors (Esses and Kostuik) have studied 80 sequential patients with burst fractures, combining early anterior decompression, grafting, and stabilization using the Kostuik-Harrington device. In patients with posterior column comminution, a second stage posterior procedure was carried out as well, a position advocated by Gertzbein et al. (80,81). The indications were: (a) acute burst injuries with or without neurologic compromise and retropulsion of bone fragments into the canal

(Fig. 29); (b) presentation of injury at greater than 7 days post injury, which was felt to be more difficult to reduce, or late injuries appearing weeks to years post injury; and (c) any burst fracture at L2 or below felt to require operative stabilization.

The age ranged from 17 to 63 years, with an average of 32. The level of injury was from T4 to L5. The timing of surgery varied. Fifty-seven of the 80 patients had neurologic lesions, with four complete and 53 incomplete. All 57 patients with neurologic injury were treated within 72 hours of injury, with an attempt to time the surgery as rapidly as possible. Four were treated within 6 hours, 35 within 48 hours, and the remaining 22 between 48 and 72 hours. None of the four patients with complete paraplegia recovered. The four patients with partial lesions at T12, L1, L2, and L3 treated within 6 hours were all Frankel Grade B, and all improved to Grade D with return of bladder and bowel function. Thirty-one incomplete lesions treated between 6 and 48 hours had neurologic improvement averaging 1.6 grades on the Frankel scale. The remaining 22 patients treated 48 to 72 hours post injury with partial paraplegia improved 1.0 grades.

Thirty-six of the 57 cases with neurologic involvement presented with loss of bowel and bladder function. The four complete lesions, as anticipated, showed no improvement. Of the remaining 32 cases, 10 patients, all with lesions in the area of the conus medullaris, have continued to require intermittent catheterization. The remainder have satisfactory bladder control which is either fully normal or requires a strict adherence to a regularly timed bladder program (see Chapter 63).

Although the trend suggests a benefit for early timing for decompression, the uncontrolled nature of the study and the numerous variables involved (age, sex, level of injury, degree of injury) makes it impossible to reach a definitive conclusion.

In the acute phase, all of the usual complications attendant to major spinal injury were observed, including urinary tract infections, atelectasis (seven cases), and pulmonary embolus (one case). No pressure sores developed during the acute hospitalization which lasted from 10 to 30 days, with an average of 24 days.

Other outcome measures include pain relief and work function. Four patients had significant incisional pain and dysathesiae (post-thoracotomy syndrome); two were relieved by extradural rhizotomies, one by phenol intercostal blocks, and one refused further treatment. Six patients had significant low back pain; in four patients this was disabling and has prevented work. All six were evaluated by discography at levels adjacent to the prior fusion. Two have undergone L5-S1 fusions, one with relief of pain, while the other has continuing symptoms.

The non-union rate was 4%. Of these, two had screw breakage. This latter complication was seen in 13 cases, and in two cases was associated with rod breakage as well. Superficial wound or donor site infection was iden-

Text continues on page 1315.

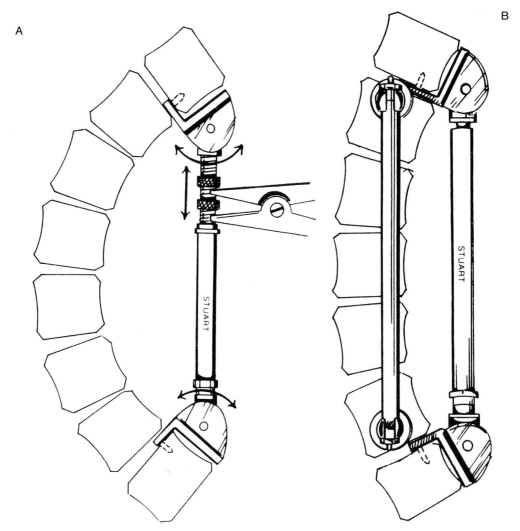

FIG. 22. Slot-Zielke device. **A:** Anterior distractive device permits correction of the kyphotic deformity. **B:** A second rod is inserted and the distractive device is then removed.

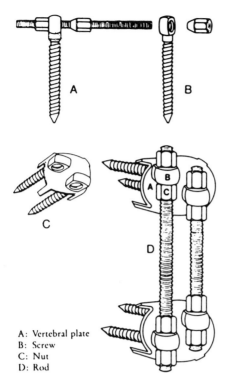

FIG. 23. Kaneda device.

A: Vertebral plate
B: Screw
C: Nut
D: Rod

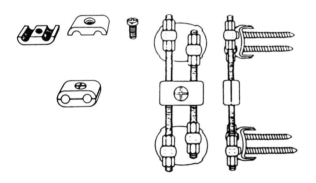

FIG. 24. Armstrong plate, which is still in the experimental stage.

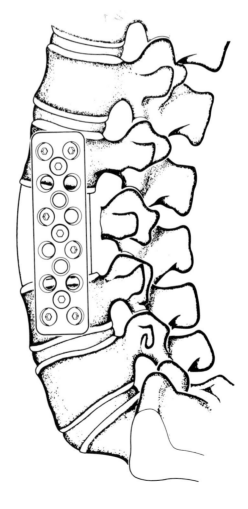

A

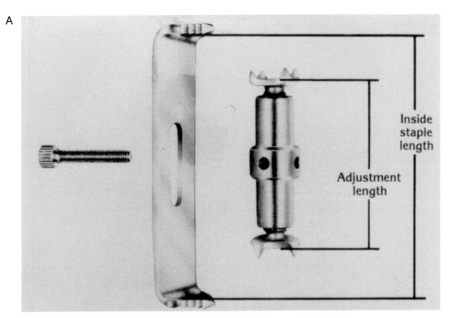

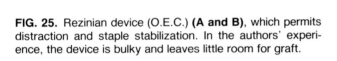

Inside
staple
length

Adjustment
length

B

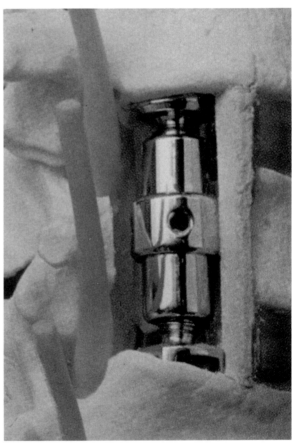

FIG. 25. Rezinian device (O.E.C.) **(A and B)**, which permits distraction and staple stabilization. In the authors' experience, the device is bulky and leaves little room for graft.

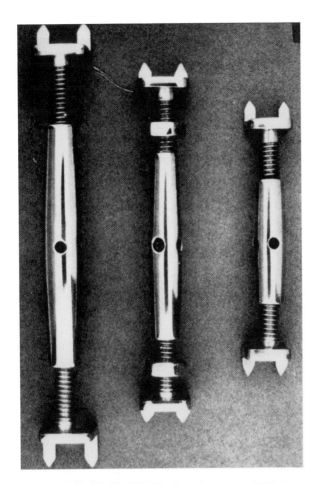

FIG. 26. Pinto Santalasa distractor. A temporary distractor to correct kyphotic deformity.

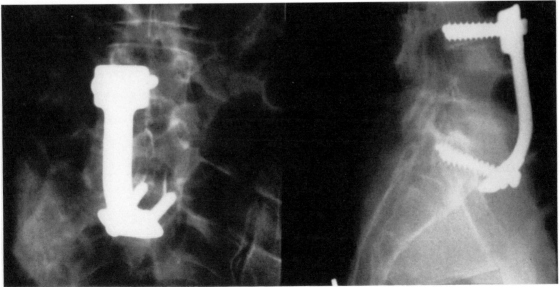

FIG. 27. Yuan Beam plate. Here used in salvage plate of posterior pseudarthrosis in a previous posterior fusion for degenerative disc disease, the plate has been contoured for the sacral promontory.

A

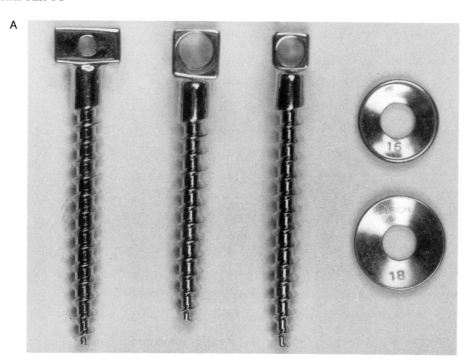

FIG. 28. A: Kostuik-Harrington apparatus used with standard Harrington round-ended rods and equipment staples are preferred to washers, as they aid in coupling.

B

FIG. 28. B: Larger-holed (distraction) screw is used for rachet end of distraction rod. Smaller-holed (collar) screws are used for collar end of distraction rod and heavy Harrington compression rods. Screw heads on compression rods are usually crimped. Nuts may be used.

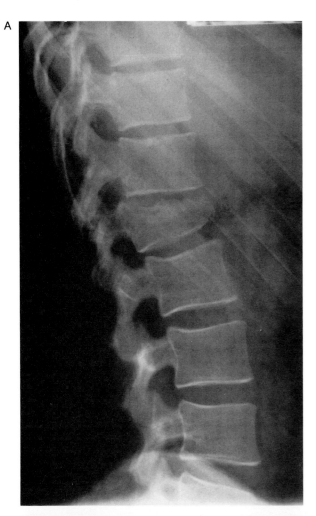

A

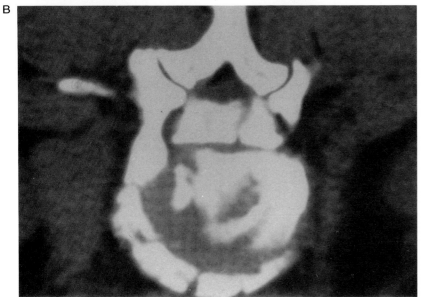

B

FIG. 29. A: Pre-operative lateral radiograph shows greater than 50% loss of anterior column height and kyphosis 34 degrees.

FIG. 29. B: Pre-operative CT scan shows marked canal occlusion, Frankel Grade B. (Figs. 29C–29E follow.)

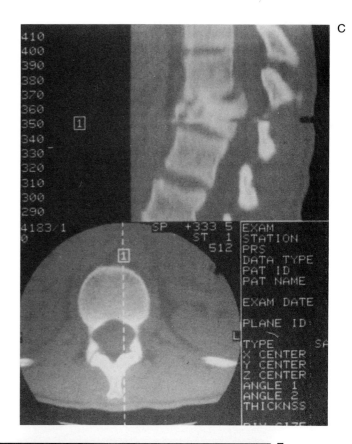

C

FIG. 29. *(Continued)* **C:** Lateral CT reconstruction. Note loss of stability. **D:** Post-operative lateral radiograph. Note complete restoration of height of vertebral body. **E:** Post-operative AP radiograph. Patient restored to Frankel Grade D. This case was done within 6 hours.

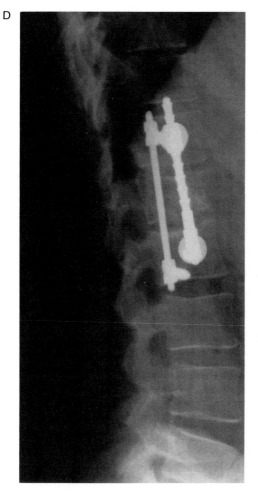

D

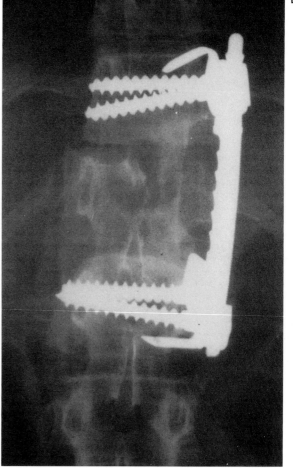

E

tified in six cases and one patient developed an osteomyelitis, necessitating removal of the fixation device once union had occurred. No patient has had a later vascular complication.

These results are comparable to those reported by other investigators. Dunn (60) concluded neurologic recovery was more certain with anterior decompression compared to a previously reported series of patients treated by posterior instrumentation or non-operative treatment. He noted particularly that the anterior approach was desirable for injuries below L2. Bradford and McBride (26) compared 20 patients treated by anterior decompression and stabilization with 39 treated by posterior or posterolateral decompression and stabilization. The neurologic recovery was greater for the anterior surgery (88% versus 64%), including recovery of bladder and bowel control (69% versus 33%). Inferior results tended to correlate with any residual bony canal stenosis identified on post-operative CT scan. Gertzbein et al. (81) combined anterior fusion with posterior fusion and instrumentation in 18 patients with over 50% canal compromise. Eighty-one percent of the incomplete lesions demonstrated neurologic improvement. They concluded that up to 35% of canal compromise and up to 20% of kyphos did not cause any pressure on the spinal cord. A prospective study in progress by the authors (Esses and Kostuik) is comparing posterior pedicle stabilization and anterior surgery. To date there has been no difference in the two groups as measured by neurologic outcome, late kyphosis, or complication. The only difference has been the degree of canal clearance which is 100% by the anterior approach and averages 80% by the posterior approach.

In summary, the optimum management of burst fractures is a source of ongoing controversy (63). For the neurologically intact patient, alternatives are conservative management which can be successful, as demonstrated by Weinstein et al. (216), initial conservative management with delayed stabilization if there is progressive deformity or pain, or early stabilization using the posterior or anterior approaches. The key to long range success is deformity correction, adequate initial stabilization, and a long-term solid bony arthrodesis. Although each surgical approach has its advocates, to date there is no certain basis for choosing one method over another. On theoretical grounds, the anterior approach or posterior approach with pedicle fixation has the advantage of incorporating only a few segments in the fusion. This is of particular importance when the injury involves the lower lumbar spine (44), where preservation of lordosis and minimization of the number of fused segments is of greater importance. However, these latter approaches and devices have a significant learning curve and are not yet readily available. Thus, more traditional

Text continues on page 1322.

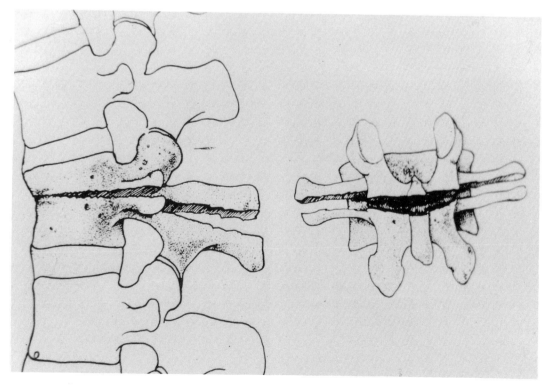

FIG. 30. A flexion-distraction fracture dislocation involving bony element. This injury will heal without operative intervention because of its pure osseous involvement. A representative case treated by Kostuik-Harrington instrumentation is shown.

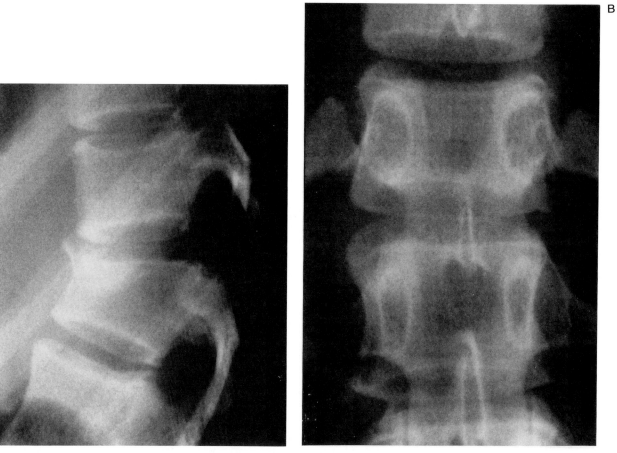

FIG. 31. AP **(A)** and lateral **(B)** x-rays of flexion-distraction lesion of T11-T12. Note the ''see through'' lesion at disc level due to dislocated facets.

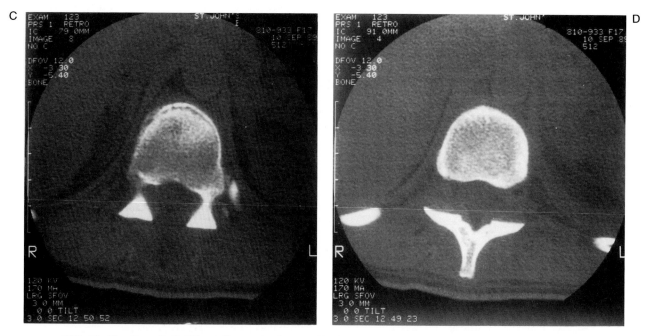

FIG. 31. *(Continued)* **C:** ''Empty'' superior facets of T12 on CT scan. **D:** ''Empty inferior facets of T11 on CT scan. (Figs. 31E–31F follow.)

E

F

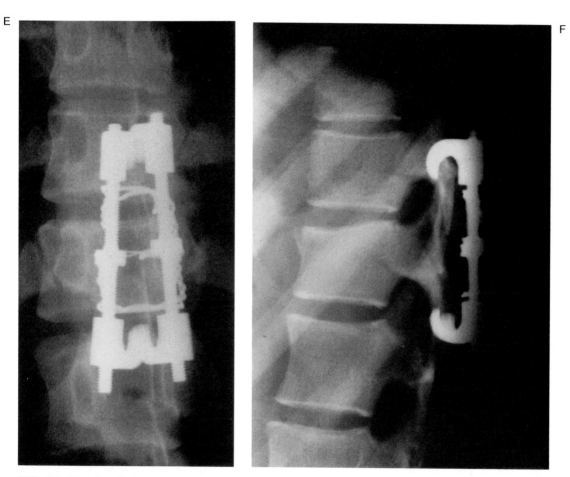

FIG. 31. *(Continued)* Post-operative AP **(E)** and lateral **(F)** x-rays of one-level compression fixation fusion.

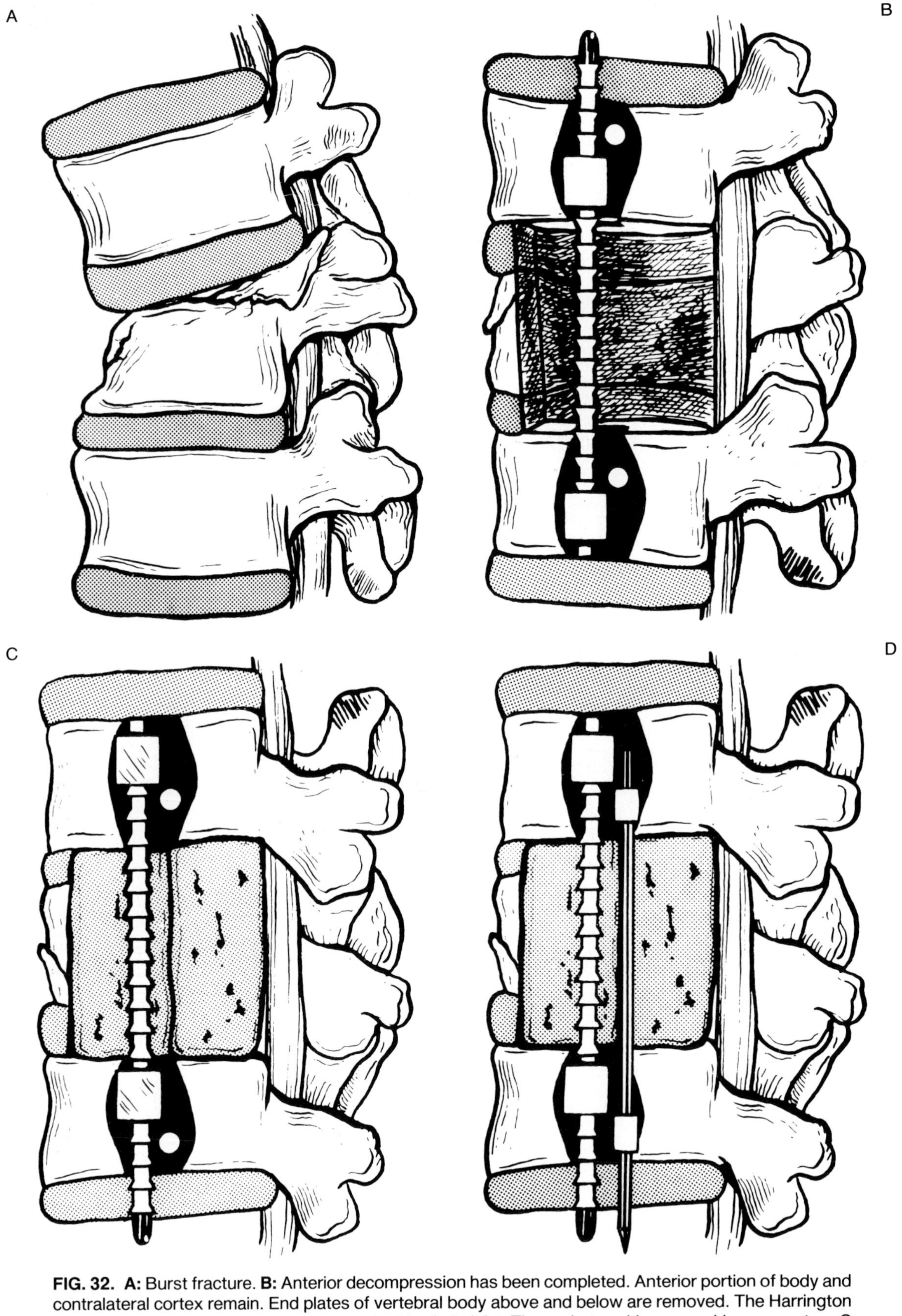

A

B

C

D

FIG. 32. A: Burst fracture. **B:** Anterior decompression has been completed. Anterior portion of body and contralateral cortex remain. End plates of vertebral body above and below are removed. The Harrington rod is used in distraction to restore vertebral body height. The rachet end is secured by one or two C clamps. **C:** Bone graft is added, usually using one iliac crest bicortical graft slightly larger than the defect (tricortical in the presence of osteopenia). **D:** In addition rib struts or small fragments of iliac crest graft are added.

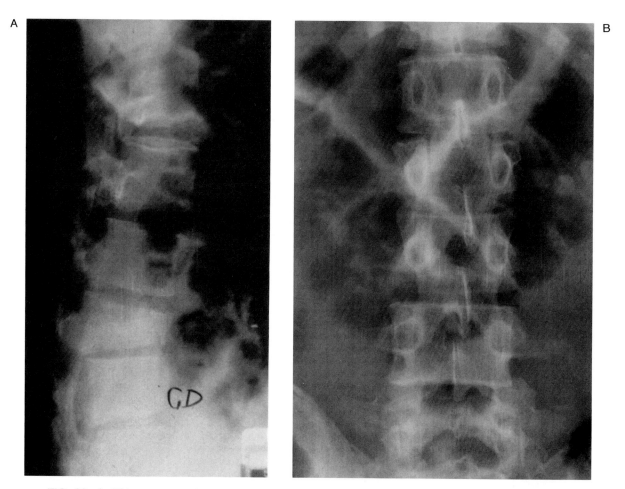

FIG. 33. A: This pre-operative lateral radiograph appears relatively innocuous, but the patient was Frankel Grade C on physical examination. **B:** Pre-operative AP radiograph. Note mild splaying of pedicles and increased spinous process distance. (Figs. 33C–33G follow.)

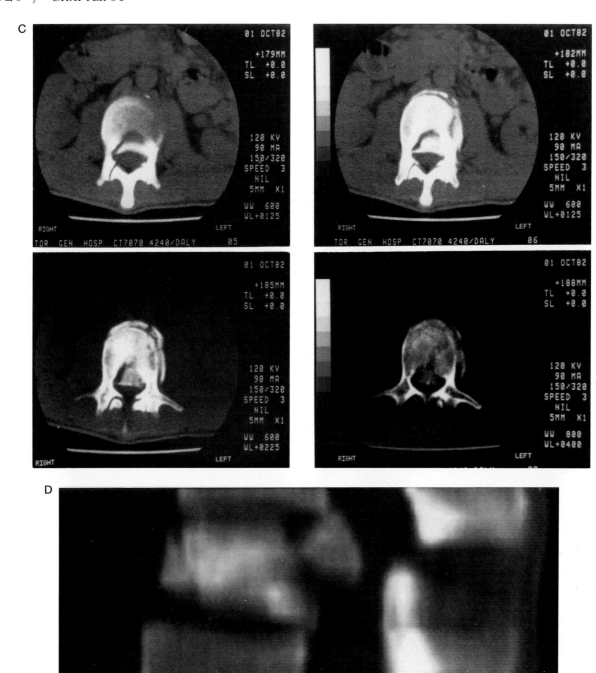

FIG. 33. *(Continued)* **C and D:** CT scan reconstruction. Note the sharp angulatory fragment unattached to soft tissue at time of surgery. Axial cuts showed marked occlusion. (Figs. 33E–33G follow.)

E

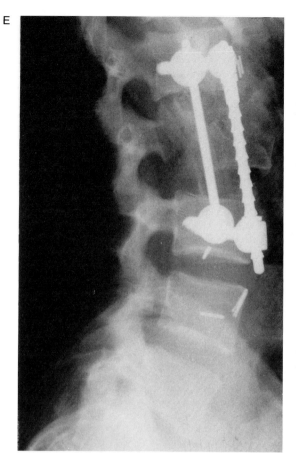

F

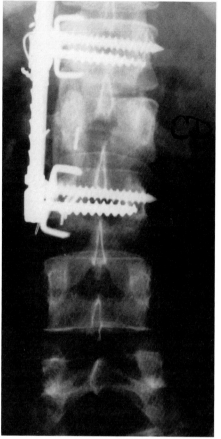

G

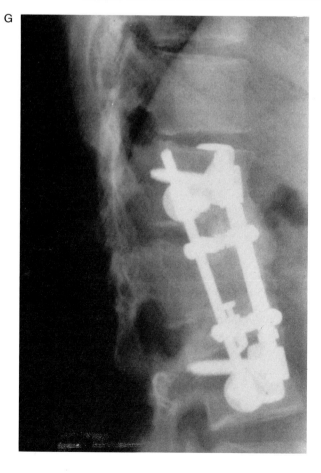

FIG. 33. *(Continued)* Post-operative lateral **(E)** and AP **(F)** radiographs. More recently **(G)**, cross linkage between the bars has been added to increase stability.

A

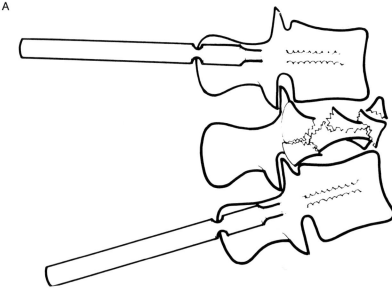

B

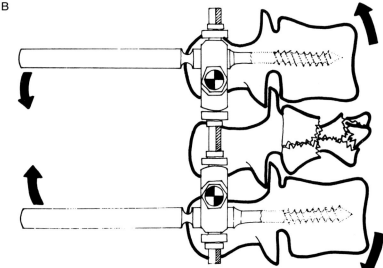

FIG. 34. Burst fracture. **A:** The Schanz pins are divergent posteriorly and convergent anteriorly due to the traumatic kyphosis. The pins are introduced through the pedicles bilaterally (4 pins) at the levels above and below the fracture. **B:** The coupling device is added to the pins and lordosis is restored by bringing the pins together posteriorly.

posterior approaches such as Harrington rods remain useful surgical techniques.

For the complete paraplegic, early surgical intervention is appropriate to promote early rehabilitation. In these instances, the surgical approach is probably less important, provided adequate stabilization is obtained. This is a place where Harrington rod constructs can be supplemented by sublaminar wire fixation.

The management of the incomplete paraplegic with a burst injury presents a major unresolved issue (26). Timing of surgery is debatable, although a trend toward earlier intervention is being identified. Complete decompression of the canal is a major issue and seems more predictable with an anterior approach with instrumentation, or possibly a posterolateral approach. Although considerable reduction is obtained with Harrington rod constructs, this seems to be less predictable than with pedicle fixation. Laminectomy alone, without stabilization, is rarely warranted, but laminectomy is important when the pre-operative status and imaging studies indicate significant neural arch comminution. In these instances, removal of entrapped neural elements from within the arch may improve neurologic status. The accompanying dural leak should be repaired and stabilization then carried out. Regardless of what form of stabilization is performed, the patient is braced by TSLO or body cast until fracture union is demonstrated to be complete.

Flexion-Rotation Injuries

The treatment considerations are identical to those for the burst injury, although the magnitude of forces in-

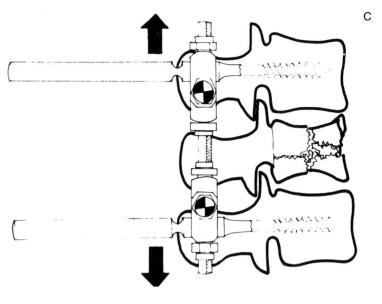

C

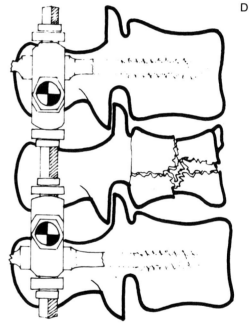

D

FIG. 34. *(Continued)* **C:** Distraction is then added and the coupling device fully tightened. Some surgeons prefer to distract prior to the motion to restore lordosis. **D:** The vertebral body height has been restored. We prefer to do a posterolateral fusion over the two disc spaces. Some surgeons bone graft the fractured vertebral body either via the pedicles or via the body directly posterolaterally and then remove the pins at one year, thus preserving motion.

volved makes it more likely that the patient has a complete neurologic injury. The posterior approach is usually advantageous to deal with facet injuries and to correct the rotational deformity. However, distraction instrumentation is not indicated if there is suspected disruption of the anterior longitudinal ligament. If gross instability is suspected, a staged anterior approach may be warranted (81).

Flexion-Distraction Injuries

The treatment choice depends on the pattern of involvement, i.e., ligamentous, osseous, or osseoligamentous. If the injury is osseous, then management with extension orthosis or cast is compatible with early

mobilization and constitutes definitive treatment (Fig. 30). Those patterns involving ligaments have less predictable capacity to be stabilized with conservative management and are best treated by operative stabilization (82) (Fig. 31). Distraction devices such as the Harrington rod are contraindicated because of the three-column involvement. Double Harrington rod compression systems remain the most common method for management.

Extension Injuries

These injuries are usually stable and can be managed with a flexion cast or orthosis for periods up to 12 weeks, dependent on the patient's comfort.

Posterior Element Fractures

These are stable and can be treated without external fixation, although the patient may be more easily mobilized and have less discomfort with light bracing.

OPERATIVE APPROACHES

Anterior Approach

The operative approach is based on the level of pathology to be treated as outlined in Chapter 60. Neural decompression is carried out first with the anterior one quarter of the body being preserved with soft tissue attachments in order to provide a viable graft (Figs. 32A–32D). The dura is completely decompressed anteriorly and to the right and left, and is allowed to float anteriorly. If neural decompression is not required, the disc space and end plates are removed on either side of the fracture back to the posterior longitudinal ligaments. The technique is then identical to that described in Chapters 64 and 65. Distractive forces are carried out sufficient to restore normal vertebral body height. Bicortical iliac grafts are harvested and if osteopenia is present, a tricortical graft is utilized. These are placed in the defect under compression. The collar-ended screws are inserted into the vertebral body above and below the fracture site if the Kostuik-Harrington instrumentation is used. The rods are inserted and the screw heads crimped to enhance stability. Staples or cross linkages are commonly used to enhance fixation (Fig. 33). If other methods of anterior fixation are chosen, the types, their indications, and their application are presented in Chapter 93.

Posterior Approach

A standard midline approach is carried out as described in Chapter 60. Depending on the fixation device to be used, the exposure may be quite extensive, particularly if a "rod long, fuse short" plan is adopted. If laminectomy or posterolateral decompression is performed, the methods are those described in Chapter 88.

Harrington Technique

Endotracheal intubation is carried out and a general anesthetic is administered. The patient is log-rolled into the prone position on the operating frame. A midline posterior incision is made, and the subcutaneous tissues are infiltrated with a 1 in 500,000 solution of adrenaline in saline. Sub-periosteal dissection of the posterior elements of the spine is carried out, beginning at either end of the incision and gradually working toward the injured area. Care is taken to ensure that the facet joints are not traumatized. With retractors in place, the fractured vertebrae can be identified. If distraction is to be effected, a 1-2-5-1 superior hook is placed two or three levels above the fracture site. The appropriate facet joint is identified, and a notch is cut with a small osteotome in the inferior portion of the inferior articular process. This allows proper purchase of the hook into the pedicle. Inferiorly, 1-2-5-3 hooks are placed in notches prepared in the lamina of the vertebra two or three levels below the fracture site. The Harrington outrigger is then purchased on the hooks, and a distraction force is gently applied. A lateral x-ray should be taken to ensure that anatomic alignment has been obtained. If the position is satisfactory, then a 1-2-5-0 distraction rod can be inserted on the contralateral side. The outrigger is now removed and replaced by a second distraction rod. Posterolateral bone grafting is recommended at each level which the instrumentation spans.

If compression is required, then 1-2-5-4 or 1-2-5-6 hooks are placed at the two levels cephalad and the two levels caudad to the injured vertebra. These hooks are placed around the transverse processes in the thoracic spine and around the lamina in the lumbar spine. They are connected by a large, threaded compression rod.

Spinal cord monitoring, if available, ensures that iatrogenic injury to the neural elements does not occur. Reduction of retropulsed fragments of bone can be ascertained by intra-operative ultrasound or by posterolateral exposure of the injured level.

Segmental Instrumentation

At the present time, the use of Luque instrumentation is primarily reserved for patients in whom there is complete spinal cord injury. In these patients, the segmental wiring can provide rigid immobilization and allow early patient mobilization.

Pedicle Screw Instrumentation

Pedicle implants can be categorized as screw-plate or screw-rod systems, which are discussed in Chapter 92. The Schanz screws provide large lever arms, and these facilitate reduction maneuvers. Posterior distraction and restoration of lordosis has been successful in adequately decompressing the spinal canal in most instances of burst fractures.

AO Spinal Internal Fixator Technique

The AO spinal internal fixator consists of Schanz screws, a coupling clamp, and fully threaded rods. The Schanz screws are 5.0 mm in diameter, and the threaded rods are 7 mm in diameter and flattened on two sides.

The coupling device is freely mobile in the sagittal plane, thus allowing for angulation of the Schanz screws before securing them to the rod. The nuts have a lug that can be crimped to secure them to the flattened rod.

The spine is exposed through a midline posterior incision. Sub-periosteal dissection is carried out at either end of the incision, gradually working toward the fractured level. Schanz screws are placed down the pedicle into the vertebral body at the level above and below the injury. These can be inserted under image intensifier control or using anatomic landmarks. Accurate screw placement must be verified before proceeding with fracture reduction.

The Schanz screws act as large level arms and can be placed in a variety of biomechanical modes including distraction, compression, or derotation.

A burst fracture is reduced first by distraction and then by correction of the kyphotic deformity. Forceful distraction can be facilitated by placing a pelvic reduction forcep over the Schanz screws and spreading the handles. The nuts on the threaded rod can then be tightened to secure their position. Lordosis is achieved by approximating the ends of the Schanz screws and tightening the coupling nut (Fig. 34).

Reduction of a flexion-distraction injury is simply effected by bringing the ends of the screws more closely together while visualizing the site of the injury.

In instances where addition rotatory stabilization is required, a Transverse Traction Device (DTT) is used to bridge the two rods. Posterolateral fusion is then carried out at the two instrumented levels.

REFERENCES

1. Abel M (1982): The exaggerated supine oblique view of the cervical spine. *Skeletal Radiol* 8:213–219.
2. Aebi M, Etter C, Kehl T, et al (1987): Stabilization of the lower thoracic and lumbar spine with the internal spinal skeletal fixation system. Indications, techniques, and first results of treatment. *Spine* 12:544–551.
3. Aebi M, Etter C, Kehl T, et al (1988): The internal skeletal fixation system. A new treatment of thoracolumbar fractures and other spinal disorders. *Clin Orthop* 227:30–43.
4. Amyes M, Vogel P, Raney R (1955): Spinal cord compression due to spontaneous epidural hemorrhage. *Bull LA Neurol Soc* 20:1–8.
5. Angtuaco E, Binet E (1984): Radiology of thoracic and lumbar fractures. *Clin Orthop* 189:43–57.
6. Ashman RB, Birch JG, Bone LB, et al (1988): Mechanical testing of spinal instrumentation. *Clin Orthop* 227:113–125.
7. Bailey S (1982): Orthopaedic injuries of the lower limb and trunk in multiple system trauma. *Can J Surg* 25:171–172.
8. Bannister J, Taylor TKF, Nade S (1975): Seat belt fractures of the spine. *J Bone Joint Surg* [Br] 57:252.
9. Bedbrook GM (1971): Stability of spinal fractures and fracture dislocations. *Paraplegia* 9:23–32.
10. Bedbrook GM (1975): Treatment of thoracolumbar dislocation and fractures with paraplegia. *Clin Orthop* 112:27.
11. Bedbrook GM (1979): Spinal injuries with tetraplegia and paraplegia. *J Bone Joint Surg* [Br] 61:267.
12. Bentley G, McSweeney T (1968): Multiple spinal injuries. *Br J Surg* 55:565–570.
13. Berquist T (1986): *Imaging of orthopaedic trauma and surgery.* Philadelphia: W.B. Saunders.
14. Betz R, Gelman A, DeFilipp G, et al (1987): Magnetic resonance imaging (MRI) in the evaluation of spinal cord injured children and adolescents. *Paraplegia* 25:92–99.
15. Binet EF, Moro JJ, Marangola JP, et al (1977): Cervical spine tomography in trauma. *Spine* 3:163–172.
16. Blumenkopf B, Juneau P (1988): Magnetic resonance imaging (MRI) of thoracolumbar fractures. *J Spinal Disord* 1:144–150.
17. Boehler L (1932): Behandlung der Wirbelbruche. *Laugenbecks Arch Klin Clin* 173:843–847.
18. Bohlman HH (1974): Traumatic fractures of the upper thoracic spine with paralysis: A study of 100 cases. *J Bone Joint Surg* [Am] 56:1299.
19. Bohlman HH, Freehafer A, DeJak J (1975): Free anterior decompression of spinal cord injuries. *J Bone Joint Surg* [Am] 57:1025.
20. Bohlman H (1979): Acute fractures and dislocations of the cervical spine. *J Bone Joint Surg* [Am] 61:114–119.
21. Bohlman H, Boada E (1989): Fractures and dislocations of the lower cervical spine. In: Sherk, HH, ed. *The cervical spine, 2nd ed.* Philadelphia; J.B. Lippincott, pp. 355–389.
22. Bonndurant F, Cotler H, Kulkarni MC, et al (1990): Acute spinal cord injury: A study using physical examination and magnetic resonance imaging. *Spine* 15:161–168.
23. Bracken MB, Webb SB, Wagner FC (1978): Classification of the severity of acute spinal cord injury: Implications for management. *Paraplegia* 15:319–326.
24. Bracken MB, Shepard MJ, Collins WF, et al (1990): A randomized, controlled trial of methylprednisolone or naloxone in the treatment of acute spinal-cord injury. Results of the second National Acute Spinal Cord Injury Study. *N Engl J Med* 322:1405–1411.
25. Bradford DS, Akbarnia BA, Winter RD, et al (1977): Surgical stabilization of fracture and fracture dislocation of the thoracic spine. *Spine* 2:185.
26. Bradford D, McBride G (1987): Surgical management of thoracolumbar spine fractures with incomplete neurologic deficits. *Clin Orthop* 218:201–216.
27. Brant-Zawadzki M, Jeffrey R, Minago H, et al (1982): High resolution CT of thoracolumbar fractures. *AJNR* 3:69–74.
28. Breig A (1972): The therapeutic possibilities of surgical bioengineering in incomplete spinal cord lesions. *Paraplegia* 9:173.
29. Broom M, Raycroft J (1988): Complications of fractures of the cervical spine in ankylosing spondylitis. *Spine* 13:763–766.
30. Brown B, Brant-Zawadzki M, Cann C (1982): Dynamic CT scanning of spinal column trauma. *AJR* 139:1177.
31. Burke D (1971): Hyperextension injuries of the spine. *J Bone Joint Surg* [Br] 53:3–12.
32. Burke D (1973): Spinal cord injuries and seat belts. *Mod J Aust* 2:801.
33. Burney R, Waggoner R, Maynard F (1989): Stabilization of spinal injury for early transfer. *J Trauma* 29:1497–1499.
34. Butt W (1988): Interpreting the spinal x-ray: 1. *Br J Hosp Med* 40:46–53.
35. Calenoff L, Chessare J, Rogers L, et al (1978): Multiple level spinal injuries: Importance of early recognition. *AJR* 130:665.
36. Cammisa FP, Eismont FJ, Green BA (1989): Dural laceration occuring with burst fractures and associated laminar fractures. *J Bone Joint Surg* [AM] 71:1044–1052.
37. Chakeres D, Flickinger F, Bresnahan J, et al (1987): MR imaging of acute spinal cord trauma. *AJNR* 8:5–10.
38. Chance GQ (1948): Note on a type of flexion fracture of the spine. *Br J Radiol* 21:452–453.
39. Christian M (1976): Non-fatal injuries sustained by seat belt wearers: A comparative study. *Br Med J* 2:1310.
40. Cochran T, Irstam L, Nachemson A (1983): Long-term anatomic and functional changes in patients with adolescent idiopathic scoliosis treated by Harrington rod fusion. *Spine* 8:576–584.
41. Cooper P, Cohen W (1984): Evaluation of cervical spinal cord injuries with metrizamide myelography-CT scanning. *J Neurosurg* 61:281.
42. Cotler JM, Vernace JV, Michalski JA (1986): The use of Harrington rods in thoracolumbar fractures. *Orthop Clin North Am* 17:87–103.

43. Cotrel Y, Dubousset J, Guillamat M (1988): New universal instrumentation in spinal surgery. *Clin Orthop* 227:10–23.

44. Court-Brown CM, Gertzbein SD (1987): The management of burst fractures of the fifth lumbar vertebra. *Spine* 12:308–312.

45. Daffner R (1988): *Imaging of vertebral trauma.* Rockville, Maryland: Aspen.

46. Dalinka M, Keszler H, Weiss M (1985): The radiographic evaluation of spinal trauma. *Emerg Med Clin North Am* 3:475.

47. Dalinka M, Boorstein J, Zlatkin M (1989): Computed tomography of musculoskeletal trauma. *Radiol Clin North Am* 27:933–944.

48. Dall B, Stauffer ES (1988): Neurologic injury and recovery patterns in burst fractures at the T12 or L1 motion segment. *Clin Orthop* 233:171–176.

49. Das De S McCreath SW (1981): Lumbosacral fracture-dislocations. A report of four cases. *J Bone Joint Surg* [Br] 63:58–60.

50. Davies E, Roylance J (1970): Aortography in the investigation of traumatic mediastinal haematoma. *Clin Radiol* 21:297–305.

51. Denis F, Armstrong G (1981): Compression fractures versus burst fractures in the lumbar and thoracic spine. *J Bone Joint Surg* [Br] 63:462.

52. Denis F (1983): The three column spine and its significance in the classification of acute thoracolumbar spinal injuries. *Spine* 8:817–831.

53. Denis F, Armstrong G, Searls F, et al (1984): Acute thoracolumbar burst fractures in the absence of neurologic deficit: A comparison between operative and nonoperative treatment. *Clin Orthop* 189:142–149.

54. Dennis LN (1989): Superior mediastinal widening from spine fractures mimicking aortic rupture on chest radiographs. *AJR* 152:27–30.

55. Dewald RL, Fister JS, Savino AW (1982): The management of unstable burst fractures of the thoracolumbar spine. Presented at the Scoliosis Research Society meeting, Denver, Colorado.

56. Dick W (1987): "The fixateur interne" as a versatile implant for spine surgery. *Spine* 12:882–900.

57. Dickson JH, Harrington PR, Erwin WD (1978): Results of reduction and stabilization of the severely fractured thoracic and lumbar spine. *J Bone Joint Surg* [Am] 60:799–805.

58. Dooley B (1975): The effect of compulsory seat belt wearing on the mortality and pattern of injury to car occupants. *J Bone Joint Surg* [Br] 57:252.

59. Ducker TB (1990): Treatment of spinal cord injury. *N Engl J Med* 322:1459–1461.

60. Dunn HK (1986): Anterior spine stabilization and decompression for thoracolumbar injuries. *Orthop Clin North Am* 17:113–119.

61. Dwyer AF (1973): Experience of anterior correction of scoliosis. *Clin Orthop* 93:191.

62. Edwards CC, Levine AM (1986): Early rod sleeve stabilization of the injured thoracic and lumbar spine. *Orthop Clin North Am* 17:121–145.

63. Esses SI (1988): The placement and treatment of thoracolumbar spine fractures. An algorithmic approach. *Orthop Rev* 17:571–584.

64. Esses SI (1989): The AO spinal internal fixator. *Spine* 14:373–378.

65. Esses S, Botsford D (1990): Development of a new neural grading scale. Presented at the Annual Meeting of the American Spinal Injury Association, Orlando, Florida.

66. Fazl M, Bilbao J, Hudson A (1981): Laceration of the aorta complicating spinal fracture in ankylosing spondylitis. *Neurosurgery* 8:712–734.

67. Feuer H (1976): Management of acute spine and spinal cord injuries: Old and new concepts. *Arch Surg* 111:638–645.

68. Fidler MW (1988): Remodelling of the spinal canal after burst fracture. A prospective study of two cases. *J Bone Joint Surg* [Br] 70:730–732.

69. Firoozina H, et al (1985): Sudden quadriplegia after a minor trauma. The role of preexisting spinal stenosis. *Surg Neurol* 23:165–168.

70. Flesch JR, Leider LL Jr, Erickson DD, et al (1977): Harrington instrumentation and spinal fusion for unstable fractures and fracture-dislocations of the thoracic and lumbar spine. *J Bone Joint Surg* [Am] 59:143–153.

71. Flynn JC, Anwarul B, Hoque MA (1979): Anterior fusion of the lumbar spine. End-result study with long-term follow-up. *J Bone Joint Surg* [Am] 61:1143–1150.

72. Fowler A. (1957): Flexion-compression injury of the sternum. *J Bone Joint Surg* [Br] 39:487–497.

73. Frankel H, Hancock D, Hyslop G, et al (1969): The value of postural reduction in the initial management of closed injuries of the spine with paraplegia and tetraplegia. *Paraplegia* 7:179–192.

74. Garfin SR, Mowery CS, Guerra J Jr, Marshall LF (1985): Confirmation of the posterolateral technique to decompress and fuse thoracolumbar spine burst fractures. *Spine* 10:218–223.

75. Gehweiler J, Osborne R, Becker R (1980): *The radiology of vertebral trauma.* Philadelphia: W.B. Saunders.

76. Gellad FE, Levine AM, Joslyn JN, Edwards CC, Bosse M (1986): Pure thoracolumbar facet dislocation: Clinical features and CT appearance. *Radiology* 161:505–508.

77. Gelman M, Unber J (1978): Fractures of the thoracolumbar spine in ankylosing spondylitis. *AJR* 130:485.

78. Gertzbein SD, MacMichael D, Tile M (1982): Harrington instrumentation as a method of fixation in fractures of the spine. A critical analysis of deficiencies. *J Bone Joint Surg* [Br] 64:526–529.

79. Gertzbein SD, Court-Brown CM (1988): Flexion-distraction injuries of the lumbar spine. Mechanisms of injury and classification. *Clin Orthop* 277:52–60.

80. Gertzbein S, Court-Brown C, Marks P, et al. (1988): The neurologic outcome following surgery for spinal fractures. *Spine* 13:641–644.

81. Gertzbein SD, Court-Brown CM, Jacobs RR, et al (1988): Decompression and circumferential stabilization of unstable spinal fractures. *Spine* 13:892–895.

82. Gertzbein SD, Eismont FJ (1990): Trauma of the lumbar spine: Classification and treatment. In: Weinstein JN, Wiesel SW, eds. *The lumbar spine.* Philadelphia: W.B. Saunders, pp. 662–698.

83. Gertzbein SD, Court-Brown CM (1988): Flexion–distraction injuries of the lumbar spine. Mechanisms of injury and classification. *Clin Orthop* 227:52–58.

84. Goldberg A, Rothfus W, Deeb Z, et al (1988): The impact of magnetic resonance on the diagnostic evaluation of acute cervicothoracic spinal trauma. *Skeletal Radiol* 17:89–95.

85. Goldner JL, McCollum DE, Urbanisk JR (1969): Anterior disc excision and interbody spine fusion for chronic low back pain. In: American Academy of Orthopaedic Surgeons. *Symposium of the spine.* St. Louis: C.V. Mosby.

86. Gordon ML, Capen DA, Zigler J, Garland D, Nelson R, Nagelberg S (1990): A comparison of operative and non-operative treatment in fractures of the high thoracic spine. *J Spinal Dis* 3.

87. Grazier KL, Holbrook TL, Kelsey JL, et al (1984): *The frequency of occurrence, impact, and cost of musculoskeletal conditions in the United States.* Chicago: American Academy of Orthopaedic Surgeons.

88. Grigolia A, Bell R, Peltier L. (1967): Fractures and dislocations of the spine complicating ankylosing spondylitis: A report of six cases. *J Bone Joint Surg* [Am] 49:339–344.

89. Guerra J, Garfin S, Resnick D (1984): Vertebral burst fractures: CT analysis of the retropulsed fragment. *Radiology* 153:769–772.

90. Gurr KR, McAfee PC, Shih CM (1988): Biomechanical analysis of anterior and posterior instrumentation systems after corpectomy: A calf-spine model. *J Bone Joint Surg* [Am] 70:1182–1191.

91. Guttman L (1954): Initial treatment of traumatic paraplegia. *Proceedings Royal Society of Medicine* 47:1103.

92. Guttman L (1966): Traumatic paraplegia and tetraplegia in ankylosing spondylitis. *Paraplegia* 4:188–203.

93. Guttman L (1969): Spinal deformities in traumatic paraplegics and tetraplegics following surgical procedures. *Paraplegia* 7:38.

94. Guttman L (1972): Spinal injuries, initial treatment of fractures and dislocations in traumatic paraplegia and tetraplegia. *Folia Traumatologica* (Geigy) 1–16.

95. Guyer DW, Yuan HA, Werner FW, et al (1987): Biomechanical comparison of seven internal fixation devices for the lumbosacral junction. *Spine* 12:569–573.

96. Hackney D, Asato R, Joseph P, et al (1986): Hemorrhage and edema in acute spinal cord compression: Demonstration by MR imaging. *Radiology* 161:387.

97. Hadden W, Gillespie W (1985): Multiple level injuries of the cervical spine. *Injury* 16:628–633.

98. Hadley M, Zabramski M, Browner R, et al (1988): Pediatric spinal trauma: Review of 122 cases of spinal cord and vertebral column injuries. *J Neurosurg* 68:18–24.

99. Hall JE, Micheli LJ (1981): The use of modified Dwyer instrumentation in anterior stabilization of the spine. Presented at the Scoliosis Research Society meeting, Montreal.

100. Hanley E, Eskay M (1989): Thoracic spine fractures. *Orthopaedics* 12:689–696.

101. Hansen S, Taylor T, Honet J, et al (1967): Fracture dislocations of the ankylosed thoracic spine in rheumatoid spondylitis. *J Trauma* 7:827.

102. Harrington PR (1962): Treatment of scoliosis. *J Bone Joint Surg* [Am] 44:591.

103. Harrington T, Barker B (1986): Multiple trauma associated with vertebral injury. *Surg Neurol* 26:149–154.

104. Harris J, Edeiken-Monroe B (1987): *The radiology of acute cervical spine trauma.* Baltimore: Williams and Wilkins.

105. Harryman DT (1986): Complete fracture-dislocation of the thoracic spine associated with spontaneous neurologic decompression. A case report. *Clin Orthop* 207:64–69.

106. Hasday CA, Passoff TL, Perry J (1983): Gait abnormalities arising from iatrogenic loss of lumbar lordosis secondary to Harrington instrumentation in lumbar fractures. *Spine* 8:501–511.

107. Hazel WA Jr, Jones RA, Morrey BF, Stauffer RN (1988): Vertebral fractures without neurological deficit. A long-term follow-up study. *J Bone Joint Surg* [Am] 70:1319–1321.

108. Hodgson AR, Stock FE (1956): Anterior spinal fusion. A preliminary communication on radical treatment of Pott's disease and Pott's paraplegia. *Br J Surg* 44:266–275.

109. Holdsworth FW (1963): Fractures, dislocations and fracture-dislocations of the spine. *J Bone Joint Surg* [Br] 45:6–20.

110. Holdsworth FW (1970): Fractures, dislocations and fracture-dislocations of the spine. *J Bone Joint Surg* [Am] 52:1534–1551.

111. Holt B (1976): Spines and seat belts: Mechanisms of spinal injury in motor vehicle crashes. *Med J Aust* 2:411.

112. Hunter T, Dubo H (1983): Spinal fractures complicating ankylosing spondylitis. *Arthritis Rheum* 26:751.

113. Jacobs RR, Asher MA, Snider RK (1980): Thoracolumbar spinal injuries. A comparative study of recumbent and operative treatment in 100 patients. *Spine* 5:463–477.

114. Jacobs RR, Schlaepfer F, Mathys R, Jr, et al (1984): A locking hook spinal rod system for stabilization of fracture-dislocations and correction of deformities of the dorsolumbar spine: A biomechanic evaluation. *Clin Orthop* 189:168–177.

115. Jones RF, Snowdon E, Coan J, King L, Engel S (1987): Bracing of thoracic and lumbar spine fractures. *Paraplegia* 25:386–393.

116. Jones K, McBride G, Memby R (1989): Sternal fractures associated with spinal injury. *J Trauma* 29:360–364.

117. Kahanovitz N, Arnoczky SP, Levine DB, et al (1984): The effects of internal fixation on the articular cartilage of unfused canine facet joint cartilage. *Spine* 9:268–272.

118. Kaneda K, Abumi K, Fujiya M (1984): Burst fractures with neurologic deficits of the thoracolumbar-lumbar spine. Results of anterior decompression and stabilization with anterior instrumentation. *Spine* 9:788–795.

119. Kauffer H, Hayes J (1966): Lumbar fracture-dislocation: A study of twenty-one cases. *J Bone Joint Surg* [Am] 48:712–730.

120. Kauffer H, Kling T (1984): Fractures and dislocations of the spine. In: Rockwood CA, Green DP, ed. *Fractures in adults, vol. 2.* Philadelphia: J.B. Lippincott, pp. 1037–1092.

121. Keene J, Goletz T, Lilleas F, et al (1982): Diagnosis of vertebral fractures. A comparison of conventional radiography, conventional tomography, and computed axial tomography. *J Bone Joint Surg* [Am] 64:586–594.

122. Keene JS (1984): Radiographic evaluation of thoracolumbar fractures. *Clin Orthop* 189:58–64.

123. Keene JS, Wackwitz DL, Drummond DS, et al (1986): Compression-distraction instrumentation of unstable thoracolumbar fractures. Anatomic results obtained with each type of injury and method of instrumentation. *Spine* 11:895–902.

124. Korres D, Katsaros A, Pantazopoulos T, et al (1981): Double or multiple level fractures of the spine. *Injury* 13:147–152.

125. Kostuik JP, Richards R (1981): Single stage anterior decompression and stabilization of thoracolumbar injuries. Presented at the Scoliosis Research Society meeting, Montreal, Quebec.

126. Kostuik JP, Richards R (1982): Single stage anterior decompression and stabilization of thoracolumbar injuries. Presented at the International Society for the Study of the Lumbar Spine meeting, Toronto, Ontario.

127. Kostuik JP (1983): Anterior spinal cord decompression for lesions of the thoracic and lumbar spine, techniques, new methods of internal fixation results. *Spine* 8:512–531.

128. Kostuik JP (1988): Anterior fixation for burst fractures of the thoracic and lumbar spine with or without neurological involvement. *Spine* 13:286–293.

129. Krompinger WJ, Fredrickson BE, Mino DE, et al (1986): Conservative treatment of fractures of the thoracic and lumbar spine. *Orthop Clin North Am* 17:161–170.

130. Kulkarni M, McArdle C, Ropanicky D, et al (1987): Acute spinal cord injury: MR imaging at 1.5T. *Radiology* 164:837–843.

131. Levine A, Edwards CC (1987): Lumbar spine trauma. In: Camins M, O'Leary P, eds. *The lumbar spine.* New York: Raven Press, pp. 193–212.

132. Louis R (1983): *Surgery of the spine.* New York: Springer-Verlag.

133. Lucas JT, Ducker TB (1979): Motor classification of spinal cord injuries with mobility, morbidity, and recovery indices. *Am Surg* 45:151–158.

134. Luque ER (1986): Segmental spinal instrumentation of the lumbar spine. *Clin Orthop* 203:126.

135. Luque ER (1986b): Interpeduncular segmental fixation. *Clin Orthop* 203:54–57.

136. Magerl F (1984): Stabilization of the lower thoracic and lumbar spine with external skeletal fixation. *Clin Orthop* 189:125–141.

137. Magerl F, Harms H, Gertzbein S, Aebi M (1989): Classification of spinal fractures. Presented at American Academy of Orthopaedic Surgeons, Vail, Colorado.

138. Maqid D, and Fishman E (1989): Imaging of musculoskeletal trauma in three dimensions: An integrated two-dimensional/three-dimensional approach with computed tomography. *Radiol Clin North Am* 27:945–956.

139. McAfee PC, Yuan HA, Lasda NA (1982): The unstable burst fracture. *Spine* 7:365–373.

140. McAfee P, Yuan H, Fredrickson B, et al (1983): The value of computed tomography in thoracolumbar fractures. *J Bone Joint Surg* [Am] 65:461–473.

141. McAfee PC, Bohlman HH (1985): Complications following Harrington instrumentation for fractures of the thoracolumbar spine. *J Bone Joint Surg* [Am] 67:672.

142. McAfee PC (1985): Biomechanical approach to instrumentation of thoracolumbar spine: A review article. *Adv Orthop Surg* 313–327.

143. McAfee PC, Farey ID, Sutterlin CE, et al (1989): Device-related osteoporosis with spinal instrumentation. 1989 Volvo Award in Basic Science. *Spine* 14:919–926.

144. McArdle C, Wright J, Prevost W, et al (1986): MR imaging of the acutely injured patient with cervical trauma. *Radiology* 159:273–274.

145. McGuire RA, Neville S, Green BA, Watts C (1987): Spinal instability and the log-rolling maneuver. *J Trauma* 27:525–531.

146. McGuire RA, Green BA, Eismont FJ, et al (1988): Comparison of stability provided to the unstable spine by the kinetic therapy table and the Stryker frame. *Neurosurgery* 22:842–845.

147. Meyer PR Jr, Cotler HB, Gireesan JT (1988): Operative neurologic complications resulting from thoracic and lumbar spine internal fixation. *Clin Orthop* 237:125–131.

148. Michaelis LS, Ungar GH, Vernon JDS, et al (1969): The value of postural reduction in the initial management of closed injuries of the spine with paraplegia and tetraplegia. Part 1. *Paraplegia* 7:178.

149. Moon MS, et al (1981): Anterior interbody fusion in fractures and fracture dislocations of the spine. *Int Orthop* 5:143.

150. Morgan TH, Wharton GW, Austin GN (1971): The results of laminectomy in patients with incomplete spinal cord injuries. *Paraplegia* 9:14.

151. Morris BD (1981): Unilateral dislocation of a lumbosacral facet. A case report. *J Bone Joint Surg [Am]* 63:164–165.

152. Murphey M, Batnitzky S, Bramble J (1989): Diagnostic imaging of spinal trauma. *Radiol Clin North Am* 27:855–872.

153. Murray B, Persellin R (1981): Cervical fracture complicating ankylosing spondylitis. *Am J Med* 70:1033–1041.

154. Myllynen P, Bostman O, Riska E (1988): Recurrence of deformity after removal of Harrington's fixation of spine fracture. Seventy-six cases followed for 2 years. *Acta Orthop Scand* 59:497–502.

155. Nachemson AL, Schultz AB, Berkson MH (1979): Mechanical properties of human lumbar spine motion segments. Influence of age, sex, disc level, and degeneration. *Spine* 4:1–8.

156. New PF, Rosen BR, Brady TJ, et al (1983): Potential hazards and artifacts of ferromagnetic and nonferromagnetic surgical and dental materials and devices in nuclear magnetic resonance imaging. *Radiology* 147:139–148.

157. Nicoll EA (1949): Fractures of the dorso-lumbar spine. *J Bone Joint Surg [Br]* 31:376–394.

158. O'Callaghan JP, Ullrich CG, Yuan HA (1980): CT of facet distraction in flexion injuries of the thoracolumbar spine: The "naked" facet. *AJNR* 1:97.

159. Olerud S, Karlstrom G, Sjostrom L (1990): Transpedicular fixation of thoracolumbar fractures. *Contemp Orthop* 20:285–300.

160. Osebold WR, Weinstein SL, Sprague BL (1981): Thoracolumbar spine fractures. Results of treatment. *Spine* 6:13–34.

161. Osgood C, Abbasy M, Mathews T (1985): Multiple spine fractures in ankylosing spondylitis. *J Trauma* 13:168–185.

162. Pang D, Pollack I (1989): Spinal cord injury with radiographic abnormality in children—The SCIWORA syndrome. *J Trauma* 29:654–664.

163. Panjabi MM, Hausfeld JN, White AA III (1981): A biomechanical study of the ligamentous stability of the thoracic spine in man. *Acta Orthop Scand* 52:315–326.

164. Parke W (1982): Applied anatomy of the spine. In: Rothman R, Simeone F, eds., *The spine,* 2nd ed. Philadelphia: W. B. Saunders, pp. 18–51.

165. Paul RL, Michael RH, Dunn JE, et al (1975): Anterior transthoracic surgical decompression of acute spinal cord injuries. *J Neurosurg* 43:299.

166. Pickett J, Blumenkopf B (1989): Dural lacerations and thoracolumbar fractures. *J Spinal Disord* 2:99–103.

167. Pitts F, Stauffer ES (1970): Spinal injuries in the multiple injured patient. *Orthop Clin North Am* 1:137–148.

168. Posner I, White AA, Edwards WT, et al (1982): A biomechanical analysis of the clinical stability of the lumbar and lumbosacral spine. *Spine* 7:374–389.

169. Post JD, Green BA, Quencer RM, et al (1982): The value of computed tomography in spinal trauma. *Spine* 7:417–431.

170. Quencer RM, Montalvo BM, Eismont FJ, et al (1985): Intraoperative spinal sonography in thoracic and lumbar fractures: Evaluation of Harrington rod instrumentation. *Am J Neuroradiol* 6:353–359.

171. Reid D, Henderson R, Saboe L, et al (1987): Etiology and clinical course of missed spine fractures. *J Trauma* 27:980–987.

172. Reid DC, Hu R, Davis LA, Saboe LA (1988): The non-operative treatment of burst fractures of the thoracolumbar junction. *J Trauma* 28:1188–1194.

173. Rennie W, Mitchell N (1973): Flexion distraction fractures of the thoracolumbar spine. *J Bone Joint Surg [Am]* 55:386–390.

174. Resnick D, Niwayama G (1976): Radiographic and pathologic features of spinal involvement in diffuse idiopathic skeletal hyperostosis (DISH). *Radiology* 119:559–568.

175. Resnik CS, Scheer CE, Adelaar RS (1985): Lumbosacral dislocation. *J Can Assoc Radiol* 36:259–261.

176. Rezaian SM, Dombrowski ET, Ghista DN (1983): Spinal fixator for the management of spinal injury (The mechanical rationale). *Eng Med* 12:95.

177. Riska EB (1977): Antero-lateral decompression as a treatment of paraplegia following a vertebral fracture in the thoracolumbar spine. *Intern Orthop* 1:22.

178. Ritchie W (1970): Combined visceral and vertebral injuries from lap type seat belts. *Surg Gynecol Obstet* 131:431.

179. Roberts JB, Curtis PH Jr (1970): Stability of the thoracic and lumbar spine in traumatic paraplegia following fracture or fracture dislocation. *J Bone Joint Surg [Am]* 52:1115.

180. Rossier AB, Cochran TP (1984): The treatment of spinal fractures with Harrington compression rods and segmental sublaminar wiring. A dangerous combination. *Spine* 9:796–799.

181. Royle ND (1928): The operative removal of an accessory vertebra. *Austral Med J* 1:467.

182. Roy-Camille R, Saillant G, Mazel C (1986): Plating of thoracic, thoracolumbar, and lumbar injuries with pedicle screw plates. *Orthop Clin North Am* 17:147–159.

183. Russman B, Kazi K (1971): Spinal epidural hematoma and the Brown-Sequard syndrome. *Neurology* 21:1066–1068.

184. Sacks S (1965): Anterior interbody fusion of the lumbar spine. *J Bone Joint Surg [Br]* 47:211.

185. Sacks S (1966): Anterior interbody fusion of the lumbar spine. Indications and results in two hundred cases. *Clin Orthop* 44:163.

186. Sapkas G, Pantazopoulos T, Efstathiou P (1985): Anteriorly displaced transverse fracture of the sacrum with fracture-dislocation at the L4-5 lumbar level. *Injury* 16:354–357.

187. Sasson A, Mozes G (1987): Complete fracture-dislocation of the thoracic spine without neurologic deficit. *Spine* 12:67–70.

188. Schaefer D, Flanders A, Northrup B, et al (1989): Magnetic resonance imaging of acute cervical spine trauma: Correlation with severity of neurologic injury. *Spine* 14:1090–1095.

189. Scher A (1983): Associated sternal and spinal fractures. *S Afr Med J* 64:98–100.

190. Shennan J (1973): Seat belt syndrome. *Br Med J* 4:786.

191. Slot GH (1981): A new distraction system for the correction of kyphosis using the anterior approach. Presented at the Scoliosis Research Society meeting, Montreal.

192. Smith W, Kaufer H (1969): Patterns and mechanisms of lumbar injuries associated with lap seat belts. *J Bone Joint Surg [Am]* 51:239–254.

193. Snyder C (1973): Bowel injuries from automobile seat belts. *Am J Surg* 123:312.

194. Soderstrom CA, McArdle DQ, Ducker TB, et al (1983): The diagnosis of intra-abdominal injury in patients with cervical cord trauma. *J Trauma* 23:1061–1065.

195. Stauffer ES (1983): Surgical management of trauma to the spine. In: Evarts CM, ed. *Surgery of the musculoskeletal system,* vol. 2. New York: Churchill Livingstone, p. 214.

196. Stauffer ES (1983b): Fractures of the lumbar spine. In: Evarts CM, ed. *Surgery of the musculoskeletal system,* vol. 2. New York: Churchill Livingstone, p. 297.

197. Stauffer ES (1984): Internal fixation of fractures of the thoracolumbar spine. *J Bone Joint Surg [Am]* 66:1136–1138.

198. Steffee AD, Biscup RS, Sitkowski DJ (1986): Segmental spine plates with pedicle screw fixation: A new internal fixation device for disorders of the lumbar and thoracolumbar spine. *Clin Orthop* 203:45–53.

199. Stevenson J (1979): Severe thoracic intra-abdominal and vertebral injury in combination in a patient wearing a seat belt. *Injury* 10:321–323.

200. Sturm J, Perry J (1984): Injuries associated with fractures of the transverse processes of the thoracic and lumbar vertebrae. *J Trauma* 24:597–599.

201. Suomalainen O, Paakkonen M (1984): Fracture dislocation of the lumbar spine without paraplegia. A case report. *Acta Orthop Scand* 55:466–468.

202. Svensson O, Aaro S, Ohlsen G (1984): Harrington instrumentation for thoracic and lumbar vertebral fractures. *Acta Orthop Scand* 55:38–47.

203. Tator CH, Rowed DW, Schwartz ML (1982): Sunnybrook cord injury scales for assessing neurologic injury and neurological recovery. In: Tator CH, ed. *Early management of acute spinal cord injury.* New York: Raven Press, pp. 7–24.

204. Tencer AF, Allen BL Jr, Ferguson RL (1985): A biomechanical study of thoracolumbar spinal fractures with bone in the canal. Part I. The effect of laminectomy. *Spine* 6:580–585.

205. Tencer AF, Ferguson RL, Allen BL Jr (1985): A biomechanical study of thoracolumbar spinal fractures with bone in the canal.

Part II. The effect of flexion angulation, distraction, and shortening of the motion segment. *Spine* 10:586–589.

206. Tracy P, Wright R, Hanigan W (1989): Magnetic resonance imaging of spinal injury. *Spine* 14:293–301.

207. Trafton P, Boyce C (1984): Computed tomography of thoracic and lumbar injuries. *J Trauma* 24:506.

208. Trent G, Armstrong G, O'Neil J (1988): Thoracolumbar fractures in ankylosing spondylitis. High risk injuries. *Clin Orthop* 227:61–66.

209. Vinters H, Barnett H, Kaufmann J (1980): Subdural hematoma of the spinal cord and widespread subarachnoid hemorrhage complicating anticoagulant therapy. *Stroke* 1:459–464.

210. Walter CL, Schmidek H, Krag MH, et al (1986): The management of thoracolumbar fractures. In: Dunsker SB, Schmidek HH, Frymoyer J, Kahn III, A, eds. *The unstable spine.* New York: Grune & Stratton, pp. 221–248.

211. Watkins R (1983): *Surgical approaches to the spine.* New York: Springer-Verlag, p. 165.

212. Watson-Jones R (1955): *Fractures and joint injuries, 4th ed.* Edinburgh: E & S Livingstone.

213. Weber SC, Sutherland GH (1986): An unusual rotational fracture-dislocation of the thoracic spine without neurologic sequelae internally fixed with a combined anterior and posterior approach. *J Trauma* 26:474–479.

214. Weinstein P, Karpman R, Gall E, et al (1982): Spinal cord injury, spinal fracture, and spinal stenosis in ankylosing spondylitis. *J Neurosurg* 57:609–616.

215. Weinstein JN, Collalto P, Lehmann TR (1987): Long-term follow-up of nonoperatively treated thoracolumbar spine fractures. *J Orthop Trauma* 1:152–159.

216. Weinstein JN, Collalto P, Lehmann TR (1988): Thoracolumbar burst fractures treated conservatively: A long-term follow-up. *Spine* 13:33–38.

217. Wenger DR, Carolla JJ (1984): The mechanics of thoracolumbar fractures stabilized by segmental fixation. *Clin Orthop* 189:89–96.

218. White AA, III, Panjabi MM, Thomas CL (1977): The clinical biomechanics of kyphotic deformities. *Clin Orthop* 128:8–17.

219. White AA, Panjabi MM (1978): *Clinical biomechanics of the spine.* Philadelphia: J.B. Lippincott.

220. White AA, Panjabi MM, Posner I, et al (1982): Spinal stability: Evaluation and treatment. In: Murray DG, ed. *Instructional course lectures.* St. Louis: C.V. Mosby.

221. Whitesides TE, Shah SGA (1976): On the management of unstable fractures of the thoracolumbar spine. Rationale for use of anterior decompression and fusion and posterior stabilization. *Spine* 1:99–107.

222. Whitesides TE (1977): Traumatic kyphosis of the thoracolumbar spine. *Clin Orthop* 128:78–92.

223. Willen J, Lindahl S, Nordwall A (1985): Unstable thoracolumbar fractures. A comparative clinical study of conservative treatment and Harrington instrumentation. *Spine* 10:111–122.

224. Wojcik WG, Edeiken-Monroe R, Harvis JH (1987): Three-dimensional computed tomography in acute cervical spine trauma: A preliminary report. *Skeletal Radiol* 16:261–269.

225. Woodring J, Dillon M (1984): Radiographic manifestations of mediastinal hemorrhage from blunt chest trauma. *Ann Thorac Surg* 37:171–178.

226. Woodring J, Lee C, Jenkins K (1988): Spinal fractures in blunt chest trauma. *J Trauma* 28:789–793.

227. Yablon I, Ordia J, Morlara R, et al (1989): Acute ascending myelopathy of the spine. *Spine* 14:1084–1089.

228. Yosipovitch Z, Robin GC, Makin M (1977): Open reduction of unstable thoracolumbar spinal injuries and fixation with Harrington rods. *J Bone Joint Surg* [Am] 59:1003–1015.

229. Zacheis HG, Condon RE (1972): Seat belts and intra-abdominal trauma: Report of two unusual cases. *J Trauma* 12:85–90.

230. Zielke K (1982): Ventral Derotation Spondylodese: Behandlungsergebnisse bei idiopathischen Lumbarskoliosen. *Orthop* 120:320–329.

The Adult Spine: Principles and Practice,
J. W. Frymoyer, Editor-in-Chief.
Raven Press, Ltd., New York © 1991.

CHAPTER 62

Late Sequelae of Thoracolumbar Fractures and Fracture-Dislocations

Surgical Treatment

Michael J. Bolesta and Henry H. Bohlman

White and Panjabi (31) define spinal instability as a loss of the ability of the spine under physiologic loads to maintain relationships between vertebrae in such a way that there is neither damage nor subsequent irritation to the spinal cord or nerve roots and, in addition, there is no development of incapacitating deformity or pain due to structural changes. Severe, unstable injuries are usually recognized in the acute phase and addressed at that time. When the initial treatment fails, instability may persist and result in deformity, pain, or increased neural deficit. In more subtle injuries, the clinician may have assessed the injury as stable but, under physiologic loading over time, problems became manifest. Each of these consequences will be considered. Similar to our previous chapter on late sequelae of cervical injuries, these consequences are divided into late deformity, pain,

neural dysfunction, and miscellaneous conditions such as infection.

DEFORMITY

Kyphosis

Normal thoracic kyphosis has a generally accepted range of 15° to 45°. A focal kyphosis may develop when there is damage to the anterior column. This is accentuated when there is posterior column disruption, with or without involvement of the middle column. If the injuries are predominantly osseous, a resulting deformity may become static. Ligamentous lesions, particularly those involving the posterior column from flexion and distraction injuries may cause late deformity. Upper thoracic fractures are more stable than fractures at the thoracolumbar junction (3,4,5).

Jodoin et al. found that deformity was associated with previous laminectomy, non-operative treatment, and short fusions of unstable injuries (13). Roberts and Cur-

M. J. Bolesta, M.D., Assistant Professor of Orthopaedics; H. H. Bohlman, M.D., F.A.C.S., Professor of Orthopaedics: Case Western Reserve University School of Medicine, The Reconstructive and Traumatic Spine Surgery Center, University Hospitals of Cleveland, Cleveland, Ohio 44106.

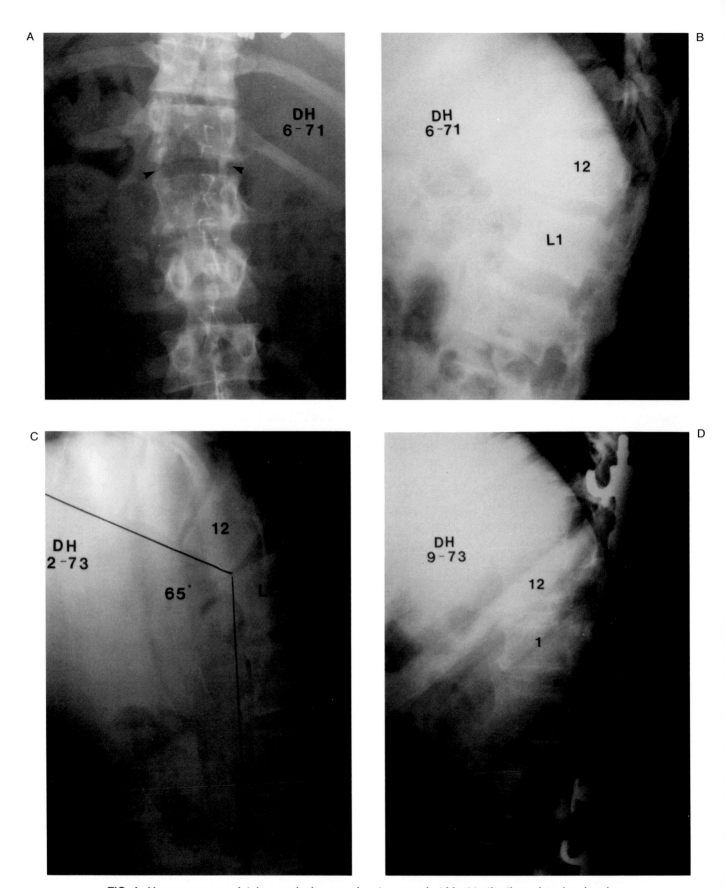

FIG. 1. Young man completely paraplegic secondary to a gunshot blast to the thoracic spine. Laminectomy produced no recovery, but he developed a kyphotic deformity. **A:** AP radiograph shortly after injury demonstrating the laminectomy. **B:** Lateral view at the same time showing a mild kyphosis. **C:** Twenty months later, the kyphosis increased to 65°. **D:** Successful reduction and stabilization with Harrington rods.

tiss found that laminectomy in association with 40° or greater kyphosis resulted in progressive deformity and paralysis (27). An absolute indication for surgical intervention is the development of a new neurologic deficit attributable to the kyphosis, or progression of an existing deficit (3,26). A second indication is the development of pain refractory to conservative measures. The management of these problems will be covered later in this chapter.

Another indication for intervention is documented progression of the deformity over time (26). In the asymptomatic patient, the goal of surgery is to obtain a stable fusion to prevent an unacceptable cosmetic deformity, and prevent development of pain or neurologic dysfunction (Fig. 1). If the kyphosis is less than 60°, posterior segmental instrumentation and arthrodesis can stabilize the spine. Some correction may be possible, depending on the flexibility of the deformity.

In kyphosis of greater than 60°, an anterior approach is usually necessary. If the posterior column is involved, this should be combined with posterior instrumentation and fusion to increase the fusion rate. Using such a combined approach, Bradford et al. (6) were able to reduce their mean kyphosis from 93° to 59° in 48 patients with kyphosis, 6 of which were due to trauma. Of the entire series, 10 lost correction (average of 19°), and 4 developed an anterior pseudarthrosis. In 9, the graft was located more than 4 cm from the apex of the deformity; of these, 5 grafts fractured.

When the kyphosis is fixed, a relative indication for operative intervention is an unacceptable cosmetic appearance, usually with pain. The same general guidelines for anterior versus posterior approach still apply, though combined approaches are necessary more often for stiffer curves to allow for better correction. The patient needs to be apprised of the risks and morbidity of these procedures. In more severe deformities, an anterior osteotomy and even corpectomy may be required to safely allow correction and posterior stabilization.

Injuries at the thoracolumbar junction in many cases can be managed according to the principles discussed above. In the lumbar spine itself, focal kyphosis greater than 30° is not well-tolerated and will commonly present with a flatback syndrome of stooped posture, fatigue, and pain. When there is documented progression and when the deformity is flexible, posterior instrumentation and fusion can correct the problem. It is becoming apparent that, unlike in the case of the thoracic spine, preservation of motion segments is very important, particularly in the lower lumbar region. This in part has led to the development of various forms of pedicular fixation. There are a variety of systems, each with unique advantages and limitations (1,12). Most systems allow for application of a correction maneuver of the spine and maintenance in the improved position. While this may

result in preservation of the lumbar motion, these techniques are technically demanding, and should be applied only by surgeons who are experienced and trained in their use. Even then, the complication rate is higher than for conventional non-pedicular systems. Conventional systems also can be associated with an increased complication rate when misapplied (20).

In fixed lumbar kyphotic deformities, anterior release and/or posterior laminectomy and osteotomy may be necessary. In the absence of symptoms, the patient and surgeon must weigh the morbidity against the anticipated result.

Scoliosis

Traumatic scoliosis is unusual, but may result from lateral compression or burst injuries and perhaps fracture-subluxations. In the absence of pain or deficit, the indication for surgical management is a documented progression or clinical deformity, which is rare. In the thoracic or thoracolumbar regions, standard posterior approaches used in other forms of scoliosis can be applied (32). In the mid-lumbar spine, an anterior approach such as that used by Zielke may be used to preserve motion segments.

Flatback Deformity

Kyphosis occurring in the lumbar spine was originally described in relation to idiopathic scoliosis of the lumbar spine treated with distraction instrumentation (see Chapter 65). The same iatrogenic problem can be generated by the injudicious use of distraction instrumentation with fusion for trauma of the lumbar spine, producing a stooped posture, pain, and fatigue secondary to loss of lumbar lordosis and a fixed kyphosis (Fig. 2). Kostuik et al. devised a combined single-stage anterior and posterior osteotomy for the correction of this deformity (16). In 54 patients, they performed an anterior opening wedge osteotomy, fixed with Kostuik-Harrington instrumentation. Posteriorly, they performed a closing extension osteotomy, fixed with a Dwyer cable-screw. They reported significant pain relief in 90% of the patients. There were three malunions, one requiring reoperation, and two neurologic deficits, one of which was permanent. Lumbar lordosis was increased from a mean of 21.5° to 49°.

Lagrone et al. had a series of 55 patients; 52 were unable to stand erect, and 49 complained of low back pain (17). Again, most were due to distraction instrumentation. They performed 66 extension osteotomies, 19 with anterior fusion. Sixty percent of the patients had at least one complication, including pseudarthrosis, dural tear, failure of hardware, and neurapraxia. At a mean 6-year

A

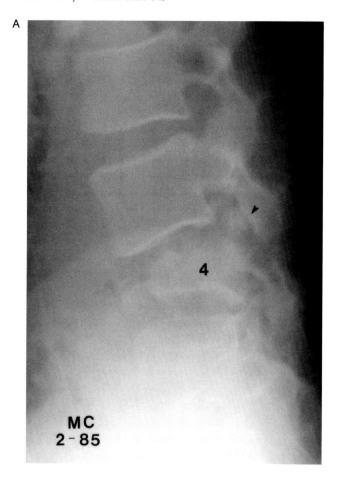

B

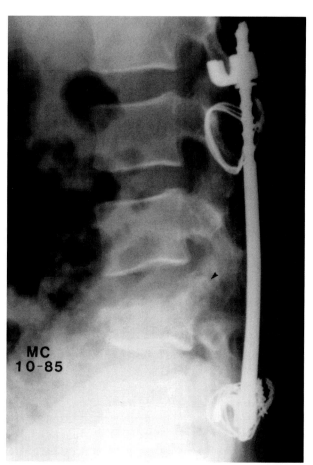

C

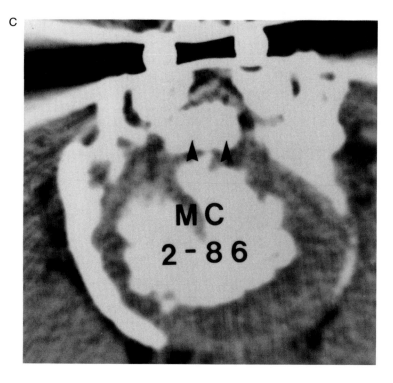

FIG. 2. Young man who sustained an L4 burst fracture and was rendered paraparetic. After laminectomy, fusion was attempted with Harrington distraction rods. The rods loosened and were replaced. He developed a solid fusion with a 30° lumbar kyphosis. Although he recovered the ability to ambulate, he was unable to stand upright because of the deformity. Four years after his injury, he underwent removal of the Harrington rods, L3 to L5 laminectomies, ventral decompression of residual L4 vertebral body, L4–L5 foraminotomies, osteotomy, and fixation with Cotrel-Dubousset instrumentation. This page: **A:** Lateral radiograph at the time of the original injury demonstrating kyphosis. **B:** A lateral film 8 months later showing the Harrington rods. Arrows demonstrate residual retropulsed bone. **C:** CT with intrathecal contrast 1 year after injury further defines the residual neural compression. (Figs. 2D–2E, opposite page.)

D
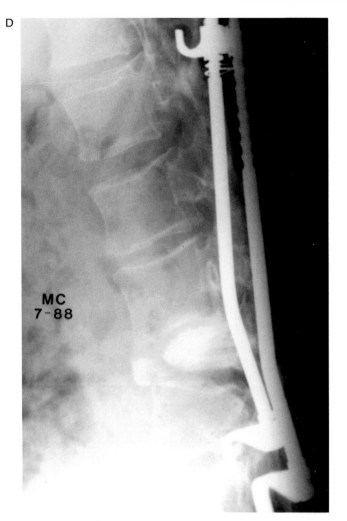

E
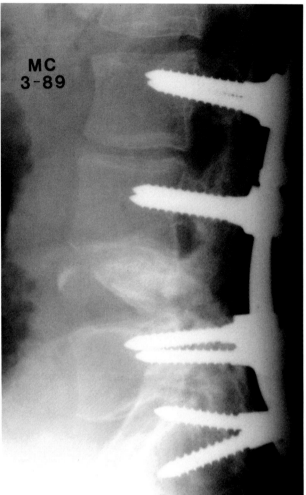

FIG. 2. *Continued.* **D:** Lateral radiograph after second Harrington instrumentation, again with lumbar kyphosis. **E:** Lateral radiograph after the third procedure, demonstrating restoration of lumbar lordosis.

follow-up, most patients felt that they had benefited from the procedure, but 26 still leaned forward, and 20 had moderate to severe low back pain. The pseudarthrosis rate was higher in those patients in which the deformity was not corrected. Circumferential fusion was more likely to maintain the correction. They concluded that treatment of this deformity was difficult, and they advised prevention by avoiding the use of distraction instrumentation in the lower lumbar region.

One potential solution has been the use of contoured rods. Casey et al. (7) reviewed 36 patients who underwent Harrington instrumentation with contouring. Regardless of this, there was a decrease in both total lumbar lordosis and lordosis above L4 as well as an increase in lordosis below L5. The improvement with contouring was not statistically significant. They concluded that contouring of distraction instrumentation was insufficient to correct the problem.

Now that this problem is recognized, we hope it will be minimized by avoiding distraction instrumentation in the lumbar spine. Stability may be attained with the newer systems, with (1,12) or without pedicle fixation (8,10,12,19,23). The unfortunate patient with this problem can generally be helped, but only with extensive surgery and with a high risk of complications.

Failure of Internal Fixation

McAfee and Bohlman (20) have reported the various late complications of Harrington instrumentation of the spine for thoracolumbar fractures. These include overdistraction, fractures and loosening of implants, infection, and lack of reduction of fractures with resultant neural deficit (Fig. 3). All of these complications have to be considered individually and addressed when they occur. Newer fixation devices may lessen these problems.

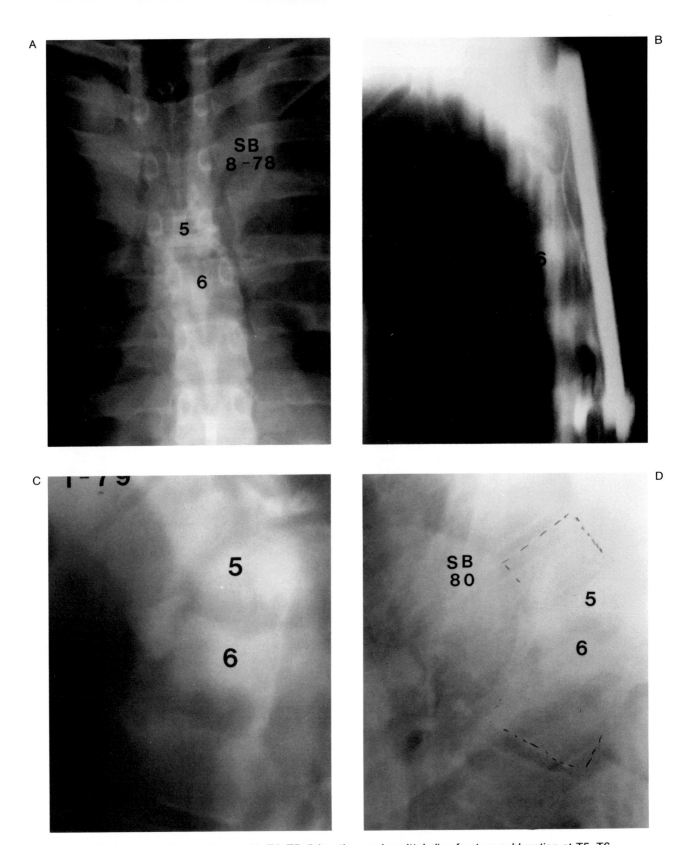

FIG. 3. Upper thoracic injury with T4–T5 dislocation, and sagittal slice fracture-subluxation at T5–T6. This was treated with laminectomy and a single Harrington distraction rod. The rod subsequently dislodged proximally and the patient's course was further complicated by *Escherichia coli* wound infection, meningitis, and osteomyelitis. He responded to debridement and a long course of intravenous antibiotics. **A:** AP radiograph at the time of injury. **B:** Lateral view 1 month after injury showing displacement of the proximal rod. **C:** Lateral tomogram revealing radiographic evidence of osteomyelitis. **D:** Thirteen months later, radiographic evidence of healing of the injuries and infection.

PAIN

Deformity

A common presentation for post-traumatic deformity is pain. At times, the etiology of the pain is elusive. With the deformity, there may be abnormal loading of the soft tissues and joints, which will produce fatigue. This may be due to excess tension posteriorly or compression anteriorly. Another component may be the overactivity of the paraspinous muscles attempting to maintain a functional posture. Direct damage to the facet joints, coupled with abnormal loading, may result in degenerative changes, which can be painful. Subtle instability without deformity can also cause pain (15).

Previous laminectomy may contribute to instability and, over time, lead to a painful deformity. On occasion, solid arthrodesis that does not span the deformity may increase stress at its junction with the mobile segments above and below.

Neural Compression

Whether or not there is a deformity, a complaint of pain should prompt further evaluation. Although there are many causes for pain, occult neural compression should be sought, even in the absence of neurologic deficit. There may be few signs when pain is due to nerve root compression. With cord involvement, there are usually reflex changes, but sensory and motor examinations may be normal (Fig. 4).

Evaluation

A thorough history should be obtained, including a detailed history of the injury, noting any associated injuries that may have an impact on the spinal problem. The physical examination will reveal clinical spinal deformity, tenderness, restriction of motion, and the presence of muscle spasm. A careful neurologic assessment should include rectal sensation and tone.

Plain radiographs remain important in terms of characterizing and localizing the lesion. Anteroposterior, lateral, and oblique views are standard, with bending films added as needed. It is valuable to review studies obtained at the time of injury and any subsequent films. Not infrequently, however, the original lateral spine x-ray performed with the patient supine on a stretcher does not allow good visualization of the posterior elements and soft tissues.

Biplane tomography is a useful technique to delineate subtle fractures and dislocations, particularly those involving the posterior elements. Unfortunately, this technology is falling into disuse; computerized tomography without intrathecal contrast may be substituted. This re-

quires contiguous slices and software reformatting in the sagittal and coronal planes. Some centers have the capability of generating three-dimensional reconstructions, which may be useful in select circumstances.

Magnetic resonance imaging gives information similar to the enhanced CT but with better definition of the spinal cord substance, and ionizing radiation is not utilized. Technical considerations limit its use in the acute setting, but this is generally not a problem when the patient is stable. Both CT and MRI can be compromised by the presence of metallic implants; despite this, useful information may still be garnered, depending on the amount, configuration, composition, and location of the metal. Sagittal and transverse images are routinely obtained using various pulse sequences, but direct imaging in virtually any plane is possible. Intravenous gadolinium, a paramagnetic contrast agent, is useful, particularly when there has been previous surgery; it is less invasive than intrathecal contrast and aids in distinguishing scar from disc material. The direct images are superior to reformatted CT, although the transverse images lack the resolution of late-generation computerized tomography. Although MRI has superior soft tissue definition compared to CT, bony detail is inferior.

The neural elements are assessed using water-soluble myelography followed by computerized tomography through the appropriate levels. This will provide excellent resolution and identify the need for decompression and the extent of decompression necessary. These techniques are readily available to most spine surgeons.

Management

When the pain is a result of demonstrable neural compression, anterior decompression with or without fusion should be included in the surgical management. For low lumbar fractures, that is, fourth and fifth levels, a laminectomy may be indicated. This will be detailed in another section. In the absence of compression, pain that can be localized to a focal area of the spine may be addressed by arthrodesis, but this is quite rare. In the absence of deformity, this is most expeditiously approached posteriorly, with an intertransverse process fusion, with or without instrumentation. Keene et al. found that instability without deformity may go on unrecognized and can lead to chronic pain. Their worst results were with wedge compression fractures treated with fusion more than 13 months after injury. Other injury patterns—flexion distraction, burst, and fracture-dislocation—all responded well to arthrodesis (15).

When there is an associated deformity, bending films will determine the amount of correction that can be expected. For kyphosis in the range of 45° to 60°, posterior segmental instrumentation and arthrodesis should give a stable spine with little or no pain. For more severe ky-

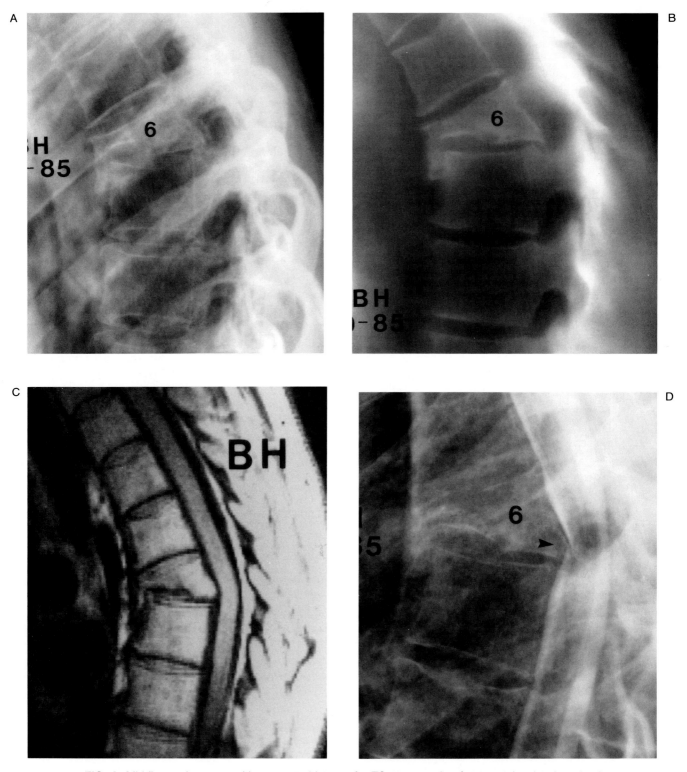

FIG. 4. Middle-aged woman with a remote history of a T6 compression fracture who developed pain without a neurologic deficit. This page: **A:** Lateral radiograph showing the compression fracture of T6. **B:** Lateral tomogram of the same area. **C:** Sagittal MRI revealing protrusion of bone from the caudal portion of T6 into the spinal canal. **D:** Lateral myelogram demonstrating indentation of the dural sac at the inferior T6 level. (Figs. 4E–4G, opposite page.)

E
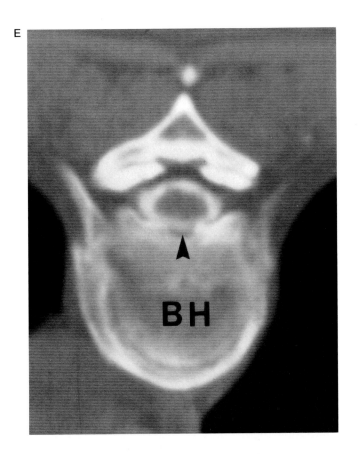

F
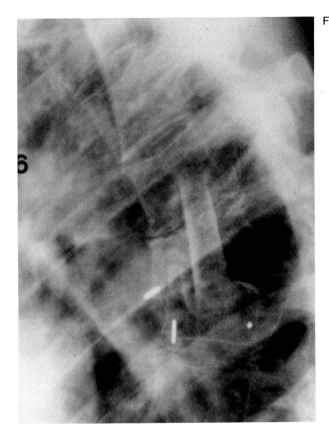

G
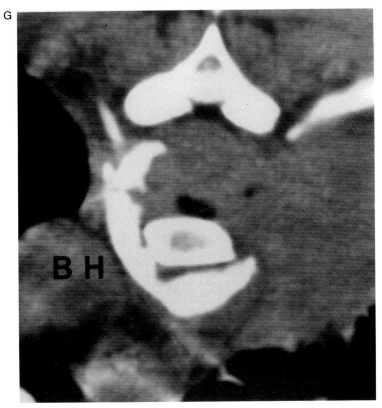

FIG. 4. *Continued.* **E:** CT through the same level demonstrating cord displacement. **F:** Lateral radiograph 4 months after transthoracic decompression and fusion demonstrating incorporation of the graft. **G:** CT confirming the decompression across the width of the canal.

phosis, circumferential fusion should be performed. Most surgeons prefer to perform this in stages, starting with anterior discectomies and fusions. Posterior segmental instrumentation and arthrodesis make up the second stage.

Although rare, lateral wedge compression fractures of the lumbar spine may produce a painful scoliotic deformity. One must attempt to localize the site of the pain, assess the flexibility of the curve with bending films, and determine the overall balance of the patient's spine and pelvis. If the individual is compensated and the deformity mild, correction may not be necessary. In the absence of neural compression, posterior instrumentation and arthrodesis with autogenous bone grafting are performed. The intertransverse process technique is utilized.

NEURAL DEFICIT

Etiology

Neurologic injury is generally evident at the time of initial presentation. In the upper thoracic spine, the canal is small, and the thoracic spine is quite stable because of the rib cage. If there is sufficient violence to disrupt this region, complete paraplegia is the general result. In fracture-dislocations, the cord is stretched and contused; in severe injuries, it may be completely disrupted. In burst fractures, the cord is impacted ventrally by bone and disc material, and occasionally disc herniation alone can produce paraplegia. In all except the last case, the etiology of the paralysis is generally evident. Furthermore, chances for meaningful recovery are very small if complete paralysis is present 48 hours after injury.

Incomplete spinal cord injury is less common in the thoracic spine. This generally occurs in individuals with large spinal canals and with less severe trauma. It may be seen with mild bursting injuries with small disc herniations and fracture-subluxations and occurs in one sixth of all patients sustaining upper thoracic fractures and paralysis.

Less commonly, a severe compression fracture that is initially associated with normal neural function may present later with pain and paraparesis. The patient's spinal cord, which is chronically draped over a rigid kyphos, may develop myelopathy, probably because of chronic ischemia and compression.

Depending on the nature of the initial insult, root compression can occur. This is generally of no functional significance in the complete paraplegic, but may be clinically relevant if intercostal pain is produced.

Another cause of late neurologic deficit in the thoracic region is a post-traumatic syringomyelia (Fig. 5). These cysts may represent liquefaction of necrotic cord or al-

tered fluid mechanics within the central spinal cord substance. Their exact incidence is unknown, but the relative ease of imaging with magnetic resonance is likely to show that they are more frequent than supposed. Significant cysts should be sought when increased pain occurs or a new neurologic deficit develops in an individual with an old incomplete cord injury.

At the thoracolumbar junction and lower lumbar region, post-traumatic neurologic deficits are frequently incomplete because this is at the level of the conus and cauda equina, and the latter tends to be more resistant to trauma. The lumbar spine is more mobile, but it is quite strong, resists rotational displacement, and has a relatively large canal. Neurologic deficits occur with disruption, contusion, compression, or stretching of the nerve rootlets. These are usually evident at the time of initial injury. In the absence of disruption, there is a tendency for varying degrees of recovery, depending on the nature and severity of the initial trauma. Late neural deficits can occur if there is continued compression, usually secondary to burst injuries producing canal stenosis. With post-traumatic scoliosis due to lateral compression or burst injuries, there may be a significant foraminal narrowing and isolated root compression. Post-traumatic degenerative changes involving the discs or facet joints may also result in post-traumatic spinal stenosis. Not only is there a direct mechanic effect, but the late presentation in these patients is likely due in part to chronic venous congestion and ischemia of the nerve roots.

In the thoracolumbar region, at the level of the conus medullaris, a mixed pattern is usually seen. There may be injury to the conus, presenting with bladder, bowel, and sexual dysfunction, which is usually evident early. Although conus injuries may occur as an isolated lesion, it is more common to have a mixed neurologic lesion of cord and root damage.

Evaluation

The patient's complaints, careful neurologic examination, and plain radiographs will focus attention on the appropriate section of the spine. Magnetic resonance imaging is our initial study in many cases. In the thoracic and thoracolumbar regions, the cord can be directly imaged in the longitudinal and transverse planes. It is currently the modality of choice for demonstrating intrinsic cord damage and post-traumatic cyst formation. Direct sagittal imaging is useful for demonstrating both central canal and foraminal compression, with complementary information obtained with the transverse slices. Long acquisition times are less of a problem in the late evaluation than in the acute setting.

Computerized tomography without intrathecal contrast is used in some centers, particularly where MRI

Text continues on page 1349.

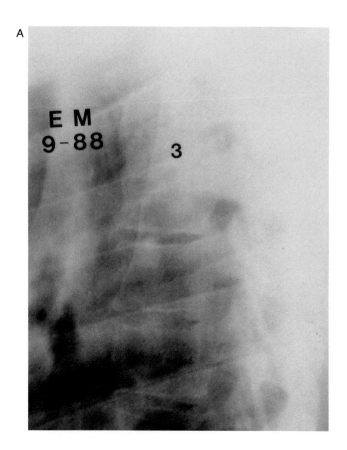

A

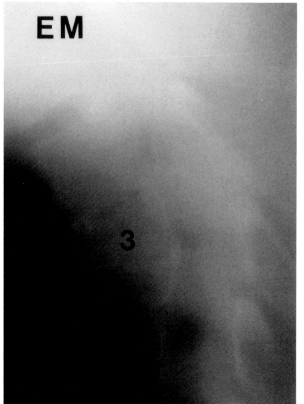

B

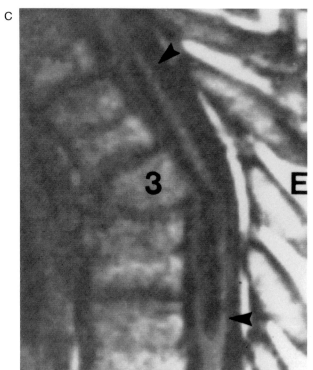

C

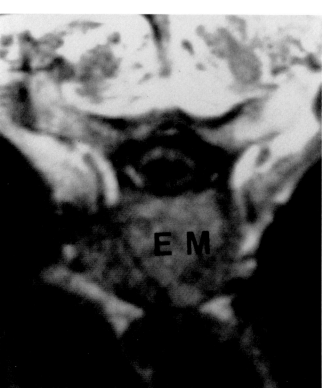

D

FIG. 5. Young man who sustained a compression fracture of T3. Although he was paraparetic initially, he recovered completely; he developed a spontaneous fusion from T2 to T4. Thirteen years later he noted weakness in his left lower extremity and was myelopathic to examination. **A:** Lateral radiograph revealing a healed T3 fracture with mild kyphosis. **B:** Lateral tomogram demonstrating the residual deformity. **C:** Sagittal MRI demonstrating residual compression at the T3 level as well as a large post-traumatic cyst. **D:** Transverse MRI revealing the large central syrinx.

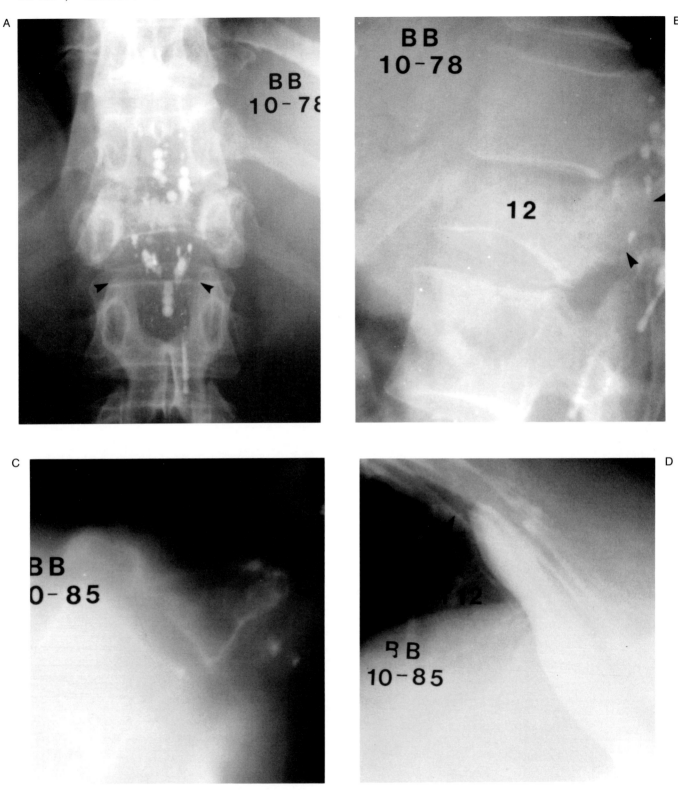

FIG. 6. Older woman who suffered a T12 burst fracture and paraparesis treated with a laminectomy. She recovered bladder and bowel function as well as ability to walk with braces. Seven years later she lost sphincter control. Bladder and bowel function again returned after anterior decompression and fusion. This page: **A:** AP view demonstrating the laminectomy shortly after injury. **B:** Lateral radiograph 1 month after injury demonstrating residual retropulsed bone (arrow). **C:** Lateral tomogram 7 years later revealing persistent bony protrusion into the canal. **D:** Lateral myelogram demonstrating deformity of the conus at this level. (Figs. 6E–6G, opposite page.)

E
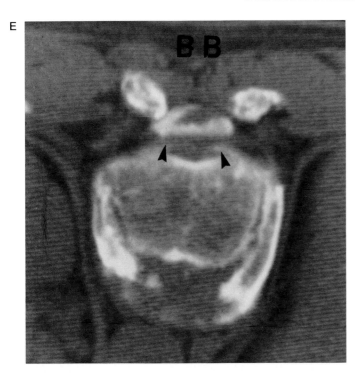

F
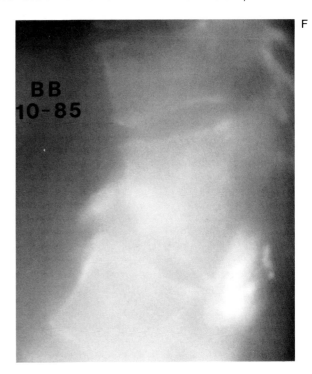

G
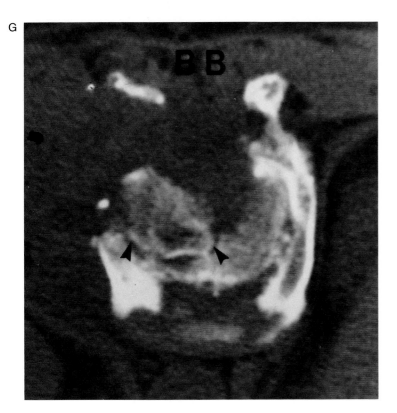

FIG. 6. *Continued.* **E:** CT revealing cord deformation. **F:** Lateral tomogram demonstrating the decompression; the graft is not visualized due to osteopenia. **G:** CT confirming decompression across the width of the spinal canal.

A

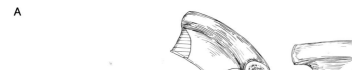

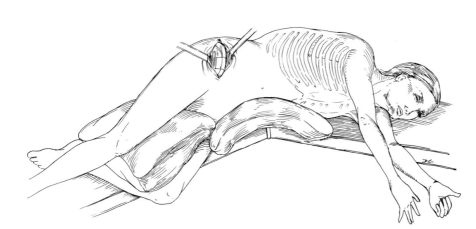

FIG. 7. Transthoracic anterior decompression and fusion. This page: **A:** Bone graft obtained. **B:** Thoracotomy performed through the rib bed of the injured segment and intercostal nerve traced toward the canal to identify the foramen. **C:** Segmental vessels identified and ligated. (Figs. 7D–7G follow.)

B

C

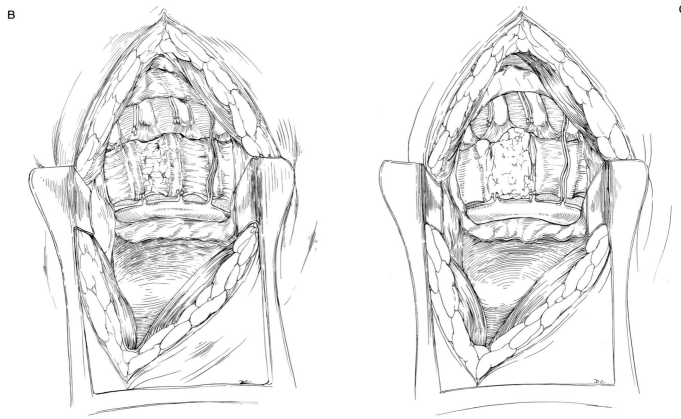

D

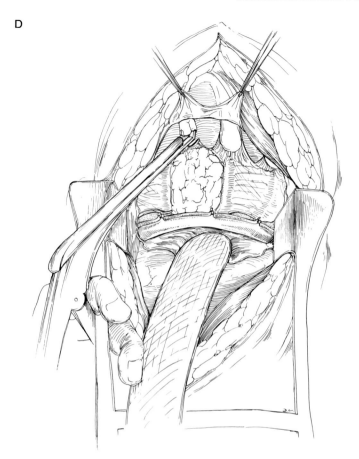

E

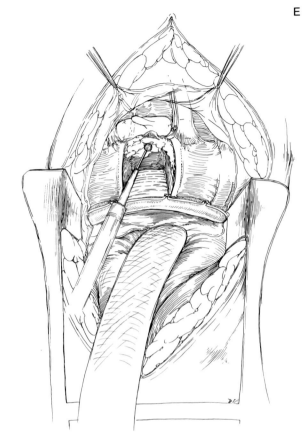

F

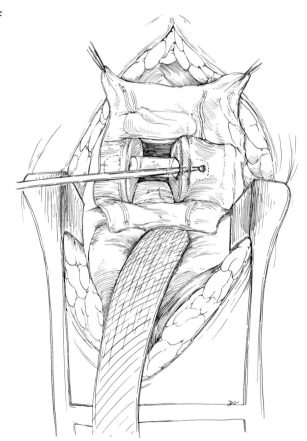

FIG. 7. *Continued.* **D:** Pedicle removed with Kerrison rongeur. **E:** Power burr removes mid-portion of the vertebral body between the discs. **F:** Interbody fusion. (Fig. 7G follows.)

G

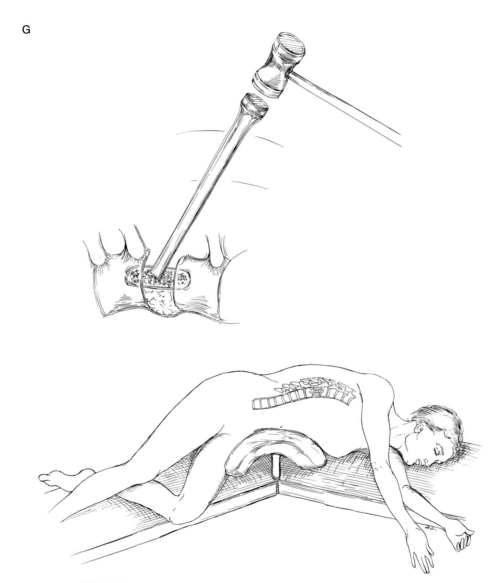

FIG. 7. *Continued.* **G:** Vertebral bodies fused with a strut of iliac crest.

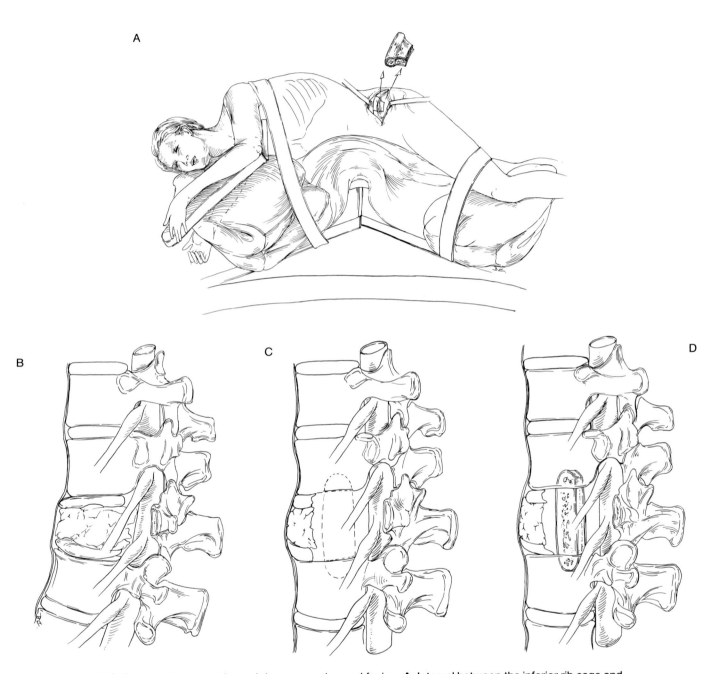

FIG. 8. Anterior retroperitoneal decompression and fusion. **A:** Interval between the inferior rib cage and the iliac crest is split. Bone graft may be harvested through the same incision. **B:** Nerve root is identified and traced into the foramen. **C:** Posterior cortex is thinned with a diamond burr and pulled anteriorly into the cavity away from the dural sac, completing the decompression. **D:** Strut is countersunk into the cranial and caudal vertebral bodies.

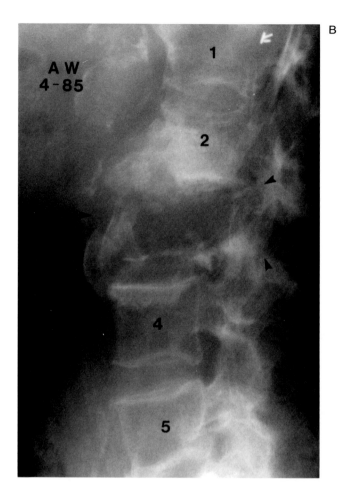

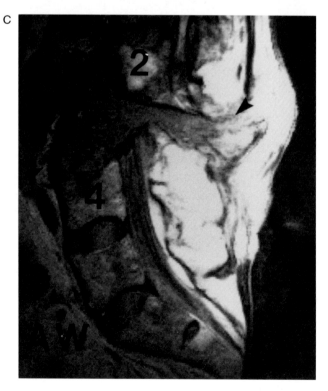

FIG. 9. Older paraplegic who underwent laminectomy 40 years previously for spinal cord injury. He presented with a draining fistula and a large pressure ulceration. This page: AP (A) and lateral (B) views demonstrating the exuberant hypertrophic changes about the spine. Sagittal MRI (C) revealing hypertrophic changes and the relationship to the spinal canal. (Figs. 9D–9E follow.)

D
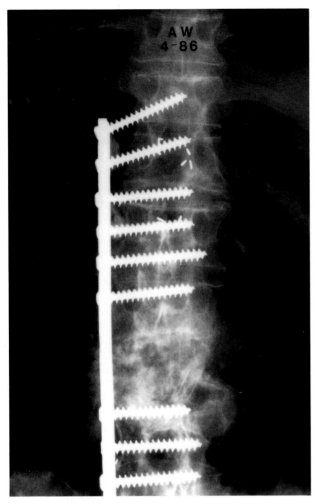

E
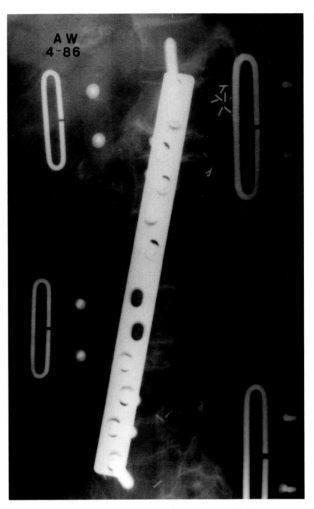

FIG. 9. *Continued.* AP (**D**) and lateral (**E**) radiographs after anterior debridement and arthrodesis with AO plates and screws.

may not be readily available. Although the bony resolution is superior to magnetic resonance, the inferior soft tissue definition limits its utility in evaluating neurologic deficit. We prefer to precede computerized tomography with water-soluble myelography. This helps the radiologist to select the appropriate levels to scan, and helps define the nature and site of the nerve and cord compression.

Management

In the upper thoracic region, root compression does not produce a functional deficit. If there is no cord compression and there is sufficient intercostal pain, hemilaminectomy and foraminotomy via a posterior approach may be utilized to decompress the nerve root; however, this is a very unusual situation in our experience.

More commonly, there is late pain or paralysis from chronic cord compression, which is anterior (Fig. 6).

Some surgeons prefer a posterolateral approach by taking down the pedicle (18), but in a late situation, the deformity is often fixed, and limited exposure by this technique makes decompression difficult. We favor an anterior transthoracic approach (2,5). Generally, the thoracotomy is performed on the right side to avoid the heart, but if the compression is at the T11–T12 levels, a left thoracotomy is performed to avoid the liver. This is generally made through the rib bed of the injured segment, and the intercostal nerve is traced toward the canal to identify the foramen (Fig. 7B). The segmental vessels are identified and ligated (Fig. 7C). The pedicle is removed with a small Kerrison rongeur (Fig. 7D). The mid-portion of the proximal and distal discs is removed. A power burr is used to remove the mid-portion of the vertebral body between the discs, taking care to preserve the anterior cortex, thus avoiding injury to the great vessels (Fig. 7E). The contralateral cortex is preserved to avoid damage to the segmental vessels. The posterior cortex is preserved initially to protect the dura and its contents. After creating a cavity the width of the spinal canal, the posterior cortex is thinned with a diamond burr. Once it is weakened on all sides, small curettes may be used to pull the remaining bone and disc into the cavity, thus decompressing the thecal sac and its contents. If the anterior third to half of the vertebral body is preserved and there is no deformity, decompression alone may be performed. If there is moderate kyphosis, an interbody fusion is performed (Fig. 7F). The intervening vertebral bodies are fused with a strut of iliac crest (Fig. 7G).

In the thoracolumbar and mid-lumbar region, the rationale for an anterior approach is very similar (2,21). Again, a lateral decubitus position is used, this time with a retroperitoneal approach. The interval between the inferior rib cage and the iliac crest is split (Fig. 8A). Generally the left side is utilized to avoid the liver, but this organ can be retracted if the major compression is right-sided. The transverse process of the affected vertebra is identified. After reflecting the muscle, the transverse process is removed. The nerve root is identified and traced into the foramen (Fig. 8B). The pedicle is removed with a small Kerrison rongeur. The spinal canal can then be identified. The segmental vessel at that level is identified and divided. The psoas muscle is reflected anteriorly. The mid-portion of the disc above and below is removed, taking care to stay out of the spinal canal. A power burr is used to create a trough across the vertebral body, taking care to span the entire spinal canal. Again, the anterior, contralateral, and posterior cortices are preserved. The posterior cortex is then thinned with a diamond burr and pulled anteriorly into the cavity away from the dural sac, completing the decompression (Fig. 8C). The iliac crest is readily available through the same incision, and a strut can be countersunk into the cranial and caudal vertebral bodies (Fig. 8D). Bone healing is enhanced by improving stability (22). A number of investigators have developed anterior devices to improve immediate stability, particularly when there has been disruption of the posterior column. The Dunn device is no longer available (9). The Kaneda device is restricted to participating centers in the United States (14). Although the anterior approach has definite advantages, complications occur, including atelectasis, pneumonia, pleural effusion, and pneumothorax (30). One complication unique to a thoracotomy is chylothorax secondary to injury of the thoracic duct. This can generally be treated conservatively with a thoracostomy tube (24,25). In our experience in over 200 anterior thoracolumbar decompressions, we have never had an increased neural deficit, and the other reported complications are rare.

At the L5 and perhaps the L4 levels, the retroperitoneal approach may be technically very difficult, so a laminectomy may be performed and the dural sac gently mobilized. Bone can then be removed from a posterior approach. Post-traumatic foraminal stenosis in the lumbar spine can be approached via laminectomy and fo-raminotomy using the same techniques used for degenerative stenosis.

OTHER SEQUELAE

Infection

Late infections generally occur in individuals treated operatively with metal implants (Fig. 3). These tend to be low-grade infections with less virulent organisms, and the most common complaint is pain. It is important to obtain an accurate history as to the nature of the original surgical procedure and elicit any problems that may have occurred, such as a documented wound infection or persistent drainage. One should also inquire about systemic symptoms such as fever, rigors, diaphoresis, diminished appetite, and weight loss. Meningitis may be a major complication of wound sepsis.

The patient with an open draining wound poses no difficulty in diagnosis. If the wound is healed, there is generally tenderness, but there may be no other signs of active infection. The white cell count is often normal, but the sedimentation rate is generally elevated.

The imaging studies are the same as for individuals with post-traumatic pain. Radionuclide studies may help distinguish between bone and soft tissue infection, but with increased bony uptake it may be difficult to discriminate between a non-union and sepsis.

The principles of managing post-traumatic sepsis are the same as elsewhere in the body. An accurate microbiological diagnosis is made by obtaining deep cultures prior to the administration of any antibiotics. The area must be thoroughly debrided of nonviable tissue. Generally, it requires the removal of all instrumentation if it is loose; however, rigid fixation can be left in place and delayed closure performed, but wound closure can be difficult. If there is a component of neural compression, that should be addressed at a later date.

If there is a non-union, the surgeon must weigh the severity of the infection against the amount of instability. If there is gross sepsis, staged debridements are performed, eventually adding bone graft enclosing the wound. Appropriate intravenous antibiotics are administered with careful monitoring of levels and toxicity. If the infection is of a lower grade and the debridement is judged to be good, one can consider primary bone grafting at the initial debridement, with closure over drains. If there is a large dead space, a plastic surgeon may have to fill the defect with a vascularized muscle flap.

The duration of antibiotic treatment depends on the nature of the organism and the bony lesion. Consultation with an infectious disease specialist is recommended. Treatment is generally monitored with serial sedimentation rates in addition to antibiotic levels. Generally, our policy in treating pyogenic osteomyelitis of the spine is administration of intravenous antibiotics until the sedimentation rate is normal, then oral administration for a total of six months.

Low energy gunshot wounds involving the spine and intestines may result in infection. Romanick (28) studied 20 patients who underwent laparotomy without debridement of the paraspinous muscle followed by a minimum of two days of intravenous antibiotics. Seven developed meningitis, paraspinous infection, or osteomyelitis of the spine. All seven had perforation of the colon. There was one colon perforation that did not lead to infection about the spine. In the four with stomach or small bowel perforation, there was no infection. There were eight individuals without evidence of gastrointestinal perforation, none of which developed infection.

Loss of Fixation

Loss of fixation is generally evident by new or persistent pain and radiographic evidence of implant dislodgment or fracture (Fig. 3). In many ways, the evaluation is similar to that outlined for pain. Plane tomography is also useful if plain radiographs do not clearly assess the status of the fusion. If the arthrodesis is solid, another cause for the pain must be found. The differential diagnosis would include persistent neural compression, malunion with secondary malarticulation and joint arthrosis, and infection. Treatment is tailored to the cause.

More commonly, there will be a non-union requiring further surgery. Deep cultures must be obtained to check for infection. Depending on the stability, re-instrumentation may or may not be necessary. Following the principles of non-union surgery, the area must be thoroughly debrided and a large amount of cancellous bone graft applied.

Neurotrophic Spine

This is an uncommon occurrence in the patient with a spinal cord injury. Bohlman et al. (29) have reported a small series of patients who developed Charcot joints many years after spinal cord injury. There is a massive destruction of the spine with a hypertrophic response (Fig. 9). The major problem that occurs is loss of sitting balance with the collapsing spine, which requires a paraplegic to utilize his or her arms continuously to sit upright in a wheelchair. Treatment consists of rigid internal fixation with a long fusion, supplemented by external support.

REFERENCES

1. Aebi M, Etter C, Kehl T, Thalgott J (1987): Stabilization of the lower thoracic and lumbar spine with the internal spinal skeletal fixation system. Indications, techniques, and first results of treatment. *Spine* 12:544–551.
2. Anderson PA, Bohlman HH (1990): Late anterior decompression of thoracolumbar spine fractures. *Semin Spine Surg* 2:54–62.
3. Bohlman HH (1985): Treatment of fractures and dislocations of the thoracic and lumbar spine. *J Bone Joint Surg* [Am] 67:165–169.
4. Bohlman HH, Ducker TB, Lucas JT (1982): Spine and spinal cord injuries. In: Rothman RH, Simeone FA, eds. *The spine.* Philadelphia: W. B. Saunders, pp. 661–756.
5. Bohlman HH, Freehafer A, Dejak J (1985): The results of treatment of acute injuries of the upper thoracic spine with paralysis. *J Bone Joint Surg* [Am] 67:360–369.
6. Bradford DS, Ganjavian S, Antonious D, Winter RB, Lonstein JE, Moe JH (1982): Anterior strut-grafting for the treatment of kyphosis. Review of experience with forty-eight patients. *J Bone Joint Surg* [Am] 64:680–690.
7. Casey MP, Asher MA, Jacobs RR, Orrick JM (1988): The effect of Harrington rod contouring on lumbar lordosis. *Spine* 12:750–753.
8. Cotler JM, Vernace JV, Michalski JA (1986): The use of Harrington rods in thoracolumbar fractures. *Orthop Clin N Am* 17:87–103.
9. Dunn HK (1986): Anterior spine stabilization and decompression for thoracolumbar injuries. *Orthop Clin N Am* 17:113–119.
10. Edwards CC, Levine AM (1986): Early rod-sleeve stabilization of the injured thoracic and lumbar spine. *Orthop Clin N Am* 17:121–145.
11. Eismont FJ, Bohlman HH, Soni PL, Goldberg VM, Freehafer AA (1983): Pyogenic and fungal osteomyelitis with paralysis. *J Bone Joint Surg* [Am] 65:19–29.
12. Gurr KR, McAfee PC, Shih C (1988): Biomechanical analysis of posterior instrumentation systems after decompressive laminectomy. An unstable calf-spine model. *J Bone Joint Surg* [Am] 70:680–691.
13. Jodoin A, Dupuis P, Fraser M, Beaumont P (1985): Unstable fractures of the thoracolumbar spine: A ten year experience at Sacre-Coeur Hospital. *J Trauma* 25:197–202.
14. Kaneda K, Abumi K, Fujiya M (1984): Burst fractures with neurologic deficits of the thoracolumbar-lumbar spine. Results of anterior decompression and stabilization with anterior instrumentation. *Spine* 9:788–795.
15. Keene JS, Lash EG, Kling TF Jr (1988): Undetected posttraumatic instability of "stable" thoracolumbar fractures. *J Orthop Trauma* 2:202–211.
16. Kostuik JP, Maurais GR, Richardson WJ, Okajima Y (1988): Combined single stage anterior and posterior osteotomy for correction of iatrogenic lumbar kyphosis. *Spine* 13:257–266.
17. Lagrone MO, Bradford DS, Moe JH, Lonstein JE, Winter RB, Ogilvie JW (1988): Treatment of symptomatic flatback after spinal fusion. *J Bone Joint Surg* [Am] 70:569–580.
18. Larson SJ, Holst RA, Hemmy DC, Sances A (1976): Lateral extracavitary approach to traumatic lesions of the thoracic and lumbar spine. *J Neurosurg* 45:628–637.
19. Lesoin F, Rousseaux M, Bouasakao N, Villette L, Thomas CE, Cama A, Jomin M (1986): Specific selection of osteosynthetic material in the treatment of thoracic or lumbar spinal injuries by the posterior approach. A review of 165 cases. *Acta Neurochir (Wien)* 81:118–124.
20. McAfee PC, Bohlman HH (1985): Complications following Harrington instrumentation for fractures of the thoracolumbar spine. *J Bone Joint Surg* [Am] 67:672–686.
21. McAfee PC, Bohlman HH, Yuan HA (1985): Anterior decompression of traumatic thoracolumbar fractures with incomplete neurological deficit using a retroperitoneal approach. *J Bone Joint Surg* [Am] 67:89–104.
22. McAfee PC, Regan JJ, Farey ID, Gurr KR, Warden KE (1988): The biomechanical and histomorphometric properties of anterior lumbar fusions: A canine model. *J Spine Disorders* 1:101–110.
23. McAfee PC, Werner FW, Glisson RR (1985): A biomechanical analysis of spinal instrumentation systems in thoracolumbar fractures. Comparison of traditional Harrington distraction instrumentation with segmental spinal instrumentation. *Spine* 10:204–217.
24. Nakai S, Zielke K (1986): Chylothorax—a rare complication after

anterior and posterior spinal correction. Report on six cases. *Spine* 11:830–833.

25. Propst-Proctor SL, Rinsky LA, Bleck EE (1983): The cisterna chyli in orthopaedic surgery. *Spine* 8:787–792.

26. Roberson JR, Whitesides TE Jr (1985): Surgical reconstruction of late post-traumatic thoracolumbar kyphosis. *Spine* 10:307–312.

27. Roberts JB, Curtiss PH (1970): Stability of the thoracic and lumbar spine in traumatic paraplegia following fracture or fracture-dislocation. *J Bone Joint Surg* [Am] 52:1115–1130.

28. Romanick PC, Smith TK, Kopaniky DR, Oldfield D (1985): Infection about the spine associated with low-velocity-missile injury to the abdomen. *J Bone Joint Surg* [Am] 67:1195–1201.

29. Sobel JW, Bohlman HH, Freehafer AA (1985): Charchot's arthrop-athy of the spine following spinal cord injury. A report of 5 cases. *J Bone Joint Surg* [Am] 67:771–776.

30. Westfall SH, Akbarnia BA, Merenda JT, Naunheim KS, Connors RH, Kaminski DL, Weber TR (1987): Exposure of the anterior spine. Technique, complications, and results in 85 patients. *Am J Surg* 154:700–704.

31. White AA III, Panjabi MM (1978): The problem of clinical instability in the human spine: A systematic approach. In: White AA III, Panjabi MM, eds. *Clinical biomechanics of the spine.* Philadelphia: J. B. Lippincott, pp. 191–192.

32. Winter RB, Anderson MB (1985): Spinal arthrodesis for spinal deformity using posterior instrumentation and sublaminar wiring. A preliminary report of 100 consecutive cases. *Int Orthop* 9:239–245.

The Adult Spine: Principles and Practice,
J. W. Frymoyer, Editor-in-Chief.
Raven Press, Ltd., New York © 1991.

CHAPTER 63

The Rehabilitation of the Patient with Neurologic Dysfunction as a Result of Injuries to the Thoracolumbar Spine

John P. Kostuik and E. Shannon Stauffer

The annual incidence of spinal cord injury is 7,000 to 10,000 cases. It is estimated that there are 150,000 to 200,000 individuals in the United States who are affected (15). Of those injured, 47% are paraplegics and 25% have functionally preserved motor power at the completion of a rehabilitation program (46,76,77). Eighty-two percent are males and over one half of the

  J. P. Kostuik, M.D., F.R.C.S.(C): Professor of Orthopaedics, University of Toronto; Director, Spinal Surgery; and Director, Biomechanics Laboratory, The Toronto Hospital, Toronto, Ontario, M5G 2C4.
  E. S. Stauffer, M.D., F.R.C.S.: Professor and Chairman, Division of Orthopaedics and Rehabilitation, Southern Illinois University School of Medicine, Springfield, Illinois 62708.

patients are between the ages of 15 and 24. In patients over age 50, far more have spinal cord dysfunction arising from non-traumatic causes such as tumors and infections, whereas in those under age 50 the vast majority are traumatic in etiology. Auto accidents, falls, and gunshot wounds are the most common causes, although there are significant regional variations in the actual percentage attributable to each category (52).

Before the era of modern rehabilitation, the outlook for a paraplegic was bleak. Ancient physicians commented in the surgical papyrus (21) that spinal cord injury was "an ailment not to be treated." The prognosis had not improved significantly by the early twentieth century when over 90% of patients succumbed to their

TABLE 1. *Life expectancies for male spinal cord injury victims by age at time of injury and impairment category*

| Age at hospital discharge (years) | General populations | Life expectancy (years) | | | |
| | | Paraplegia | | Quadriplegia | |
		Incomplete	Complete	Incomplete	Complete
10	59.09	57.22	42.20	49.88	28.60
20	49.65	47.85	33.73	40.88	21.57
30	40.61	38.95	26.29	32.57	16.45
40	31.53	29.98	18.55	24.13	10.49
50	23.08	21.70	11.96	16.61	5.90
60	15.75	14.65	7.08	10.61	2.97
70	9.72	9.00	3.95	6.29	1.50

With permission from ref. 15.

TABLE 2. *Life expectancies for female spinal cord injury victims by age at time of injury and impairment category*

| Age at hospital discharge (years) | General populations | Life expectancy (years) | | | |
| | | Paraplegia | | Quadriplegia | |
		Incomplete	Complete	Incomplete	Complete
10	65.59	64.09	50.94	58.05	37.81
20	55.85	54.41	41.75	48.55	29.56
30	46.24	44.82	32.85	39.24	21.83
40	36.80	35.47	24.40	30.27	14.77
50	27.84	26.64	17.03	22.06	9.29
60	19.50	18.52	10.94	14.86	5.37
70	11.84	11.15	6.02	8.68	2.55

With permission from ref. 15.

injuries (2). The major advance was pioneered during World War II by Guttmann (26,35–37), who established many modern concepts for the rehabilitation of spinal cord injury. Today spinal cord injury centers optimize care. Despite these advances, paraplegics still have a diminished life expectancy with genitourinary tract infections resulting in renal failure, pulmonary embolism, and suicide as significant causations (16) (Tables 1 and 2).

Given all of the complexities of acute and chronic management of paraplegia, the purpose of this chapter is limited to providing the reader with a broad overview of thoracolumbar injuries rather than a detailed analysis of all aspects of the rehabilitation process, a topic to which major textbooks are devoted (1,4,14,17).

GENERAL APPROACH TO A PATIENT WITH PARAPLEGIA

A systematic approach to this process requires a clear understanding of the neural anatomy and function as it is affected by the level of injury. More specifically, it is important to determine if the neurologic lesion affects the spinal cord, conus medullaris, or cauda equina. This can usually be determined by the level of the fracture, the extent of paralysis, and the presence or absence of reflex activity. Sacral sparring is an important clue to the potential for later neurologic recovery (51).

The spinal cord usually terminates caudally at the conus medullaris at the L1 vertebral body. An injury from T1 to T11 usually causes spinal cord injury, which behaves similarly to cervical injury except that recovery of root function is more important in the latter condition. An injury at T12–L1 may result in neurologic lesions affecting the conus (sacral segments) accompanied by lumbar nerve root injuries within the caudal equina. Injuries below L1 usually affect the cauda equina or present as an isolated root injury.

Thoracic Cord Injuries (T1-T11)

Fractures of the upper six levels of the thoracic spine are distinctly less frequent than fractures below that level. However, certain cohorts seem susceptible, particularly motorcyclists (45) (Fig. 1). The determination of complete versus incomplete lesions and the description of incomplete cord syndromes is basically the same as for cervical injuries, and is quantified by Frankel's classification (24) (Table 3). Complete paralysis which persists following return of the bulbocavernosus reflex has a poor prognosis. Incomplete lesions are less common in the thoracic than in the cervical region because of the smaller bony canal dimensions relative to the size of the thoracic cord. However, an incomplete lesion at the thoracic level often has a better prognosis for some neurologic recovery.

T11-T12 Injuries

These injuries occur just above the conus medullaris, sometimes referred to as the supraconus region of the spinal cord. Because only the T11 and T12 roots are involved, the diagnosis and prognosis of these injuries is very similar to the more proximal lesions. The patient may recover function of the T12, L1, and occasionally L2 roots. Because the neurologic injury is upper motor neuron, reflex bladder emptying may be expected to develop even though voluntary bladder and bowel control will not return in a complete lesion.

T12-L1 Injuries

Injuries at the T12-L1 vertebral levels are most complex and difficult to diagnose with accuracy. However, once the diagnosis is established, the prognosis can be predicted. The lesion is a combination of cord injury involving the conus medullaris and sacral segments, and a cauda equina injury variably affecting the first through fifth lumbar nerve roots. Therefore the patient may have an initial complete paraplegia at the T12 level, accompanied by flaccid paralysis of bowel and bladder which will not recover due to upper motor neuron nerve cell injury. However, the lower extremity paralysis due to nerve root injury may show progressive recovery over a period of 6 to 12 months.

L1 Injuries

The prognosis for recovery of neurologic deficits at the L1 level is also difficult to predict. The lower end of the conus medullaris and all or some of the nerve roots from L2 to S4 may be involved. The loss of bladder control may be due to upper motor neuron injury in which case recovery will not occur. Conversely, it may be due to

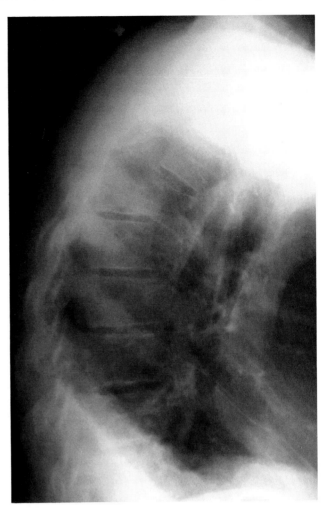

FIG. 1. A rare upper thoracic fracture dislocation in a motorcyclist. The proposed mechanism of injury is a catapulting ejection over the handlebars and axial loading of the upper thoracic spine (45).

root damage within the cauda equina, in which case recovery may occur over time. As a general rule of thumb, the longer the bladder and bowel paralysis persists, the less the likelihood of progressive recovery. Similar to T12-L1 injuries, lower extremity function may recover over time since it is due to nerve root rather than upper motor neuron damage.

Injuries Below L1

Injuries to the lumbar spine below the L1 vertebral level do not cause injury to the spinal cord, but often are associated with neurologic deficits resulting from nerve root damage within the cauda equina. In general, these patients more commonly present with an incomplete motor paralysis because roots are more resistant to injury than is the spinal cord. These injuries also have a better prognosis for progressive recovery, even when there is no sign of function for several weeks. Progressive

TABLE 3. *Frankel Scale (24)*

A. *Complete.* The lesion is found to be complete both motor and sensory below the segmental level marked. If there is an alteration of level but the lesion remains complete below the new level, then the arrow would point up or down the complete column.
B. *Sensory only.* There is some sensation present below the level of the lesion but the motor paralysis is complete below that level. This column does not apply when there is a slight discrepancy between the motor and sensory levels, but does apply to sacral sparring.
C. *Motor useless.* There is some motor power present below the lesion but it is of no practical use to the patient.
D. *Motor useful.* There is useful motor power below the level of the lesion. Patients in this group can move the lower limbs and many can walk with or without aids.
E. *Recovery.* The patient is free of neurologic symptoms (i.e., no weakness, no sensory loss, no sphincter disturbance). Abnormal reflexes may be present.

A 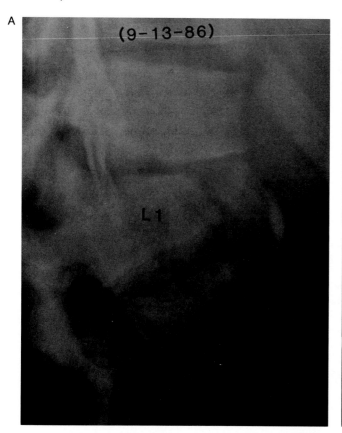 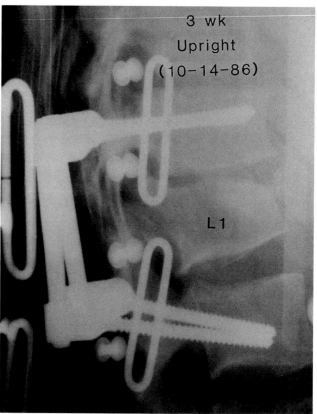 B

FIG. 2. This patient had a complete neurologic lesion **(A)**. Reduction and fixation with the Vermont Spinal Fixator and fusion allowed rapid mobilization **(B)**.

improvement may occur over an interval of 6 to 18 months as regeneration progresses down the axonal tubes, more often in patients who have initial greater motor deficits accompanied by relative sparing of dorsal sensory function. In general, these patients' motor functions ultimately progress to match the root level of the initial sensory sparing. In comparison, the recovery of bladder and bowel function is virtually impossible to predict, although fortunately many patients will recover. The bulbocavernosus reflex is not a useful guide because it is absent in a lower motor neuron injury. Because the prognosis is variable and many patients recover, the value of surgical versus non-surgical treatment is difficult to establish from uncontrolled, non-randomized clinical studies.

IMAGING STUDIES

Imaging studies have been of minimal use in establishing the prognosis, particularly in the lumbar spine where severe encroachment on the canal by bony fragments may nevertheless have no associated neurologic deficits. Currently there is information suggesting that magnetic resonance imaging may have some value in predicting recovery, particularly when the spinal cord is injured (7).

PRINCIPLES OF REHABILITATION

An overriding principle for all patients with thoracic, thoracolumbar, and lumbar fractures is early mobilization (Fig. 2), although whether this requires operative stabilization or can be accomplished by conservative methods remains a topic for debate (51). The principle of early mobilizations is very important to prevent medical complications; decrease hospitalization time; promote functional independence; and prevent muscular atrophy, joint contractures, pressure sores, and deep venous thrombosis. As a principle, the greater the extent of initial paralysis, the greater the need for early mobilization. The indications for surgical intervention are also based on neurologic deterioration with incomplete lesions and the stability of the fracture. In general, thoracic fractures are inherently stable because of rib cage support, and the patient often can be mobilized with an orthosis or cast (18,51). Fractures at the thoracolumbar junction and lumbar spine, which are more likely to be unstable, more often warrant early surgical intervention to promote early mobilization and prevent later deformities.

The three key goals for patients with paraplegia are complete independent living, ambulation, and pursuit of their occupation. A fourth key goal, management of bladder and bowel function, will be discussed later in this chapter.

Independent Living

With modern rehabilitation techniques and assistive devices, patients, regardless of the level of injury, are expected to achieve the goal of mastering all aspects of daily living including dressing, wheelchair transfers, homemaking, cooking, cleaning, and driving. This goal is facilitated by a variety of aids and architectural adaptations (32).

Although almost all patients with paraplegia who have functional upper extremities may have a goal to become independent ambulators, the achievement of that goal depends on the level of neurologic function. With complete thoracic cord injuries, it is unlikely that the patient will be ambulatory. The key to functional community ambulation is active control of at least one quadriceps muscle to provide active knee extension control. For example, the patient who can actively extend one knee yet needs an ankle-foot orthosis on the same side and a knee-ankle-foot (KAFO) orthosis on the other side, theoretically can become a community ambulator. In practicality, most patients who require at least one long leg brace will select a wheelchair for most of their activities, reserving crutches and braces for getting in and out of the automobile or going up and down steps. If the patient does not have adequate knee control and requires two KAFOs, it is likely that he will be neither a functional household nor community ambulator, but may use braces for exercise. In that regard, it is important to stress the high level of athletic performance of many types achieved by the paraplegic (63). At this time the use of powered exoskeletons has not reached the level of sophistication to be practical for most patients, despite the considerable media attention these devices have received. However, these devices remain an exciting prospect for the future.

VOCATIONAL REHABILITATION

The vocational rehabilitation of the patient must start as soon as possible following injury, with the goal of return to work. Since many patients with spinal cord injury have antecedent manual jobs, the goal of returning them to their original occupation may be difficult. However, when the patient is neurologically intact, the goal should be achievable. Huler et al. (42) prospectively studied patients with unstable thoracolumbar burst fractures who were neurologically intact. Eighty-two percent who were employed prior to injury returned to gainful employment, but 22% required a less physically demanding occupation. When neurologic injury is present significantly, greater efforts are required to achieve the goal of return to work.

Fortunately, laws to protect the disabled have resulted in a far greater hope for return to work. Today 75% of paraplegics return to some form of gainful employment and every effort should be made to achieve that goal. This requires an early team effort by psychologists, occupational therapists, rehabilitation counselors, physicians, and prevocational counseling which should begin within 6 to 8 weeks of hospital admission. Factors to be considered in prevocational counseling are the previous level of education and job training, the place of the home relative to employment, the geographic area and the work availability, motivation, personality, and physical performance. Psychologic assessment provides an understanding of the patient's present education level and future potential, and gives some measure of motivation. Our experience suggests that one third of patients have little desire to return to work, particularly when there is pending litigation. As in all spinal conditions, lack of motivation is a difficult barrier to overcome but must be addressed.

Work assessments can measure potential performance. The rehabilitation counselor helps patients to understand their skills and physical injuries, and arrive at the most suitable type of training or education. Usually the motivated patient with a previous sedentary occupation can return to former work, provided the physical barriers are overcome. Where this is not possible, job retraining may suffice. Sheltered workshops may also provide an opportunity for gainful employment. Potential employers must be educated in the problems of disability, and in the fact that disabled workers will not have an adverse effect on safety records or endanger insurance premiums.

In addition to vocational rehabilitation, the rehabilitative effort includes the medical, social, and educational domains.

MEDICAL REHABILITATION

Medical rehabilitation includes attention to medical, surgical, bacteriologic, and pharmacologic management, as well as orthotic, prosthetic, and wheelchair care. Of greatest importance is psychologic support and compassion, while at the same time helping the patient to realistically face the injury and its prognosis. A patient with complete paraplegia from a thoracic injury can usually be told within hours that the prognosis is poor for neurologic recovery. As already noted, establishing the prognosis may be difficult in thoracolumbar and lumbar injuries, as well as in incomplete lesions. Although the majority of neurologic recovery occurs within the first to 6 weeks, incomplete neurologic deficits may continue to improve for many years, particular with lumbar injuries involving the cauda equina. The importance of progressing kyphosis to deteriorating neurologic function and its reversal by anterior decompressive surgery should be stressed (6) (see Chapter 62).

Frequently the patient develops a significant depression often associated with anger, which should be managed through psychologic support of the patient and family. As already noted, these psychologic problems may be ongoing and result in a significant increase in the risk of later suicide (14,70). The issues of sexual function also should be addressed as part of this process (to be discussed in greater detail later in this chapter). If available, the local Paraplegia Association may be an invaluable support group.

As part of this process, acute hospital care should be minimized and the patient transferred to an active rehabilitation unit as soon as possible. There is little question that complications have been avoided and the ultimate functional outcome has been favorably influenced by such rehabilitation units (51).

Many of the other medical problems the patient will face during rehabilitation and as ongoing issues will be presented later under the "Education" heading. Inclusion in that section rather than here emphasizes the critical importance of education in medical problems not only to patients but to all members of the rehabilitation team.

SOCIAL REHABILITATION

The counseling process should include a social worker who can be involved early in working with the patient and family. An overriding concern is the loss of physical independence. Multiple issues need to be addressed such as family care, modifications of home environment, financial problems, sickness benefits, and worker's compensation. Frequently the social worker has to serve as guardian of the patient's rights and is invaluable in overcoming the bureaucracy related to disability benefits, worker's compensation, and other forms of insurance. When necessary, the social worker can assist the patient in obtaining legal help.

Both the family and patient must be prepared to accept periods of prolonged hospitalization and the resulting stress of separation. The patient who has a pre-existing, unstable social environment is more difficult to manage than the patient who comes from a strong family unit. Another issue which must sometimes be addressed is the potential rejection by friends, spouses, sexual partners, and relatives.

Prior to discharge from the rehabilitation unit, the home environment must be assessed by an occupational therapist for physical barriers. Community assistance programs may be required to provide financial, physical, nursing, and home care support. If the patient does not have a family unit, it may be necessary to make arrangements for discharge to a center for the handicapped.

TABLE 4. *Occurrence of related medical complications*

Disease category	Occurrence per patient
Genitourinary system	1.3
Respiratory system	0.8
Circulatory system	0.7
Integumentary system	0.4
Musculoskeletal system	0.4
Digestive system	0.4

Data obtained from the National Spinal Cord Injury Data Research Center, Phoenix, Arizona.

A total of 739 paraplegic patients were admitted to the model system SCI hospitals between 1972 and 1981. The data reflect the risk of complications to paraplegic patients.

EDUCATIONAL REHABILITATION

Educational rehabilitation requires the use of vocational guidance, experts in educational psychology, and adult education specialists. Many spinal cord injury centers employ an educator whose function it is to educate patients and relatives. The nursing, physiotherapy, occupational therapy, social workers, and rehabilitation staff must be coordinated to educate patients about the multiple issues they will face. In addition to the vocational, psychological, and social issues, very specific attention should be directed to physical care and the prevention of medical problems and complications (Table 4). These medical problems vary as a function of patient age (20).

BLADDER MANAGEMENT

Management of the bladder is a central part of both medical management and education. Repeated urinary tract infections, later renal failure, and secondary amyloidosis are all sequelae of altered bladder function (13).

Phase I Bladder Management

Following the acute injury, an indwelling catheter is left in situ because overhydration due to intravenous fluids and secondary bladder distention must be controlled. As quickly as possible intermittent catheterization should be initiated. The underlying rationale for early catheter removal is the very high rate of associated urinary infection, bladder calculi, urethral stricture and fistulae, and prostatitis and epididymitis in the male. It is also thought that indwelling catheters delay the return of the reflex detrusor activity if the spinal reflex arc is present.

Intermittent catheterization has been associated with a much lower incidence of infection and other complications, as well as a shorter period when catheterization is necessary. In the acute phase this activity is best done by nurses or a catheter team. Daily urine cultures are taken and the team may perform cystometry as necessary, follow bladder reflexes, and if necessary, perform bladder lavage.

Phase II Bladder Management

Bladder training depends on the specific level of neurologic injury and resultant type of neurogenic bladder. Injuries proximal to the conus medullaris involve the upper motor neurons, therefore the spinal reflex arc is intact. When the injury is at or below the conus medullaris, a lower motor neuron injury results and the reflex arc is lost. An exception may be when the level of injury is distal, but thrombosis of spinal arteries results in cephaladly directed spinal cord degeneration (25,51).

To determine if the patient has an upper or lower motor neuron injury, the bulbocavernosus reflex, superficial anal reflex, and historically the ice water test provide the most clinically accessible and useful information, although the ice water test may cause damage to the bladder through overdistention. More sophisticated tests may be required and include urodynamic studies to study urethral pressure profiles and measure pressure and flow. Electromyography may also be employed (as discussed in Chapter 26).

Once the type of bladder function is established, different training programs are employed.

Upper Motor Neuron Bladder Training

In this situation, the reflex arc returns within 2 to 8 weeks after the injury. At this point, bladder training may commence. The patient is taught to stimulate the reflex arc by tapping the superpubic region with fingers every 2 hours during the daytime. Initially, night stimulation is done by the nursing staff.

During the early part of this phase, the need for intermittent catheterization, fluid intake, and residual urine volumes are monitored. Residual urine volumes of less than 80 ml are compatible with a minimal risk of urinary tract infection. It should also be noted that measurements of residual urines are reliable only when the initial bladder volume is greater than 200 ml.

Once the residual urines are less than 50 ml, the need for controlling fluid intake and measuring urine volumes can be eased. The stimulation of the reflex arc also can be reduced to once every 3 to 4 hours during the day and once during the middle of the night.

Adjuncts to this basic process include cholinergic drugs when the bladder is hypoactive, such as carbachol or bethanechol chloride. Oral baclofen and newer therapeutic agents (40,47) are useful in decreasing spasm of the external urethral sphincter which may retard bladder emptying. If this medication is not effective, a transurethral division of the external urethra may be necessary.

Often this surgical intervention results in uncontrolled incontinence and the need for condom drainage in the male. Unfortunately, there is not a comparably effective device for the female. Thus, it is a less desirable procedure in the ambulant patient, particularly those with incomplete cord lesions. In these instances, bilateral pudendal nerve blocks may be a preferable alternative.

Lower Motor Neuron Bladder Training

Training may start as soon as 2 weeks after injury by straining unparalyzed abdominal muscles and the diaphragm and by suprapubic manual compression. Initially these maneuvers are done every 2 hours during the day by the patient and at night by the nursing staff. The same procedures are used to monitor the increasing effectiveness as previously described for upper motor neuron lesions. Similarly, intermittent catheterization is discontinued when residual urines are less than 50 ml. The protocol of stimulation every 3 to 4 hours during the day and once in the middle of the night is then progressively instituted.

In both upper and low motor neuron lesions, failure to achieve the goals for bladder training should lead to a careful re-evaluation of bladder and kidney function and possible outflow obstruction. Radiologic investigations may include voiding cystourethrograms, intravenous pyelograms, and retrograde urethrograms to determine the need for relief of obstruction.

Late Phase Bladder Management

Prior to the advent of antibiotics and a better understanding of bladder function, 90% of paraplegics died most commonly from septicemia, secondary to urinary tract sepsis (2) or uremia. In male patients who use condom drainage, the normal urethral bacteria, such as *Staphylococcus epidermidis, Streptococci,* and diphtheroids are replaced by gram negative bacilli. During the era when long-term indwelling catheters were used, prophylactic antibiotic therapy was recommended. Today, with better bladder training and short-term use of indwelling catheters, antibiotic prophylaxis is often unnecessary, except in the subset of patients who are unusually prone to recurrent infections. The issue of whether one should treat asymptomatic bacteriuria is debated (18). Instead, urinary acidification is promoted through oral intake of cranberry juice.

In addition to these general measures, it is important that urinary studies be conducted at the time of discharge from the rehabilitation unit, followed by regular periodic re-evaluations of urinary function. These initial studies include routine urinalysis and culture, serum blood urea nitrogen (BUN) and creatinine, observation of the urinary stream, measures of residual volume, voiding cystourethrograms, urethral pressure profiles, intravenous pyelograms, and bladder and kidney ultrasound. Later, urinalysis, culture, and residual volumes are determined on a periodic basis, and the other studies are performed as indicated. Of primary importance is detecting early the development of large residual volumes which will promote infections, hydronephrosis, and later renal failure.

Despite the ideal approach outlined here, many patients do not achieve this objective and require intermittent catheterization as their ongoing treatment. Some authorities do not believe such an idealized residual volume can be achieved, and that 200 cc is reasonable (18). Similarly, urinary tract infections are common, estimated by some to involve 100% of patients with complete paraplegia (18) if asymptomatic bacteruria is used as the criterion.

BOWEL MANAGEMENT

Spinal neurologic injury affects mainly the left colon and rectum, and anal sphincter. Constipation is the essential feature of all spinal injuries resulting from recumbency, decreased general activity, inadequate fluid intake, and improper diet. Conversely, constipation can be controlled through dietary measures such as foods with adequate roughage, appropriate hydration, early mobilization, and the judicious use of bulk expanding laxatives or stool softeners (50).

Upper Motor Neuron Lesions

In the upper motor neuron lesions, reflex function of the anus and rectum will return and at this point bowel re-education can be instituted. A strict regimen is encouraged including proper diet with appropriate roughage, adequate fluid intake, the use of mild laxatives at night, and rectal stimulation by digital distension, suppositories, or small enemas at a set time each morning. The gastrocolic reflex can be cultivated as well by drinking hot fluids or massaging the lower abdomen to promote colonic contraction. Adherence to this program is essential since the patient has no awareness of when the rectum is full. Impaction must be suspected when the patient's normal bowel routine breaks down or when there is diarrhea without apparent cause. In this instance high enemas and re-establishment of the bowel program is necessary.

This overall program may be particularly difficult in patients with T6 or higher neurologic levels and hyperreflexia. Severe headaches and perfuse sweating may occur when there is rectal distention as part of the overall problem of autonomic dysreflexia (see page 1362).

Lower Motor Neuron Lesions

In lower motor neuron lesions the rectum behaves as receptacle, and there may be some or no reflex activity, depending on the degree of neurologic involvement. The same overall principles apply as for the upper motor neuron lesions, but manual evacuation may be necessary if straining bowel and abdominal muscles is inadequate.

SEXUALITY

The spinal cord segments responsible for sexual function include S2, S3, and S4, which control ejaculation in the male. There is also involvement of T11 and L2, where parasympathetic, and sympathetic afferents synapse with efferents which are important to erection and emission in the male and genital lubrication in the female.

Most spinal injuries occur after sexual maturity has been reached, thus the perceived loss of sexual function is a major consideration. Management of this issue requires education, understanding, and the encouragement of sexual interactions. The patients need to understand that they have retained the cerebral component of sexual function, despite the alteration in peripheral function. However, later loss of libido is not uncommon. In one study, only 26% of male paraplegics with complete upper motor neuron lesions retained libido (69).

Initially, a complete neurologic lesion is accompanied by loss of sexual function because of the gross disturbance of autonomic nervous function.

In the female, sensory and motor sexual function is lost in the early stages, although the ability to conceive remains (38). The menstrual cycle is interrupted, frequently for months, but then is re-established. Autonomic dysreflexia is more likely to occur with pregnancy in paraplegics with high thoracic lesions. If the patient becomes pregnant, delivery usually can be accomplished normally unless there are significant perineal contractions. When there is an upper motor neuron lesion, deep sexual sensations may occur with stimulation, accompanied by clitoral erection. However, the female paraplegic rarely recovers the ability to reach orgasm when the neurologic lesion is complete; patients with incomplete lesions may achieve orgasm with adequate stimulation.

In the male, high cord lesion results in priapism initially, which is viewed as one component of spinal shock. Later priapism may be associated with intermittent catheterization, which may result in urethral trauma and require diazepam for relief. The reflex priapism may remain in a significant number of patients, estimated to be as high as 74% (43). Thus, patients with upper motor neuron lesions are capable of reflexogenic but not psychogenic erections, and few normally ejaculate or attain orgasms. In comparison, the male with a lower motor neuron lesion usually has penile flaccidity. Some lower motor neuron patients may have psychogenic erections, and ejaculation is estimated to occur in 7% to 11% (44).

Incomplete paraplegics often have better preservation of sexual function, particularly if posterior column sensation is preserved. Penile implants have been used for the inability of both complete and incomplete paraplegics to obtain an erection, although the use of intrapenile papaverine injection often is used as a substitute.

To overcome these difficulties, understanding, counseling, and encouragement are important, as is involving the patient with the sexual partner or spouse. They should be encouraged to participate in any type of sexual activity that is physically and mentally pleasurable and gratifying.

SKIN CARE

Insensate skin may break down rapidly at any time after neurologic injury (12,67,68). In the early phase, prevention is achieved through log rolling the patient every 2 hours, the use of oscillating mattresses, and padding of bony prominences. Pressure points should be inspected every time the patient's position is altered, which is initially the responsibility of the nursing staff. Subsequently, the patient and family must be instructed to examine for and prevent pressure sores. The maintenance of good nutrition, skin cleanliness, and proper maintenance of clothing are essential. Urinary tract infections, in particular, contribute to perineal pressure sores. Wheelchairs must be constructed to reduce pressure over insensitive areas such as the ischial tuberositas. This need has been greatly facilitated by the use of silicone gels, and newer methods of designing cushions (62,78).

Despite these efforts, pressure sores may develop commonly over the ischial tuberositates, sacrum, greater trochanters, lateral and medial malleoli, and os calces. Less commonly, vertebral deformities such as a kyphos serve as a site for abnormal pressure.

Two distinct types of pressure sores occur, the acute and chronic. Two morphologic subdivisions are also identified: the direct, which results from skin pressure and anoxia; and the bursal, which results from shearing forces creating an underlying bursitis. In this latter type, stage 1 is characterized by bursal swelling with or without an inflammatory component. Stage 2 follows when a sinus develops between the overlying skin and bursal cavity. Stage 3 is characterized by a frank ulcer. When these lesions are chronic, infection by multiple organisms may occur and further complicate the management of the local lesion. Other possible sequelae include osteomyelitis and/or septic arthritis, which may lead to joint destruction. In long-standing, chronic decubitis ulcers, malignant transformation of the adjacent skin is also a known, but fortunately rare complication.

When decubitus ulcers occur, conservative management and secondary healing often does not provide a satisfactory solution because it results in an unstable scar which has a lessened ability to withstand stress even at lower tissue pressures. Thus, surgical repair of all but small sores, particularly over the trochanters and ischium, is usually the preferred course of action.

OSTEOMYELITIS AND JOINT INFECTION

The most common cause of osteomyelitis is secondary to decubitus, most frequently located over the ischial tuberosities and trochanters. However, it can occur without a decubitus, often secondary to septicemia from urinary tract infection. Unfortunately, the underlying osteomyelitis often remains undetected and is only discovered later. When a patient has a recurring decubitus ulcer or sinus which fails to heal following adequate local treatment, osteomyelitis must be assumed to be present until proven otherwise. As with osteomyelitis in the nonparaplegic, treatment consists of local debridement, antibiotics, partial or complete ostectomies, excision of joints (33), and, in extreme cases, amputation (Fig. 3).

SPASMS

Spasms are the result of upper motor neuron injury where intact neuro reflex arc in the spinal cord occurs without the influence of higher cerebral centers. The result is uncontrolled activity of muscles in response to multiple stimuli, which may include skin pressure sores, joint contractures, bowel or bladder dysfunction, infections or visceral dysfunction, premenstrual tension, extreme temperatures, and local irritation, including tight clothing or shoes. The spasms may be either extensor or flexor. Sometimes extensor spasms may be useful and help the patient to stand. In contrast, flexor spasms produce disability and may significantly interfere with rehabilitation, subsequent life-style, and also contribute to decubitus ulcers and infections (Figs. 3A and 3B).

In treating spasms, relief from any of the numerous potential stimulators is important. Other treatments include the antidepressants diazepam and baclofen. In severe and untreatable spasms, the patient may require intrathecal injections of phenol, or in extreme cases, anterior and posterior rhizotomies, or cordotomies. The latter operations are now facilitated by percutaneous techniques.

In addition to managing the neurologic causation, local measures may be useful: including tenotomies, myotomies, peripheral neurectomies, and tendon transfers.

CONTRACTURES

Contractures typically are flexor in nature, but may occur as the result of incorrect positioning in extension.

A

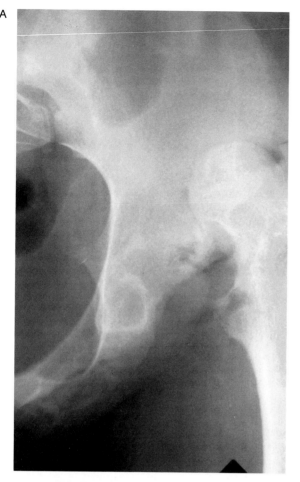

B

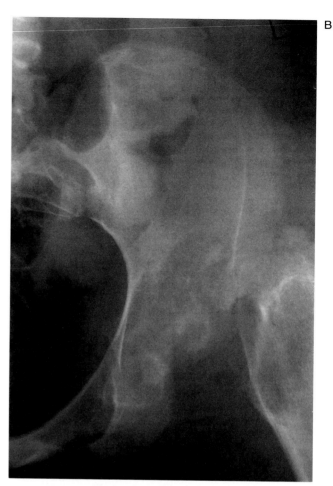

FIG. 3. A 16-year-old female with thoracolumbar junction fracture and severe adductor spasm, combined with recurrent urinary tract infection (A). She developed dislocation of the left hip with associated decubitus over the ischium and trochanter. Recurrent fevers and septicemia led to the diagnosis of osteomyelitis and pyarthrosis of the left hip (B). The infection was controlled by Girdlestone procedure, intravenous antibiotics, and plastic surgical reconstruction.

Often spasms lead to contractures and may even mask the contracture which then is only discovered when the patient is examined under anesthesia. Other causations include fracture, minor repetitive trauma produced by overzealous stretching, or inadequate attention to posturing. Ectopic bone formation is also contributory. The most common type is a hip flexion contracture, but all joints below the neurologic level may be involved. In addition to contributing to pressure sores, contractures affecting the hip associated with pelvic obliquity may result in secondary spinal deformity, and particularly in the growing child, either a kyphosis, scoliosis, or kyphoscoliosis. This is to be differentiated from the kyphos which results from inadequate initial fracture management. It may progress and be associated with increasing loss of neurologic function. In the latter instance, anterior decompression and fusion has been associated with a significant neurologic improvement (6) (see Chapter 62).

The treatment of such contractures is directed to relief of spasm when this is the underlying causation by gentle stretching, splitting, and when required, tendon releases. In extreme cases, osteotomies, fusions, or joint excision may be required.

AUTONOMIC DYSREFLEXIA

Autonomic dysreflexia (hyperreflexia) rarely affects patients whose neurologic level is below the sixth thoracic vertebra. Characteristically, affected patients have acute onset of headache and hypertension, associated with flushing, piloerection, sweating, dilated pupils, blurred vision, and bradycardia. Multiple noxious stimuli may promote these events such as rectal stimulation, impactions, decubitus ulcers, pregnancy, bladder distention, and renal calculi. Unrecognized, this condition may lead to death, therefore it is important to monitor blood pressure closely when this condition arises. Acute episodes may be managed by nitroglycerin and amyl nitrite, although long-term prevention may require a variety of antihypertensive medications. In extreme or uncontrolled hypertension, intravenous antihypertensives and occasionally spinal anesthesia may be required for control.

PAIN

Pain following spinal fracture with paraplegia has been classified in a variety of ways (58). We identify three types:

1. Neurologic pain occurs at the root level, usually from injuries to the conus, cauda equina, or nerve roots. Such pain generally is paroxysmal in nature, is more common in partial lesion, and tends to occur early after injury.
2. Central pain is characterized by intolerable, persistent, burning dysesthesia, intensified by varying stimuli including change in mood (49). Phantom pain is one variant, which may be influenced by the position and posture of the limbs immediately preceding the onset of paralysis. In these instances, amputation (when it has been performed for some other reason or as treatment) has not been successful in relieving the symptom.
3. Psychologic pain tends to occur later, and may be associated with narcotic abuse and other manifestations of psychologic dysfunction such as depression.

In addition to these three general pain problems, a number of pain-specific syndromes are identified, including post-traumatic syringomyelia as a late complication of spinal cord injury (see Chapter 53), local vertebral pain due to persisting instability, viscerally mediated pain (58), and truncal pain associated with dorsal lesions. The most common distribution of pain is the sacral coccygeal region, perineum, and adductor region of the thighs.

The management of the pain depends on an accurate diagnosis. In the early phase, analgesics can be used liberally, but soon other strategies must be introduced. Modulation of sensory input and psychologic management including antidepressants and local anesthetic agents may all be useful, depending on the cause. Central pain may sometimes respond to sympathectomy, but this should be preceded by a series of stellate blocks to determine the likely efficacy. Today, intrathecal and extradural blocks are felt to be of little lasting benefit, but percutaneous stimulation is thought to have a role. In severe and intractable cases a variety of neurosurgical interventions may be considered, similar to the approach outlined by Wilkinson in Chapter 99.

FRACTURES

Disuse osteoporosis makes the paraplegic more susceptible to long bone fractures (10,64) which are reported to occur in 4% of adult patients with paraplegia (19). Precipitating causes may include catching a lower extremity in bedclothing while turning, falls from wheelchairs, overzealous physical stretching, and uncontrolled spasm. It has long been recognized that patients with neurologic injury heal with abundant callus formation (11,27,28,59), a finding duplicated in experimental animals (30) (Fig. 4). Although neurologic mediation of callus formation has been hypothesized, a simpler explanation is that uncontrolled motion in the paraplegic is the cause (3). Support for this latter theory is derived from

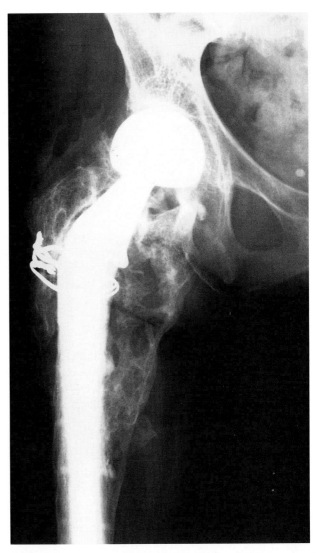

FIG. 4. This patient with a complete lesion of T10 sustained intertrochanteric fracture of the hip, treated initially by compression hip screw. The device was cut out and a prosthesis was inserted with cement. Note the massive heterotopic ossification and associated osteopenia.

the observation that exuberant callus formation is not seen when rigid internal fixation is used. However, it is observed that rigid external fixation is also associated with exuberant callus, lending less credence to the theory.

Most fractures in the paraplegic can be treated non-operatively, particularly when the foot, tibia, and supracondylar region of the femur are involved (27,48,55). The presence of pre-existent or subsequent spasm may alter this approach, particularly in the femoral shaft and hip. In general, fractures in those locations, whether spasm is present or not, are better treated by internal fixation devices to permit more rapid mobilization (31).

ECTOPIC BONE FORMATION

In addition to the exuberant callus formation observed with fractures, paraplegics also tend to form ectopic bone, particularly about the hip joint. The most

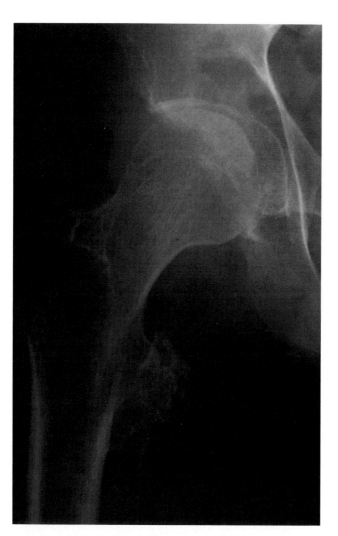

FIG. 5. A 26-year-old male with complete lesion at T11 and no symptoms referable to the hip. A benign finding is the ectopic bone adjacent to the trochanter.

commonly affected are younger, previously muscular males in whom the incidence is variously reported as 0.5% to 53.3% (28,29,39,51,71). In addition to a postulated neurologic mechanism, other contributing factors are thought to include spasms, overzealous stretching causing hemorrhage, and infection (23,41). In many instances, the finding may be of no greater significance than as an incidental observation made during radiographs for some other purpose (Fig. 5). However, the ectopic bone may contribute to contracture and, in the extreme result, in partial or complete ankylosis of the joint (75). In these instances, excision is not considered until bone scan shows no further activity (26). Then, surgical removal is followed by prophylaxis such as local irradiation and the use of anti-inflammatory agents or diphosphonates (65,66). Occasionally the acute phase of ectopic bone formation is accompanied by redness and swelling sufficient to lead to a misdiagnosis of thrombophlebitis.

VENOUS THROMBOSIS AND PULMONARY EMBOLUS

Venous thrombosis, with possible pulmonary embolization, most commonly occurs within the first 40 days of injury, typically in patients with complete neurologic dysfunction. The incidence varies as a function of the criteria used for diagnosis, but deep vein thrombosis is probably extremely common in complete paraplegics, and pulmonary emboli may occur in as many as 13% of patients (8,22,53,56,57,61,72,73). For that reason most patients are now prophylactically anticoagulated until they are mobilized completely. Other preventive measures include the use of antiembolic stockings and intermittent pneumatic pressurization of the lower extremities (34). The reasons for this high rate of DVT are variously speculated to be venous congestion, absence of muscular pumping of peripheral veins, or abnormal clotting mechanisms (60). In the chronic phase of spinal cord injury, peripheral edema and post-phlebitic syndrome are common. It is advisable to consider prophylactic anticoagulation when patients with chronic paraplegia undergo elective major surgical interventions. In doing so it is to be recognized that there may be an increased risk of bleeding, particularly into lower extremity muscles.

OBESITY

Weight loss is common in the acute phase of paraplegia because of nitrogen imbalance and decreased caloric intake (9). Later, loss of physical activity and overeating contribute to obesity, which can be prevented through maintenance of physical activity, dietary counseling, and when needed, psychologic counseling.

UPPER EXTREMITY SYMPTOMS

The paraplegic who uses either a wheelchair or crutches is an increased risk for shoulder and elbow pain, ulnar nerve entrapments, and carpal tunnel syndrome. One or another of these conditions affects 50% of patients, and the incidence continues to rise as a function of the number of years the assistive devices are used (5,54,74).

OTHER MEDICAL PROBLEMS

Problems such as hypertension and recurrent pulmonary infections are less of a problem for patients with thoracic, thoracolumbar, and lumbar neurologic injuries than they are for the quadriplegic. The exception is the very high thoracic lesion. In most injuries the phrenic nerve control of diaphragmatic function is retained, and the majority of patients have preservation of the lower thoracic spine intercostal muscles.

SUMMARY

The advent of modern rehabilitation has improved dramatically the survival and function of patients with neural injuries of the thoracic, thoracolumbar, and lumbar spine. However, careful adherence to the principles of early and later rehabilitation remains critical, as is the careful monitoring of psychologic status. Although mortality has decreased, later dysfunction and even suicide remain more prevalent in this population. To manage these patients, regional spinal cord injury centers are vital and can both improve functional outcomes and minimize complications. Continued close surveillance is necessary, using a team approach to prevent and manage the complex medical problems faced by these patients.

REFERENCES

1. Adkins HV (1985): *Spinal cord injury.* New York: Churchill Livingstone.
2. Allen AR (1908): Injuries of the spinal cord. *JAMA* 50:941.
3. Anderson LD (1965): Compression plate fixation and the effect of different types of internal fixation on fracture healing. *J Bone Joint Surg* [Am] 47:191–208.
4. Bedbrook GM (1981): *The care and management of spinal cord injuries.* New York: Springer-Verlag.
5. Blankstein A, Shmueli R, Weingarten I, et al (1985): Hand problems due to prolonged use of crutches and wheelchairs. *Orthop Rev* 14:735–740.
6. Bohlman H (1986): Late anterior decompression for spinal cord injury: Review of 131 patients with long-term results of neurologic recovery. *Am Spinal Injury Assoc Abstr Dig* 205–208.
7. Bondurant FJ, Cotler HB, Kulkarni MV, et al (1990): Acute spinal cord injury. *Spine* 15(3):161–168.
8. Bors E, Conrad CA, Massell TB (1954): Venous occlusion of lower extremities in paraplegic patients. *Surg Gynecol Obstet* 99:451–454.
9. Clarke KS (1966): Caloric costs of activity in paraplegic persons. *Arch Phys Med Rehabil* 47:427.
10. Claus-Walker J, Halstead LS, Rodriquez GP, et al (1982): Spinal cord injury hyperclacemia: Therapeutic profile. *Arch Phys Med Rehabil* 63:108–115.
11. Comarr AE, Hutchinson RH, Bors E (1962): Extremity fractures of patients with spinal cord injuries. *Am J Surg* 103:732–739.
12. Crenshaw RP, Vistnes LM (1989): A decade of pressure sore research: 1977–1987. *J Rehabil Res Dev* 26(1):63–74.
13. Dalton JJ Jr, Hackler RH, Bunts RC (1965): Amyloidosis in the paraplegic: Incidence and significance. *J Urol* 93:553.
14. DeLisa JE (1988): *Rehabilitation medicine: Principles and practice.* Philadelphia: J.B. Lippincott.
15. DeVivo MJ, Fine PR, Maetz HM, et al (1980): Prevalence of spinal cord injury: A reestimation employing life table techniques. *Arch Neurol* 37:707–708.
16. DeVivo MJ, Kartus PL, et al (1989): Cause of death for patients with spinal cord injuries. *Arch Intern Med* 149:1761–1766.
17. Donovan WH, Bedbrook GM (1982): Comprehensive management of spinal cord injury. *CIBA Clin Symp* 34:1.
18. Donovan WH, Dwyer AP (1984): An update on the early management of traumatic paraplegia (nonoperative and operative management). *Clin Orthop* 189:12–21.
19. Eichenholtz SN (1963): Management of long bone fractures in paraplegic patients. *J Bone Joint Surg* [Am] 45:299–310.
20. Eisenberg MG, Tierney DO (1985): Changing demographic profile of the spinal cord injury population: Implications for health care support systems. *Paraplegia* 23:335–343.
21. Elsberg CA (1931): The Edwin Smith surgical papyrus, and the diagnosis and the treatment of injuries to the skull and spine 5,000 years ago. *Am Med Hist* 3:271.
22. Flinn WR, Peterson LK, Harris JP, et al (1981): Recognition and prevention of deep venous thrombosis in acute spinal cord injured patients. *Am Spinal Injury Assoc Abstr Dig* 61–62.
23. Forrest L, Cohen P, Staas W (1985): Recurrent ischial decubitus ulceration and underlying heterotopic ossification as a late complication of spinal cord injury (abstr.). *Arch Phys Med Rehabil* 66:536.
24. Frankel HL, Hancock DO, Hyslop G, et al (1969): Value of postural reduction in the initial management of closed injuries of the spine with paraplegia and tetraplegia. *Paraplegia* 7:179–192.
25. Frankel HL (1969): Ascending cord lesion in the early stages following spinal injury. *Paraplegia* 7:111.
26. Freed JH, Hahn H, Menter R, et al (1982): The use of the three-phase bone scan in the early diagnosis of heterotopic ossification and in the evaluation of Didronel therapy. *Paraplegia* 20:208–216.
27. Freehafer AA, Hazel CM, Becker CL (1981): Lower extremity fractures in patients with spinal cord injury. *Paraplegia* 19:367–372.
28. Freehafer AA, Mast WA (1965): Lower extremity fractures in patients with spinal cord injury. *J Bone Joint Surg* [Am] 47:683–694.
29. Freehafer AA, Yurish R, Mast WA (1966): Para-articular ossification in spinal cord injury. *Med Serv J Can* 22:471–478.
30. Frymoyer JW, Pope MH (1977): Fracture healing in the sciatically denervated rate. *J Trauma* 17(5):355–361.
31. Garland DE, Rieser TV, Singer DI (1985): Treatment of femoral shaft fractures associated with acute spinal cord injuries. *Clin Orthop* 197:191–195.
32. Garland SR (1987): Mobility and mobility devices for the spinal cord injured person. *Clin Prosthet Orthot* 11:215–224.
33. Girdlestone GR (1943): Acute pyogenic arthritis of the hip. Operation giving free access and effective drainage. *Lancet* 1:419.
34. Green D, Rossi EC, Yao JS, et al (1982): Deep vein thrombosis in spinal cord injury: Effect of prophylaxis with calf compression, aspirin, and dipyridamole. *Paraplegia* 20:227–234.
35. Guttmann L (1966): Initial treatment of traumatic paraplegia and tetraplegia. In: *Spinal injuries.* Edinburgh: The Royal College of Surgeons.
36. Guttmann LJ (1969): Spinal deformities in traumatic paraplegics and tetraplegics following surgical procedures. *Paraplegia* 7:38.
37. Guttmann L (1976): *Spinal cord injuries—Comprehensive management and research, 2nd ed.* Boston: Blackwell Scientific Publications, pp. 137–141.
38. Guttmann LJ, Robertson S (1963): The paraplegic patient in pregnancy and labour. *Proc R Soc Med* 56:380.

39. Hardy S, Dickson J (1963): Pathologic ossification in traumatic paraplegia. *J Bone Joint Surg* [Br] 45:76–87.
40. Hassan N, McLellan DL (1980): Double blind comparison of single doses of DS103-282, baclofen and placebo for suppression of spasticity. *J Neurol Neurosurg Psychiatry* 43:1132–1136.
41. Hassard GH (1975): Heterotopic bone formation about the hip and unilateral decubitus ulcers in spinal cord injury. *Arch Phys Med Rehabil* 56:355–358.
42. Huler RJ, Esses SI, Botsford DJ (1990): Work status after posterior fixation of unstable but neurologically intact burst fractures of the thoracolumbar spine. Presented A.S.I.A., Orlando, Florida, May 1990.
43. Jacobson SA, Bors E (1970): Spinal cord injury in Vietnamese combat. *Paraplegia* 8:263.
44. Jochheim KA, Wahle H (1970): A study of sexual function in 56 male patients with complete irreversible lesions of the spinal cord and cauda equina. *Paraplegia* 8:166.
45. Kupferschmid JP, Weaver ML, Raves JJ, Diamond DL (1989): Thoracic spine injuries in victims of motorcycle accidents. *J Trauma* 29(5):593–596.
46. Kurtzke JF (1975): Epidemiology of spinal cord injury. *Exp Neurol* 48:163–236.
47. Mathias CJ, Luckitt J, Desai P, et al (1989): Pharmacodynamics and pharmacokinetics of the oral antispastic agent tizanidine in patients with spinal cord injury. *J Rehabil Res* 26(4):9–16.
48. McMaster W, Stauffer E (1975): The management of long bone fracture in the spinal cord injury patient. *Clin Orthop* 112:44–52.
49. Melzack R, Loeser JD (1978): Phantom body pain in paraplegics: Evidence for a central "pattern generating mechanism" for pain. *Pain* 4:195–210.
50. Meshkinpour H, Nowroozi F, Glick ME (1983): Colonic compliance in patients with spinal cord injury. *Arch Phys Med Rehabil* 64:111–112.
51. Meyer PR Jr (1978): Complications of treatment of fractures and dislocations of the dorsolumbar spine. In: Epps CH Jr, ed. *Complications of orthopaedic surgery.* Philadelphia: J.B. Lippincott, pp. 643–709.
52. Meyer PR Jr, Raffensperger JG (1973): Special centers for the care of the injured. Midwest regional spinal cord injury care system. *J Trauma* 13:308.
53. Naso F (1974): Pulmonary embolism in acute spinal cord injury. *Arch Phys Med Rehabil* 55:275–278.
54. Nicholas P, Norman P, Ennis J (1979): Wheelchair users' shoulder. *Scand J Rehabil Med* 11:29–32.
55. Nottage W (1981): A review of long bone fractures in patients with spinal cord injuries. *Clin Orthop* 155:65–70.
56. Perkash A (1980): Experience with management of deep vein thrombosis in patients with spinal cord injury. *Paraplegia* 18:2.
57. Phillips RS (1963): The incidence of deep venous thrombosis in paraplegia. *Paraplegia* 1:116.
58. Pollack LJ, et al (1951): Pain below the level of injury of the spinal cord. *Arch Neurol Psychiatry* 5:319.
59. Ragnarsson KT, Sell GH (1981): Lower extremity fractures after spinal cord injury: A retrospective study. *Arch Phys Med Rehabil* 62:418–423.
60. Rossi EC, Green D, Rosen JS, et al (1980): Sequential changes in factor VIII and platelets preceding deep vein thrombosis in patients with spinal cord injury. *Br J Haematol* 45:143–151.
61. Shull JR, Rose DL (1966): Pulmonary embolism in patients with spinal cord injury. *Arch Phys Med* 47:444.
62. Sprigle S, Chung K-C, Brubaker CE (1990): Reduction of sitting pressures with custom contoured cushions. *J Rehabil Res* 27(2):135–140.
63. Staas WE Jr, Formal CS, Gershkoff AM, et al (1988): Rehabilitation of the spinal cord-injured patient. In: DeLisa JE, ed. *Rehabilitation medicine: Principles and practice.* Philadelphia: J.B. Lippincott, pp. 635–659.
64. Stewart AF, Adler M, Byers CM, et al (1982): Calcium homeostasis in immobilization: An example of resorptive hypercalciuria. *N Engl J Med* 306:1136–1140.
65. Stover SL, Hahn HR, Miller JM III (1976): Disodium etidronate in the prevention of heterotopic ossification following spinal cord injury (preliminary report). *Paraplegia* 14:146–156.
66. Stover SL, Neimann KM, Miller JM III (1976): Disodium etidronate in the prevention of post-operative recurrence of heterotopic ossification in spinal cord injury patients. *J Bone Joint Surg* 58:683–688.
67. Sugarman B (1984): Osteomyelitis in spinal cord injury. *Arch Phys Med Rehabil* 65:132–134.
68. Sugarman B (1985): Infection and pressure sores. *Arch Phys Med Rehabil* 66:177–179.
69. Talbot HS (1949): A report on sexual function in paraplegics. *J Urol* 61:265.
70. Tribe CR (1963): Causes of death in early and late stage of paraplegia. *Paraplegia* 1:19.
71. Venier LH, Ditunno JF Jr (1971): Heterotopic ossification in the paraplegic patient. *Arch Phys Med Rehabil* 52:475–479.
72. Walsh JJ, Tribe C (1965): Phlebo-thrombosis and pulmonary embolism in paraplegia. *Paraplegia* 3:209.
73. Watson N (1968): Venous thrombosis and pulmonary embolism in spinal cord injury. *Paraplegia* 6:13.
74. Weiss M (1983): Subclinical medial and ulnar nerve compression neurolopathy in acute paraplegia. *Am Spinal Injury Assoc Abstr Dig* 316.
75. Wharton GW, Morgan TH (1970): Ankylosis in the paralyzed patient. *J Bone Joint Surg* [Am] 52:105–112.
76. Young JS, Burns PE, Bowen AM, McCutchen R (1982): *Experience of the regional spinal cord injury system.* Phoenix: Good Samaritan Medical Center, p. 32.
78. Young JS, Burns PE, Bowen AM, McCutchen R (1982): *Spinal cord injury statistics: Experience of the Regional Spinal Cord Injury Systems.* Phoenix: Good Samaritan Medical Center.
79. Zacharkow D (1984): *Wheelchair posture and pressure sores.* Springfield, IL: Charles C Thomas.

Adult Spine Deformities

The Adult Spine: Principles and Practice,
J. W. Frymoyer, Editor-in-Chief.
Raven Press, Ltd., New York © 1991.

CHAPTER 64

Adult Kyphosis

John P. Kostuik

The majority of kyphotic deformities treated are those seen in childhood years, primarily congenital deformities and some developmental deformities such as spondylolisthesis and Scheuermann's disease (see Table 1). Today, however, with the increasing age of our population and the increasing use of the automobile, kyphotic deformities form a major component of any spinal deformity surgeon's practice. Deformity secondary to osteoporosis, post-traumatic kyphosis, Scheuermann's kyphosis, tumor, and, more recently, the iatrogenic deformity secondary to wide laminectomy combined with increasing incidence of pyogenic infections of the spine have resulted in numerous cases treated by this author in recent years. A new subtype has been proposed, called "lumbar

degenerative kyphosis," which etiologically relates to disc space narrowing, wedged or collapsed vertebral bones due to osteoporosis, or atrophy of lumbar spinal muscles (32).

This chapter provides a basic explanation of the morphology of the adult deformity and a working classification of deformity based on etiology. A brief description of the major types is provided and methods of treatment are reviewed. The reader is referred to other texts for specifics of kyphotic deformities seen in osteochondral dysplasia and other forms of kyphosis, including congenital deformities.

METHODOLOGICAL CLASSIFICATION OF KYPHOSIS

There are three morphological types (Table 2). The first is pure kyphosis where the deformity is uniquely in

J. P. Kostuik, M.D., F.R.C.S.(C): Professor of Orthopaedics, University of Toronto, Toronto, Ontario; Director, Spinal Surgery; Director, Biomechanics Laboratory, The Toronto Hospital, Toronto, Ontario, M5G 2C4.

TABLE 1. *Classification of kyphosis*

1. Congenital
   Defects of segmentation
   Defects of formation
   Fixed
2. Developmental
   Scheuermann's kyphosis
   Developmental round back
   Spondylolisthesis
3. Inflammatory
   Infective
      Pyogenic
      Tuberculosis
   Rheumatoid
   Ankylosing spondylitis
4. Metabolic
   Osteoporosis
   Osteomalacia
5. Post-traumatic
6. Tumor
   Metastatic
   Neurofibromatosis
   Other
7. Chondrodystrophic kyphosis
   Achondroplastic dwarf
   Mucopolysaccharidoses
   Spondylo-epiphyseal dysplasia
8. Iatrogenic
   Post laminectomy
   Post irradiation

the sagittal plane and the vertebral canal continues to face anteriorly. Examples are Scheuermann's kyphosis and some cases of post-traumatic kyphosis (Figs. 1A and 1B). The second is kyphotic subluxation. On the lateral x-ray, the deformity gives an appearance of a staircase, while in the frontal view it has the appearance of a bayonet-like deformity (Figs. 2A and 2B). Symmetrical loss of radiological landmarks (i.e., pedicles) also is found most often in congenital subluxations (Fig. 2C). The third is an angular kyphoscoliosis where on the lateral view the angulation is greater than the angulation on the frontal view (Figs. 3A and 3B). Two particular types of kyphoscoliosis are of concern. The first is kyphosis associated with rotatory dislocation or subluxation, which may result in a severe deformity (Fig. 3A). The vertebral bodies give an appearance of being cuneiform in both planes, which may be noted in a single vertebra or a group of adjacent vertebrae. The second is a hairpin kyphosis (Fig. 3B). In this extreme case, a very severe kyphosis is accompanied with an increasing scoliosis. On

TABLE 2. *Morphological classification of kyphosis*

1. Pure kyphosis
2. Kyphosis with vertebral subluxation
3. Angular kyphoscoliosis—severe types
   Kyphosis with rotatory subluxation
   Hairpin kyphosis

the lateral view the anterior border of the vertebral body above appears to be below the body of adjacent vertebra. This deformity is often associated with neurofibromatosis.

ETIOLOGIES

The etiology of kyphosis is diverse and the prevalence and incidence vary depending upon the population studied. Post-infectious kyphosis secondary to tuberculosis is more common in the less developed nations, whereas post-traumatic kyphosis is more common in those parts of the world where high speed motor vehicle accidents are more likely to occur. Generally, congenital, post-infective secondary to tuberculosis, neurofibromatosis, and post-traumatic etiologies predominate.

Congenital Kyphosis

The congenital kyphoses are frequently confused with those secondary to tuberculosis. In 1955, James (9) first described the problem, and subsequently Moe (17) demonstrated the possibility of correction by the anterior approach. In 1977, Winter (35) proposed a classification (Fig. 4) including Type I, absence of segmentation resulting in an anterior block of bone; Type II, defects of formation of one or more vertebral bodies; and Type III, mixed, associating both Types I and II.

Defects of Segmentation

Kyphotic deformities secondary to the defects of segmentation are far less common than lateral defects of segmentation resulting in scoliosis. Anterior defects in the presence of continued posterior growth result in kyphosis. The severity depends on the length of the area involved and the discrepancy in growth between the anterior and posterior columns. Complete failure of formation results in a less severe deformity than if the disc is absent in only the anterior part of the vertebral body. Some defects of segmentation do not manifest themselves until later during growth. For several years there may be a normal or near normal appearance of disc and end plates, yet a severe deformity may develop by the end of growth. Kyphotic deformities secondary to defects of segmentation are usually less severe than those that result from anterior defects of formation. Paraplegia usually does not ensue.

Defects of Formation

The deformities range from mild to extremely severe. The mild deformities show failure of development of the anterior one quarter to one third of the vertebral body.

A

B

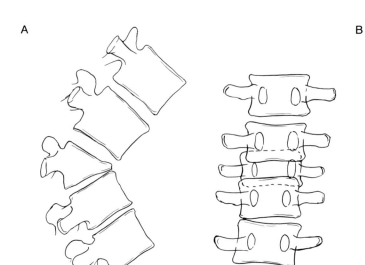

FIG. 1. A and B: Pure kyphosis.

A

B

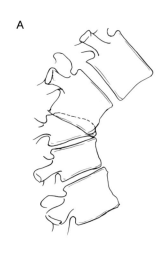
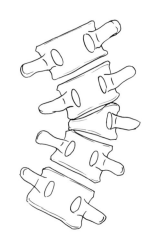

FIG. 2. A and B: Kyphoscoliosis.

C

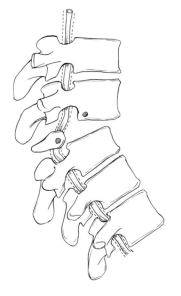

FIG. 2. C: Congenital subluxation.

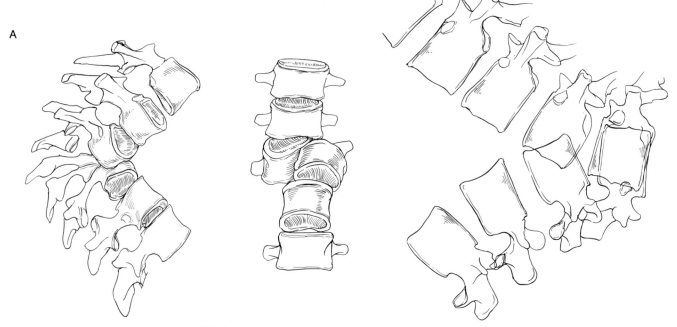

FIG. 3. A: Rotatory dislocation. **B:** Hairpin turn kyphosis.

Severe types may have total absence of vertebral body. The deformity may be symmetrical, and result in a pure kyphosis, or asymmetrical, in which case a kyphoscoliosis develops. These deformities increase with growth, resulting in significant and severe deformity and may lead to paraplegia. Indeed, they are the most common cause of paraplegia other than kyphosis associated with tuberculosis. These deformities tend to occur more commonly in the thoracolumbar junction. Progression at an average rate of seven degrees per year was noted by Winter (36). In children, paralysis may occur at any age, but more commonly in adolescence.

Developmental Kyphosis

Two basic types occur: Scheuermann's kyphosis and postural round back.

The etiology of Scheuermann's kyphosis is not well understood. Scheuermann (25) proposed a disease process caused by avascular necrosis of the cartilage ring of the vertebral body. He thought that growth inhibition occurred and subsequent kyphotic deformity developed. This hypothesis has been refuted in more recent work. Schmorl in 1930 (26) suggested that herniation of the vertebral disc through the growth plate initiated the process; abnormal enchondral ossification ultimately produced the kyphosis. This theory has not been widely accepted.

Mechanical factors have been implicated in the development of kyphosis. Scheuermann himself noted that the deformity occurred in young agricultural workers who were involved in heavy labor and frequently bent over. This theory seems unlikely, since the deformity often occurs in individuals with no history of physical labor.

Muscle causes have been implicated as well, without proof. There is no doubt that familial clusterings of Scheuermann's disease occur, implicating genetic predisposition, but frequently, there is no relevant family history. Endocrine or nutritional abnormalities have been advocated as well. The deformity has been noted with Turner's syndrome, but it is recognized that these patients often have severe osteoporosis. Pathologically, it is noted that the anterior longitudinal ligament is frequently thickened in Scheuermann's kyphosis. It is thought that the ligament may act as a drawstring and cause the vertebral bodies to develop a wedge shape.

Radiological criteria are three contiguous vertebral bodies that are wedge shaped. In adolescents the disc width is maintained, but the bodies may fuse spontaneously later in life, particularly if the deformity is severe.

The reported prevalence of Scheuermann's disease varies. Some studies have found a male to female ratio of 2 to 1. The changes of Scheuermann's are rarely noted before the age of 10 or 11. The long-term natural history is not well known. It is suspected that females with a significant deformity between 60 and 65 degrees at the end of growth may later develop an increased deformity due to post-menopausal osteoporosis. Scheuermann's disease must be distinguished from developmental round back deformity. In the latter, kyphosis is rarely severe and the deformity is usually more mobile. Verte-

ity at the apical deformity. The presence of a rigid apex is more ominous than if the deformity is mobile. At the moment of surgical reduction, the tension on the neural structures is greater when a rigid deformity is corrected.

Individual Factors. Patients vary, and not all respond to initial treatment, particularly non-operative treatment. Neurological complications may develop during the course of traction or may become more severe. In the course of correcting a kyphotic deformity, the application of traction should be slow and gentle with initial low loads. Deformities are more easily corrected when the apex is flexible. Similarly, better results are obtained with traction and immobilization with braces or cast in the case of a flexible deformity than with a rigid defor-

mity. In the presence of a kyphosis, it is also important to recognize that posterior procedures such as osteotomies, laminectomies, or decompression may result in increased instability and increasing deformity (Fig. 5).

BIOMECHANICS OF KYPHOTIC DEFORMITIES

Definition

In the thoracic spine, angulation in the sagittal plane greater than 40 degrees is considered abnormal. In the cervical and lumbar spines, 5 degrees or more of fixed posterior angulation is defined as a kyphotic deformity.

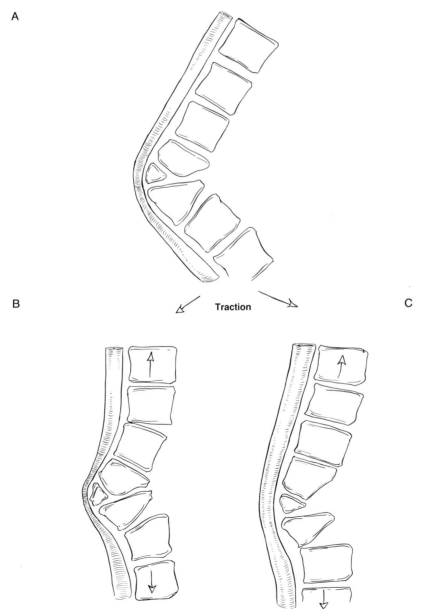

FIG. 5. A: Congenital kyphosis. **B:** Rigid apex not reducible; spinal cord at risk. **C:** Flexible apex; traction may be beneficial.

Anatomical Considerations

The spinal column is essentially divided into two parts, consisting of the anterior elements and the posterior elements. Everything anterior to the posterior longitudinal ligament is considered in the former category. This conceptualization differs from that of Denis (6), which is important to an understanding of burst fractures of the spine but less relevant to kyphosis. Muscles that apply loads to the spine can temporarily alter the spatial arrangement of the vertebrae, but the resting positions of the spine are dictated by the osseous and ligamentous components. The physiological thoracic kyphosis is determined primarily by osseous structures, and the lordotic curves of the cervical and lumbar spines are determined more by ligamentous structures.

The posterior elements are under tension and the anterior elements are under compression. Kyphosis may occur when either of these two components is disrupted. Posteriorly, the laminae and yellow ligaments are major structures resisting tension, while anteriorly the vertebral body and disc are the major structures that carry compressive loads.

Unphysiological loads, both in magnitude and direction (Fig. 6), may also result in a kyphotic deformity. An increase in the moment arm (Fig. 6) also plays an important role in the production of kyphosis. The more angulation there is, the greater the chance of additional angulation under a given load.

As the result of an increasing angulation, an increase in the moment arm results in further eccentric loading and can result in more wedging and a subsequent increase in angulation. A vicious cycle ensues when further wedging accentuates angulation and effectively increases the moment arm, which in turn increases eccentric loading.

Biomechanical Considerations Involved with Treatment

The treatment of severe kyphosis involves one or more steps including, if necessary, adequate decompression of the spinal cord and the application of forces to correct deformity (Fig. 7). These corrective forces consist of axial traction and sagittal plane bending moments (transverse loading). Axial loading is greater than transverse loading when the Cobb angle is greater than 53 degrees. These correctional forces reverse the roles of the anterior and posterior structures. The biomechanical concepts of creep and relaxation also play a role in the treatment of spinal deformities (see Chapter 68). Creep plays a particular role in axial correction with the patient erect, a concept used in halo-gravity or halo-pelvic traction.

Pathomechanics of Fusion (Grafts)

Posterior fusions are generally under tension and are usually thin and susceptible to stress fractures and indeed may bend (Figs. 8 and 9). A posterior fusion is usually considered more stable the greater its length. Despite this apparent stability, pseudarthrosis rates and failure to maintain correction are as high as 40% (11). Conversely, the anterior fusions are under compression and therefore ideal in the presence of these deformities.

A kyphotic deformity can also be considered a bent column, and the middle of the column the neutral axis. The more forces move away from this neutral axis toward the concavity, the more the moment arms are reduced and the more effective the support. Ideally, bone grafts for fusion kyphosis should be placed as close as feasible to the neutral axis on the compressive side and include all vertebrae that are in the deformity (Fig. 10).

In analyzing a uniform kyphotic curve (Fig. 11A), there exists a neutral line L (dotted line, Fig. 11A) that is in neither compression nor distraction. If this line is displaced toward the outside concavity of the curve, tension decreases; if the line L is displaced toward the concavity, compressive forces decrease.

If the curve is instrumented on its convexity (Fig. 11B), the neutral line L displaces toward the convexity. Compressive forces in the concavity then displace toward the center of the curve but maintain their same value with respect to their distance from the neutral line.

The instrumentation on the convexity (Fig. 11B) (or posterior side of the spine) acts as a tension band, and the tension on the bone is in fact decreased.

Based on these principles, there exists an optimal zone for a bone graft (Figs. 11C and 11D). With an anterior graft the optimal zone is directly under force F (Fig. 11C). With a posterior tension band (posterior compression instrumentation) the neutral line L is displaced toward the convexity of the curve. As a result, forces are displaced toward the convexity, and the optimal zone for the anterior graft is more toward the center of the concavity of the curve (Fig. 11D). It is necessary to place the graft in the mechanical axis under compression. If the graft is too close to the center of the curve, compression may be too excessive and the graft may have a tendency to resorb over the long term. If the graft is too far from the curve, it will have the same tendency, and the construct will not be sufficient for good osteosynthesis.

Bone that ideally can incorporate quickly is best. On this basis, autograph interbody grafts, obtained from the iliac crest, are preferable, but these cannot withstand the loads encountered in the erect position. Fibular grafts are sufficiently strong, but take up to six months to begin incorporation and revascularization unless a vascularized graft is used. For this reason, internal fixation devices are used anteriorly to enhance stability.

Text continues on page 1381.

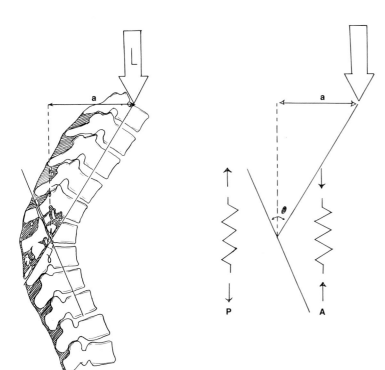

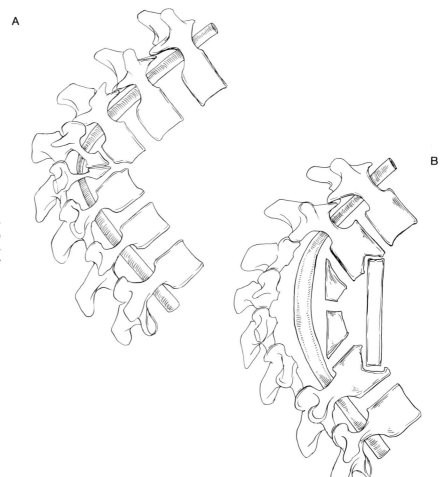

FIG. 6. Kyphosis may be progressive due to 1) and increase in load and an increase in duration of the load (1), and 2) the amount of angulation present (γ). With an increase in angulation, the moment increases and the kyphosis tends to increase.

FIG. 7. A and B: Congenital defects of formation with spinal cord compression. The cord has been decompressed anteriorly allowing it to translate anteriorly. An anterior strut graft arthrodesis is also performed.

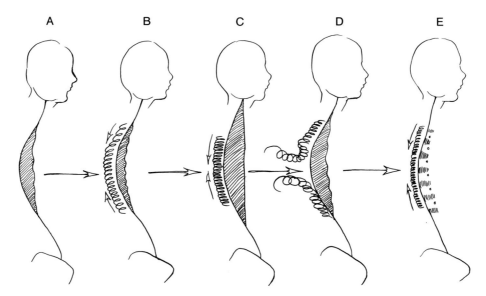

FIG. 8. A: Posterior fusion for severe kyphosis may **(B)** fail even with the use of posterior instrumentation (tension band) although initially successful **(C)**. The anterior structures are rigid and the posterior fusion is under tension **(D)**. Failure may occur **(E)**. Anterior release together with anterior fusion and anterior instrumentation or posterior fusion and instrumentation will produce a satisfactory result.

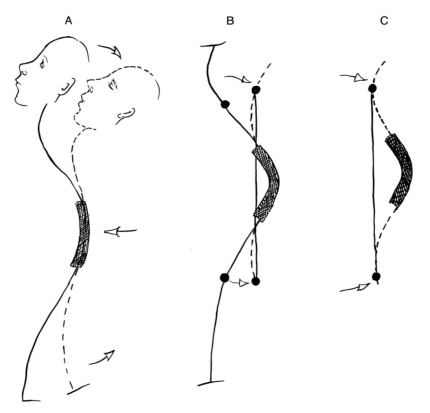

FIG. 9. Kyphotic deformities are best corrected anteriorly. Fusion on the posterior or tension side may fail. The extent of anterior fusion depends upon the flexibility of the kyphosis, which can be judged by hyperextension x-ray of the spine **(A)**. Anterior fusion should include at least the rigid and inflexible portion of the kyphosis **(heavy lines in B)**. In deformities with less flexibility, anterior fusion must include a greater area **(heavy lines in C)**. A posterior spine fusion should include the full extent of the kyphosis, regardless of the degree of flexibility.

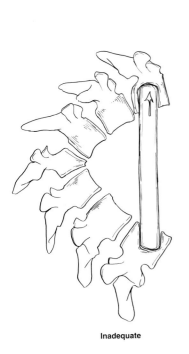
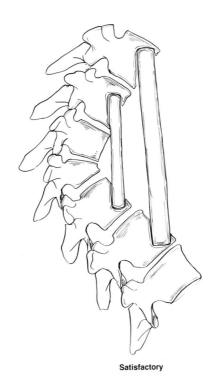

Inadequate

Satisfactory

FIG. 10. Bone graft close to the neutral axis of the spine and involving most vertebral levels is the most satisfactory.

A

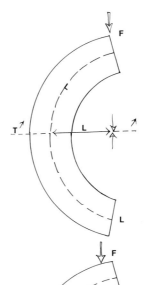

B

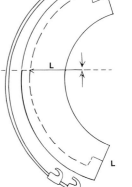

C

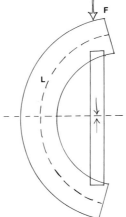

D

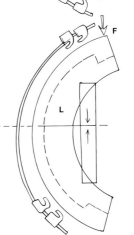

FIG. 11. A: Neutral line *L* (dotted line) is neither in compression nor distraction. **B:** Posterior instrumentation causes the neutral line to displace toward the convexity. **C:** Optimal zone for bone graft is directly under force *F.* **D:** With posterior instrumentation, the optimal zone is displaced toward the concavity of the curve.

TABLE 3. *Treatment options: Kyphosis—no neurological compromise*

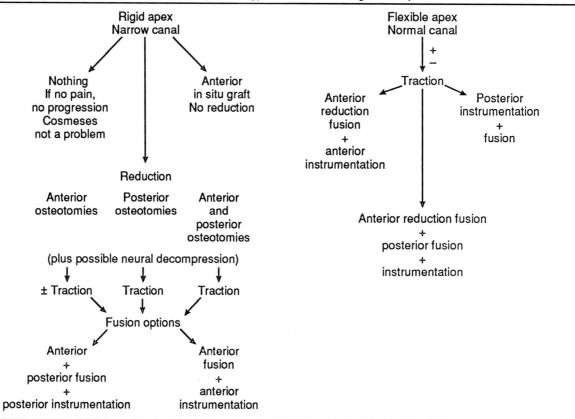

TABLE 4. *Treatment options: Kyphosis—neurological compromise*

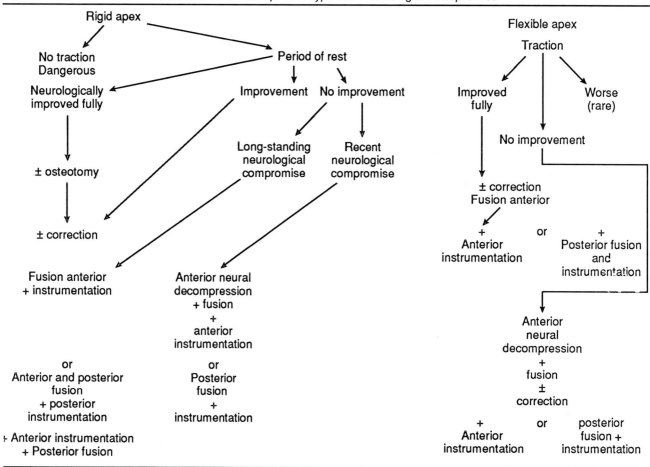

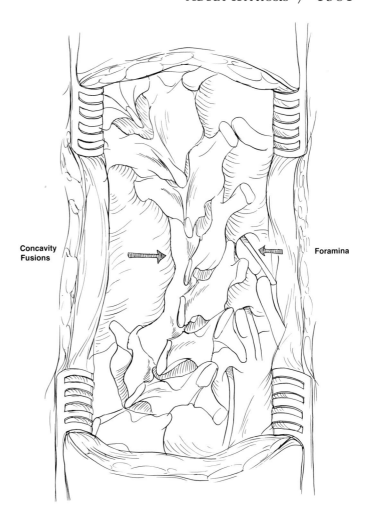

Concavity
Fusions

Foramina

FIG. 12. Thoracolumbar kyphoscoliosis.

Traction

Traction may play a role in the presence of a rigid or a mobile deformity. If the apex of the deformity is rigid, particularly in a congenital scoliosis, significant danger exists to compromise the spinal cord (Tables 3 and 4). In contrast, traction is particularly beneficial with a mobile deformity. In the presence of a rigid deformity, the neural elements should be decompressed prior to the application of traction and the curve made mobile. Both rigid or mobile kyphoses, particularly in the thoracic spine, may significantly affect respiratory ventilation. This may be significantly improved by correction of the kyphosis. Prior to surgery, application of traction in the presence of a mobile kyphosis may show significant improvement in ventilation, thus signifying the importance of surgical correction.

TREATMENT

Congenital Kyphosis (Kyphoscoliosis)

In the treatment of kyphoscoliosis, the kyphosis is more significant than the scoliosis. The basic principles consist of freeing any spontaneous or congenital fusions in the concavity of the deformity, applying distractive force in the concavity of the deformity, and using compression forces on the convexity combined with a posterior fusion (Figs. 12 and 13).

Operative Approach

Posterior transverse osteotomies are made through any spontaneous fusions. On the convex side, the osteotomies pass through the articular facets to the intervertebral foraminae (Fig. 12). In severe cases, Stagnara (27–31) described applying a distraction rod in the concavity of the deformity anterior to the ribs that are resected or osteotomized (Fig. 14). More recently, posterior liberation has been accomplished through osteotomies and rib releases; the deformity is then approached anteriorly using distraction with a Kostuik-Harrington system (Fig. 15).

In anterior approaches for kyphoscoliosis, the approach may be from either the concavity or the convexity. An approach from the concavity allows for easier placement of bone grafts from a mechanical point of view. However, the one problem encountered is that the

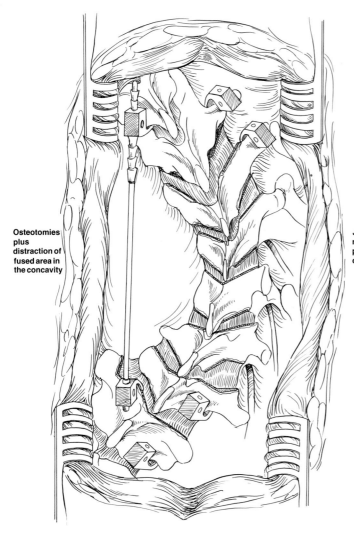

Osteotomies
plus
distraction of
fused area in
the concavity

Joint
resection
plus
compression

FIG. 13. Posterior surgery for kyphoscoliosis.

depth to the center of the curvature may be considerable and may present difficulties in decompression and graft placement.

In cases of severe kyphoscoliosis, the convex approach would appear to be preferable (Fig. 16). As an alternative, Bradford et al. (3) described a subperiosteal dissection in the concavity of the vertebral body, a so-called osteoplasty technique. Stagnara (29) subsequently expanded on this concept (Figs. 17A and 17B).

I have found in severe cases that the approach from the convexity can be easily performed, including decompression (Fig. 18). In cases of kyphoscoliosis, where the scoliotic component is moderate, an approach from the concavity is preferable, whereas in severe cases of decompression it is best performed from the convexity.

In congenital spine deformities, specific principles must be adhered to in their management. These principles depend on the etiology of the problem defects.

With anterior segmentation defects, posterior surgery alone can be used to stabilize the deformity but not correct the deformity. In a young child, posterior arthrodesis with instrumentation may correct deformity. However, in adults the choice lies between a posterior arthrod-

esis to only stabilize the deformity or a more extensive procedure, including anterior releases, osteotomies, posterior releases and osteotomies, traction, and subsequent fusion with instrumentation. Indications for treatment in the adult are progression of the deformity, intractable pain, and/or neurological signs and symptoms. As noted, the risks of neurological problems are high in a rigid deformity; thus, surgery for purely cosmetic reasons is a rare indication.

Defects of Formation
Anterior With Increasing Kyphosis

Early detection and fusion are the keys to treatment in most patients. These problems are best treated in childhood, because the risk of subsequent paralysis is high in these particular defects.

In the adult, treatment cannot be carried out by posterior approaches. Again, anterior releases and cord decompression together with posterior releases are necessary, followed by a period of traction and subsequent fusion with instrumentation. An alternative is to per-

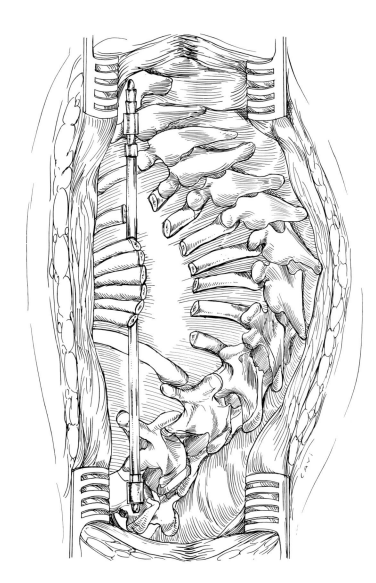

FIG. 14. Severe kyphoscoliosis: extrapleural rod.

FIG. 15. Kostuik-Harrington screw. Distraction screws for rachet end of Harrington distraction rod. Collar-ended screws for butt (distal) end of a standard round-ended Harrington compression rod. The same screw is used for heavy Harrington compression rods. Screws are available in three lengths and can be coupled with washers or staples.

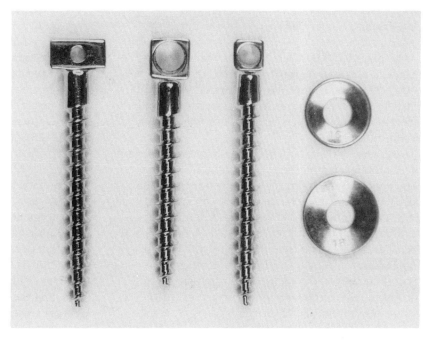

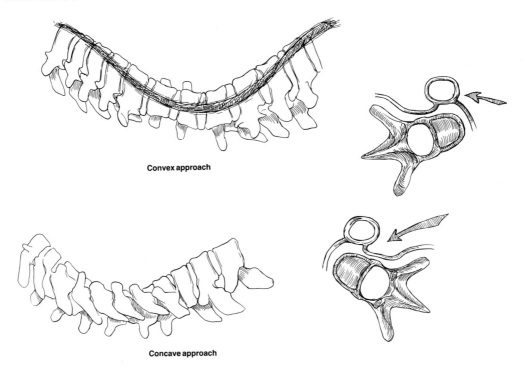

Convex approach

Concave approach

FIG. 16. Convex and concave approaches.

form posterior releases and then subsequent anterior decompression and releases, and anterior instrumentation, which may accomplish the same goal (Figs. 17, 18, 19, 20, 21, and 22) (Tables 3 and 4).

A technique currently achieving increasing popularity for the correction of kyphoscoliosis and congenital kyphosis is the "eggshell" procedure as described by Heinig (personal communication) (see Chapter 88.)

Post-Laminectomy Kyphosis

The majority of post-laminectomy kyphotic spine deformities occur in children, generally in those treated with posterior decompression for spinal cord tumors. This problem is rare in adults but can occur, particularly when a laminectomy has been done in the presence of severe osteoporosis.

As a result of my experience with progressive deformities that follow laminectomy in the presence of osteoporotic bone and/or scoliosis, I have recommended the addition of fusion in such cases. However, not everyone agrees. My indication for fusion after laminectomy is involvement of two or more levels in the female, regardless of etiology (spinal stenosis, scoliosis). If decompression is done for spinal stenosis in the presence of a scoliosis, stabilization at the very least must be carried out for the entire curve. Otherwise, the curve is at risk to progress significantly (Figs. 23A–23D).

Scheuermann's Kyphosis

Scheuermann's kyphosis in a growing child can often be controlled by the use of a Milwaukee brace. If the deformity reaches 65 degrees in the thoracic spine, many authors advocate posterior arthrodesis and compression instrumentation (36).

In the adult, the problems are somewhat different. Adults frequently present with pain in conjunction with a possibly psychological handicap. The pain may be difficult to control except by spinal fusion. The kyphosis accompanying Scheuermann's disease rarely results in neurological problems. Therefore, the indications for the surgical treatment of Scheuermann's kyphosis in the adult are (a) significant progressive deformity reaching 70 to 75 degrees or greater, (b) psychological handicap with a curve of about 75 degrees or greater, and (c) pain in the presence of a significant deformity of 70 to 75 degrees in the thoracic spine unresponsive to non-operative methods of treatment.

Long-term studies of the surgical treatment of Scheuermann's kyphosis in the adult by posterior instrumentation now indicate the progressive loss of correction that occurs in long-term follow-up (11). This loss of correction is due to the fusion being on the tensile side of the spine, high pseudarthrosis rates with posterior fusion, and the development of late stress fractures due to repetitive cycling on the tensile side of the spine (Fig. 24).

Text continues on page 1389.

A

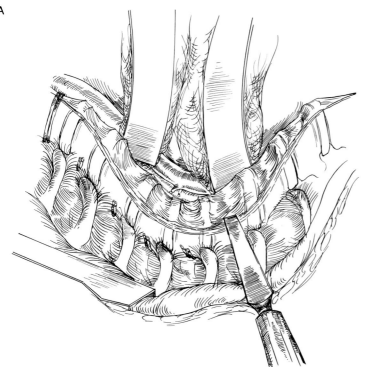

FIG. 17A. Subperiosteal dissection.

B

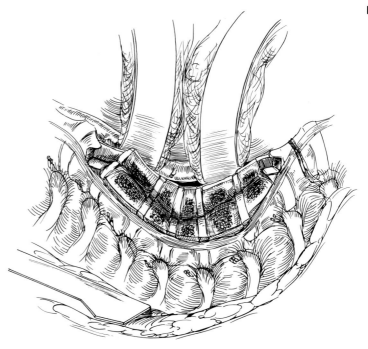

FIG. 17B. Subperiosteal dissection completed; a layer of bone disc has been elevated.

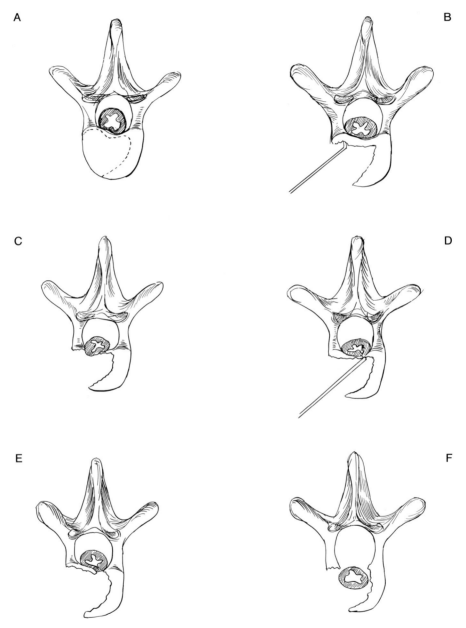

FIG. 18. A–F: Anterior cord decompression.

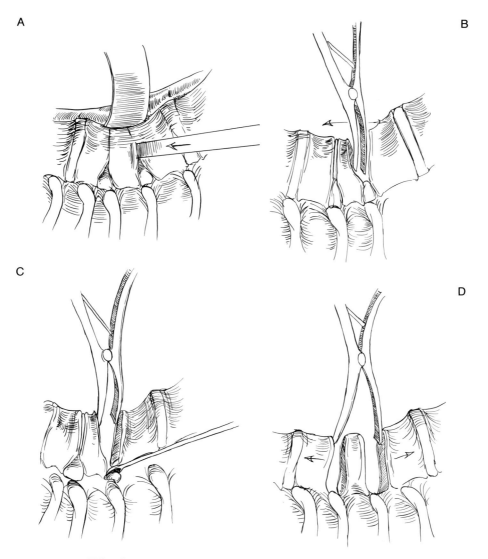

FIG. 19. A–D: Anterior osteotomies in congenital kyphosis.

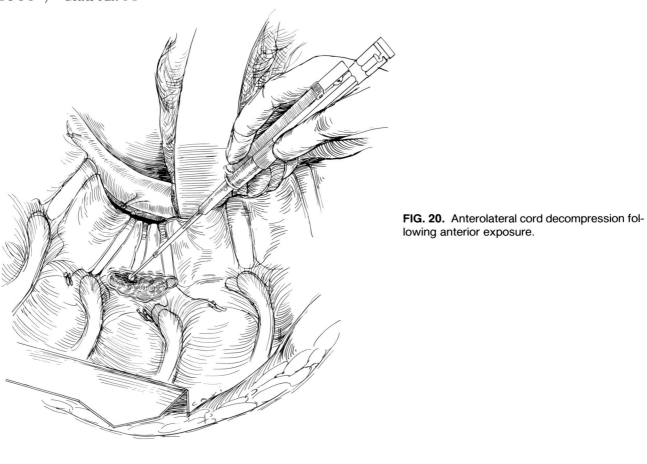

FIG. 20. Anterolateral cord decompression following anterior exposure.

FIG. 21. Following completion of the cord decompression, an anterior graft is added.

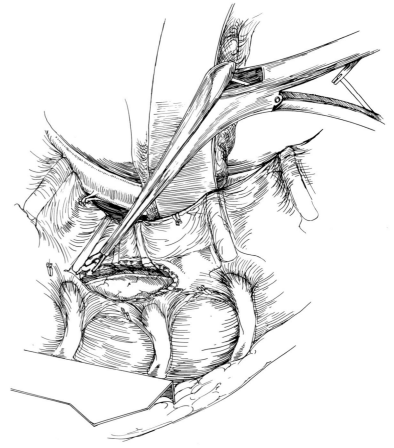

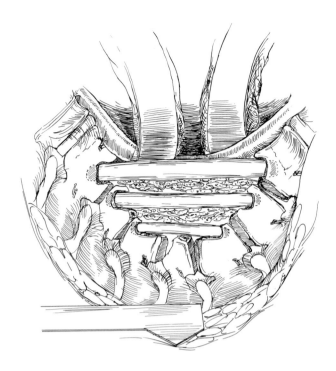

FIG. 22. Anterior grafting using strut grafts starting at the apex and including all levels in the kyphosis.

For that reason, anterior techniques are often used (Fig. 25).

Since the graft is on the tensile side of the spine it may, with repetitive cycling, become thinner with time and develop late stress fractures. My report to the Scoliosis Research Society in 1981 showed an incidence of pseudarthroses of 40% with a minimum of six-year follow-up. Late stress fractures also followed posterior instrumentation or the combination of anterior releases and posterior instrumentation. The pseudarthrosis rate at two years was 20%. More recently, Ogilvie and Bradford (20) have shown almost complete loss of correction despite the use of anterior interbody fusion and posterior arthrodesis with Luque sublaminar wires and instrumentation. No long-term results in adults are yet available with the use of Cotrel-Dubousset instrumentation.

The adult is somewhat different from the child in that the deformity is usually rigid. The magnitude of the rigidity is determined by obtaining a hyperextension radiograph of the patient with the apex of the deformity placed over a sand bag. A lateral radiogram is then taken and compared to the non–hyperextended radiograph.

ANTERIOR APPROACH TO KYPHOTIC DEFORMITIES

My experience has shown that a poor outcome often follows posterior instrumentation, and there is a high pseudarthrosis rate even when combined with anterior fusion. I have also encountered complications and the need for subsequent surgical procedures performed for loss of correction. This experience has led to the development of techniques of anterior instrumentation and interbody fusion. The general aim is to stabilize and

correct the kyphotic deformity by a mechanically sound procedure, with minimal immobilization and minimal complications, that will not deteriorate over time within either the fusion mass or adjacent vertebral segments.

The biomechanical aims are to stabilize and correct the kyphotic deformity by providing axial distraction and reducing bending moments and producing a fusion mass that is (a) under compression, (b) long, (c) far from the neutral axis, and (d) interbody.

Rationale for Anterior Instrumentation

Iliac crest grafts (bicortical or tricortical in older, more osteopenic people) incorporate well but cannot withstand the loads encountered in the erect position in the lumbar spine, which is three to four times body weight, according to White and Panjabi (33). The same is true of most rib grafts in adults. Fibular grafts are sufficiently strong but do not incorporate and revascularize quickly enough. Internal fixation devices enhance stability (Fig. 23).

Anterior Instrumentation

The Kostuik-Harrington instrumentation provides adequate rigidity and stability, provided it is used in a rectangular or parallelogram configuration (Figs. 26A and 26B).

The system is versatile and allows for correction of deformity and early ambulation. A standard Harrington distraction instrumentation is all that is required, together with a crimper for the screw heads when heavy compression rods are used in conjunction with distrac-

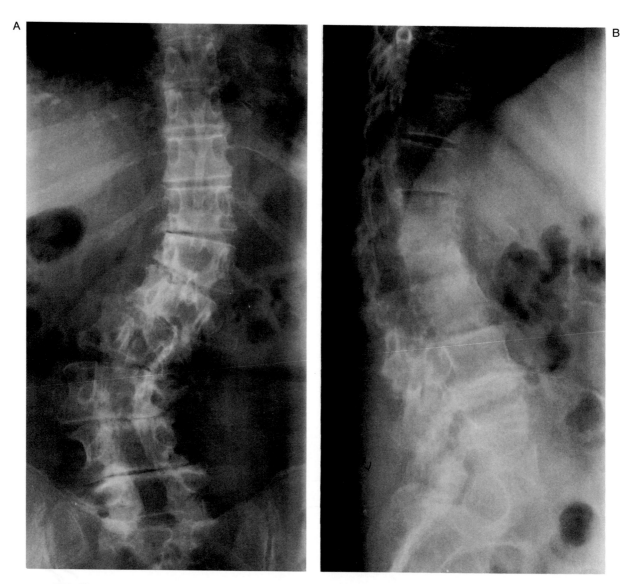

FIG. 23. A: Following decompression for spinal stenosis in this 63-year-old female, the curve increased 50%. No stabilization had been carried out. **B:** Marked post-laminectomy kyphosis developed following loss of posterior supporting structures in an already potentially unstable spine. (Figs. 23C–23D follow.)

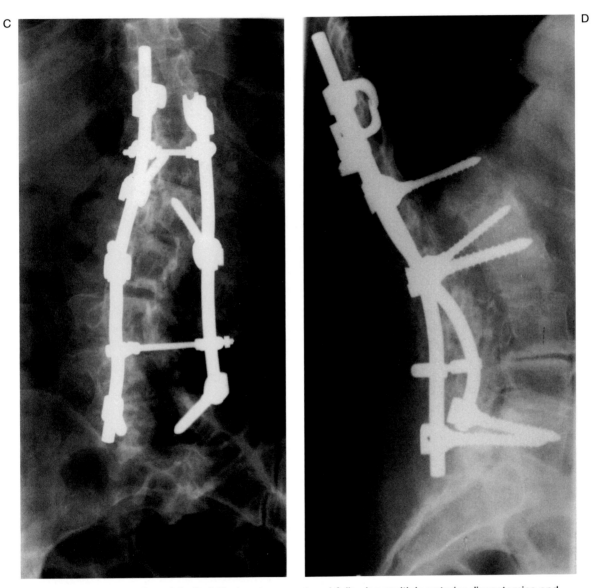

FIG. 23. *Continued.* **C and D:** Stability has been restored following multiple anterior discectomies and bone grafting followed by a second stage posterior Cotrel-Dubousset instrumentation and fusion.

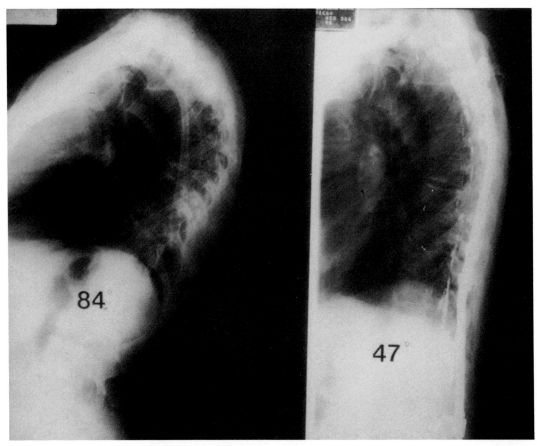

FIG. 24. A 24-year-old female who underwent correction of kyphosis secondary to Scheuermann's disease. The kyphosis was reduced from 84 to 47 degrees following traction and posterior instrumentation. Fortunately, 15 years later, she remains unchanged.

tion rods (i.e., burst fractures). Crimping the collar-ended heads over the heavy compression rod avoids the need for nuts and is as effective. Equipment consists of collar-ended screws and a distraction screw. The heads of either screws are compatible with the standard round end of the Harrington rods. The screw heads are attached to cancellous threads that come in three lengths. The depth of insertion required is measured with a depth gauge to which 2 to 3 mm are added in order to assure penetration of the contralateral cortex of the vertebral body. The length to bridge all defects to be incorporated in the construct plus this small extra measured amount determines rod length, which can be cut to size.

Indications

I use the anterior Kostuik-Harrington system for all forms of kyphotic deformities, both acute and chronic. The following are the specific indications: acute burst injuries, post-traumatic kyphosis, Scheuermann's disease, rigid round back, rigid kyphosis, post-laminectomy kyphosis and instability, iatrogenic lumbar kyphosis (flat back syndrome), kyphosis secondary to tumor, and kyphosis secondary to osteoporosis with fracture.

Surgical Techniques

For thoracic deformities a thoracotomy is performed through the fifth and sixth ribs. The scapula is mobilized. If there is an associated right thoracic scoliosis, a left-sided approach is preferred. The segmental vessels are clipped and the spine is exposed over an appropriate length, usually from T3 to T12. All discs and end plates back to the posterior annulus are removed. Rachet and collar-ended screws are inserted. The screws must pierce both cortices of the body and are placed as far posterior as possible. The rods are inserted and, if necessary, may be contoured. Distraction of both rods is carried out concurrent with application of manual pressure applied posteriorly. Clamps are used to secure the rods. Bicortical iliac crest grafts are inserted under compression (Figs. 26A and 26B). The grafts should be slightly larger than the interspace. Supplementary rib is also used. In osteoporotic bodies cement may be used to hold the screws in place. In some thoracic kyphotic deformities, the fusion and instrumentation may have to extend to L1 or L2 in order to prevent the development of secondary junctional kyphosis. In this instance, the diaphragm must be partially detached, usually through a separate flank inci-

A

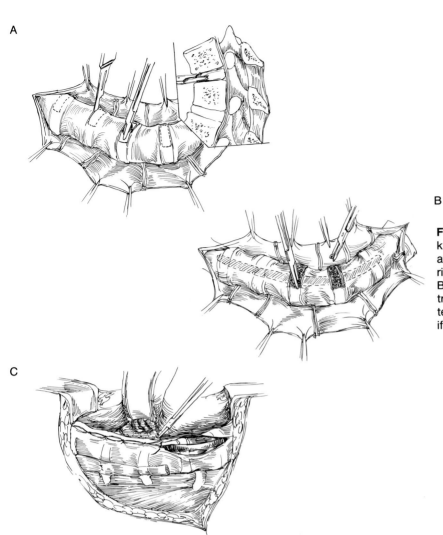

B

FIG. 25. Surgery for severe Scheuermann's kyphosis. **A:** Multiple disc excisions are done after exposure. This must be done as far posteriorly as the posterior longitudinal ligament. **B:** Bone graft can be added either as a rib graft in a trough or as interbody grafts. **C:** The periosteum and pleura are closed over the fusion area if possible.

C

sion along the eleventh rib.

For thoracolumbar deformities, the standard thoraco-abdominal transpleural, retroperitoneal approach is used, taking down the diaphragm. The procedure is then carried out as described above.

The preliminary experience with anterior interbody fusion and modified Kostuik-Harrington anterior instrumentation took place from 1982 to 1987 and included 36 patients with an average age of 27.5 years. Post-operatively, patients were immobilized in a plastic orthosis for six months. The average hospital stay was twelve days. All patients had a minimum follow-up of two years. The average pre-operative curve was 75.5 degrees, which was reduced to 56 degrees with instrumentation. After the two-year follow-up the average curve was 60 degrees. Six patients (16%) had progression of their curves within their fusions. One patient underwent subsequent surgery and two patients had a pseudarthrosis. The complications were minimal, with four screw fractures (Figs. 27A, 27B, 28A, and 28B).

Surgical Results in Adult Scheuermann's Kyphosis

The results are tabulated in Table 5. It is now generally accepted that posterior instrumentation and fusion do not suffice. In one series, the two-year results were acceptable, but at six years a 40% pseudarthrosis rate was identified (12).

The evolution of my treatment protocol began with posterior instrumentation and fusion using long Harrington compression rods. This was followed by anterior release of the disc spaces over 9 to 10 levels plus or minus fusion over 3 to 4 spaces at the apex followed by 10 days of halo-femoral traction and then posterior instrumentation using long Harrington compression rods or $\frac{1}{4}$-inch diameter heavy Luque rods with sublaminar wiring. Although initial correction appeared better, long-term results revealed no improvement over posterior instrumentation and fusion. Ogilvie and Bradford (20) found similar results using Luque instrumentation.

Although the experience is still preliminary, anterior

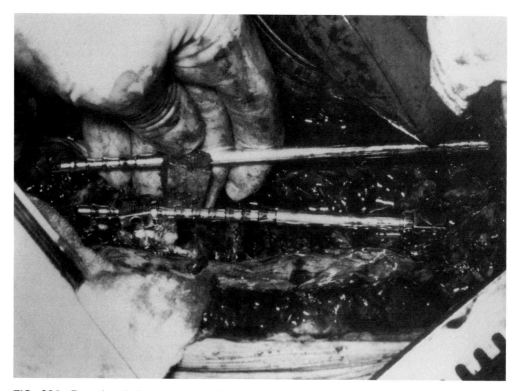

FIG. 26A. Round-ended standard Harrington rods have been inserted; distraction has been carried out. Bicortical iliac crest blocks of bone are then inserted into each disc space.

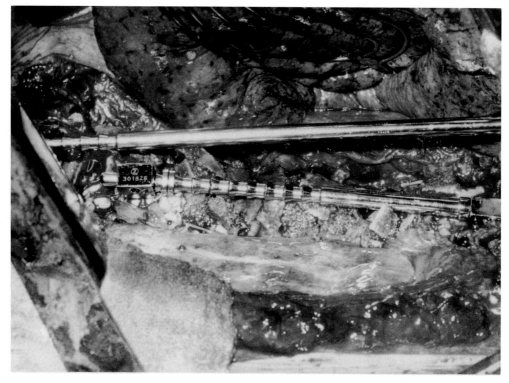

FIG. 26B. Grafting is complete prior to closing.

A

B

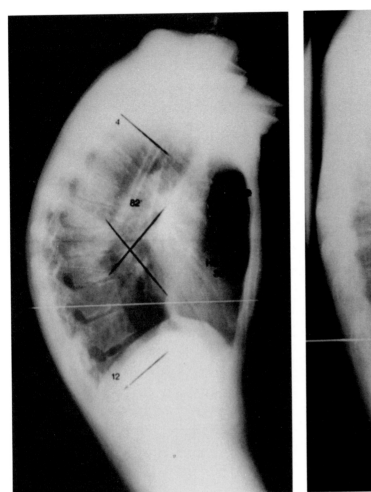
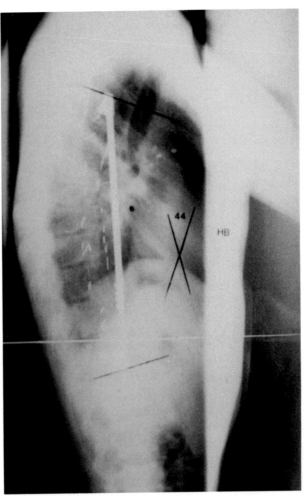

FIG. 27. Male age 32, pre **(A)** and post **(B)** anterior Kostuik-Harrington instrumentation and fusion. Patient remains well 7 years later. Curve has been corrected from 82 to 44 degrees. Pain has been alleviated. In the first few cases, a single rod was used.

Kostuik-Harrington instrumentation and anterior interbody fusion appear to be an improvement over the previously described techniques. Initial post-operative correction is less but appears to be better maintained. The pseudarthrosis rate (Table 5) is 2 of 36 (5.5%). There have been no early or long-term vascular or pulmonary problems. Another alternative, the use of Cotrel-Dubousset instrumentation, has recently been advocated.

My use to date has been limited to four cases, all successful.

Two patients treated by Kostuik-Harrington instrumentation developed a late junctional kyphosis at the level below the distal end of the anterior instrumentation. This has been noted to occur following posterior instrumentation by Ogilvie and Bradford (20) and by Lowe (14). In both my anteriorly instrumented cases, as

TABLE 5. *Results of surgical treatment in adult Scheuermann's kyphosis*

Procedure	No.	Patient's age	Pre-op curves (degrees)	Post-op curves (degrees)	Late post-op curves (degrees)	Follow-up	Pseud-arthrosis	Compli-cations	Prog degrees
Post fusion with HR	6	23	74	46	59	7 yrs	6	7	7
Ant. release post fusion with HR	9		81	42	62				
Ant. release post fusion with SSI	5	23	70	41	43	3 yrs	1	3	3
Ant. release ant. fusion with K-H rod	36	31	79	56	60	2 yrs	2	4	4

HR = Harrington rods. SSI = Luque or Harrington-Luque rods. K-H = Kostuik-Harrington instrumentation

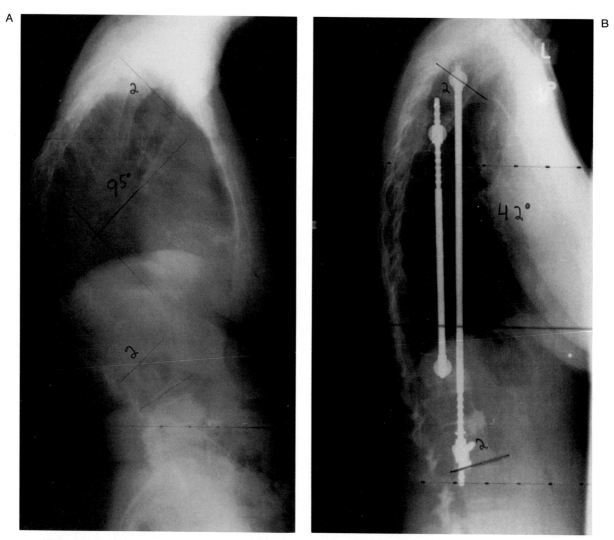

FIG. 28. Female age 62. **A:** Progressive painful kyphosis secondary to Scheuermann's disease first noticed in adolescence. Curve 95 degrees. **B:** Three years following single stage anterior Kostuik-Harrington instrumentation the patient remains corrected to 42 degrees and is pain free. Methylmethacrylate bone cement was used to help support the screws. Instrumentation was extended to L2 to avoid development of a junctional kyphosis.

well as those cases reported to occur following posterior instrumentation, the cause was a failure to extend the fusion and instrumentation far enough distally.

POST-TRAUMATIC KYPHOSIS

Kyphosis is recognized as a common sequelae to the fracture of the lumbar or thoracolumbar spine (1,8). The sequelae of post-traumatic kyphosis are either mechanical or neurological in nature. These include pain, progression of deformity, and abnormal movement. In the neurologically impaired, additional problems include difficulties in sitting, standing, and balance and skin ulceration. Neurological sequelae may include increasing deficits or potentially correctable but persisting deficits associated with anterior compression of the spinal canal contents. The goals of treatment of an established post-traumatic kyphosis are the improvement of the neurological status, correction of deformity, and establishment of spinal stability.

Previous reports (16,22) have indicated that the outcome of anterior decompression is better than that obtained by a posterior approach when there is a post-traumatic kyphosis. Posterior approaches have generally been associated with significant loss of correction or prolonged post-operative immobilization. Recognizing the inadequacies of posterior approaches, my approach in recent years has been to treat symptomatic post-traumatic kyphosis in the thoracic and lumbar spine by anterior correction of the kyphotic deformity, stabilization with Kostuik-Harrington instrumentation and fusion, and, where necessary, decompression of the neural elements.

Thirty-seven such patients have been treated since 1984 with long-term follow-up. All patients had burst fractures. The age range was from 19 to 57, with an average age of 42 years. The time interval from initial injury to surgery ranged from 6 months to 20 years, with an average of 4.2 years. All patients presented with pain, usually localized to the apex of the deformity and/or at levels below the injury. The levels ranged from as high as T4 in the thoracic spine to L2 in the lumbar spine. Seventeen cases were located at L1. Six patients had multiple levels of injury, ranging from two to three contiguous levels.

Eight patients exhibited residual neurologic problems related to their initial injuries with paraparesis. Another 9 patients developed spinal stenosis secondary to their injuries. Symptom onset in these patients occurred from a minimum of one year post-injury to as long as 20 years. Symptoms of spinal stenosis included pain, radicular symptoms with inability to walk more than a few blocks, and development of stress incontinence in females. Physical signs in patients with late development of spinal stenosis included progressive weakness as exhibited on physical examination after walking and sluggish or absent reflexes.

Radiographic investigation included plain x-rays as well as myelography in all patients, followed by CT scanning when this became available.

The indications for discography or facet injections were pain not accurately localized to the apex of the deformity by the patient or examiner or a history of pain below the apex of the deformity. In these cases, discography was done at the level immediately below the old fracture.

If the level adjacent to the fracture reproduced the patient's pain and showed evidence of dye leakage, then the next adjacent level was done until a normal level was reached.

Discography was done in 17 of the 37 cases. The level immediately below the fracture was identified as the source of pain in 12 cases. In 5 cases degenerative and painful discs were identified, two to three levels distal to the fracture.

In patients who had not had previous posterior surgery, facet blocks also were used to ascertain and localize the level of pain. This technique was used in 12 cases. In 10 of the 12 cases, the block caused relief of the patient's pain.

Initial treatment consisted of non-operative management in 23 patients, posterior instrumentation consisting of Harrington rods in 10 patients, 4 of whom had an associated laminectomy. Four additional patients had laminectomy alone. Two patients had undergone previous anterior decompression and interbody fusions using iliac crest grafts, but had gone on to late collapse and recurrence of the deformity. One of these two patients had recurrence of her initial paraparesis. The second had had anterior graft collapse and late development of spinal stenosis. Minimum follow-up was 3 years, and the maximum follow-up was 10 years for the first 37 patients.

The number of levels fused range from three to nine. Twenty patients had fusion over three levels anteriorly.

Surgical Technique

The technique is that employed by the author (11) in the anterior treatment of acute burst injuries with or without neurological involvement. If the patient has had previous posterior fusion he should always be positioned so that a simultaneous posterior approach may be performed if necessary, if anterior correction cannot be adequately obtained at a single stage. This has not been necessary in any of my cases to date, including the 37 in this series and cases performed in the last three years.

Anterolateral approach is made from the left side. Following exposure of the spine, the segmental vessels are divided in the midline to avoid any trauma to the intravertebral foramina and possible embarrassment to the blood supply of the spinal cord. In order to avoid impingement of the vascular structures against any subsequent metallic implants, it is important to ligate the in-

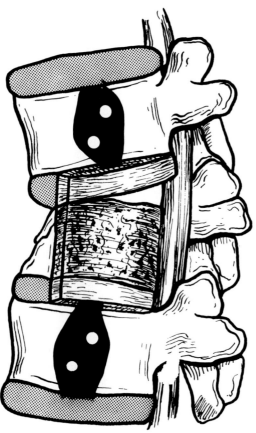

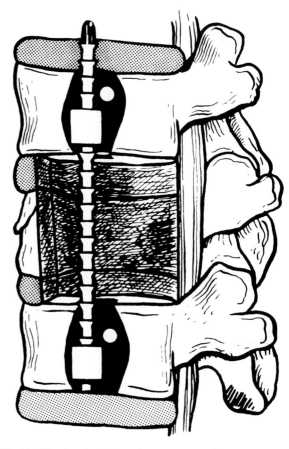

FIG. 29. Post-traumatic kyphosis following neural decompression. The anterior vertebral body and contralateral cortex are left.

FIG. 30. The kyphosis has been corrected by anterolateral Kostuik-Harrington distraction instrumentation.

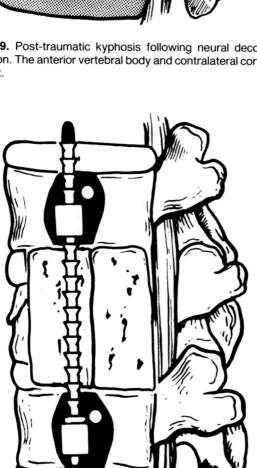

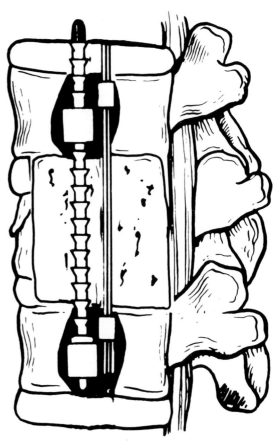

FIG. 31. Iliac graft (strut–interbody) has been added.

FIG. 32. A second lateral heavy Harrington compression rod is added and the graft is slightly compressed.

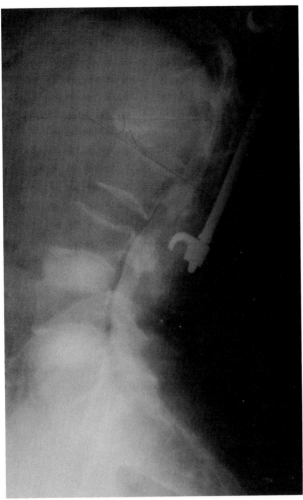

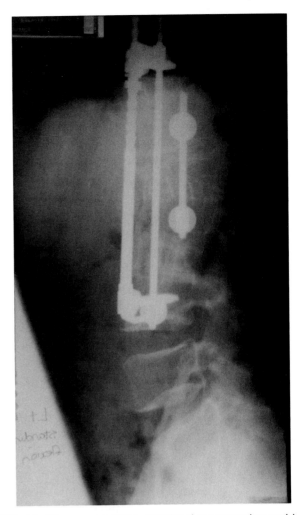

FIG. 33. A 21-year-old with burst fracture L1. Initially there were no neurological symptoms or signs. Because of pain one year later, posterior instrumentation and fusion were carried out with no relief despite a solid fusion. She later developed signs and symptoms of spinal stenosis.

FIG. 34. Three years later, anterior decompression and instrumentation were done. The fusion was extended to L3 as the L2-L3 disc was also damaged.

tersegmental vessels two levels above and if possible two levels below the planned area of instrumentation. This maneuver allows the aorta to fall away to the contralateral side. Using this technique in over 350 cases of anterior instrumentation done for various causes, I have not experienced any late vascular sequelae. Decompression is carried out, extending from the anterior aspect of the vertebral body posteriorly, exposing the contents of the spinal canal. A cortical shell may be left on the contralateral side (Fig. 29). Whitesides (34) has stated that it is easier to decompress starting anteriorly and removing the entire vertebral body rather than simply removing the posterior half of the vertebral bodies in the affected area. Following decompression of the canal, the kyphosis is corrected with anterior Kostuik-Harrington instrumentation. An anterior distraction rod of appropriate length and screws using the rachet-ended screw for the rachet ends, and the collar end of the screw for the butt

end of the round and Harrington rod are used (Fig. 30). In older patients, it may be necessary if any degree of osteopenia is present to use a tricortical graft. This may be supplemented by rib graft if the thoraco-abdominal approach is used. In the upper thoracic spine, rib alone is used as multiple small struts.

A second rod for rotational control is applied somewhat posterior to the anterior placed rod. Care is taken to angle the screws away from the canal (Fig. 32). A heavy Harrington compression rod is used with two collar-ended screws. Slight compression is applied through the rod to lock the grafts in place. The screw ends on the compression rod are crimped. Nuts may be used as an alternative.

Blood loss averaged 1.414 ccs, with a range from 300 ccs to 2,800 ccs. Post-operative immobilization consisted of a molded plastic orthosis. Plaster-of-paris cast immobilization was used in seven cases when it was felt

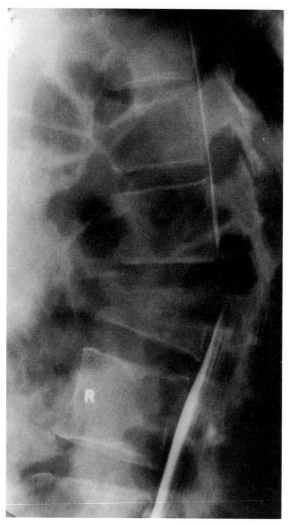

FIG. 35. A 38-year-old female with burst fracture L1.

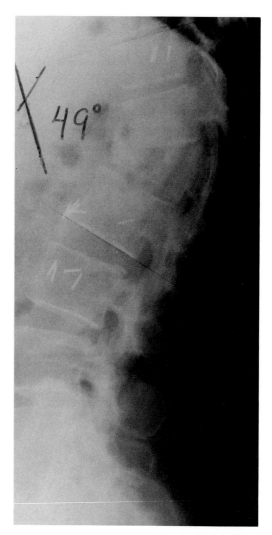

FIG. 36. Anterior decompression and iliac crest grafting were done with resolution of signs and symptoms. Six months later the graft had collapsed with recurrence of pain and neurological signs.

that the patient might not be reliable in wearing the orthosis. Patients were allowed to ambulate a few days post-operatively. In no patients, despite previous posterior laminectomy, was a second-stage procedure carried out. However, the posterior instrumentation was removed in eight of the ten patients prior to anterior surgery. In no patients was posterior osteotomy of a previous fusion performed.

Presentation

Case 1

A female aged 21 sustained a burst fracture of L1 without neurologic involvement. One year following her injury the patient developed symptoms of spinal stenosis and weakness in her legs on walking more than six city blocks (Fig. 33). She underwent a three-level posterior fusion from T11 to L3 without instrumentation and

without correction of her kyphos. Her symptoms persisted despite her solid fusion, which was verified by tomography and later re-exploration of her fusion mass. Three years later she underwent anterior decompression as well as correction of her kyphosis with anterior instrumentation and interbody grafting without posterior osteotomy. Her curve was corrected from 34 degrees to 18 degrees (Fig. 34). She has had successful resolution of her symptoms with relief of back pain and no neurological findings. She has returned to gainful employment.

Case 2

A 38-year-old woman sustained an L1 burst injury with Frankel Grade C neurologic involvement (Fig. 35). She underwent decompression within 24 hours with resolution of her symptoms. Over the ensuing six months her

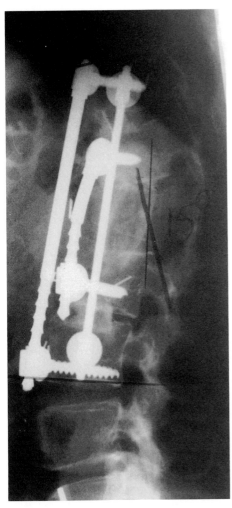

FIG. 37. Post-operative Kostuik-Harrington instrumentation and fusion. Deformity has been corrected and symptoms and signs resolved.

graft collapsed (Fig. 36) with recurrence of her neurological problems. An anterior decompression was performed, followed by continued pain. Discography revealed two affected discs below her initial fracture. She underwent anterior decompression of L1 and anterior interbody fusion from T11 to L3 with instrumentation with complete resolution of her symptoms and relief of her back pain. She returned to full-time work as a factory worker with normal neurological findings (Fig. 37). Her curve was corrected from 49 degrees to 15 degrees.

Case 1 serves to indicate that pain is rarely relieved in posterior fusions for post-traumatic kyphosis unless that deformity is corrected. Posterior osteotomy of an intact fusion mass is not generally required to correct the kyphos, since posterior fusions over a period of time in the presence of a continuing kyphosis become thin with repetitive cycling.

The second case serves to illustrate that anterior decompression may relieve neurological symptoms in acute burst injuries, but graft collapse may ensue. The addition of anterior instrumentation may prevent this complication.

Results

Union

Union was achieved in 36 of 37. One non-union occurred in a patient who had had a previous laminectomy. A screw broke anteriorly with subsequent graft collapse. Four patients had an average loss of 11 degrees of correction. All but one patient obtained and maintained correction of their kyphosis.

Pain Relief

Eighteen patients reported little or no pain requiring analgesics or other therapeutic pain modalities.

Eleven patients continued to have mild pain requiring the use of mild analgesics such as acetylsalicylic acid or extra-strength acetaminophen. One patient had increasing pain for reasons that could not be determined. Three other patients continued to have pain. Subsequent discography at levels below their fusions found other discs to be affected. To date, none of these patients has undergone subsequent treatment.

Neurological Results

Three of eight patients with residual paraparesis improved. Two patients who were initially wheelchair bound subsequently were able to ambulate with the aid of below-knee orthoses and canes. One recovered bowel and bladder function. Two patients showed mild improvement of motor power, but not enough to make a functional difference. Three patients showed no neural improvement.

The nine patients who subsequently developed spinal stenosis secondary to their initial injuries improved following anterior decompression, correction of their kyphosis, and stabilization. There was no deterioration of neurological status in any case.

Complications

Complications included one Horner's syndrome in a female who underwent anterior decompression at T4. One patient developed a hemothorax and required chest tube drainage. One patient developed an incisional post-thoracotomy syndrome that required intercostal blocks. Three patients developed adult respiratory distress syndrome that necessitated ventilatory assistance for an average of three days post-operatively. One patient, who had undergone anterior decompression with subsequent collapse of her graft, had recurrence of her deformity. She underwent repeat anterior correction of her deformity with instrumentation, but ruptured her diaphragm three months post-operatively, which required repair using Marlex graft. It is now four years since her surgery and she works full time. One patient, as noted, sustained screw breakage, loss of correction of his deformity, and developed a non-union.

Residual pain in post-traumatic kyphosis is not uncommon. Nicoll (19) indicated that 43% of his patients had pain at the injured motion segment and 57% had low back pain. He did not differentiate the type of spinal injury these patients had sustained. Roberts and Curtiss (23) reported a 40% incidence of pain with residual instability. In the series of Malcolm and Bradford (16), 85% of the 48 patients who had been managed non-operatively had pain.

In this series, 23 of 37 patients were treated non-operatively. All had incapacitating pain. A review of over 500 patients following spinal surgery (15) revealed a high incidence of continuing pain and disability that followed fracture as a result of post-traumatic kyphosis.

As with Malcolm and Bradford's series (16), early surgical stabilization of the spine in 10 patients in this series with posterior instrumentation, properly performed, failed to prevent late development of deformity. Seven of these were associated with laminectomies. One patient had a pseudarthrosis that was repaired before the subsequent treatment of her late anterior cord compression and post-traumatic kyphosis.

I have had no experience with the use of laminectomy and intradural lysis of adhesions (21) for improvement of incomplete or increasing neural deficit in post-traumatic kyphosis or with posterolateral decompression (4,5,13).

VASCULARIZED RIB GRAFTS FOR STABILIZATION OF KYPHOSIS

The use of autografts in structural kyphosis and resection for tumor or other causes is a standard procedure. It is well documented that such grafts may take up to two years to incorporate. Johnson and Robinson (10) noted that a vascularized fibular graft could avoid the difficulties encountered with allografts or autografts by providing immediate stability and rapid healing.

Rose, Owen, and Sanderson (24) proposed transposition of the rib with its intact blood supply. Bradford (2) independently proposed a similar technique and reviewed the results of vascularized rib transfer in 25 patients. Radiographs showed early and rapid incorporation of the grafts in 4 to 16 weeks, with an average of 8.5 weeks. He felt that this was a useful alternative to allografts or autografts, since it prompted rapid healing without requiring the microsurgical techniques necessary for a vascularized fibular graft.

Indications for surgery were progression of kyphosis, a painful kyphosis, or both. He used the grafts as inlay grafts and onlay grafts as struts. A thoracotomy is planned so that the blood supply and rib removal will not be compromised. For a kyphosis proximal to T5 in a patient without neurologic involvement, a rib one or two segments below the distal vertebra of the kyphosis is removed. The distal end of the rib is rotated to reach the proximal vertebra. Internal stabilization may be used. If the kyphosis does not extend proximal to T5, a rib one or two levels above the distal vertebra of the kyphosis is removed, rotating its distal portion to reach the distal vertebral body.

If, on the other hand, anterior cord decompression is to be done, it is preferred to remove the rib corresponding to the level of the apex of kyphosis in order to facilitate the exposure for the decompression. For arthrodesis of the thoracolumbar or lumbar spine, the tenth rib containing its vascularized pedicle is sufficient graft material.

Coagulating cautery is used after exposure of the rib, cutting the intercostal muscle along the superior part of the rib. A margin of approximately 4 to 5 mm should be left attached to the inferior aspect of the rib in order to avoid damaging the intercostal vessels. The rib is cut distally at the sternocostal junction and the distal vessels

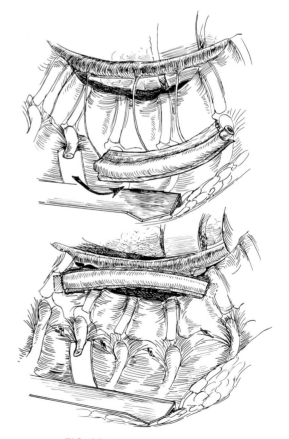

FIG. 38. Vascularized rib graft.

ligated. Identification of the intercostal vessel on the inside of the chest facilitates proximal dissection. The rib is divided at its posterior angle after careful subperiosteal dissection. The intercostal vessels are mobilized over the anterior longitudinal ligament, facilitating a more mobile vascular pedicle. The rib may be shortened at either end, depending on the length needed. Great care must be taken to avoid damaging the intercostal vessels (particularly during anterior decompression). Circulation of the rib may be checked by making an incision one to two centimeters in the periosteum overlying the rib to see whether bleeding occurs. Stabilization may be enhanced by anterior or posterior internal fixation.

The use of vascularized rib struts allows the grafts to lie more anterior than non-vascularized struts (Fig. 38). If a non-vascularized strut lies more than four centimeters anterior to the apical vertebral body, the likelihood of fracture during bone consolidation and revascularization is possible, whereas with the vascularized rib strut, this does not occur. The procedure of a vascularized rib strut is uniquely suited for stabilization in-situ, but may be utilized during the correction of kyphosis as well. In the growing child, the use of a vascularized rib is undesirable, as this might produce an anterior tether. If its use is essential, a second-stage posterior arthrodesis is advisable.

REFERENCES

1. Bohlman HH (1976): Late progressive paralysis and pain following fractures of the thoracolumbar spine. *J Bone Joint Surg* [Am] 58:728.
2. Bradford DS (1980): Anterior vascular pedicle grafting for the treatment of kyphosis. *Spine* 5:318–323.
3. Bradford DS, Winter RB, Lonstein JE, Moe JH (1977): Techniques of anterior spinal surgery for the management of kyphosis. *Clin Orthop* (128):129–139.
4. Capener N (1954): The evolution of lateral rhachotomy. *J Bone Joint Surg* [Br] 36:173–179.
5. Chou SN (1978): Treatment of thoracic spinal deformity with neurological deficit. In: Shou SN, Seljeskog EL, eds. *Spinal deformities and neurological dysfunction.* New York: Raven Press, pp. 131–137.
6. Denis F (1983): The three column spine and its significance in the classification of acute thoracolumbar spinal injuries. *Spine* 8:817–831.
7. Dubousset J (1982): Cyphoses et cyphoscolioses angulaires. SOFCOT, Reunion annuelle, November.
8. Guttmann L (1969): Spinal deformities in traumatic paraplegics and tetraplegics following surgical procedures. *Paraplegia* 7:38–58.
9. James JIP (1955): Kyphoscoliosis. *J Bone Joint Surg* [Br] 37:414–426.
10. Johnson JTH, Robinson RA (1968): Anterior strut grafts for severe kyphosis. *Clin Orthop* (56):25–36.
11. Kostuik JP (1988): Anterior Kostuik-Harrington distraction systems for the treatment of kyphotic deformities. *The Iowa Orthopaedic Journal* 69:77.
12. Kostuik JP, Carl A, Ferron S (1989): Anterior Zielke instrumentation for adult spinal deformity. *J Bone Joint Surg* [Am] 71:898–912.
13. Leidholt JD, Young JJ, Hahn HR, Jackson RE, Gamble WE, Miles JS (1969): Evaluation of late spinal deformities with fracture-dislocations of the dorsal and lumbar spine in paraplegics. *Paraplegia* 7:16–28.
14. Lowe TG (1987): Double L-rod instrumentation in the treatment of severe kyphosis secondary to Scheuermann's disease. *Spine* 12:336–341.
15. Macnab I, Tile M, Chapman H, Kostuik JP: Unpublished data.
16. Malcolm BW, Bradford DS, Winter RB, et al. (1979): Post-traumatic kyphosis. A review of 48 surgically treated patients. American Academy of Orthopaedic Surgeons, San Francisco, Feb. 25.
17. Moe JH (1965): Treatment of adolescent kyphosis by non-operative and operative methods. *Manitoba Med Rev* 45:481–484.
18. Moe JH, Winter RB, Bradford DS, Lonstein JE (1978): *Scoliosis and other spinal deformities.* Philadelphia: W.B. Saunders.
19. Nicoll EA (1949): Fractures of the dorsal-lumbar spine. *J Bone Joint Surg* [Br] 31:376–394.
20. Ogilvie J, Bradford D (1988): Luque instrumentation in adults with Scheuermann's kyphosis. North American Spine Society, Colorado Springs.
21. Ransohoff J (1970): Lesions of the cauda equina. *Clin Neurosurg* 17:331–344.
22. Roberson JR, Whitesides TE Jr (1985): Surgical reconstruction of the late post-traumatic thoracolumbar kyphosis. *Spine* 10:307–312.
23. Roberts JB, Curtiss PH Jr (1970): Stability of the thoracic and lumbar spine in traumatic paraplegia following fracture or fracture-dislocation. *J Bone Joint Surg* [Am] 52:1115–1130.
24. Rose GK, Owen R, Sanderson JM (1975): Transposition of rib with blood supply for the stabilisation of a spinal kyphos. *J Bone Joint Surg* [Br] 57:112.
25. Scheuermann J (1920): Kyphosis doralis. *Juvenilis Ugeskr Laeger* 82:384–393.
26. Schmorl G, Junghan H (1956): Clinique et radiologie de la colonne verteral normal et pathologique. Doin Editeurs.
27. Stagnara P (1971): Radiologie des deformatins vertebrales: Les scolioses in radiodiagnostic. Paris: EMC.
28. Stagnara P (1977): Arthrodeses transthoraciques dans le traitement des cyphoses et cyphoscolioses. *Int Orthop* (SICOT) 199–214.
29. Stagnara P (1978): Scolioses cyphosantes de l'adulte et greffes anterieures. *Int Orthop* (SICOT) 149–165.
30. Stagnara P (1985): Les deformations du rachis: Scolioses, cyphoses, lordoses. Paris: Masson.
31. Stagnara P, Gounot J, Fauchet R, Jouvinroux P (1974): Les greffes anterieures par voie thoracique dans le traitement des deformations et des dislocations vertebrales en cyphose et cyphoscolioses. *Rev Chir Orthop* 60:39–56.
32. Takemitsu Y, Harada Y, Iwahara T, Miyamoto M, Miyatake Y (1988): Lumbar degenerative kyphosis: Clinical, radiological and epidemiological studies. *Spine* 13:1317–1326.
33. White AA III, Panjabi MM, Thomas CL (1977): The clinical biomechanics of kyphotic deformities. *Clin Orthop* (128):8–17.
34. Whitesides TE Jr, Shah SGA (1976): On the management of unstable fractures of the thoracolumbar spine. Rationale for use of anterior decompression and posterior stabilization. *Spine* 1:99–107.
35. Winter RB (1977): Congenital kyphosis. *Clin Orthop* (128):26–32.
36. Winter RB, Hall JE (1978): Kyphosis in childhood and adolescence. *Spine* 3:285–308.

The Adult Spine: Principles and Practice,
J. W. Frymoyer, Editor-in-Chief.
Raven Press, Ltd., New York © 1991.

CHAPTER 65

Adult Scoliosis

John P. Kostuik

Adult scoliosis has been defined as a presentation of that deformity following skeletal maturity. Some definitions have specified that the age must be 20 years or older when the patient first presents for treatment.

Adult scoliosis can further be classified as a curve that starts prior to skeletal maturity, but only later is treatment sought; or a deformity that arises *de novo* after skeletal maturity. The former usually are idiopathic, but may be due to congenital or paralytic causes. The latter are secondary to degeneration, osteoporosis, or osteomalacia, or follow extensive surgical decompression, usually for spinal stenosis. In addition, patients may present as adults who have a later complication of spinal fusion. The most common problems are iatrogenic flat back and accelerated degeneration of mobile adjacent vertebral segments.

Thirty years ago most experts felt that surgical treatment of these conditions was not warranted, with few exceptions, most commonly a thoracic curve in patients in their third decade of life. Conservative care was advocated by such authorities as Nachemson (48), who reported the risks for scoliosis surgery in the adult. For complicated adult curves he estimated the respective risks were death 5%, neurologic damage 6%, significant loss of correction 20%, deep infection 10%, and medical problems 40%. Numerous clinical investigators (4,9,12, 13,38,53,56,63,64,65,66,67,68,70,76) showed not only that idiopathic curves could progress in the adult, but also that they might become the source of significant clinical symptoms.

A more aggressive surgical approach to these adult deformities became possible, first with the advent of Harrington rods (24), followed by many subsequent improvements in spinal instrumentation such as the devices designed by Dwyer (16,23,75), Luque (28,43, 44,69), Zielke (32,77), and Cotrel-Dubousset (10,11,14). These fixation devices have overcome many of the tech-

J. P. Kostuik, M.D., F.R.C.S.(C): Professor of Orthopaedics, University of Toronto; Director, Spinal Surgery; and Director, Biomechanics Laboratory, The Toronto Hospital, Toronto, Ontario, M5G 2C4.

nical obstacles to successful surgical treatment. At the same time, improvements in pre-operative assessment, advances in anesthetic techniques and intra-operative management, and spinal cord monitoring (8), combined with better understanding of post-operative care, have markedly improved the ability to deal with the complex problems of adult spinal deformities (33). Today, this capability is recognized not only by orthopedists, but also by family physicians and paramedical personnel.

SCOLIOSIS BEGINNING BEFORE SKELETAL MATURITY AND PRESENTING IN THE ADULT

The three basic types are: (a) an idiopathic curve, which is by far most common; (b) a congenital curve, usually associated with marked rigidity and kyphosis; and (c) a paralytic curve.

Magnitude of the Current Problem

Kostuik and Bentivoglio (35) found that the prevalence of curves involving the adult thoracolumbar and lumbar spine was 3.9% in a review of 5,000 intravenous pyelograms. These curves were truly structural and appeared to have commenced in adolescence and later progressed in adult life, rather than arising de novo. This figure was similar to that reported by Dewar (unpublished data reported by Shands [60]), who analyzed 10,000 consecutive chest radiographs done for routine hospital admission. The prevalence of true structural

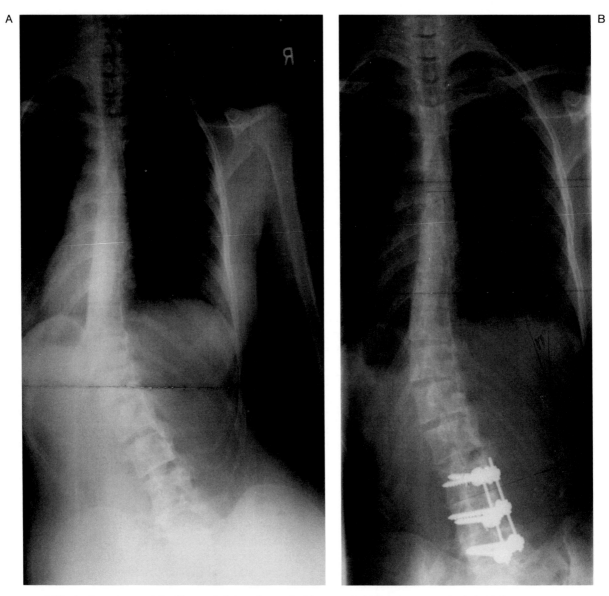

FIG. 1. Female age 26 with a painful scoliosis. **A:** Note marked imbalance to the left. Pain was reproduced on discography at both L4-L5 and L1-S1 discs. **B:** Rebalanced with relief of pain secondary to lateral closing wedges. Note double Zielke rods to control rotational forces.

curves in that sample was 4%. These figures parallel a classic study by Shands and Eisberg (60), who studied a representative sample of 194,060 chest radiographs made in the state of Delaware in 1953. This represented 82.2% of the entire population over the age of 14 years. They found that 1.9% of the population had a spinal curvature; 1.4% had mild curves (10 to 19 degrees), 0.3% had moderate curves (20 to 29 degrees), and only 0.2% had significant curves of 30 degrees or more. The age distribution was fairly consistent. Shands and Eisberg reported that their results were similar to those reported by Niebauer (personal communication reported by Shands and Eisberg [60]), where the prevalence was 2.5/100, but in the age group 20 to 65 years this rose to 4.2/100.

Weinstein and Ponsetti (73) determined those factors that are responsible for continued progression in adult life. Thoracic curves between 50 and 75 degrees at skeletal maturity increased an average of 30 degrees over a lengthy follow-up interval. Thoracolumbar curves 50 to 75 degrees at skeletal maturity increased 22.3 degrees over the next 40 years. Progression was the greatest when there was a lumbar curve, the fifth lumbar vertebra was not well seated, and the apical rotation was greater than 33%. These findings are similar to our observations (35). An adolescent patient with the worst prognosis for later difficulty as an adult is the one who presents with an imbalanced lumbar or thoracolumbar curve, the fifth lumbar vertebra not parallel with the sacrum, and the curve emanating from the lumbosacral junction (Fig. 1). This curve pattern also presents the greatest technical difficulty for correction in the older adult, and is best treated surgically at an earlier age, if possible.

Other curves with a poorer prognosis include those that have a pattern where the apex falls at L2-L3 or L3-L4, have a grade III rotation, are unbalanced, and have a secondary compensatory curve that is sharp and angular at L4-L5 and L5-S1. These curves, as will be seen later, can often be treated in the young adult or adolescent by dealing with the compensatory curve at 1 or 2 levels, rather than dealing with the entire and more proximal curve, which often extends over 5 to 7 levels.

Despite the increased knowledge about risk factors for progression, it is not uncommon for the spinal surgeon to be presented with an adult patient with scoliosis, increasing pain, loss of lumbar lordosis, or truncal imbalance. Accompanying these deformities may be the problems associated with osteoporosis and spinal stenosis. These conditions, too, can be treated (Fig. 2). The question then is how often do these problems occur and, in particular, how common is significant axial pain?

In a review of adult patients with lumbar and thoracolumbar scoliosis, Kostuik and Bentivoglio (35) found 60% complained of pain. This was similar to the prevalence in 100 age-matched patients without curvature, and also to the figures reported in numerous population studies of low back pain (see Chapter 8). When the curves were greater than 45 degrees, the prevalence and severity of pain complaints increased significantly. These findings are in contrast to those of Nachemson (46,47,48) and Nilsonne (52) who found a similar prevalence of pain, but noted that it was rarely a significant clinical problem. All studies seem to agree that thoracic curves are rarely a source of pain, although a hyperlordotic curve may cause significant pulmonary dysfunction.

A variety of factors have been analyzed to determine which may be important in pain complaints. Age is relevant, similar to all spinal disorders. Pain appears to reach its maximum between the ages of 40 and 60 years and then, in general, is less of a problem.

The effects of occupation are less well understood, but a patient with a pre-existing adolescent curve may self-select less physically demanding occupations (35,58). If a patient has scoliosis and has a physically demanding occupation, he or she is more likely to miss time from work or become disabled (35).

Pain is also associated with curves greater than 45 degrees at skeletal maturity. When the apex of the curve shows radiographically evident degeneration, this is associated with both greater pain and greater degeneration at the lumbosacral joint (35).

PATIENT EVALUATION

History

Obviously, it is important to obtain a complete history, as it is for any patient with a spinal disorder (see Chapter 15). A family history of progressive deformity may give some clue to prognosis. The date of onset of the deformity should be elicited but usually is not, in itself, important. However, the history of curve progression is important. Some measure of progression may be surmised from changes in how clothes fit, an observed increase in rib hump, loss of height, or altered waistline. Ideally, a more precise definition of curve progression can be obtained from serial radiographs; unfortunately, these often have been lost or never taken.

It is also important to discuss and understand how the deformity affects the patient's life. Many adults are reluctant to discuss the aesthetic consequences of their curve unless asked directly. Many have learned to cope with the deformity, but for others it is a source of major concern. This problem was identified in 10% of the patients we surveyed (35).

A careful pain history should also be elicited, which can be aided by the use of pain drawings. Pain at the apex of the curve should be differentiated from pain remote from the apex. Important information is pain duration and how it affects activities of daily living, occupation, social function, recreation, and sexual activities.

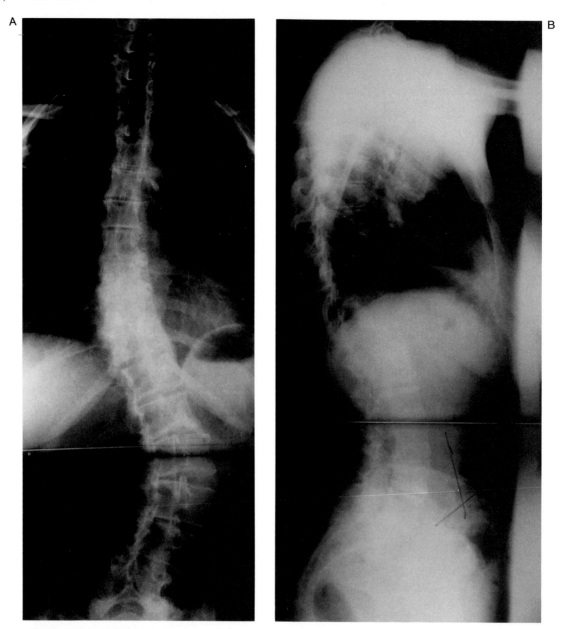

FIG. 2. Female age 65. **A:** Documented progressive painful curve 44 degrees. L4-L5 and L5-S1 discs not painful on discography; L4-S1 and L5-S1 facet blocks did not relieve pain. Note previous total hip. **B:** Pre-operative lateral 66 degrees.

Often a radicular or referred component of the axial pain will be present. Sometimes this is related to the apex of the curve. A thoracic or thoracolumbar curve may present with intercostal neuralgia. Leg symptoms may relate to the primary or compensatory curve and either be scleratomal in nature or have the characteristics of frank sciatica. Any associated bladder or bowel dysfunction is an important diagnostic and prognostic clue. Incontinence, particularly in the elderly female, should not be assumed to be secondary to myogenic causes until proven otherwise. Often, spinal stenosis can be causative.

In addition to the history of the deformity and associated pain, the general impact on health needs to be evaluated. Respiratory malfunction may be a presenting symptom with adult scoliosis, but is far more common in paralytic or severe congenital curves, and relatively rare in old idiopathic curves. We reviewed (unpublished data) 200 consecutive adults with idiopathic scoliosis. Functionally important, respiratory dysfunction was not observed even in curves of 100 degrees or more. However, ventilation was often decreased to as low as 25% of normal predicted values. Arterial blood gases were generally normal. Exceptions to this overall favorable picture

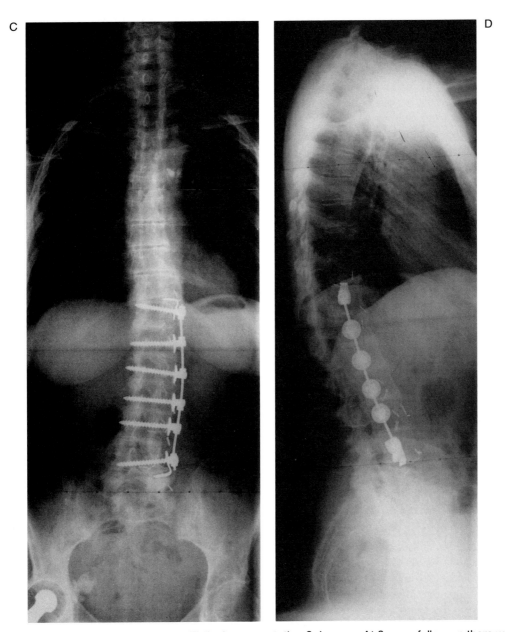

FIG. 2. *(Continued)* **C:** Post-operative Zielke instrumentation 2 degrees. At 6 years follow-up there was no pain. **D:** Lordosis has been fully preserved.

are patients with idiopathic scoliosis associated with marked thoracic lordosis.

Physical Examination

Again, the elements of the physical examination are comparable to the evaluation of all patients with spinal disorders (see Chapter 15). Curve assessment includes the following: the three-dimensional characteristics, including kyphosis and lordosis; the rib hump; the degree of decompensation; and flexibility.

The neurologic examination should be complete, and subtle neurologic findings assessed. For example, left tho-racic idiopathic curves are sometimes associated with syringomyelia. Mild clawing of the toes may indicate a tethered cord.

Imaging Studies

The initial radiographic analysis includes three: foot, standing posteroanterior, and lateral films. Focal, coned views may be useful in patients with pain to evaluate facets, congenital anomalies, and disc narrowing. Oblique radiographs are taken using Stagnara views, to assess the rotational deformity, particularly when a kyphosis is present.

Lateral bending radiographs will indicate the curve's flexibility, but do not predict positively or negatively the degree of surgical correction that might be obtained. For example, we found the amount of correction obtained by anterior Zielke instrumentation was twice that predicted by the pre-operative bending films. Extension views may have greater value in determining whether an associated kyphosis is flexible, while flexion views may give similar information about lordotic deformities. Traction films occasionally may be of value in determining whether distraction will overcome decompensation.

Once the routine radiographs are obtained, a variety of ancillary imaging studies may be considered. Bone scans are rarely indicated, except in the younger adult with pain and a minor curve. In this instance, the bone scan may reveal an alternative cause, most particularly osteoid osteoma.

If there are neurologic findings or surgical correction is contemplated, we still use myelography as our imaging modality of choice. Its particular importance is to determine any areas of actual or potential compression, which would become important when corrective forces are applied. CT scans have little use, except when combined with myelographic enhancement. The role of magnetic resonance imaging appears promising, but its usefulness remains uncertain for the evaluation of spinal deformities.

Other Ancillary Tests, Discography, and Facet Blocks

One of the major issues in the adult with scoliosis and pain is to determine the source of symptoms. This issue is of major importance when surgery is contemplated to accurately assess what spinal levels to include in the fusion. In my early experience with adult deformities, 30% to 35% of patients had persisting pain after attaining a solid fusion. Since that time, my results (see surgical results section) appear to have improved, which I attribute in part to the use of discography (33,38). Specifically, I evaluate the L3-L4, L4-L5, and L5-S1 levels, but rarely perform the test at the apex of the curve. Although the ideal approach is posterolateral, the rotational deformity may necessitate a transdural approach.

Facet blocks are also employed (see Chapter 25), usually at the same lower lumbar levels. If discography produces pain and facet blocks relieve it, my opinion is that the fusion should incorporate that level. I believe this is particularly important when the lumbosacral level fulfills these criteria. Conversely, should discogram not reproduce the patient's pain and facet block not relieve it, then this level is not incorporated.

NON-OPERATIVE CARE

The basic approach to non-operative care is similar to the treatment for all chronic, painful spinal disorders

(see Chapters 71 and 72) and includes exercise and non-steroidal, anti-inflammatory drugs. It is important to stress that modalities and exercises will not prevent curve progression, but may serve to maintain flexibility. Low-thrust aerobics, cycling, and swimming are useful adjuncts and are particularly important to preventing osteoporosis. It is also important to utilize the other preventive measures for osteoporosis as outlined in Chapter 32.

The role of orthotics is unknown, and there is no evidence to suggest that they will prevent curve progression in the adult (see Chapter 74). However, orthotics seem to be useful in elderly patients, but must be rigid and fitted carefully to the patient's deformity.

SURGICAL INDICATIONS

The indications for surgery in an adult with an idiopathic curve are: (a) to obtain pain relief; (b) to prevent further progression of deformity; (c) to manage current significant neurologic dysfunction or to prevent later dysfunction in a patient at risk; and (d) to improve upon cosmetic appearance.

Pain

Pain is the most common indication. Determining the sources of pain and predicting its surgical relief are a great challenge. The prevalence of pain and the use of a variety of testing techniques, such as discography, have been discussed. Like any spinal disorder, the more certain the causation of pain, the more likely is a successful outcome.

Progressing Deformity

An even greater question than who to fuse for pain relief is who to fuse to prevent further progression of deformity. It is my opinion that two groups of patients are candidates. First, I fuse an obviously increasing deformity in young adults below the age of 35, in particular those patients with lumbar or thoracolumbar curves that measure 45 degrees or greater. Inevitably these curves seem to progress and develop pain. In the female, the secondary degenerative changes may convert a scoliosis with retention of lumbar lordosis to a kyphoscoliosis. If this later deformity becomes rigid, it requires a two-stage surgical correction. In comparison, the younger adult can be treated by a one-stage anterior correction and fusion with Zielke instrumentation with minimal morbidity (Fig. 3).

Second, I fuse the younger patient with truncal imbalance, whose major curve of 40 degrees or more extends to L3 or L4, accompanied by a compensatory curve at

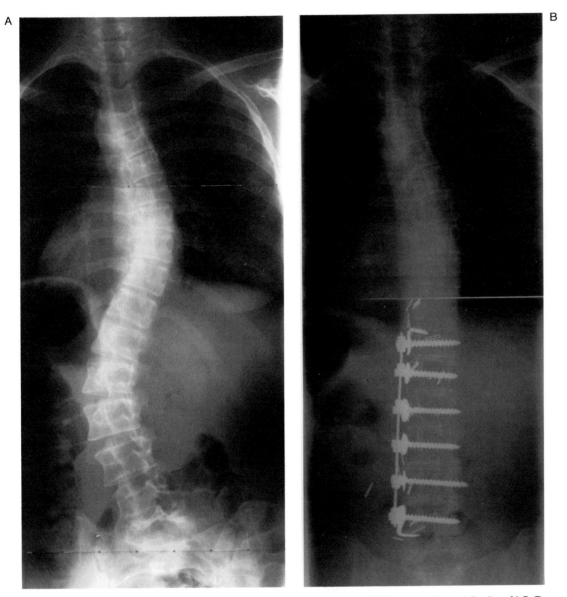

FIG. 3. Female age 24. **A:** Lumbar curve 60 degrees, thoracic curve 52 degrees. Note obliquity of L5. **B:** Post-operative lumbar curve 25 degrees, thoracic curve reduced to 40 degrees. L5 is more parallel to the horizontal.

A

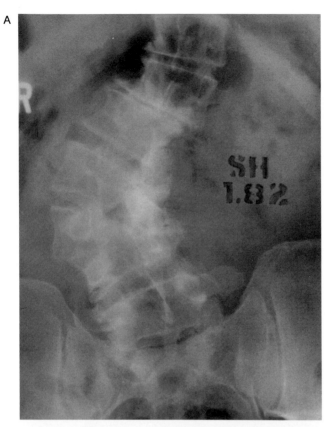

B

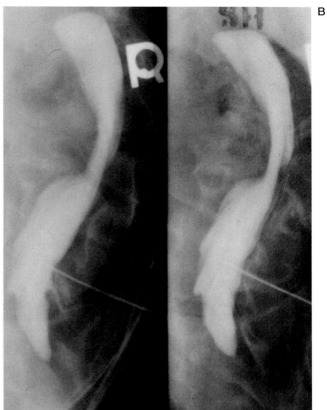

C

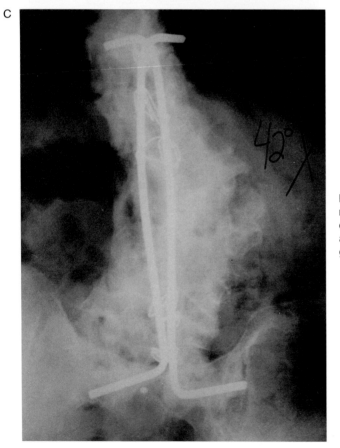

FIG. 4. Male age 56. **A:** Curve 68 degrees. Patient had marked symptoms and mild signs of spinal stenosis. **B:** Pre-operative myelogram indicates severe compromise of canal at the apex of the curve. **C:** Post-operative AP curve 42 degrees. Five years later patient is pain free and working.

L4, L5, or the sacrum. The primary curve in this instance may be reduced significantly by rebalancing only the lower compensatory curve. This approach should be employed if the lower curve is painful. The patient should be aware that extension of the fusion may be required at a later date. To date, I have used this technique in 6 patients. The average degree of correction of the major curve has been more than 40%.

Neurologic Deficit

Neurologic deficits are occasionally an indication for surgical intervention in an individual with pre-existent curvature, who presents as an adult. In one review, only 5 out of 227 patients treated surgically required decompression (33). However, with an increasingly aged population, it is possible that a greater number of patients will be seen with an associated spinal stenosis (Fig. 4).

Jackson and Simmons (29) described a subset of patients who had radicular symptoms arising from a compensatory rather than a primary curve. They noted significant improvement of these symptoms following anterior stabilization of the major curve. This approach has been less successful in my experience.

Cosmesis

Cosmesis is generally thought to be an uncommon indication in the adult scoliotic, with the exception of the young adult who has an unbalanced curve. However, this may be an underestimation. We followed 100 patients for more than 10 years after spinal fusion (41). Retrospectively, they reported that body image and cosmesis had played a greater role in their decision to have surgery than was evident at the time of the operation.

If a patient's goal is predominantly cosmetic, surgical intervention may be warranted after repeated discussions with the patient and his or her close relatives. Cotrel-Dubousset instrumentation is particularly helpful, especially if the patient is hypokyphotic, and excellent cosmetic correction can be obtained. The use of thoracoplasty (partial rib excision over 4 to 6 levels) may be used as an additional means to improve that outcome.

SURGICAL TECHNIQUES

Today, Harrington posterior instrumentation is rarely indicated in the treatment of adult scoliosis. Loss of lumbar lordosis inevitably occurs with this distracting device, even with the use of sacroalar hooks, contouring, or square-ended rods. Three basic strategies are available: anterior fusion using internal fixation (32,45,77), posterior fusion using Cotrel-Dubousset instrumentation (11), and combined anterior posterior approaches (5,30).

I treat the majority of lumbar and thoracolumbar curves with anterior instrumentation using the Zielke technique (77). However, this method is not useful if there is an associated true kyphosis, which will increase with this approach. This possibility is best evaluated by oblique Stagnara views.

In that latter group of patients, pain relief and restoration of balance should be accompanied by restoration of lumbar lordosis. This objective at present is best achieved in rigid curves by a two-stage procedure. An anterior approach is done, followed by multiple-level discectomies and fusion with instrumentation. Two weeks later, a posterior fusion is performed using Cotrel-Dubousset instrumentation (Figs. 5 and 6).

On the other hand, if the kyphoscoliosis is mobile, correction can be achieved by a single-stage procedure using the Cotrel-Dubousset technique (CDI). The advantage of this instrumentation is its ability to derotate the spine and restore lordosis when there is curve mobility. An alternative is the use of contoured Luque rods, combined with the Galveston technique (1,8,22,27, 28,31,34,43,44,51,59,69). Although this technique initially showed great promise, pain related to the sacroiliac joint has been reported in the presence of a solid lumbar fusion. There is also a risk of neurologic damage associated with passage of the sublaminar wires. For these reasons, I have abandoned this technique.

Anterior Zielke Instrumentation

The primary indication for this approach is a thoracolumbar or lumbar curve that does not require a lumbosacral fusion, is mobile on bending films, and where lordosis is preserved (32,36,39,45,54). The entire curve should be spanned in the adult. In comparison, the adolescent spine may require a fusion of lesser extent.

Once the levels to be fused have been exposed (see Chapter 60), the disc spaces are cleared, including the end plates, back to the posterior longitudinal ligaments. This exposure is essential so that an accurate angle of insertion can be obtained for the screws. If at all possible, the screws should be angled towards the contralateral junction of the pedicle with the vertebral body. In order to ensure that the opposite cortex is penetrated, a depth gauge is placed on the exposed disc space to determine the pathway and length of the screw. Arbitrarily, I add 2 mm of additional length, which is particularly important when there is lipping of the vertebral margins, secondary to degeneration. If there is significant osteoporosis, methylmethacrylate is used (see Chapter 33). In these instances, the screw hole is enlarged with a curette to retain the cement and enhance screw fixation (Fig. 7). The use of low-viscosity or cooled cement will increase the working time. This technique is particularly useful in the most proximal screw. Rather than adding an extra

Text continues on page 1418.

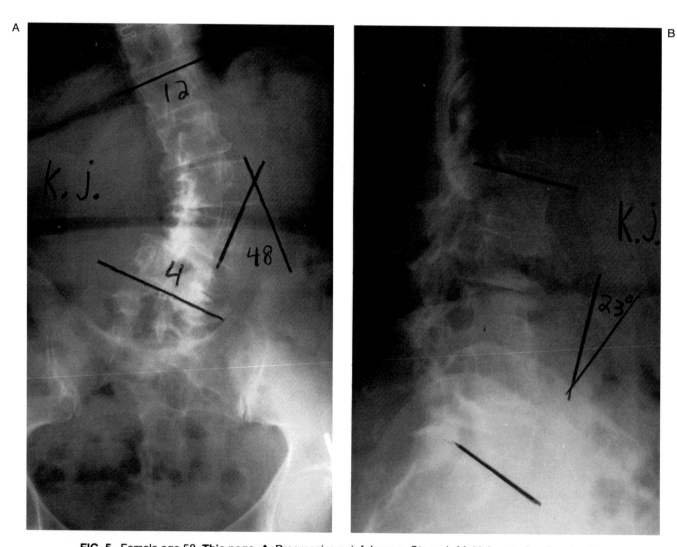

FIG. 5. Female age 58. **This page. A:** Progressive painful curve. Stage 1: Multiple anterior discotomies with morcellized bone graft. Stage 2: Cotrel-Dubousset instrumentation and fusion. **B:** Pre-operative lateral view. Note significant loss of lordosis (minus 23 degrees L1-S1). **Opposite page. C:** Post-operative AP view. **D:** Post-operative lateral view. Note significant return of lumbar lordosis due to derotation and anterior release (increase of 48 degrees).

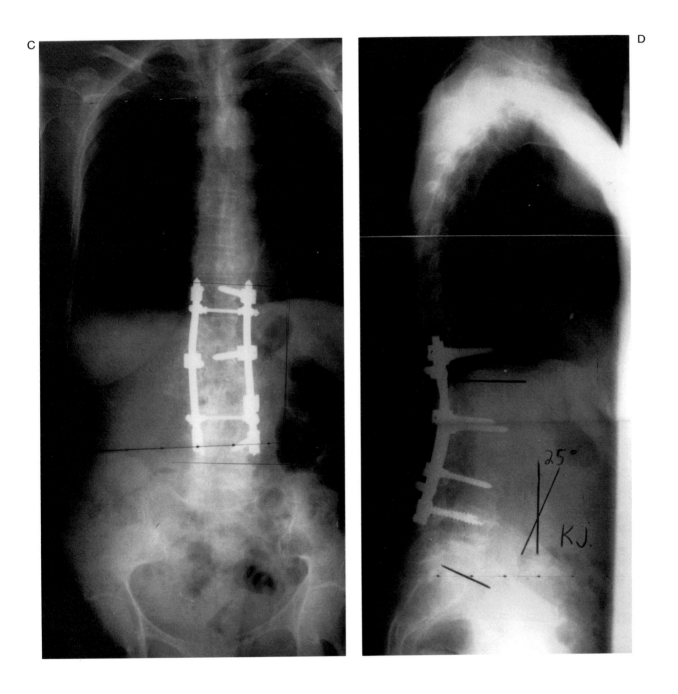

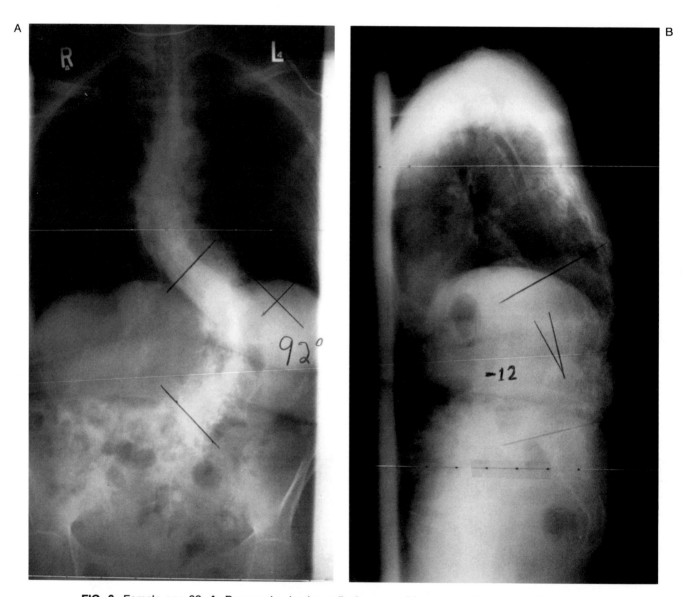

FIG. 6. Female age 63. **A:** Progressive kyphoscoliosis, curve 92 degrees. Stage 1: Multiple anterior discotomies with morcellization of L2-L3. Stage 2: Cotrel-Dubousset instrumentation and fusion. **B:** Pre-operative lateral view. Minus 12 degrees lordosis.

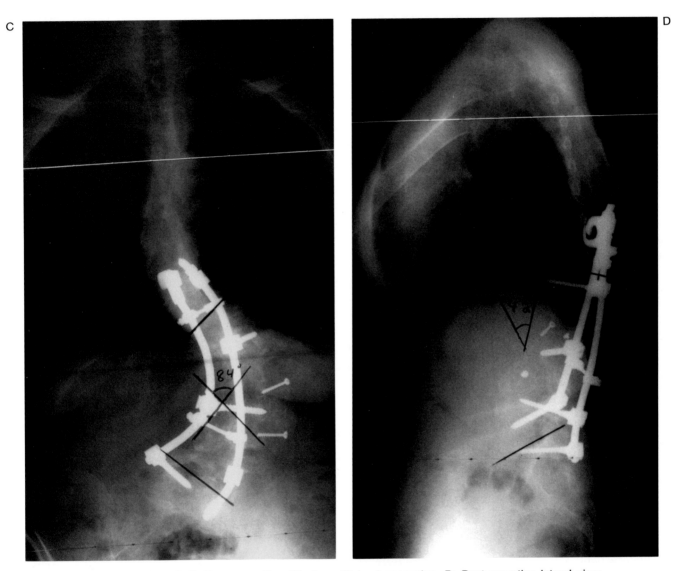

FIG. 6. *(Continued)* **C:** Post-operative AP view. Minimal correction. **D:** Post-operative lateral view. Marked restoration of lordosis to 42 degrees (gain 54 degrees).

level across an unfused level, I now routinely use cement at the upper level (Fig. 8). The use of a derotator is now almost routine, because it has the capability to reproduce lordosis in the lumbar spine or reduce kyphosis in the thoracolumbar spine.

Autogenous bone graft is used, usually consisting of excised ribs cut up into very small fragments. In order to increase the lordosis, block or minced grafts are selectively placed anteriorly in the disc space. The average blood loss with this technique has been 1,750 cc.

Limitations of Technique. The technique is possible from L5 to T9 or T10. Further extension above that level is rarely of value, since the disc spaces are so narrow that little correction can be obtained. Although fusion can be extended across the lumbosacral junction, I routinely combine this with a posterior fusion.

Post-Operative Care. Prolonged recumbency is not required; patients usually become ambulatory by the third or fourth post-operative day. Patients with thoracolumbar curves are fitted to a total contact orthosis, modular Boston overlap-type brace, or molded plastic corset. Thoracic curves require no exterior support.

Surgical Results. The results obtained with the Zielke instrumentation have markedly improved upon the results obtained with Dwyer and other posterior instrumentation techniques. We have reviewed our first 57 patients and found that the average correction was 70%, compared with 45% obtained with Dwyer instrumentation (36,39). Moreover, there were no pseudarthroses. In double idiopathic curves, the average correction was 62% initially. Twenty-four months post-operatively, the mean loss of initial correction was 3.4 degrees (4%). The non-instrumented proximal thoracic curves improved 28%, and there was no deterioration during the 2-year follow-up.

The use of the derotation devices has further improved curve correction in the sagittal and anteroposterior planes. Rotational deformity improved by 1 grade, based on the Nash-Moe method (50).

As previously noted, we have also used Zielke instrumentation in 6 patients with imbalance and pain on the distal convex side of a fractional lumbosacral curve. This has resulted in a 40% correction of the proximal, uninstrumented major curve. In these cases, the distal fractional curve was thought to be the source of pain, the patients were unbalanced, and the balance was not restored on bending radiographs of the major curve. The follow-up duration of 4 years is too short to determine whether they will require further surgery for their major curves at a later date.

Complications. No major complications or deaths were encountered in the 57 patients. General complications were limited to 10 cases of atelectasis and pleural effusion, which resolved without major treatment. Short-term local complications included 3 lateral femoral cutaneous nerve entrapments, 1 of which required

later surgical decompression, and 2 post-thoracotomy syndromes (see Chapter 66). Later complications were: 1 case of instrument failure, which required later posterior surgery; proximal staple pullout at 2 levels, and an additional 5 patients had partial staple disengagement, none of which required treatment; the nuts backed out of the screw head in 10 cases without loss of correction or rod displacement; and rod disengagement from the screw head was present in 6 cases without loss of correction.

Cotrel-Dubousset Instrumentation

The Cotrel-Dubousset instrumentation is the other major option for patients with scoliosis or mobile kyphoscoliosis. This device combines the rigidity of segmental fixation with derotation. Between 1985 and 1986, I treated 49 patients who had developed their deformities secondary to idiopathic scoliosis (41). The surgical indications were disabling back pain with or without neurologic symptoms in 44 patients (Figs. 9 and 10). Curve progression was the indication for surgery in 5 patients.

The surgical technique for this instrumentation has been described in detail elsewhere (10,11). Adjuncts to this basic approach were anterior releases in rigid curves, posterior releases when there had been prior posterior surgery, and rib excision to improve upon cosmetic outcome when there was significant curve rigidity and a rib hump.

There were 43 females and 6 males. The average age of the patients was 43, with a range of 21 to 75. There were 19 patients older than 50 years at the time of surgery.

The curves included 16 primary thoracic, 15 primary lumbar, 14 double major, and 4 thoracolumbar patterns. Twelve patients had undergone previous spinal fusions.

Four of these patients had a severe, rigid thoracic curve greater than 90 degrees or a previous fusion. Prior to the CDI, an anterior or posterior release was performed. In the interval between the two stages, halo-pelvic dependent traction was used to improve curve flexibility and correction.

Similarly, the treatment of certain thoracolumbar and lumbar curves often involved staged surgery. The goal in these instances was to reduce the high rate of complications, reduce the rate of pseudarthrosis and poor curve correction, improve upon truncal imbalance, and improve the lumbar lordosis to a degree greater than could be achieved with posterior surgery alone. Specifically, this strategy was employed in the following conditions:

1. The patient had a rigid lumbar kyphoscoliosis, in which case an initial anterior release, accompanied by morcellized bone grafting of the interspace, was performed. This was followed by a second-stage CDI to derotate the curve and restore the lumbar lordosis. In these cases the average curve correction was 63%.

2. The pre-operative discograms and facet blocks sug-

Text continues on page 1425.

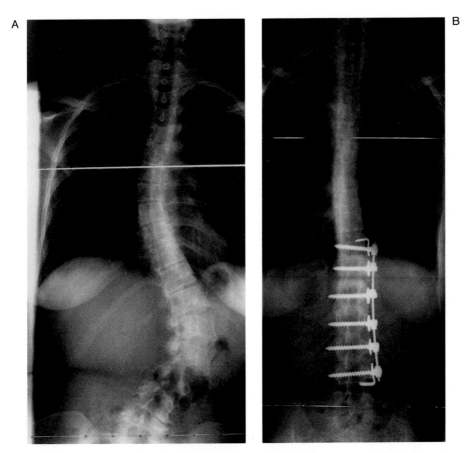

FIG. 7. Female age 77. **A:** Severe incapacitating painful curve of 75 degrees. **B:** Post-operative curve 15 degrees. Methylmethacrylate used to hold the screws. Pain free 1 year post-operative.

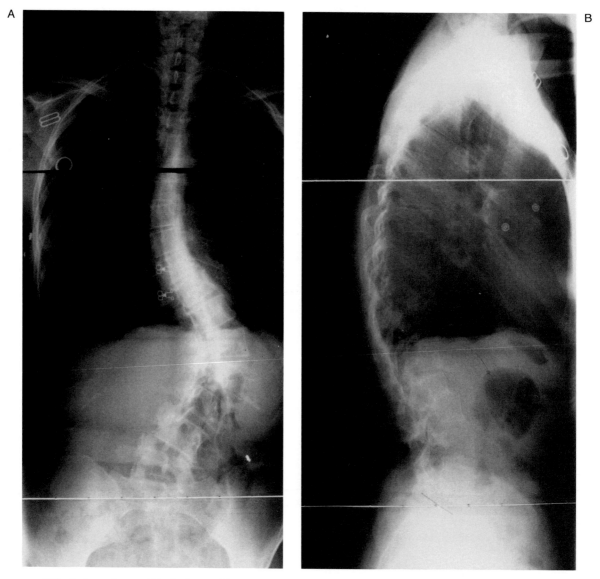

FIG. 8. Female age 52. **A:** Curve 68 degrees, painful, progressive, rigid. **B:** Pre-operative lordosis 50 degrees L1-S1.

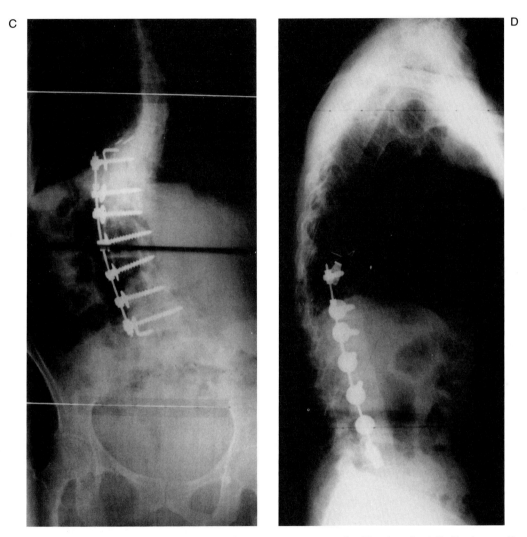

FIG. 8. *(Continued)* **C:** Post-operative curve 34 degrees, note proximal hook pullout. **D:** Post-operative lateral 38 degrees, good long-term result.

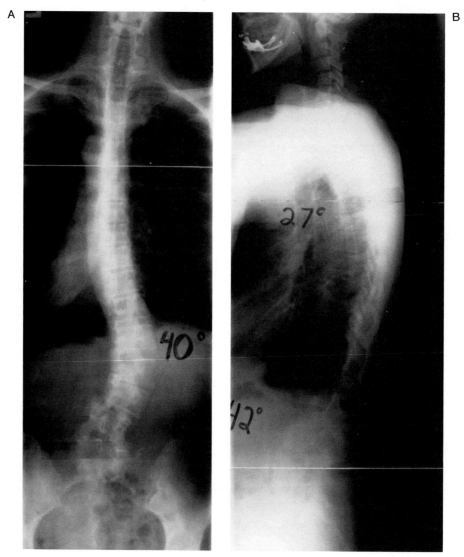

FIG. 9. Female age 53. **A:** Progressive painful scoliosis 40 degrees. **B:** Curve was flexible. Pre-operative discography revealed painful degenerative L4-L5 and L5-S1 discs.

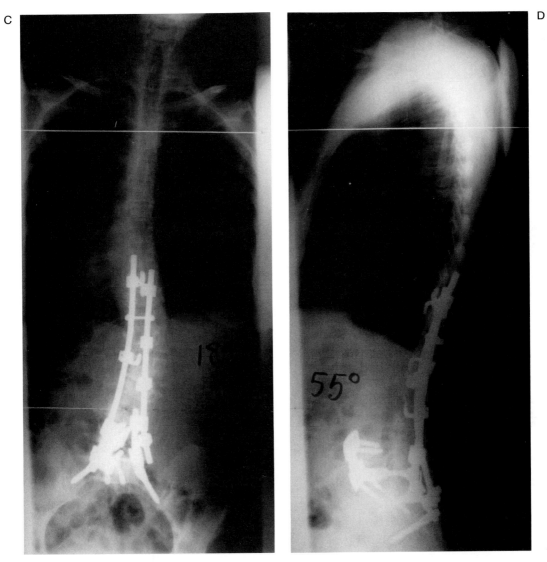

FIG. 9. *(Continued)* **C and D:** In order to achieve solid fusion, two-stage surgery was performed. First stage consisted of anterior L4-L5 and L5-S1 discectomies, interbody iliac crest grafts, and internal fixation with a Yuan I beam plate at L4-S1 and 2 AO 6.5 mm screws at L5-S1. The second stage Cotrel-Dubousset instrumentation and fusion derotated the spine and increased lordosis. Pain was relieved.

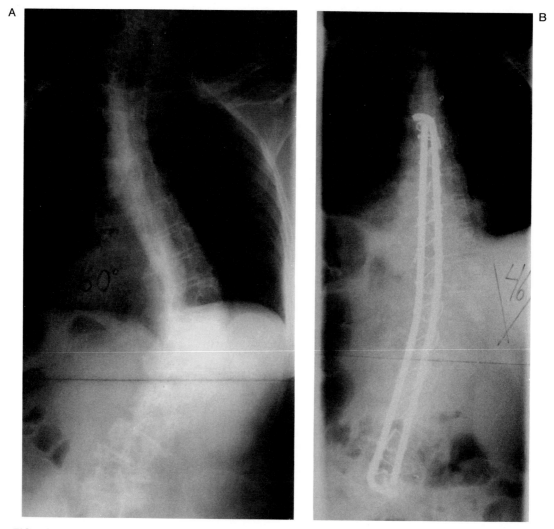

FIG. 10. Female age 58. **A:** Progressive painful thoracolumbar kyphoscoliosis. **B:** Luque instrumentation. The kyphosis precluded the use of Zielke instrumentation. Today Cotrel-Dubousset instrumentation with derotation would be used.

gested the need to extend the fusion to the sacrum because of painful degeneration, associated with a rigid kyphoscoliosis. In this instance, an anterior release was performed over the length of the curve. The L4-L5 and L5-S1 interspaces were excised, and a wedge-shaped bone block was placed to improve lumbar lordosis and the rate of fusion. This technique was often supplemented by anterior internal fixation at these two levels. The remaining levels were grafted anteriorly with morcellized bone. Two weeks later, a second-stage CDI was performed extending to the sacrum, if necessary.

A total of 19 patients had staged or associated surgery, including 2 anterior thoracic releases, 2 posterior thoracic releases, 10 anterior thoracolumbar or lumbar releases, and 1 thoracoplasty. Four patients underwent nerve root decompression.

The post-operative treatment usually did not include braces, except in 14 elderly, osteoporotic patients in whom the fixation was felt to be at risk.

Surgical Results. The curves measured 60 degrees pre-operatively, with a range of 13 to 115 degrees. Post-operatively, the average curve was 35 degrees, and for previously unoperated patients, the curve correction averaged 50%. The results by curve type were: primary thoracic curves 48 degrees; primary lumbar curves 55 degrees; thoracolumbar curves 55 degrees. In double major curves, the thoracic component averaged 76 degrees, and the lumbar curve 66 degrees.

The loss of correction was negligible for 42 of 49 patients. Seven patients lost greater than 5 degrees, with an average of 13 degrees, and a range of 6 degrees to 28 degrees. The average lost correction for these 7 patients was 49%, with a range of 19% to 93%.

The correction obtained in the sagittal planes was a function of the pre-operative magnitude of deformity. When the spine was relatively kyphotic (less than 20 degrees), the improvement averaged 133%. The pre-operative average was 15 degrees, while post-operatively it improved to 35 degrees. When there was greater kyphosis the results were less dramatic. Patients who had pre-operative kyphos in the range of 20 to 50 degrees (average 38 degrees) improved their sagittal curves only 32% and averaged 47 degrees. In the relatively hyperlordotic lumbar spine, the post-operative lordosis declined an average of 11%.

The results in the lumbar spine for sagittal plane correction were relatively similar. In the hypokyphotic spine (less than 20 degrees, average 11 degrees), the thoracic kyphosis improved an average of 173%, or 30 degrees. In the 20- to 60-degree range, the change was insignificant. In the excessively kyphotic spine (average 73 degrees), the deformity decreased an average of 11 degrees.

The apical rotational deformity improved an average of one-half grade; it was 2.5 pre-operatively, and 2.0 post-operatively, based on the Nash and Moe method. Pre-operatively, 41 patients were imbalanced, while post-operatively, 36 were rebalanced; 5 had significant residual imbalance greater than 2 centimeters.

Pain Relief. Significant or disabling pain was present in 44 of the 49 patients. Post-operatively, 30 were pain free, 6 had significant improvement, and 8 were the same or worse. Three of the unimproved patients were thought to have a pseudarthrosis, 2 of which have been repaired. One required extension of the fusion to incorporate a painful lumbosacral level.

Complications. The rate of complication was significant. Twenty patients had 28 complications. The general problems were 2 pneumothoraxes, 1 pancreatitis, and 3 urinary tract infections. Local complications included 1 dural tear closed primarily without sequelae; 1 superficial wound infection that responded to local care; and 1 hemothorax that required a repeat thoracotomy, and the patient later developed post-thoracotomy pain syndrome. Neurologic complications included 3 neuropraxias (2 followed anterior approaches); an L4 nerve root lesion with quadriceps weakness that resolved; and 1 with persistent pain in the genitofemoral nerve distribution, which resolved after nerve resection. The only injury attributable to the CDI was another L4 neuropraxia, which resolved with no treatment.

The later failures included 8 patients (16%) who complained of prominent rods, 5 of whom have undergone rod removal. Five patients had hook pullout; 4 of the 5 occurred in the lumbar region at the distal fixation site; all patients were over 50 years of age and had undergone a preliminary anterior lumbar release. One patient had fixation failure in the thoracic region. She had undergone multiple previous operations and, prior to CDI, an anterior release had been performed. Four of the 5 were reinstrumented in the early post-operative period, and 2 have had a good result. Another patient was revised 10 months later. Loss of lumbar lordosis had occurred, with the development of a flat-back deformity. This was corrected with lumbar extension osteotomy, and she now has a good result. The 2 patients with no additional surgery have fused with loss of lumbar lordosis. Both have continued pain, and 1 is considering an extension osteotomy.

Based on this experience, I believe that it is important to supplement the distal lumbar fixation with pedicle screws when possible, instead of relying on laminar hooks. In 10 subsequent cases, this approach has been used and, to date, there are no failures.

One patient required extension of her fusion to the sacrum 18 months after fusion with CDI. She had undergone Harrington instrumentation at age 16, but later developed pain attributed to multiple pseudarthroses in the lumbar region. Continued pain after CDI led to re-evaluation by discography, which revealed a painful L5-S1 disc. This has resolved following the extension of her fusion.

Three pseudarthroses occurred in the 49 patients: 1 patient had fusion failure at L4-L5 despite having a combined anterior/posterior approach at that level; 1 patient had multiple failures in the lumbar region, which have been repaired; and the third patient had a pseudarthrosis in the thoracic region identified by loss of correction, persistent pain, and increased uptake with bone scan.

This experience, which is ongoing, suggests that CDI is a versatile device, which provides a means to deal with complex adult structural deformity. However, there is a steep learning curve, a real "fiddle-factor," and the rate of complication is significant. These disadvantages, which can be overcome with experience, are outweighed by the ability it provides to deal with the complex three-dimensional anatomy of scoliosis in the adult.

SPECIAL PROBLEMS IN THE ADULT SCOLIOTIC

There is a group of special problems that will be encountered in the adult scoliotic, which will influence both the approach and the results. These include the problems of severe rigidity, paralysis, and the patient over 50 years of age.

Severe Rigid Scoliotic Deformities

Patients with severe rigid structural deformities may present as a consequence of an idiopathic or, much less commonly, a congenital curve, usually associated with significant or severe kyphosis (see Chapter 64). My initial experience with 85 patients with these challenging deformities was reported in 1979 (33). The age range was from 20 to 55. The curves ranged from 75 to 180 degrees, and all were rigid, based on bending radiographic criteria. Of these 85 patients, 15 were primarily kyphotic, 42 had idiopathic curves, and 28 had congenital curves. In addition to the 28 patients with congenital curves due to failures of segmentation, 4 additional patients had spontaneous fusions. An additional 20 patients had undergone previous arthrodeses and, thus, 52 had rigidity from a congenital or previous surgical fusion.

The approach in all patients was a posterior release including, if necessary, osteotomies of surgical or congenital fusion. The usual number of osteotomies required was 4, often associated with rib releases over 3 to 4 levels on the curve concavity, transverse process osteotomies, and rib resections on the convexity, usually involving 5 to 6 ribs. Forty patients required anterior osteotomies as well.

Once the preliminary releases were accomplished, traction was applied. In the first 32 patients halo-femoral traction was used. Later, halo-pelvic distraction became the method of choice. Most recently, we have tended to use halo-dependent traction in either the Circoelectric bed positioned for 30 degrees of dependency or the halo-wheel chair device.

The second-stage procedure, done 2 weeks later, first used Harrington instrumentation, superseded first by sublaminar wiring techniques, and most recently by Cotrel-Dubousset instrumentation.

Results. The initial degree of correction obtained after anterior and/or posterior releases and traction was 40% with halo-pelvic, and 32% with halo-femoral distraction. In those patients treated by Harrington instrumentation, a further 8% correction occurred. The overall correction obtained was 40%. As expected, the improvement was less for congenital curves, which averaged a total of 33% correction, as compared with idiopathic curves, which corrected an average of 48%. The more recent experience with the Cotrel-Dubousset instrumentation will be reported in Chapter 64.

Paralytic Curves

The patient who has a paralytic curve may find sitting at a desk or in a wheelchair difficult because of marked pelvic obliquity, accompanied by either kyphosis or hyperlordosis (Fig. 11). The latter problem is encountered particularly in patients who have had peritoneal shunts. In addition, collapsing curves are often associated with respiratory dysfunction, which can be improved by correction and stabilization. The mechanism by which this pulmonary function is improved is by lifting the diaphragm out of the abdomen, which results in improved diaphragmatic breathing. A pre-operative trial of halo-dependent traction will help estimate the degree of improvement in pulmonary function that might be anticipated.

Surgical Approach. I have advocated a combined anterior and posterior approach to eliminate the need for post-operative immobilization and to facilitate a rapid return to wheelchair function. At the present time, there is insufficient information to use a posterior approach alone, even with the availability of Cotrel-Dubousset instrumentation.

Spinal Deformities Over Age Fifty

The adult over the age of 50 presents special challenges: The deformity is often rigid and may be associated with significant imbalance and loss of normal

A

B

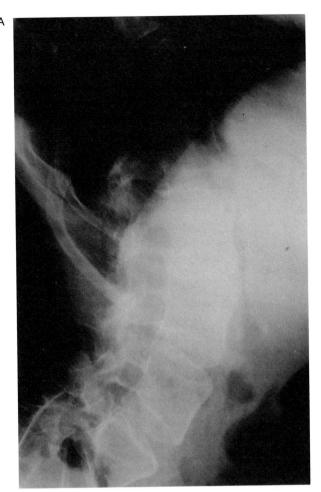
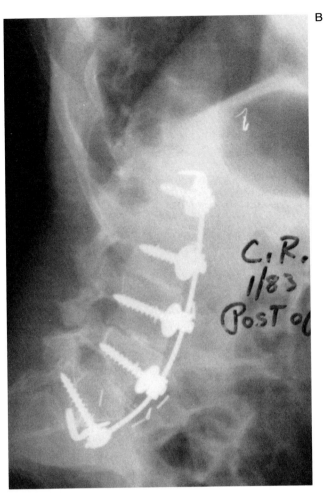

FIG. 11. A: Marked paralytic hyperlordosis. **B:** Lordosis has been reduced to 60 degrees L1-S1 by anterior Zielke instrumentation. Note the anterior-posterior orientation of the screws.

lumbar lordosis; the bone is more apt to be osteopenic, and spinal stenosis is more often present. Because of these problems, and the greater risk of neurologic or even vascular injury, these later adult deformities were usually stabilized posteriorly, without any effort at correction. The approach I use is basically similar to that for younger patients with curve rigidity. When there is good preservation of lordosis, the anterior Zielke approach is used. In the presence of a rigid kyphoscoliosis, a two-stage procedure is preferable, as described previously in this chapter. Methylmethacrylate is used to enhance screw fixation for the anterior devices, but is avoided in the pedicle with posterior screw fixation because of the risk of cement extrusion and potential neurologic injury (see Chapter 33).

Surgical Results. I have reviewed a subset of 80 patients undergoing surgery for spinal deformity after the age of 50 (41). Fifty had idiopathic curves and the remainder had a congenital curve, paralytic curve, or pure kyphotic deformity. Of the 50 idiopathic curves, 12 were

thoracic, 9 thoracolumbar, 17 lumbar, and 12 were double primary curves.

The major indication for all 80 patients was pain; all patients had a significant element of back pain and 16 had associated nerve root pain. Additional factors were progressive pulmonary dysfunction, usually related to an increasing kyphosis (8 patients) or evidence of progression of greater than 10 degrees in the preceding 3 years, which was found in 46 patients (57%).

The 80 patients underwent 100 procedures. Twenty (25%) had staged anterior and posterior surgery for enhanced stabilization, and 12 had simultaneous anterior and posterior operations. This latter group was largely in patients who had a flat-back deformity (discussed later in this chapter).

The overall results obtained were 12.5% excellent, 56.5% good, 6% fair, and 25% poor. Complete pain relief occurred in 27 of the 80 patients (34%), but root pain was relieved in all patients. The curve correction obtained was analyzed with respect to type of instrumentation used. The results were: Harrington instrumentation 22%, sublaminar wired Harrington rods 22%, Harrington rods combined with L rods 21%, double L rods 33%, Cotrel-Dubousset 50%, Dwyer 42%, and Zielke 67%. Although the numbers in each category are small and the indications for the various devices somewhat different, the Zielke correction appears to be the greatest. Moreover, the results obtained with the Zielke devices in the patients over age 50 were similar to the results obtained in all adults over the age of 20 (36,39).

The general complications included 24% who had pulmonary problems such as pneumonia, atelectasis, and adult respiratory distress syndrome. Infection occurred in 1%. One patient became paraparetic with partial but incomplete recovery.

The local complications observed were significant and to some degree dependent on the approach and device. Thirteen of the patients treated with Harrington instrumentation alone developed flat-back deformity. Four have undergone later single-stage anterior and posterior osteotomy. Intra-operative fracture of either lamina or vertebral bodies occurred in an additional 7 cases, which was overcome by using methylmethacrylate.

Later instrument failures occurred in 11 of the 80 patients and included 6 Harrington rod fractures and 1 rod displacement, 2 L rod migrations, 1 anterior screw breakage, and 1 other rod failure. An additional 9 patients later had increased kyphosis above the fusion secondary to osteoporotic compression fractures.

The pseudarthrosis rate was 21%, most of which occurred in the Harrington rod constructs. By vertebral level, fusions carried to L5 had a 25% failure, and those carried to the sacrum a 24% failure. All of these pseudarthroses occurred prior to the two-stage approach now used when fusion is carried to the sacrum. To date, Zielke and Cotrel-Dubousset devices have not been associated with pseudarthrosis.

It appears that a successful outcome can be obtained in the patient over the age of 50, but that great care must be taken to improve or preserve lumbar lordosis, osteopenia must be managed, and the operative approach has to be specifically tailored, often utilizing combined approaches. Moreover, there is a high rate of potential complication, both generally and locally, although major neurologic problems and death fortunately have not been a significant issue to date.

PROBLEMS RELATED TO ADJACENT MOTION SEGMENTS FOLLOWING OLD FUSION FOR SCOLIOSIS

Patients who have had previous fusions for scoliosis are at risk for degeneration in adjacent motion segments. The risk increases proportional to the extent of the prior fusion into the lumbar spine (7,17,26). These patients may require extension of their fusions if non-operative means fail to control symptoms. It is also common for the problem to be progressive and associated with some degree of spinal stenosis (Fig. 12).

Evaluation. After history and physical examination, investigative studies may include myelography, CT scanning, and MRI, as well as discography and facet blocks. The plain radiographic and bending films frequently show abnormal translational motion, which varies according to the fusion extent. The presence of retrolisthesis correlates with pain, but little relationship has been reported to the degree of lordosis or disc space height (26). The choice of test will depend on the pattern of referred pain, neurologic involvement, and the extent of back pain.

Operative Approach. The approach is dictated by whether or not the lumbosacral joint must be included in the fusion. When the lumbosacral joint is not involved, an anterior or posterior fusion with instrumentation will suffice. However, extension of the fusion to the sacrum, I believe, requires a combined approach (5). Today, this is done with anterior instrumentation and posterior pedicle fixation. In order to improve lordosis, some of the posterior laminae at L3-L4, L4-L5, or L5-S1 may be removed, and compression applied to the pedicles to increase lordosis. The important principle in the anterior approach is to use interbody grafts applied at the front of the disc space to further increase lordosis. Anterior instrumentation may improve upon the rate of fusion.

Surgical Results. A review of 24 cases treated by a variety of methods has confirmed this perspective (Kostuik, unpublished data) (Fig. 13). Six patients had posterior fusion with Harrington rods; 5 of the 6 failed due to pseudarthrosis or flat-back deformity. Nine patients were fused *in situ* by an anterior approach with interbody graft, followed by posterior instrumentation and fusion. Three of the 9 failed because of pseudarthrosis and flat back. A far more favorable result was obtained in 10 patients treated by posterior decompression through the pars interarticularis, and an anterior interbody fusion. Nine of these 10 patients have gone on to solid fusion and restoration of their lordosis.

IATROGENIC FLAT BACK DEFORMITIES

Fusions to the sacrum using Harrington instrumentation result in a 50% loss of lumbar lordosis. Many of these patients will require later restorative surgery (15,19,37,42). This may not be apparent in the early years following fusion in an adolescent, but becomes a significant problem when the patient reaches his or her third, fourth, or fifth decade of life. Onset of symptoms is heralded by complaints of low back fatigue, followed by increasing pain despite a solid fusion. The increasing loss of lordosis causes the patient to walk with a hip and knee

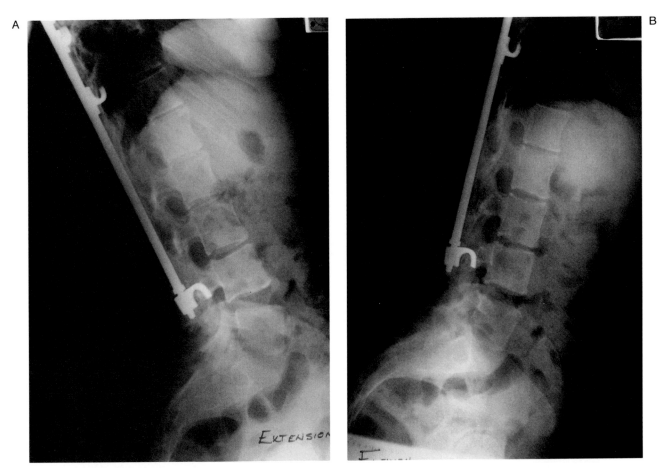

FIG. 12. Extension **(A)** and flexion **(B)** views demonstrate marked instability at the L4-L5 disc space. The patient had undergone Harrington instrumentation 12 years earlier.

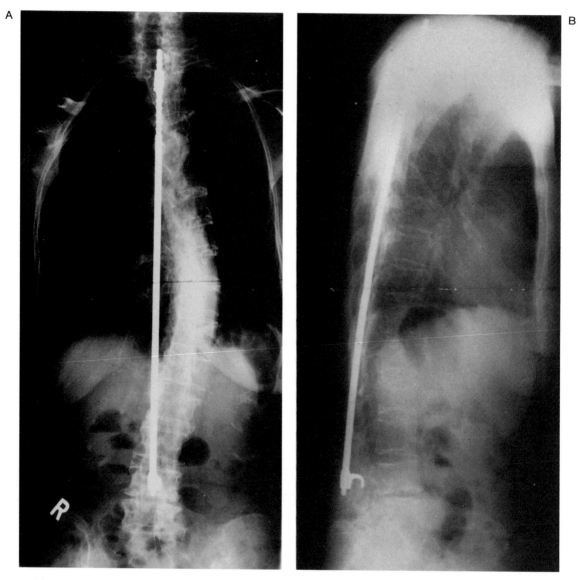

FIG. 13. Female age 56. **A and B:** Previous fusion 25 years ago. AP view demonstrates marked degenerative changes at L4-L5 and L5-S1 with a flat back.

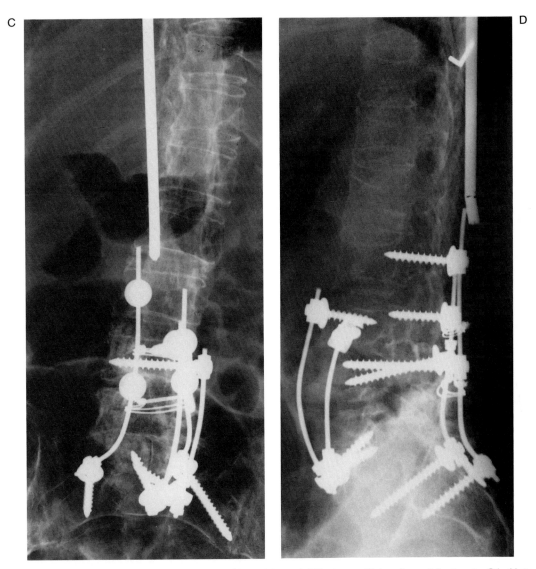

FIG. 13. *(Continued)* Post-operative AP **(C)** and lateral **(D)** views. Extension of fusion to S1. Note restoration of lordosis. Pre-operative discography had reproduced pain at L4-L5 and L5-S1. Relief was obtained with facet blocks.

flexion contracture (25). The deformity that results may be striking and disabling (Fig. 14).

The etiologic factors that are causative in descending order of frequency are distraction instrumentation of the lumbar spine that ends caudally at the L5 or S1 level; a thoracolumbar junction kyphosis of greater than 15 degrees, especially if associated with a hypokyphotic thoracic spine; or degenerative changes above and/or below the previous fusion. If pseudarthrosis is a component of the deformity, repair without correction of lordosis will not relieve the symptoms.

There are two approaches to deal with this problem: one preventative, the other restorative.

Prevention. Throughout this chapter I have emphasized the importance of maintaining lumbar lordosis when dealing with adult scoliosis. A review in 1978 revealed that 4% of all fusions in adolescents for scoliosis resulted in significant loss of lumbar lordosis when posterior instrumentation was used (33). When the fusions extended into the lumbosacral joint, this figure rose to 50%, and one half required later surgery (2). In the his-

toric perspective, attempts to overcome this risk included contouring of the Harrington rod (6), together with use of square-ended Moe rods and sacral-alar hooks. However, the rate of pseudarthrosis remained at 40%. The Luque rod appeared to offer an improvement and reduced the rate of pseudarthrosis to 15%, and flat-back deformities to 15% (34,40). The Cotrel-Dubousset instrumentation appears to have further improved these results. However, I still prefer in general a two-stage procedure that varies according to the curve mobility.

If the curve is mobile, the first stage includes Zielke instrumentation with anterior fusion. Care must be taken to avoid impingement of the screw heads against the adjacent vessels. Occasionally two rods are necessary in order to control rotation at the lumbosacral junction. A second-stage posterior fusion is then done. Although Luque rods were used historically, they have been replaced with CDI. The alternative is to correct the scoliosis and restore the lordosis with a first-stage posterior Cotrel-Dubousset device and posterior fusion, followed by a second-stage interbody fusion and instrumentation.

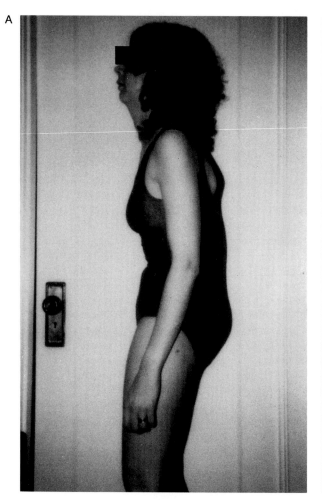 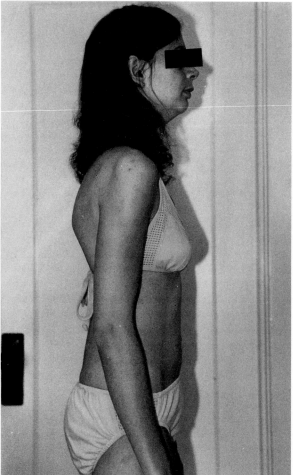

FIG. 14. Female age 24. **A:** Previous lumbar fusion. Note marked kyphosis (flat back) secondary to distraction. **B:** Post-operative. Note restoration of lordosis.

A

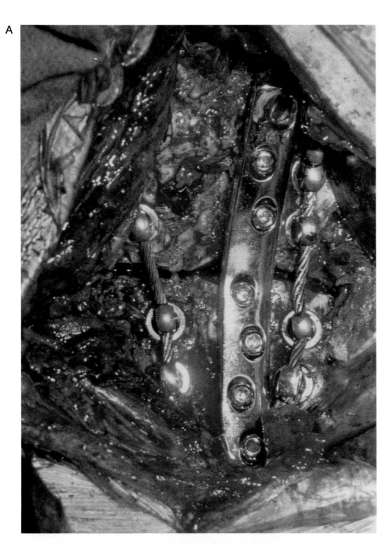

B

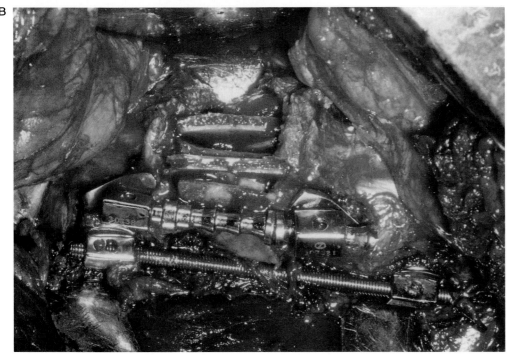

FIG. 15. A: Posterior osteotomy has been closed by the application of Dwyer screws in the lateral fusion mass and an AO plate has been added in the mid line to help control rotation. **B:** Simultaneous to posterior closure, the anterior osteotomy site is opened with Kostuik-Harrington instrumentation. Iliac crest grafts are added and a second Kostuik-Harrington compression rod is added to enhance stability.

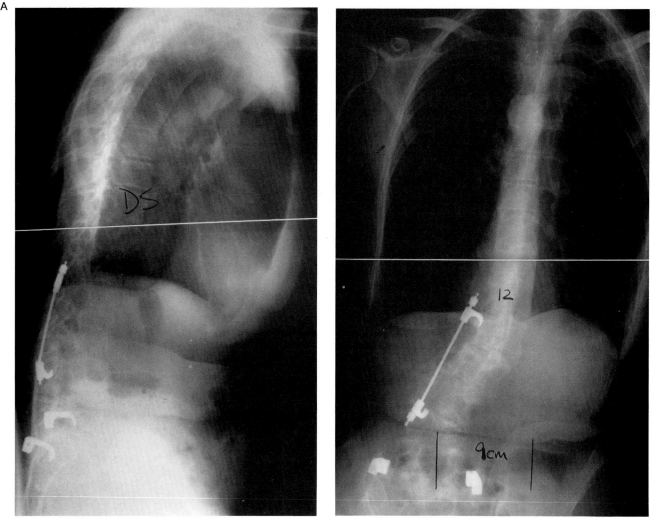

FIG. 16. Female age 45. **A:** Note loss of lordosis and marked flat back secondary to distraction and fusion of lumbar spine. **B:** AP view shows imbalance 9 cm to the right. Harrington distraction rod has been removed.

In the past 4 years, I have used the rigid contoured I plate designed by Yuan (see Chapter 93).

If the patient has a rigid curve, the first stage consists of multiple anterior discectomies and chip grafts in the upper lumbar levels. In the L4-L5 and L5-S1 levels, an interbody bicortical or tricortical graft is used to maximally fill the disc space and increase the lordosis. Two weeks later a posterior fusion is done with the CDI to increase the lordosis.

Using these approaches, the rate of pseudarthrosis has been reduced to 5% in my experience with the last 30 cases (Kostuik, unpublished data).

Restoration of Lordosis in Patients with Iatrogenic Flat Back. A combined approach is necessary, utilizing anterior and posterior osteotomies, as opposed to solely a posterior osteotomy (40,42) (Fig. 15). This is because greater correction can be obtained, and it is unnecessary to immobilize the patients post-operatively. Moreover, I

have encountered cases treated by posterior osteotomy alone that have had recurrence of deformity.

Surgical Indications. The indications are a patient with pain and loss of lordosis, particularly when the symptoms and deformity are increasing. As previously indicated, a pseudarthrosis if present, cannot be assumed to be the cause of symptoms.

Surgical Approach. The approaches used are varied according to the type of deformity. If the patient is imbalanced in the anteroposterior plane, a quadrilateral wedge osteotomy is done anteriorly and posteriorly to correct that deformity (Fig. 16). The technique used is similar to that described by Smith-Peterson for the treatment of ankylosing spondylitis (see Chapter 36). When the fusion is solid, this is usually done at the L3-L4 level. If a pseudarthrosis is present, this is simply enlarged. The nerve roots at the level of osteotomy must be clearly identified. Currently we use the Dwyer screws inserted

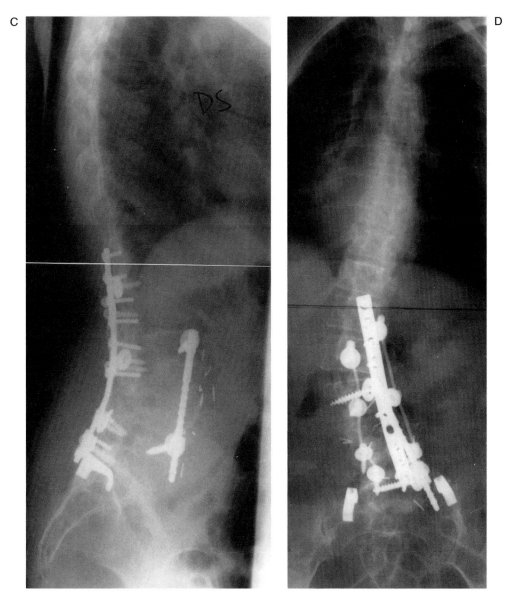

FIG. 16. *(Continued)* **C and D:** Lordosis and balance have been restored by a single-stage anterior and posterior osteotomy.

into the lateral fusion mass, combined with cables to close the osteotomy. Four screws are placed proximal and 4 screws are placed distal to the osteotomy. However, the cables are not tightened at this time. Following the posterior approach, an anterior approach is immediately carried out correspondent in level to the posterior osteotomy. An opening wedge osteotomy is done through the disc or a previous anterior fusion mass, if present. Simultaneous with the anterior opening of the osteotomy, the posterior cables are tightened and a bicortical or tricortical graft then impacted. A posterior, midline, contoured AO plate may be added to control rotation, with at least 2 screws proximal and distal to the osteotomy (Fig. 16).

Surgical Results. We have treated 54 patients with this technique. Pain was relieved in 48 (90%). Non-

union occurred in 3 patients due to anterior graft collapse, 1 of whom requested re-operation. Neurologic complications occurred in 2 patients, 1 with permanent dorsi and plantar flexion weakness and inconsistent bladder control.

The minimum follow-up interval has been 4 years. The average pre-operative lordosis was 21.5 degrees and was restored to 49 degrees. The average correction was 29 degrees, and ranged from 24 to 64 degrees.

DEGENERATIVE ADULT SCOLIOSIS

The other major category of adult scoliosis is deformity presenting de novo in the adult. This has been referred to as "collapsing scoliosis" (62), and "senescent lumbar scoliosis" (18). Exactly how often this occurs is unknown. The only certain proof that a patient has a new curve, rather than progression in a previously unrecognized curve, is a normal spinal radiograph sometime in the past. For this reason, a precise estimate is not possible to determine the prevalence in the population. Vanderpool, James, and Wynne-Davies (72) were the first to study this problem carefully. The control group, which averaged 61.4 years of age, had a prevalence of 6%, but most curves were mild (7 to 16 degrees). A similar finding was observed in adult relatives of patients with scoliosis. An osteoporotic group showed 36% with curvature. The average age was 71 years. They were able to identify 14 of the 36 patients who had unequivocal evidence of having been free of scoliosis at an earlier age. The average age of onset was 40 years. An episode of back pain was usually the identified point at which scoliosis began, and had usually been secondary to an osteoporotic compression fracture. The curves were, in general, mild and ranged from 7 to 53 degrees. The distribution in the spine involved all levels equally. A similar finding was present in 24 patients with osteomalacia; 38% had a curvature, but it was generally mild, and had little or no rotation. On the basis of this analysis, they concluded that adult-onset curves were secondary to osteomalacia and osteoporosis.

A quite different perspective was advanced by Robin et al. (57). They followed a group of 554 subjects for intervals of 8 to 13 years. Some degree of scoliosis was found in 70% of subjects, and 30% had curves of greater than 10 degrees. Ten percent of their patients developed scoliosis in the follow-up interval. However, they concluded that there was little relationship to progression, osteoporosis, or degenerative changes in the spine. Their conclusion is intriguing: "Since scoliosis in the elderly seldom becomes a clinical problem of significance, there would appear to be no valid reason for more extensive study of this condition at this time."

Their conclusion is striking in its contrast to the experience of Epstein (18), Benner and Ehni (3), and Grubb et al. (21). Their conclusion is that scoliosis can arise de novo in the adult, is probably degenerative in etiology, and can be the source of severe symptoms.

Attempts to differentiate the adults with pre-existent but progressing scoliosis from those with a new curve have been made by Grubb (20). Significant differences and similarities were identified:

Demographics. All of the idiopathic group were females with a mean age of 42, whereas the sex distribution was equal in the degenerative group, and the mean age was 60 years.

Pain. Low back pain was equivalent in both groups, radiating into the buttock and upper thighs. However, 90% of the degenerative cases had symptoms indicative of spinal stenosis, compared to 31% of the idiopathic group. The major attribute of the stenotic pain was aggravation by spinal extension. Unlike typical degenerative stenosis, patients often were not relieved by sitting down. Rather they had to support body weight with their arms.

Radiologic Findings

Magnitude of Curve. The curve was greater in the idiopathic group and averaged 52 degrees, and ranged from 34 to 78 degrees. The degenerative group curve average was 28 degrees, with a range of 15 to 53 degrees. However, the average 9-degree deformity per vertebral level was the same in both groups. An additional finding in the degenerative group was lateral translation, a finding emphasized by Epstein (18).

Myelographic Defects. Myelographic defects were most commonly seen within the compensatory lumbosacral curve in the idiopathic group. In comparison, the degenerative group showed most myelographic defects within the primary curve.

Discography. The adult-onset group had grossly degenerate changes within the curve, but pain frequently was not produced by discography. In comparison, reproduction of pain by discography was common in the idiopathic group, an observation made earlier (33). It is speculated that when degeneration is so advanced, injection does not distend the disc, and pain does not result.

Conservative Management

The management is similar to that described for patients who have idiopathic curves presenting in adulthood, and consists of non-steroidal anti-inflammatory medications, exercise (usually with avoidance of extension), as well as general aerobic conditioning. Braces and corsets may offer temporary relief, but there are no studies to prove their efficacy over time. Treatment of existent osteoporosis and prevention of further bone loss are encouraged, particularly in the female patient.

Operative Indications

The most common indication for surgery in adult-onset scoliosis is nerve root symptoms and spinal stenosis. Back pain is currently a less common indication. The debate about who can be treated by decompression alone and who requires decompression with fusion is unresolved. I believe decompression without fusion can be done when it is limited to one nerve root and the facets can be preserved. If greater decompression is necessary or facets are sacrificed, the operation should include a fusion *in situ* or correction of the deformity plus fusion. Otherwise, progression and increasing pain are a major future problem (Fig. 17). This perspective is not shared by others. For example, Epstein (18) thought that patients with significant osteophytes might be treated by decompression alone, a perspective advocated by Nachemson (48).

Pre-Operative Evaluation

All of the pre-operative tests recommended for the idiopathic group may be necessary for the degenerative scoliotic. However, pulmonary dysfunction is rarely an issue, unless the patient has some other coexistent disease.

If fusion is to be done, the question is how many vertebrae to include in the fusion. Nash, Goldstein, and Wilham (49) have analyzed whether the criteria for fusion extent in the adolescent are applicable to the adult. The criteria selected were the stable zone, central sacral line, neutrally rotated vertebra, degenerative arthritis, displaced wedging, rotatory subluxation, and hemisacralization. They concluded that multiple factors needed to be considered in selecting the extent of fusion, and that no single measurement had particular predictive value. The stable zone and the central sacral line were of little use in comparison to the adolescent patient with scoliosis. However, it was relevant when the fusion included L2, L3, and L4.

The most important factors were the magnitude of degeneration and its extent into the lower lumbar levels. Incorporation of vertebral levels with rotatory subluxation, disc space narrowing, and wedging seemed to be of importance. All of these findings were common and seen in at least 50% of patients. An oblique L5 takeoff and hemisacralization were seen in 25% of patients and were relevant to the decision to include the lumbosacral joint. When all criteria were applied, Nash et al. (49) reported significant pain improvement in 89% of patients. It is my opinion that the important factor is to incorporate all painful areas into the fusion, which is best accomplished by pre-operative discography and facet blocks.

Surgical Approaches

The first important decision is whether decompression is necessary, as assessed by the pre-operative findings and imaging studies. Unfortunately, there is no one criterion to establish that adequate decompression has been accomplished, unless the patient presents with very specific nerve root findings localized to one or two levels. The criteria that are considered are: the levels of involvement seen by myelography and the myelographically enhanced CT scan; the restoration of pulsatile dura; and the patency of the foramina. Intra-operative evoked somatosensory potentials have also been reported to be useful (see Chapter 27). Some surgeons often take a radical approach, including removal of facets, pars, and por-

tions of the pedicles to ensure adequate decompression (61).

When decompression is a necessary part of the operation, the posterior approach is used, and the technique is identical with that described by Spengler in Chapter 86.

If fusion is selected, many of the same basic strategies apply as described previously in this chapter. Fusion *in situ* may be done, although it seems likely, but not yet proven, that a lower rate of pseudarthrosis will result with instrumentation. In general, pedicle systems that incorporate rigid linkages, particularly plates, are less suitable because they are less adaptable to the three-dimensional curve characteristics. This difficulty can be overcome with the CDI or posterior Zielke apparatus as described by Simmons and Capicotto (61). Using that technique, a 100% fusion rate was obtained in a patient cohort with a mean age of 62 years, which included a variety of conditions, including degenerative scoliosis. I remain convinced that it is still important to combine anterior and posterior approaches, particularly at unstable levels and particularly at the lumbosacral junction.

Degenerative Scoliosis Following Decompression for Spinal Stenosis

There is no question that an increased curve can follow decompression in a patient with previous degenerative scoliosis. The question is how common is scoliosis after decompression of spinal stenosis where there were normal spinal curves pre-operatively. At present, there is no information to give a precise answer (see Chapter 90).

SUMMARY

Adult scoliotics comprise a diverse group of patients, whose commonality is their presentation in adulthood. Regardless of etiology, the important issues are back pain as well as neurologic symptoms, which are more common in those with degenerative curves. These two symptoms serve as the most common indications for surgery, although curve progression and occasionally cosmesis may be important issues. If surgery is necessary, a critical issue is the restoration or maintenance of lumbar lordosis. The surgical management of an iatrogenic flat back is a major undertaking. Fusion often may have to extend into the lumbosacral joint; I believe it is important to assess that need not only from plain radiographs and other imaging studies, but also by discography. In general, I advocate a combined anterior-posterior approach, when the lumbosacral joint is included in the fusion. The addition of internal fixation devices adds to the predictability of fusion, and properly selected devices allow the maintenance of lumbar lordosis. Using these techniques and principles, a high rate of symptomatic relief and fusion can be achieved. However, the

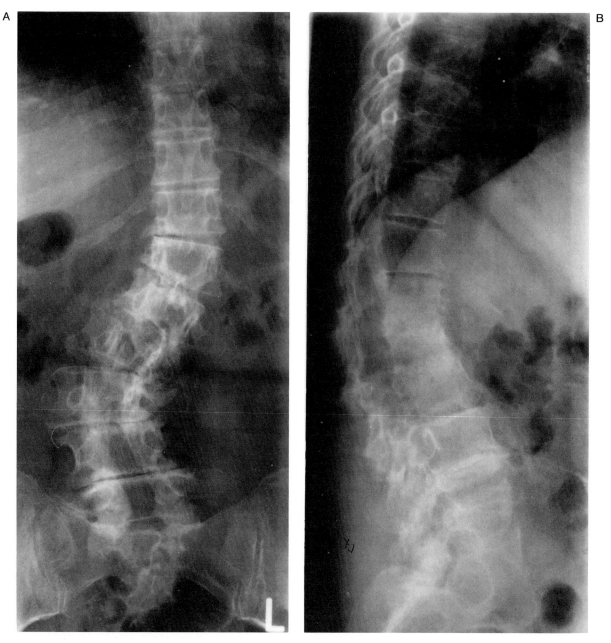

FIG. 17. Female age 68. **A and B:** Pre-laminectomy scoliosis measured 22 degrees. Following decompression, the deformity increased to 32 degrees, together with totally disabling back pain, and subsequently to 50 degrees. Note loss of lumbar lordosis post decompression.

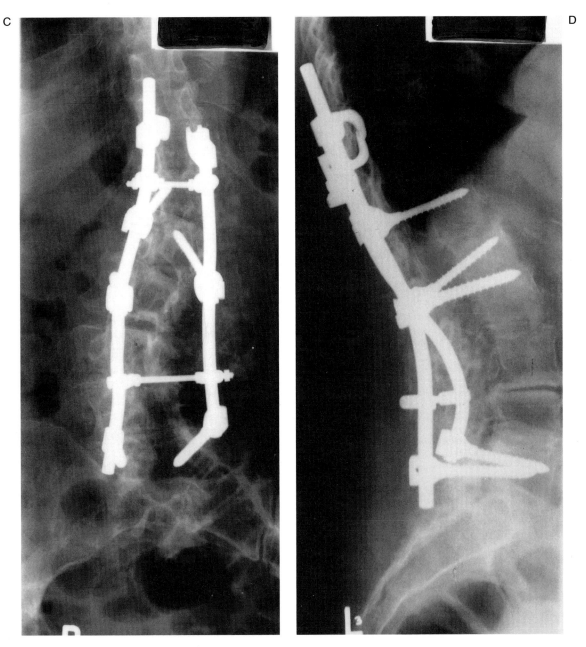

FIG. 17. *(Continued)* **C and D:** Two stage surgery restored lordosis and relieved pain. First stage consisted of multiple anterior discectomies and bone graft. The second stage Cotrel-Dubousset instrumentation and fusion corrected the deformity and restored lordosis.

complication rate is significant. With continued refinements in technique, the rate of success and the reduction of complications can be predicted.

REFERENCES

1. Allen BL Jr, Ferguson RL (1982): The Galveston technique for L-rod instrumentation of the scoliotic spine. *Spine* 7:276–284.
2. Balderston RA, Winter RB, Moe JH, Bradford DS, Lonstein JE (1986): Fusion to the sacrum for nonparalytic scoliosis in the adult. *Spine* 11:824–829.
3. Benner B, Ehni G (1979): Degenerative lumbar scoliosis. *Spine* 4:548–552.
4. Bradford DS (1988): Adult scoliosis: current concepts of treatment. *Clin Orthop* 229:70–87.
5. Byrd JA III, Scoles PV, Winter RB, Bradford DS, Lonstein JE, Moe JH (1987): Adult idiopathic scoliosis treated by anterior and posterior spinal fusion. *J Bone Joint Surg* [Am] 69:843–850.
6. Casey MP, Asher MA, Jacobs RR, Orrick JM (1987): The effect of Harrington rod contouring on lumbar lordosis. *Spine* 12:750–753.
7. Cochran T, Irstam L, Nachemson A (1983): Long-term anatomic and functional changes in patients with adolescent idiopathic scoliosis treated by Harrington rod fusion. *Spine* 8:576–584.
8. Coe JD, Becker PS, McAfee PC, Gurr KR (1989): Neuropathology with spinal instrumentation. *J Orthop Res* 7:359–370.
9. Collis DK, Ponsetti IV (1969): Long term follow-up of patients with idiopathic scoliosis not treated surgically. *J Bone Joint Surg* [Am] 51:425–445.
10. Cotrel Y (1986): *Instrumentation for surgery of the spine*. Freud Publishing House, Ltd.
11. Cotrel Y, Dubousset J, Guillaumat M (1988): New universal instrumentation in spinal surgery. *Clin Orthop* 227:10–23.
12. Cummine JL, Lonstein JE, Moe JH, Winter RB, Bradford DS (1979): Reconstructive surgery in the adult for failed scoliosis fusion. *J Bone Joint Surg* [Am] 61:1151–1161.
13. Dawson EG, Caron A, Moe JH (1973): Surgical management of scoliosis in the adult. *J Bone Joint Surg* [Am] 55:437.
14. Denis F (1988): Cotrel-Dubousset instrumentation in the treatment of idiopathic scoliosis. *Orthop Clin North Am* 19:291–311.
15. Doherty JH (1973): Complications of fusion in lumbar scoliosis. *J Bone Joint Surg* [Am] 55:438.
16. Dwyer AF (1973): Experience of anterior correction of scoliosis. *Clin Orthop* 93:191–214.
17. Edgar MA, Mehta MH (1982): A longterm review of adults with fused and unfused idiopathic scoliosis. *Orthop Trans* 6:462–463.
18. Epstein JA, Epstein BS, Jones MD (1979): Symptomatic lumbar scoliosis with degenerative changes in the elderly. *Spine* 4:542–547.
19. Grobler LJ, Moe JH, Winter RB, Bradford DS, Lonstein JE (1978): Loss of lumbar lordosis following surgical correction of thoracolumbar deformities. *Orthop Trans* 2:239.
20. Grubb SA, Lipscomb HJ, Coonrad RW (1988): Degenerative adult onset scoliosis. *Spine* 13:241–245.
21. Grubb SA, Lipscomb HJ, Coonrad RW (1989): Diagnostic findings in painful adult scoliosis. Presented at the Scoliosis Research Society meeting, Amsterdam.
22. Haher JE, Devlin V, Freeman B, Rondon B (1987): Long-term effects of sublaminar wires on the neural canal. *Orthop Trans* 11:106.
23. Hall JE (1981): Dwyer instrumentation in anterior fusion of the spine. *J Bone Joint Surg* [Am] 63:1188–1190.
24. Harrington PR, Dickson JH (1973): An eleven-year clinical investigation of Harrington instrumentation. A preliminary report on 578 cases. *Clin Orthop* 93:113–130.
25. Hasday CA, Passoff TL, Perry J (1983): Gait abnormalities arising from iatrogenic loss of lumbar lordosis secondary to Harrington instrumentation in lumbar fractures. *Spine* 8:501–511.
26. Hayes MA, Tompkin SF, Herndon WA, et al (1988): Clinical and radiological evaluation of lumbosacral motion below fusion levels in idiopathic scoliosis. *Spine* 13:1161–1167.
27. Herndon WA, Sullivan JA, Yngve DA, Gross RH, Dreher G (1987): Segmental spinal instrumentation with sublaminar wires. *J Bone Joint Surg* [Am] 69:851–859.
28. Herring JA, Wenger DR (1982): Segmental spinal instrumentation. A preliminary report of 40 consecutive cases. *Spine* 7:285–298.
29. Jackson RP, Simmons EH, Stripinis D (1983): Incidence and severity of back pain in adult idiopathic scoliosis. *Spine* 8:749–756.
30. Johnson JR, Holt RT (1988): Combined use of anterior and posterior surgery for adult scoliosis. *Orthop Clin North Am* 19:361–370.
31. Johnston CE II, Happel LT Jr, Norris R, Burke SW, King AG, Roberts JM (1986): Delayed paraplegia complicating sublaminar segmental spinal instrumentation. *J Bone Joint Surg* [Am] 68:556–563.
32. Kaneda K, Fujiya N, Satoh S (1986): Results with Zielke instrumentation for idiopathic thoracolumbar and lumbar scoliosis. *Clin Orthop* 205:195–203.
33. Kostuik JP (1979): Decision making in adult scoliosis. *Spine* 4:521–525.
34. Kostuik JP (1988): Treatment of scoliosis in the adult thoracolumbar spine with special reference of fusion to the sacrum. *Orthop Clin North Am* 19:371–381.
35. Kostuik JP, Bentivoglio J (1981): The incidence of low back pain in adult scoliosis. *Spine* 6:268–273.
36. Kostuik JP, Carl A, Ferron S (1989): Anterior Zielke instrumentation for spinal deformity in adults. *J Bone Joint Surg* [Am] 71:898–912.
37. Kostuik JP, Hall BB (1983): Spinal fusions to the sacrum in adults with scoliosis. *Spine* 8:489–500.
38. Kostuik JP, Israel J, Hall JE (1973): Scoliosis surgery in adults. *Clin Orthop* 93:225–234.
39. Kostuik JP, Maurais GR, Richardson WJ (1989): Primary fusion to the sacrum using Luque instrumentation for adult scoliotic patients. *Orthop Trans* 13:30.
40. Kostuik JP, Maurais GR, Richardson WJ, Okajimay (1988): Combined single stage anterior and posterior osteotomy for correction of iatrogenic lumbar kyphosis. *Spine* 13:257–266.
41. Kostuik JP, Worden HR, Salo P (1990): Long term functional outcome following surgery for adult scoliosis. Presented at the American Orthopaedic Association meeting, Boston.
42. Lagrone MO, Bradford DS, Moe JH, Lonstein JE, Winter RB, Ogilvie JW (1988): Treatment of symptomatic flatback after spinal fusion. *J Bone Joint Surg* [Am] 70:569–580.
43. Luque ER (1982): The anatomic basis and development of segmental spinal instrumentation. *Spine* 7:256–259.
44. Luque ER (1982): Segmental spinal instrumentation for correction of scoliosis. *Clin Orthop* 163:192–198.
45. Moe JH, Purcell GA, Bradford DS (1983): Zielke instrumentation (VDS) for the correction of spinal curvature. Analysis of results in 66 patients. *Clin Orthop* 180:133–153.
46. Nachemson A (1968): A longterm follow-up study of non-treated scoliosis. *Acta Orthop Scand* 39:466–476.
47. Nachemson A (1969): A longterm follow-up study of non-treated scoliosis. *J Bone Joint Surg* [Am] 50:203–204.
48. Nachemson A (1979): Adult scoliosis and back pain. *Spine* 4:513–517.
49. Nash CL, Goldstein JM, Wilham MR (1989): Selection of lumbar fusion levels in adult idiopathic scoliosis patients. Presented at the Scoliosis Research Society meeting, Amsterdam.
50. Nash CL Jr, Moe JH (1969): A study of vertebral rotation. *J Bone Joint Surg* [Am] 51:223–229.
51. Nicastro JF, Hartjen CA, Traina J, Lancaster JM (1986): Intraspinal pathways taken by sublaminar wires during removal. An experimental study. *J Bone Joint Surg* [Am] 68:1206–1209.
52. Nilsonne U, Lundgren KD (1968): Longterm prognosis in idiopathic scoliosis. *Acta Orthop Scand* 39:455–465.
53. Nuber GW, Schafer MF (1986): Surgical management of adult scoliosis. *Clin Orthop* 208:228–237.
54. Ogiela DM, Chan DPK (1986): Ventral derotation spondylodesis. A review of 22 cases. *Spine* 11:18–22.
55. Ponder RC, Dickson JH, Harrington PR, Erwin WD (1975): Results of Harrington instrumentation and fusion in the adult idiopathic scoliosis patient. *J Bone Joint Surg* [Am] 57:797–801.
56. Ponsetti IV (1968): The pathogenesis of adult scoliosis. In: Zorab

PA, Cansation E, Livingstone S, eds. *Proceedings of the second symposium on scoliosis.* Edinburgh.

57. Robin GC, Span Y, Steinberg R, et al (1982): Scoliosis in the elderly. A follow-up study. *Spine* 7:355–359.

58. Rogala EJ, Drummond DS, Gurr J (1978): Scoliosis: Incidence and natural history. A prospective epidemiological study. *J Bone Joint Surg* [Am] 60:173–176.

59. Schrader WC, Bethem D, Scerbin V (1987): The chronic local effects of sublaminar wires—an animal model. *Orthop Trans* 11:106.

60. Shands AR Jr, Eisberg HB (1955): The incidence of scoliosis in the state of Delaware. *J Bone Joint Surg* [Am] 37:1243–1249.

61. Simmons EH, Capicotto WN (1989): Posterior transpedicular Zielke instrumentation of the lumbar spine. *Clin Orthop* 236:180–191.

62. Simmons EH, Jackson RP (1979): The management of nerve root entrapment syndromes associated with the collapsing scoliosis of idiopathic lumbar and thoracolumbar curves. *Spine* 4:533–541.

63. Sponseller PD, Cohen MS, Nachemson AL, Hall JE, Wohl ME (1987): Results of surgical treatment of adults with idiopathic scoliosis. *J Bone Joint Surg* [Am] 69:667–675.

64. Stagnara P (1969): Scoliosis in adults. Surgical treatment of severe forms. *Excerpta Med Found Int Cong* 192.

65. Stagnara P (1973): *Utilization of Harrington's device in the treatment of adult kyphoscoliosis above 100 degrees. Fourth International Symposium, 1971.* Stuttgart: George Thieme Verlag.

66. Stagnara P, Fleury D, Fauchet R, et al (1975): Major scoliosis over 100 degrees, in adults. 183 surgically treated cases. *Rev Chir Orthop* 61:101–122.

67. Stagnara P, Jouvinoux P, Peloux J, et al (1969): Cyphoscoliosis essentielles de l'adulte. Formes severe de plus de 100. Redressment partial et arthrodese. Presented at the XI SICOT Congress, Mexico City, Mexico.

68. Swank S, Lonstein JE, Moe JH, Bradford DS (1981): Surgical treatment of adult scoliosis. A review of two hundred and twenty-two cases. *J Bone Joint Surg* [Am] 63:268–287.

69. Thompson GH, Wilber RG, Shaffer JW, Scoles PV, Nash CL Jr (1985): Segmental spinal instrumentation in idiopathic scoliosis. A preliminary report. *Spine* 10:623–630.

70. van Dam BE (1988): Nonoperative treatment of adult scoliosis. *Orthop Clin North Am* 19:347–351.

71. van Dam BE, Bradford DS, Lonstein JE, et al (1987): Adult idiopathic scoliosis treated by posterior spinal fusion and Harrington instrumentation. *Spine* 12:32–36.

72. Vanderpool DW, James JIP, Wynne-Davies R (1969): Scoliosis in the elderly. *J Bone Joint Surg* [Am] 51:446–455.

73. Weinstein SL, Ponsetti IV (1983): Curve progression in idiopathic scoliosis. *J Bone Joint Surg* [Am] 65:447–455.

74. Wilber RG, Thompson GH, Shaffer JW, Brown RH, Nash CL (1984): Postoperative neurological deficits in segmental spinal instrumentation. A study using spinal cord monitoring. *J Bone Joint Surg* [Am] 66:1178–1187.

75. Winter RB (1978): Combined Dwyer and Harrington instrumentation and fusion in the treatment of selected patients with painful adult idiopathic scoliosis. *Spine* 3:135–141.

76. Winter RB, Lonstein JE, Denis F (1988): Pain patterns in adult scoliosis. *Orthop Clin North Am* 19:339–345.

77. Zielke K, Stunkat R, Beaujean F (1976): Ventrale derotationsspondylodese. *Arch Orthop Unfallchir* 85:257–277.

The Adult Spine: Principles and Practice,
J. W. Frymoyer, Editor-in-Chief.
Raven Press, Ltd., New York © 1991.

CHAPTER 66

Thoracic Pain Syndromes and Thoracic Disc Herniation

John W. Skubic and John P. Kostuik

Pain in the thoracic region is a common presenting complaint whose source is too often enigmatic. Like most back symptoms, these obscure maladies are usually fleeting, benign, and respond to tincture of time. There are, however, some patients whose symptoms remain a source of disability and frustration. More ominous are those thoracic pain syndromes that are not benign and demand rapid diagnosis so that delay in treatment does not lead to unnecessary harm.

The objective, then, in treating thoracic pain syndromes is to identify those patients who have an underlying serious disease. For those patients with persistent yet benign symptoms, the source, if possible, needs to be located so that specific treatment, when available, may be applied.

CLASSIFICATION

Many classification schemes could be devised for this problem (Table 1). This chapter concentrates on the syndromes related to the spinal column and associated

J. W. Skubic, M.D.: Assistant Professor, Department of Orthopaedics, Loma Linda University Medical Center, Loma Linda, California, 92350.
J. P. Kostuik, M.D., F.R.C.S.(C): Professor of Orthopaedics, University of Toronto, Toronto, Ontario; Director, Spinal Surgery; Director, Biomechanics Laboratory, The Toronto Hospital, Toronto, Ontario, M5G 2C4.

structures. However, the discussion would be dangerously incomplete if mention were not made of those sources of thoracic pain not spinal in origin. Since the spinal cord is potentially involved, we have subdivided thoracic pain syndromes into those with and without neurologic involvement. Among those without neurologic involvement, potential sources might be labeled viscerogenic and costospondylogenic. Those patients with neurologic involvement usually fall into the category of extrinsic compression such as thoracic disc herniations, tumorous conditions (which are dealt with elsewhere), and intrinsic spinal cord problems. Finally, a short discussion of what has been labeled post-thoracotomy syndrome is included. This last condition is the iatrogenic result of increasingly popular anterior approaches to thoracic spinal pathology.

THORACIC PAIN SYNDROMES WITHOUT NEUROLOGIC DEFICIT

Viscerogenic Thoracic Pain

A discussion of thoracic pain syndromes must mention those causes that are visceral in origin. This is to avoid the catastrophic consequences attendant in their omission from the differential diagnosis. Table 2 outlines some of the disorders to provide a general framework and to emphasize the importance of visceral causes

TABLE 1. *Classification of thoracic pain syndromes*

I. Thoracic pain syndromes without neurologic impairment
  A. Viscerogenic and miscellaneous
  B. Costospondylogenic
    1. Costochondral
    2. Costovertebral
    3. Facetal
    4. Discogenic
  C. Neoplastic
  D. Infectious
  E. Structural
    1. Scoliosis
    2. Kyphosis
      a. Scheuermann's
      b. Post-traumatic
      c. Osteoporotic
  F. Cervical spondylogenic
II. Thoracic pain syndromes with neurologic impairment
  A. Neoplastic
    1. Extradural
      a. Primary
      b. Metastatic
    2. Intradural-extramedullary
    3. Intramedullary
  B. Infectious
  C. Thoracic disc herniation
III. Post-thoracotomy syndrome

TABLE 2. *Visceral conditions simulating thoracic spondylogenic pain*

I. Intrathoracic
  A. Cardiovascular
    1. Angina pectoris
    2. Myocardial infarction
    3. Mitral valve prolapse
    4. Pericarditis
    5. Aortic aneurysm
  B. Pulmonary
    1. Pneumonia
    2. Carcinoma
    3. Pneumothorax
    4. Pleurisy
    5. Infarction, embolus
  C. Mediastinal
    1. Esophagitis, tumor
    2. Mediastinal tumors
II. Intra-abdominal
  A. Hepatobiliary
    1. Hepatitis
    2. Abscess
    3. Cholecystitis, biliary colic
  B. Gastrointestinal
    1. Peptic ulcer disease
    2. Hernia—hiatal, inguinal, other
    3. Pancreatitis
III. Retroperitoneal
  A. Pyelonephritis
  B. Ureteral colic
  C. Aneurysm
  D. Tumor
IV. Miscellaneous
  A. Herpes zoster
  B. Polymyalgia rheumatica
  C. Hyperventilation syndrome
  D. Rib fracture, neoplasm

of thoracic pain. Suffice it to say that the diagnosis cannot be made unless the treating physician considers the condition. Therefore, prior to zeroing in on a musculoskeletal or neurogenic diagnosis, these other conditions should be considered and excluded in a systematic fashion. A careful history and physical examination, ancillary tests, and consultation with colleagues are essential.

Costospondylogenic Pain Syndromes

Just as the physician involved in the treatment of spinal pathology must recognize the possible visceral origin of seemingly musculoskeletal complaints, it is apparent that musculoskeletal disorders may masquerade as cardiac or abdominal in nature (4,6,30). Oille (35), in 1937, reported 600 cases of new onset chest pain referred for cardiac consultation, of which one third were spondylogenic in origin. Rawlings (44) details an extensive differential diagnosis of chest pain, and includes the "rib syndrome" as a very common cause, with spondylogenic sources also prominent.

Costochondritis (Tietze's Syndrome)

In 1921, Tietze (53) described a syndrome that consists of painful swelling of the costal cartilage and usually involves the second rib. Others have stressed the importance of palpation of the chest wall in the diagnosis of thoracic pain complaints to detect costochondral pain mistaken for cardiac symptoms (44,56). Relief was usually obtained by steroid injection or the use of non-steroidal anti-inflammatory medication.

Rib-Tip Syndrome

McBeath (31) called attention in the orthopedic literature to the rib-tip syndrome. This syndrome involves the lower four ribs with pain radiating from anterior around the flank to the back. He noted that the pain could be reproduced by palpating the painful rib tip. The condition could easily be mistaken for a thoracic radiculopathy of discogenic origin if a careful physical examination were not performed. The patient's symptoms were permanently relieved by excision of the offending rib in two cases and by steroid injection in one.

Costovertebral Pain Syndromes

The anatomy of the costovertebral joint is complex (20) (Figs. 1–4 and 6). There are two costovertebral joints per rib, one between the rib tubercle and transverse process, and one between the rib head and adjacent vertebral bodies. Ribs two through ten have two facets to articulate with adjacent vertebral bodies. Separating the facets is a ligament attaching to the crest of the head and to the intervertebral disc. The articular capsule is thickened anteriorly by a radiate ligament that attaches to the disc and adjacent vertebral bodies. Rib heads one, eleven, and twelve usually have a single facet to articulate with the corresponding vertebra.

The costotransverse joints are synovial joints with thin articular capsules that are strengthened by costotransverse ligaments. These ligaments extend between articulating rib and transverse process and to the transverse process above.

Nathan et al. (34) documented the incidence of osteoarthritis involving the costovertebral joints. The highest incidence was in the first, eleventh, and twelfth ribs, i.e., those with single rib head/vertebral body articulations, and at the sixth through eighth ribs, i.e., the longest ribs. Arthritic changes began appearing in the third decade, and by age forty affected 50% to 60% of the spines examined.

Raney in 1966 reported 156 patients that he felt had symptomatic costovertebral arthritis (41). The pain was often unilateral and described as aching or burning, radiating to or from the back, often associated with hyperalgesia. He described tenderness over the costovertebral junction, with the patient's pain reproducible by manipulation of the rib. Injection of a local anesthetic into the joint was felt to be a helpful diagnostic test, although the location of the intercostal nerve in close proximity calls into question the specificity of the injection. He reported the results of surgical excision of the affected joint in 35 patients: 29 had good or excellent relief of pain, 5 fair, and 1 poor. Injection of corticosteroid into the area has also been reported to be of benefit (34).

Thoracic Facet Arthropathy

The fact that painful degenerative arthrosis occurs in the spinal facet joints whether they are cervical, thoracic, or lumbar is accepted by most physicians. The debate is over the diagnostic criteria, the most appropriate form of treatment, and especially whether or not facet arthrosis is a surgically correctable lesion. Most attention regarding facet arthropathy has naturally been directed to the lumbar region, given the greater incidence of low back pain. The diagnostic specificity and therapeutic effectiveness of lumbar facet blocks remain controversial. Surgical approaches to presumed primary lumbar facet arthrosis by various forms of facet denervation procedures, synovectomies, or fusions appear to have met with mixed results at best. It appears that circumstances in the thoracic spine are not substantially different.

Shore has documented the incidence of degenerative facet arthrosis in the thoracic spine and has found the highest frequency at C7-T1, T3-T4-T5, and T11-T12-L1 (50). In the evaluation of intractable thoracic back pain,

thoracic facet blocks have played a useful role in further defining the origin of the pain. The evaluation is usually combined with thoracic discography, as will be discussed in the following section. A patient with primary facet arthropathy would have relief of thoracic back pain following the facet block and painless thoracic discography at the same level. However, isolated facet arthropathy appears to be exceedingly uncommon, and most patients have combined facet and disc pathology.

We have encountered only three such patients who have been treated surgically for primary thoracic facet arthropathy at Toronto General Hospital since 1973. The procedure was a posterior fusion and instrumentation with Luque rods. All appeared to obtain a solid fusion that extended over the length of the symptomatic facets as determined by the facet blocks. Two patients had complete relief of pain and one patient failed to obtain any relief. Exploration of the fusion mass and rod removal in that patient did not improve the symptoms.

Based on this small number of cases, it is impossible to endorse this procedure without reservation. Our experience does show that despite the relatively frequent occurrence of thoracic back pain and the number of patients evaluated for such complaints, only a very small number of patients have an isolated facet arthropathy for which surgery is a consideration.

Thoracic Discogenic Pain

As a source of thoracic back pain and other referred pain symptoms, the thoracic disc itself has been a fairly well documented culprit (1,3,7,9,12,17,15,16,19,23, 24,27,33,36,42,49,51,52). Most of these cases have been in association with an actual herniation of the disc resulting in varying degrees of spinal cord compression and myelopathy, the thoracic back pain being considered, quite properly, of secondary importance.

Not as well recognized are the cases of thoracic disc pathology in which pain is the major complaint with objective neurologic findings being absent. The absence of a disc herniation as documented by myelogram or CT scan does not exclude the possibility that the thoracic disc is a source of pain. We have found thoracic discography to be most helpful in identifying the painful disc, although we recognize the controversial nature of this test.

The disc levels to be studied by discography are identified on the basis of where the patient localized the back pain and by the referral pattern if present. Prior to discography, water-soluble myelography followed by CT scanning is performed. If a disc herniation is present that corresponds anatomically to the patient's pain origin, then this disc is chosen as a starting point for discography. Our use of magnetic resonance imaging in this condition has been limited. As experience is gained, it

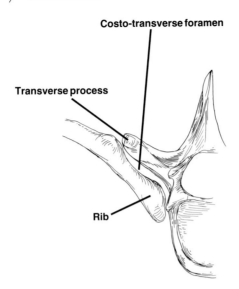

Costo-transverse foramen

Transverse process

Rib

FIG. 1. Articulation of rib with transverse process and vertebral body.

appears that MRI may supplant myelography and CT scanning as the procedure of choice to diagnose thoracic disc herniation (46). The status of disc hydration, as seen on the T2-weighted images, in identifying a pain-provoking disc remains unclear. At present, we believe discography remains the diagnostic procedure of choice.

The technique of thoracic discography is much the same as that of lumbar discography. Because the spinal cord is present, the only available approach is posterolateral. Proper disc levels are identified by counting disc spaces proximally from the sacrum with the fluoroscope. An entry point six to eight centimeters from the midline is chosen. The needle should pass above the rib at the desired disc space, as this is technically easiest and also avoids inadvertent injury to the neurovascular bundle located beneath the rib. For example, at the T6-T7 disc space, the needle will be passed above the seventh rib (Figs. 5 and 6).

The angle of approach is slightly steeper than in lumbar discography because the distance to the disc from the posterior body surface is usually less in the thoracic region than in the lumbar region. Also, by choosing a slightly steeper angle and starting farther away from the midline instead of a flatter angle and closer to the midline, advantage can be taken of the rib's natural downward course, making it easier to pass the needle above the rib and into the disc.

A 22-gauge spinal needle is used. It is important that the stylet remain in place during needle passage so that air is not introduced into the pleural space, thereby creating a pneumothorax. The other way to create a pneumothorax would be by lacerating the visceral pulmonary pleura and parenchyma, thus allowing air into the pleural cavity via the small bronchioles. The patient must, of course, be warned of this complication prior to the procedure, and facilities for its management must be readily available. Fortunately, this complication has been infrequently encountered in our use of discography.

Once the needle is within the desired disc space as confirmed by biplanar fluoroscopy, standard discography is performed. In a non-degenerate disc, the volume of fluid accepted is often quite small, sometimes less than one milliliter. Radiographic appearance, dye ex-

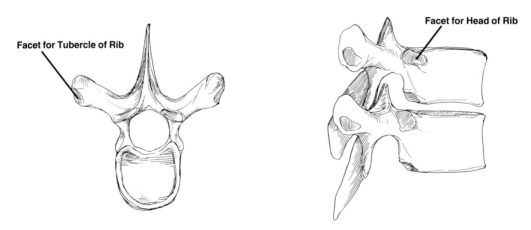

Facet for Tubercle of Rib

Facet for Head of Rib

FIG. 2. Facets for tubercle of rib and rib head on the thoracic vertebrae.

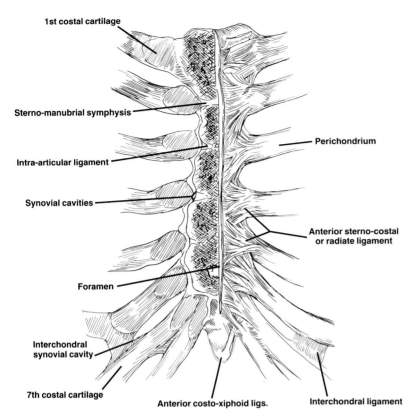

1st costal cartilage

Sterno-manubrial symphysis

Intra-articular ligament

Synovial cavities

Foramen

Interchondral
synovial cavity

7th costal cartilage

Anterior costo-xiphoid ligs.

Perichondrium

Anterior sterno-costal
or radiate ligament

Interchondral ligament

FIG. 3. Ligaments of the chondrosternal joints.

FIG. 4. Lateral costotransverse ligament attaching the tubercle of the rib to the thoracic transverse process.

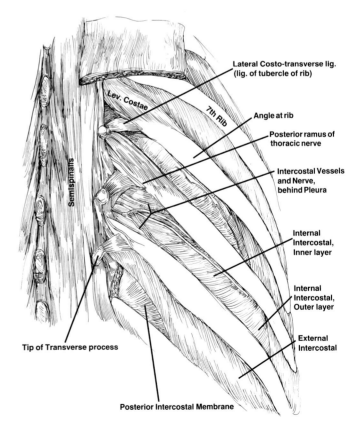

Lateral Costo-transverse lig.
(lig. of tubercle of rib)

Angle at rib

Posterior ramus of
thoracic nerve

Intercostal Vessels
and Nerve,
behind Pleura

Internal
Intercostal,
Inner layer

Internal
Intercostal,
Outer layer

External
Intercostal

Lev. Costae

7th Rib

Semispinalis

Tip of Transverse process

Posterior Intercostal Membrane

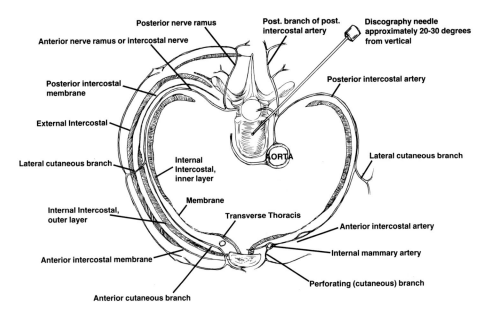

FIG. 5. Coronal view to demonstrate angle of entry for thoracic discography. The head of the rib may interfere on occasion with direct access to the disc space (see Fig. 6).

travasation, and, most important, pain response is recorded.

If the patient's typical pain is reproduced, then the discs above and below the symptomatic disc are examined. The goals are to isolate the symptomatic disc and determine that surrounding contiguous discs are asymptomatic. Typically three or four discs are examined. If, however, the number of symptomatic discs exceeds three, the procedure is abandoned, as the pain-causing process appears more generalized and will not be helped by a local fusion. Similarly, if a pain-reproducing disc is not identified after two or three discograms, the procedure is also terminated pending further evaluation. In doing thoracic discography, there have been no neurologic complications and no disc space infections; the very rare occurrences of pneumothorax have been easily managed with a small chest tube.

The vast majority of patients presenting with com-

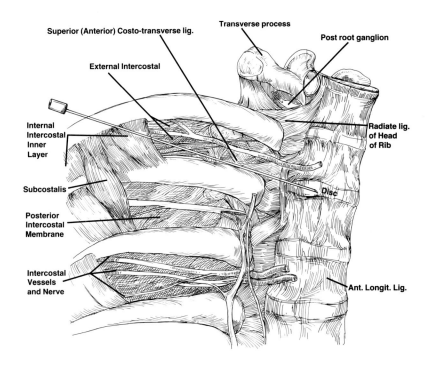

FIG. 6. Discography needle in a thoracic disc. Note the costovertebral ligaments.

plaints of thoracic back pain without neurologic deficit (and assuming the absence of a significant visceral cause) are treated non-operatively. Physical therapeutic and anti-inflammatory drug regimens are employed, resulting in a positive response in most patients. Only when conservative measures have failed and the patient persists in having disabling pain that prevents normal employment and social activities is further investigation with discography suggested.

Since 1973, thirteen patients have undergone anterior thoracic fusion for the treatment of thoracic discogenic pain without neurologic impairment. The duration of symptoms prior to surgical treatment ranged from two to seven years, with an average of three and one-half years. Trauma in the form of either an industrial accident or motor vehicle accident was felt to be the provocative factor in four patients. The remaining patients felt that their symptoms were of spontaneous onset. Our experience with these thirteen patients underscores the difficulty in making the diagnosis of thoracic discogenic pain because of the wide variety and sometimes anatomically distant complaints patients may manifest.

Three of the thirteen patients in this series had been treated for visceral complaints prior to the discovery that their pain was the result of thoracic disc derangement. The difficulty in the diagnosis was that the referred pain complaint seemed more severe than the thoracic back complaint. One patient was treated for pyelonephritis, one underwent an inguinal herniorrhaphy, and a third patient had a cholecystectomy prior to the diagnosis of thoracic discogenic pain. Following anterior thoracic discectomy and fusion, the patients' complaints were relieved.

Patients were also mistakenly diagnosed as having lumbar disc derangement as a source of their pain. Two had undergone previous lumbar laminectomies prior to the treatment of their thoracic discogenic pain. Review of available myelograms of these patients demonstrated a lack of correlation between the lumbar myelographic defect and the patients' complaints.

Most of the patients complained primarily of back pain originating in the thoracic region with variable degrees of referral. Quite often the pain was felt to radiate anteriorly around the trunk, frequently, but not always, in a dermatomal pattern. Occasionally, the referred pain was more predominant than the local thoracic back pain, as in the patients in whom a misdiagnosis of visceral causes was initially made. Rarely, the pain was felt to radiate straight anteriorly through the chest instead of around the trunk.

The quality of the pain as reported by the patients was not consistent, being variously described as sharp, dull, aching, electric, and burning. In all the patients, the pain was incapacitating and prevented or interfered with normal occupational or social activities. All had been treated with various combinations of physical therapy, chiropractic, drug therapy, or bracing in an attempt to control their symptoms, to no avail.

Physical examination of all thirteen patients failed to disclose an objective neurologic deficit. Plain radiographs showed diffuse thoracic degenerative changes in seven, and local degenerative changes in six. Myelography and CT scanning revealed small centrolateral disc herniations in two and a small disc bulge in three. The remaining eight had no myelographically discernible disc pathology.

Discography was performed in all the patients to localize their symptoms. In six patients, one level was positive; in another six, two levels were positive; and in one patient, three levels were positive. Interestingly, one patient with a small disc herniation had two positive levels on discography, underscoring the importance of discography in determining the operative levels.

All patients underwent an anterior thoracic discectomy and fusion via a thoracotomy approach. A complete discectomy was performed back to the posterior longitudinal ligament (PLL). If a herniated disc fragment was present, the PLL was incised and the fragment carefully removed. The fusion was performed using the excised rib as graft material. Internal fixation with a Kostuik-Harrington compression device was routinely performed (Figs. 7 and 8).

The results were as follows: Of the thirteen patients, two had fair or poor results due to failure to obtain pain relief and inability to return to work. Both of these patients were workers' compensation cases; there were a total of three compensation cases in this group. The remaining eleven patients experienced improvement or complete relief of their pain such that they could return to work or engage in their normal activities of daily living. All thirteen patients obtained a solid arthrodesis.

Other authors have reported patients treated for symptomatic thoracic disc degeneration without motor or bladder involvement (9,16,30,36,37). These cases were usually in association with a documented thoracic disc herniation. Bohlman (9), in his review of nineteen patients with thoracic disc herniation, found three had no motor or bladder involvement. All three were treated by a costotransversectomy approach and disc excision, and one also had fusion. A good result was obtained in two, and a poor result occurred in a workers' compensation case.

O'Leary (36) reported two patients without disc herniation but with thoracic discogenic pain. He also emphasized the value of discography in isolating the involved discs. Treatment by anterior discectomy and fusion successfully alleviated the pain in both patients.

Finally, the differentiation of pain arising from the cervical spine from that arising from the upper thoracic spine is sometimes difficult. This is particularly true

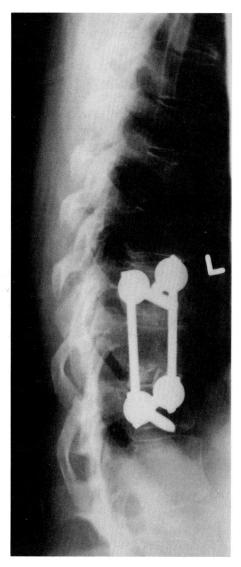

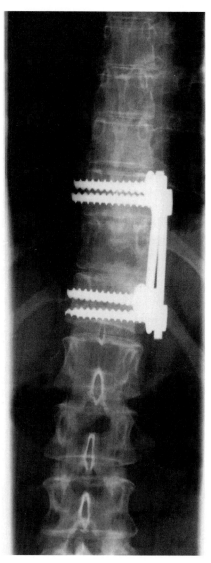

FIG. 7. Male age 34. Chronic pain reproduced on discography at T9-T10 and T10-T11. Following disc excision the fusion (rib struts) was stabilized with an anterior Kostuik-Harrington compression device.

FIG. 8. Same patient as in Figure 7.

when cervical spine pain is referred to the medial border of the scapula and the upper interscapular area. Some of the important differentiating points are:

1. Thoracic pain does not produce brachialgia and is not aggravated by neck rotation, which are common when the pain arises from the cervical spine.
2. Thoracic pain syndromes are rare in the upper part of the thoracic spine and occur much more frequently in the distal thoracic spine, when the neck is one early suspect.
3. If there is difficulty differentiating between pain arising from the thoracic and cervical spine, discography and facet blocks may be of help.

THORACIC PAIN SYNDROMES WITH NEUROLOGIC DEFICIT

Thoracic Disc Herniation

The previous section discussed the syndrome of thoracic discogenic pain without motor or bladder involvement, which can occur in the absence of a disc herniation. If a disc herniation is present in such a case, it is usually lateral or centrolateral in location and is not causing sufficient pressure on the spinal cord to cause a myelopathy, and pain is the only manifestation. However, if the herniation is large enough or located in a critical position, spinal cord impingement can occur, resulting in various forms of myelopathy.

The anatomy of the thoracic spinal canal makes it predisposed to spinal cord impingement from even relatively small disc herniation. This is due to the large ratio of spinal cord area to thoracic canal area found in the thoracic spine. This leaves little room for an extradural mass to be present without compressing the cord (Figs. 9 and 10). The tenuous blood supply to the thoracic cord, termed the "critical vascular zone of the spinal cord" by Dommisse (14), may also predispose the thoracic cord to damage by a disc herniation.

The first report of a thoracic disc herniation was by Key in 1838 (24). Middleton and Teacher (32), in 1911, described a patient with acute paraplegia after lifting a heavy metal plate. The patient died sixteen days later due to urinary sepsis. At autopsy, a large thoracic disc herniation was found to have compressed the spinal cord. The first report of surgery being performed to treat a thoracic disc herniation was by Adson in 1922, as reported by Love and Schorn (27).

The incidence of thoracic disc herniation in 2,000 autopsy studies by Schmorl (47) revealed 737 cases of either intravertebral herniation (Schmorl's nodes) or posterior thoracic disc herniation. The vast majority of the posteriorly directed herniations were small, one to two millimeters in size, and contained beneath the posterior

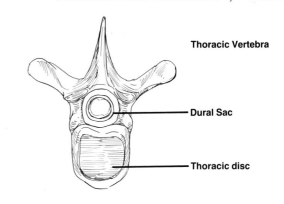

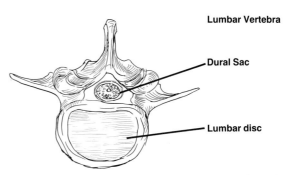

FIG. 10. Axial views of the thoracic and lumbar vertebrae indicate the smaller thoracic column largely occupied by the spinal cord in contrast to the lumbar spine.

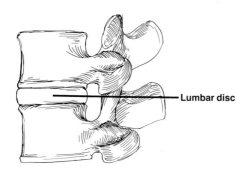

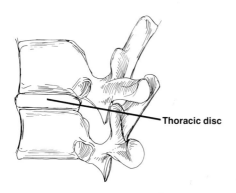

FIG. 9. Diagrammatic view of the thoracic and lumbar vertebrae. Note the relative narrowness of the thoracic disc.

longitudinal ligament. Andrae (2) found in 368 autopsies a 15% incidence of posterior disc herniation, again with the majority being small and contained beneath the posterior longitudinal ligament.

Thus, although the space available for the cord is comparably small in the thoracic spine, there appears to be enough room for the vast majority of these very small disc herniations such that neurologic symptoms are absent. The incidence of clinically significant thoracic disc herniation has been variously estimated to be between one patient per million population (12) or about 0.2% to 1.8% of total disc operations (27,37).

The patient usually presents in the fourth to sixth decade of life, although there are reports of thoracic disc herniation in children (28,39). Cases in which Scheuermann's disease has been associated, in both adolescents and adults, have been detailed (10,55). The herniation usually involves the lower third of the thoracic spine, but all levels have been reported. It is possible that the rib cage provides a stabilizing influence and protects the upper thoracic spine from disc herniation. Intradural erosion by the disc herniation has been described (17), as has two-level disc herniation (8). Trauma in the past was reported to be a common causative factor, but more recent reports have de-emphasized the importance of traumatic antecedents.

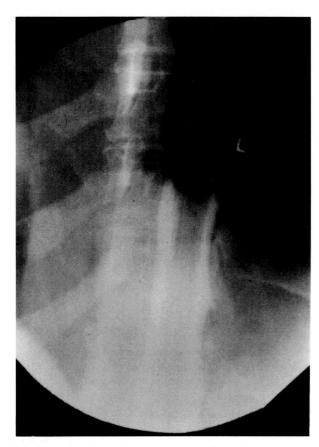

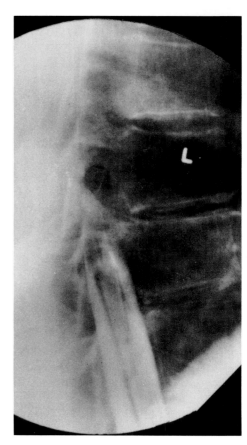

FIG. 11. Anteroposterior thoracic metrizamide myelogram. Note the complete block.

FIG. 12. Lateral view indicates a complete block at the level of the disc.

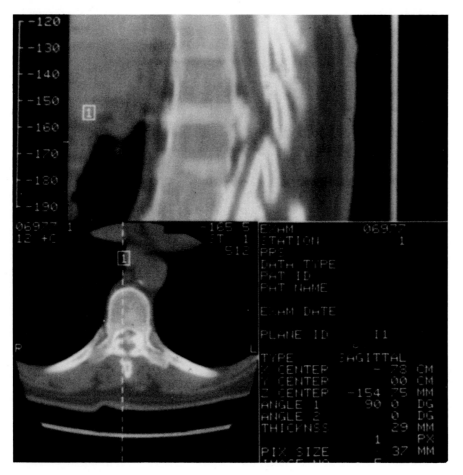

FIG. 13. Sagittal reconstruction of CT scan demonstrates a large thoracic disc herniation with cord compression.

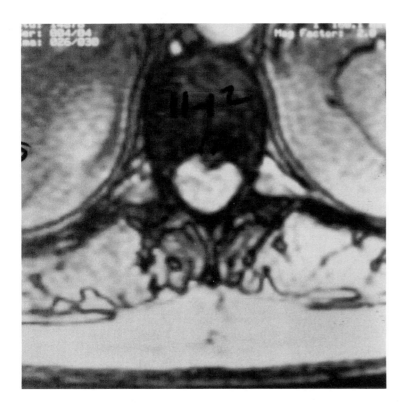

FIG. 14. Axial view using MRI portrays a central thoracic disc herniation.

From the low incidence of clinically important cases, it is apparent that the diagnosis will be difficult to make, since any physician's personal experience with thoracic disc herniation will be quite limited. Further complicating the difficulty in making the diagnosis are the varied symptoms with which the syndrome can present. As discussed in the previous section on thoracic discogenic pain, pain can be variously described and located in the thoracic region, referred to the lumbar area, and radiate anteriorly around the trunk, into the groin, or to the lower extremities.

Neurologic findings may include non-specific lower-

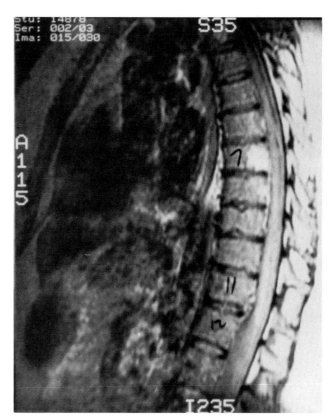

FIG. 15. Sagittal MR image demonstrates thoracic disc herniation with cord compression.

extremity weakness, spasticity, ataxia, numbness, and bowel and bladder disturbance with associated sphincter dysfunction. One or more of these symptoms and signs may present in any combination. For example, the patient may present with only bladder dysfunction or gait ataxia with very little localizing pain, or pain may be the predominant feature, as discussed in the preceding section. Neurologic complexes such as a Brown-Sequard or a Horner's syndrome may be present (18).

Depending on the combination of symptoms, the differential diagnosis can be quite large and include the various diagnoses in Table 1 as well as demyelinating diseases and spinal cord infarction.

Prior to the advent of computerized tomography, the radiologic diagnosis of thoracic disc herniation was often inaccurate. Disc calcification or a calcified mass within the canal gives a clue to the diagnosis, if present. Oil-based myelography allows visualization of large herniations, but these are frequently considered primary tumors, and only at surgery is the true pathology revealed. With the combination of water-soluble myelography and computerized axial tomography, the diagnosis, once suspected, can be made with a high level of sensitivity and specificity (Figs. 11, 12, and 13). As experience is gained and techniques improve, magnetic resonance imaging will likely displace myelographically enhanced CT scanning as the procedure of choice (46) (Figs. 14, 15, 16, and 17). Caldwell has described the use of intercostal motor conduction time in the diagnosis of intercostal nerve root compression (11), but its clinical usefulness was limited by the requirement for general anesthesia due to pain induced by the procedure.

The surgical treatment of the thoracic disc herniation, in terms of the most advantageous approach, has, in the past, been somewhat controversial. The first reported series of surgical treatment utilized thoracic laminectomy followed by extradural or transdural disc fragment excision (3,17,23,25,26,33,35,43,52,54). The results were often disastrous, frequently inducing a greater neurologic deficit. Perot (40) reviewed 91 cases treated by laminectomy; 29 patients were cured, 22 improved, 18 remained unchanged, 16 developed paraplegia post-operatively, and 6 died. As might be expected, the results were far worse for central herniations, in which 15 of 57 cases were rendered paraplegic. This disastrous complication is apparently due to the excessive retraction of the cord that must occur when an anterior and central disc lesion is approached posteriorly or posterolaterally.

Anterolateral approaches using variations of the costotransversectomy have been employed with improved success. First advocated by Hulme (22) in 1960, variations include pedicle excision (38) and division of the erector spinae muscle mass (12) to improve approaches to the thoracic and thoracolumbar spine.

The transthoracic approach appears to be gaining in-creasing popularity as its benefits are recognized. The first report of this approach concerned an anterolateral disc fenestration, wherein the majority of the affected disc was excised, but the actual herniated disc fragment was not removed. The patient made a good recovery. In 1969, Ransohoff et al. (42) and Perot and Munro (40) reported their successful use of a transthoracic approach to remove the disc, including the herniated fragment. Otani (37) reviewed the literature and found 23 cases treated by anterior thoracic approaches up to 1977, all giving a good result. He believed that an anterior extrapleural approach was useful to lessen the morbidity associated with a transpleural approach. Bohlman and Zdeblick's (9) recent review of their experience with thoracic disc herniation, comparing anterior approaches via either a costotransversectomy or a thoracotomy, also concluded that a thoracotomy approach seemed best. Interestingly, they did not routinely perform a fusion following the discectomy (Figs. 18,19,20,21,22, and 23).

Reviewing the experience with thoracic disc herniation at Toronto General Hospital would also seem to indicate that improved results with less morbidity are obtained by employing a transthoracic route to perform the discectomy rather than either a laminectomy or an anterolateral costotransversectomy approach. A total of twenty-four patients have undergone treatment, with a follow-up of from three to twelve years.

The sex distribution was equal and the average age was fifty-two years, with a range of thirty to eighty years. Symptom duration prior to diagnosis ranged from four weeks to eight years, with seventeen patients not diagnosed for at least one year. Twenty-three of twenty-four complained of thoracic or thoracolumbar back pain. Thirteen complained of referred or radiating pain into the legs or girdle-like pain about the trunk. All patients complained of varying degrees of leg weakness or gait disturbance. Bladder dysfunction was present in six. Physical signs included motor weakness in the legs in all patients. Upper motor neuron signs such as spasticity with resultant gait disturbance, hyperreflexia, and a positive Babinski sign were present in fifteen. Sensory changes were present in fifteen, and changes in rectal sphincter tone were present in six.

Radiographs revealed diffuse degenerative changes in the thoracic spine in two thirds. More localized changes such as end-plate wedging suggesting previous Scheuermann's disease, Schmorl's nodes, or local degenerative changes were observed in one third. In only one patient was there calcification of the involved disc space. Calcification of the affected disc space has been emphasized by other authors in the past, but was not found in our patients.

Sixteen of the twenty-four patients underwent oil-based myelography. This led to a correct pre-operative diagnosis in only six; the remaining ten were initially felt

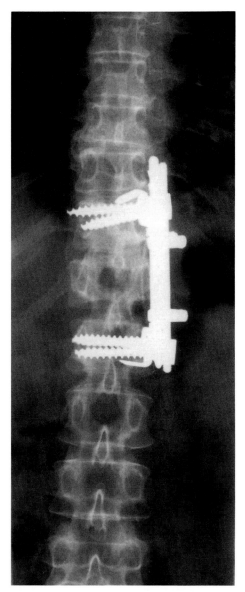

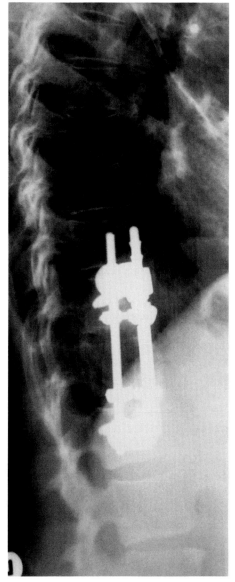

FIG. 16. The patient shown in Figures 14 and 15 presented with paraparesis and signs of an upper motor neuron lesion. An anterior approach consisting of discotomy, fusion, and stabilization with Kostuik-Harrington instrumentation was successfully done. The T12-L1 level was also found to be degenerate and painful (typical) on discography and was included in the fusion.

FIG. 17. Same patient as in Figure 16.

to have either intradural or extradural tumors. Later in the series, water-soluble contrast combined with CT scanning was used in eight patients. This led to the correct pre-operative diagnosis in six, but two patients were initially diagnosed as having lymphoma.

Eighteen of the herniations involved the lower third of the thoracic spine, with the location being centrolateral in eleven, lateral in four, and central in three. The re-maining involved levels above T8 and were centrolateral in location.

Results of surgical treatment can be divided into categories based on the surgical procedure performed. Twelve patients had disc excision via a laminectomy approach, two by a costotransversectomy approach, and ten by a thoracotomy and anterior disc excision, including an interbody fusion. Pre-operatively, there did not

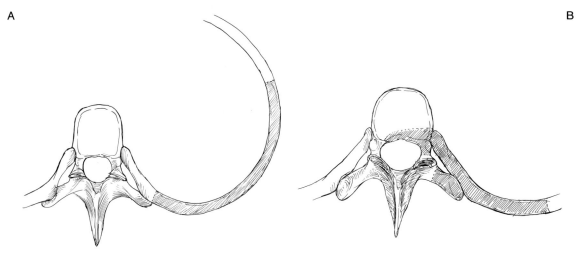

FIG. 18. Removal of thoracic disc. A: Costotransversectomy. B: The anterolateral transthoracic approach is preferred to the costotransversectomy since it permits better access to both anterior and lateral aspects of the thoracic vertebrae.

appear to be major differences in the age or sex distribution or in the degree of neurologic impairment among the groups.

A slightly modified Frankel scale was used to assess motor function before and after surgery. The traditional Frankel grade D was subdivided into a D+ category if bowel and bladder function was normal, and into a D− category if there was bowel and bladder dysfunction. All patients with Frankel grade C had bowel or bladder dysfunction, thus obviating the need to subdivide this class.

In the laminectomy group, nine patients were D+ pre-operatively, one was D−, and two were grade C. Post-operatively, five of the D+ patients improved to grade E, two of the D+ patients remained unchanged, and two D+ patients deteriorated to grade C. Both patients who were grade C pre-operatively and the one patient who was D− deteriorated to grade A. Thus, five patients were improved, two were the same, and five were worse.

The results were equally dismal in the costotransversectomy group, with one patient grade D+ and one patient grade C pre-operatively, deteriorating to grade A post-operatively.

In general, the patients operated on by a laminectomy or costotransversectomy approach were done earliest in the series. Of the ten patients in whom a thoracotomy approach was used, eight were grade D+ pre-operatively, one was D−, and one was grade C. Six of the grade D+ and the one D− patients improved to grade E post-operatively. The one grade C patient improved to grade D+ with recovery of ambulatory ability and bladder function. One D+ patient was unchanged. Unfortunately, one of the D+ patients was made worse and deteriorated to grade B post-operatively. In total, seven patients had complete resolution of their weakness, one was dramatically improved to a functional status, one was unchanged, and one was worse.

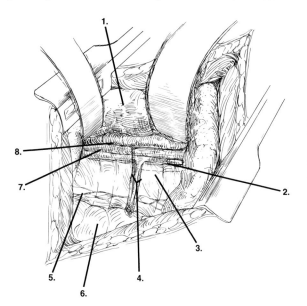

FIG. 19. Transthoracic approach. Area of pleural incision is indicated by the dotted line (right sided approach). 1: Lung. 2: Pleura over azygos vein. 3: Incision of parietal pleura. 4: Segmental vessels. 5: Paravertebral ganglion. 6: Pleura over medial end of rib. 7: Pleura over esophagus. 8: Pleura over aorta. From the left side, the aorta replaces the azygos veins. The esophagus is not seen.

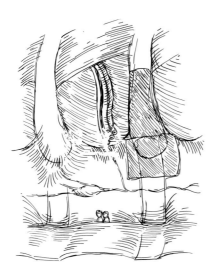

FIG. 20. Area of bone resected.

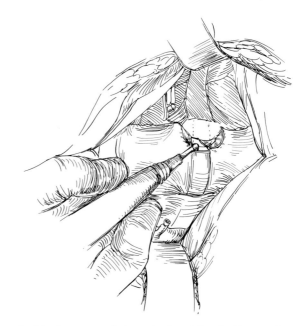

FIG. 21. Removal of thoracic disc (after Bohlman). Bone is resected and a drill is used to remove vertebral body posteriorly on either side of the disc space.

Relief of pain complaints for the entire group was difficult to assess, as complete data were not available for the laminectomy group. All the patients in the thoracotomy group had an interbody fusion performed using the excised rib as bone graft, often supplemented with internal fixation using a Kostuik-Harrington device. Relief of pain in this group was in general excellent, with no patient having significant pain complaints post-operatively. Fusion was added as a result of having previously observed two cases of transthoracic decompression develop an increasing kyphosis and back pain requiring referral to the second author (Kostuik) for correction and fusion with a subsequent good result (Figs. 24, 25, 26, 27, and 28).

Associated complications were about equal in both groups, with one deep vein thrombosis occurring in the laminectomy group and two in the thoracotomy group; one urinary tract infection in the laminectomy group and five in the thoracotomy group. There was one superficial wound infection in the thoracotomy group. Pulmonary complications were not seen in the thoracotomy group.

Although the number of cases in the costotransversectomy group was too small for comparison, it would seem that the thoracotomy approach and anterior disc excision is far safer and results in more frequent neurologic improvement than a laminectomy approach. Because of the poor results reported here and found in the literature,

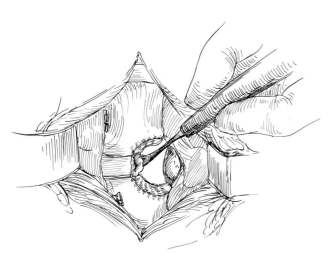

FIG. 22. Curettes are used to remove disc material.

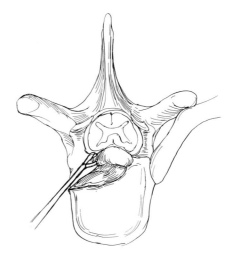

FIG. 23. Posteriorly projecting osteophytes are also removed with curettes.

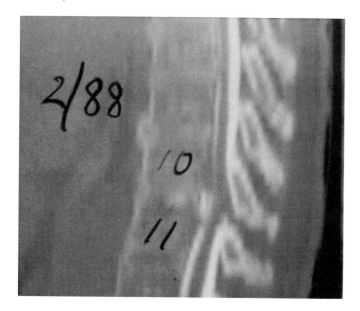

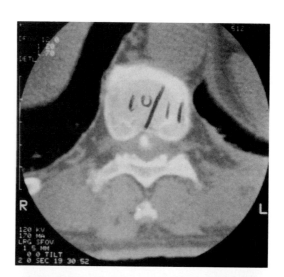

FIG. 24. CT–myelography demonstrates a thoracic disc herniation at T10-T11 with paraparesis.

FIG. 25. CT-myelography.

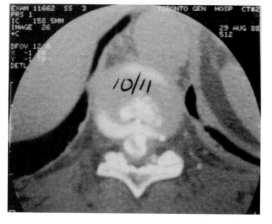

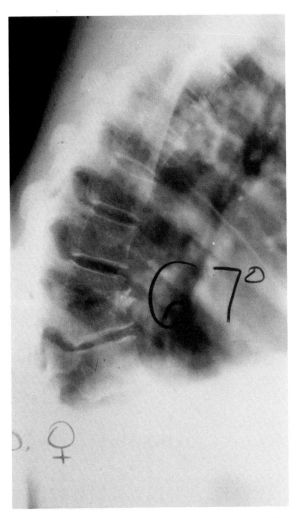

FIG. 26. Patient underwent anterior decompression with relief of her neurological problem but developed severe mechanical back pain with a localized kyphosis.

a laminectomy approach for excision of a central thoracic disc herniation seems contraindicated.

Two techniques are available for disc removal with the transthoracic approach. Bohlman (9) has advocated bone resection from the body posteriorly on either side of the disc space and then removal of the disc material and any projecting osteophytes with curettes (Figs. 18A, 18B, 19, 20, 21, 22, and 23).

We prefer, after proper identification of the level, to excise the disc in its entirety, including bone from the vertebral body posteriorly on either side of the disc space. This produces a reverse V. The final disc fragments are removed with forceps, including, if necessary, spreading and opening the posterior longitudinal ligament. The space is then slightly distracted with the Kostuik-Harrington instrumentation, and bone graft, either rib struts or bicortical iliac crest, is added (Figs. 24, 25, 26, 27, and 28). We feel this latter technique is easier and safer.

POST-THORACOTOMY PAIN SYNDROME

After a thoracotomy (performed for whatever reason), a small percentage of patients (approximately 5%) subsequently report disturbing or painful sensations in or about their thoracotomy incisions. The sensations often follow a dermatomal pattern and seem to be due to irritation of the intercostal nerve. In patients in whom the thoracotomy was performed for treatment of a spinal disorder, e.g., fracture, scoliosis, or disc herniation, about 5% subsequently complain of post-thoracotomy pain. The majority of these patients gradually improve with time and reassurance. A small minority persist in having dysesthetic complaints.

Initially, these patients are treated with an intercostal block consisting of a long-acting local anesthetic and an injectable corticosteroid. This is usually quite helpful in providing long-term if not permanent relief of the pain. If pain relief is obtained by the block initially but returns, the block may be repeated or a more permanent rhizotomy attempted by using 1% phenol in oil or absolute alcohol. This will sometimes create a permanent area of numbness, but based on the local anesthetic injection, the patient often finds this sensory loss more tolerable than the pain.

Very rarely, the symptoms do not respond to the above measures; in this instance, the patient is offered a surgical intercostal rhizotomy, which is performed preganglionic but extradural. This has proven effective in about 80% of the cases.

In general, this complication is usually correctable, and concern about its occurrence should not prevent advantage being taken of the excellent surgical exposure of the thoracic spine provided by a thoracotomy approach.

SUMMARY

Although thoracic pain is a common presenting complaint, determining its exact origin can be quite difficult. It is important to determine quickly whether a significant visceral source for the pain exists so that appropriate treatment may be rendered. Musculoskeletal causes for thoracic back pain are quite varied, but most respond to routine non-operative modalities. It is only in the rare patient in whom all non-operative measures have failed that surgical intervention is attempted. Most of these patients are in the thoracic discogenic pain category and, if properly evaluated, can be successfully treated by a localized anterior fusion.

The presence of significant neurologic deficit implies spinal cord involvement. The cause will usually be either a neoplastic or infectious process. If these are excluded, then a thoracic disc herniation should be considered, as it is a lesion that is often surgically correctable, preferably by an anterior thoracic approach.

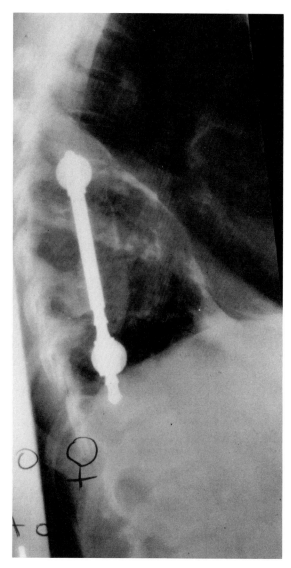

FIG. 27. Kyphosis corrected by a repeat thoracotomy with anterior grafting and Kostuik-Harrington instrumentation.

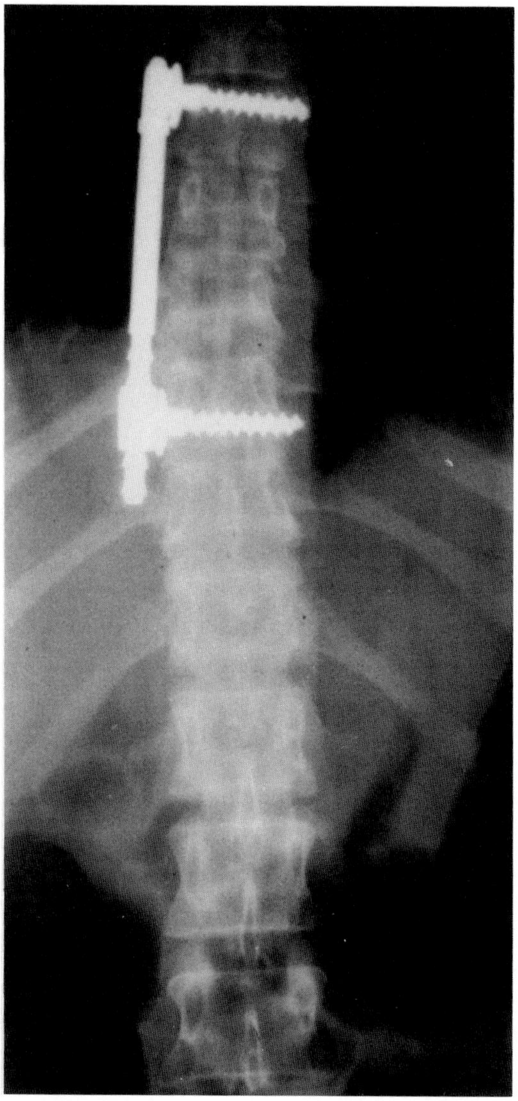

FIG. 28. Same patient as in Figure 27.

REFERENCES

1. Albrand OW, Corkill G (1979): Thoracic disc herniation: Treatment and prognosis. *Spine* 4:41–46.
2. Andrae R (1929): *Beit path anat allg path* 82:464.
3. Arseni C, Nash F (1960): Thoracic intervertebral disc protrusion. A clinical study. *J Neurosurg* 17:418–430.
4. Ashby EC (1977): Abdominal pain of spinal origin. Value of intercostal block. *Ann Roy Col Surg Eng* 59:242–246.
5. Baker HL, Love JG, Uihlein A (1965): Roentgenologic features of protruded thoracic intervertebral disks. *Radiology* 84:1059–1065.
6. Banyai AL (1976): Anterior chest pain. *Chest* 70:69.
7. Benson MKD, Byrnes DP (1975): The clinical syndromes and surgical treatment of thoracic intervertebral disc prolapse. *J Bone Joint Surg* [Br] 57:471–477.
8. Bhole R, Gilmer RE (1984): Two-level thoracic disc herniation. *Clin Orthop* (190):129–131.
9. Bohlman HH, Zdeblick TA (1988): Anterior excision of herniated thoracic discs. *J Bone Joint Surg* [Am] 70:1038–1047.
10. Bradford DS, Garcia A (1969): Neurological complications in Scheuermann's disease. *J Bone Joint Surg* [Am] 51:567–572.
11. Caldwell JW, Crane CR, Boland GL (1968): Determinations of intercostal motor conduction time in diagnosis of nerve root compression. *Arch Phys Med Rehab* 24:515–518.
12. Carson J, Gumbert J, Jefferson A (1971): Diagnosis and treatment of thoracic disc protrusions. *J Neurol Neurosurg Psychiat* 34:68–77.
13. Crafoord C, Hiertonn T, Lindblom K, Olsson SE (1958): Spinal cord compression caused by a protruded thoracic disc. *Acta Orthop Scand* 28:103–107.
14. Dommisse GF (1974): The blood supply of the spinal cord. *J Bone Joint Surg* [Br] 56:225–235.
15. Edgren W, Karaharju EO, Snellman O (1973): Intervertebral disc calcification with complete protrusion interspongially. *Acta Orthop Scand* 44:663–667.
16. Epstein JA (1973): The syndrome of herniation of the lower thoracic intervertebral discs with nerve root and spinal cord compression. *J Neurosurg* 11:525–538.
17. Fisher RG (1965): Protrusions of thoracic disc. The factor of herniation through the dura mater. *J Neurosurg* 22:591–593.
18. Gelch MM (1978): Herniated thoracic disc at T1-2 level associated with Horner's syndrome. Case report. *J Neurosurg* 48:128–130.
19. Hawk WA (1936): Spinal compression caused by ecchondrosis of the intervertebral fibrocartilage: With a review of the recent literature. *Brain* 59:204–224.

20. Hollinshead WH (1974): *Textbook of anatomy, 3d ed.* Hagerstown, Maryland: Harper and Row, pp. 492–500.
21. Hochman SM, Pena C, Ramirez R (1980): Calcified herniated thoracic disc diagnosed by computerized tomography. Case report. *J Neurosurg* 52:722–723.
22. Hulme A (1960): The surgical approach to thoracic intervertebral disc protrusions. *J Neurol Neurosurg Psychiat* 23:133–137.
23. Jefferson A (1975): The treatment of thoracic intervertebral disc protrusions. *Clin Neurol Neurosurg* 1:1–9.
24. Key CA (1838): On paraplegia depending on disease of the ligaments of the spine. *Guy's Hosp Rep* 3:17–34.
25. Logue V (1952): Thoracic intervertebral disc prolapse with spinal cord compression. *J Neurol Neurosurg Psychiat* 15:227–241.
26. Love JG, Kiefer EJ (1950): Root pain and paraplegia due to protrusion of thoracic intervertebral disks. *J Neurosurg* 7:62–69.
27. Love JG, Schorn VG (1965): Thoracic-disk protrusions. *J Am Med Assn* 191:627–631.
28. MacCartee CC Jr, Griffin PP, Byrd EB (1972): Ruptured calcified thoracic disc in a child. Report of a case. *J Bone Joint Surg* [Am] 54:1272–1274.
29. Maiman DJ, Larson SJ, Luck E, El-Ghatit A (1984): Lateral extracavitary approach to the spine for thoracic disc herniation: Report of 23 cases. *Neurosurgery* 14:178–182.
30. Marinacci AA, Courville CB (1962): Radicular syndromes simulating intra-abdominal surgical conditions. *Amer Surg* 28:59–63.
31. McBeath AA, Keene JS (1975): The rib-tip syndrome. *J Bone Joint Surg* [Am] 57:795–797.
32. Middleton GS, Teacher JH (1911): Injury to the spinal cord due to rupture of an intervertebral disc during muscular effort. *Glasgow Med J* 76:1–6.
33. Mixter WJ, Barr JS (1934): Rupture of the intervertebral disc with involvement of the spinal canal. *N Eng J Med* 211:210–215.
34. Nathan H, Weinberg H, Robin GC, Avaid I (1964): The costovertebral joints. Anatomical-clinical observations in arthritis. *Arth Rheum* 7:228–240.
35. Oille JA (1937): Differential diagnosis of pain in the chest. *Can Med Assn J* 37:209–216.
36. O'Leary PF, Camins MB, Polifroni NV, Floman Y (1984): Thoracic disc disease: Clinical manifestations and surgical treatment. *Bull Hosp Joint Dis Orthop Inst* 44:27–40.
37. Otani K, Shunichi M, Shibasaki K, Nomachi S (1977): The surgical treatment of thoracic and thoracolumbar disc lesions using the anterior approach. *Spine* 2:266–275.
38. Patterson RH Jr, Arbit E (1978): A surgical approach through the pedicle to protruded thoracic discs. *J Neurosurg* 48:768–772.
39. Peck FC Jr (1957): A calcified thoracic intervertebral disk with herniation and spinal cord compression in a child. Case report. *J Neurosurg* 13:105–109.
40. Perot PL Jr, Munro DD (1969): Transthoracic removal of midline thoracic disc protrusions causing spinal cord compression. *J Neurosurg* 31:452–458.
41. Raney FL (1966): Costovertebral-costotransverse joint complex as the source of local or referred pain. *J Bone Joint Surg* [Am] 48:1451–1452.
42. Ransohoff J, Spencer F, Siew F, Gage L Jr (1969): Transthoracic removal of thoracic discs. Report of three cases. *J Neurosurg* 31:459–461.
43. Ravichandran G, Frankel HL (1981): Paraplegia due to intervertebral disc lesions: A review of 57 operated cases. *Paraplegia* 19:133–139.
44. Rawlings MS (1963): Differential diagnosis of painful chest. *Geriatrics* 18:139–150.
45. Reeves DL, Brown HA (1968): Thoracic intervertebral disc protrusion with spinal cord compression. *J Neurosurg* 28:24–28.
46. Ross JS, Perez-Reyes N, Masaryk TJ, Bohlman H, Modic MT (1987): Thoracic disk herniation: MR imaging. *Radiology* 165:511–515.
47. Schmorl G (1929): *Fort Geb Rony* 40:629.
48. Sekhar LN, Jannetta PJ (1983): Thoracic disc herniation: Operative approaches and results. *Neurosurgery* 12:303–305.
49. Shaw NE (1975): The syndrome of the prolapsed thoracic intervertebral disc. *J Bone Joint Surg* [Br] 57:412.
50. Shore LR (1935): On osteo-arthritis in the dorsal intervertebral joints. *Brit J Surg* 22:833–839.
51. Simmons EH, Evans DC, Bailey SI (1975): Thoracic disc disease. *J Bone Joint Surg* [Am] 57:475.
52. Terry AF, McSweeney T, Jones HWF (1981): Paraplegia as a sequela to dorsal disc prolapse. *Paraplegia* 19:111–117.
53. Tietze A (1921): Uber eine eigenartige haufung von fallen mit dystrophie der rippenknorpel. *Berl Klin Wochenschr* 58:829–831.
54. Tovi D, Strang RR (1960): Thoracic intervertebral disk protrusions. *Acta Chir Scand* (Suppl) 267.
55. Van Landingham JH (1954): Herniation of thoracic intervertebral discs with spinal cord compression in kyphosis dorsalis juvenilis (Scheuermann's disease). Case report. *J Neurosurg* 11:327–329.
56. Wolf E, Stern S (1976): Costosternal syndrome. *Arch Intern Med* 136:189–191.

PART VI

Lumbar Spine

The Adult Spine: Principles and Practice,
J. W. Frymoyer, Editor-in-Chief.
Raven Press, Ltd., New York © 1991.

CHAPTER **67**

Anatomy and Pathology of the Lumbar Spine

Wolfgang Rauschning

This chapter contains a selection of images illustrating some important normal anatomical features of the lumbar spine and sacrum (Figs. 1 to 3) as well as examples of degenerative changes, traumatic and neoplastic pathology (Figs. 4 to 9).

The nomenclature used here is consistent with the glossary on spinal terminology issued by the American Academy of Orthopaedic Surgeons' Committee on the Spine (1) with two exceptions: The term "spinous process" is used instead of "spine" and the correct anatomical designation "vertebral canal" is used synonymously with the clinically established term "spinal canal."

At the thoracolumbar junction, the intervertebral discs rapidly increase in height. The anterior wall of the vertebral canal is straight; the intervertebral discs show no tendency of bulging into the canal. The lower lumbar vertebrae are slightly wedge-shaped, accounting in part for the lumbar lordosis and lumbosacral angulation. Similarly the discs in the lower lumbar spine are slightly wedge-shaped. The pedicles of the lumbar spine are strong and project posteriorly behind the vertebral bodies. An important exception is the pedicle of L5 which is broader and takes an oblique posterior and lateral course from the posterolateral aspect of the vertebra.

The lower borders of the laminae terminate at the level of the inferior disc and in most cases lumbar spinous processes are heavy and rectangular (Fig. 1B). The

superior articular processes diverge both superiorly and posteriorly, which on axial CT or MR scans renders a biplanar or curvilinear configuration of the lumbar facet joints in that their anterior portions are oriented toward the coronal plane and the posterior ones oriented more sagittally (7,12,19,23).

The transverse processes are flattened anteroposteriorly and run slightly dorsally and upward. They represent attachment sites for the intertransverse ligaments and muscles. The former are continuous with a strong aponeurosis, the lumbodorsal fascia. At the base of the transverse processes, small spike-formed accessory processes emerge to which the accessory-mamillary ligament attaches. These processes are typically located at the recommended entrance point for pedicle screw insertion and may cause insertion problems, especially in percutaneous pedicle fixation. The transverse processes of L5 are attached to the medial portion of the iliac crest by several strong strands of the iliolumbar ligament. Transitional bone and soft-tissue form variations are common in the lumbosacral region and may be quite treacherous both with respect to the identification of the appropriate surgical level as well as for the surgical procedure itself (Figs. 1 and 2).

Depending on the shape and size of the vertebral bodies, the pedicles, and the laminae and articular processes of each vertebra, which together form the bony vertebral foramen, the lumbar vertebral canal may be more ovoid or triangular. Short pedicles entail an inverted teardrop shape and slitlike anteroposterior narrowing of the intervertebral foramen in sagittal cross-section (Fig. 2B), leav-

---

W. Rauschning, M.D., Ph.D.: Department of Orthopaedic Surgery, Uppsala University Academic Hospital, Uppsala, Sweden; Swedish Medical Research Council.

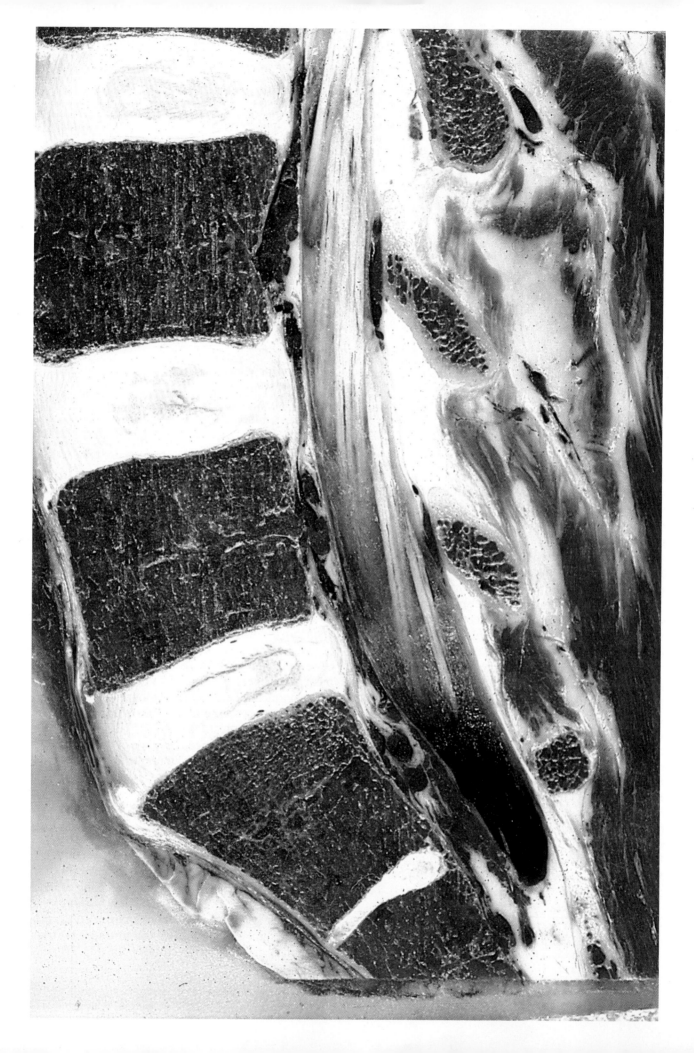

ing less reserve for space-occupying offending lesions (6,8,10,11,25). The transverse diameter of the spinal canal increases from L1 to L5, whereas the sagittal diameter decreases.

The thecal sac is normally wide and occupies the entire vertebral canal. Its size is inversely related to the amount of epidural tissue and also varies widely between individuals. The location of the roots of the cauda equina depends on the position of the patient (prone versus supine) and the postures such as flexion and extension (3,10,13,15,20,24). My studies indicate the roots do not seem to follow a strict pattern, except for the fact that roots bound to exit lie anterolaterally within the thecal sac (Fig. 2).

Posteriorly in the spinal canal, a triangular pad of fat, which is virtually devoid of blood vessels, occupies the space behind the dura between the two ligamenta flava (17,20,21,26). Dissection between the interlaminar ligamenta flava rarely entails hemorrhage; the posterior internal spinal veins lie clustered underneath the lamina and rarely extend under the ligamentum flavum (Fig. 1A). This is of significance both for the surgical exposure, especially the detachment of the ligamentum flavum from the laminae as well as for sublaminar wiring and the insertion of lamina hooks.

The posterior longitudinal ligament attaches to the endplate portion of the vertebrae and to the posterior circumference of the intervertebral discs where it fans out to a thin fibrous layer of diverging collagenous strands, indistinguishably interwoven with the outermost lamellae of the annulus fibrosus. At the midvertebral level this ligament measures barely 1 mm square in axial cross-section; several biomechanical studies have shown that it is not particularly strong. It bridges the concavity behind the vertebral bodies in a bowstring fashion, creating an osseomembranous compartment for the voluminous ventral internal venous plexus.

Ventral internal veins communicate with a system of venous channels which transgresses the midportion of each vertebra through vascular foramina (Fig. 2) which commonly are referred to as the outlet of the Batson vein plexus (4,5,13,14). The fact that the posterior longitudinal ligament is a suspensory ligament for the thecal sac to which it is closely attached, also means that spinal movements influence the position of the thecal sac and the retrovertebral venous plexus space. The posterior longitudinal ligament is one component of the suspensory system of Hofmann ligaments (3,9,14,18,20,24). The ligament also has a rich supply of sensory nervous fibers and probably acts more as a strain gauge type of positional control device than a mechanical restraint.

The thick lumbar spinal ganglia occupy the upper portion of the intervertebral foramen (subpedicular notch), surrounded by connective tissue and fat which is interspersed with foraminal veins. These veins are less voluminous than in the thoracic and cervical spine. The spinal branch of the segmental radicular artery and the recurrent sinuvertebral nerve also traverse the upper portion of the foramen. The lower foramen is bounded by the intervertebral disc anteriorly and the ligamentum flavum joint capsule posteriorly (Figs. 1B and 5) and normally is a narrow slit containing small veins and some lymphatics.

The thickest portion of the conus medullaris usually lies at the T11 and T12 levels. Anterior and posterior bundles of cauda equina roots emerge from the anterolateral and posterolateral sulcus of the spinal cord and of the conus on each side. Contrary to the cervical and upper thoracic roots, which form by stepwise fusion of small filaments or rootlets, the lumbosacral roots emerge directly from the cord without intermittent rootlets. In axial cross-section and on contrast enhanced CT scans and on MR images, the conus area with the dorsal and ventral root bundles take the shape of a butterfly. In the lumbar spine (7,15,16,18,22), the intervertebral discs further increase in thickness relative to the height of the vertebrae. Whereas the discs of L1 and L2 have a straight posterior margin, the discs of L3, L4, and L5 have a distinctly posteriorly convex, bulging configuration.

Contrary to the discs in the thoracic spine, where the peripheral layers of the annulus fibrosus insert into the apophyseal ring, the lower lumbar discs feature insertion of the outer annular lamellae beyond the assimilated ring apophysis into the periosteum and Sharpey's fibers of the vertebral body. This normal architecture of the discs can be seen in sagittal CT and MR scans and should not be confused with pathological bulging of the discs as a result of their degeneration or instability (7,19,22).

In horizontal cross-section, the vertebral bodies of the cervical, thoracic, and the upper lumbar spine as well as their intervening discs have a more or less distinct concave configuration posteriorly. The only exception is the L5 body and the lumbosacral disc which always have a posteriorly convex or at least straight posterior border. Only at the L5 disc a small amount of areolar soft tissue may be interposed between the dura and the annulus; at all other levels the dura is firmly attached to the disc, although the dura can be dissected from the disc without much difficulty. At the disc level the ventral internal veins have merged into one vertically running major vein which connects adjacent retrovertebral veins in a ropeladder fashion (2,4,13,15). This vascular architecture is beautifully outlined in ascending epidural phlebograms. In the lumbar spine, the thecal sac is normally round. The location of the roots in the thecal sac varies with posture and movement as described for the cervical spinal cord.

Normal movement in the lumbar spine entails less anterior posterior translatory movement than in the cervical spine because the facet joints have a less pronounced slope (Fig. 5). Considerable inter-individual variations are found. In spines with developmentally short pedicles and borderline dimensions of the vertebral canal, even slight hypermobility or compromise by functional or structural degenerative lesions, fracture fragments, or segmental translation may cause compromise of the intraspinal blood vessels and nerve structures (10,25).

The thick lumbar roots with their voluminous ganglia and the thick postganglionic lumbar spinal nerves invariably and snugly follow the medial and inferior aspect of the pedicles. Owing to their size, they normally occupy a large proportion of the lumbar root canals (foramina). Hypermobility and/or reduction of the intervertebral disc height (e.g., following chemonucleolysis) may cause a relatively sudden decrease in foramen dimensions and compression of the root which may be further accentuated in extension and/or rotation (10). Figure 5 shows the undistorted relationships between the nerve roots and the vertebral column in a specimen which had been frozen in moderate extension.

The sacrum is a composite bone which has formed by fusion of five vertebral segments. Its upper surface bares the endplate for the lumbosacral disc and the superior articular processes. The thick pars lateralis (ala sacri) has ear-shaped articular surfaces of hyaline cartilage which articulate with the wings of the ilium anteriorly. Posteriorly a meshwork of very strong ligaments contributes to the stability of the sacroiliac joint which in an anatomical sense more resembles an ampharthrosis (like a discovertebral junction or the symphysis pubis) than a diarthrodial articulation. At its anterior, concave surface transverse ridges indicate the site of the disc remnants. They terminate at the trumpet-shaped pelvine foramina which transmit the sacral ganglia and nerves and small blood vessels. At the convex posterior surface much smaller dorsal foramina carry the small dorsal sacral nerves. The sacral canal is triangular in horizontal cross-section, with narrower sagittal than transverse dimensions.

Figure 4 shows a cross-section at the disc level in an inveterated thoracolumbar compression fracture. Analysis of the specimen clarified that the bone of the vertebral body had healed and was stable although there was a marked loss in the anterior height of the vertebra. Fissures of the upper endplate of the fractured vertebra were found. An old hematoma was occupying the entire center portion of the disc. This raises the question whether and to what extent traumatically injured intervertebral discs can heal and if traumatic disc and endplate lesions develop into late spondylosis, i.e., degenerative changes of the "disc joint" with progressive instability of the injured segment, reactive circumferential enthesopathic ridge formation at the insertion of the

outer annulus, and eventually endplate sclerosis and fusion of the cartilaginous endplates (Fig. 7).

Degenerative changes of the spine occur at the level of the mobile portion of the segment and only in rare cases at the level of the bony ring (pedicles and lamina). Figures 6A, 6B, and 7 illustrate advanced degenerative lumbar spinal stenosis. At the disc level the ballooning of the disc anteriorly and the marked thickening of the ligamenta flava in combination with the hypertrophy of the superior articular processes compress the vertebral canal to a small triangular conduit in which the thecal sac is compressed to a small tube in which the roots lie tightly packed. In the same specimen, the subpedicular portion of the foramen is severely encroached on by arthrosis-type osteophytes at the insertion areas of the ligamentum flavum. The various components of the nerve roots are compressed from inferiorly by the protruding disc and posteriorly by the large facet joint osteophytes and pressed and flattened against the unyielding pedicle.

In spondylolisthesis, a highly complex pathoanatomical situation is found. The instability owing to the insufficient restraint of the posterior elements inevitably entails early and severe degeneration of the disc which allows pathological translatory and rotatory movements. The "beak" of the pars interarticularis is typically dislodged anteriorly and inferiorly and plunges into the interlaminar ligamentum flavum, pushing it anteriorly against the upper endplate of the vertebra below and the thin remnants of the posterior annulus fibrosus, both compressing the root components from inferiorly (Fig. 8).

Weakening of the lumbar vertebral column by disseminated metastatic disease occurs where the venous channels connect the external and internal anterior spinal vein system through the waist-shaped midportion of the vertebral bodies. Cancer metastases spread along venous channels to the subchondral collecting venous system (4) and eventually weaken the cancellous bone which supports the endplates. In early stages of vertebral column collapse the upper and later the lower endplate yield (Fig. 9A), which causes tilting of the endplate fractures and central protrusion of cancellous vertebral material interspersed with tumorous masses into the vertebral canal. In some cases, pathological fractures severing fragments resemble those found in traumatic thoracolumbar fractures (Fig. 9B). In other cases the vertebral bodies "implode," allowing the discs to expand into the midportion of the vertebral body which then assumes the shape of a fish vertebra. The posterior elements are less commonly affected by metastatic lesions.

Acknowledgments and references follow on page 1486.

FIG. 1. A (page 1470). Sagittal section through a normal lower lumbar spine and upper sacrum of a young female adult at the level of the lateral portion of the thecal sac. This level displays the segmental root bundles converging towards each intervertebral level. The L3, L4, and L5 discs all display a slight posterior convexity and attachment of the peripheral layers of the annulus fibrosus into the border of the vertebral bodies some millimeters beyond the apophyseal ring. The vertebral bodies all display concavities posteriorly and at L5 a large venous vascular foramen (arrow). These concavities are occupied by epidural fat and the ventral internal venous plexus which communicates with the veins crossing the vertebral body through the vascular foramina. Note that the posterior vertebral body wall is weak at the level of these foramina and that fractures usually run through these channels (see Fig. 9B). The laminae have a characteristic shape in sagittal cross-section. Towards the vertebral canal only a narrow vertical band of cortical bone is exposed. Superiorly the laminae have a sharp ridge. The lamina is sloping postero-inferiorly and the ligamentum flavum attaches to a large area of its inferior, posteriorly receding surface. At the infrajacent lamina the ligamentum flavum attaches to the sharp upper ridge and a small area posterior to this ridge. Note that the ligamentum flavum at the lumbosacral level is much thinner than at the levels above. Anomalies and variations are common in the transitional lumbosacral segment. In this specimen a very thin "ligamentum flavum membrane" bridges the posterior arch equivalents of the first and second sacral segment (open arrow). The cul de sac (here filled with blood-tinted CSF) terminates slightly below the S1-S2 level which is delineated by the vestige of the S1 disc.

FIG. 1. B (page 1471). Sagittal section through the pedicles of the same specimen. The discs display the texture of the lamellae of the lateral portion of the annulus fibrosus. Some of the endplates show markedly concave configuration. The pedicles are relatively short, causing an inverted teardrop shape of the foramina. The important neurovascular structures are located in the "subpedicular notch" which corresponds to the deep incisura vertebralis inferior of the vertebral body. The foramen cross-section can be divided into a subpedicular (vertebral) portion and a disc- or retrodiscal portion. The former is bounded by bone anteriorly and superiorly and by ligamentum flavum/joint capsule posteriorly. The latter is frequently obliterated (especially at L4-L5) because the disc inserts into the upper aspect of the pedicle and physiologically "bulges" and because the joint capsule/ligamentum flavum broadly attaches to the anterior surface of the superior articular process. This attachment usually extends to the upper surface of the pedicle. At L4 and L5 the dorsal root ganglia can be distinguished from the whiter and smaller ventral roots.

FIG. 2 (page 1472). Axial section through a typical vertebra at the level of the mid-pedicle. The cancellous bone is coarse and strong. Venous vascular channels traverse the vertebral body and transgress the cortical bone posteriorly in the midline and anterolaterally on the right side. Anteriorly, the vertebra is braced by the thick and wide anterior longitudinal ligament (1). The posterior longitudinal ligament is narrow and thin and always attached to the dura (2). Behind the base of the transverse processes a pointed bony spike, the accessory process (closed arrows), lies exactly in the trajectory along which screws typically are inserted into the pedicle. This explains occasional difficulties encountered during percutaneous insertion of pedicle screws which tend to slide out of the "bulls-eye" image of the pedicle. Posteriorly, the upper sharp margin of the lamina and of the spinous process are visualized. The thecal sac is displayed at the level of the axillary outpouchings of the dura which constitute the steeply inferiorly directed offset of the root sleeves. Posteriorly the thecal sac is bounded by the sublaminar veins. These dorsal internal veins are far less voluminous than the ventral internal veins.

FIG. 3 (page 1473). Coronal section through the mid-portion of the pedicles of L2, L3, and L4 showing the course of the nerve roots. The thecal sac is wide and accommodates the thick lumbar cauda equina nerve roots. Owing to the lumbar lordosis, the roots run slightly posteriorly in the lower portion of this figure. The thinner sacral roots lie more posteriorly in the midline. The shallow root sleeve pouches are situated at the lower medial aspect of the pedicles. Still intrathecally, the dorsal and ventral roots snugly follow the medial surface of the pedicles. The cancellous and cortical bony constituents as well as the cross sectional shape of the pedicles vary within wide ranges. At the L2-L3 level large veins lie lateral to the dura, at L3-L4 the dura is predominantly bordered by fat interspersed with smaller veins. At L2-L3 the section is closer to the base of the pedicles and therefore shows the ventral internal venous plexus whereas at L3-L4 the posterior, less vascularized portion of the foramen is displayed. At two levels the entire course of the "roots" can be followed. It consists of (1) the intrathecal root, (2) the root sheath, (3) the dorsal root ganglion and the ventral root, and (4) the postganglionic lumbar nerve. The long, cylindrical ganglions of the lumbar spine take a steep obliquely inferiorly directed course towards the upper lateral corner of the infrajacent pedicle. Lateral to the ganglion and close to the inferior-lateral margin of the pedicle the segmental arteries are situated (arrows). The lumbar nerve curves around the lateral aspect of the pedicle below, firmly held by the deep portions of the iliopsoas muscle.

Figures 4, 5, 6A, and 6B follow on pages 1476–1479.

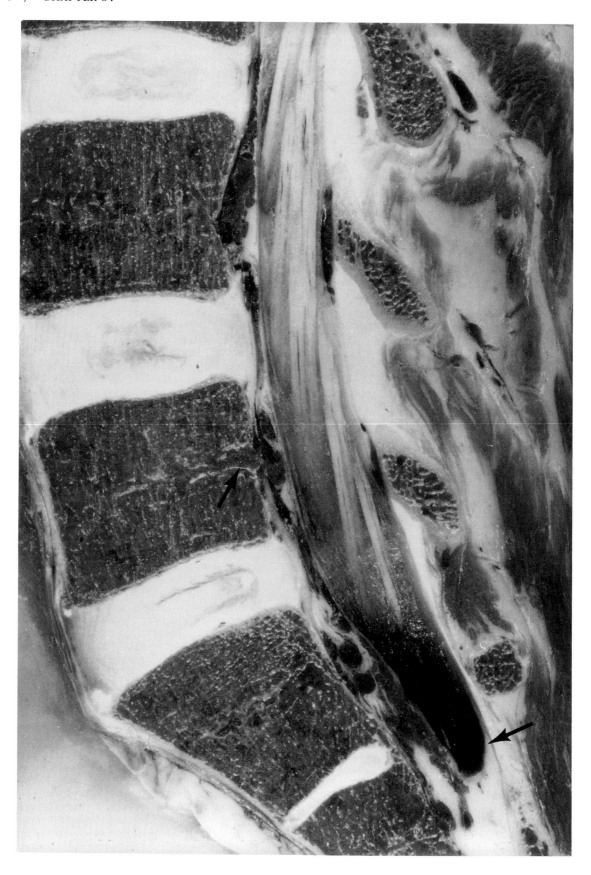

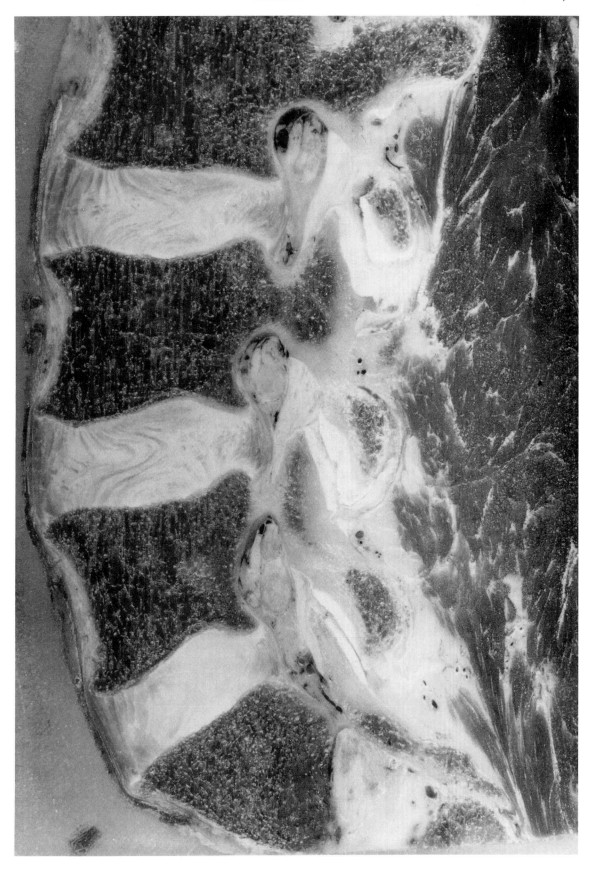

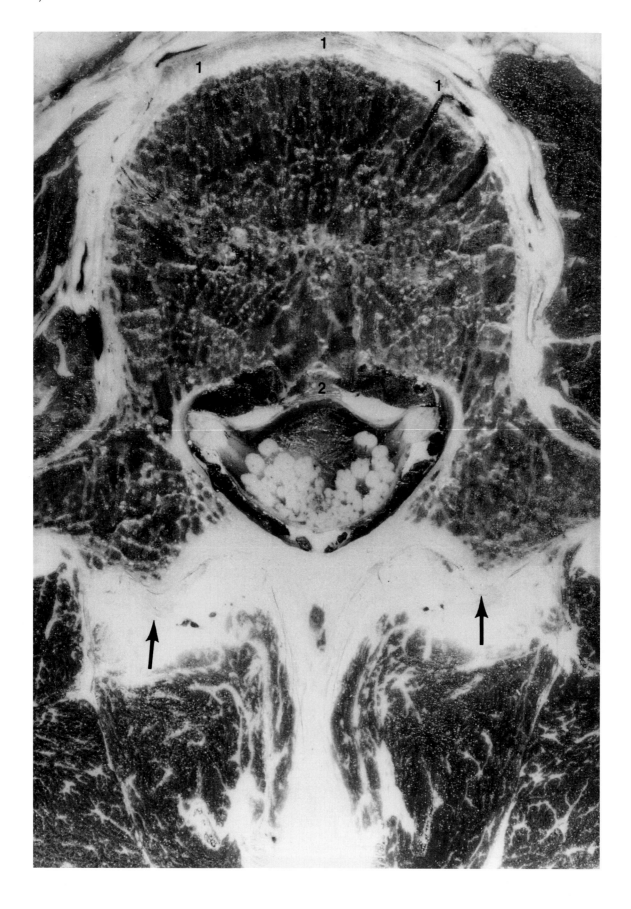

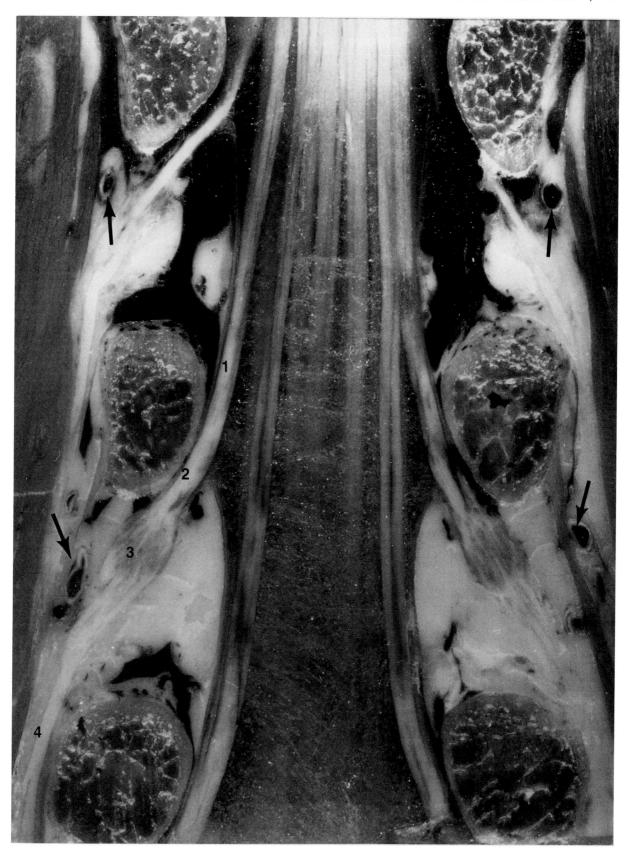

FIG. 4 (page 1476). This specimen is from a 32-year-old male who had sustained a typical burst fracture of L1 ten years ago. The fracture was treated conservatively. He committed suicide because he had relentless and increasing back pain and was denied monetary compensation. Serial sections and radiographs showed that the vertebral body had healed with kyphotic angulation but there was practically no encroachment on the size of the vertebral canal. This axial section through the lower endplate of L1 and the L1-L2 disc shows an inveterated hematoma (black center area) in the injured disc. There is marked disruption of the inner annular lamellae. The cartilaginous endplate and the lateral annulus are sectioned tangentially and display no gross abnormalities. The thecal sac is rounded-triangular and shows a perfectly normal arrangement of the postero- and anterolateral cauda equina root bundles surrounding the distal conus medullaris.

FIG. 5 (page 1477). Sagittal high power photograph of the L4-L5 facet joint and foramen in a spine which was positioned in extension in the intact cadaver and frozen in situ to maintain the undistorted soft tissue-bone relationships. The extension was done without axial loading. The extension induces a sagittal rotation of L4 posteriorly on L5. In addition, the slight obliquity of the facet joint forces a slight posterior translation of L4. Extension causes the tip of the inferior articular process to hit the pars interarticularis of L5 which also is hugged from inferiorly by the superior articular process (SAP) of S1. The joint capsule is elongated and severely compressed against the interarticular pars. The degree of angulation is obvious from the wedge-shaped opening of the superior joint space into which a loose areolar meniscoid synovial tag is projecting (1). The ligamentum flavum joint capsule attaches broadly to the anterior surface of the SAP. It is pushed into the subpedicular notch and compresses and flattens the dorsal root ganglion (2) posteriorly. Anterior to the ganglion the separate ventral roots are discernible (arrows).

FIG. 6. A (page 1478). Severe degenerative spinal stenosis at the L4-L5 level in a 70-year-old man who had a history of intermittent claudication. The central and lateral stenosis is most pronounced at this motion segment level. The encroachment is almost exclusively caused by soft tissues. Anteriorly, the circumferentially "ballooning" disc narrows the thecal sac anteriorly and also completely obliterates the retrodiscal portion of the root canals (compare with Fig. 2B). The facet joints, especially the superior articular processes (1) are moderately hypertrophied, rendering a ball-and-socket configuration of the facet joints. Note the effusion posteriorly of the left facet joint and the sclerotic meniscoid tag posteriorly into the right facet joint (arrows). The thecal sac is severely compressed posterolaterally by the thick ligamentum flavum (2) and assumes a triangular slit-shaped configuration in which the roots of the cauda equina are tightly packed without any cerebrospinal fluid surrounding them. The two ligamenta flava are continuous posteriorly with the thick and degenerated interspinous ligament (3).

FIG. 6. B (page 1479). A few millimeters above the level of Figure 6A the morphology changes dramatically. The posterior contour of the vertebral body appears beveled and slightly V-shaped. From posteriorly large enthesopathic insertion-site osteophytes of the ligamentum flavum into the superior articular processes (1) cause complete obliteration of the subpedicular notch and of the lateral recess. The ganglia are seen laterally (2), flattened against the inferior surface of the pedicles by the disc underneath (see Fig. 6A). Anteriorly in the vertebral canal, thick and congested veins are visible (black). The thecal sac is flattened from the sides but has a much wider diameter in this less mobile portion of the motion segment and the thin cauda equina roots are surrounded by CSF.

Figures 7, 8, 9A, and 9B follow on pages 1482–1485.

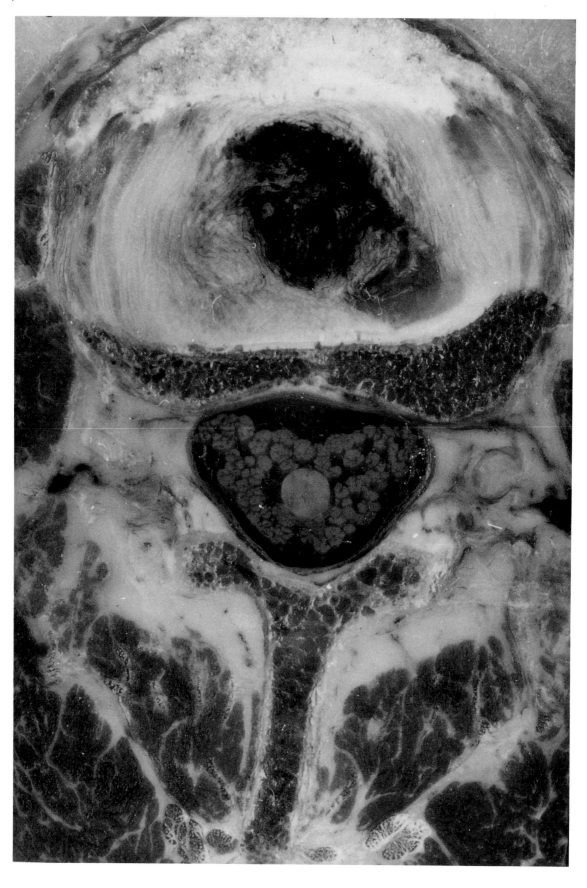

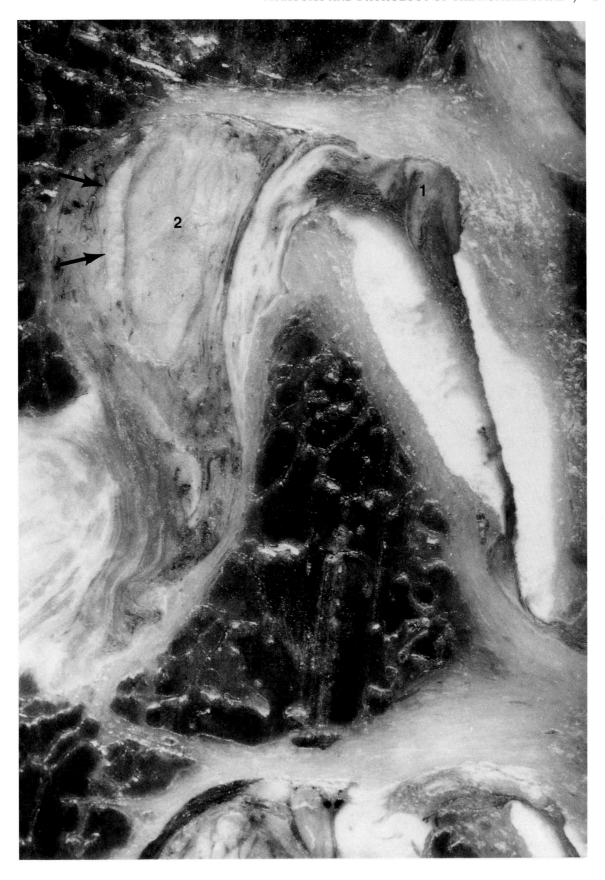

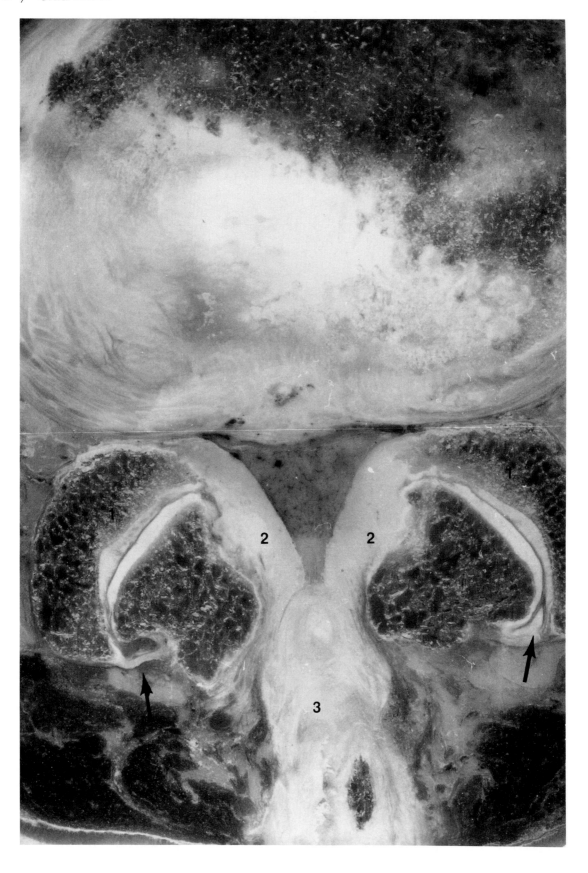

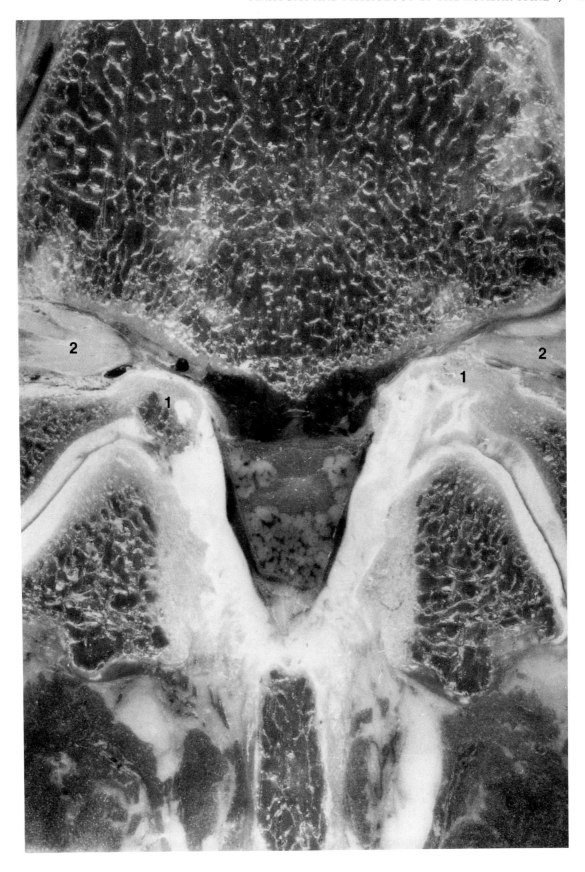

FIG. 7 (page 1482). Sagittal section through a degenerated lower lumbar spine of a 68-year-old man with no history of back pain or radiculopathy. At L5-S1 there is complete resorption of the intervertebral disc and stable fusion of the cartilaginous endplates (1). A 1.5 cm wide band of subchondral endplate sclerosis borders this fusion area (2). Posteriorly in the disc, hard and dark outer annular layers are extruded into the midzone or pedicle portion of the radicular canal in which the relatively small dorsal root ganglion (3) snugly follows the pedicle. The radicular artery anterior to the ganglion (arrow) is very small and so are the segmental veins which, however, are not entirely collapsed. The total resorption of the disc also entails a severe shortening in the posterior elements as demonstrated here by the axial shortening subluxation of the facet joint. Its vertical, apparently less loaded facet carries macroscopically normal hyaline cartilage (4) whereas the superior tip of the upper articular process erodes into the inferior aspect of the pars interarticularis of L5 (arrow). There is osteoarthrosis with osteophyte formation of the tip of the SAP.

FIG. 8 (page 1483). Isthmic spondylolisthesis of L4-L5 in a 44-year-old male. In this sagittal section through the medial border of the pedicle the "beak" of the pars interarticularis (1) plunges into the interlaminar ligamentum flavum and causes it to mushroom anteriorly into the lateral recess (2). L4 is markedly rotated posteriorly which is facilitated by the severe internal disruption of the L4 disc. Its posterior annulus is partially detached superiorly from the apophyseal rim (arrow) and allows the posterior annulus fibrosus to project posteriorly, virtually closing the lateral recess inferiorly. The extension-rotation of L4 causes the sharp lower rim of the pedicle to "fall" down on the ganglion like a guillotine. Subchondral endplate sclerosis appears to designate areas of particular axial stress exposition (3).

FIG. 9. A (page 1484). Pathological fracture of a midlumbar vertebra weakened by a hypernephroma metastasis. Both the upper and the lower endplates have yielded in an almost symmetrical fashion and triangular bone fragments are tilted so as to create the appearance of a "fish vertebra." The overall height of this vertebral segment is slightly decreased but no major sagittal kyphotic angulation has yet occurred. The adjacent discs seem to have exploded into the collapsed vertebra. Posteriorly in the vertebra, infiltrative cancerous growth at the site of the Batson plexus venous outlet causes the periosteum and the dura to bulge posteriorly into the vertebral canal (1). Note that the disc margins are almost straight anteriorly and posteriorly. The vertebra below displays normal anatomy with natural texture of the cancellous bone and macroscopically normal red bone marrow. In the center of its posterior wall a normal basivertebral vein outlet is seen (asterisk).

FIG. 9. B (page 1485). Partial collapse of the L1 vertebra due to a superior endplate failure in the same spine. The inferior part of the vertebra is macroscopically normal. At the level of the basivertebral vein a focal osteolytic metastasis has caused a compression-fracture type of failure of the upper endplate, detaching a triangular upper posterior fragment to rotate posteriorly into the vertebral canal. The stroma of the nucleus pulposus tracks into the weakened vertebra giving the impression of a volcanic eruption. The fragment is attached to the entire posterior annulus which serves as a soft tissue hinge together with the posterior longitudinal ligament.

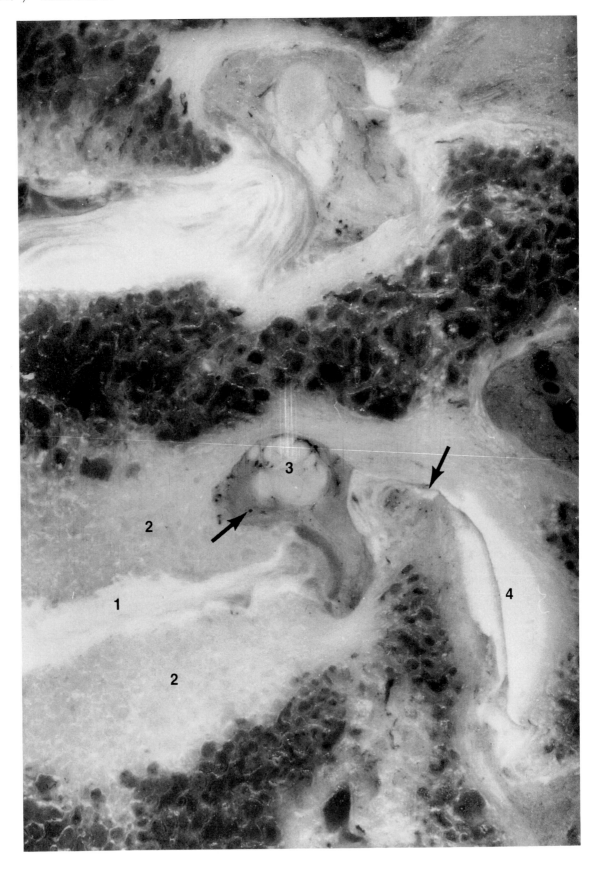

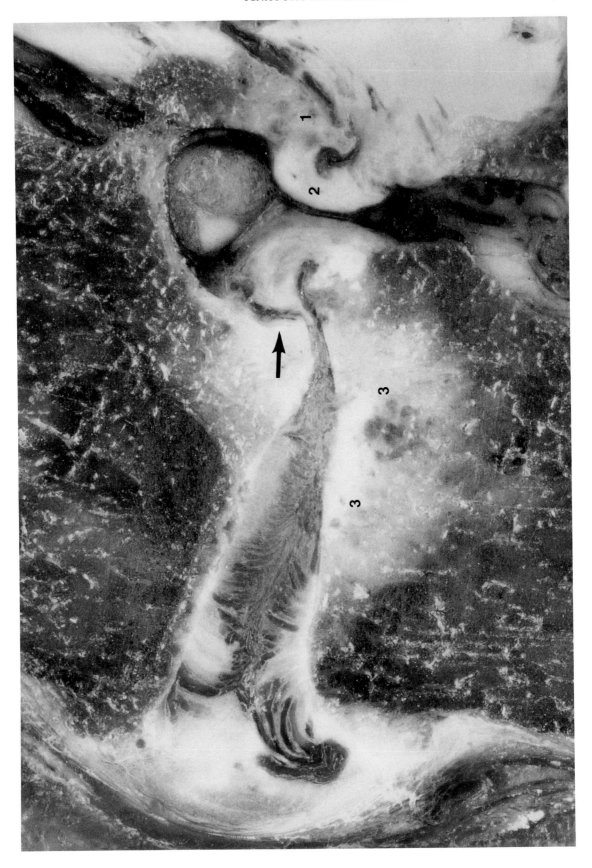

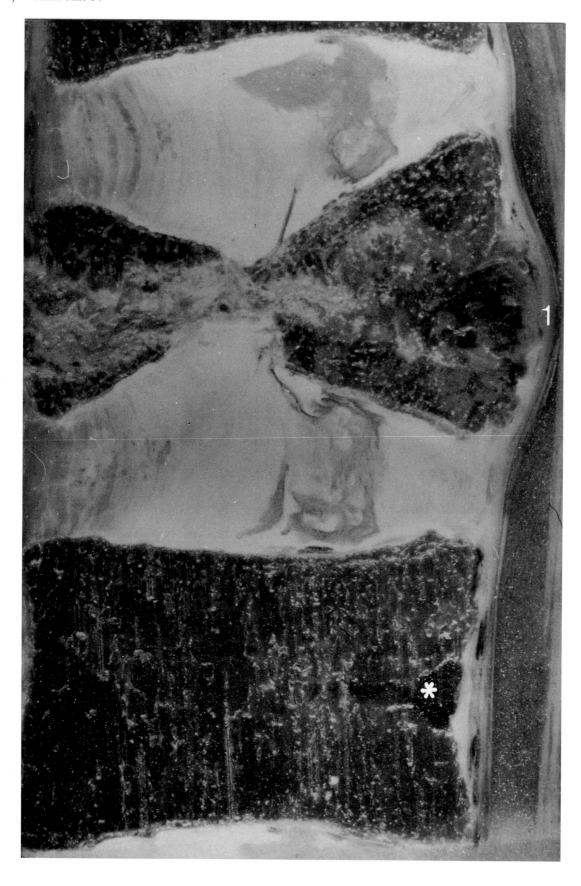

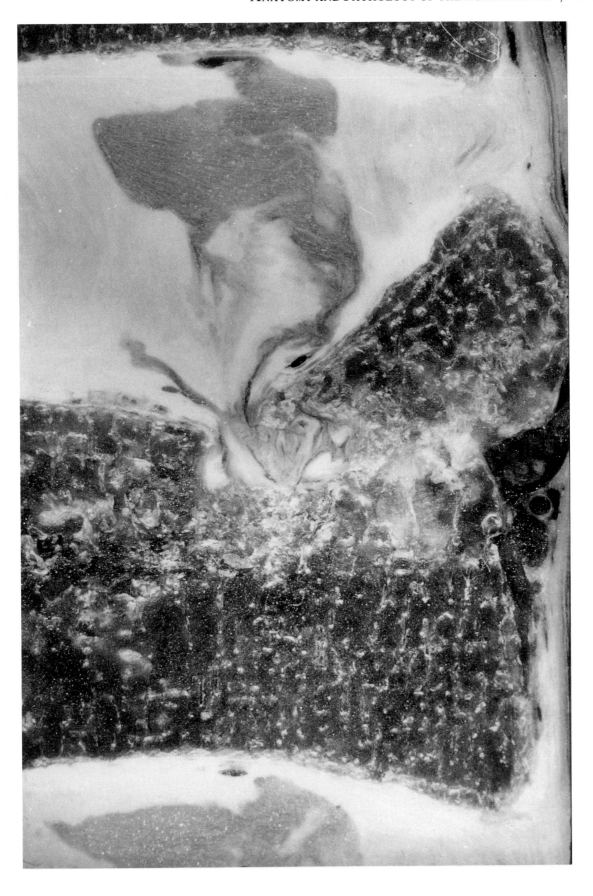

ACKNOWLEDGMENTS

The author wishes to thank the Swedish Medical Research Council, the Swedish Cancer Research Foundation, and the Trygg Hansa Insurance Company, Stockholm.

REFERENCES

1. American Academy of Orthopaedic Surgeons (1980): *Glossary of spinal terminology.* Document 675–80.
2. Batson OV (1957): The vertebral vein system. *Am J Roentgenol* 78:195–212.
3. Breig A (1978): *Adverse mechanical tension in the central nervous system: An analysis of cause and effect: Relief by functional neurosurgery.* New York; John Wiley.
4. Crock HV, Yoshizawa H (1981): *The blood supply of the vertebral column and spinal cord in man.* New York: Springer Verlag.
5. Emery I, Hamilton G (1980): Epidurography using metrizamide. An outpatient examination. *Clin Radiol* 31:643–649.
6. Farfan HF (1980): The pathological anatomy of degenerative spondylolisthesis. A cadaver study. *Spine* 5:412–418.
7. Glenn WV, Burnett K, Rauschning W (1986): *Magnetic resonance imaging of the lumbar spine: Nerve root canals, disc abnormalities, anatomic correlations, and case examples.* Milwaukee: General Electric Medical Systems.
8. Hadley LA (1961): Anatomico-roentgenographic studies of the posterior spinal articulations. *Am J Roentgenol* 86:270–276.
9. Hofmann M (1898): Die Befestigung der Dura Mater im Wirbelkanal. *Arch Anat Physiol (Anat Abteilung)* 403:1898–1911.
10. Kirkaldy-Willis WH, Wedge JH, Yong-Hing K, Reilly J (1978): Pathology and pathogenesis of lumbar spondylosis and stenosis. *Spine* 3:319–328.
11. Lee CK, Rauschning W, Glenn WV (1988): Lumbar lateral spinal canal stenosis. Classification, pathologic anatomy and surgical decompression. *Spine* 13:313–320.
12. Lewin T (1964): Osteoarthritis in lumbar synovial joints: A morphologic study. *Acta Orthop Scand (Suppl)* 73:1–112.
13. Lewit K, Sereghy T (1975): Lumbar peridurography with special regard to the anatomy of the lumbar peridural space. *Neuroradiology* 8:233–240.
14. Louis R (1978): Topographic relationships of the vertebral column, spinal cord and nerve roots. *Anat Clin* 1:3–12.
15. McCormick CC (1978): Radiology in low back pain and sciatica: An analysis of the relative efficacy of spinal venography, discography and epidurography in patients with a negative or equivocal myelogram. *Clin Radiol* 29:393–406.
16. Monajati A, Wayne WS, Rauschning W, Ekholm SE (1987): The cauda equina: MR imaging considerations. *Am J Neuroradiol* 8:893–900.
17. Ramsey RH (1966): The anatomy of the ligamenta flava. *Clin Orthop* 44:129–140.
18. Rauschning W (1983): Computed tomography and cryomicrotomy of lumbar spine specimens. A new technique for multiplanar anatomic correlation. *Spine* 8:170–180.
19. Rauschning W (1984): Detailed sectional anatomy of the spine (chapter 3). In: *Multiplanar CT of the spine,* SLG Rothman, WV Glenn, eds. Baltimore: University Park Press, pp. 33–85.
20. Rauschning W (1987): Normal and pathologic anatomy of the lumbar root canals. *Spine* 12:1008–1019.
21. Rauschning W (1989): Pathomorphology of lumbar spinal stenosis (chapter 5). In: *Lumbar spinal stenosis,* F Postacchini, ed. New York: Springer Verlag, pp. 87–99.
22. Reicher MA, Gold RH, Halbach VV, Rauschning W, Wilson GH, Lufkin RB (1986): MR imaging of the lumbar spine: Anatomic correlations and the effects of technical variations. *Am J Roentgenol* 147:891–898.
23. Schmorl G, Junghanns H (1971): *The human spine in health and disease, 2nd Amer ed.* New York: Grune and Stratton.
24. Spencer DL, Irwin GS, Miller JA (1983): Anatomy and significance of fixation of the lumbosacral nerve roots in sciatica. *Spine* 8:672–679.
25. Verbiest H (1975): Pathomorphologic aspects of developmental lumbar stenosis. *Orthop Clin North Am* 6:177–196.
26. Yong-Hing K, Reilly J, Kirkaldy-Willis WH (1976): The ligamentum flavum. *Spine* 1:226–234.

The Adult Spine: Principles and Practice,
J. W. Frymoyer, Editor-in-Chief.
Raven Press, Ltd., New York © 1991.

CHAPTER 68

Biomechanics of the Lumbar Spine

A. Basic Principles

Malcolm H. Pope, David G. Wilder, and Martin H. Krag

OVERVIEW AND DEFINITIONS

The spine can be considered a flexible multi-curved column. Hirsch and Nachemson (52) have reported that the shape is important in absorbing energy and protecting against impact.

The spine has four major interrelated and somewhat disparate functions: (a) support, (b) mobility, (c) housing and protection, and (d) control. The spine supports the internal organs, the upper and lower extremities, the trunk, the head, and external load moments. Mobility is required for the many physical tasks of daily living and work which tend to complicate the spine structure. The basic functional unit of the spine is termed the motion segment as shown in Figure 1. The motions of the individual spinal segments are important in contributing to the total motion of the lumbar spine. The biomechanics of the motion segment will be described subsequently. The spine architectures also serve to protect the spinal

cord and nerves as they pass from the head to their point of departure to either the upper or lower extremities. The spinal cord terminates at the first or second lumbar vertebra and beyond this point is the cauda equina.

The facet (or zygoapophyseal) joints are essential to the control of normal motion, and they also serve as a constraint because of their orientation. Thus, the motion of each segment is controlled actively by muscles and passively by ligaments. These tissues attach to the spinous and transverse processes which act as lever arms.

Important terms are defined as follows:

Motion segment: The basic anatomic unit of the spine as shown in Figure 1.

Stress: The force normalized by the area over which it acts. Normal stress is perpendicular to the cross section and sheer stress is parallel to it.

Strain: Deformation divided by the original length of the specimen.

Stiffness: The ratio of a load to the deformation it causes.

Compliance: The inverse of stiffness.

Creep: The continued deformation of a viscoelastic material with time under a constant load.

Viscoelastic material: One that shows a sensitivity of its mechanical properties to rate of loading or deformation.

M. H. Pope, Dr. Med. Sc., Ph.D., Professor; D. G. Wilder, Ph.D., P.E., Research Assistant Professor; M. H. Krag, M.D., Associate Professor: McClure Center for Musculoskeletal Research, Vermont Rehabilitation Engineering Center, Department of Orthopaedics and Rehabilitation, University of Vermont, Burlington, Vermont 05405.

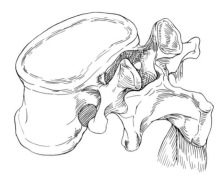

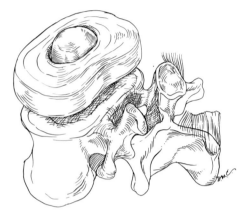

FIG. 1. The basic functional unit of the spine, usually termed "the motion segment."

Kinematics: The description of a geometry of motion of the spinal segments.

MOTION SEGMENT BEHAVIOR

Compliance and Stiffness

Extensive studies have been performed assessing the mechanical characteristics of the spinal motion segments. Reviews of this work show that the motion segment is viscoelastic, absorbs energy, moves with six degrees of freedom (three translations and three rotations), exhibits coupled motion (motion in one direction affects motion in others), has limited fatigue tolerance, and depends upon its bony and ligamentous components for mechanical tasks.

Early work concentrated on the effects of single loads or torques applied to the motion segment. Recently, researchers have been studying the three-dimensional effects of loads and torques applied in three dimensions (16,34,65,78,92,93,95–98,104,118,130–132,140). Testing of this type is important, as it is difficult to assess directly all the loads and torques experienced by the motion segment in vivo (31). The coupled motion is normally presented in the form of a flexibility or stiffness matrix which describes the motion in three dimensions with respect to imposed forces and moments.

Three groups have studied the six degree-of-freedom (three translations and three rotations) response to applied loads and torques of the minimally constrained vertebral body (16,82,97,114,118,130–132). These studies have defined the mechanical response by means of main and coupled stiffness characteristics. Loads and torques applied to motion segments along or about the anterior-posterior, lateral, and axial axes have produced main and coupled translations and rotations with which to generate the motion segments' complex flexibility characteristics. One limitation of these works is that there is no description of a mechanically based reference at which the specimens are loaded. Except for the point of application of preload in the study by Panjabi et al. (96) and the description of the balance point in the work by Tencer (130) and Tencer and Ahmed (131), loads are applied to the motion segment over geometrically based reference locations. All of the above-mentioned unconstrained testing methodologies applied loads either in line with the geometric center of the upper vertebral body or along an axis co-linear with the line segment connecting the geometric centers of both centra of the upper and lower vertebral bodies of the motion segment.

A limitation in the use of the flexibility matrix for reporting the mechanical characteristics of the motion segment is that it is specific to the point at which the load was applied to obtain it. Therefore, it is possible to obtain different flexibility matrices in response to different load rates, magnitudes, orientations, and point of load applications. A way to solve the problem of load application location is to find a point which demonstrates a consistent mechanical response (31). Both Rolander (112) and Lin et al. (67) found these points and called them "a balanced position of the load" and an "operational centroidal axis" respectively. They were both defined as that point where, when a vertical load was applied, the segment would move only vertically. More recently, Wilder et al. (144) studied the vertical balance point in great depth. These data show that the vertical balance point axis is at a reasonably reproducible location. The balance point was found to be sensitive to three loading parameters: (a) vector magnitude, (b) orientation, and (c) load rate. Loads of different magnitudes cause different deflections in the motion segment and thus may increase or decrease the role of the segment's bony elements. The presence of a balance point raises intriguing questions regarding the neuromuscular control system. Does the system apply the generalized load and torque to each motion segment using the minimization of the segment's six degree-of-freedom motion as its objective function?

Obvious rotations occur in the segment as it is loaded further from its balance point. The physical implications of such a position change could be that muscles in the spine need to adjust their activity strategy to accommodate the new segment response characteristics. Further questions are raised, for example, would a fatigued muscle produce a deleterious motion segment loading condition by a mismatch of the application point of the muscle load vector and the load application point where minimum coupled motion occurs?

Effect of Interventions

Markolf and Morris (73) compressed motion segments minus the posterior elements. Removal of the nucleus did not significantly change the stiffness. The disc was said to be self-sealing after injury. This view was disputed by Posner et al. (105) and Tencer et al. (132) who included the posterior elements. An injury to a disc did affect the mechanical properties. Panjabi et al. (94) studied the disc after a window was cut in the annulus and after nucleotomy. Main and coupled stiffness were decreased and the disc was clearly shown not to be self-sealing. However Goel et al. (45) suggested that the change in coupled stiffness was due to the unusual location of the annular cuts. These workers emphasized that little of the nucleus should be removed in surgery so as to maintain stability.

Several workers have shown that many physical changes and disc herniations have been caused in lumbar motion segments by exposure to cyclic loading (2,20,69,143). Brown et al. (20) produced a tear throughout the annulus after 1,000 cycles of a 63.6 N compression load and 5.0 degrees of forward flexion at a frequency of 1,100 cycles/minute. Adams and Hutton (2) simulated a day of heavy labor involving flexion and torsion at a rate of 40 times/minute, and produced visible distortions of the lamellae of the annulus fibrosus. Liu et al. (69) found facet or vertebral body failures or facet capsular ligament tears as a result of a 0.5 hertz cyclic torque with a 445 N axial preload. Generally, failures occurred in segments subjected to more than 1.5 degrees of axial rotation.

These findings may be explained by the fact that the body's building blocks such as biopolymers are affected by cyclic loading. For example rat and human medial collateral ligaments (41) have been shown to become softer and weaker due to vibration loading (139), a fatiguing type response (51).

In vivo whole body vibration studies have established the motion characteristics and natural frequency of the lumbar region during vibration exposure (32,91,94, 103,107,121,141,145). These studies suggest that the soft tissues may be under a risk of injury at the 5 Hz natural frequency.

Wilder et al. (144) have reported the effects of load rate and load history on the mechanical properties of the motion segment and demonstrated the sensitivity of the human lumbar motion segment to load applicator point, load vector, load rate, and load magnitude. These tests have also shown a mechanical cause and effect relationship between application of conservative, combined flexion-compression (vibration or static) loading, as found in static or vibrating seating environments, and mechanical changes in the motion segment. In addition, the lumbar motion segment has a potential for sudden, large rotation bending. Such observations indicate the motion segment depends strongly upon the generalized load and torque provided by the surrounding musculature for its proper support and function. In some loading cases the segment rotated to a certain point, it then rotated rapidly to a new equilibrium orientation near its physiological limit. When this occurred, at times it would rotate in a combination of flexion and lateral bend, thus imposing large, rapidly occurring, tensile deflections in the postero-lateral region of the disc. This suggested itself as a viable mechanism for acute disc herniation or chronic, cumulative trauma.

Wilder et al. (142) found that overload of motion segments exhibited the immediate tendency to produce a large-rotation response of the segment. It revealed that the balance point is sensitive to load magnitude in addition to the load vector, application point, and load rate. It increased the compliance of the motion segments, and increased the means and standard deviations of the coupled lateral bend rotation exhibited upon follow-up mechanical testing. This occurred after exposure to a prolonged flexion-compression static or vibration loading environment.

Later, Wilder et al. (143) found a response which they suggested may coincide with patients' reporting of a sudden "giving way" in the spine as a flexion or lateral bend is performed. These responses were designated either stable or unstable depending on the amount of translation or rotation exhibited. A segment response was defined as stable for these series of experiments as long as it exhibited coupled translation less than 1.0 mm and coupled rotation less than 1.0 degree. Wilder et al. (144) defined larger responses as exhibiting instability since there was a sudden shift to a new orientation. Plots of typical stable and unstable responses are shown in Figure 2. Note that in this case the unstable response occurs after exposure to sustained vibration loading.

Creep

The motion segment suffers time-dependent motion under load, or creep, due to the morphology of the disc itself. In the younger person the nucleus is nearly 90% water, with the remaining structure being comprised of fibrous materials termed collagen and proteoglycans, which are specialized materials that bind water. In the young healthy disc, a positive pressure is present within

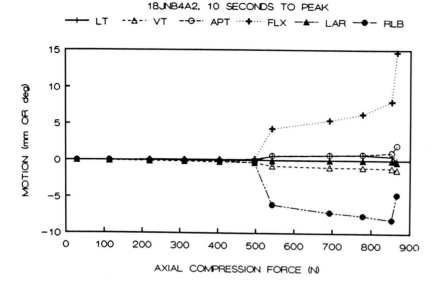

18JNB4A2, 10 SECONDS TO PEAK

—+— LT --△-- VT --⊝-- APT ····+···· FLX --▲-- LAR --●-- RLB

FIG. 2. Plots of typical stable (0–500 N) and unstable (500–870 N) responses of an L4 motion segment tested using a 10 second load ramp. The individual responses are noted as LT: Left lateral translation; VT: Vertical translation; APT: Anterior translation; FLX: Flexion rotation; LAR: Left axial rotation; RLB: Right lateral bend. This segment was exposed to an hour of vibration and a subsequent overload event.

the nucleus pulposus at rest and increases as the loads are applied to the spine. This pressure approximates to 1.5 times the mean applied pressure.

Hirsch and Nachemson (52) were the first to report creep. They found that higher loads not only produced greater deformation but also fostered creep. Kazarian (55,56) reported creep tests on degenerated motion segments and found that the non-degenerated discs creep slowly as compared to the degenerated discs. Thus in degeneration the discs have less ability to absorb shocks. Virgin (137) found that the disc's hysteresis varies with the magnitude of the load applied, the age of the disc, and its level. It increases with load magnitude and decreases with age. Keller et al. (57) used rheological models to mathematically characterize the compressive creep-relation behavior of the discs before and after alteration by either chemonucleolysis (chymopapain injection) or denucleation. Partial denucleation primarily increased the initial stiffness behavior of the disc whereas chemonucleolysis increased the creep rate and elastic modulus. Likewise Kazarian (56) and Wakano et al. (138) found increased creep rates for degenerated and chemonucleolyzed discs respectively, characteristic of structures that can no longer maintain internal hydrostatic pressures. Wilder et al. (144) also found that motion segments tested exhibited a significantly higher creep rate during vibration loading than during static loading. They also absorbed significantly more energy. The energy absorbed probably contributed both to fluid migration from the disc, similar to that shown by Adams and Hutton (2) and cyclic plastic strain of the composite material comprising the disc. The response of the segment to sustained loading showed not only a creep response, but also demonstrated softening (increased compliance) in one or more of its degrees of freedom of motion.

The exact location and mechanism of the fatigue needs closer inspection, but these tests indicate that regional changes were occurring in the disc. The posterior movement of the balance point and the increased flexion response of the segment seemed to prove this point.

Disc Mechanics

Nachemson et al. (80,81) conducted a number of experiments that measured intradiscal pressure by means of a needle, connected to a pressure gauge, placed directly in the nucleus in vivo. They clearly showed that intra-discal pressure (IDP) is higher in sitting than in standing. At the L3 disc the in vivo experiments revealed a load in standing corresponding approximately to body weight. In the supine position the load was about 50% lower, whereas the load while coughing or laughing was about 20% higher than the load in standing position. Lifting a 20 kg weight can result in a load of more than three times the load in standing position. Insight can also be gained by IDP measurements in seating. For example, an increase of the back-rest inclination in a seat led to a decreased pressure, as did an increase in lumbar support; whereas a thoracic support increased the disc pressure (3–5,7,8) (Fig. 3). Such techniques have shown that intra-discal pressures are significantly greater in the flexed posture in both cervical and lumbar discs. This has a tension increasing effect on the disc collagen fibers analogous to increasing the tension in a taut wire by pushing on it from the side (3–5,7,8,15,50,64,78,81,84,117).

Although most in vitro studies have analyzed the disc as a single unit, some in vitro work has been done on parts of the disc. For example, tensile testing of lamellae of the annulus fibrosus (42,89), motion segment flexibility changes induced by cutting of various ligaments (98)

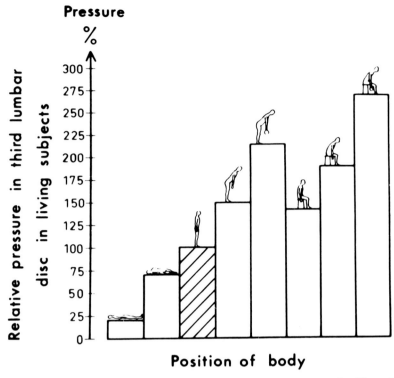

FIG. 3. Relative increase and decrease in intra-discal pressure in different supine, standing, and sitting postures compared to the pressure in upright standing (100%) (81).

or denucleation (18,94,136), annulus surface fiber strain with motion segment loading (120,125), or intra-discal pressure measurements have all been investigated.

Several workers have injected a radio-opaque fluid (discography) into the center of the disc (36,37,108) to detect movement of the nucleus pulposus. This injection, however, significantly changes the stiffness of the disc (10). Krag et al. (62,63) reported a method for obtaining quantitative data describing the internal displacements of the intervertebral discs, with only minimal disruption of normal function.

We have previously alluded to the changes that occur in the aging, degenerated, or denucleated disc. As extensions of that work, for example, Horst and Brinckmann (53), using lateral bend loads, found asymmetry and symmetry in end plate pressure distributions for degenerated and normal discs respectively: upon denucleation the normal pressure distribution became asymmetric (degenerative in character), and upon injection with silicone rubber it returned to a symmetric "normal" state.

As shown in Table 1, we can find reports of decreased disc height, increased bulge, reduced pressure, and increased mobility.

In Vivo Studies

There is a great deal of clinical interest in the accurate measurement of intervertebral motion. Most studies have used radiographic techniques and most have measured coupled motions at the end points of normal clinical motions. For example, Knutsson (58) found abnormal translations during spinal flexion and extension. During forward flexion, anterior shear was found to be related to disc degeneration by Frymoyer et al. (40), Arkin (11), Lindahl (68), and Dupuis et al. (33).

Panjabi (90) pointed out the reliability and accuracy problems inherent in radiographically determining the instant center of rotation in any joint. Gertzbein et al. (43) have shown a technique for finding the instantaneous center of rotation of a lumbar motion segment (in flexion-extension rotation) by means of Moire fringe. Their kinematic results indicate that, in normal discs, the instant center is located in the posterior portion of the disc during flexion-extension rotations. Six degree-of-freedom movements of the in vivo motion segment can be obtained by biplanar or stereo radiography (40,104,126,127). The authors have relied on the identification of bony landmarks as reference points and have developed optimization techniques to minimize the errors due to the localization of such landmarks (126,127). Olsson et al. (85–87) have increased the accuracy of this method by the implantation of discrete metallic markers, which permit accuracies within the range of 0.1 mm to 0.2 mm, a resolution far greater than that possible with bony landmarks. More recently, Krag et al. (61) have used K-wires implanted in the spinous process

TABLE 1. *Reported characteristics of degenerated and denucleated discs: Comparison to normal disc mechanics*

Type of disc	Decreased disc weight	Increased lateral bulge	Inward bulge of inner annulus	Reduced internal pressure	Increased mobility
Degenerated	Generally accepted	Hirsch and Nachemson (52) Lin et al. (67) Reuber et al. (109)	Ritchie and Fahrni (110)	Erlacher (36) Nachemson (78) Andersson and Schultz (115)	Knutsson (58) van Akkerveeken et al. (136)
Mechanically denucleated	Brinckmann and Horst (119) Bradford et al. (17)	Brinckmann and Horst (119)	Krag et al. (62)	—	Harris and Macnab (48) Roaf (111)
Chemonucleolysis (before regeneration)	Takahashi et al. (128) Tsuchida et al. (135)	—	Takahashi et al. (128)	Takahashi et al. (128)	—
Possible clinical relevance	Increased loading to facet joints	Nerve root compression	Separation of lamellae: Pain or physical disruption	Change in end plate loads (osteophyte formation ?)	Increased load on adjacent structures

to measure intersegmental motion. The method has been proven in the laboratory but has yet to receive clinical trials.

TRUNK MECHANICS

Muscle Mechanics

The spine is unstable without the support of the muscles. Gregersen and Lucas (46) showed how an excised spine with the ligaments intact, but without the muscles, buckles under very small compressive forces. The muscles power the trunk and position the spinal segments. Generally the muscles act in an efficient manner but in asymmetric postures marked antagonistic activity may occur. A convenient division is that between the flexors and extensor.

The flexor muscles are made up of the psoas, which attaches directly to the vertebral bodies anterolaterally, and the abdominal muscles, which flex the spine through their attachments to the rib cage and pelvis.

The abdominal muscles consist of the midline and anterior rectus abdominus muscles, internal and external obliques, and transverse abdominal muscles. The extensor muscles (erector spinae, multifidi, and intertransversarii) attach intrasegmentally (between adjacent vertebrae only) or intersegmentally (bridging multiple motion segments). The lumbar erector spinae consists of the iliocostalis lumborum and longissimus thoracis. The lumbar fibers arise from the accessory processes and the L1-L4 transverse processes and insert in the ileum (70) (Fig. 4).

Several workers have investigated the role of the trunk musculature by the use of electromyography. For example, Flint and Gudgell (38) showed that increased myo-electric activity of the external obliques occurs during a pelvic tilt, with the subject erect. Partridge and Walters (99) showed that both the external obliques and the rectus abdominus exhibit little myoelectric activity in this posture unless some resistance is added. They also found that the internal oblique does not exhibit much activity during the pelvic tilt.

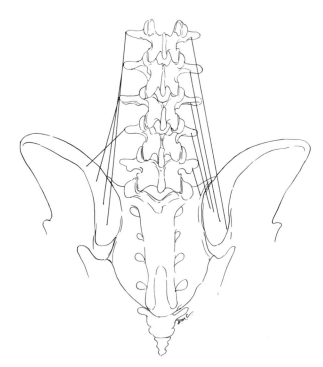

FIG. 4. Schematic illustration. **Left:** Lumbar fascicles of iliocostalis lumborum. **Right:** Fascicles of the longissimus thoracis pars lumborum. Fascicles L1 to L4 have long caudal tendons.

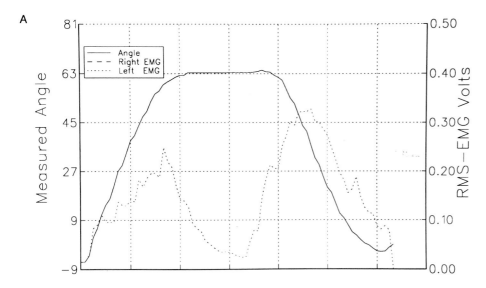

FIG. 5A. Flexion-relaxation phenomenon. Pre-injury measured angle vs. RMS-EMG.

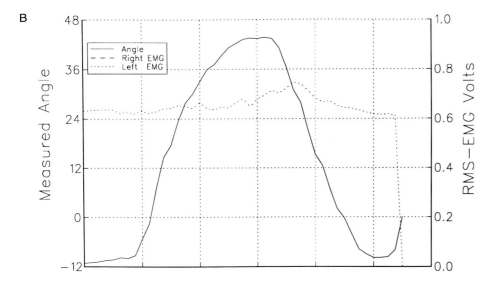

FIG. 5B. Flexion-relaxation phenomenon. Post-injury measured angle vs. RMS-EMG.

Floyd and Silver (39) found that a Valsalva maneuver contracts the internal and external obliques, but the rectus abdominus contracts to a much lesser degree. De-Sousa and Furlani (30) have investigated the role of the rectus abdominus in different activities. It was found that the rectus abdominus contracts during flexion. The rectus abdominus infrequently showed activity in twisting. The rectus abdominus usually contracted during abdominal efforts.

Antagonistic muscle activity is an important consideration in many activities. Basmajian (13) found antagonistic activity of the deep lumbar trunk muscles during axial rotation. Morris et al. (76) noted activity in the rotatores and multifidi during ipsilateral rotation. Pope

et al. (102) reported high levels of antagonistic activity in isometric twist efforts. Andersson et al. (9) noted high levels of activity on the contralateral side when positions of lateral bend and rotation are combined with an external load.

Schultz et al. (117), in an experiment involving sagittal plane loading, found little antagonistic muscle activity whereas more complicated loadings demonstrated such activity (116). The erector spinae muscles are largely responsible for sagittal plane lifts. If the load gets off center the supporting obliques quickly become active (119). Ekholm et al. (35) studied the erector spinae, rectus, and oblique abdominis muscles during four different types of lifts. They presented descriptions of the sequential activity of various trunk muscles throughout lifting and demonstrated that kinetic lifts reduce the loads on the spine. It is clear that coordination of muscle activity plays as important a role in the dynamics of lifting as strength of the individual muscles.

It has been reported by several groups that the dorsal muscle activity is usually absent in full flexion. Floyd and Silver (39) demonstrated that, in the extreme-flexed position of the back, the erector spinae remain relaxed in the initial stages of heavy weight lifting. It is movement at the hip joint that accounts for the earliest phase of apparent extension of the trunk. Tanii and Masuda (129) found that marked changes of erector spinae activity during flexion-extension movements were closely related to the flexibility of the vertebral column. We have recently used this "flexion-relaxation" response in the evaluation of low back pain patients. Figure 5 shows a subject prior to and following a herniated disc. The absence of the flexion relaxation response can be clearly noted after herniation.

An important contribution to our understanding of the behavior of the trunk muscles comes from mathematical modeling. Such models have demonstrated a generally good correlation between predicted muscle contraction forces and measured levels of myoelectric activity of the same muscles. In modeling flexion-extension effects, an objective function of minimization of compression of the disc has been used. The models usually assume that antagonistic muscle activity is absent. Schultz et al. (115–117) report that in the modeling of extension efforts, the latissimus dorsi, which has a larger moment arm than the erector spinae, reaches maximum contraction levels before the erector spinae starts to contract. This is in spite of the fact that the physiologic or effective cross-section of the latissimus dorsi in the lumbar region is minimal since only the thoracolumbar fascia, part of the origin, is there. Andersson et al. (9) found that the prediction of loads is better in the symmetric postures as compared to the asymmetric ones.

Strength Measurement

Snook et al. (122) found that approximately one half of all compensable LBP episodes are associated with manual lifting tasks. Chaffin and Park (23), Magora (71) and Chaffin (21) have demonstrated that workers with inadequate lifting strength working in relatively stressful lifting tasks have higher low back injury rates than workers with less stressful lifting tasks. Apparently, when lifting near the strength limit of these muscles, excessive strain may be transmitted to other soft tissues (e.g., the ligaments and discs). Not all studies have confirmed these relationships, for example Battié et al. (14) found that strength was not related to time lost due to LBP. The

majority of the literature does support the hypothesis of higher strength being prophylactic against LBP. For example Chaffin et al. (22), Paulson and Jergenson (100), and Rowe (113) have conducted studies, based on isometric strength testing, which suggested that individuals with good strength capabilities are less prone than their weaker coworkers to low back injuries when performing manual materials handling tasks in industry.

The strength of and strength testing of LBP patients remain controversial areas. While most studies indicate a weakness of some muscle groups among low back pain patients, there has been disagreement about the results (25,123). Rowe (113) found a relative weakness in the abdominal muscles, as compared to the dorsal muscles. A few authors, for example Pedersen et al. (101) investigating back muscle strength, did not find any differences between back patients and controls. Thorstensson et al. (133), studying the imbalance in strength of muscles controlling the trunk movements, reported high extension-flexion ratios of trunk muscle strength among low back patients. Onishi and Nomina (88) found by examining the strength of low back patients versus healthy controls in different occupations strength differences for some

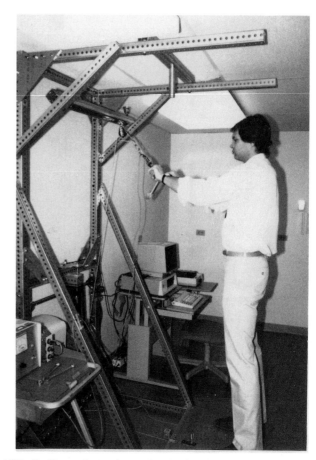

FIG. 6. Strength testing using an isokinetic pulling apparatus.

occupations (e.g., teachers) but not for others (e.g., cleaning workers).

We have recently developed a new device to determine the isokinetic strength of workers and patients alike in different planes of motion. Figure 6 shows the subject lifting vertically in an isometric pull in the sagittal plane. Figure 7 shows a pulling test at 45 degrees to the vertical. Figure 8 shows a typical ISO strength test, in the sagittal plane, for isokinetic lifting. These contour plots are used to identify uniformity between lifting and pulling demands in industry and the patients' ability to meet those demands. The isokinetic strength in flexion extension has also been reported by Hasue et al. (49).

Intra-Abdominal Pressure

Intra-abdominal pressure (IAP) is widely believed to have a beneficial role in spine biomechanics. The force generated by IAP is thought to help unload the back muscles and spine during trunk effort. Davis (27,28), Bartelink (12), and Morris, Lucas, and Bresler (77) measured IAP and found that IAP increases with trunk ef-

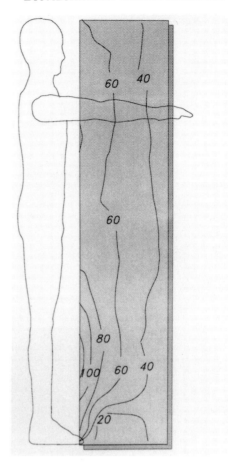

FIG. 8. Contour plot of isokinetic lifting capability as a function of position (force in pounds).

fort. In lifting, there is a linear relationship between the amount of weight lifted and the intra-abdominal pressure that can be measured in the stomach or rectum (6,47). The observed correlation between IAP and trunk effort formed the basis for their conclusion that IAP reduces loads in the trunk.

In fact, both the abdominal and thoracic cavities have been shown to become pressurized during strenuous activity. The abdominal cavity is pressurized by mechanical contraction of the muscles of the abdominal wall, together with the diaphragm. Concomitant closing of the glottis (Valsalva maneuver) results in further pressurization (28). This increased pressure tends to force the pelvic wall (floor of abdominal cavity) and the lung's diaphragm (roof of the abdominal cavity) apart. Bartelink (12) and Morris, Lucas, and Bresler (77) suggest that this mechanism tends to extend the spine and thus reduce the contraction force required in the extensor muscles. In turn, this force rebalancing is said to reduce the compressive load bearing of the disc. Gilbertson et al. (44) have shown that the abdominal muscles must contract, producing a flexion moment in order to produce the IAP increase.

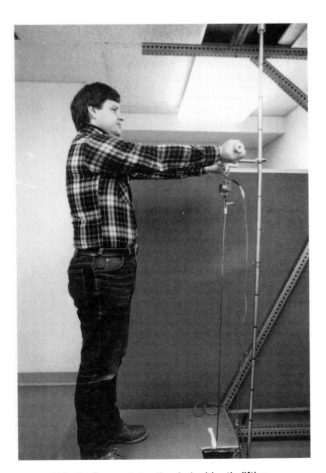

FIG. 7. Strength testing in isokinetic lifting.

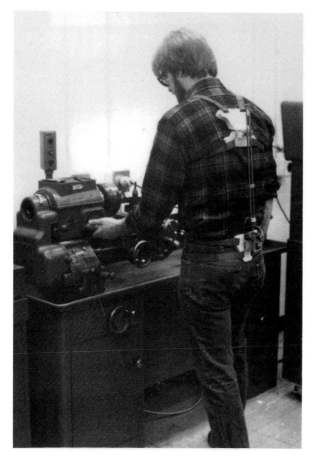

FIG. 9. Goniometer to measure and record flexion-extension, lateral bend, and axial rotation.

The broad conclusion of this study is that there is still no direct evidence to support the hypothesis that intra-abdominal pressure reduces back muscle tension and disc compressive loads during trunk effort. Likewise, Schultz et al. (117) found intra-abdominal pressures to

be low and to have little effect on trunk mechanics. Farfan (37) has suggested that the lumbodorsal fascia can shorten the dorsal ligament by means of a laterally directed force from the oblique musculature. Farfan postulated that this is the mechanism by which intra-abdominal pressure creates extension moments about the spine and thus assists in compressive load bearing. However, the importance of the lumbodorsal fascia has recently been disputed by McGill and Norman (75).

The general concept of spinal support from the abdomen has led to a rationale for flexion exercises, the wearing of corsets, and the protection of the spine by a belt for weight lifters. Davis (29) has used this concept in the determination of safe loads to be used in industry.

ERGONOMICS

Ergonomics is the study of work and working environments. An ergonomically designed workplace will avoid excessive loads on the body due to lifting, pulling, and pushing, and will avoid prolonged static postures, excessive postures, or excessive vibrational exposure. The important factors in lifting along with a guideline are given by NIOSH (83).

Nachemson and Elfstrom (80) and Andersson et al. (3–5,7,8) have extensively evaluated seating postures by electromyographic and intra-discal pressure methods. Their work may explain why both sedentary and other workers get LBP. The disc pressure is similar in the worker bending forward at 20 degrees and the worker sitting unsupported. In any posture, lifting raises the disc pressure and muscle forces. Damkot et al. (26) found significant differences in the incidence of LBP as a function of stretching versus reaching demands. Forty percent of the group without LBP and 36 percent of the moderate LBP group were required to stretch and reach,

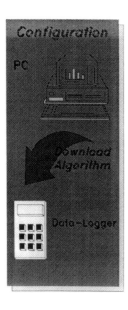
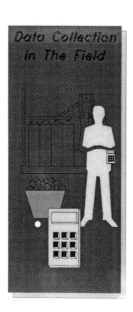
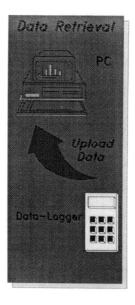

FIG. 10. System design for recording postural data.

whereas 59 percent of the severe LBP group had these job requirements. Furthermore, those with severe LBP were more likely to reach with their arms fully extended than were the other two groups. Bending and twisting, when combined with a lifting task, was reported to be related to LBP by Troup et al. (134).

Traditional work analysis systems break down the task into elements. These elements are about the same length of time for most subjects. An example is the method time system which relies on film. Unfortunately such systems are designed to improve efficiency and not to enhance safety. Corlett et al. (24) designed an observational method purely with posture in mind. The method is called posture targeting and permits observations of body segment position and task.

We have tended toward an automated system that does not require observation but at the end of the day gives a summary of postures held. Figure 9 shows a subject wearing the goniometer (Work Recovery Systems, Tucson, Arizona) while working at a lathe. The worker is slightly forward flexed. The system design (Fig. 10) consists of a data logger which is down loaded with data collection instructions by the PC. The goniometer gives postural information (at 0.5 Hz) to the data logger, which is worn on the belt. At the conclusion of the sampling period the data from the data logger are downloaded to the PC for data retrieval. These data (see Fig. 11) can be plotted in a variety of forms (i.e., flexion versus lateral bend, flexion versus axial rotation) and with different time bins. These displays are invaluable in identifying excessive or prolonged postures and can be used for job task modification and for matching job requirements to worker capacities.

BIOMECHANICS OF SURGERY

Extensive studies of the effects of surgery have been carried out in motion segment preparations. These studies have evaluated the effects of different interventions such as fusion. For example, Lee and Langrana (66) tested lumbosacral spines under simulated fixation with polymethylmethacrylate. Anterior fusion gave the highest stiffness increase. This was accompanied by a cephalad shift of the center of rotation of L5-S1. This shift was largest in the bilateral-lateral fusion and in the posterior fusion.

Other workers have evaluated different spinal instrumentation schemes. Kornblatt et al. (59) applied combined flexion and compression to lumbosacral spines. The intact spine stiffness was non-linear. Internal fixation doubled the stiffness. Facet screws were 20 times stiffer but all systems had similar strength. Similarly, Purcell et al. (106) created a posterior ligamentous defect at T12-L1 in T5-T5 preparation. Flexion created an unstable fracture. The fractured spines were instrumented with Harrington distraction rods and then retested in flexion. The rodded spines were not significantly stronger than the uninstrumented. Hook placement at T12 and L2 increased the strength and changed the mode of failure.

Stauffer and Neil (124) used four point bending to compare Harrington rods to Weiss springs to isolated thoracolumbar spines. The rods were found to be significantly stronger than the springs. It should be noted that those tests were on the old springs without internal rods. This work was complemented by Jacobs et al. (54), who compared Roy Camille plates and Harrington rods to

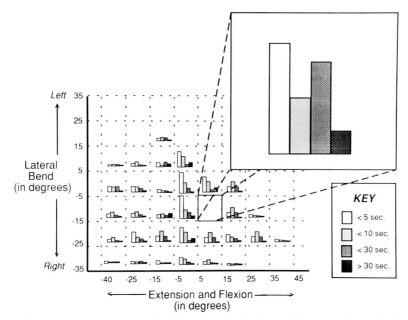

FIG. 11. Postural data retrieved at the conclusion of the sampling period plotted as a function of time spent in a given posture.

Weiss springs under bending and concluded that the original Weiss springs were too elastic.

In a more sophisticated and realistic approach, Maiman et al. (72) mounted spines on an MTS and loaded them in flexion-compression. The specimens ranged from T3-S1 and C2-L5 to complete cadavers. Most spines fractured at T11 and T12. The fractures were then fixed by a variety of devices and reloaded to failure by the same method. Compared to the instrumented unbroken specimen, the Harrington distraction rod failed at an average of 42% of control; the Weiss springs failed at 54%, and the Luque rods failed at 82%. The Weiss spring system permitted much more deformation without catastrophic failure. Other loading modes have also been investigated. McAfee et al. (74) investigated the mechanical behavior of thoracolumbar specimens under torsion with axial preload. In normal specimens failure of the Harrington system occurred at the bone clamp interface while the Luque system failed elsewhere in the motion segment. With experimental burst fractures the segmentally wired Harrington system was the most stable. In the translational fracture dislocations the Luque was the stiffest system.

More recently, the accuracy of such investigations have been improved by Abumni (1) who utilized a stereophotogrammetry approach to establish the role of the Harrington rod, Luque system, Roy-Camille system, Dunn device, and Kaneda device. Pure moments were applied to each vertebra by pneumatic cylinders. Axial rotation was the most severe loading mode but it was concluded that transpedicular external fixation and the Kaneda device provided the best fixation.

Krag et al. (60) have conducted extensive studies of the biomechanics of pedicle screw fixation leading to the design of the Vermont Spinal Fixator. This is discussed in great detail in Chapter 92.

SUMMARY

The lumbar spine is a complex structure with the function of support, mobility, housing, and control. Kinematics are generally specified for the functional spinal unit (FSU), which is defined as the superior body, the inferior body, the intervertebral disc, and the associated ligaments. The FSU can be fatigued, is viscoelastic, absorbs energy, and exhibits coupled motion. A balance point can be defined as the point where coupled motion is minimized. The balance point is found to change with exposure to cyclic loading and to mechanical overload. The FSU is susceptible to creep due to the composition of the disc. Degenerated discs and discs subjected to chemonucleolysis are found to have increased creep rates. Cyclic loading also increases the creep rate.

Intra-discal pressure (IDP) measurements reveal that the nucleus pressure is increased in sitting as compared to standing. IDP is reduced if the backrest is inclined and if lumbar support is provided. IDP is also increased if a forward flexed posture is adopted.

Most in vivo studies have relied upon radiographic techniques. Accuracy has been improved by the use of certain bony landmarks, however the accuracy necessary for diagnostic purposes can only be achieved by the use of implanted spheres. Electromyographic tests can reveal a great deal about muscle forces and by means of mathematical models can be utilized to compute joint forces. The flexion relaxation response has promise as a method to assess recovery following injury or surgery. Isometric and isokinetic strength measurements are widely used both in industry and in the clinic, but questions remain about their reliability and their ability to simulate "real" lifts. Ergonomics can be used by industry to minimize the disc pressure and to avoid awkward and uncomfortable postures.

FSU preparations have been extensively used to evaluate different spinal instrumentations. This approach, along with finite element analysis, will be used in the future to optimize designs.

ACKNOWLEDGMENT

We wish to acknowledge support from the National Institute of Disability and Rehabilitation Research through the Vermont Rehabilitation Engineering Center.

REFERENCES

1. Abumni K (1988): A biomechanical study on stability of injured thoracolumbar spine fixed with spinal instrumentation. *J Japanese Orthop Assoc* 62:205–216.
2. Adams MA, Hutton WC (1983): The effect of fatigue on the lumbar intervertebral disc. In: Proceedings of the International Society for the Study of the Lumbar Spine, Cambridge, England, April 8, 1983.
3. Andersson GB (1974): On myoelectric and back muscle activity and lumbar disc pressure in sitting postures. Doctoral dissertation, Gothenburg University, Gothenburg, Sweden.
4. Andersson GB, Ortengren R (1974): Lumbar disc pressure and myoelectric back muscle activity during sitting. II. Studies on an office chair. *Scand J Rehab Med* 6:115–121.
5. Andersson GB, Ortengren R (1974): Lumbar disc pressure and myoelectric back muscle activity during sitting. III. Studies on a wheelchair. *Scand J Rehab Med* 6:122–127.
6. Andersson GB, Ortengren R, Nachemson A (1977): Intradiscal pressure, intra-abdominal pressure and myoelectric back muscle activity related to posture and loading. *Clin Orthop* (129):156–164.
7. Andersson GB, Ortengren R, Nachemson A, Elfstrom G (1974): Lumbar disc pressure and myoelectric back muscle activity during sitting. IV. Studies on a car driver's seat. *Scand J Rehab Med* 6:128–133.
8. Andersson GB, Ortengren R, Nachemson A, Elfstrom G (1974): Lumbar disc pressure and myoelectric back muscle activity during sitting. I. Studies on an experimental chair. *Scand J Rehab Med* 6:104–114.
9. Andersson GB, Ortengren R, Nachemson AL, Schultz AB (1983): *Biomechanical analysis of loads on the lumbar spine in sitting and standing postures,* Biomechanics VIII-A. Champaign: Human Kinetics Publishers.

10. Andersson GB, Schultz AB (1979): Effects of fluid injection on mechanical properties of intervertebral discs. *J Biomech* 12:453–458.

11. Arkin AM (1950): The mechanism of rotation in combination with lateral deviation in the normal spine. *J Bone Joint Surg* [Am] 32:180–188.

12. Bartelink DL (1957): The role of abdominal pressure in relieving the pressure on the lumbar intervertebral discs. *J Bone Joint Surg* [Br] 39(4):718–725.

13. Basmajian JV (1978): *Muscles alive. Their functions revealed by electromyography.* Baltimore: Williams and Wilkins.

14. Battié MC, et al (1989): The reliability of physical factors as predictors of the occurrence of back pain reports. A prospective study within industry. Thesis, University of Goteborg, Goteborg, Sweden.

15. Belytschko T, Kulak RF, Schultz AB, Galante JO (1974): Finite element stress analysis of an intervertebral disc. *J Biomech* 7:277–285.

16. Berkson MH, Nachemson AL, Schultz AB (1979): Mechanical properties of human lumbar spine motion segments. Part II: Responses in compression and shear; influence of gross morphology. *J Biomech Eng* 101:53–57.

17. Bradford DS, Swedenburg SM, Carpenter RJ, Hofmeister F, Oegema TR (1987): Facet joint changes after surgical excision of the nucleus pulposus of mature dogs. In: *Trans Orthop Res Soc,* San Francisco, California, January, 1987.

18. Brinckmann P (1986): Injury of the annulus fibrosus and disc protrusions. An in vitro investigation on human lumbar discs. *Spine* 11:149–153.

19. Brinckmann P, Horst M (1985): The influence of vertebral body fracture, intradiscal injection, and partial discectomy on the radial bulge and height of human lumbar discs. *Spine* 10:138–145.

20. Brown T, Hansen RJ, Yorra AJ (1957): Some mechanical tests on the lumbosacral spine with particular reference to the intervertebral discs: A preliminary report. *J Bone Joint Surg* [Am] 39:1135–1164.

21. Chaffin DB (1974): Human strength capability and low back pain. *J Occup Med* 16(4):248–254.

22. Chaffin DB, Herrin GD, Keyserling WM (1978): Pre-employment strength testing—An updated position. *J Occup Med* 20:403–408.

23. Chaffin DB, Park KS (1973): A longitudinal study of low back pain as associated with occupational weight lifting factors. *Am Ind Hyg Assoc J* 34:513–525.

24. Corlett EN, Bishop RP (1976): A technique for assessing postural discomfort. *Ergonomics* 19(2):175–182.

25. Dalen A (1971): Back muscle training of military personnel at L3. *Def Med J* [Suppl 1] 10:57.

26. Damkot DK, Pope MH, Lord J, Frymoyer JW (1984): The relationship between work history, work environment and low back pain in men. *Spine* 9:395–399.

27. Davis PR (1956): Variations of the human intra-abdominal pressure during weight-lifting in different postures. *J Anatomy* 90:601.

28. Davis PR (1959): Posture of the trunk during the lifting of weights. *Brit Med J* 1:87–89.

29. Davis PR (1981): The use of intra-abdominal pressure in evaluating stresses on the lumbar spine. *Spine* 6:90–92.

30. deSousa OM, Furlani J (1974): Electromyographic study of the m. rectus abdominus. *Acta Anat* 88:281–298.

31. Dimnet J, Dumas GA, Pope MH, Wilder DG (1984): The laws of behavior of the intervertebral segment. A mechanical analysis and experiment protocol. Eleventh meeting of the International Society for the Study of the Lumbar Spine, June 3–7, 1984, Montreal.

32. Dupuis H (1974): Belastung durch mechanische Schwingungen und moegliche Gesundheitsschaedigungen im Bereich der Wirbelsaeule [Impact through mechanical vibrations and possible damage to health in the area of the spine]. *Fortschritte der Medizin* 92(14):618–620.

33. Dupuis PR, Yung-Hing K, Cassidy JD, Kirkaldy-Willis WH (1985): Radiologic diagnosis of degenerative lumbar spinal instability. *Spine* 10:262–276.

34. Edwards WT, Hayes WC, Mann RW, White AA (1983): The mechanical stiffness of human lumbar functional spinal units. In: *1983 Advances in Bioengineering.* Winter Annual Meeting of American Society of Mechanical Engineers, November 13–18, 1983, Boston, New York: ASME.

35. Ekholm J, Arborelius UP, Nemeth G (1982): The load on the lumbosacral joint and trunk muscle activity during lifting. *Ergonomics* 25:145–161.

36. Erlacher PR (1952): Nucleography. *J Bone Joint Surg* [Br] 34:204–210.

37. Farfan HF (1973): *Mechanical disorders of the low back.* Philadelphia: Lea and Febiger.

38. Flint MM, Gudgell J (1965): Electromyographic study of abdominal muscular activity during exercise. *Res Quart* 36:29–37.

39. Floyd WF, Silver PH (1955): The function of erectores spinae muscles in certain movements and postures in man. *J Physiol* 129:184–203.

40. Frymoyer JW, Hanley EN Jr, Howe J, et al (1979): A comparison of radiographic findings in fusion and non-fusion patients ten or more years following lumbar disc surgery. *Spine* 4:435–440.

41. Fung YC (1981): *Biomechanics: Mechanical properties of living tissues.* New York: Springer-Verlag.

42. Galante JO (1967): Tensile properties of the human lumbar annulus fibrosus. *Acta Orthop Scand* [Suppl] (100):1–91.

43. Gertzbein SD, Holtby R, Tile M, Kapasouri A, Chan KH, Cruickshank B (1984): Determination of a locus of instantaneous centers of rotation of the lumbar disc by Moire fringes. A new technique. *Spine* 9:409–413.

44. Gilbertson LG, Krag MH, Pope MH (1983): Investigation of the effect of intra-abdominal pressure on the load bearing of the spine. *Trans Orthop Res Society* 8:177.

45. Goel VK, Nishiyama K, Weinstein JN, Liu YK (1986): Mechanical properties of lumbar spinal motion segments as affected by partial disc removal. *Spine* 11(10):1008–1012.

46. Gregersen GG, Lucas DB (1967): An in-vivo study of the axial rotation of the human thoracolumbar spine. *J Bone Joint Surg* [Am] 49(2):247–262.

47. Grew ND (1980): Intraabdominal pressure response to loads applied to the torso in normal subjects. *Spine* 5(2):149–154.

48. Harris RI, Macnab I (1954): Structural changes in the lumbar intervertebral discs. *J Bone Joint Surg* [Br] 36:304–322.

49. Hasue M, Fujiwara M, Kikuchi S (1980): A new method of quantitative measurement of abdominal and back muscle strength. *Spine* 5(2):143–148.

50. Hattori S, Oda H, Kawai S, Oka S (1982): Intradiscal pressure of the cervical spine. Presented at the 10th Cervical Spine Research Society Meeting, New York. *Orthop Transactions* (spring 1983):121.

51. Hertzberg RW, Manson JA (1980): *Fatigue of engineering plastics.* New York: Academic Press, p. 64.

52. Hirsch C, Nachemson A (1954): New observations on the mechanical behavior of lumbar discs. *Acta Orthop Scand* 23:254–283.

53. Horst M, Brinckmann P (1981): Measurement of the distribution of axial stress on the endplate of the vertebral body. *Spine* 6:217–232.

54. Jacobs RR, Nordwall A, Nachemson A (1980): Stability and strength provided by internal fixation systems for dorso-lumbar spinal injuries. *J Biomech* 13:802.

55. Kazarian LE (1972): Dynamic response characteristics of the human vertebral column. *Acta Orthop Scand* [Suppl] (146):1–186.

56. Kazarian LE (1975): Creep characteristics of the human spinal column. *Orthop Clin N Am* 6:3–18.

57. Keller TW, Hansson TH, Holm SH, Pope MH, Spengler DM (1989): In-vivo creep behavior of the normal and degenerated procine intervertebral disk: A preliminary report. *J Spinal Disord* 1(4):267–278.

58. Knutsson F (1944): The instability associated with disk degeneration in the lumbar spine. *Acta Radiol* 25:593–609.

59. Kornblatt MD, Casey MP, Jacobs RR (1986): Internal fixation in lumbosacral spine fusion. *Clin Orthop* (203):141–150.

60. Krag MH, Beynnon BD, Pope MH, Frymoyer JW, Haugh LD, Weaver DL (1986): An internal fixator for posterior application to short segments of the thoracic, lumbar, or lumbosacral spine: Design and testing. *Clin Orthop* (203):75–98.

61. Krag MH, Pope MH, Miller D, Fenwick J (1989): Intervertebral 3-D motion detection: Description of method. Presented at 1989 International Conference on Spinal Manipulation (FCER), Washington, DC.
62. Krag MH, Seroussi RE, Wilder DG, Pope MH (1987): Internal displacement distribution from in vitro loading of the human lumbar spinal motion segments: Experimental results and theoretical predictions. Spine 12:1001–1007.
63. Krag MH, Trausch I, Wilder DG, Pope MH (1983): Internal strain and nuclear movements of the intervertebral disc. Proceedings International Society for Study of the Lumbar Spine, 10th Annual Meeting, Cambridge, England.
64. Kraus H, Farfan HF, Jones TJ (1972): Stress analysis of human intervertebral discs. 25th Annual Conference on Engineering in Medicine and Biology, Bal Harbour, Florida, October 1–5, 1972.
65. Laborde JM, Burstein AH, Song K, Brown RH, Bahniuk E (1981): A method of analyzing the three-dimensional stiffness properties of the intact human lumbar spine. J Biomech Eng 103:299–300.
66. Lee CK, Langrana NA (1984): Lumbosacral spinal fusion. A biomechanical study. Spine 9(6):574–581.
67. Lin HS, Liu YK, Adams KH (1978): Mechanical response of the lumbar intervertebral joint under physiological (complex) loading. J Bone Joint Surg [Am] 60:41–55.
68. Lindahl O (1966): Determination of the sagittal mobility of the lumbar spine. Acta Orthop Scand 37:241–254.
69. Liu YK, Goel VK, DeJong A, Njus GO, Wu HC (1983): Torsional fatigue of the lumbar intervertebral joints. Proceedings International Society for the Study of the Lumbar Spine, Cambridge, England, April 8, 1983.
70. Macintosh JE (1988): The biomechanics of the lumbar musculature. Thesis, Department of Anatomy, University of Queensland, St. Lucia, Australia.
71. Magora A (1974): Investigation of the relation between low back pain and occupation. VI. Medical history and symptoms. Scand J Rehab Med 6:81–88.
72. Maiman DJ, Sances A, Larson SJ, Myklebust JB, Chilbert MA, Nesemann SP, Flatley TJ (1985): Comparison of the failure biomechanics of spinal fixation devices. Neurosurgery 17(4):574–580.
73. Markolf KL, Morris JM (1974): The structural components of the intervertebral disc: A study of their contributions to the ability of the disc to withstand compressive forces. J Bone Joint Surg [Am] 56:675–687.
74. McAfee PC, Werner FW, Glisson RR (1985): A biomechanical analysis of spinal instrumentation systems in thoracolumber fractures. Spine 10(3):204–217.
75. McGill SM, Norman RW (1986): Partitioning of the L4-L5 dynamic moment into disc, ligamentous and muscular components during lifting. Spine 11(7):666–678.
76. Morris JM, Benner G, Lucas DB (1962): An electromyographic study of the intrinsic muscles of the back in man. J Anat 96:509–520.
77. Morris JM, Lucas DB, Bresler B (1961): Role of the trunk in stability of the spine. J Bone Joint Surg [Am] 43:327–351.
78. Nachemson A (1960): Lumbar intradiscal pressure. Acta Orthop Scand [Suppl] 43:1–104.
79. Nachemson A (1976): Lumbar intradiscal pressure. In: The lumbar spine and back pain, Jayson M, ed. New York: Grune and Stratton, p. 261.
80. Nachemson A, Elfstrom G (1970): Intravital dynamic pressure measurements in lumbar discs. A study of common movements, maneuvers and exercises. Scand J Rehab Med [Suppl] 1:1–40.
81. Nachemson AL, Morris JM (1964): Lumbar intradiscal pressure. Acta Orthop Scand [Suppl] (43).
82. Nachemson AL, Schultz AB, Berkson MH (1979): Mechanical properties of human lumbar spine motion segments: Influence of age, sex, disc level and degeneration. Spine 4:1–8.
83. NIOSH (National Institute for Occupational Health and Safety) (1981): A work practices guide for manual lifting. Technical Report No. 81-122, U.S. Dept. of Health and Human Services (NIOSH), Cincinnati, Ohio.
84. Okushima H (1970): Study on hydrodynamic pressure of lumbar intervertebral disc. Arch Jap Chir 39:45–57.
85. Olsson TH, Selvik G, Willner S (1976): Kinematic analysis of posterolateral fusion in the lumbosacral spine. Acta Radiol (Diagn) 17:519–530.
86. Olsson TH, Selvik G, Willner S (1976): Kinematic analysis of spinal fusions. Investigative Radiol 11:202–209.
87. Olsson TH, Selvik G, Willner S (1977): Mobility in the lumbosacral spine after fusion studied with the aid of roentgen stereophotogrammetry. Clin Orthop (129):181–190.
88. Onishi N, Nomura H (1973): Low back pain in relation to physical work capacity and local tenderness. J Human Ergol 2:119–132.
89. Panagiotacopulos ND, Knauss WG, Bloch R (1979): On the mechanical properties of human intervertebral disc material. Biorheology 16:317–330.
90. Panjabi MM (1979): Centers and angles of rotation of body joints: A study of errors and optimization. J Biomech 12:911–920.
91. Panjabi MM, Andersson GBJ, Jorneus L, Hult E, Mattson L (1983): In vivo measurement of spinal column vibrations. Proceedings of American Society of Biomechanics, Rochester, Minnesota, September 28–30, 1983.
92. Panjabi MM, Andersson GBJ, Jorneus L, Hult E, Mattson L (1986): In vivo measurements of spinal column vibrations. J Bone Joint Surg [Am] 68(5):695–702.
93. Panjabi MM, Brand RA Jr, White AA III (1976): Three-dimensional flexibility and stiffness properties of the human thoracic spine. J Biomech 9:185–192.
94. Panjabi MM, Krag MH, Chung TQ (1984): Effects of disc injury on mechanical behavior of the human spine. Spine 9:707–713.
95. Panjabi MM, Krag MH, Goel VK (1981): A technique for measurement and description of three-dimensional six degree-of-freedom motion of a body joint with an application to the human spine. J Biomech 14:447–460.
96. Panjabi MM, Krag MH, White AA III, Southwick WO (1977): Effects of preload on load displacement curves of the lumbar spine. Orthop Clin N Am 8:181–192.
97. Panjabi MM, White AA III (1978): Physical properties and functional biomechanics of the spine. In: Clinical biomechanics of the spine, White AA III, Panjabi MM, eds. Philadelphia: J.B. Lippincott.
98. Panjabi MM, White AA III, Johnson RM (1975): Cervical spine mechanics as a function of transection of components. J Biomech 8(5):327–336.
99. Partridge MJ, Walters CE (1959): Participation of the abdominal muscles in various movements of the trunk in man. An electromyographic study. Phys Ther Rev 39(12):791–800.
100. Paulson E, Jergenson K (1971): Back muscle strength, lifting and stooped working postures. Applied Ergon 2:133–137.
101. Pedersen O, Petersen R, Staffeldt E (1975): Back pain and isometric back muscle strength of workers in a Danish factory. Scand J Rehab Med 7:125–128.
102. Pope MH, Andersson GB, Broman H, Svensson M, Zetterberg C (1986): Electromyographic studies of the lumbar trunk musculature during the development of axial torques. J Orthop Res 4:288–297.
103. Pope MH, Svensson M, Broman H, Andersson GB (1986): Mounting of the transducers in measurement of segmental motion of the spine. J Biomech 19(8):675–677.
104. Pope MH, Wilder DG, Matteri RE, Frymoyer JW (1977): Experimental measurements of vertebral motion under load. Orthop Clin N Am 8:155–167.
105. Posner I, White AA, Edwards WT, et al (1982): A biomechanical analysis of the clinical stability of the lumbar and lumbosacral spine. Spine 7:374–389.
106. Purcell GA, Markolf KL, Dawson EG (1981): Twelfth thoracic-first lumbar vertebral mechanical stability of fractures after Harrington-rod instrumentation. J Bone Joint Surg [Am] 63(1):71–78.
107. Quandieu P, Pellieux L (1982): Study in-situ and in-vivo of the acceleration of lumbar vertebrae of a primate exposed to vibration in the Z-axis. J Biomech 15:985–1006.
108. Quinnell RC, Stockdale HR (1983): The use of in-vivo lumbar discography to assess the clinical significance of the position of the intercrestal line. Spine 8:305–307.
109. Reuber M, Schultz A, Denis F, Spencer D (1982): Bulging of lumbar intervertebral disks. J Biomech Eng 104:187–192.

110. Ritchie JH, Fahrni WH (1970): Age changes in the lumbar intervertebral discs. *Canad J Surg* 13:65–71.
111. Roaf R (1960): A study of the mechanics of spinal injuries. *J Bone Joint Surg* [Br] 42:810–823.
112. Rolander SD (1966): Motion of the lumbar spine with special reference to the stabilizing effect of posterior fusion. An experimental study on autopsy specimens. *Acta Orthop Scand* [Suppl] 90:1–144.
113. Rowe ML (1971): Low back disability in industry: Updated position. *J Occup Med* 13:476–478.
114. Schultz AB (1974): Mechanics of the human spine. *Applied Mechanics Rev* 27(11):1487–1497.
115. Schultz AB, Andersson GBJ, Ortengren R, Bjork R, Nordin M (1982): Analysis and quantitative myoelectric measurements of loads on the lumbar spine when holding weights in standing postures. *Spine* 7:390–397.
116. Schultz AB, Andersson GBJ, Ortengren R, Haderspeck K, Nachemson A (1982): Loads on the lumbar spine, validation of a biomechanical analysis by measurement of intradiscal pressures and myoelectric signals. *J Bone Joint Surg* [Am] 64:713–720.
117. Schultz AB, Andersson GB, Haderspeck K, Ortengren R, Nordin M, Bjork R (1982): Analysis and measurement of lumbar trunk loads in tasks involving bends and twists. *J Biomech* 15:669–675.
118. Schultz AB, Warwick DN, Berkson MH, Nachemson AL (1979): Mechanical properties of human lumbar spine motion segments. Part I: Responses in flexion, extension, lateral bending and torsion. *J Biomech Eng* 101:46–52.
119. Seroussi RE, Pope MH (1987): The relationship between trunk muscle electromyography and lifting moments in the sagittal and frontal planes. *J Biomech* 20(2):135–146.
120. Shah JS, Hampson WG, Jayson MI (1978): The distribution of surface strain in the cadaveric lumbar spine. *J Bone Joint Surg* [Br] 60:246–251.
121. Slonim AR (1984): Some vibration data on primates implanted with accelerometers on the upper thoracic and lower lumbar spine: Results in baboons. Air Force Aerospace Medical Research Laboratory, Technical Report: TR-83-091.
122. Snook SH, Campanelli RA, Hart JW (1978): A study of three preventive approaches to low back injury. *J Occup Med* 20:478–481.
123. Sparup KH (1960): *Late prognosis in lumbar disc herniation.* Copenhagen: Munksgaard.
124. Stauffer ES, Neil JL (1975): Biomechanical analysis of structural stability of internal fixation in fractures of the thoracolumbar spine. *Clin Orthop* (112):159–164.
125. Stokes IAF, Greenapple DM (1985): Measurement of surface deformation of soft tissue. *J Biomech* 18:1–7.
126. Stokes IA, Medlicott PA, Wilder DG (1980): Measurement of movement in painful intervertebral joints. *Med Biol Eng Comput* 18:694–700.
127. Stokes IA, Wilder DG, Frymoyer JW, Pope MH (1981): Assessment of patients with low back pain by biplanar radiographic measurement of intervertebral motion. 1980 Volvo Award for Spine Research. *Spine* 6:233–240.
128. Takahashi K, Inoue S, Takada S, Nishiyama H, Mimura M, Wada Y (1986): Experimental study on chemonucleolysis with special reference to the change of intradiscal pressure. *Spine* 11:617–620.
129. Tanii K, Masuda T (1985): A kinesiologic study of erectores spinae activity during trunk flexion and extension. *Ergonomics* 28(6):883–893.
130. Tencer A (1981): *The mechanical properties of the human lumbar spine.* Doctoral dissertation, Department of Mechanical Engineering, McGill University, Montreal, Quebec.
131. Tencer AF, Ahmed AM (1981): The role of secondary variables in the measurement of the mechanical properties of the lumbar intervertebral joint. *J Biomech Eng* 103:129–137.
132. Tencer AF, Ahmed AM, Burke DL (1982): Some static mechanical properties of the lumbar intervertebral joint, intact and injured. *J Biomech Eng* 104:193–201.
133. Thorstensson A, Oddsson L, Andersson E, Arvidson A (1987): Balance in muscle strength between agonist and antagonist muscles of the trunk. Department of Physiology III, Lidinguvagen 1, Karolinska Institute, Stockholm, Sweden.
134. Troup JG, Rountree WB, Archibald RM (1970): Survey of cases of lumbar spinal disability. A methodological study. Med offices broadsheet, National Coal Board.
135. Tsuchida T, Suguro T, Inoue S, Kondoh Y, Nagai Y (1987): Regeneration of the nucleus pulposus after experimental chemonucleolysis: Collagenase. *Trans Orthop Res Soc,* San Francisco, California, January, 1987.
136. van Akkerveeken PF, O'Brien JP, Park WM (1979): Experimentally induced hypermobility in the lumbar spine. *Spine* 4:236–241.
137. Virgin WJ (1951): Experimental investigations into the physical properties of the intervertebral disc. *J Bone Joint Surg* [Br] 33:607–611.
138. Wakano K, Kasman R, Chao EY, Bradford DS, Oegema TR (1983): Biomechanical analysis of canine intervertebral discs after chymopapain injection: A preliminary report. *Spine* 8:59–68.
139. Weisman G, Pope MH, Johnson RJ (1980): Cyclic loading in knee ligament injuries. *Am J Sports Med* 8:24–30.
140. White AA III (1969): Analysis of the mechanics of the thoracic spine in man. *Acta Orthop Scand* [Suppl] 127:1–105.
141. Wilder DG, Frymoyer JW, Pope MH (1985): The effect of vibration on the spine of the seated individual. *Automedica* 6:5–35.
142. Wilder DG, Pope MH (1988): The biomechanics of lumbar disc herniation and the effect of overload and instability. *J Spinal Disorders* 1:16–32.
143. Wilder DG, Pope MH, Frymoyer JW (1982): Cyclic loading of the intervertebral motion segment. Proceedings of Tenth Northeast Bioengineering Conference, March 15–16, 1982, Dartmouth College, Hanover. New York: Institute Electrical and Electronic Engineers.
144. Wilder DG, Pope MH, Seroussi RE, Dimnet J, Krag MH (1989): The balance point of the intervertebral motion segment. *Bulletin Hosp Joint Dis Orthop Inst* 49(2):155–169.
145. Zagorski J, Jakubowski R, Solecki L, Sadlo A, Kasperek W (1976): Studies on the transmission of vibrations in human organism exposed to low-frequency whole-body vibration. *Acta Physiol Polonica* 27:347–354.

The Adult Spine: Principles and Practice,
J. W. Frymoyer, Editor-in-Chief.
Raven Press, Ltd., New York © 1991.

CHAPTER 68

Biomechanics of the Lumbar Spine

B. Surgical Principles

Vijay K. Goel, James N. Weinstein, and T. Okuma

The human spine is a complex columnar structure. It consists of vertebrae, discs, and ligaments, whose intricate interaction provides flexibility of motion, spinal cord protection, and distribution of body forces. In the diseased (or injured) state, this delicate equilibrium is disturbed. Low back pain presents one such disturbance and is one of the most common ailments afflicting Western society. While there are many accepted causes of low back pain, degeneration of the spinal segment is considered the most common cause (34). The degenerative process, which proceeds slowly with age, is generally asymptomatic, but in certain individuals it proceeds at a rapid rate with recurring or chronic pain. The changes in the vertebral bodies, intervertebral discs, facets, and ligaments of a spinal motion segment have been observed clinically to be associated with the degenerative process. As a result, it is not surprising to note an increase of intersegmental spinal mobility as an early symptom of

spinal degeneration. Although the exact mechanism is not known, epidemiological studies (13,17,35) have shown that mechanical factors of various kinds (inappropriate work habits, poorly designed chairs, repetitive loading (flexion and/or twisting) of the spine in an industrial setting) imposed during daily living do play a significant role in the onset of chronic low back pain.

Since mechanical factors play a significant role in the onset of low back pain, in vitro biomechanical studies may be undertaken to provide a basic understanding of the proportional resistance offered by the various spinal elements in response to external loading. These experiments may be undertaken on the "normal" (intact) specimens and then specimens artificially injured (to mimic clinical injuries and degenerative processes) and subsequently stabilized. This part of Chapter 68 reviews the recent work accomplished by various authors, as well as our own, in this direction. This presentation, therefore, complements the material presented by Pope, Wilder, and Krag in Part A of this chapter.

   V. K. Goel, Ph.D.: Professor, Department of Biomedical Engineering, University of Iowa, Iowa City, Iowa, 52242.
   J. N. Weinstein, D.O.: Associate Professor, Department of Orthopaedics; Director, Spine Diagnostic and Treatment Center, University of Iowa Hospitals and Clinics, Iowa City, Iowa, 52242.
   T. Okuma, M.D.: Orthopaedic Surgeon, Koganel-Shi, Tokyo, Japan.

TYPES OF SURGICAL PROCEDURE

Discectomy describes one of the surgical procedures used to remove a herniated disc. During this procedure the herniated, extruded, or sequestered fragments are removed. Partial excision of the bony lamina is sometimes necessary for good visualization. In spinal stenosis, partial facetectomy, dissection of the medial aspect of the superior facet of the involved apophyseal joint, may be indicated. In some cases with central stenosis, bilateral (total) laminectomy and facetectomy at the involved level(s) may be required.

Depending on the amount of bony and soft tissue decompression required, these surgical procedures may lead to spinal instability. Fusion of the lumbar spine segments to restore stability following some surgical procedures is undertaken using bone chips (mass) and/or spinal instrumentation. Internal fixation through instrumentation is done primarily to augment spinal stability and enhance post-operative mobilization of the patient. A number of devices—Harrington rods, Knodt rods, Kaneda device, Luque D-loops, and screw plates—for spinal fusion are currently in use (15, 28,38,44,45,74). Selection of a proper internal fixation system for a given clinical situation depends on the type of injury, the capabilities of the fixation system, and the preferences of the surgeon.

Despite a plethora of literature comparing results of discectomy to discectomy with lumbar fusion, there is a relative paucity of quantitative information on the long-term results of these surgical procedures (16,18,30,-39,40,41,49,59,67,68,69,71,73). However, the following biomechanical problem areas have been identified:

1. The extent of injury to spinal elements, which may lead to instability of a magnitude requiring further stabilization.
2. The effects of various internal fixation devices on the adjacent segments, since the clinical follow-ups indicate an increase in motion one to two levels above the fusion.
3. Biomechanical investigation of various currently available spinal instrumentation, to provide an objective assessment of their effects on instrumented and non-instrumented levels.

Results of biomechanical investigations addressing these questions are covered in the following paragraphs. The literature is subdivided into the following three categories: biomechanics of intact motion segment, effects of injured motion segments, and effects of stabilization.

BIOMECHANICS OF INTACT MOTION SEGMENT

A knowledge of the load-displacement (kinetic) behavior of the spine segments or its individual components (Fig. 1) allows an understanding of the relative contributions of various components in resisting the applied external load. The data base is also essential for inves-

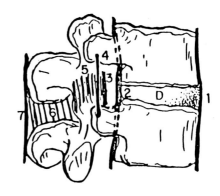
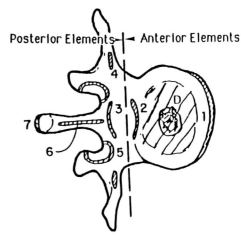

FIG. 1. The motion segment. It consists of two adjacent vertebrae and the interconnecting soft tissues. The ligaments are: anterior longitudinal **(1)**, posterior longitudinal **(2)**, ligamentum flavum **(3)**, transverse **(4)**, capsular **(5)**, interspinous **(6)**, and supraspinous **(7)**. Disc is represented by **D.** The line of demarcation separating the spinal elements into anterior and posterior elements is also shown.

tigating spine behavior using more sophisticated biomechanical models. Both in vivo investigations on humans and in vitro testing of ligamentous spine segments may be undertaken for generating the biomechanical data. This section reviews the techniques used for undertaking biomechanical studies and is followed by a summary of the results, reported in the literature, for the intact human lumbar spinal motion segments.

Measurement Techniques

In Vitro Biomechanical Studies

Both the experimental and analytical approaches have been used for this purpose. The experimental testing protocol varies, depending on the spinal component and the size and flexibility of the specimen used for testing. The vertebral body, the disc (whole or a section taken from a particular region), the ligaments, the two vertebrae intact motion segments, or a spine segment with more than two vertebrae are some of the spinal structures that would need different experimental protocols for testing. The following subsections describe representative testing protocols relevant for understanding the effects of injury and stabilization (surgical procedures) on the spine.

Spine Segments

The spinal elements of a motion segment impart the much-needed stability/flexibility to the segment. Their relative contributions, in resisting various load types, can be estimated by determining the load-displacement behaviors of intact specimens and specimens with a particular element (for example, facets) dissected. A number of experimental protocols have been developed with these objectives in mind.

The motion segments are dissected from cadavers at autopsy. Anteroposterior and lateral radiographs or computer tomographic scans are taken to identify structural abnormalities. The physiological data of the cadaver (age, sex, height, cause of death, degree of degeneration) are also recorded. This enables an investigator to discard specimens that may be highly degenerated. This data base also provides a basis for studying correlations, if any, among the biomechanical properties, degree of degeneration, sex, age, specimen size, and a host of other parameters (4). Since it is not practical to prepare and test the specimen while it is fresh, the specimen is preserved for future use by deep freezing at $-20°C$. It has been shown that deep freezing at this temperature does not alter, to a significant extent, the biomechanical characteristics of the bone (62), annulus (31), longitudinal ligament (72), or the motion segment as a single unit itself (55). A number of techniques have been used to prepare a specimen and test for its load-displacement behavior data (2,19,20,21,26,46,52,54,57,61,70,75,76).

The general methodology consists of freeing the specimen of all musculature tissue, leaving the ligamentous structure intact. Fixtures of some type are appropriately secured to the vertebral body at either end of the specimen (Fig. 2). The desired loads are applied through one

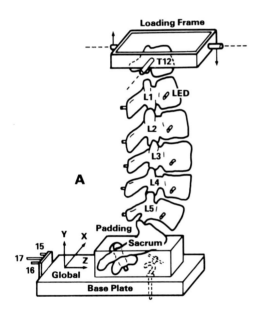

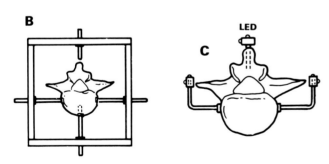

FIG. 2. The steps involved in preparing a specimen for testing are shown schematically. **A:** The relative positions of the loading frame, LEDs, Plastic Padding base, baseplate, and the directions of the global axes. The arrows at the loading rods indicate arrangement of load lines to apply flexion moment to the specimen. **B:** Details of the loading frame and rods. **C:** Method to attach three LEDs to a vertebra.

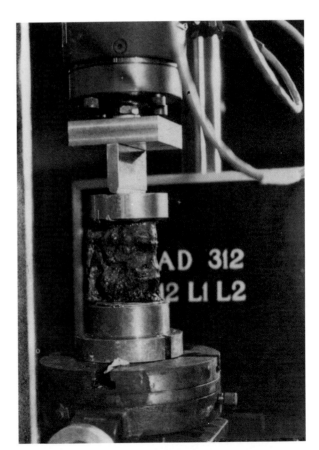

FIG. 3. The two vertebrae motion segment placed within an Instron testing machine (adapted from ref. 76).

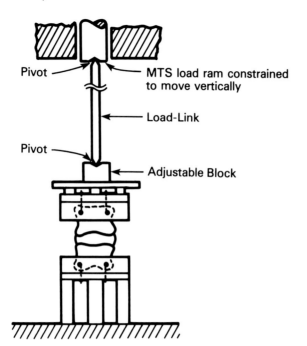

FIG. 4. The placement of a load link between the MTS load ram and the specimen permits application of axial load while letting the specimen move in any direction (adapted from ref. 75).

of the fixtures, while the other one is fixed to a base. The resulting displacements of the vertebral bodies with respect to the base are recorded. The methods of applying loads and measuring the resulting motion vary. For example, Yang and King (76) used an Instron machine to apply the loads and measure the resulting motion (Fig. 3). The axial load exerted on the specimen was recorded through the load cell, and the corresponding axial displacement of the moving fixture was taken as the dis-

placement experienced by the superior vertebra itself. In this set-up the vertebra was constrained, due to its rigid mounting to the top fixture, to move in the axial direction only. Thus only the load-displacement behavior of a motion segment in the axial direction was investigated. However, in response to an applied load the specimen exhibits displacements in the three-dimensional space (19). A modification of the loading system for use with an MTS system that would permit an unconstrained motion of the specimen is shown in Figure 4 (75). These authors placed a long rigid rod (load-link with a pivot on either end) between the MTS cross-head and the loading frame attached to the superior vertebra. This enabled the specimen to move in space in response to the applied axial load. Panjabi et al. (52) developed a technique to measure the three-dimensional load-displacement behavior of a two vertebrae motion segment. This technique has been used by a number of other investigators as well (20). The technique allows investigation of changes in the relative motion between the two adjacent vertebrae as a function of injury/stabilization. However, the effects of induced injury/stabilization on the adjacent levels cannot be investigated. For this purpose, multilevel spine segment studies are mandated. Techniques, based on the principles of stereophotogrammetry, have been used to investigate three-dimensional load-displacement behaviors of individual vertebral bodies of a whole spine specimen tested as one unit. A real time data acquisition technique, based on the Selspot II system, has been developed by the authors (21,25). In this system, light-emitting diodes (LEDs), attached to the vertebral bodies, are used to define the location of the vertebra in space. The system is an optoelectronic device in which the infrared light emitted by an LED is picked up by two cameras, located at different positions with respect to the

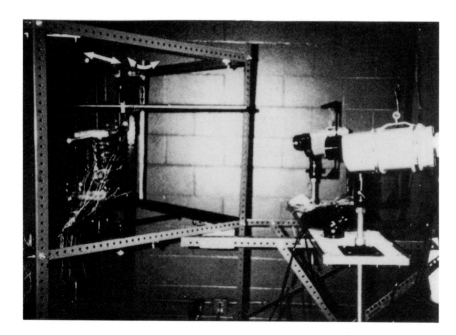

FIG. 5. The prepared specimen, with LEDs mounted, housed in the testing rig. The two Selspot II cameras are visible. The specimen may be subjected to various loads through pulleys. These pulleys could be moved in space with the aid of horizontal and vertical rods shown.

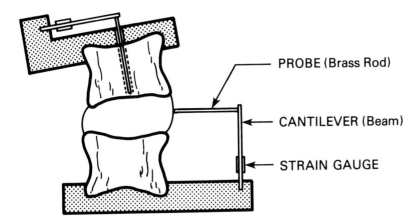

FIG. 6. Schematic diagram of the transducers used to measure transverse disc and endplate bulges (adapted from ref. 58).

LED. The principles of stereophotogrammetry are then applied to convert the voltage outputs from the two cameras into the spatial location of the LED. The system, with the LEDs mounted on a spine specimen and placed in the view of the cameras, is shown in Figure 5.

Disc and End-Plate Bulge

The source of pathology in cases of intervertebral disc prolapse is fairly clear. The extruded nuclear material presses on a nerve root, causing pain. This may happen due to excessive disc bulge, although true prolapse may not be apparent. Thus it would be of value to quantify disc bulge in response to an external load. An elegant technique to determine disc bulge at a few discrete points has been reported by Reuber et al. (58). The strain-

gauge-mounted cantilevers are used to measure disc bulge at five locations along the disc periphery: two lateral, two points along posterolateral, and one posterior. The transducer consists of a small-diameter brass rod (probe) attached to the tip of a strain-gauged cantilever flexure (Fig. 6). The free end of the rod was made to rest against the disc surface and the flexure was oriented to sense transverse disc bulge as a function of the applied load. The same device was used by the authors to record axial displacement of the bony end plate above the nucleus (Fig. 6). The tip of the rod butts against the top of the end plate and the cantilever end is fixed to the vertebral body. Thus the relative displacement between the body and the end plate is recorded by the transducer. Typical variations in disc bulge along lateral, posterolateral, and posterior regions in compression (COMP), right lateral bending (RLB), extension (EXT), flexion (FLX), and right axial rotation (RAR) are shown in Figure 7.

Intradiscal Pressure

Intradiscal pressure measurements are taken as an indicator of the axial load imposed across a motion segment during various physical activities. Such measurements may be used in teaching patients to avoid activities that are likely to increase loads on the spine. Consequently, the quantification of intradiscal pressure would be of immense value in the conservative treatment of low back pain patients. Nachemson and associates were the first to develop a technique for recording pressures within the disc in vivo (50). It consists of a pressure transducer attached to the tip of a needle (Fig. 8) (11). The operation of the transducer is based on the piezoresistive effect of a semiconductor strain gauge embedded in rigid resin in an elastic tube. When a uni-axial load is applied to this "strain tube" in the axial direction, the load is transmitted to the gauge through the rigid resin. The frequency response of the pressure needle allows measurements of pressure changes up to at least

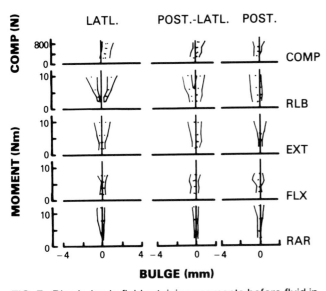

FIG. 7. Disc bulge in fluid-retaining segments before fluid injection. Mean compressive motion at 800 N was 1 mm, mean vertebral tilt values were approximately 5 degrees for a 10 Nm moment in flexion (FLX), extension (EXT), or lateral bending (RLB). Mean twist was approximately 2 degrees for a 10 Nm torsional moment (adapted from ref. 58).

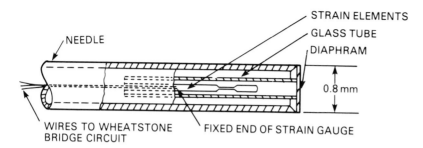

NEEDLE

STRAIN ELEMENTS
GLASS TUBE
DIAPHRAM

0.8 mm

WIRES TO WHEATSTONE
BRIDGE CIRCUIT

FIXED END OF STRAIN GAUGE

FIG. 8. Intradiscal pressure transducer on end of needle as developed by Nachemson and associates (adapted from ref. 11).

5,000 hertz. The intradiscal pressure approximates to 1.5 times the mean applied pressure over the entire area of the vertebral end plate (48).

Results

By use of techniques similar to the ones described above, the contributions of various spinal elements in resisting the external load and their roles in stabilizing the spinal column have been delineated by a number of investigators, including the authors. These studies also help in identifying the structures that may be overloaded and consequently be the source of low back pain. The findings are summarized below.

The simple compression test of the disc-body unit (motion segment without posterior elements) has been the most popular experiment in the past. The compression and tension tests revealed that the disc is stiffer in compression than in tension (46). This may be attributed to the buildup of fluid pressure within the nucleus under compression loading. The response of the disc-body unit to high-speed dynamic loads was investigated by Perey (56). The specimens failed due to either end-plate failure or the compression of the vertebra. The rupture of the end plate may be due to the intradiscal pressure buildup during compressive loading. However, no disc herniations ever took place. Brown et al. observed that flexion bending of about 15 degrees leads to a failure of the disc-body unit by means of avulsion of a triangular piece of bone from the vertebra in the postero-inferior region (8). The presence of posterior elements during testing protected the segment to the extent that the flexion angles reduced to 6 to 8 degrees and no failures at all could be observed. In their study as well no disc failure ever occurred. More recent studies have looked at the motion behavior of intact motion segments and segments with sequential cutting of elements in an effort to understand the role of various spinal elements in resisting external loads. Adams and Hutton (1) found that the osteoligamentous lumbar spine was most at risk in the lordotic posture and when bending forward. Sustained lordotic posture can produce abnormal loading of the apophyseal joints. Bending forward wedges the lumbar discs, rendering them vulnerable to fatigue injuries during heavy la-

bor. Excessive flexion can cause posterior ligament damage which, followed by a strong contraction of the back muscles, can lead to a prolapsed intervertebral disc. Axial torsional load applied to failure caused fractures adjacent to the facets and ultimately failure of the interspinous ligaments. These may be another cause of low back pain. Reduced torsional strength may result if the fracture produces facet asymmetry, thus rendering the individual more susceptible to later torsional stresses.

Posner et al. (57) examined the role of spinal elements in producing instability by testing 18 motion segments subjected to an antero-posterior (extension) or postero-anterior (flexion) shear force and a preload. The preload forces corresponded to the axial compressive force experienced at a motion segment of a person lying supine (66% to 73% of body weight) or standing (132% to 146% of body weight). Likewise the maximum shear force applied was 50% to 90% of body weight. The specimens, under these loads, were found to fail in flexion when all the posterior components plus one anterior component had been destroyed; in extension when all the anterior components plus two posterior components had been destroyed. The preload appeared to protect the motion segments from excessive sagittal rotation in extension, but increase it in flexion.

Schultz et al. (61), Berkson et al. (4), and Tencer et al. (70) undertook studies to investigate the effects of various injuries—sequentially sectioning both facets, posterior ligaments, excision of the disc annulus and the anterior longitudinal ligament—on the motion behavior of the lumbar motion segments. The joint was most flexible in anterior shear and least flexible in axial compression. The disc was found to be the major load-bearing element in lateral and anterior shears and axial compression and flexion. In lateral and anterior shears and axial compression, with high displacements, the facets may transmit part of the load. However, in posterior shear (extension) and axial torque, facets were the major load-bearing structures.

A number of studies using saline solution to increase nucleus fluid within the disc revealed an increase in intradiscal pressure and disc height. Andersson and Schultz (3), however, studied the changes in motion behavior as a function of fluid content and found that fluid injection uniformly reduced (i.e., led to an increase in stiffness) mean motions, but less so in compression, extension, and torsion (5% to 20% less) than in flexion and lateral bending (25% to 52% less). Mean intradiscal pressure increased with loading after injection but was smaller than before injection in flexion and torsion, nearly the same in compression, and larger in extension and lateral bending. The total pressure in every case was considerably greater, by as much as 83%. These studies show that state of hydration of the nucleus is an important determinant of biomechanical behavior of the motion segment.

Reuber et al. (58) found that under compressive loads of up to 800 N with and without bending moments of up to 11.8 Nm, mean disc bulge of up to 2.7 mm beyond the unloaded states may occur, but the end-plate bulge was not noticeable. Degenerated discs bulged more than nondegenerated discs under the same load. Posterior element removal did not have much effect on disc bulge. The posterolateral disc bulge was seen to be larger than the posterior bulge. There was no clear relationship between intradiscal pressure and disc bulge. Brinckmann et al. (6) found that at higher loads, the deformations experienced by the bony parts may not be negligible and would contribute (especially knowing that the vertebral body is filled with blood) towards the load-sharing mechanism. For example, the bulge in the vertebral end plates at higher loads (>2,500 N) would reduce straining of the disc fibers. This mechanism also explains the fracture of end plates frequently observed as a result of axial overloading.

Lorenz et al. (43) presented experimental data on the facet loads, contact areas, and peak pressure across the apophyseal joints of L2-L3 and L4-L5 motion segments. The capsular ligaments were excised and a strip of Fuji Prescale pressure-sensitive film was inserted across the joint. The loads borne by facets were higher in extension posture (141 N) in comparison to neutral posture (58 N) for an axial load of about 1,000 N. The effect of unilateral facetectomy was that the loads on the remaining facet were reduced substantially after facetectomy (15.5 N in neutral and 21.8 N in extension). This implies some kind of wedging mechanism in which both facet joints are responsible for the force transmission. Thus all of the load-resistance characteristics can be altered when the facets are maloriented.

Analytical Models

Mathematical models of a motion segment are essential for a number of reasons. These help systemize thinking, make predictions, and therefore, suggest experiments that might otherwise not have come to mind. The mathematical models, based on the biomechanical properties of individual components described above, can simulate behavior of the spine in situations in which other means of investigation are not feasible. Further-

more, certain parameters cannot be measured experimentally and one has to resort to mathematical models to find an answer. For example, a knowledge of state of stress and strain and the forces acting throughout the lumbosacral joint may be helpful to a proper understanding of some of the mechanical causes of low back pain. Technical difficulties either preclude direct measurements of such parameters or make experiments very time-consuming, cumbersome, and error prone. A mathematical model may be one of the alternative approaches to overcome these hurdles. The unusual complexity of the spinal structure, however, demands a stepwise approach, i.e., at each step of model development, its prediction should be validated in terms of those parameters amenable to experimental measurement. The finite-element technique has been used to determine the state of stress and strain within all of the spinal elements of a given motion segment. A review of the use of the finite-element technique for modeling a spine motion segment and development of the models is provided by Liu and Goel (42). Some of the pertinent results obtained from an intact motion segment model are described here.

The effects of a number of variables—variation in intradiscal pressure, nucleus removal, disc degeneration, variation of fiber angles and shape variations of the disc (on its posterior aspect) on the axial compressive displacement, disc and end-plate bulges, and stress distribution within the structures—were investigated by Shirazi-Adl et al. (64) using a finite-element model of the disc-body unit subjected to an axial compressive load. Comparison of the predicted gross response characteristics (such as load-displacement behavior, intradiscal pressure, strains in ligaments) with available experimental measurements indicated satisfactory agreements. The stress-distribution results, which cannot be determined experimentally, revealed the following.

In the cancellous bone of the vertebral body with a normal disc, the maximum compressive stress occurred at the regions adjacent to the nucleus space, while in the disc void of the nucleus, this stress occurred adjacent to the annular attachment region. The authors also found that under compressive load, the most vulnerable elements in a normal disc were the cancellous bone and the end plate adjacent to the nucleus space. This prediction appears to correlate with the frequent occurrence of Schmorl's nodes in nondegenerated discs. For the disc void of the nucleus, however, the most vulnerable element appeared to be the annulus ground substance that was predicted to undergo large radial tensile strain. This result correlates with the occurrence of circumferential clefts in degenerated discs. Also, the stresses in the cancellous bone and the end plate, although markedly reduced, still remained sufficiently high to cause failure in regions adjacent to the annulus attachment zone. The annular fibers of the disc did not appear to be particularly susceptible to rupture under compressive load.

The disc-body unit model, described above, has been extended by Shirazi-Adl and associates (63) and at the authors' laboratory (36) to include the anterior and posterior elements: ligaments and facets. The results indicate that the load-transfer path through the posterior elements of the joint in flexion is different from that in extension.

In flexion, the ligaments are the means of load transfer. Consequently, the ligaments experience large strains (as high as 25% in the supraspinous and interspinous ligaments for 30 Nm of flexion with no preload) and are vulnerable to rupture. The cancellous bone adjacent to the disc may fracture under large loads, being in compression (1.81 MPa for 60 Nm and magnitude being comparable to the yield strength of the bone). In the extension mode, load is transmitted through the pedicles, laminae, and articular processes. In this mode, the anterior longitudinal and capsular ligaments are highly strained (about 25% for 30 Nm). The strain in the anterior longitudinal ligament increases upon removal of the facets. The stress analysis results indicate that the cancellous bone adjacent to the disc undergo large tensile stresses (1.81 MPa for 60 Nm). Large compressive stresses in the tips of the inferior facets and large tensile stresses in the articular surfaces of the inferior facets (113.5 MPa) are found, which point to the possibility of fracture failure at these locations under hyperextension.

The computation of facet forces in various load types revealed the following. In pure compression, the force is transmitted primarily by the intervertebral disc. The application of compression, depending on the point of application, produces axial displacement and the accompanying flexion rotation. For the case in which the flexion rotation takes place (about 2.5 degrees under 5,000 N), each facet carries only a small percentage (1% to 4%) of load. When the load is applied at a point such that the accompanying flexion rotation is minimum (called the balance point of the specimen), this percent-

age may increase to 10%. In extension with no preload applied, each facet resists a considerable amount of force (Fig. 9). For example, the axial component of the force on each facet for 6.9 Nm is about 58 N. The capsular ligaments, although in tension, carry a negligible load. In extension, with a preload applied, the load across each facet may be 10% to 30% of the preload value. This percentage is higher at smaller preload values (about 35% at 120 N load and 12 Nm) and goes down at higher preloads. In flexion with a preload, facets do not carry any load until 7 degrees of rotation. The major load-bearing elements are the disc and the ligaments. Beyond 7 degrees of flexion, however, some load (as large as in extension) may be borne by the facets.

These studies reinforce the concept that stress analysis, concurrent with experimental measurements, is an appropriate approach toward the elucidation of the mechanical causes of the disorders affecting the human lumbosacral spine. The finite-element model can be used to assess the biomechanical effects of injuries (which mimic surgical procedures) and stabilization on the motion segment. The results of such models developed by the authors are described at appropriate places within the text (36).

BIOMECHANICS OF INJURY

Both the experimental and analytical tools have been used to analyze the effects of injury/surgery on the spine behavior. These two approaches are complementary to each other. For example, the effect of injury on the three-dimensional motion behavior, using a multispine segment, in response to applied loads can be investigated through an experiment. However, it is neither practical to test a specimen subjected to complex loads seen in vivo nor possible to estimate the stresses and strains within the motion segment as a function of injury. It is

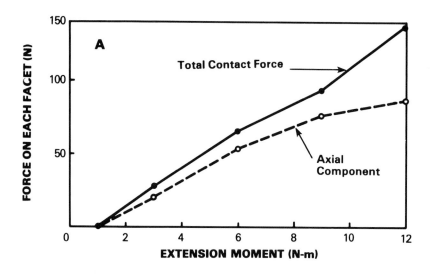

FIG. 9. Predicted variation of the contact force on each facet with extension (adapted from ref. 63).

also not practical to quantify the loads being imposed on spinal elements. For these reasons, an analytical model, however crude it may be, would be helpful. The results of both types of studies are described below.

Experimental Studies

Markolf and Morris (46) characterized the load-displacement behaviors of lumbar discs (motion segments with posterior elements removed) subjected to axial compression. These tests were repeated after partial and total nucleus removal in one series of experiments, while in another series the vertebral end plates were also scraped off. A comparison of the data for mechanically altered specimens with those of intact specimens revealed insignificant changes in the compressive stiffness of the disc with nucleus removal. This suggests that there exists a self-sealing mechanism within the disc that negates the effects of injury inflicted on the structure. The response of the injured specimens to other load types (flexion, extension, lateral bending, and axial rotation) was not studied. Also, the effect of the injury in the presence of posterior elements of a motion segment may be different.

Investigators improved upon the Markolf and Morris model by including the posterior elements of the motion segment during testing of intact as well as injured motion segments (4,61,70). The sequential disc injuries induced in these studies included the following: cutting of annulus layers and transection of the anterior or posterior half of the disc. The main conclusion was that the injury to the disc results in an alteration of the motion behavior even though none of the disc injuries mimicked clinical situations.

Panjabi et al. (53) undertook a detailed three-dimensional investigation of the mechanical behavior of the lumbar motion segments as affected by injuries to the two components of the disc. The sequential injuries considered were (a) cutting a square window (5 × 5 mm) in the annulus on the right posterolateral side lateral to the neural foramen, and (b) total removal (as much as possible) of the nucleus material. A significant increase in the primary as well as secondary/coupled motion components with disc injuries was observed for almost all loading modes. The results clearly showed that the self-sealing effect of annulus, as observed by Markolf and Morris, did not hold true. The observed increase in secondary motion in flexion and extension modes meant that the characteristic symmetric motion about the mid-sagittal plane, usually exhibited by an intact motion segment, was no longer present after the injury. The authors rightly hypothesized that this would lead to an asymmetric movement of the apophyseal joints. This movement, in turn, may lead to facet degeneration. However, clinical follow-up studies of patients who underwent disc ex-

cision surgery did not report any problems specific to facets over time at the injury site (29,67,73). The excessive increases in secondary motions observed by Panjabi et al. may be due to the unusual location of the injury site in their model. Disc herniations usually occur in the posterolateral margins within the vertebral canal. Discectomy usually involves removing the ligamentum flavum and then partially removing the nucleus, with small pituitary rongeurs. A small bony laminotomy is sometimes necessary for good visualization. We, therefore, initiated an in vitro biomechanical study to investigate the effect of clinically realistic disc injuries induced at the most common site of herniation within a motion segment (24).

The load-displacement behaviors of intact specimens were obtained. The experiment was repeated after each of the two disc injuries shown in Figure 10. The first injury simulated disc protrusion or herniation (HRN), an injury associated with low back pain prior to surgery. The disc herniation was created on the left side posterolaterally (within the vertebral canal) by cutting the left ligamentum flavum and the annulus horizontally. The nucleus pulposus was then gently teased out of the annulus. The teased nucleus was therefore not totally separated from its remaining part. The second sequential injury was a partial discectomy (PDS), as suggested by Spengler (67). A small amount of nucleus pulposus was removed with the aid of a pituitary rongeur inserted into the incision already made during the first injury. The

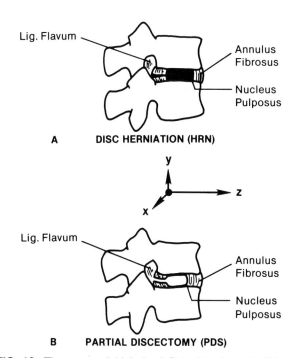

FIG. 10. The sequential injuries inflicted to simulate **(A)** disc herniation (HRN), and **(B)** partial discectomy (PDS). The injuries were located within the vertebral canal and close to the mid-sagittal plane.

results indicate that the most significant increase in motion, for specimens with partial discectomy, occurs in the flexion mode followed by axial rotation and lateral bending. Our results are in agreement with Panjabi et al. (53) that the self-sealing mechanism of the injured disc, as observed by Markolf and Morris (46), is not present in loading modes investigated in the present study. The results, however, differ from those of Panjabi et al. with respect to the effect of discectomy on the secondary/coupled motions. We did not observe any significant increases in these components after injury. These differences, we believe, may be due to the following: the unusual injury sight chosen by Panjabi et al. and the large size of the annulus cut and the greater amount of nucleus material removed in comparison to our study.

Goel et al. (21), using whole lumbar spine specimens (T12-sacrum), also investigated the effects of partial laminectomy and facetectomy along with denucleation of the disc on the motion behavior of the involved as well as adjacent segments. The three-dimensional load-displacement behaviors of the five vertebral bodies (L1 through L5) of a specimen in flexion (FLX), extension (EXT), lateral bending (RLB, LLB), and axial twist (LAR, RAR), for a maximum of 3.0 Nm were obtained through the use of the Selspot II system. To study the effect of injury on the motion behavior of the specimens, in Group I, four clinically relevant injuries (Fig. 11) were artificially induced at the L4-L5 disc level on the right side (21). In Group II, bilateral nerve root decompression clinically indicated for lateral and central spinal ste-

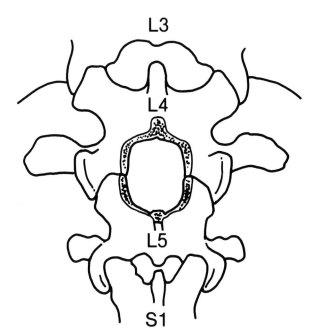

FIG. 12. Schematic of spinal decompression surgery. It involves cutting of the supraspinous and interspinous ligaments and the ligamentum flavum. Bilateral laminectomy and facetectomy complete the procedure.

nosis was performed at the L4-L5 level (Fig. 12). The specimen was loaded and tested to determine the changed motion behavior after each injury. Discectomy, partial or total, led to an increase in motion at the injury site, especially in flexion. In extension, the change in the motion post-injury was the least. Subtotal discectomy, however, was found to induce significantly less motion at the injury site than total discectomy. At the L3-L4 level, the motion segment above the injury level, anteroposterior translation in flexion and lateral translation in left lateral bending showed an increase with the removal of the nucleus.

If one pools together the results of the studies described above, the relationship between the extent of disc excision and the likely effects on the motion behavior of the lumbar spine may be that increase in motion is directly related to the amount of nucleus excised at surgery and the extent and location of injury to the disc annulus fibers. The studies lend support to the clinical practice for management of patients with low back pain, i.e., as little as possible of the nucleus is excised at surgery. Furthermore, patients are advised to do extension exercises following herniation and discectomy, which is in agreement with the findings of this study in which extension was found to be the stablest loading mode, especially after subtotal discectomy. They are also advised to avoid lateral bending and axial rotation following discectomy, which were found to be possible modes of instability.

The results for the injury protocol of Group II (bilateral decompression) revealed that the motion at the in-

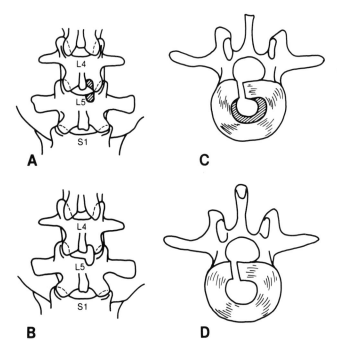

FIG. 11. The clinically relevant injuries artificially created at the L4-L5 level. **A:** Partial laminectomy. **B:** Partial facetectomy. **C:** Subtotal discectomy. **D:** Total discectomy.

jured level after injury, in comparison to the normal state, increased significantly in flexion, extension, and axial rotation modes. In flexion, the increase in motion is primarily due to the cutting of the ligaments, while a damage to the facets contributed to the observed increase in motion in extension and axial rotation. Since the lateral aspects of the facets that are involved in resisting lateral bending were more or less left intact, no significant instability was observed in this mode. A total excision of facets or disc, if indicated in a patient, would induce instability in a lateral bending mode also (27).

Effects of Chymopapain

Chemonucleolysis is an alternative approach to discectomy. The intradiscal injection of chymopapain dissolves the nucleus without disrupting any other spinal structures. The exact mechanism by which enzymatic dissolution of the nucleus relieves the pain associated with the disc prolapse is not known (7). It is proposed that by destroying the proteoglycan core the water-binding capacity of the disc is lost, reducing intradiscal pressure and hence pressure on the entrapped nerve root (5,7,66). A direct anti-inflammatory effect or a chemical effect also has been suggested. The role of reduced intradiscal pressure, however, in relieving the entrapped nerve root has been challenged (7).

Brinckmann and Horst (7), using cadaver lumbar motion segments, monitored the changes in disc height, intradiscal pressure, end-plate pressure distribution, and motion segment flexibility in various loading modalities that may occur up to 8 hours after the injection of chymopapain in one group of specimens and isotonic solution in the control group. All specimens increased in height after intradiscal injection (saline or chymopapain). The restoration of height to the starting value took an average of 3 hours. A further 0.8 mm decrease in height was seen after 8 hours. The axial stiffness decreased (creep behavior) continuously during the 8-hour period. However, no difference could be noticed between the two groups. The bending stiffness for both groups increased, although marginally. In conclusion, these authors did not find any significant differences between the chymopapain and saline injected groups.

One hundred twenty-two lumbar intervertebral discs from 43 mongrel dogs were used by Spencer et al. (66) to study the effect of chemonucleolysis on the flexion, torsion, and lateral bending flexibilities of the disc (motion segments with posterior elements removed). The dogs were killed 2, 4, 12, 26, and 52 weeks following injection with 0.1 to 0.15 ml of either crude collagenase, semipurified collagenase, or chymopapain. Controls consisted of saline-injected and uninjected discs. The bending and torsional properties of each disc were determined by applying incremental moments (up to 0.8 Nm) and mea-

suring the resultant rotations. The discs were then sectioned for morphologic evaluation. Increases in disc flexibilities ranging from 1.4 to 5.8-fold were found two weeks after injection with all three enzymes. The largest increase was noted in flexion in discs injected with chymopapain. By three months, all lateral bending flexibilities had returned to control values. In general, however, flexion and torsion flexibilities did not return to control values six months following chemonucleolysis. The extent of the gross morphologic changes produced by each of the three enzyme preparations did not correlate with the acute increases in disc flexibilities. At six months, there was an apparent replacement of the nuclear material by the fibrotic tissues. This finding is in contrast to the disc regeneration reported by Bradford et al. (5). The discrepancy may be dose-related: lower dosage may promote nuclear regeneration.

As is obvious from the above-described studies, no explanations, based on mechanical grounds, could be offered to explain the immediate efficacy of therapeutic intradiscal chymopapain injections. We believe, however, that the effectiveness of chymopapain injection in relieving pain comes from the decrease in disc bulge, which results from the dissolution of the nucleus as discussed in the following section (22,37). The above studies did not document the effect of chymopapain on the disc bulge per se.

Analytical Studies

The biomechanical effects of total denucleation of the disc with and without partial laminectomy and facetectomy (to mimic chemonucleolysis (CHM) and total discectomy (TDS), respectively) and disc degeneration on a ligamentous motion segment were investigated by the authors using the finite-element models (22,36,37).

The axial translation and flexion rotation of the center of the superior vertebral body of the L3-L4 model as a function of the applied load are shown respectively in Figures 13A and 13B. The motion behavior of the intact (INT) model is included for the sake of comparison. For chemonucleolysis (CHM) and total discectomy (TDS) models, the axial displacement and rotation angle are almost double that of an intact case. The increase in axial displacement is larger for the TDS model compared to the CHM model. The two-fold decrease in stiffness of the denucleated specimen is compatible with the clinical observation of decrease in disc space height following surgery. The total contact force across the two facet joints for three models is shown in Figure 13C. The contact force for the CHM model is higher than for the INT model. For 1,160 N axial compressive load, the total force for the CHM model was found to be 25.9% of the applied axial load. This represents a two-fold increase, compared to the intact model. This shows clearly that

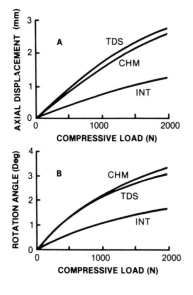

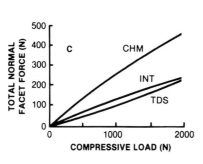

FIG. 13. The computed variation in the **(A)** axial displacement, **(B)** flexion rotation angle, and **(C)** total force across the two facets due to chemonucleolysis (CHM) and total discectomy (TDS). The corresponding parameters for the intact model (INT) are also provided for a comparison.

the denucleation of the disc would induce abnormal stresses across the facet joint. Our results of von Mises stresses in the region of pedicles indicate this to be true (1.8 MPa in intact vs. 2.6 MPa in CHM model). Denucleation also altered the disc bulging pattern and strains in the annulus fibers. In the posterior region, the disc bulge was less for the CHM model as compared to an intact model (0.74 mm vs. 1.26 mm under 1,160 N compressive load). This decrease may be sufficient to relieve pressure on the entrapped nerve roots. We believe that the immediate relief in pain as a result of chymopapain injection comes from the decrease in disc bulge in the posterior region. The undesirable effects of increased load on the facets and stresses in the adjacent regions over time may be offset by the regeneration of nucleus, which has been reported to occur. In the TDS model the contact force is similar to that in the INT model, but the stresses induced would still be very high, since the contact area is reduced as a result of facetectomy.

The results of the two motion segments/three vertebrae model in which the L4-L5 disc nucleus was replaced by a fibrosus material—to simulate disc degeneration and its effects on the adjacent levels—indicate that for the same displacement of the L3-L4 superior end plate the nucleus pressure in the L3-L4 disc, compared to the intact model, showed an 8% to 10% increase. The increase in the disc pressure and other parameters support the clinical observation that injury (disc degeneration) at one level affects the adjacent levels as well.

BIOMECHANICS OF SPINAL INSTRUMENTATION

Spinal stabilization and spinal fusion have been used since early in this century to treat a variety of spinal problems, including disc degeneration, fracture, spondylolisthesis, and tumors. As described earlier, a number of

devices are currently in use. These instrumentations are either used alone or in combination with bone grafts and/or external support (such as casts or braces). The results of the experimental and analytical studies reported in the literature are summarized in the following.

Experimental Investigations

The in vitro experimental investigations reported in the literature may best be described under three categories. The studies in the first category deal with the design of the "nuts and bolts" of the system itself. For example, what should be the shape and size of the screws and the dimensions of the plate in the Steffee plate system? This requires a thorough knowledge of (a) vertebral and spinal functional anatomy, and (b) techniques that may be used for mechanical testing of the individual components of the system once those have been fabricated out of an appropriate material. Krag et al. and a few other investigators have published detailed experimental protocols that were developed and used by the authors for various fixation systems (9,12,38,65) (see Chapter 92).

In the second category are investigations dealing with the overall strength afforded by the use of a particular instrumentation (10,28,32,78). In these studies, ligamentous spine segments (say T12-sacrum) are injured to mimic a clinically relevant injury and then stabilized. The stabilized spine segments are subjected to flexion, extension, lateral bending, or axial twist loads until failure. The load and resulting overall displacement at failure, for example, are compared with similar data obtained for a group of intact spines. This helps to characterize the overall stiffness of the stabilized spines. The results of such studies have shown that most of the devices currently in use are effective in restoring the stability to the injured specimens in flexion/extension, although the degree of effectiveness varies among different devices. These studies do not, however, provide an insight into the displacement behavior between the injured/stabilized level and the levels adjacent to it. These two aspects, as described earlier, are important from a clinical standpoint. Experiments elucidating these aspects constitute the last category (14,25,27,51,77). The characteristic testing and evaluation protocol, as described in studies undertaken by the authors (14,25,27) and adopted, are as follows.

Fresh cadaveric ligamentous spines (T12-sacrum) were acquired and prepared for testing as per the protocol described earlier. The three-dimensional load-displacement behaviors of intact specimens in flexion (FLX), extension (EXT), right and left lateral bending (RLB, LLB), and left and right axial rotation (LAR, RAR) were recorded. The specimens were then divided into four groups of ten specimens each for further testing as described below.

Group I. The specimens first were destabilized at the L4-L5 level to create bilateral nerve root decompression clinically indicated for spinal stenosis (central and lateral) (Fig. 12). The supraspinous and interspinous ligaments were transected at the L3-L4 and L5-S1 levels, and two 19-gauge stainless-steel wires were placed one on either side of the midline from the L3-L4 to the L4-L5 interspace and similarly from the L4-L5 to the L5-S1 interspace. A small amount of the ligamentum flavum was also removed at the median raphe to allow passage of the wires. The specimens were stabilized with Luque loops, shown schematically in Figure 14C, of appropriate sizes. A 5 cm Luque closed-loop system was then secured with the four wires. The inferior portion of each wire was placed on the lateral aspect of the ring. The wires were then twisted and tightened using a wire tightener.

Group II. The specimens in this group were injured by creating bilateral laminectomy, bilateral facetectomy, and total discectomy across the L4-L5 motion segment (Fig. 14A). The injury model was an extension of the Group I injury in which total discectomy was not undertaken. A bone graft was inserted into the disc space and then further stabilized sequentially using the Luque loop and then the Steffee plates (Figs. 14B and 14C). This group provided a comparison between the two fixation devices.

Group III. The specimens in this group were used to assess the efficacies of the Luque loop and Steffee plates while stabilizing the L5-S1 level in place of the L4-L5 level. The injury model was similar to that of Group II.

Group IV. In this group, the injuries and stabilizations of Groups II and III were combined to determine the stabilization characteristics for the Luque loop and the Steffee plates used to stabilize the L4-S1 segment instead of one segment only.

The specimens were tested after each injury and after each stabilization procedure in an entirely analogous manner to that of the intact state; the position information of all the LEDs was stored. The LED spatial location data of the intact, injured, and stabilized specimens were reduced further to yield percent change in displacements (or motions) after injury or stabilization in comparison to the intact cases as functions of load magnitude, load type, and the vertebral levels (stabilized segments or the adjacent segments). The results obtained for the various injury models have already been described. The effects of stabilization are described below.

Group I: Luque Loop Across the L4-L5 Motion Segment

In the flexion mode the relevant primary motions involved are the rotation about the X axis (R_X) and the translation along the Z axis (T_Z). At the L4-L5 motion segment (Fig. 15) the rotation decreased after stabilization (-39.6%, $P < 0.01$). The translation demonstrated decreasing trends but not at a significant level, decreasing after stabilization (-10.0%, $P < 0.2$). Above the injured/stabilized level at the L3-L4 (Fig. 16), the rotation increased after stabilization (25%, $P < 0.05$). No significant changes were observed in the translation. Below the

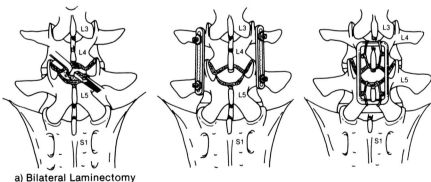

a) Bilateral Laminectomy
b) Bilateral Facetectomy
c) Total Discectomy
d) Bone Graft
A

Steffee Plates
B

Luque Loop
C

FIG. 14. The injury to achieve spinal decompression is shown **(A)**. The injured specimen is stabilized sequentially using **(B)** Steffee plates, and then **(C)** Luque loop.

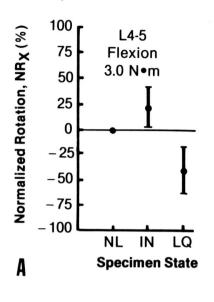

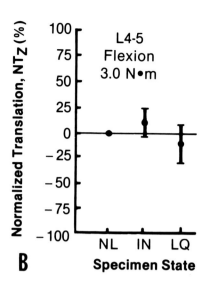

FIG. 15. Normalized primary motion components at the L4-L5 level corresponding to 3.0 Nm of flexion moment as a function of a specimen state. **A:** Normalized rotation NR$_x$. **B:** Normalized translation NT$_z$. NL, normal state; IN, injured state; and LQ, Luque closed-loop state.

injury level at the L5-S1, the rotation increased after stabilization but not significantly. At the L4-L5 motion segment, the rotation in extension decreased after stabilization (-36.0%, $P < 0.05$). The use of a closed loop to stabilize the segment restored the translation motion back to normal (no significant change). In lateral bending, left as well as right, the changes in motion components at the stabilized level (L4-L5), as well as adjacent levels, were found to be less than 10%. Thus, no definite conclusions can be made regarding the degree of instability induced after injury or the effectiveness of the closed loop. This also was found to be the case in the axial loading mode.

After stabilization with a closed loop, the motion at the L3-L4 motion segment, the level above the injured/stabilized level, increased significantly in flexion. This

increase in motion may be due to the use of the closed loop at the L4-L5 and/or the cutting of the supraspinous and interspinous ligaments and, to some extent, the ligamentum flavum at the L3-L4 to install the closed loop appropriately. In extension, the closed loop impinged against the L3 spinous process upon loading. Obviously this would lead to a decrease in motion at the L3-L4 level in the extension mode, as observed. The posterior ligaments at the L5-S1 were also transected to accommodate the closed loop, but the increase in motion after stabilization was marginal, suggesting that these ligaments do not play a significant role in resisting flexion. This is primarily due to differences in the orientation of facets across the L3-L4 and L5-S1 segments. The facets exhibit a more sagittal disposition at the L3-L4 level, whereas an almost coronal placement exists at the lumbosacral junction. The facet orientation at the L5-S1 is thus suited to resist flexion/extension loads better, as has been shown to be the case by Jepson et al. (33).

The closed-loop system seems to provide stability based on the following principles. In flexion/extension, the tension induced in the wire during twisting helps to transmit loads from the L4, the closed loop, and then to the L5 vertebra. The stability provided against the axial and lateral bending loads is primarily due to frictional force between the loop and the laminae of the L4 and L5. (This frictional force is a function of the tension in the wires.) With time, in vivo the wires would become loose and so would the stabilizing effect. The frictional force being small would help explain the lack of stability in the axial and/or lateral bending modes.

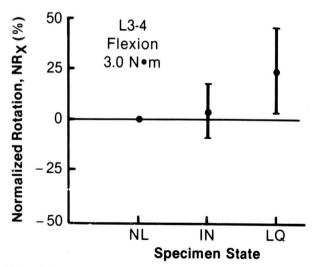

FIG. 16. Normalized primary rotation, NR$_x$ at L3-L4 corresponding to 3.0 Nm of flexion moment as a function of specimen state. NL, normal state; IN, injured state; and LQ, Luque closed-loop state.

Groups II–IV Results

The inability of the closed loop to provide significant fixation for the Group I model raises questions about its ability to impart a definite stability in cases of spinal decompression when stability in response to lateral bending loads is also present. Relevant cases include the application of the closed loop for patients suffering low back pain due to disc herniation and spinal stenosis and/or patients in need of total facetectomy. The situation may be further compromised if more than one motion segment needs to be stabilized, because obtaining a solid fusion may become even more difficult in such cases. The studies in Groups II, III, and IV were designed with these questions in mind. Data analyses similar to the ones undertaken for Group I were accomplished for the specimens tested in these groups also. The effectiveness of the Luque loop in stabilizing the injured models in all groups seems to be similar. It provides stabilization to the tune of 50% in flexion and extension and is not very effective in other load types. The Steffee system is very effective in restoring stability to the injured level(s) in all loading modalities. Reductions in motion as large as 85%, in comparison to the intact motion data, were seen.

Analytical Investigations

Experimental investigations like the ones described above have enabled the investigators to understand the effects of instrumentation on the levels adjacent to the stabilized levels during the physiological range of motion of the spine. This is an important contribution from a clinical viewpoint.

A number of other clinical issues still need to be addressed, such as the loosening/breakage of screws, redistribution of loads, and stresses and strains within both the stabilized and adjacent segments. An investigation of these factors will not only further our understanding of

the interaction between the spine and the instrumentation, but may afford us an opportunity to improve the designs. This mandates development of analytical models. The authors have developed extensive three-dimensional nonlinear finite-element models of the lumbar spine segments (one motion segment/two vertebrae, and two motion segments/three vertebrae) to investigate the effects of an interbody bone graft and a fixation device like the Steffee plate-screw system on the spine (23,36). The following paragraphs describe only the responses of the stabilized model (Steffee system, Fig. 17) in compression, flexion, and extension.

Response in Axial Mode

The injury and subsequent stabilization of the model using the interbody bone graft and the Steffee plates resulted in a localized increase in stresses (von Mises) in the cortical bone region immediately below the screws for 405 N of axial compressive load (Table 1). In the cancellous region a decrease of about 36% was observed following stabilization (Table 1). The average stress in the bone graft was 1.12 MPa. The load transmitted across the bone graft (compressive stress × area of cross section) was 320 N and was 80% of the applied load, compared to the 96% transmitted by the disc in the intact model. Thus, the plates transmitted 20% of the applied load as opposed to 4% by the facets in the intact model. The load-transmission path in the stabilized model with the intervertebral disc and bone graft totally removed would be entirely through the screws and the plates. The model computed that stresses in the screw (223 MPa) were quite high. This suggests that in the ab-

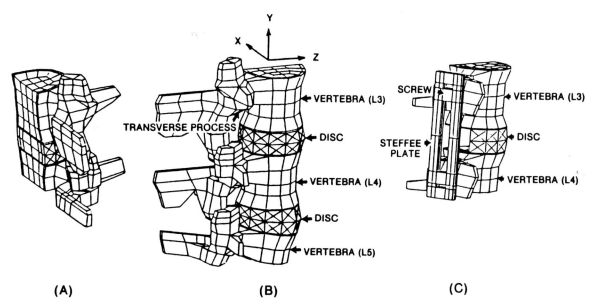

(A)   **(B)**   **(C)**

FIG. 17. The finite element models used for analyses are shown. **A:** The half one motion segment model. **B:** The half two motion segments model. **C:** The stabilized half one motion segment model (SPH1S) simulating the Steffee plate and screw system. The bone graft is not shown for the sake of clarity.

TABLE 1. *von Mises stresses (MPa) in various structures of intact and stabilized models in compression, flexion, and extension modes*

Load type (Magnitude)		Cortical bone		Cancellous bone		Bone graft	Plate	Screw
		Stabilized	Intact	Stabilized	Intact	Stabilized	Stabilized	Stabilized
Axial comp	Maximum	4.98	2.21	0.137	0.22	2.58	3.57	1.52
(405 N)	Average	2.18	1.98	0.104	0.12	1.12	1.53	0.89
Flexion	Maximum	3.37	1.1	0.11	0.024	1.62	3.07	1.58
(2.05 Nm)	Average	0.67	0.86	0.018	0.017	0.96	2.02	0.98
Extension	Maximum	3.01	1.62	0.059	0.034	2.26	3.53	1.68
(2.05 Nm)	Average	0.95	1.09	0.032	0.02	1.04	2.3	1.02

sence of bone graft, the screws may experience stresses very close to their failure limit. The disc annulus was found to experience a negligible stress.

Response in Flexion and Extension Modes

The trend in stresses in the cortical bone region in flexion and extension modes was similar to that in the axial load case (Table 1). The stresses in the cancellous bone region for the stabilized model showed an increase. However, these magnitudes are lower than those for the compression case. The average stress in the bone graft was about 1.0 MPa in both cases. The stresses in the plates and screws for the three load types analyzed are also shown in Table 1.

To interpret the results presented here properly, the following aspects must be noted. The model has been developed using the Steffee plates. However, the results presented will be true for any of the screw-plate devices currently available on the market because a perfect bond has been assumed at the bone/screw interface, and also across the screw/plate interface. This represents an ideal situation. In reality some motion will always be present, especially at the bone/screw interface. The amount of motion will depend on the quality of the bone, the characteristics of a particular device, and the technique used for implanting the device. The presence of motion is likely to alter the load-transfer mechanism across the stabilized motion segment.

The stabilized model may be treated as a linear model because of the absence of soft tissues. The response of the model to loads other than the ones used here can be obtained by a linear extrapolation of the stress results for the load magnitudes reported here. Similarly, the response of the stabilized model to complex loads would be a linear combination of the cases analyzed in this chapter. For example, the stress distributions within the structures for 2.05 Nm of flexion moment and a preload of 405 N can be obtained by adding the von Mises stress values for the 405 N axial case and 2.05 Nm flexion case from Table 1. Last, it is essential to estimate the loads experienced by a stabilized spine in order to identify, in conjunction with the stresses, the structures most likely to experience failure over time.

Present knowledge of the forces within the trunk muscles and spinal elements of a motion segment of a normal subject is primarily based on the quantitative biomechanical models of the human spine (47,60). Most of the in vivo experimental data have been accumulated by monitoring loads on the spinal instrumentation used to stabilize an injured lumbar spine (38). The results of the biomechanical models suggest that a motion segment may experience axial compressive loads ranging from 400 N (during quiet standing) to as high as 7,000 N (during lifting) (47,60). The flexion acting across a motion segment during lifting, according to these publications, is primarily balanced by the restorative generated by the back muscles. Thus the disc, per se, in a normal subject does not generate any flexion in resisting the external bending. In vivo measurement of loads on an external fixation device used for human lumbar spine fractures indicates that the implant is also very largely shielded from bending by the trunk muscles (38). In vivo bending of spine plates has not been reported to be a problem. Mechanical testing in vitro has shown that a plastic deformation of the Roy-Camille plates occurs at 11.3 Nm (38). Thus, the bending across a stabilized motion segment in vivo must be lower than this value. Keeping in mind that (a) the stabilized segment may be protected further by the use of braces following surgery and (b) the patient is not expected to undertake strenuous activities immediately after surgery, the stabilized motion segment may experience about 400 N of preload and a bending less than 10 Nm. It is also evident as the patients recover from surgery that, with time, the primary load on the spine would be the axial component.

The stress results of Table 1 when linearly extrapolated to 10 Nm of flexion bending and a preload of 405 N show that none of the structures experience large stresses in comparison to the corresponding failure strength (Table 2). Furthermore, the average stresses in the cancellous bone below the screw level in the stabilized model for the compression and flexion cases are lower than the corresponding values in the intact case. Since compressive load is the main component of the load exerted on the spine, this suggests that the bone is stress-shielded by the screw-plate system and more load is being transmitted through the fixation device as compared to the posterior elements in an intact model (20% vs. 4%, as stated

TABLE 2. *Von Mises stresses extracted from Table 1 for a complex load of 10 Nm flexion moment and 405 N of preload (the failure strength of various structures is also listed for comparison)*

	Computed stress (MPa)	Yield stress (MPa)
Cortical bone	21.42	138
Cancellous bone	0.67	1–10
Bone graft	10.5	—
Plate	18.54	698
Screw	9.22	698

earlier). The use of interbody bone graft plays an active role in transmitting the applied loads. This is further corroborated by the results of the model in which the disc space between the vertebrae was kept void. The stresses in the screws in that case increased greatly.

The decrease in stresses in the cancellous bone region and localized increase in stresses in the cortical shell (pedicles) around the screw are supportive of the clinical observations that screws become loose with time. This may in turn lead to screw breakage at the pedicles because of the cumulative effects of high stresses, stress concentration due to the screw threads, and fatigue loading in the presence of body fluids. However, our finding that the interbody bone graft is a weight-bearing structure from the time of its implantation suggests that the bone healing may take place by the time screws become loose or break. Clinical follow-ups are supportive of this observation. The results of a two-motion-segments finite-element model with the L4-L5 disc degenerated indicate that the nucleus pressure in the adjacent L3-L4 disc, compared to the nondegenerated two-motion-segments model, shows an 8% to 10% increase. The replacement of the intact L4-L5 disc nucleus with a fibrosus material to simulate disc degeneration leads to an increase in the stiffness of the segment. The use of bone graft and plates to achieve stabilization of the L4-L5 motion segment, from a mechanical viewpoint, will also increase the stiffness/rigidity of the segment. The increase would be more than that obtained by replacing the disc nucleus with a fibrosus material. The stiffness will also be higher in a case in which the bone graft has healed and the plates have been removed—stabilization without the use of any instrumentation. Under these circumstances, it may be realistic to extrapolate our findings of the disc degeneration model and to predict that the adjacent discs are likely to experience higher stresses as a result of stabilization. It is also tempting to suggest that the use of the bone graft alone for restoring the spinal stability, upon its healing, may also have similar adverse effects on the adjacent segments. We feel, based on these results, that the adverse iatrogenic effects seen clinically are not entirely due to the use of instrumentation itself. The healed bone graft alone may also induce similar effects. Consequently, efforts may be directed to the development and use of more compliant materials in place of the bone graft and the plates.

In summary, our results indicate that the interbody bone graft is a weight-bearing structure from the day of its implantation. The use of a fixation device stress-shields the vertebral body. More load, as compared to the load through the posterior element in the intact case, is transmitted through the screw-plate system. As a result of this, the screws are also likely to become loose with time. The use of interbody bone graft alone or in combination with any of the currently available fixation devices is likely to induce higher stresses across the adjacent segments. This in turn may trigger disc degeneration and other adverse iatrogenic effects as seen in clinical follow-ups.

SUMMARY

The biomechanical literature dealing with the effects of surgery (e.g., discectomy, with and without fusion) on the "mechanical" behavior of a ligamentous lumbar spine is reviewed. The results of both the experimental and the analytical studies are included to understand clinical relevance of the changes in motion, loads transmitted through various structures, and stresses and strains induced within the structures, in comparison to the corresponding parameters for the intact spines.

ACKNOWLEDGMENT

Preparation of this chapter was supported in part by grants AM R01-32954-4 (NIH), 395-85 (OREF), and a grant from AcroMed Co., Cleveland, Ohio.

REFERENCES

1. Adams MA, Hutton WC (1982): Mechanical factors in the etiology of low back pain. *Orthopedics* 5:1461.
2. Adams MA, Hutton WC (1983): The effect of fatigue on the lumbar intervertebral disc. *J Bone Joint Surg* [Br] 65:199–203.
3. Andersson GB, Schultz AB (1979): Effects of fluid injection on mechanical properties of intervertebral discs. *J Biomech* 12:453–458.
4. Berkson MH, Nachemson A, Schultz AB (1979): Mechanical properties of human lumbar spine motion segments—Part II: responses in compression and shear, influence of gross morphology. *J Biomech Engrg* 101:53–57.
5. Bradford DS, Oegema TR Jr, Cooper KM, Wakano K, Chao EY (1984): Chymopapain, chemonucleolysis, and nucleus pulposus regeneration—A biochemical and biomechanical study. *Spine* 9:135–147.
6. Brinckmann P, Horst M (1985): The influence of vertebral body fracture, intradiscal injection, and partial discectomy on the radial bulge and height of human lumbar discs. *Spine* 10:138–145.
7. Brinckmann P, Horst M (1985): Short term biomechanical effects of chymopapain injection—An *in vitro* investigation on human lumbar motion segments, ISSN 0721-264X no. 24. Orthopadische Universitatsklinik Munster, West Germany, Aug.
8. Brown T, Hansen RJ, Yorra AJ (1957): Some mechanical tests on the lumbosacral spine with particular reference to the interverte-

bral discs. A preliminary report. *J Bone Joint Surg* [Am] 39:1135–1164.

9. Brunski JB, Hill DC, Moskowitz A (1983): Stresses in a Harrington distraction rod: their origin and relationship to fatigue fractures in vivo. *J Biomech Engrg* 105:101–107.

10. Casey MP, Jacobs RR (1984): Internal fixation of the lumbosacral spine: a biomechanical evaluation. XI Proceedings of International Society for the Study of the Lumbar Spine, Montreal, Canada, June 3–7.

11. Chaffin DB, Andersson GB (1984): *Occupational biomechanics.* New York: John Wiley & Sons.

12. Cook SD, Barrack RL, Georgettee FS, Whitecloud TS 3d, Burke SW, Skinner HB, Renz EA (1985): An analysis of failed Harrington rods. *Spine* 10:313–316.

13. Damkot DK, Pope MH, Lord J, Frymoyer JW (1984): The relationship between work history, work environment and low-back pain in men. *Spine* 9:395–399.

14. Du W (1989): Biomechanics of spinal instrumentation—An experimental investigation. MS Thesis, University of Iowa.

15. Fidler MW (1985): Posterior and anterior instrumentation of the spine. XII Proceedings of International Society for the Study of the Lumbar Spine, Sydney, Australia, April 14–19.

16. Frymoyer JW (1981): The role of spine fusion. *Spine* 6:289.

17. Frymoyer JW, Pope MH, Clements JH, Wilder DG, MacPherson B, Ashikaga T (1983): Risk factors in low back pain. *J Bone Joint Surg* [Am] 65:213–218.

18. Frymoyer JW, Selby DK (1985): Segmental instability: rationale for treatment. *Spine* 10:280–286.

19. Goel VK (1987): Three-dimensional motion behavior of the human spine—A question of terminology. *J Biomech Engr* 109:353–355.

20. Goel VK, Fromknecht S, Nishiyama K, Weinstein J, Liu YK (1985): The role of spinal elements in flexion. *Spine* 10:516–523.

21. Goel VK, Goyal S, Clark C, Nishiyama K, Nye T (1985): Kinematics of the whole lumbar spine—effect of discectomy. *Spine* 10:543–554.

22. Goel VK, Kim YE (1989): Effects of injury on the spinal motion segment mechanics in the axial compression mode. *Clin Biomech* 4:161–167.

23. Goel VK, Kim YE, Lim T-H, Weinstein JN (1988): An analytical investigation of the mechanics of spinal instrumentation. *Spine* 13:1003–1011.

24. Goel VK, Nishiyama K, Weinstein J, Liu YK (1986): Mechanical properties of lumbar spinal motion segments as affected by partial disc removal. *Spine* 11:1008–1012.

25. Goel VK, Nye TA, Clark CR, Nishiyama K, Weinstein JN (1987): A technique to evaluate an internal spinal device by use of the Selspot system—An application to the Luque closed loop. *Spine* 12:150–159.

26. Goel VK, Weinstein JN (1990): *Biomechanics of spine surgery–Clinical and surgical perspective.* Boca Raton: CRC Press, Inc.

27. Goel VK, Weinstein J, Liu YK, Okuma T, et al. (1987): Comparative biomechanical evaluation of the Steffee and Luque loop systems. XIV Proceedings of The International Society of the Study of the Lumbar Spine, Rome, Italy, May 24–28.

28. Guyer DW, Yuan HA, Werner F, Frederickson BE, Murphy D (1987): Biomechanical comparison of seven internal fixation devices for the lumbosacral junction. *Spine* 12:569–573.

29. Hazlett JW, Kinnard P (1982): Lumbar apophyseal process excision and spinal instability. *Spine* 7:171–176.

30. Hirabayashi K, Maruyama T, Wakano K, Ikeda K, Ishii Y (1981): Postoperative lumbar canal stenosis due to anterior spinal fusion. *Keio J Med* 30:133–139.

31. Hirsch C, Galante J (1967): Laboratory conditions for tensile tests in annulus fibrosis from human intervertebral discs. *Acta Ortho Scand* 38:148–162.

32. Jacobs RR, Nordwall A, Nachemson A (1982): Reduction, stability and strength provided by internal fixation systems for thoracolumbar spinal injuries. *Clin Orthop Rel Res* (171):300–308.

33. Jepson KM, Miller JA, Schultz AB, Andersson GB (1985): Mechanical properties of L5-S1 motion segments. Presented at the ASME-WAM Bioengineering Symposium, Miami Beach, Florida, Nov. 17–22.

34. Keim HA, Kirkaldy-Willis WH (1980): Low back pain. *Clin Symp* 32:1–35.

35. Kelsey JL, Githkens PB, White AA, et al. (1984): An epidemiologic study of lifting and twisting on the job and risk for acute prolapsed lumbar intervertebral disc. *J Ortho Res* 2:61–66.

36. Kim YE (1989): An analytical investigation of the ligamentous lumbar spine mechanics. PhD dissertation, University of Iowa.

37. Kim YE, Goel VK, Weinstein J (1988): The role of facets in denucleated discs—An analytical biomechanical study. 34th Orthopedic Research Society, Atlanta, Georgia, Feb. 1–4.

38. Krag MH, Beynnon BD, Pope MH, Frymoyer JW (1986): An internal fixator for posterior application to short segments of thoracic, lumbar, or lumbosacral spine. *Clin Orthop Rel Res* (203):75–98.

39. Lee CK (1983): Lumbar spinal instability (olisthesis) after extensive posterior spinal decompression. *Spine* 8:429–433.

40. Lehmann TR, Tozzi JE, Weinstein JN, Reinarz SJ, El-Khoury G (1987): Long term follow up of lower lumbar fusion patients. *Spine* 12:97–104.

41. Lipson SJ (1983): Degenerative spinal stenosis following old lumbosacral fusions. *Orthopaedic Transactions* 7:143.

42. Liu YK, Goel VK (1987): Mathematical models of the spine and their experimental validation. In: Jayson MIV, ed. *The lumbar spine and low back pain.* New York: Churchill Livingstone, pp. 177–190.

43. Lorenz M, Patwardhan A, Vanderby R Jr (1983): Load-bearing characteristics of lumbar facets in normal and surgically altered spinal segments. *Spine* 8:122–130.

44. Louis R (1985): Single-staged posterior lumbo-sacral fusion by internal fixation with screw plates. 12th International Society for the Study of the Lumbar Spine, Sydney, Australia, April 14–19.

45. Luque ER (1982): The anatomic basis and development of segmental spinal instrumentation. *Spine* 7:256–259.

46. Markolf KL, Morris JM (1974): The structural components of the intervertebral disc. A study of their contributions to the ability of the disc to withstand compressive forces. *J Bone Joint Surg* [Am] 56:675–687.

47. McGill SM, Norman RW (1986): Partitioning of the L4-L5 dynamic moment into disc, ligamentous, and muscular components during lifting. *Spine* 11:666–678.

48. Nachemson A (1966): The load on lumbar disks in different positions of the body. *Clin Orthop* (45):107–122.

49. Nachemson A (1981): The role of spine fusion. *Spine* 6:306.

50. Nachemson A (1987): Lumbar intradiscal pressure. In: Jayson MIV, ed. *The lumbar spine and back pain.* London: Churchill Livingstone, p. 191.

51. Panjabi MM, Abumi K, Duranceau JS (1987): Three-dimensional stability of thoraco-lumbar fractures stabilized with eight different instrumentations. 33rd Annual Meeting, Orthopaedic Research Society, San Francisco, Jan. 19–22.

52. Panjabi MM, Brand RA Jr, White AA 3d (1976): Mechanical properties of human thoracic spine as shown by three-dimensional load-displacement curves. *J Bone Joint Surg* [Am] 58:642–652.

53. Panjabi MM, Krag MH, Chung TQ (1984): Effects of disc injury on mechanical behavior of the human spine. *Spine* 9:707–713.

54. Panjabi MM, Krag MH, Goel VK (1981): A technique for measurement and description of three-dimensional six degree-of-freedom motion of a body joint with an application to the human spine. *J Biomech* 14:447–460.

55. Panjabi MM, Krag M, Summers D, Videman T (1985): Biomechanical time-tolerance of fresh cadaveric human spine specimens. *J Ortho Res* 3:292–300.

56. Perey O (1957): Fracture of the vertebral end-plate in the lumbar spine. *Acta Orthop Scan* (Suppl.) 25:1–101.

57. Posner I, White AA, Edwards T, Hayes WC (1982): A biomechanical analysis of the clinical stability of the lumbar lumbosacral spine. *Spine* 7:374–389.

58. Reuber M, Schultz A, Denis F, Spencer D (1982): Bulging of the lumbar intervertebral disks. *J Biomech Engrg* 104:187–192.

59. Rothman SLG, Glen WV (1985): CT evaluation of interbody fusion. *Clin Res Rel* 193:47–56. (See also other articles of the symposium *Posterior lumbar interbody fusion* in this issue.)

60. Schultz AB (1987): Loads on the lumbar spine. In: Jayson MIV,

ed. *The lumbar spine and back pain.* New York: Churchill Livingstone, p. 204.

61. Schultz AB, Warwick DN, Berkson MH, Nachemson AL (1979): Mechanical properties of human lumbar spine motion segments—Part I: Responses in flexion, extension, lateral bending and torsion. *J Biomech Engrg* 101:46–52.

62. Sedlin ED, Hirsch C (1966): Factors affecting the determination of the physical properties of femoral cortical bone. *Acta Orthop Scand* 37:29–48.

63. Shirazi-Adl A, Drouin G (1987): Load-bearing role of facets in a lumbar segment under sagittal plane loadings. *J Biomech* 20:601–613.

64. Shirazi-Adl SA, Shrivastva SC, Ahmed AM (1984): Stress analysis of the lumbar disc-body unit in compression. *Spine* 9:120–134.

65. Skinner R, Maybee J, Venter R, Chalmers W (1986): Experimental testing and comparison of variables in transpedicular screw fixation: A biomechanical study (personal communications).

66. Spencer DL, Miller JA, Schultz AB (1985): The effects of chemonucleolysis on the mechanical properties of the canine lumbar disc. *Spine* 10:555–561.

67. Spengler DM (1982): Lumbar discectomy results with limited disc excision and selective foraminotomy. *Spine* 7:604–607.

68. Stokes IAF, Wilder DG, Frymoyer JW, Pope MH (1981): Assessment of patients with low-back pain by biplanar radiographic measurement of intervertebral motion. *Spine* 6:233–240.

69. Sypert GW (1986): Low back pain disorders—lumbar fusion. *Clin Neurosurg* 33:457–483.

70. Tencer AF, Ahmed AM, Burke DL (1982): Some static mechanical properties of the lumbar intervertebral joint, intact and injured. *J Biomech Engrg* 104:193–201.

71. Tibrewal SB, Pearcy MJ, Portek I, Spivey J (1985): A prospective study of lumbar spinal movements before and after discectomy using biplanar radiography, correlation of clinical and radiographic findings. *Spine* 12:455–460.

72. Tkaczuk H (1968): Tensile properties of human lumbar longitudinal ligaments. *Acta Orthop Scan* (Suppl.) 115:1–69.

73. Weber H (1983): Lumbar disc herniation. A controlled, prospective study with ten years of observation. *Spine* 8:131–140.

74. White AH, Wynne G, Taylor LW (1983): Knodt rod distraction lumbar fusion. *Spine* 8:434–437.

75. Wilder DG, Pope MH, Frymoyer JW (1987): The biomechanics of lumbar disc herniation and the effect of overload and instability, University of Vermont, Burlington, VT (personal communication).

76. Yang KH, King AI (1984): Mechanism of facet load transmission as a hypothesis for low back pain. *Spine* 9:557–565.

77. Yang SW, Langrana NA, Lee CK (1986): Biomechanics of lumbosacral spinal fusion in combined compression-torsion loads. *Spine* 11:937–941.

78. Zindrick MR, Wiltse LL, Holland RR, Widell EH, Thomas JC, Spencer CW (1985): A biomechanical study of intrapeduncular screw fixation in the lumbosacral spine. XII Proceedings of International Society for the Study of the Lumbar Spine, Sydney, Australia, April 14–19.

The Adult Spine: Principles and Practice,
J. W. Frymoyer, Editor-in-Chief.
Raven Press, Ltd., New York © 1991.

CHAPTER 69

Surgical Approaches to the Lumbar Spine

Ernest M. Found, Jr., and James N. Weinstein

Surgical approaches to the lumbar spine allow for complete exposure and visualization of all portions of that structure, as well as the contents within the spinal canal. The choice of approach is dictated by the site of the primary pathologic condition. If the disease process or deformity primarily involves the vertebral bodies, then it is usually best to approach them anteriorly through the abdomen or flank. On the other hand, the posterior elements of the lumbar spine are best approached directly through a vertically oriented posterior midline incision. This allows direct accessibility to the spinous processes, laminae, and facets. By extending the dissection more laterally through the posterior approach, adequate exposure to the transverse processes and pedicles can be attained without difficulty. As an alternative, the posterolateral muscle-splitting approach provides direct access to the transverse processes and pedicles, but a more limited exposure of the vertebral bodies themselves.

As in any surgical procedure, the anatomy of the proposed operative site needs to be reviewed and understood prior to embarking on surgery. The surgeon should carefully study a skeletal model in conjunction with plain films, CT scan, MRI, and other imaging modalities to create a three-dimensional mental image of the structures that will be treated surgically. In planning the procedure, particularly anteriorly about the lumbar spine, the approach should be made so that it can be extensile if needed at the time of the operative proce-

dure. The principles of any surgical procedure must be strictly adhered to when operating upon the lumbar spine. These considerations include patient positioning and comfort, visibility related to the size of the incision, retraction, illumination, visual contact, and maneuverability of instrumentation. The surgeon should not be constrained by poor positioning or draping.

POSTERIOR APPROACH

The posterior approach to the lumbar spine is by far the most common and widely used surgical exposure. It is generally made through a longitudinal midline incision, providing direct access to the spinous processes, laminae, and facets of all levels of the lumbar spine. Through the direct posterior approach, the surgeon can remove some or all of the posterior osseous structures (laminotomy or laminectomy) and obtain access to the posterior aspect of the cauda equina, conus medullaris, lumbar vertebral disc, and vertebral body. Via this approach, removal of an extruded portion of herniated disc and exploration of the thecal sac and nerve roots can usually be performed. With further dissection and retraction of the paraspinal muscles laterally, the facet joints and full extent of the transverse processes can be easily exposed.

After satisfactory installation of anesthesia, the patient is gently log rolled and positioned prone on a spine frame. Proper positioning will allow the abdomen to hang free to reduce abdominal pressure, allowing for diminished venous engorgement and intra-operative bleeding at the operative site. Using a midline posterior

E. M. Found, Jr., M.D., Assistant Professor and Assistant Director; J. N. Weinstein, D.O., Associate Professor and Director: Spine Diagnostic and Treatment Center, Department of Orthopaedics, University of Iowa Hospitals and Clinics, Iowa City, Iowa, 52242.

A

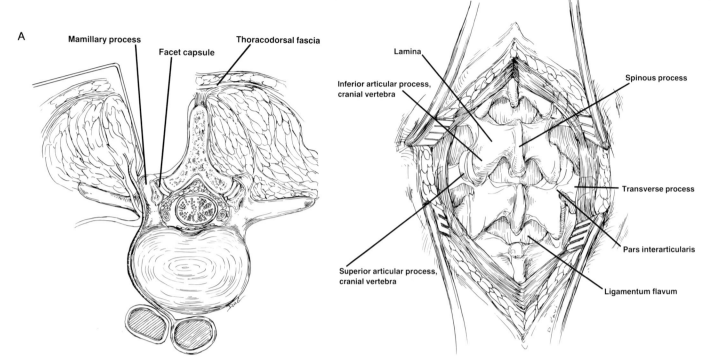

FIG. 1. A: Midline posterior approach in axial plane. B: Posterior osseous exposure of the lumbosacral spine (redrawn from Hoppenfeld S, *Surgical Exposures in Orthopaedics*).

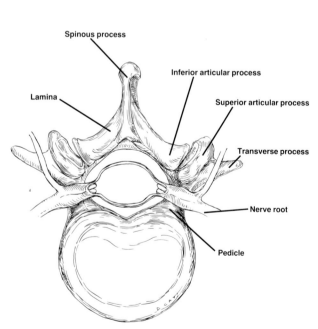

FIG. 2. Transverse (axial) plane section of a lumbar segment emphasizing orientation of spinous process bulbous tip, facet articular processes, pedicle, and neuromotor elements (redrawn from Watkins R, *Surgical Approaches to the Spine*).

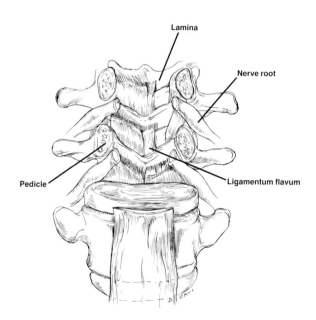

FIG. 3. View from inside the canal looking posteriorly demonstrates the anatomy of the ligamentum flavum. The ligamentum flavum inserts approximately midway under the cephalad lamina and inserts into the cephalad edge of the caudal lamina below. The ligamentum flavum is thinnest in the midline, providing for easiest point of entry into the spinal canal (redrawn from Watkins R, *Surgical Approaches to the Spine*).

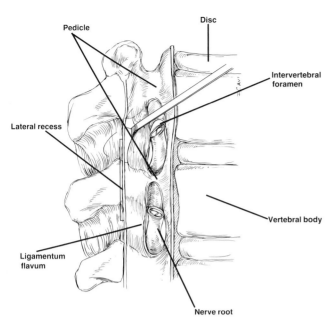

FIG. 4. The boundaries of the neural foramen as viewed from inside the spinal canal looking out (see text) (redrawn from Watkins R, *Surgical Approaches to the Spine*).

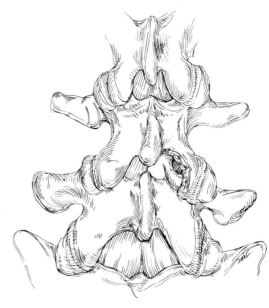

FIG. 5. Laminotomy with partial (hemi) facetectomy on the right side to expose underlying nerve root and disc pathology.

approach (Fig. 1), an incision is made longitudinally over the palpable spinous processes. Prior to incision, skin bleeders can often be controlled with the subdermal injection of 1-500,000 dilution of epinephrine. Sharp dissections by scalpel or electrocautery are carried through subcutaneous tissue in line with the midline skin incision, and hemostasis is obtained with electrocoagulation. The thoracolumbar fascia (thoracodorsal

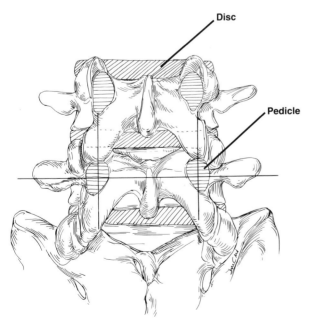

FIG. 6. Localization of the pedicle, with posterior elements intact (redrawn from Watkins R, *Surgical Approaches to the Spine*).

fascia) is identified in the midline as it merges with the supraspinous ligaments. All efforts should be made to maintain the integrity of the supraspinous and interspinous ligaments. The thoracolumbar fascia can be incised just lateral to the supraspinous ligament and the paraspinal muscles subperiosteally elevated laterally off the spinous processes, laminae, and facet joints with a Cobb elevator and gauze packing. The tip of the spinous processes has a bulbous configuration (see Fig. 2). The internervous plane lies directly in the midline between the two paraspinal (sacrospinalis) muscles, each of which receives its segmental nerve supply from the posterior primary rami of the lumbar nerves of its corresponding side. The dissection can continue laterally, exposing the capsule of the facet joint, which should be protected if fusion is not planned. In preparation of the posterior elements for fusion, the lateral aspect of the superior articular facet may then be cleared and the dissection continued laterally to expose the transverse processes by dissecting down the lateral side of the ascending facet and onto the transverse process itself.

The ligamentum flavum (yellow ligament) fanning between the lumbar laminae originates cranially approximately midway under the cephalad laminae and inserts under the cephalad edge of the caudad laminae (Fig. 3). The ligamentum flavum has a superficial portion and a deep portion and is thinnest in the midline. The ligamentum flavum extends down to form the anterior capsule of the facet joint (Fig. 4). Variable portions of the laminae can be removed (laminotomy or laminectomy) to expose the underlying thecal sac, nerve roots, and surrounding soft tissue structures. The removal of bone can continue laterally to involve the medial aspect of the pedicle or the medial aspect of the facet joint (hemifac-

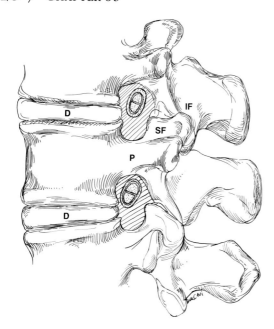

FIG. 7. The neural foramen and its boundaries viewed laterally. **SF:** Superior facet. **IF:** Inferior facet. **SF + IF:** Facet joint. **P:** Pedicle. **D:** Disc.

etectomy) (Fig. 5), or the facet joint may be completely removed (total facetectomy).

The key to the intracanal anatomy in lumbar spine surgery is the pedicle. Three-dimensional thinking is vital to accurate spinal surgery and requires the ability to orient the intracanal structures from visualization of the posterior elements. The center of the pedicle is at a point formed by the intersection of three lines: the axes of the transverse process, superior facet, and pars inter-articularis (Fig. 6). With identification of the pedicle, the cephalad disc and caudal nerve root can be accurately located. Immediately cephalad within 1 centimeter of the pedicle is the intervertebral disc; immediately caudad to the pedicle is the exiting nerve root. Meticulous probing is man-

FIG. 8. The muscular branches of the lumbar arteries in relation to the operative exposure. Note rich and abundant blood supply about the facet joint, pars interarticularis, and transverse process. **1:** Interarticular artery, found immediately lateral to the pars interarticularis. **2 and 3:** The two superior articular arteries lie immediately lateral to the tip of the superior articular facet. **4:** Communicating artery is a large vessel lying immediately lateral to the superior articular facet and extending onto the dorsum of the transverse process. **5:** Inferior articular artery lies in the angle formed by the transverse process and superior articular facet (redrawn from ref. 8).

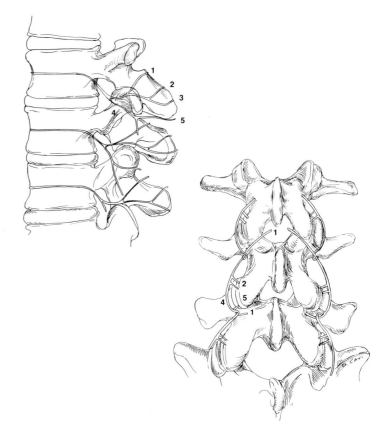

datory in the pedicular portion of the canal, as the pedicular vascular plexus in this region can be a source of troublesome bleeding. As the dissection progresses, it is important to remember the nerve root above, and its relationship to the interlaminar space. The L5-S1 disc is approximately at the level of the interlaminar space between L5-S1, whereas the L2-L3 disc space is well cephalad under the laminae of L2 rather than directly at the level of the interlaminar space between L2-L3. Bipolar electrocautery is very useful in dealing with the epidural venous plexus.

Decompressive laminectomy and foraminotomies are performed via the posterior approach. The neural foramen is a canal whereby the nerve root and its accompanying vascular structures are located. The margins of the canal are formed anteriorly by the disc and vertebral body; posteriorly by the facet joint; inferiorly by the pedicle of the level below; and superiorly by the pedicle of the level above (Figs. 4 and 7). Neural foramen by definition are canal(s) or tunnel(s) with three dimensions (height, width, depth), rather than just open holes or foramen.

The blood supply about the facet joints and pars interarticularis is rich with multiple muscular branches (Fig. 8). The arterial supply has been found to be remarkably constant in its anatomical distribution. Knowledge of the anatomical location of these articular and muscular branches allows the surgeon to identify and cauterize these vessels in an attempt to minimize intra-operative bleeding.

POSTEROLATERAL APPROACH

This is a popular approach used for posterolateral lumbosacral fusions (10). The posterolateral approach can provide direct access to the transverse processes, as well as the mammillary processes of the facets. Through this approach the transverse process may be removed, exposing nerve root from the level above. This approach also provides access to the pedicle. The lateral aspects of the vertebral body may be exposed in a limited fashion.

Two types of skin incisions may be used. A midline incision may be made with elevation of a subcutaneous tissue flap to expose the thoracodorsal fascia. Then, bilateral paraspinous incision(s) may be made through the thoracodorsal fascia to expose the sacrospinalis muscle groups. Muscle splitting between the multifidus and longissimus provides direct access to the facet joint(s) and transverse processes (Fig. 9). Alternatively, bilateral paraspinal skin incisions may be made (Fig. 10), approximately three finger breadths lateral to the midline, followed by a muscle-splitting division of the sacrospinalis group. This provides a direct approach to the facet joint(s) and transverse processes. This approach has been popularized by Wiltse (12,13) and colleagues, who feel it is advantageous because it provides less muscle mass re-

traction medially and may decrease operative bleeding. Additional advantages of this approach are access to far lateral disc herniations, some intraforaminal discs (see Chapters 83 and 84), decompressions of the "far out syndrome," and access to the iliac crest for harvesting bone graft.

ANTERIOR APPROACHES

Although the majority of operative procedures in the lumbar spine are performed by means of classic posterior approaches, selective indications arise for anterior approaches at single or multiple levels (Fig. 11). The anterolateral retroperitoneal flank approach can usually provide visualization of all lumbar vertebrae. However, the exposure that it provides at its cranial and caudal extents is limited. For full access and exposure to L1, a thoracoabdominal approach is recommended (see Chapter 60). For satisfactory anterior exposure of the L5 and S1 vertebrae, the transperitoneal approach is often required.

Anterolateral Transperitoneal Flank Approach to the Lumbar Vertebrae

The anterolateral approach to the lumbar vertebrae is an extension of the standard flank incision used for years by general surgeons for lumbar sympathectomy (Fig. 11). It provides excellent exposure for complete debridement and/or reconstructive bone grafting, which can include L2, L3, and L4. The access is more limited to L5. By dividing portions of the insertion of the arcuate ligament of the diaphragm on the first lumbar transverse process, this approach can provide limited access to as high as T12. However, if an extensive reconstructive procedure or grafting is planned for L1 or T12, it is recommended that consideration be given to the thoracoabdominal T10 retroperitoneal approach (see Chapter 60).

Generally, the lumbar vertebrae are approached retroperitoneally from the left side if all other considerations are equal and the pathologic condition can be resected from this side. The liver, located on the right side, is large and difficult to retract without injury. Additionally, the vena cava and its associated veins are often difficult to locate and are more fragile than the left-sided arterial system. Inadvertent vena cava hemorrhage can be very difficult to control. The spleen, on the left, is fragile, but is much smaller than the liver, more mobile, and easily retracted, and can be sacrificed in an emergency. Hodge and DeWald (6) reported a splenic injury with an anterior approach from the left side.

The patient is placed on the operating room table in the right lateral decubitus position. The kidney rest or inflatable roll is elevated and the table flexed to open the left flank. The left hip should be slightly flexed to relax

A

Multifidus

Longissimus

Iliocostalis

Psoas major

B

Longissimus

Iliocostalis

Multifidus

Psoas major

Facet joint

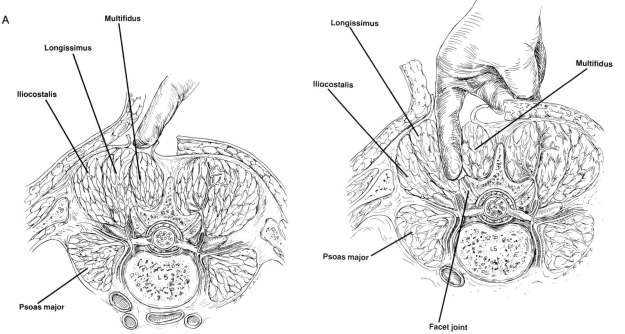

FIG. 9. A: Paraspinal approach through midline incision and muscle splitting exposure to facets and transverse processes (12,13). An interval is made between the multifidus and longissimus muscle groups. **B:** Further digital dissection places the surgeon's finger easily into the facet joint. Multifidus, longissimus, and iliocostalis muscles are often collectively termed the sacrospinalis group (redrawn from ref. 13).

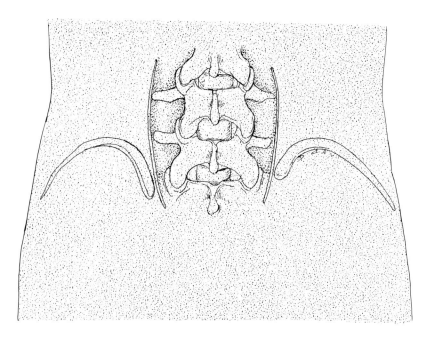

FIG. 10. Skin incisions for bilateral paraspinous approach to lower lumbar spine, followed by muscle splitting to visualize facet joints, transverse processes, and ala of sacrum (redrawn from Watkins R, *Surgical Approaches to the Spine*).

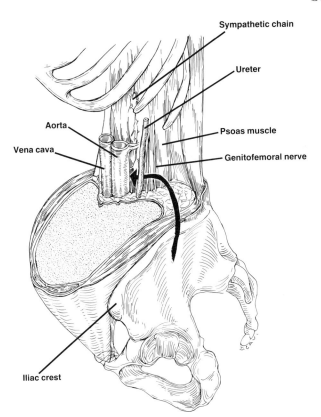

FIG. 11. With removal of abdominal viscera and muscles, the anatomy of the flank is depicted. The arrow directs the surgical route to approach the anterolateral portion of the lumbar spine between the peritoneum anteriorly and the retroperitoneal structures posteriorly (redrawn from Hoppenfeld S, *Surgical Exposures in Orthopaedics*).

psoas and the quadratus lumborum muscle. The genital femoral nerve must be identified and protected as it exits through the iliopsoas muscle belly, variably, at approximately L3. The lumbar spine is immediately medial to the psoas, and is often partially obscured by the psoas muscle, while the paravertebral sympathetic chain lies just medial to that muscle (Fig. 11). The ureter is reflected medially with the under surface of the peritoneum within the contents of the retroperitoneal fat. Digital palpation medial to the psoas will lead directly to the vertebral bodies, and the raised white soft discs can be palpated directly. An intra-operative x-ray should then be obtained to identify the appropriate level. The psoas is then retracted laterally to expose the anterolateral aspect of the vertebral bodies (Fig. 13C). At the mid-level of each lumbar vertebra are the segmental vessels that must be identified. When necessary, these vessels should be ligated to control potential bleeding. Their inadvertent injury can cause significant bleeding. After satisfactory control of segmental vessels, the aorta can then be mobilized more medially to fully expose the anterior aspect of the lumbar vertebrae (Fig. 13D). At the L4-L5 level, the ascending iliolumbar vein crosses the left L4-L5 disc level and must be identified and ligated for satisfactory exposure to the L4-L5 disc space and L5 vertebral body. The anterior longitudinal ligament may be elevated and/or resected from the mid-portion of the vertebral body as desired for the indicated reconstructive surgery about the vertebral body.

the psoas muscle, an important landmark in the retroperitoneal approach. The level of incision varies according to the level of the lumbar spine requiring treatment (see Fig. 12). This approach employs a muscle-splitting dissection and starts with electrocautery transection of the external oblique muscle and fascia, followed by the internal oblique muscle and fascia (Fig. 13A). The transverse abdominis muscle is often very thin or an absent muscle layer. Deep to the transverse abdominis muscle is the transversalis fascia. The transversalis fascia in the midline is adherent to the underlying peritoneum. In order to safely enter the retroperitoneal space, the transversalis fascia should be opened in the posterior aspect of the wound (Fig. 13B). The peritoneum is thickest laterally and easiest to separate from the transversalis fascia laterally; the peritoneum then thins toward the midline. If it is inadvertently entered, it should be closed before proceeding. The retroperitoneal fat and retroperitoneal contents, including the ureter, are then gently elevated off the quadratus lumborum and psoas muscle, the key to the retroperitoneal space. One must avoid entering the retropsoas space, which is a blind pouch between the

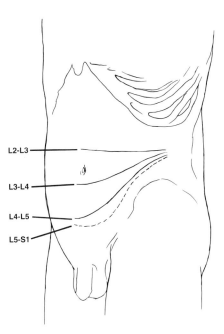

FIG. 12. Patient in lateral decubitus position, right side down. Levels of incision for anterior retroperitoneal approach according to the level of the spine to be approached (redrawn from Watkins R, *Surgical Approaches to the Spine*).

A

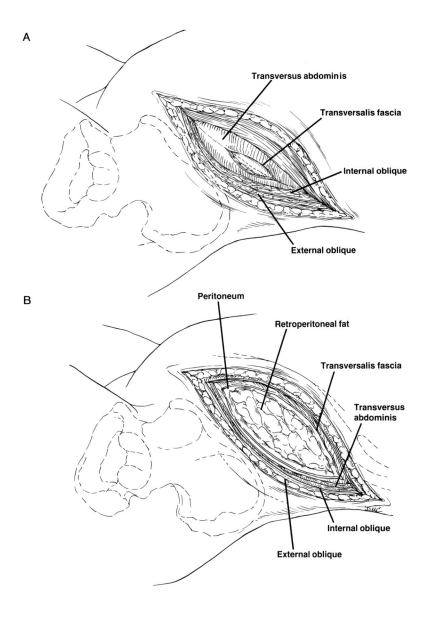

Transversus abdominis

Transversalis fascia

Internal oblique

External oblique

B

Peritoneum

Retroperitoneal fat

Transversalis fascia

Transversus abdominis

Internal oblique

External oblique

FIG. 13. A: Sequential division of abdominal muscles exposes the transversalis fascia. **B:** The retroperitoneal cavity with its retroperitoneal fat (especially in posterior aspect of wound) is entered. (Figs. 13C-13D follow.)

C

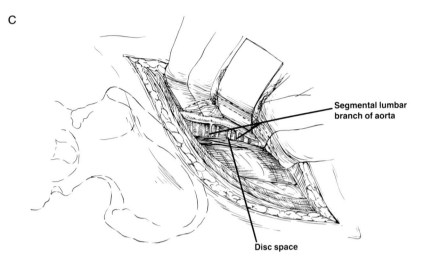

Segmental lumbar
branch of aorta

Disc space

FIG. 13. *Continued.* **C:** Psoas muscle exposed. **D:** Ligation of segmental vessels, aorta mobilized medially to reach the anterior and anterolateral positions of the vertebral body (redrawn from Watkins R, *Surgical Approaches to the Spine*).

D

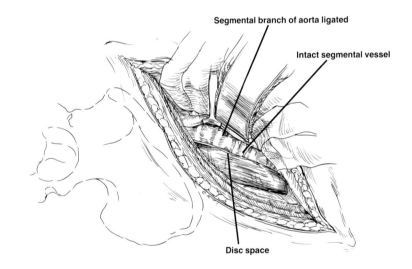

Segmental branch of aorta ligated

Intact segmental vessel

Disc space

The described retroperitoneal approach can be combined with the transthoracic retroperitoneal approach for complete anterior exposure from L5 to the upper thoracic level, as required.

Anterior Approach to the Lumbosacral Spine Through a Paramedian Incision

In some cases, L4, L5, and the sacrum can best be approached anteriorly through the anterior abdominal wall in the midline. This is particularly advantageous for procedures about L5-S1, but can be employed for L4-L5, although it involves significant mobilization of the great vessels. This approach may require the assistance of a general or vascular surgeon, a urologist, or a colleague more familiar with the area to be exposed.

The patient is placed supine on the operating table and slight hyperextension is employed. A paramedian incision is made (Fig. 14) over the abdomen extending from the umbilicus to the pubis. The rectus fascia beneath is identified and opened longitudinally in line with the incision. The rectus abdominis muscle is mobilized laterally to expose the underlying posterior rectus fascia. The peritoneum is then encountered and a decision then made whether to proceed transperitoneally (4,7) or retroperitoneally (9).

Transperitoneal Approach

The peritoneum can then be opened longitudinally in line with the skin incision, with care to protect the bowel beneath from injury. The intra-abdominal contents are then packed cranially to expose the posterior peritoneum overlying the great vessels and vertebral body (Fig. 15). The posterior peritoneum is then incised longitudinally in the midline over the sacral promontory. Presacral and parasympathetic nerve fibers should be preserved. The deep surgical dissection consists of freeing the distal ends of the aorta and vena cava from the vertebrae in the L4-L5 vertebral area. The aorta divides on the anterior surface of the L4 vertebra into the two common iliac arteries. The common iliac vessels then generally divide at approximately the S1 level into the internal and external iliac vessels (Fig. 16). Note that the left common iliac vein lies below the left common iliac artery, whereas the right common iliac artery lies below and medial to the right common iliac vein. The parasympathetic nerves in the presacral area exist as a diffuse plexus of nerves running around the aorta, and then heading inferiorly from the bifurcation along the anterior surface of the sacrum beneath the posterior peritoneum. This should be protected if at all possible to preserve adequate sexual function and prevent retroejaculation in men (3).

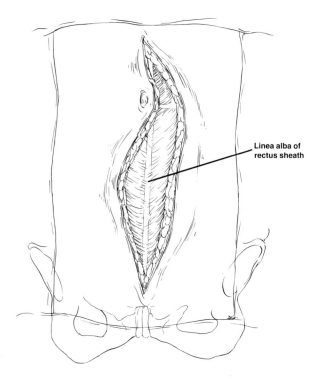

FIG. 14. Longitudinal midline incision with identification of the rectus sheath (redrawn from Hoppenfeld S, *Surgical Exposures in Orthopaedics*).

Linea alba of rectus sheath

The middle sacral artery (Fig. 16) is often adherent to the vertebral bodies, and some difficulties may be encountered in its mobilization. In this situation, the artery can be ligated with vascular clips.

Retroperitoneal Approach

Once the exposure through the anterior abdominal wall is complete, the spine may still be approached using a retroperitoneal plane of dissection rather than transperitoneal. The left side is again preferred, staying posterior on the renal fascia plane posterior to the ureter. The retroperitoneal dissection provides a less direct route to the spine, but if the tissue planes are well developed by blunt dissection and the abdominal contents are packed away, satisfactory exposure is obtained with less risk to the visceral and to the hypogastric plexus.

The midline anterior approaches are often utilized for spondylolisthesis, tumors, or pseudarthrosis or failures from prior posterior surgery. They are commonly used for anterior interbody fusions. Complications in male patients include impotence or sterility, although the incidence is reported to be less than 1% (3). Care must be taken not to extend the dissection well below the pelvic brim, as the parasympathetics or pudendal nerve may be prone to injury.

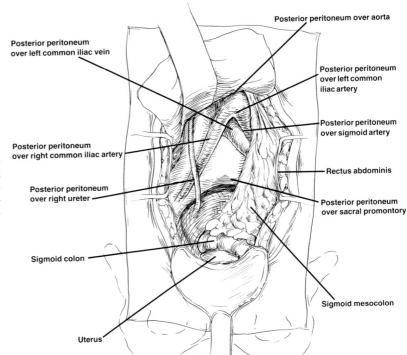

FIG. 15. The posterior peritoneum is incised to reveal the bifurcation of the aorta and vena cava, parasympathetic nerve fibers, and anterior longitudinal ligament, and sacral promontory (redrawn from Hoppenfeld S, *Surgical Exposures in Orthopaedics*).

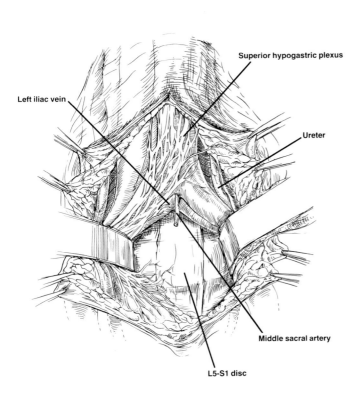

FIG. 16. Mobilization of the great vessels, ligation of the middle sacral artery, and gentle retraction of hypogastric plexus for adequate exposure of L5-S1 or L4-L5 internals (redrawn from Watkins R, *Surgical Approaches to the Spine*).

REFERENCES

1. Burrington JD, Brown C, Wayne ER, Odom J (1976): Anterior approach to the thoracolumbar spine—technical considerations. *Arch Surg* 111:456–463.
2. Cauthen JC (1988): *Lumbar spine surgery.* Baltimore: Williams & Wilkins.
3. Flynn JC, Price CT (1984): Sexual complications of anterior fusion of the lumbar spine. *Spine* 9:489–492.
4. Freebody D, Bendall R, Taylor RD (1971): Anterior transperitoneal lumbar fusion. *J Bone Joint Surg* [Br] 53:617–627.
5. Gill GG, Manning JG, White HL (1955): Surgical treatment of spondylolisthesis without spine fusion. Excision of the loose lamina with decompression of the nerve roots. *J Bone Joint Surg* [Am] 37:493–494.
6. Hodge WA, DeWald RL (1983): Splenic injury complicating the anterior thoracoabdominal surgical approach for scoliosis. A report of two cases. *J Bone Joint Surg* [Am] 65:396–397.
7. Lane JD Jr, Moore ES Jr (1948): Transperitoneal approach to the intervertebral disc in the lumbar area. *Ann Surg* 127:537–551.
8. Macnab I, Dall D (1971): The blood supply of the lumbar spine and its application to the technique of intertransverse lumbar fusion. *J Bone Joint Surg* [Br] 53:628–638.
9. Southwick WO, Robinson RA (1957): Surgical approaches to the vertebral bodies in the cervical and lumbar regions. *J Bone Joint Surg* [Am] 39:631–635.
10. Watkins MB (1953): Posterolateral fusion of the lumbar and lumbosacral spine. *J Bone Joint Surg* [Am] 35:1014–1018.
11. White AH, Rothman RH, Day CD (1987): *Lumbar spine surgery: Techniques and complications.* St. Louis: C.V. Mosby.
12. Wiltse LL, Bateman JG, Hutchinson RH, Nelson WE (1968): Paraspinal sacrospinalis-splitting approach to the lumbar spine. *J Bone Joint Surg* [Am] 50:919–926.
13. Wiltse LL, Spencer CW (1988): New uses and refinements of the paraspinal approach to the lumbar spine. *Spine* 13:696–706.

Low Back Disorders
Diagnosis and Conservative Treatment

The Adult Spine: Principles and Practice,
J. W. Frymoyer, Editor-in-Chief.
Raven Press, Ltd., New York © 1991.

CHAPTER 70

Natural History of Low Back Disorders

John W. Frymoyer and Alf Nachemson

The natural history of any disorder or disease is critical to determining the time-dependent morbidity and/or mortality of untreated individuals who have the condition in question, as well as the intrinsic and extrinsic factors which influence disease progression favorably or unfavorably. This information obviously is of great importance to performing prospective treatment outcome studies. The practicing clinician also needs this information to counsel the patient about an anticipated prognosis, particularly when a viable treatment option is "wait and see." An understanding of the natural history may also be very relevant to health policy decisions, including the allocation of resources from the government and the insurance industry for diagnosis and treatment.

This chapter focuses on natural history, which is largely derived from epidemiologic surveys. Some of the material will overlap with the extensive data presented by Andersson in Chapter 8 and the reader should consult that chapter for additional data.

J. W. Frymoyer, M.D.: Professor of Orthopaedics; Director, McClure Musculoskeletal Research Center, Department of Orthopaedics and Rehabilitation, University of Vermont, Burlington, Vermont, 05405.

A. Nachemson, M.D., Ph.D.: Professor and Chairman, Department of Orthopaedics, Gothenburg University, Gothenburg, Sweden.

METHODOLOGIC PROBLEMS IN THE STUDY OF THE NATURAL HISTORY OF LOW BACK DISORDERS

The analysis of the natural history of most low back disorders is particularly difficult in comparison to studies of diseases which have more measurable outcomes or a shorter natural history. Often the outcome measure utilized in studies of spine disorders has been an assessment of pain reduction. Other, more objective measures which may be used to quantify the natural history are return to work, reduced requirements for medication, or assessment of the activities of daily living. Because so many different criteria have been used in low back disorders research, many of the useful comparisons which might be made between studies and populations are not possible. The choice of outcome measure used may of itself significantly influence the reported severity of residual symptoms or functional capacity (40).

Yet another problem in analyzing the natural history of back disorders is the stability of the patients' or subjects' self-reported symptoms with the passage of time. In his 1 year, prospective study of low back pain, Biering-Sorensen (13) noted accurate reporting in only 84% of patients. Other epidemiologic studies have reported greater stability of patient recall, including the perception of pain intensity (32). These same difficulties with subject recall are a greater problem when attempts are made to quantify factors which may influence the natural history, such as "exposures" to cigarette smoke, hours spent driving, or sports participation history.

Additional methodological problems which negatively influence the ability to collect reliable natural history data include:

1. Stability of the population. It is rare that 100% of a population can be followed either in retrospective or prospective studies. A sample of 80% is usually considered the threshold for scientific validity. It is noteworthy that patients or subjects that cannot be located easily often are the individuals who have had a less favorable outcome.

2. Comparability of the populations. It is typical of retrospective study designs to compare two groups; one treated and the other untreated (the natural history group), and attempt to insure their comparability for all relevant factors. Typically, there are significant differences between groups despite these efforts, which often include age variation and different socioeconomic and occupational grouping. Stratification of the sample in the statistical analysis is often employed to overcome this problem.

3. Missing data. This is a particular problem to retrospective studies which depend often on medical records.

4. "Can the results from a study be generalized to other populations?" In low back disorders research much of the information has been garnered from the Swedish population which has a very different social system than the United States. Similarly, research conducted in rural populations with relative cultural and ethnic stability may not easily be generalized to urban societies with marked population heterogeneity.

METHODS TO STUDY NATURAL HISTORY

There is no single, idealized strategy to study natural history, although in general the meticulously conducted, prospective study design has the greatest scientific validity. Because multiple epidemiologic study designs have been used in low back pain research, the following material is presented as general background information and is not intended to be a detailed analysis of epidemiologic methodology (76).

Prospective

The prospective study design gives the investigator the greatest opportunity to control all of the relevant variables, which may influence the natural history. If the study includes a treatment group, randomization also creates the greatest likelihood that all relevant variables will be comparable between the natural history and treatment groups. Common pitfalls are attempting to amass too much information about the subjects; the absence of an a priori, clear statistical approach to data analysis; well-constructed outcome measures, and a strategy for the management of "drop-outs." Most of these problems can be overcome by good statistical design. A number of strategies are available to reduce the number of variables, such as the use of "expert panels." A subtler problem is the "Hawthorne effect." Simply stated, the Hawthorne effect occurs when repetitive questioning or testing of the individual contributes to producing the symptom being studied. This phenomenon occurs most frequently in pain and behavioral research. For example, studies of low back industrial injuries may heighten the workers' awareness of their back problems and lead to an increased reporting of symptoms. Changes in public policy or regional or national economics may also influence the results. For example, the Boeing studies (7–9,14) were significantly influenced by an unexpected reduction in the labor force which occurred mid-term in the prospective surveillance.

Retrospective

The retrospective study design has the benefit that a much longer observational period is possible at the expense of much less certain entry data, greater problems in recall of events by the subjects, and often loss of significant numbers of individuals from the follow-up evaluations. One of the major benefits of these studies is to provide essential input into the design of prospective studies.

Cross-Sectional

The cross-sectional study design simply evaluates a population or cohort at a given point in time. As such, it does not give longitudinal data regarding individuals. Stratification of the sample, for example, by age, will give some information about the expected natural history. Data can also be obtained about possible risk factors, although the problems of recall and exposure are significant barriers. Retrospective or cross-sectional studies, however, never prove anything from a pure scientific point of view (76).

Case Control

Case control can be used in either prospective or retrospective study designs. In this strategy subjects are matched for important demographic, occupational, and socioeconomic variables, so as to minimize the differences between the groups. This methodology is quite applicable to very specific populations or conditions. Kelsey et al. (49–51) used this strategy to characterize predictor variables for lumbar disc herniation. However, the selection of an appropriate case control is often difficult.

Survivorship Analysis

This statistical technique allows clinical experience gained over a short time interval to be used to predict future outcomes of a disease process or treatment. Validation of the prediction then occurs as the actual results become known over time. This technique has been used most successfully when the outcome can be measured discretely, such as expected versus actual deaths occurring with malignant tumors. It has also been used successfully to measure ongoing results of surgical interventions which have a fairly linear rate of failure over time, such as loosening of total hip replacements. This technique has been employed to predict the risk of a second disc prolapse following an initial operation for lumbar disc herniation (20).

NATURAL HISTORY OF LOW BACK PAIN

The early research into the natural history of low back pain was performed in Sweden (24,39,41,72), Great Britain (46), and within the Eastman Kodak plant of Rochester, New York (61). The early Swedish and English studies were cross-sectional and established the commonality of low back complaints, the age-relationship of the complaint, the radiographic changes which occurred with aging and in association with low back pain, and some estimate of the effects of occupation on symptoms and disability. In contrast, Rowe's Eastman Kodak analysis was truly prospective. He placed great credence on the radiographic evidence of degeneration as the dominant causation of low back symptoms. Since that time, several cross-sectional studies and a few prospective studies have given important information about the natural history and associated risk factors, which unfavorably influence recovery.

Figure 1 presents the natural history of an acute low back pain episode as measured by subjects' self-reports of pain and by return to work. The first important conclusion to be derived from this graph is the acute episodes are self-limited for the vast majority of individuals. In most studies the mean duration for return to work ranges from 20 to 30 days, while the duration of symptoms is slightly longer (4,81).

The second important observation is that there is a small subset of patients whose symptoms or disability becomes chronic. What constitutes the acute, subacute, or chronic phases has been variously classified. The Que-

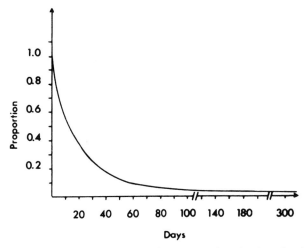

FIG. 1. The natural history of an acute low back episode measured by return to work (with permission from ref. 3).

bec study (69) concluded symptoms were chronic when they persisted beyond 7 weeks, while another review concluded symptoms of 3 months or more constituted the chronic phase (28). The question as to what constitutes a chronic pain is far less significant than the chronic disability. As will be seen, this latter issue has major socioeconomic consequences and appears to define a population subset with distinct psychosocial attributes.

Acute Low Back Pain

Prevalence and Incidence

The prevalence of any condition usually refers to a specific point in time (point prevalence) when the question is asked: Are you currently having low back pain? Incidence introduces time-dependency, and commonly is based on the annual occurrence of low back symptoms (annual incidence) or less often the lifetime incidence. As shown in Chapter 8 there is a high point prevalence, annual incidence, and lifetime incidence of acute low back pain symptoms. The observation that a lower lifetime incidence occurs in non-industrialized countries (19) has led to the unproven hypothesis that low back pain is the result of the industrial revolution. Obviously these epidemiologic data give an incomplete picture of symptom severity, which can range from a minimal backache with little or no functional incapacity to symptoms which are severe and temporarily disabling. The severity can be described by the subject's self-reports or the functional outcome, both of which influence the duration (32).

Self-reports of pain are usually analyzed by visual analogue scales which provide anchor points ranging from no pain, to the most severe pain imaginable, or by pain descriptors that scale severity (McGill Pain Questionnaire) (55).

The second approach is to describe the functional consequences of a low back pain episode. Here many approaches can be used including time lost from work, impairments of daily living or utilization of health services. For example, the National Health and Nutrition Examination Survey (NHANES) demonstrated a significant relationship between the utilization of health care services (a proxy for severity) and the duration of symptoms (26). Those studies also show significant variations in use and type of health service as a function of age and geography.

The third approach is to describe the duration of symptoms. Deyo (26) has analyzed the NHANES which represents a probability sample of the adult, non-institutionalized, civilian population of the United States. Low back pain of greater than 2 weeks duration was identified in 1,355 of the 10,404 subjects, and 161 additional subjects reported low back pain accompanied by sciatica. In this sample of 10,404 subjects, 1,516 (13.8%) had back symptoms of greater than 2 weeks. This lifetime incidence of more severe symptoms, as measured by duration, reasonably approximates the lifetime incidence of symptoms described as significant in another survey (32).

The conclusion which can be drawn from all of this data is that acute low back pain is an extremely common occurrence, but that the natural history for recovery is favorable for the majority of patients and results in modest utilization of health care services.

Factors That Influence the Natural History of Acute Low Back Pain

Two broad categories of factors will affect any symptom or health condition: (a) factors over which the individual has no control (age, sex, and race) and (b) factors which may be modified or controlled (occupation, health habits [smoking, physical fitness]). The latter group of factors are appropriately termed risk factors. Often, the increased risks are quantified by "odds ratio" determination. The results of an odd ratio analysis determines the chances are X times greater when a particular factor is present.

Age

The early studies of Hult, Horal, and others demonstrated that the usual onset of low back pain occurred during the third decade of life, and the peak prevalence during the fifth decade. It has been generally thought that low back symptoms continue to increase throughout life, although a number of studies indicate this traditional wisdom may be inaccurate. Biering-Sorenson (13) observed a reduction in the point prevalence of low back pain after age 55 years in males, but not in females. A hypothesis to explain the differences is the continued increase in the point prevalence of low back complaints in women results from osteoporosis. There is little data which clarify the effect of age on the natural history of an acute episode.

Sex

Traditional wisdom has suggested males have greater risk of acute back pain than females, attributed to the greater physical and occupational demands made on men. This belief is not confirmed by cross-sectional surveys which show little or no difference between males and females in the prevalence or incidence of back pain. As will be seen, gender differences may influence the treatment options chosen, particularly in those patients whose symptoms include sciatica due to lumbar disc herniation. However, gender does not influence the natural history of recovery.

A second factor of importance is pregnancy. Complaints of non-functionally, disabling low back pain are common during pregnancy (3). It is speculated this occurrence might be the result of demands made on paraspinal muscles resulting in muscle fatigue, increases in the lumbar lordosis to accommodate the shift in the center of gravity, or due to ligamentous strain as the pelvic ligaments undergo changes in their biochemistry and mechanical properties. However, measures of lumbar lordosis indicate little or no change, and direct stereoradiographic measurements in early post-partum women show no evidence of sacroiliac instability (64).

Regardless of causation, the increased complaint of low back pain during pregnancy is followed by an increased likelihood of later symptoms with multiparous females reporting 3 times more symptoms than their non-parous counterparts.

Race/Genetics

Pain research demonstrates significant differences in the behavioral manifestations of many different types of painful conditions between different ethnic groups (see Chapter 12). In general, individuals of southern European extraction, particularly populations bordering the Mediterranean, have more outward expressions of pain (pain behavior) than their northern European counterparts, who are often described as stoic. Whether these cultural differences might explain the lower lifetime incidence of back complaints in non-industrialized societies remains speculative. There is little information to determine if the expression of pain influences the natural history of low back pain symptoms. However, some pathologic conditions of etiologic significance to low back pain appear to have genetic antecedents as will be shown later in this chapter.

Anthropometric Factors

A variety of anthropometric factors have been studied, primarily as they influence the incidence and prevalence of back pain complaints as opposed to how they influence the natural history. Body habitus, including weight and height (26,58) have variously been reported to be or not to be related to back pain complaints. The most complete data was derived from the NHANE survey, which showed adults in the upper fifth quintile of height and weight had a greater prevalence of low back pain lasting more than 2 weeks duration. This would suggest an unfavorable effect of these factors on recovery. The effect of leg length discrepancy is also controversial. There is no convincing evidence that equalizing subtle differences in leg lengths favorably impacts on the natural history of acute (or chronic) symptoms. Similarly, normal variations in posture including lumbar lordosis and minor degrees of scoliosis appear to have no impact on occurrence or natural history of low back pain (29), although not everyone agrees (27) with this conclusion.

Risk Factors

A variety of risk factors for low back disorders have been studied including physical fitness, smoking, and occupation.

Physical fitness is currently a major area of interest in both the epidemiology and treatment of low back disorders. Stimulus for this interest has come from basic biochemical and biomechanical research which demonstrates the beneficial effects of aerobic exercise on the intervertebral disc, articular cartilage, ligaments, and muscles, and the adverse effects of inactivity on these same tissues (33). Prospective, randomized treatment outcome studies also strongly indicate that aerobic exercise has the same beneficial effects on the rate of recovery from acute low back pain episodes and also subacute (2 months duration) low back pain in blue collar workers (56). Extended bedrest has been shown to have no beneficial effects (25). As a subset of physical fitness, muscular strength has also been evaluated, a topic extensively discussed in Chapter 16. There is also little information to confirm whether muscle strength or muscle imbalance influences the natural history of acute back pain. Studies of patients with chronic/disabling back pain, undergoing chronic rehabilitation have shown little correlation between isokinetically, measured flexor and extensor strength and the rate of recovery or outcome of rehabilitation 1 year after the intervention (54).

Cigarette smoking has been shown to be a significant risk factor for low back pain, as well as low back pain with sciatica due to lumbar disc herniation, and cross-sectional surveys (28) indicate smokers self-report more severe symptoms and sciatica (51), suggesting smoking

may unfavorably influence the natural history of recovery (28,72). The hypotheses advanced to explain the effects have included: (a) a direct effect of smoking on the nutrition of the lumbar intervertebral disc, (b) an indirect mechanical effect of coughing, or (c) differences in the behavior or physical fitness of smokers (see Chapter 31).

Occupational risk factors comprise yet another major influence on both the occurrence of acute low back pain and recovery. Although this topic is extensively reviewed in Chapter 8, it is worth re-emphasizing that heavier job requirements do influence recovery (2,41,53,65).

Understanding the effects of occupation on the occurrence and recovery from back pain symptoms has also been analyzed in specific occupational cohorts. Snook (65) has summarized data regarding the point prevalence of low back pain symptoms, as it is affected by specific occupations which show the impact of both static mechanical requirements and vibration. How occupation also influences the natural history of a back disorder and impacts on chronic disability will be discussed later in this chapter.

The second major category of occupational risk factors relates to work environment and how the individual interacts with that environment. These data have been derived largely from cross-sectional studies (7,8,11,12, 14–16,74,78), although one prospective study (16) now has offered additional confirmatory evidence. A summary of these studies is that the following factors are associated with an increased risk of acute low back pain and adversely favor the recovery:

1. Worker's perception of the job. The jobs are viewed by the worker as dissatisfying, repetitious, and boring. Since heavy manual labor often has this attribute, there are probably interactions between mechanical factors and job perception.
2. Employer's perception of the worker. The supervisors view the worker as less competent and give poorer job evaluations.
3. Interaction between worker and employer. The worker finds less social support in his work environment, as measured by the "work APGAR" test instrument (see Chapter 9).
4. Work environment. The environment is described as unpleasant and noisy.

In summary, the occurrence of low back pain and the generally favorable natural history of acute low back pain is significantly influenced by a variety of factors, some of which are inherent to the individual, and some of which can be controlled.

Chronic Low Back Pain

The chronic phase of low back pain is variously classified as beginning at 7 to 12 weeks. It is particularly im-

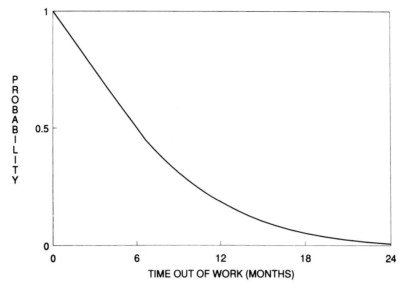

FIG. 2. The natural history of chronic low back pain as measured by return to work. Note the increasingly unfavorable outlook as time progresses.

portant to differentiate 2 patient groups: those with symptoms of chronic back pain from those patients whose symptoms result in continued work loss. There is little information about the former group, whereas a great deal of knowledge has been gained about the chronically disabled subset. Figure 2 shows the natural history of chronic low back disability. Six months after an episode, the likelihood of ever returning to work is 50%, by 1 year that figure is 20%, and at 2 years the probability approaches zero. Two studies have compared recovery in a treatment group receiving intensive rehabilitation and a comparison group (the natural history cohort) (54) (see Chapter 13). The comparison group was chosen by the refusal of their insurance carriers to pay for the rehabilitation program, but were similar to the treatment group in all other significant parameters. The average duration of disability in both studies was 1 year; based on historic surveys, the expected probability for return to work would have been 20% (10). In fact, the return to work rate in the northeast cohort was 17% 1 year later, whereas the comparable rate was 40% in the Texas cohort. The cause of the Texas deviation from the historic and northeast experience remains unclear, but may have been the result of adverse entitlement programs or a very favorable job market. Nevertheless, it is clear that the natural history for recovery with chronic low back pain disability remains distinctly unfavorable and is a problem of major socioeconomic importance for the following reasons:

1. The number of chronically, low back pain disabled individuals is large; in the United States the point prevalence of disability is 5.2 million individuals, of which one-half (2.6 million) are permanent and the other one-half temporary. In Sweden (population 8.5 million) the figure is even more staggering; in 1988, 240,000 workers were permanently disabled due to low back pain.

2. The chronic low back pain disabled population is growing in the United States and other industrialized countries at a rate disproportionate to population growth or the increase in disability due to other health conditions. An example of this increase is shown in Table 1 for the Swedish population.

3. The chronic low back pain disabled subset produces the vast majority of the costs for low back diseases as a whole—most surveys indicate 80% to 90% of costs relate to this patient population (65,68). Although many of the costs are indirect (lost work, cost of replacing the disabled employee), the direct medical costs are high be-

TABLE 1. *Low back pain sick listing and the resulting increase in permanent disability*

Low back sick listing		
Year	% of insured	Duration (days)
1970	1	20
1975	3	22
1980	7	25
1987	8	34
Permanent disability due to back pain		
Total sum of persons in Sweden		
1952	850	
1982	37,100	
1987	51,700[a]	

With permission from ref. 56a.
[a] Population base 8.5 million.

cause of a disproportionate utilization of health care services. (Note: In the United States, 30% of the total is in direct costs, while in Sweden only 7% of health dollars goes to direct costs.)

Risk Factors for Chronic Low Back Pain

In the preceding section, and in other chapters, many of the risk factors which unfavorably alter the natural history of recovery from an acute low back pain episode, have already been presented. The weight of the evidence suggests the determinants are primarily psychosocial rather than physical disease process, based upon retrospective, cross-sectional, and prospective analyses. These data can be summarized as follows:

1. Cross-sectional surveys indicate chronic disability is associated with psychosocial dysfunction, multiple other painful conditions (such as headache), and psychologic profiles indicative of hysteria, hypochondriasis, and depression (10,17,30). The results of one survey are shown in Table 2. It has been speculative if these observed psychosocial dysfunctions were the cause or the result of the disability. Two prospective surveys have yielded somewhat conflicting results. The Boeing study showed HY and HS scales of the Minnesota Multiphasic Personality Inventory (MMPI) were predictive of later disability, whereas a Predictive Risk Model demonstrated little value of these same scales (22). In both stud-

TABLE 2. Indicators measuring psychosocial dysfunction and poor health habits for subjects with and without significant low back disability

Symptom checklist response rates by pain group (% answering yes)			
	Asymptomatic	Moderate	Severe
Unhappy	5.2	10.4	15.4
Hopeless	8.0	12.3	18.8
Worried	15.6	31.0	42.0
Scared	7.4	19.1	19.4
Nervous	11.2	28.8	23.9
Annoyed	32.3	51.1	59.7
Temper	8.0	19.0	21.2
Lonely	21.1	23.2	26.9
Touchy	7.8	14.6	14.9
Hurt	4.2	8.5	11.8
Unsympathetic	9.1	15.3	21.3
Headaches	6.1	21.4	20.9
Sleep	28.3	54.6	55.1
Medical care	79.1	83.5	65.6
Handicapped	0.0	8.5	11.8
Miserable	6.1	22.1	35.3
Alcohol and drugs	7.1	9.4	4.4
Nervous breakdown	3.0	1.4	3.0
Psychiatric help	8.9	7.2	11.9
Counseling	8.6	16.2	11.9

With permission from ref. 30.

ies, certain commonalities were observed, most particularly in measures of work satisfaction, consistent with another long-term retrospective analysis (11).

2. The work environment, as already discussed, appears to be a potent predictor of future disability, particularly when there is a perception that the work environment caused an injury. When this perception is combined with the presence of a lawyer or threatened legal action, the return-to-work rate is significantly diminished (21,34,35).

3. The potential for successful treatment is significantly reduced in this patient population, regardless of the method chosen, although the aggressive functional restoration programs outlined in Chapter 13 have significantly improved upon the historic experience.

A variety of other demographic factors also appear to have an impact on chronic disability, as determined from NHANE survey data. In that survey, the questionnaire utilized did not permit a precise definition of chronic low back disability, but it was argued that other questions served as reasonable proxies for low back pain disability. These data are displayed in Figures 3, 4, and 5 and show the effects of age, income, and educational level on disability rates (23).

The summary statement about chronic low back pain is that the condition is not self-limiting when disability is present; and the determinants of chronic disability and its continuation are significantly based on psychosocial, occupational, and demographic factors, rather than by the clinical diagnosis or its treatment.

Recurrent Low Back Pain

The rate of recurrence following an acute low back pain episode has been calculated to range from 40%, to as high as 85% (79,80). Retrospective and cross-sectional surveys give limited information in this regard because patient recall of the episodes and their severity is often poor. It is also difficult to establish what constitutes a true recurrence, as opposed to a continuation of symptoms with intermittent, acute exacerbations. In the historic surveys, such as those of Hult and Horal, it was generally thought that the onset of low grade backache (termed muscular insufficiency) in the third decade of life was commonly followed by symptoms of greater severity in the fifth decade due to disc disease. Prospective studies have been limited in their duration, and thus, a complete picture of the natural history is yet to be available. These studies do suggest the following: (a) the determinants of recurrence are greater if the back pain is accompanied by sciatica and nerve root tension signs; (b) occupational factors including requirements for heavy manual labor are adverse factors; and (c) if the recurrent episodes are accompanied by significant periods of dis-

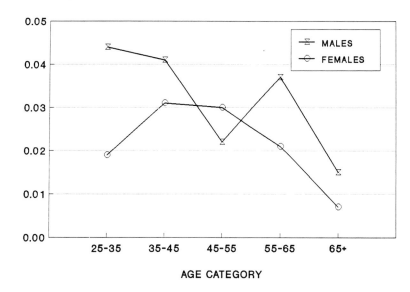

FIG. 3. Effect of age on disability calculated from the NHANES II survey data. The vertical gives the prevalence, i.e., 0.01 indicates that 1% of that age group has had a period of disability (with permission from ref. 23).

ability, many of the same psychosocial determinants of chronic disability can be identified.

NATURAL HISTORY OF SCIATICA

The point prevalence and lifetime incidence of sciatica vary widely between epidemiologic surveys (3,36). Some cross-sectional studies indicate a lifetime incidence of sciatica of 40% in males (28,72), while others suggest a significantly lower incidence which ranges from 1.5% to 13.8%. The lowest lifetime incidence recorded is 1.5% in the NHANE survey. However, in the subset who had reported low back pain of greater than 2 weeks duration the lifetime incidence rose to 11%. These conflicting data point to significant differences in surveillance techniques and the definition of sciatica. In one cross-sectional study, reporting a lifetime incidence of 40% (31), significant associations were identified between the complaint of sciatica and other signs of neurologic dysfunction as shown in Table 3.

The natural history of sciatica appears to be favorable as measured by the need for surgery. Evidence to that point is derived from the cross-sectional, as well as prospective, survey data. In the cross-sectional studies demonstrating a lifetime incidence of 40%, the lifetime incidence of lumbar disc surgery ranged from 1% to 2% (28). These figures also appear concordant with other cross-sectional data (72). However, the subset of patients who described their pain as severe, had a lifetime incidence of 10% (30). A clearer picture of the natural history is derived from other retrospective surveys and one prospective survey of lumbar disc excision, which will be reviewed in Chapter 80.

FIG. 4. Effect of income on disability calculated from the NHANES II survey data (with permission from ref. 23).

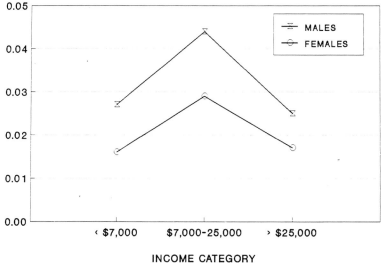

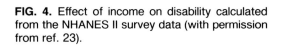

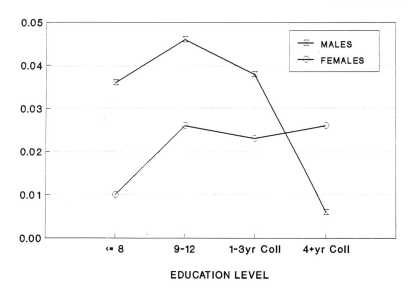

FIG. 5. Effects of educational level on disability calculated from the NHANES II survey data (with permission from ref. 23).

Risk Factors for Sciatica

Age

As previously noted, the cross-sectional survey data have indicated an increased risk for more severe back symptoms in the fifth decade of life. The best information about age is derived from Spangfort's data (67), although his analyses were limited to the subset of patients with lumbar disc herniation which required surgery. These data are displayed in Figure 6 and show that the peak age is 42 years for both men and women, and the need for surgical intervention after 42 years of age then rapidly declines. An important additional observation made by Spangfort (67) was that age also was a determinant of the level of herniation, with younger patients more commonly affected by L5–S1 herniations, somewhat older patients by L4-L5, and a small, but distinctive subset of considerably older patients with disc herniations at the L3–L4 and higher levels.

How age affects the natural history of sciatica once the symptoms occur is less certain. Comparisons of young and old patients indicate the younger population more frequently has more positive nerve root tension signs and reflex alteration, but how this affects the long-term prognosis is uncertain. Furthermore, the clinical evidence suggests the older patient with sciatica often has spinal stenosis affecting the lateral nerve root canal as the major or associated determinant of sciatica (38). How this influences recovery with non-operative treatment has not been analyzed.

Sex

Most cross-sectional surveys indicate the incidence and prevalence of sciatica are similar in males and females, although a greater prevalence of sciatica has been recorded in males in some studies (47,49,73). However, most clinical studies show a distinct difference between

TABLE 3. *Relationship of sciatic-like symptoms and self-reported symptoms of neurologic dysfunction for a cohort of males 18 to 55 years of age (Significant relationships identified)*

	Men with low back pain (%)	
Symptoms in the lower limbs[a]	Moderate (N = 565)	Severe (N = 288)
Pain	28.9	54.5[b]
Numbness	14.0	37.4[b]
Weakness	17.9	44.0[b]

With permission from ref. 28.

[a] A subject may have reported one or more of these symptoms.

[b] p < 0.001, chi-square analysis.

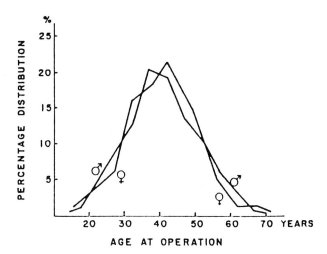

FIG. 6. Age of occurrence of lumbar disc excision for males and females. Note that the highest surgical rates occur early in the fifth decade (with permission from ref. 67).

males and females in the rate of subsequent surgical intervention, ranging from a two- to threefold increase in males (50,75). A superficial evaluation of this data would suggest males have a less favorable recovery potential. However, it is speculated that males are less tolerant of the symptoms or social and occupational factors are the primary determinants of treatment choice, rather than symptom or disease severity.

Genetic Factors

A genetic predisposition to sciatica has been suggested by Lawrence (52), in his analyses of degenerative conditions. but the data are limited. The most convincing evidence for a genetic determinant is Varlotta and Brown (82). They demonstrated a significant increased risk of lumbar disc herniation in the first degree relatives of adolescents who had lumbar disc herniation. Whether these data can be generalized to the population of patients with sciatica or lumbar disc herniation is unproven. A smaller subset of patients with a genetic predisposition to sciatica are achondroplastic dwarfs, where the presentation of lumbar disc herniation is often associated with major caudal dysfunction resulting from small spinal canal dimensions.

Anthropometric Factors

The anthropometric data have not been analyzed with respect to how these factors influence the natural history. Alterations in spinal canal dimensions, as measured by plane radiographs and ultrasound, indicate a smaller canal size increases the risk of sciatica (38,59). Increased body height, but not weight, has been shown as a significant factor (36). There is little evidence that posture influences the risk or recovery from sciatica. However, diabetes is a factor of importance in two respects. First, sciatic-like symptoms may be due to diabetic neuropathy in this population. Moreover, there is also experimental evidence that diabetes in laboratory animals is associated with an increased rate of disc degeneration (see Chapter 31). As yet, no evidence is available in humans. Second, there is a fourfold increase in degenerative spondylolisthesis in diabetics, and thus, there is a specific increased risk of sciatica from that condition (60). How diabetes influences the recovery from sciatica due to lumbar disc herniation is uncertain, although some of us have a clinical impression that diabetic patients fare less well.

Other Risk Factors

Many of the risk factors associated with acute low back pain have been associated with sciatica including occupational requirements for heavy lifting, particularly when this includes twisting, exposure to vibration caused by motor vehicles, poorer physical conditioning, and cigarette smoking (37). However, information is limited on how these factors affect the recovery once sciatica has occurred. The influence of psychosocial factors will be presented elsewhere in this book, but the summary statement is that these factors are of major importance in the success of surgical and non-surgical interventions in the treatment of patients with sciatica.

Effects of Surgery on the Natural History of Sciatica

It has been shown that surgery hastens the initial recovery as measured by symptom reduction and return to work, but has minimal influence on the later risk of recurrence, residual symptoms, or ultimate functional status (83). Surgery is necessary in a relatively small percent of patients, and the lifetime incidence of low back surgery ranges from 1% to 3%. However, there is some speculation that this rate is increasing. It should also be emphasized that there are significant variations in this rate between countries, and even between regions of the United States. Pokras and associates (57) reported that 69.5 individuals per 100,000 of the United States population undergo a disc excision annually. An additional 31 individuals per 100,000 undergo some other lumbar procedure, for a combined rate of approximately 100 individuals per 100,000. Recently, the annual incidence of lumbar disc surgery has been carefully analyzed. A population-based study was conducted in Olmsted County, Minnesota for the years 1950 through 1979. The age and sex specific incidence rates were determined. These incidence rates adjusted to the age and sex distribution of the United States white population were 52.3 person years per 100,000 individuals for all such operations and 46.3 person years per 100,000 individuals for initial operations. Over the 30 year study interval, these rates remained fairly constant. The age at operation was quite similar to that reported by Spangfort (67) (Fig. 6). The most important finding of the study was that patients with a surgically-proven lumbar disc prolapse had about 10 times the risk of another operation for that same condition within the first ten years after their initial operation, when compared with the general population (20).

The figure for other countries indicates a lower surgical rate, such as 31 to 41 individuals per 100,000 in Finland, 20 individuals per 100,000 in Sweden, and 10 individuals per 100,000 in Great Britain (42). Kane (44) estimated as much as a tenfold variation in the annual rate of surgery across the United States. This type of variation has been observed for other surgical procedures such as prostatectomy and hysterectomy (86). These studies indicate that regional variations have little to do with differences in the prevalence of disease, but are significantly associated with physician behavior, and the local prevailing opinion as to what constitutes optimum treatment (45).

NATURAL HISTORY OF CLAUDICATION

There is limited information about the natural history of claudication as distinct from sciatica. It is known that neurogenic claudication more frequently occurs in the older age group; that the radiologic correlates of claudication, such as degenerative spinal stenosis are also more common (80); and that there may be an increased risk of this symptom in those who have done heavy labor. However, the recovery from claudication is unknown, except in patients who are severely affected and have required surgical treatment. This issue will be discussed in Chapter 85. The effect of surgical intervention, including instability which results from overzealous decompression, will be discussed in Chapters 89 and 90. Johnsson (43) demonstrated in a retrospective study comparing non-operated to operated patients, followed for 2 to 10 years, that 60% of the non-operated cases improved.

NATURAL HISTORY OF SPECIFIC DISEASE PROCESSES

Degenerative Spinal Conditions

The natural history of spinal degeneration from a pathoanatomic and clinical perspective has been discussed extensively in previous chapters, as has the difficulty in separating age-related degeneration from degenerative conditions that produce symptoms (see Chapter 31). Thus, degeneration, as seen pathologically and radiographically, is an almost inevitable consequence of the aging process, whereas degeneration causing symptoms occurs in association with specific disease entities such as spinal stenosis, degenerative spondylolisthesis, and lumbar disc herniation.

Scoliosis

The effects of scoliosis on low back pain have been alluded to earlier in this chapter, and it has been noted that minor degrees of scoliosis appear to have little or no impact on either risk of occurrence or natural history. The natural history of idiopathic scoliosis, and its progression in the adult, have been studied extensively over long time intervals. Although the results are somewhat conflicting, they offer important insights into the natural history and how this is favorably or unfavorably influenced.

Weinstein (84,85) studied 219 patients (84% female, 16% male) whose average age was 53 years (range 38–70)

at follow-up evaluation, with an average duration of follow-up of 40 years (range 31–52 years). The prediction of progression of the curve varied by the level and curve pattern (see Chapter 65). The higher degree of curves (greater than 60) were associated with pain, particularly when the curve involved the lumbar spine. Ascani and associates (5) performed a similar survey in 187 "random cases," 15 to 47 years after they attained skeletal maturity. The average curve progression, as measured by the Cobb angle, was 0.40 degrees per year. Pain was present in 61% and was more likely in females, particularly after pregnancy. He also observed cardiopulmonary dysfunction in 22%, psychologic disturbances in 49%, and a mortality of 17%, which he concluded was two times greater than the Italian population without scoliosis. Other long-term follow-ups have reached essentially similar conclusions, but it is debated whether or not scoliosis produces back pain in the adult. This debate, in part, relates to the absence of adequate comparison groups. The consensus opinion is that curves greater than 60 degrees are associated with an increased risk of back pain, particularly when they involve the lumbar spine, the curve is unbalanced, or there is anomalous lumbosacral take-off for the curve. There is also a consensus that if prior fusion has been done, the risk of back pain increases dramatically as the fusion extends lower into the lumbar spine.

Scheuermann's Disease

Scheuermann was a Danish radiologist who demonstrated in the early 1920s that the changes seen in the vertebra often ascribed to an earlier tuberculosis of the spine, in fact, were a specific disease entity (62,63). Since that time, various pathoanatomical studies have been performed, without conclusive results, although the latest finding is a collagen weakness in the vertebral end plates (1,6,18).

Also, genetic factors have been implicated because the disease very often clusters in families.

In a recent study, Svard (71) could not corroborate the earlier proposition by Alexander (1) that Scheuermann changes were more common in athletes than in non-athletes.

There are various studies of the normal range of kyphosis in different populations, all of which point to 35–45 degrees of kyphosis to be normal in the 15- to 20-year-old (71). Stagnara (70) has demonstrated a rather wide variation in his population from France and Italy and in his view the range is 20–50 degrees.

The Scoliosis Research Society has defined kyphosis of less than 20 degrees as abnormal and has coined the term *hypo-kyphosis.*

According to the definition first proposed by Sorensen (66), and thereafter adopted by most authors, patients with Scheuermann's disease should exhibit at least three wedge-shaped vertebrae with irregularities of the end plates and the wedging exceeding 5 degrees.

Sorensen also in his thesis gave a rather optimistic prognosis for those exhibiting Scheuermann's disease in the thoracic area, moderately good for those in the thoracolumbar area, and relatively poor in the lumbar region, all with regard to work capacity. His findings have been corroborated by later authors, including Travaglini from Italy and the epidemiologic studies by Valkenburg and Haanan (80).

Scheuermann's disease afflicts nearly 10% of the population but only 1% ever seeks medical attention during their youth.

The symptoms usually are tiredness and rather little ache, but then gradually more deformity, which in some areas is called "unsightly." In the adult, severe pain in conjunction with Scheuermann's disease is uncommon.

SUMMARY AND CONCLUSIONS

Analyses of the natural history of low back disorders still present significant challenges in experimental design, particularly in the measurements of pain and function. Despite these limitations, there is a body of evidence which supports the following conclusions:

1. Acute low back pain is an extremely common, age-related symptom affecting 70% of all adults sometime during their life. For the majority of individuals, the condition is of mild severity, is a self-limiting problem whose occurrence and recovery are influenced by a variety of anthropometric and occupational factors, many of which can be favorably controlled. In contrast, chronic low back pain, when associated with disability, is not a self-limiting problem and is largely determined by complex psychosocial, demographic, and occupational factors, many of which are not easily controlled. This unfavorable natural history, combined with the major socioeconomic implications and the continued uncontrolled growth in the rate of disability, makes this problem a focus for national policy and a critical area for research. Although low back pain is often recurrent, the major impact relates to the subset of patients whose recurrent episodes are associated with disability.

2. Sciatica is a common, age-related occurrence, although there are wide variations in the reported incidence and prevalence. The recovery rate from sciatica, in general, appears also to be favorable and only a minority require surgical intervention. The impact of surgery is primarily a reduction in short-term disability and symptoms, with the exception of those patients with major neurologic dysfunction. The impact of specific operations, such as disc excision alone, versus disc excision combined with fusion, also appears to have little impact on the natural history, although the pattern of failures are distinctly different between the two operations. Many of the factors which influence both the risk of sciatica and recovery are identical with the factors influencing low back pain alone. Similar to the problem of low back pain disability, the most potent indicators are psychosocial and occupational, rather than physical.

3. There are few data regarding the natural history of neurologic claudication or spinal stenosis, other than its age relationships and association with conditions such as diabetes. Idiopathic scoliosis has a slow rate of progression in the adult and produces only a minimal risk of low back pain when the curve is less than 60 degrees. An increased risk is associated with certain curve patterns, particularly those which involve an anomalous lumbar takeoff, or when there has been prior fusion extending into the lower lumbar spine.

4. There is an ongoing need to gather prospective, longitudinal data to better understand those factors which can be influenced by the health care profession, versus those which will require the development of national policies or changes in the work environment. The tremendous social and monetary implications of low back pain symptoms will tend to drive this need for additional information, and with it will come an increased understanding of low back diseases, their cause and natural history. As the population ages, specific focus on spinal stenosis will also become of greater importance.

REFERENCES

1. Alexander CJ (1977): Scheuermann's disease. A traumatic spondylodystrophy? *Skeletal Radiol* 1:209–221.
2. Andersson GBJ (1981): Epidemiologic aspects on low-back pain in industry. *Spine* 6:53–60.
3. Andersson GBJ, Svensson H-O, Oden A (1983): The intensity of work recovery in low back pain. *Spine* 8:880–884.
4. Andersson GBJ (1990): Personal communication.
5. Ascani E, Salsano V, Giglio G (1977): The incidence and early detection of spinal deformities. A study based on the screening of 16,104 schoolchildren. *Ital J Orthop Traumatol* 3(1):111–117.
6. Aufdermaur M, Spycher M (1986): Pathogenesis of osteochondrosis juvenilis Scheuermann. *J Orthop Res* 4:452–457.
7. Battié MC, Hansson TH, Engel JM, et al (1986): The reliability of measurements of the lumbar spine using ultrasound B-Scan. *Spine* 11:144–148.
8. Battié MC, Bigos SJ, Sheehy A, Wortley MD (1987): Spinal flexibility and individual factors that influence it. *Phys Ther* 67:653–658.
9. Battié MC, Bigos SJ, Fisher LD, et al (1989): A prospective study of the role of cardiovascular risk factors and fitness in industrial back pain complaints. *Spine* 14:141–147.
10. Beals RK, Hickman NW (1972): Industrial injuries of the back and extremities: Comprehensive evaluation—An aid in prognosis and management. A study of one hundred and eighty patients. *J Bone Joint Surg* [Am] 54:1593–1611.
11. Bergenudd H, Nilsson B (1988): Back pain in middle age; occupational workload and psychologic factors: An epidemiologic survey. *Spine* 1:58–60.
12. Bergenudd H (1989): Talent, occupation and locomotor discomfort. Malmo, Sweden: Thesis, Lunds Universitet.
13. Biering-Sorensen F (1982): Low back trouble in a general population of 30-, 40-, 50-, and 60-year-old men and women: Study design, representativeness and basic results. *Dan Med Bull* 29:289–299.

14. Bigos SJ, Spengler DM, Martin NA, Zeh J, Fisher L, Nachemson A, Wang MH (1986): Back injuries in industry: A retrospective study. II. Injury factors. *Spine* 11:246–251.
15. Bigos SJ, Spengler DM, Martin NA, Zeh J, Fisher L, Nachemson A (1986): Back injuries in industry: A retrospective study. III. Employee-related factors. *Spine* 11:252–256.
16. Bigos SJ, Battié MC, Spengler DM, et al (submitted for publication): A prospective study of work perceptions and psychosocial factors affecting the report of back injury. *Spine.*
17. Blumer D, Heilbronn M (1982): Chronic pain as a variant of depressive disease: The pain-prone disorder. *J Nerv Ment Dis* 170:381–406.
18. Bradford DS (1981): Vertebral osteochondrosis (Scheuermann's kyphosis). *Clin Orthop* 158:83–90.
19. Bremner JM, Lawrence JS, Miall WE (1968): Degenerative joint disease in a Jamaican rural population. *Ann Rheum Dis* 27:326–332.
20. Bruske-Hohlfeld I, Merritt JL, Onofrio BM, et al (1990): Incidence of lumbar disc surgery. A population-based study in Olmsted County, Minnesota, 1950–1979. *Spine* 15(1):31–35.
21. Carron H, DeGood DF, Tait R (1985): A comparison of low back pain patients in the United States and New Zealand: Psychological and economic factors affecting severity of disability. *Pain* 21:77–89.
22. Cats-Baril WL, Frymoyer JW (in press): Identifying patients at risk of becoming disabled due to low back pain: The Vermont Rehabilitation Engineering Center predictive model. *Spine.*
23. Cats-Baril WL, Frymoyer JW (in press): Demographic factors associated with the prevalence of disability in the general population: Analysis of the NHANES I database. *Spine.*
24. Choler U, Larsson R, Nachemson A, Peterson L-E (1985): Ont i ryggen—Forsok med vardprogram for patienter med lumbala smarttillstand. *Spri rapport 188.*
25. Deyo RA, Diehl AK, Rosenthal M (1986): How many days of bed rest for acute low back pain? A randomized clinical trial. *N Engl J Med* 315:1064–1070.
26. Deyo RA, Tsui-Wu YJ (1987): Descriptive epidemiology of low-back pain and its related medical care in the United States. *Spine* 12:264–268.
27. Fahrni WH, Trueman GE (1965): Comparative radiological study of the spines of a primitive population with North Americans and northern Europeans. *J Bone Joint Surg [Br]* 47:552–555.
28. Frymoyer JW, Pope MH, Clements JH, Wilder DG, MacPherson B, Ashikaga T (1983): Risk factors in low-back pain. *J Bone Joint Surg [Am]* 65:213–218.
29. Frymoyer JW, Newberg A, Pope MH, Wilder DG, Clements J, MacPherson B (1984): Spine radiographs in patients with low-back pain. An epidemiological study in men. *J Bone Joint Surg [Am]* 66:1048–1044.
30. Frymoyer JW, Rosen JC, Clements J, Pope MH (1985): Psychologic factors in low-back pain disability. *Clin Orthop* 195:178–184.
31. Frymoyer JW, Cats-Baril W (1987): Predictors of low back pain disability. *Clin Orthop* 221:89–98.
32. Frymoyer JW (1988): Back pain and sciatica. *N Engl J Med* 318:291–300.
33. Frymoyer JW, Gordon SL (1989): *New perspectives on low back pain.* Chicago: American Academy of Orthopaedic Surgeons.
34. Garron DC, Leavitt F (1983): Chronic low back pain and depression. *J Clin Psychol* 39:486–493.
35. Greenough CG, Fraser RD (1989): The effects of compensation on recovery from low back injury. *Spine* 14:947–955.
36. Heliovaara M, ed (1988): *Epidemiology of sciatica and herniated lumbar intervertebral disc.* Helsinki, Finland: Social Insurance Institution, ML:76.
37. Heliovaara M (1988): Body height, obesity, and risk of herniated lumbar intervertebral disc. In: Heliovaara M, ed. *Epidemiology of sciatica and herniated lumbar intervertebral disc,* Helsinki, Finland: Social Insurance Institution.
38. Heliovaara M, Vanharanta H, Korpi J, et al (1988): Herniated lumbar disc syndrome and vertebral canals. In: Heliovaara M, ed. *Epidemiology of sciatica and herniated lumbar intervertebral disc.* Helsinki, Finland: Social Insurance Institution, pp. 433–435.
39. Horal J (1969): The clinical appearance of low back disorders in the city of Gothenburg, Sweden: Comparisons of incapacitated probands with matched controls. *Acta Orthop Scand Suppl* 118:1–109.
40. Howe J, Frymoyer JW (1985): The effects of questionnaire design on the determination of end results in lumbar spinal surgery. *Spine* 10:804–805.
41. Hult L (1954): The Munkfors investigation: A study of the frequency and causes of the stiff neck-brachialgia and lumbago-sciatica syndromes, as well as observations on certain signs and symptoms from the dorsal spine and the joints of the extremities in industrial and forest workers. *Acta Orthop Scand Suppl* 16.
42. Hurme M, Alaranta H, Torma T, et al (1983): Operated lumbar disc herniation: Epidemiological aspects. *Ann Chir Gynaecol* 72:33–36.
43. Johnsson K-E (1987): *Lumbar spinal stenosis. A clinical, radiological and neurophysiological investigation.* Thesis. Lund University, Malmo General Hospital, Malmo, Sweden.
44. Kane W (1989): Personal Communication.
45. Keller RB, Soule DM, Wennberg JE, Hanley DF (in press): Dealing with geographic variations in hospital use: The experience of the Maine medical assessment program's orthopaedic study group. *J Bone Joint Surg [Am].*
46. Kellgren JH, Lawrence JS (1958): Osteo-arthrosis and disk degeneration in an urban population. *Ann Rheum Dis* 17:388–397.
47. Kelsey JL, Ostfeld AM (1975): Demographic characteristics of persons with acute herniated lumbar intervertebral disc. *J Chronic Dis* 28:37–50.
48. Kelsey JL, Hardy RJ (1975): Driving of motor vehicles as a risk factor for acute herniated lumbar intervertebral disc. *Am J Epidemiol* 102:63–73.
49. Kelsey JL (1978): Epidemiology of radiculopathies. *Adv Neurol* 19:385–398.
50. Kelsey JL (1982): *Epidemiology of musculoskeletal disorders.* New York: Oxford University Press, pp. 145–167.
51. Kelsey JL, Githens PB, O'Connor T, et al (1984): Acute prolapsed lumbar intervertebral disc: An epidemiologic study with special reference to driving automobiles and cigarette smoking. *Spine* 9:608–613.
52. Lawrence JS (1977): *Rheumatism in populations.* London: Heinemann.
53. Magora A (1970): Investigation of the relation between low back pain and occupation. 2. Work history. *Ind Med Surg* 39:504–510.
54. Mayer TG, Gatchel RJ, Kishino N, et al (1985): Objective assessment of spine function following industrial injury: A prospective study with comparison group and one-year follow-up. *Spine* 10:482–493.
55. Melzack R (1975): The McGill Pain Questionnaire: Major properties and scoring methods. *Pain* 1:277–299.
56. Nachemson A, Eek C, Lindstrom IL, et al (1989): Chronic low back disability can largely be prevented: A prospective randomized trial in industry. Presented at AAOS 56th Annual Meeting, Las Vegas.
56a. Nachemson A (1990): Ont i ryggen–ett samhällsproblem. Statens beredning för utvärdering av medicinsk metodik. Stockholm.
57. Pokras R, Graves EF, Dennison CF (1982): *Surgical operations in short-stay hospitals: United States, 1978, Series 13, No. 61.* Hyattsville, Maryland: DHEW publication (PHS) 82–1722.
58. Pope MH, Bevins T, Wilder DG, et al (1985): The relationship between anthropometric, postural, muscular, mobility characteristics of males ages 18–55. *Spine* 10:644–648.
59. Porter RW, Hibbert CS, Wicks M (1978): The spinal canal in symptomatic lumbar disc lesions. *J Bone Joint Surg [Br]* 60:485–487.
60. Rosenberg NJ (1975): Degenerative spondylolisthesis: Predisposing factors. *J Bone Joint Surg [Am]* 57:467–474.
61. Rowe ML (1969): Low back pain in industry: A position paper. *J Occup Med* 11:161–169.
62. Scheuermann H (1920): Kyphosis dorsalis juvenilis. *Ugeskr Laeger* 82:384–393.
63. Scheuermann H (1934): Roentgenologic studies of the origin and development of juvenile kyphosis, together with some investigations concerning the vertebral epiphyses in man and in animals. *Acta Orthop Scand* 5:161–216.
64. Selvik G (1974): *A roentgen stereophotogrammetric method for the study of the kinematics of the skeletal system.* Thesis. AV-Centralen, Lund, Sweden.

65. Snook SH (1982): Low back pain in industry. In: White AA III, Gordon SL, eds. *American Academy of Orthopaedic Surgeons symposium on idiopathic low back pain.* St. Louis: Mosby, pp. 23–38.

66. Sorensen KH (1964): *Scheuermann's juvenile kyphosis. Clinical appearances, radiography, aetiology, and prognosis.* Thesis. Munksgaard, 1–273, Copenhagen, Denmark.

67. Spangfort EV (1972): The lumbar disc herniation: A computer-aided analysis of 2,504 operations. *Acta Orthop Scand* 142 (Suppl.):1–95.

68. Spengler DM, Bigos SJ, Martin NA, Zeh J, Fisher L, Nachemson A (1986): Back injuries in industry: A retrospective study. I. Overview and Cost Analysis. *Spine* 11:241–245.

69. Spitzer WO, LeBlanc FE, Dupuis M, et al (1987): Scientific approach to the assessment and management of activity-related spinal disorders: A monograph for clinicians. Report of the Quebec Task Force on Spinal Disorders. *Spine* 12:S1–S59.

70. Stagnara P, De Mairoy JC, Dran G, et al (1982): Reciprocal angulation of vertebral bodies in a sagittal plane: Approach to references for the evaluation of kyphosis and lordosis. *Spine* 7:335–342.

71. Svard L (1990): *The back of the young top athlete. Symptoms, muscle strength, mobility, anthropometric and radiological findings.* Thesis. Gothenburg University, Goteborg, Sweden.

72. Svensson H-O, Andersson GBJ (1982): Low back pain in forty to forty seven year old men: Frequency of occurrence and impact on medical services. *Scand J Rehabil Med* 14:47–53.

73. Takala J, Sievers K, Klaukka T (1982): Rheumatic symptoms in the middle-aged population in southwestern Finland. *Scand J Rheumatol* 47(Suppl.):15–29.

74. Taylor PJ (1968): Personal factors associated with sickness absence. A study of 194 men with contrasting sickness absence experience in a refinery population. *Br J Ind Med* 25:106–118.

75. Thomas M, Grant N, Marshall J, et al (1983): Surgical treatment of low backache and sciatica. *Lancet* 2:1437–1439.

76. Troidl H, Spitzer WO, McPeek B, Mulder DS, McKneally MF (1986): *Principles and practice of research: Strategies for surgical investigators.* New York: Springer-Verlag.

77. Troup JD, Martin JW, Lloyd DC (1981): Back pain in industry: A prospective survey. *Spine* 6:61–69.

78. Troup JDG (1984): Causes, prediction and prevention of back pain at work. *Scand J Work Environ Health* 10:419–428.

79. Troup JDG, Foreman TK, Baxter CE, Brown D (1987): The perception of back pain and the role of psychophysical tests of lifting capacity. *Spine* 12:645–657.

80. Valkenburg HA, Haanen HCM (1982): The epidemiology of low back pain. In: White AA III, Gordon SL, eds. *American Academy of Orthopaedic Surgeons symposium on idiopathic low back pain.* St. Louis: Mosby, pp. 9–22.

81. Vallfors B (1985): Acute, subacute and chronic low back pain: Clinical symptoms, absenteeism and working environment. *Scand J Rehabil Med* 11(Suppl):1–98.

82. Varlotta GP, Brown MD (1988): Familial predisposition for adolescent disc displacement. Presented at the meeting of the International Society for the Study of the Lumbar Spine, Miami, Florida.

83. Weber H (1983): Lumbar disc herniation. A controlled, prospective study with ten years of observation. *Spine* 8:131–140.

84. Weinstein SL, Zavala DC, Ponseti IV (1981): Idiopathic scoliosis. Long-term follow-up and prognosis in untreated patients. *J Bone Joint Surg* [Am] 63:702–712.

85. Weinstein SL, Ponseti IV (1983): Curve progression in idiopathic scoliosis. *J Bone Joint Surg* [Am] 65:447–455.

86. Wennberg J, Gittelsohn A (1973): Small area variations in health care delivery. *Science* 182:1102–1108.

The Adult Spine: Principles and Practice,
J. W. Frymoyer, Editor-in-Chief.
Raven Press, Ltd., New York © 1991.

CHAPTER 71

Differential Diagnosis of Low Back Disorders

Principles of Classification

Vert Mooney

A valid pathoanatomic diagnosis for any symptom ideally should fulfill certain rigorous criteria: the clinical signs should be identifiable and reproducible between experienced clinicians; the laboratory and imaging studies should be congruent; and tissue samples, if obtained, should fulfill specific histologic criteria. Fulfillment of these rigorous criteria are the basis on which the clinician can advise the patient regarding the likely outcome, based on a known natural history, as well as planning specific therapy. By these rigorous criteria, a verifiable medical diagnosis is available in fewer than 15% of patients who present with low back pain (54).

A wiser approach to the categorization of low back disorders is to classify the syndrome when the findings are non-specific, and to render a pathoanatomic diagnosis only when objective documentation is certain.

THE QUEBEC STUDY CLASSIFICATION

The conclusion given above was reached by a committee commissioned and funded by the Institute for Worker's Health and Safety of Quebec. The consensus

report reflects the rigorous evaluation of the medical literature and the wisdom of an experienced group of medical experts representing numerous disciplines (68). This classification is shown in Table 1.

The implications of the Quebec Study are far reaching. First, it clearly acknowledges that the majority of patients who present with low back disorders do not have a verifiable structural abnormality. Second, it recognizes that the majority of low back symptoms are time-limited and will resolve relatively quickly. Before sophisticated diagnostic tests were available, this favorable, time-limited natural history was demonstrated. Dillane (17) found that for those seeking medical care for low back pain, 44% were better within one week, 92% were better within one month, and only 8% had pain persisting greater than two months. It is interesting to speculate that these results were so favorable because the experience of back pain was less perturbed by sociopolitical and litigious confounders. However, this same favorable natural history has been demonstrated by many other studies (2) (Fig. 1). Thus, the passage of time rewarded by remission for most patients and structural verification is usually unnecessary.

The third major conclusion of the consensus report is the recognition of the limited benefit of the physical examination in determining the diagnosis in the majority

V. Mooney, M.D.: Division of Orthopaedic Surgery, University of California, Irvine, Irvine, California, 92714.

TABLE 1. *Quebec classification for disorders of the lumbar spine (with permission from ref. 68)*

Classification	Symptoms	Duration of symptoms from onset	Working status at time of evaluation
1	Pain without radiation		
2	Pain + radiation to extremity, proximally	a (<7 days)	W (working)
3	Pain + radiation to extremity, distally*	b (7 days–7 weeks)	I (idle)
4	Pain + radiation to upper/lower limb neurologic signs	c (>7 weeks)	
5	Presumptive compression of a spinal nerve root on a simple roentgenogram (i.e., spinal instability or fracture)		
6	Compression of a spinal nerve root confirmed by Specific imaging techniques (i.e., computerized axial tomography, myelography, or magnetic resonance imaging) Other diagnostic techniques (e.g., electromyography, venography)		
7	Spinal stenosis		
8	Postsurgical status, 1–6 months after intervention		
9	Postsurgical status, >6 months after intervention 9.1 Asymptomatic 9.2 Symptomatic		
10	Chronic pain syndrome		W (working)
11	Other diagnoses		I (idle)

* Not applicable to the thoracic segment.

of patients. They conclude that the most useful information is derived from the patient's description of pain location, about which all observers should be able to agree. Thus, the consensus report separates the pain complaint into three categories: (1) represents low back pain alone; (2) is pain in the back referable to the upper buttocks or thigh; and (3) is referral of pain below the knee. The

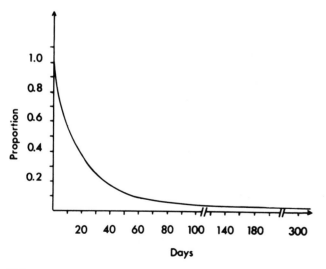

FIG. 1. The recovery from an acute low back pain episode is generally favorable (with permission from ref. 2).

categorization also delineates two important modifiers, the duration of the pain and the patient's work status. As emphasized throughout Section I of this volume, the duration of symptoms and the work capability of the patient have important implications to the eventual treatment outcome, and the socioeconomic costs of back disorders. Categories 4, 5, 6, and 7 delineate specific, suspected, or verifiable clinical disorders, which are predominantly of degenerative or traumatic etiology. For example, Category 4 calls for specific neurologic signs indicative of nerve root compression, which becomes verifiable either by plane radiography (Category 5) or by imaging studies (Category 6). Category 7 delineates the subset of patients with symptoms (neurologic claudication), signs, and imaging studies, who have spinal stenosis.

As emphasized by the authors, this classification has the attractive feature of permitting the diagnosis to be updated continuously with respect to possible, probable, or definite causation, while monitoring the duration of symptoms and their effects on work. For example, a patient might present with Category 3 pain, later develop neurologic signs and move to Category 4, and still later, if not improving, have a confirmed lumbar disc herniation and be reclassified into Category 6. Still later, disc surgery might be performed and the patient reclassified with a successful or unsuccessful result.

From the perspective of the Quebec study, it seems

TABLE 2. *Indications for spinal radiographs in acute low back pain (adapted from refs. 15 and 46)*

Indication	Significance
Age greater than 50 years	Risk of tumor, severe degeneration
History of severe trauma	Fracture likely
History of osteoporosis	Compression fracture
Known primary cancer	Suggest spinal cancer or possible infection
Unrelenting pain at rest	
Unexplained weight loss	
History of corticosteroids	Risk factors for spinal infection
Organ recipient	
AIDS	
Diabetes mellitus	
Drug abuse	
Alcohol abuse	Greater risk for fractures
Findings suggestive of spondylitis	
Neurologic defect	Risk of bony tumor or infectious cause

inappropriate to make a major pathoanatomic diagnosis for most patients in the early stages of their low back problem. Conversely, deterioration of neurologic function as a patient moves into Category 4, or a patient's unaltering pain in spite of rational treatment, should lead to vigorous efforts to determine the cause. This perspective has been advocated by others, who have delineated the features of the clinical history and physical examination, which should lead to a high suspicion of a serious pathoanatomic causation for symptoms and direct the clinician to urgently perform diagnostic studies. Hadler (29) delineated these clinical symptoms and signs:

If the patient is writhing in pain, a vascular condition or intra-abdominal cause is possible.

If the back pain is not modified at rest and is unrelenting, a neoplasm or infection is possible, such as osteomyelitis, discitis, or epidural abscess.

If the neurologic findings are rapidly evolving, or if there is caudal anesthesia or urinary or bowel incontinence or retention, epidural hemorrhage, epidural abscess, neural tumors, or massive central disc prolapse should be considered and urgently evaluated.

If the patient has had major trauma or is at risk for pathologic fracture (osteoporosis, known primary tumor).

These same considerations were used by Liang and Komaroff (46) and Deyo and Diehl (15) to outline specific indications for early spinal radiography. Their indications and their rationale are given in Table 2. They calculated the risk of missing a significant diagnosis, i.e., Category 11, if these historical and clinical indications were followed, and they concluded that it was extremely safe to wait one month before obtaining radiographs in the majority of patients.

POSSIBLE SOURCES OF PAIN IN CATEGORIES 1, 2, AND 3

Although the Quebec Classification acknowledges that certain pathoanatomic causation is impossible, it is nevertheless important to consider the tissues which might be injured and cause symptoms before proceeding to a description of the specific known pathoanatomic causes of low back pain.

Implicit in the Quebec Study is the time-dependency of soft tissue healing. Clinical experience indicates peripheral joint soft tissue injuries usually have an acute duration of one week and a sub-acute phase of one to seven weeks. The selection of a seven week duration to denote the end of the sub-acute phase of low back pain thus tacitly implies an unknown soft tissue "injury" would be expected to heal during this time interval. From a structural and mechanical perspective, there seem to be three potential sources of low back pain; the soft tissues, the joints, and the intervertebral disc. Of course there are alternatives: non-traumatic pathologic conditions such as inflammatory, neoplastic, and metabolic diseases can affect these same structures, but only rarely in the broad perspective of low back disorders.

Injury to Soft Tissues

The tissues of interest in low back pain are the supportive soft tissues including muscles, fascia, and ligaments. When considering a mechanically-induced disorder of the spine, injury to soft tissues is commonly assumed to have occurred as the result of acute or repetitive mechanical overload. To a certain extent, the severity of the injury should be identifiable from the patient's history. It could be expected that a significant soft tissue tear would result in immediate pain, similar to that seen elsewhere in the musculoskeletal system. These events follow an ankle or knee sprain and should be similar in the spine. Pain which occurs one or two days later, after an assumed injury, would not seem to fit the well known clinical criteria for soft tissue injury. However, there is pathologic evidence that ligamentous tears do occur and increase as a function of age. Because the tissue is poorly vascularized and relatively acellular, repair may be slow, but would be expected to occur within a seven-week time interval. Because Category 1 and 2 low back pain does not seem to fulfill the usual clinical attributes of soft tissue injury elsewhere in the human body, it has been generally assumed that pain must arise from injury or overuse of the paraspinal muscles. In the extremities overuse is associated with aching discomfort, often hours after the inciting cause. In extreme cases, continued overuse results in a compartment syndrome. A paraspinal muscle compartment can be identified in human

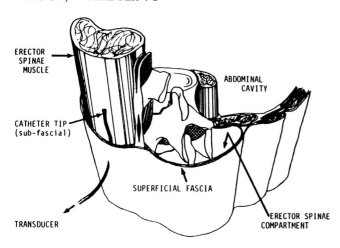

FIG. 2. The anatomic boundaries of the lumbar paraspinal compartment are shown as determined from cadaveric dissections (with permission from ref. 13).

dissections (13) (Fig. 2), and pressures as high as 175 mm of mercury have been measured in paraspinal muscles. These pressure values are far greater than observed in the extremities. Also, a few cases (13) have been reported with extreme low back pain and evidence of rhabdomyolysis, suggesting an acute compartment syndrome. This has led to the speculation that low back pain in some instances could be a chronic compartment problem. In an extensive search, Styf (69) could identify only 12 patients whom he could categorize as possible paraspinal compartment syndrome. In these patients, pain was induced by exercise, relieved by rest, and there were no neurologic or radiologic abnormalities. In only 1 of these 12 patients was there a persistent elevation of compartment pressure which could be associated with pain. A fasciotomy of lumbodorsal fascia in this patient did return the muscle pressure to normal and relieve his pain. The other 11 patients had normal pressures. Thus, on rare occasions, a specific cause of low back pain due to compartment syndrome can be identified. The diagnosis should be made by measurements of compartment pressure, although the precise criteria for abnormalities are not yet established.

What are the other potential causes of muscle-induced pain? All of us who have challenged muscles unprepared for extensive exercise recognize that muscle aching and even pain do occur, usually of short duration. Clinical studies have shown maximal eccentric exercise causes the release of large quantities of proteins, but the presence of these proteins is not correlated with symptoms (39). Painful muscles demonstrate no unusual electrical activity and are silent at rest, similar to non-painful muscles (9). It is also proposed that ischemia might be a cause of back muscle pain, yet there is no direct evidence to support that contention, nor is there evidence of unusual buildup of lactic acid in the muscles of patients with low back pain. To date, histologic evidence of chronic isch-

emia within the muscles of patients with low back pain has not been identified.

Recent evidence does show partial denervation in the paraspinal musculature of people with chronic low back pain, particularly those with known disc herniations and previous lumbar surgery (44). These conditions might produce denervation by direct involvement of the efferent branches of the posterior primary rami, either surgically or by local compression. Thickening of the connective tissues surrounding the muscles in these patients is another finding, but no evidence of tears per se are identified. In that regard, MRI has been thought to be a new and exciting means to identify the patient with a tear (23). In other muscles of the human body, such tears usually occur at the myotendinous junction (77). It is, therefore, of note that the erector spinae muscles and multifidi have rather indistinct myotendinous junctions, the significance of which is uncertain as to the location or likelihood of tearing.

All of the data regarding muscles suggest they are an unlikely source for sub-acute pain, particularly when the onset is gradual. As an alternative explanation, the syndrome termed fibromyalgia and fibromyositis has been considered. Validation of this clinical diagnosis is problematic (29). Making a presumptive diagnosis requires the presence of specific persistent tender sites known as trigger points. Patients thought to have this condition generally complain of stiffness and a sense of fatigue (Table 3). Attempts to define the syndrome by pathoanatomic criteria have not been successful, although many

TABLE 3. Signs and symptoms associated with fibromyalgia compared to non-specific low back pain and normal subjects (with permission from ref. 76)

Symptoms and signs	Patients with fibromyalgia (%)	Patients with low back pain (%)	Normal subjects (%)
No.	155	48	58
Low back or hip pain	71	58	10
"Aches all over"	64	29	0
Awakened at night by pain	46	40	3
Pain in muscles, joints	83	57	5
Pain in neck, shoulders	74	63	14
Tires easily	75	74	14
Stiff in morning	83	67	7
Feels unrefreshed in morning	80	81	31
Tender points			
4 or more	96	23	0
7 or more	94	15	0
12 or more	54	6	0

Note that many of the symptoms occur with equal frequency in fibromyalgia and low back pain and the major differences are in night pain and the presence of tender points.

practitioners feel local anesthetic injections do hasten recovery and provide pain relief. Biopsies from patients with this diagnosis have demonstrated "mothy fibers" and inflammatory infiltrates in degenerating and regenerating muscles (6). Unfortunately, similar findings have been identified in control subjects without back pain.

Others have suggested the entire syndrome can be reproduced merely by sleep deprivation (50). More significant was the finding that 95% of the patients with fibromyositis had an acceptable psychiatric diagnosis (20). Most significant is the observation that clinical symptoms are reduced by aerobic exercise (48). In that study, a group of patients who fulfilled the clinical criteria for fibromyositis were randomly divided into groups who received stretching exercises and those who received aerobic exercise on a bicycle ergometer. Twice as many of the patients treated by the aerobic regimen improved significantly when compared to the stretching group.

In summary, the role of ligaments and muscles remains uncertain in the causation of low back pain, particularly in explaining persistent and chronic pain over greater than seven weeks duration.

Injury to the Facet Joints

It is well known that arthritic conditions can follow acute traumatic events, as well as evolve without significant antecedent trauma. Thus, it has been logical to focus attention on the facet joints, as first suggested by Goldthwait in 1911 (25). This view was expounded by Putti (61) and Ghormley (24). The enormous interest generated by Mixter and Barr's 1934 description of lumbar disc herniation (49) deferred attention from the facet joints until 1941, when Badgley (4) pointed out what is still evident today; most patients with low back problems have no clinical evidence of nerve root irritation. He reported neuroanatomic dissections which identified a nerve supply to the facets joints, making them a plausible source of pain. Equally important was the concept that all extremity pain need not be distributed in a dermatomal pattern (21) and could be referred to locations remote from the presumed source of mechanical or chemical irritation. Additional clinical confirmation was derived from the clinical studies of Lewis and Kellgren (45) and Inman (36). Injection of irritation solutions into spinal structures caused pain which was referred to the legs. The location of pain radiation varied according to the spinal level and structure injected. This same phenomenon was shown by Hirsch in 1963 (33), but unlike his predecessors, these studies were done with benefit of radiographic control. Using fluoroscopy as a method to localize the structure being injected, this author (51) was able to demonstrate more specifically the patterns of pain referral, and the relationship between the amount of noxious stimulus and the location of pain. By slowly increasing the volumes of injected hypertonic saline, the area of referred pain was progressively enlarged. Injection of local anesthetics into the facet joints never produced motor or sensory deficits. In a small number of individuals the noxious injection produced pain far into the calf, which was relieved promptly by anesthetic injection. Thus, the facets can be implicated in the production of Category 1, 2, and 3 back pain.

Although the facets can be the source of back pain, the mechanisms by which this occurs are not entirely clear. There is no question that they form an important component of spinal stenotic syndromes (Category 7), and Category 4, 5, and 6 pain either through their contribution to lateral recess narrowing or less commonly by the production of degenerative cysts which impinge on the nerve root. Their role in Category 1, 2, and 3 back pain is less certain. Abnormality of alignment has long been considered a major source of pain by those who are enthusiasts for manipulation. It must be recognized that there exists no radiographic confirmation of "malalignment" associated with clinical pain, nor has clinical relief of symptoms been associated with clear evidence for "realignment." Mechanical blockage of the joint by some structural abnormality such as impinged synovial folds has been advanced, and pathologic dissections indicate their presence in some specimens (40). However, the presence of these folds in patients with low back pain and the subsequent manipulative removal from the joint have not been shown.

Another explanation for low back pain arising from the facets has been sub-clinical, non-radiographically visible, degenerative change, conceptualized as similar to chondromalacia patellae. Eisenstein (19) studied patients with long-standing back pain, no neurological deficit, and normal spinal radiographs and imaging studies. He performed spinal fusion on a small sub-set of these patients. Histologic evaluation demonstrated vascularization and cystic changes in the deeper layers of the cartilage similar to the changes seen in chondromalacia. This small group of patients apparently fared well after the fusion. Attempts to provide clinical criteria for facet-caused low back pain have met with far less success. Jackson (37) evaluated 454 patients with Category 1, 2, and 3 low back pain, attempting to identify those clinical variables which would predict a response to anesthetic injections. This meticulously performed study included facet joint arthrograms to assure accurate needle placement, and also to identify pathologic change within the joint. Although initial relief occurred in 29% of the patients, the clinical distribution of pain and relief/aggravation patterns for that pain were not identified, nor was the relief related to muscle spasm. These investigators reluctantly concluded that facet-caused low back pain cannot be diagnosed with certainty. It recently has been shown that pain relief occurs equally as well with intra-articular and peri-articular injections (47), indicating the pain may be of capsular origin rather than synovial inflammation.

In other studies, attempts have been made to focus on the alternative source of lower leg pain (Category 3 in the Quebec Classification). Porter (60) analyzed 2,360 patients with persistent pain seen in a referral clinic. The clinical diagnosis of nerve root entrapment was made if there was single-sided leg pain extending into the lower calf, which was more severe in the leg than the back. His clinical criteria for the diagnosis of nerve root entrapment were somewhat vague. There was no straight leg raising restriction in the majority of patients, but there was a lack of spinal extension in 88%. Despite the leg pain, 85% had normal reflex, 82% had normal sensation, and 95% had normal muscle strength. Eighty percent of the patients had radiographic evidence of spinal degeneration. Ultimately, 10.5% of the patients had sufficient evidence to make a clinical diagnosis of nerve root entrapment not due to disc herniation. Eventually 9.6% (n = 24) of his patients with the clinical diagnosis of nerve root entrapment underwent surgical intervention. Eighteen of the 24 patients improved. As one attempts to determine the role of the facet joints, their contribution to sciatica seems uncertain. It can be concluded, based simply on patient numbers, that the contribution was small.

Another possible articular cause of pain is the sacroiliac joint. Because the nerve supply to the sacroiliac joint overlaps with that innervation of the facet joint, the contribution of the sacroiliac is even harder to evaluate. It is obvious the sacroiliac joint can degenerate, and this condition is identified in 67% of patients over the age of 55 (78). Whether these changes produce pain is more difficult to define, particularly since some studies show the joint has little or no capacity to move under normal loads (71). One carefully controlled injection study (7) indicated that 25% of patients with non-specific low back pain were possible candidates for a sacroiliac-caused symptom. Epidemiologic analyses of post-partum women (3) also strongly implicate the sacroiliac joint as a plausible source of their pain. The popularity of the diagnosis of "sacroiliac syndrome" is high among physical therapists. However, the specificity of clinical tests which involve manipulating the joint are suspect because it is impossible to stress that joint without stressing adjacent spinal structures. The controversies surrounding the diagnosis and the evidence favoring a sacroiliac syndrome will be further discussed in Chapter 101.

Injury to the Discs

Injury to the disc seems the most likely source of persisting low back pain. Although this anatomic structure is apparently no more or less vulnerable to injury than any other spinal structure, its limited potential for repair makes it a prime candidate for pain that persists.

The capacity for repair potential is significant. The nucleus has the smallest number of cells of any tissue in the body, which is uniform across the entire structure except at the margins of the outer annulus. In the human nucleus there are fewer cells (4,000 to 6,000/cubic millimeter) than other animal discs (35). The small cell population, the barriers to rapid nutrition, and the absence of blood supply lead to the potential for delayed or absent repair. This is reflected by a significant increase in the lactate concentrations in the middle portion of the nucleus (34). Despite these experimental findings in animals, the normal and asymptomatic degenerative disc in live humans show a pH near neutral. When the patient is symptomatic, the pH may be quite acid (16), but the decrease in pH is not consistent throughout the disc. Our experiments have shown that within the same disc at the same time, a variation in acid pH of .3 to .4 below neutral may occur (52). I have proposed that the injured disc, for a yet undefined reason, may have a greater focal concentration of proteoglycan, dependent on the location within the disc. If we imagine the proteoglycans to be like a fluid filled balloon, encapsulated by a "fishnet" of collagen, the variable size of the proteoglycan "balloons" might influence the metabolic exchange potentials and account for these local variations in pH. In the injured disc these "balloons" might be larger, which is plausible because injured chondroblasts manufacture larger proteoglycan moieties (12).

These hypothetical considerations are presented to conceptualize one mechanism which might cause the disc to be painful in one individual and not another. The mechanism by which injury occurs is better understood. A peripheral tear in the annulus may be initiated by torsional overload (57). Centralized annular tears can also occur, which gradually progress to the periphery and communicate with pre-existent peripheral tears when the latter are present (32). Such tears are identified in pathologic specimens obtained from apparently normal people (57). Whether these tears produce pain is uncertain. In a discography study that compared asymmetrical radial tears with symmetrical degeneration, those tears which were asymmetric and deep were more likely to be associated with reproduction of pain (64) (Table 3).

A second question is whether there is a specific set of pathologic or mechanical events which initiate the eventual herniation of the disc. Watts (72) proposed the concept of intradiscal lumbar herniation, whereby the nucleus symptomatically displaces within the substance of the disc. A chance case report provides some rationale for this concept. Murphy (53) observed a soldier who had back and leg pain without neurologic deficit, and whose myelogram was normal. Post-myelogram meningitis led to death. At the autopsy, a posterolateral tear was identified which extended halfway through the annulus of the L4-L5 disc. Buried in this rent was a fragment of nucleus and annulus, which he surmised was the cause of the patient's pain. Later, he performed lumbar discectomies under local anesthesia and could observe patterns of pain provocation. Stimulation of the posterior longitudinal ligament and posterior annulus produced what he called "true referred pain" as differentiated from the more classic sciatic distribution which resulted from stimulation of the nerve root. The significance of these observations is that they define the potential for the deteriorating disc to be a source of pain with radiation into the thigh and legs, without directly implicating the anterior primary ramus. When the pain is truly persistent and chronic, is worse in the back than the legs, there has been a significant traumatic overload, and spinal radiographs are normal, then an alternative diagnosis is considered, termed the disc disruption syndrome (14). This clinical syndrome will be presented in detail in Chapter 97, but the extent to which it is prevalent in the population remains controversial. In one series (18), 87 patients were referred to a spinal clinic and categorized as having disc displacement (see Chapter 76 by Donelson and McKenzie), but only one eventually fulfilled the criteria outlined by Crock. This study suggests the rarity of this type of syndrome. Currently, we can conclude there is no way to define with precision the role of the intervertebral disc in the production of acute or subacute low back pain, although the absence of healing potential, combined with pathologic data, suggest it may be of significance. At present, discography is the only test which might answer this question, but it cannot be used routinely in acute or sub-acute low back pain, with or without radiation, except in a very small sub-set of patients. Although abnormalities in the water content and morphology of the disc seen by MRI are of importance to research, equating these changes with spinal pain is not currently possible.

CATEGORIES 4 AND 6

There is no question that the clinical syndrome of lumbar disc herniation can be reliably identified if the patient's history and physical examination reveal typical symptoms and findings which are then confirmed by a correlated imaging study. These patients, who are classified as Category 6 in the Quebec Study, constitute a minority of patients, estimated to be 1% of individuals who have acute low back pain and 10% of patients who have pain persisting after six weeks (2). In other clinical studies similar frequencies are noted. In 1293 patients referred to a spinal clinic, 14% had the clinical feature of lumbar disc herniation (7), while in 2,360 patients re-

ferred to a British orthopedic consultant, 8.7% fulfilled these same clinical criteria (60).

The most important clinical findings are the production of sciatica by nerve root tension signs. When the contralateral straight leg raising test is positive, the probability that a disc herniation is present is 98% (65). The other findings, such as reflex alterations, sensory deficits, and diminished motor function are confirmatory and help localize the specific level of nerve root involvement. Although these findings are clinically important, their functional significance is usually minimal. For example, a dropped foot is identified in only 5% of patients who fulfill the clinical and myelographic criteria for lumbar disc herniation (73). The presence of a narrowed disc by spinal radiography is non-predictive, contrary to popular belief (30).

The clinical syndromes associated with specific nerve root lesions are well known and are presented in Figs. 3, 4, and 5. Variations in these classic clinical patterns can lead to misdiagnosis and surgery at an inappropriate level with failure. The important determinants are segmentation abnormalities such as lumbralization and sacralization, the intraforaminal disc, which may cause

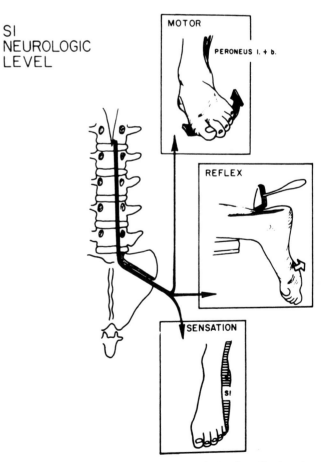

FIG. 3. The physical findings of an L5-S1 lumbar disc herniation.

L5
NEUROLOGIC
LEVEL

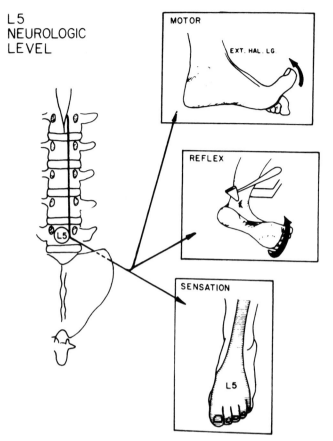

FIG. 4. The physical findings of an L4-L5 lumbar disc herniation.

L4
NEUROLOGIC
LEVEL

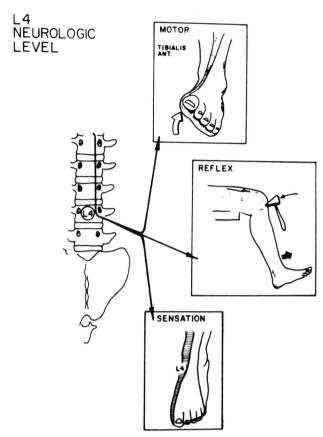

FIG. 5. The physical findings of an L3-L4 lumbar disc herniation.

symptoms one level proximal to that usually expected for that level, and the extraforaminal disc which may produce symptoms as much as two levels higher than expected (Fig. 6). It must also be kept in mind that other pathologic conditions can produce similar signs and symptoms, but are rare causes of sciatica. Included in this category are degenerative synovial cysts (56), congenital abnormalities of lumbar nerve roots (59), benign and malignant nerve root tumors, and epidural abscesses (5). Branches of the lumbosacral plexus and peripheral nerve entrapments may also be associated with clinical pain syndromes which mimic the nerve root entrapment of lumbar disc herniation. These causes include involvement of the lumbosacral plexus by retroperitoneal tumors, endometriosis, and viral infections, direct pressure on the sciatic nerve from external pressure ("hip-pocket sciatica," "toilet seat neuritis"), local tumors of the sciatic nerve, peroneal nerve compression commonly confused with an L5 nerve root lesion, and the neuropathies associated with metabolic diseases, particularly diabetes mellitus. A particularly controversial cause is the piriformis syndrome, which is thought to be produced by local abnormalities or inflammations of the pryriformis tendon which anatomically relates to the sciatic nerve in the

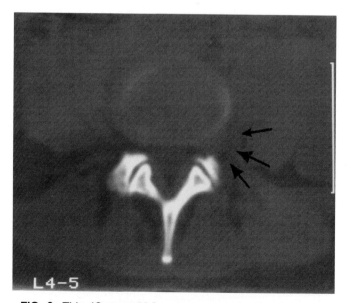

FIG. 6. This 48-year-old female presented with left anterior thigh pain, absent knee jerk, quadriceps weakness, and a positive femoral stretch test. The CT scan here demonstrates a far lateral disc at L4-L5, which mimics the physical findings of a patient with a more central L3-L4 lesion.

buttock (55) (Fig. 7). Most of these conditions can be suspected from the detailed history or physical examination and comprise a distinct minority of patients who present with sciatica.

The other syndrome which is rare but requires special attention, is the cauda equina syndrome due to massive lumbar disc prolapse. This condition is rare. In patients with confirmed disc herniations subjected to surgery, the cauda quina syndrome is reported in 1% to 3% of patients (41,67). We know that 250,000 lumbar disc operations are performed annually (63) in the United States population of 250 million, and therefore as few as 2,500 or as many as 7,500 operations could be expected to be done for cauda equina syndrome. Based on that entire population, the range of 1 in 100,000 to 1 in 33,000 seems reasonable. The important features of this syndrome are (1) the rapid progression of neurologic signs and symptoms in a patient with a known disc herniation; (2) the bilateral leg pain and neurologic symptoms which frequently accompany it; (3) the presence of caudal anesthesia; (4) the presence of genitourinary dysfunction manifested by overflow incontinence or retention; and (5) loss of rectal sphincter tone, sometimes accompanied by fecal incontinence (Fig. 8).

The importance in recognizing this condition is its time-dependent course. Although delays in surgical in-

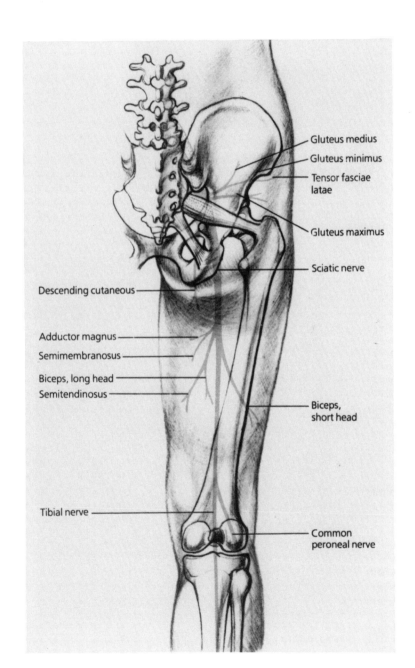

Gluteus medius
Gluteus minimus
Tensor fasciae latae
Gluteus maximus
Sciatic nerve
Descending cutaneous
Adductor magnus
Semimembranosus
Biceps, long head
Semitendinosus
Biceps, short head
Tibial nerve
Common peroneal nerve

FIG. 7. The relationships of the pyriformis tendon to the sciatic nerve. Compression of the nerve may produce sciatica, as well as buttock pain, easily confused with a lumbar disc herniation (with permission from ref. 55 and with permission and appreciation to the artist, Mr. Paul Singh-Roy).

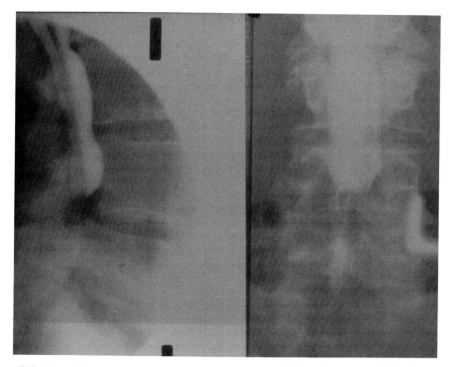

FIG. 8. A 60-year-old female had acute onset of back pain, incontinence, and bilateral lower dorsiflexor weakness. A complete myelographic block is shown. At surgery she had a low grade degenerative spondylolisthesis, modest spinal stenosis, upon which was superimposed a significant midline bulge, all creating an acute cauda equina syndrome.

tervention are not inevitably associated with persistent neurologic dysfunction, the time-dependency of caudal compression to recovery makes it prudent to perform diagnostic studies and surgical interventions rapidly (41).

CATEGORY 5

The issues surrounding the diagnoses of acute spinal trauma and segmental instability will be presented in Chapters 61 and 90.

CATEGORY 7

Category 7 includes patients with all forms of spinal stenosis affecting both the central spinal canal, the lateral nerve root canal, or combinations thereof (Fig. 9). Typically, these conditions do not appear as acute or subacute low back pain, but rather are diagnosed when symptoms have been chronic or recurrent. An exception is the patient with stenosis who has a superimposed disc herniation, in which case the sciatica may be profound. The central spinal canal stenotics are classically characterized by the symptom of neurologic claudication. The pain, which may be either a mono- or polyradiculopathy, increases with walking and is relieved by rest. Un-

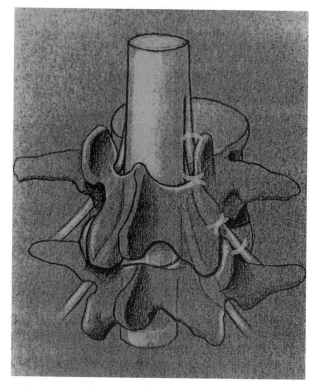

FIG. 9. The anatomic boundaries of the nerve root canal and the points where nerve root compression can occur (with permission from ref. 43).

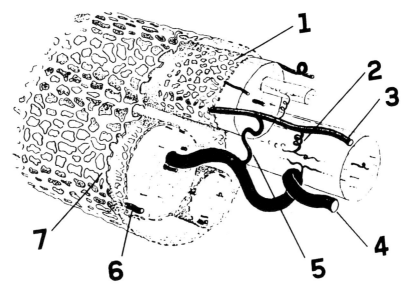

FIG. 10. The basic elements of a spinal nerve root and its intrinsic vasculature. The fasicular pia (1) is relatively thicker and less open-meshed than the radicular pia (7). A major longitudinal radicular artery (3) is accompanied by several collateral radicular arteries (6), which give rise to interfasicular and intrafasicular branches that show compensating coils (2) before supplying precapillary arterioles. The slowly spiraling major radicular vein (4) receives frequent and relatively larger arteriovenous anastomoses (5) (with permission from ref. 57).

like the pain of vascular claudication, symptom relief usually requires the patient to sit. The pathoanatomy of this condition has been reviewed in depth recently (22) and will only be briefly highlighted here. The underlying vascular causation seems to be related to the unique vascular supply of the nerve roots and cauda equina which is characterized by arteriovenous anastamoses (Fig. 10). These anastamoses may explain why patients with venous hypertension have exacerbation of their symptoms (42). Elegant research also has characterized the effects of chronic compression, not only on the vascular supply, but also on the neurophysiology of the cauda equina. It is thought that the pain may have two components: one is the vascular cause which is reversible by decompression; the second is intrinsic damage to the neurophysiologic function which may be irreversible.

The other major feature of spinal stenosis is the relief that occurs with sitting. It is generally accepted that the mechanical events that underlie relief are the increased canal dimensions, which occur with spinal flexion.

When the lateral spinal canal is the site of greater compression, the clinical syndrome is more variable, and may range from sciatica, which is indistinguishable from lumbar disc herniation, to predominantly a monoradiculopathy with claudication.

The physical findings reflect the extent of the stenosis, but characteristically are not those of single nerve root involvement. In fact, the multiple, and sometimes spotty nerve root involvement, a "stocking-glove" distribution of sensory loss, and the frequent absence of nerve root tension signs sometimes suggest an underlying psychologic disturbance. On rare occasions, a cauda equina syndrome may occur, although its onset is usually less dramatic than an acute lumbar disc sequestration. The recovery of caudal function following decompression also seems more favorable in the stenotic sub-group (41).

The diverse etiologies which are causative are given in Figure 11 and Table 4 (1). There are not yet sufficient

TABLE 4. *A comprehensive classification of spinal stenosis based on etiology (with permission from ref. 1)*

1. Congenital–Developmental stenosis
   a. Idiopathic
   b. Achondroplastic
2. Acquired Stenosis
   a. Degenerative
      i. Central portion of spinal canal
      ii. Peripheral portion of canal, lateral recesses and nerve root canals (tunnels)
      iii. Degenerative spondylolithesis
   b. Combined
      Any possible combinations of congenital/developmental stenosis, degenerative stenosis and herniations of the nucleus pulposus
   c. Spondylolisthetic spondylolytic
   d. Iatrogenic
      i. Post laminectomy
      ii. Post fusion (anterior and posterior)
      iii. Post chemonucleolysis
   e. Post-traumatic, late changes
   f. Miscellaneous
      i. Paget's Disease
      ii. Fluorosis

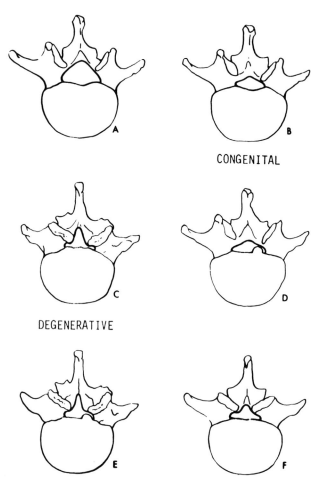

CONGENITAL

DEGENERATIVE

FIG. 11. A schematic diagram of the various types of spinal stenosis. A. Normal spinal anatomy; B. Congenital stenosis; C. Degenerative stenosis; D. Congenital stenosis in association with lumbar disc bulge; E. Degenerative stenosis in association with disc bulge, and F. A trefoil configuration (with permission from ref. 1).

epidemiologic data to determine the frequency of these conditions. It is known that 10% of patients over the age of 65 have radiographic evidence of degenerative spondylolisthesis, but many of these patients are asymptomatic (70). There is also clear evidence that females are more commonly involved than males (4:1) and that diabetics are at particular risk (62).

CATEGORIES 8, 9, AND 10

The specific issues relating to spinal surgery and the "chronic pain syndrome" will be presented in other chapters in this section.

CATEGORY 11

This represents the small but important sub-set of patients other than lumbar disc herniations, fractures, and stenotics, who have a pathoanatomic cause for their symptoms. It is this category which is most important to

keep in mind when evaluating an individual with back/leg pain, in the acute and sub-acute phases. It is for these patients—who may have tumors, infections, inflammatory, or metabolic diseases—that sophisticated evaluation and expert medical care are necessary. The probability of these conditions occurring is fairly small. For example, Wiesel (75) evaluated 5,362 patients with low back pain over a five-year interval. At the end of six months, 109 (2%) had failed to improve, and yet had a diagnosis. After extensive re-evaluation, 14 of the 109 patients were found to have a medical causation for their symptoms, such as multiple myeloma, metastatic disease, and intrapelvic causations. The most commonly overlooked cause was a spondyloarthropathy which was identified in 7 of the 14.

Although the detailed clinical presentation, physical findings, laboratory and radiologic features, and treatment for these conditions are presented in other chapters, it is worthwhile emphasizing certain important clinical features.

As previously noted, Hadler (28), Liang and Komaroff (46), and Liang have given important clinical information which alerts the examining health professional to these conditions. Others have emphasized how the history of pain suggests certain diagnoses (22). In the usual "mechanical back pain," i.e., Category 1, 2, or 3, mechanical loading of the spine occurring during the day is associated with increasing pain, which then is usually relieved by rest. Although stiffness and discomfort are common in patients when they first awaken, these complaints usually diminish with activity. In patients with suspected tumors or infections, the pain pattern is often characterized by rest pain, which is particularly evident at night, often awakening the patient. Although patients with mechanical pain may awaken when they change position, it is uncommon for their symptoms to be unchanged or worsened persistently. In patients with suspected spondyloarthropathies, morning pain and stiffness which persists are common complaints. Unlike mechanical pain, these patients are often awakened at an hour earlier than their accustomed time (10).

SPONDYLOLISTHESES

The numerous etiologies, diagnostic criteria, and treatments will be presented in Chapter 78.

TUMORS

Primary tumors are relatively uncommon, and calculated by Liang and Komaroff (46) to occur annually in 0.07% of the population. By far the most common primary malignancy is multiple myeloma. Metastatic tumors are more common and occur in 0.12/1,000. Obviously, this condition should be suspected in a patient with a known primary site, which is most commonly lung, breast, kidney, and thyroid. In Kirkaldy-Willis's series, only 0.13% of patients presenting to a low back clinic had primary or metastatic lesions. The tumors most often involve the vertebral body, rather than the posterior elements or epidural space. Thus, back pain rather than leg pain is the more common presentation. Age also helps determine the likelihood of primary malignant and benign lesions. In Weinstein's patients, the mean age of patients with malignant tumors was 49 years, and 21 for those with benign lesions (74). Because benign tumors more often involve the lamina and pedicle, these will more commonly produce leg pain. Occasionally, a sacral tumor will present with a change in bowel habits and pain, which is predominantly peroneal (66).

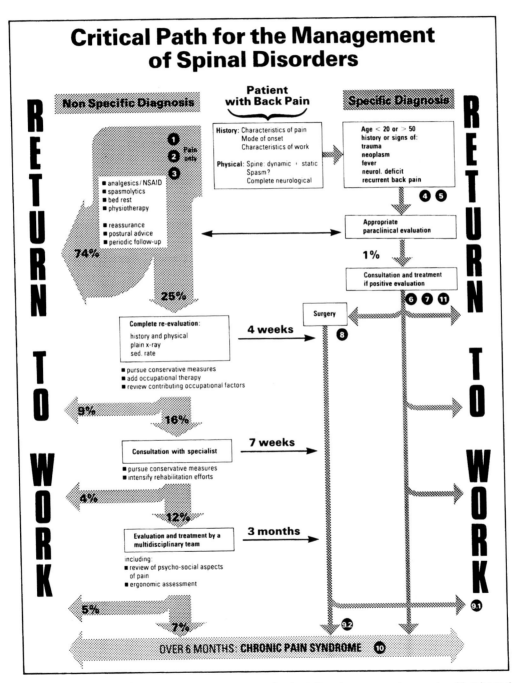

FIG. 12. The "critical path" for the management of spinal disorders suggests one algorithm based upon the Quebec Classification and that group's analysis of current effective treatment. The percentages refer to the proportion of patients with acute low back pain, who will enter into a particular phase of treatment (with permission from ref. 68).

INFLAMMATORY LESIONS

Chapter 35 covers this subject in depth. The spondyloarthropathies are more common and are estimated to involve 2 to 40/1,000 population (8,11,31). To some degree, the variation is produced by whether serologic criteria are used, or whether serologic criteria are combined with strict clinical criteria. In his spinal clinic Kirkaldy-Willis identified these conditions in 0.27% of his patients. Included under the broad title of spondyloarthropathies are ankylosing spondylitis, Reiter's syndrome, and the arthritis associated with inflammatory bowel disease and psoriatic arthritis. All of these diseases share a variety of clinical, radiographic, and genetic features (38). Typically, they affect younger males, but are often easily confused with non-specific (Category 1, 2, or 3) back disorders. In addition to the suggestive history of morning pain and stiffness, the simple estimation of chest expansion is an important diagnostic clue. Restriction of expansion to less than 2 centimeters in the male and 1 centimeter in the female is a suggestive finding (11). All of these conditions have a high association with the HLA-B27 antigen.

The specific diagnoses which comprise the spondyloarthropathies can be identified from the clinical history and examination. Thus, Reiter's is associated with uveitis and urethritis, there may be skin lesions on the palm and sole, and the patient is typically a young male. The spondyloarthropathies associated with inflammatory bowel disorders may antedate the gastrointestinal manifestations. The skin and nail involvement of psoriasis usually identifies that sub-set of patients although, here too, the skin involvement may lag by years. Stiffness seems less common with psoriasis, and the sacroiliac joints are less frequently involved (27).

In comparison to spondyloarthropathies, true infections are uncommon, particularly in the industrialized countries of the world. The estimated annual frequency is 0.037 for epidural abscess, 0.037 for pyogenic vertebral osteomyelitis, and 0.037 for disc space infection, exclusive of patients with post-operative discitis, which occurs in 1 of 100 disc operations (67). In less industrialized countries, spinal tuberculosis still is frequent and commonly overlooked. A delay in diagnosis of two months is typical (26) because the condition is unsuspected. As previously noted, the population at particular risk are drug addicts; the immunosuppressed, either from acquired immunodeficiency syndrome or medical treatment for tumors, arthritis, and organ transplantation; diabetics; or those who have undergone recent urinary tract instrumentation. The delay in diagnosis relates to the subtle presentation, failure to appreciate the unrelenting pain which often occurs, and often the absence of systemic signs such as temperature elevation. The laboratory studies may be misleading: normal leukocyte counts are common, radiographs often show no abnormalities early in the course of the illness, and even more sensitive diagnostic testing such as bone scans may not become positive for a week. When the diagnosis is suspected, the MRI now seems to be the most reliable early confirmatory test, while elevations of sedimentation rate are the most valuable screening test.

In addition to these causes, referred pain sources should be kept in mind and a complete examination performed.

Figure 12 presents the algorithm which summarizes this diagnostic approach, and how the Quebec Classification can be effectively used to stage diagnostic studies in a rational sequence. In Chapter 5, this same information has been used to demonstrate how this approach can be used to improve the quality of low back care as measured by outcome and cost effectiveness.

CONCLUSION

A pathoanatomic diagnosis is unavailable for the vast majority of patients with low back pain using today's clinical and technical knowledge. In this chapter, I emphasize how the Quebec Classification is a rational approach to diagnosis, rather than fooling ourselves that we have diagnoses which can stand rigorous scrutiny. The emphasis is that the clinical history and physical examination will suggest the small sub-set of patients who need urgent further diagnostic evaluation. For the vast majority, a delay in diagnosis is justifiable and the natural history will favor recovery. However, when symptoms persist beyond normal expected healing time, a rigorous evaluation is then warranted with studies selected according to the suspected clinical diagnosis, rather than a fishing expedition. Although we do not have complete knowledge about the causes of Category 1, 2, and 3 back pain, the disc remains the most suspect structure.

REFERENCES

1. Arnoldi CC, Brodsky AE, Cauchoix J et al (1976): Lumbar spinal stenosis and nerve root entrapment syndromes: Definition and classification. *Clin Orthop* (115):4–5.
2. Andersson GB, Svensson HO, Oden A (1983): The intensity of work recovery in low back pain. *Spine* 8:880–884.
3. Andersson GJB (1989): Unpublished data.
4. Badgley CE (1941): The articular facets in relation to low-back pain and sciatic radiation. *J Bone Joint Surg* [Am] 23:481–496.
5. Baker, AS, Ojemann RG, Swartz MN, Richardson EP Jr (1975): Spinal epidural abscess. *N Engl J Med* 293:463–468.
6. Bengtsson A, Henriksson KG, Larsson J (1986): Muscle biopsy in primary fibromyalgia. Light-microscopical and histochemical findings. *Scand J Rheum* 15:1–6.
7. Bernard TN Jr, Kirkaldy-Willis WH (1987): Recognizing specific characteristics of nonspecific low back pain. *Clin Orthop* (217):266–280.
8. Bluestone R (1985): Ankylosing spondylitis. In: *Arthritis and Allied Conditions,* Philadelphia: Lea and Febiger, pp. 819–840.
9. Bobbert MF, Hollander AP, Huijing PA (1986): Factors in delayed onset of muscle soreness of man. *Med Sci Sports Exerc* 18:75–81.
10. Calin A, Porta J, Fries JF, Schurman DJ (1977): Clinical history as a screening test for ankylosing spondylitis. *JAMA* 237:2613–2614.
11. Calin A, Kaye B, Sternberg M, et al (1980): The prevalence and nature of back pain in an industrial complex: A questionnaire and radiographic and HLA analysis. *Spine* 5:201–205.

12. Carney SL, Billingham ME, Muir H, Sandy SD (1985): Structure of newly synthesised (35S)-proteoglycans and (35S)-proteoglycan turnover products of cartilage explant cultures from dogs with experimental osteoarthritis. *J Orthop Res* 3:140–147.

13. Carr D, Gilbertson L, Frymoyer J, Krag M, Pope M (1985): Lumbar paraspinal compartment syndrome. A case report with physiologic and anatomic studies. *Spine* 10:816–820.

14. Crock HV (1970): A reappraisal of intervertebral disc lesions. *Med J Australia* 1:983–989.

15. Deyo RA, Diehl AK (1986): Lumbar spine films in primary care: Current use and effects of selective ordering criteria. *J Gen Intern Med* 1:20–25.

16. Diamant B, Karlsson J, Nachemson A (1968): Correlation between lactate levels and pH in discs of patients with lumbar rhizopathies. *Experientia* 24:1195–1196.

17. Dillane JB, Fry J, Kalton G (1966): Acute back syndrome - a study from general practice. *Br Med J* 2:82–84.

18. Donelson R (1986): Centralization phenomenon: Its usefulness in evaluating and treating sciatica. *Orthop Trans* 10:533.

19. Eisenstein SM, Parry CR (1987): The lumbar facet arthrosis syndrome: Clinical presentation and articular surface changes. *J Bone Joint Surg* [Br] 69:3–7.

20. Fishbain DA, Goldberg M, Steele R, Rosomoff H (1989): DSM-III diagnosis of patients with myofascial pain syndrome (fibrositis). *Arch Phys Med Rehab* 70:433–438.

21. Foerster (1933): The dermatomes in man. *Brain* 56:1–39.

22. Frymoyer JW, Gordon SL, eds. (1989): *New perspectives on low back pain.* Park Ridge, Illinois: American Academy of Orthopaedic Surgeons.

23. Garrett W Jr, Bradley W, Byrd S, Edgerton VR, Gollnick P (1989): Muscle. Part B. Basic science perspective. In: *New Perspectives on Low Back Pain,* JW Frymoyer and SL Gordon, eds. Park Ridge, Illinois: American Academy of Orthopaedic Surgeons, pp. 335–372.

24. Ghormley RK (1933): Low back pain: With special reference to the articular facets, with presentation of an operative procedure. *JAMA* 101:1773–1777.

25. Goldthwait JE (1911): The lumbosacral articulation: An explanation of many cases of "lumbago," "sciatica" and paraplegia. *Boston Med Surg J* 164:365–372.

26. Griffiths HE, Jones DM (1971): Pyogenic infection of the spine. A review of twenty-eight cases. *J Bone Joint Surg* [Br] 53:383–391.

27. Habif TP (1985): *Clinical dermatology.* St. Louis: Mosby.

28. Hadler NM (1986): Regional back pain. [editorial] *N Engl J Med* 315:1090–1092.

29. Hadler NM (1986): A critical reappraisal of the fibrositis concept. *Am J Med* 81(Suppl 3A):26–30.

30. Hakelius A, Hindmarsh J (1972): The comparative reliability of preoperative diagnostic methods in lumbar disc surgery. *Acta Orthop Scand* 43:234–238.

31. Hawkins BR, et al (1981): Use of the B27 test in the diagnosis of ankylosing spondylitis: A statistical evaluation. *Arthritis Rheum* 24:743–746.

32. Hirsch C, Schajowicz F (1953): Studies on structural changes in the lumbar annulus fibrosus. *Acta Orthop Scand* 22:184–231.

33. Hirsch C, Ingelmark B, Miller M (1963): The anatomical basis for low back pain. *Acta Orthop Scand* 33:1–17.

34. Holm S, Maroudas A, Urban JP, Selstam G, Nachemson A (1981): Nutrition of the intervertebral disc: solute transport and metabolism. *Connective Tissue Research* 8:101–119.

35. Holm SH, Urban SPG (1987): The intervertebral disc: Factors contributing to its nutrition and matrix turnover. In: *Joint Loading,* Hjhelminen, ed., Wright Bristol, publisher.

36. Inman VT, Saunders JB (1944): Referred pain from skeletal structures. *J Nev Ment Dis* 99:660–667.

37. Jackson RP, Jacobs RR, Montesano PX (1988): 1988 Volvo award in clinical sciences. Facet joint injection in low-back pain. A prospective statistical study. *Spine* 13:966–971.

38. Jayson MIV (1986): Spinal diseases and back pain. In: *Atlas of Clinical Rheumatology,* PA Dieppe et al, eds. Philadelphia: Lea and Febiger, pp. 13–17.

39. Jones DA, Newham OG, Giamberaridino MA (1987): Nature of exercise-induced muscle pain. *Advances in Pain Research and Therapy* 10:207–218.

40. Kirkaldy-Willis WH (1983): *Managing low back pain.* New York: Churchill Livingstone.

41. Kostuik JP, Harrington I, Alexander D, Rand W, Evans D (1986): Cauda equina syndrome and lumbar disc herniation. *J Bone Joint Surg* [Am] 68:386–391.

42. LaBan MM (1984): "Vespers curse": Night pain—the bane of Hypnos. *Arch Phys Med Rehabil* 65:501–504.

43. Lee CK, Rauschning W, Glenn W (1988): Lateral lumbar spinal canal stenosis: Classification, pathologic anatomy and surgical decompression. *Spine* 13:313–320.

44. Lehto M, Hurme M, Alaranta H et al (1989): Connective tissue changes of the multifidus muscle in patients with lumbar disc herniation. An immunohistologic study of collagen types I and III and fibronectin. *Spine* 14:302–309.

45. Lewis T, Kellgren JH (1939): Observations relating to referred pain, visceromotor reflexes and other associated phenomena. *Clin Sci* 4:47–71.

46. Liang M, Komaroff AL (1982): Roentgenograms in primary care patients with acute low back pain: a cost-effectiveness analysis. *Arch Intern Med* 142:1108–1112.

47. Lilius G, Laasonen EM, Myllynen P, Harilainen A, Gronlund G (1989): Lumbar facet joint syndrome. A randomised clinical trial. *J Bone Joint Surg* [Br] 71:681–684.

48. McCain GA (1986): Role of physical fitness training in the fibrositis/fibromyalgia syndrome. *Am J Med* 81(3A):73–77.

49. Mixter WJ, Barr JS (1934): Rupture of the intervertebral disc with involvement of the spinal canal. *N Engl J Med* 211:210–215.

50. Moldofsky H, Scarisbrick P, England R, Smythe H (1975): Musculoskeletal symptoms and non-REM sleep disturbance in patients with "fibrositis syndrome" and healthy subjects. *Psychosomatic Med* 37:341–351.

51. Mooney V, Robertson J (1976): The facet syndrome. *Clin Orthop* (115):149–156.

52. Mooney V (1989): A perspective on the future of low back research. In: *Spine, state of the art reviews,* vol. 3, RD Guyer, ed. Philadelphia: Hanley and Belfus.

53. Murphey F (1968): Sources and patterns of pain in disc disease. *Clin Neurosurg* 15:343–351.

54. Nachemson AL (1985): Advances in low-back pain. *Clin Orthop* (200):266–278.

55. Nakano KK (1987): Sciatic nerve entrapment: the piriformis syndrome. *Musculoskeletal Med* 4:33–37.

56. Onofrio BM, Mih AD (1988): Synovial cysts of the spine. *Neurosurgery* 22:642–647.

57. Park WM, McCall IW, O'Brien JP et al (1979): Fissuring of the posterior annulus fibrosus in the lumbar spine. *Br J Radiol* 52:382–387.

58. Parke WW, Watanabe R (1985): The intrinsic vasculature of the lumbosacral spinal nerve roots. *Spine* 10:508–515.

59. Peyster RG, Teplick JG, Haskin ME (1985): Computed tomography of lumbosacral conjoined nerve root anomalies: potential cause of false-positive reading for herniated nucleus pulposus. *Spine* 10:331–337.

60. Porter RW, Hibbert C, Evans C (1984): The natural history of root entrapment syndrome. *Spine* 9:418–421.

61. Putti V (1927): New conceptions in the pathogenesis of sciatic pain. *Lancet* 2:53–60.

61a. Quebec Task Force on Spinal Disorders (1987): see ref. 68.

62. Rosenberg NJ (1975): Degenerative spondylolisthesis: Predisposing factors. *J Bone Joint Surg* [Am] 57:467–474.

63. Rutkow IM (1986): Orthopaedic operations in the United States, 1979 through 1983. *J Bone Joint Surg* [Am] 68:716–719.

64. Sachs BL, Vanharanta H, Spivey MA et al (1987): Dallas discogram description: A new classification of CT/Discography in low-back disorders. *Spine* 12:287–294.

65. Scham SM, Taylor TK (1971): Tension signs in lumbar disc prolapse. *Clin Orthop* (75):195–204.

66. Sim FH, Dahlin DC, Stauffer RN, Laws ER (1977): Primary bone tumor simulating lumbar disc syndrome. *Spine* 2:65–74.

67. Spangfort EV (1972): The lumbar disc herniation. A computer-aided analysis of 2,504 operations. *Acta Orthop Scand* [Suppl], 142:1–95.

68. Spitzer WO et al [Quebec Task Force on Spinal Disorders] (1987): Scientific approach to the assessment and management of activity-related spinal disorders. A monograph for clinicians. Report of the Quebec Task Force on Spinal Disorders. *Spine* 12:S1–S59.

69. Styf J (1987): Pressure in the erector spinae muscle during exercise. *Spine* 12:675–679.

70. Valkenburg HA, Haanen HCM (1982): The epidemiology of low back pain. In: *American Academy of Orthopaedic Surgeons symposium on idiopathic low back pain,* edited by AA White, SL Gordon, eds. St. Louis: Mosby, pp. 9–22.

71. Walheim GG, Selvik G (1984): Mobility of the pubic symphysis: In vivo measurements with an electromechanic method and a roentgen stereophotogrammetric method. *Clin Orthop* (191):129–135.

72. Watts C (1988): Syndrome of intradiscal lumbar herniation: Clinical presentation and management. *Surg Neurol* 30:263–267.

73. Weber H (1983): Lumbar disc herniation. A controlled, prospective study with ten years of observation. *Spine* 8:131–140.

74. Weinstein JN, McLain RF (1987): Primary tumors of the spine. *Spine* 12:843–851.

75. Wiesel SW, Feffer HL, Borenstein DG (1988): Evaluation and outcome of low-back pain of unknown etiology. *Spine* 13:679–680.

76. Wolfe F, Hawley DJ, Cathey MA et al (1985): Fibrositis: Symptom frequency and criteria for diagnosis. An evaluation of 291 rheumatic disease patients and 58 normal individuals. *J Rheumatol* 12:1159–1163.

77. Woo SL, Buckwalter JA (1988): Injury and repair of the musculoskeletal soft tissue. *Am Academy of Orthop Surgeons* Chapter 5, pp. 171–207.

78. Yagan R, Khan MA, Marmolya G (1987): Role of abdominal CT, when available in patients' records, in the evaluation of degenerative changes of the sacroiliac joints. *Spine* 12:1046–1051.

The Adult Spine: Principles and Practice,
J. W. Frymoyer, Editor-in-Chief.
Raven Press, Ltd., New York © 1991.

CHAPTER 72

Non-Operative Treatment of Low Back Disorders

Differentiating Useful from Useless Therapy

Richard A. Deyo

A wide variety of non-operative treatments are advocated in the management of low back pain, and the list grows continuously. Unfortunately, the multiplicity of treatment methods implies the absence of a clearly superior treatment program. Although these treatments are less expensive and less invasive than surgical interventions, their use should be carefully scrutinized. All entail some expense, some require hospitalization or work loss, and all have occasional side effects. Furthermore, while nearly 80% of adults will experience back pain at some point in their lives, only 1%–2% will undergo lumbar spine surgery (16,27). Thus, treatment of the vast majority of patients will exclusively involve conservative therapy.

Conflicting claims exist for nearly every form of conservative therapy. It seems likely that many of the controversies are a result of studies performed among widely differing types of patients with back pain, or of methodologic problems which create a potential for unconscious patient or investigator bias. Furthermore, while competing treatment programs generally have some basis in physiologic observations or theories, evaluating their actual success in clinical practice requires carefully controlled clinical observation.

CRITERIA FOR EVALUATING RESEARCH ON CONSERVATIVE THERAPY

In order to resolve conflicting or competing claims, it is important to evaluate published evidence according to the likelihood of its internal validity, and also its probable applicability to one's own patients. Based on the

R. A. Deyo, M.D., M.P.H.: Departments of Medicine and Health Services, University of Washington; Northwest Health Services Research and Development Field Program, Seattle VA Medical Center, Seattle, Washington, 98108.

work of a number of methodologists (19,20), we have previously suggested use of the following criteria for evaluating evidence for therapeutic efficacy (22).

Criteria for Validity

Randomization

This is the best way to eliminate many of the biases that can produce misleading results (11). Even among study subjects with seemingly uncomplicated mechanical low back pain, there is wide heterogeneity in prognosis according to the method and site of recruitment, medical history, economic factors, and psychosocial traits. The natural history of acute low back pain includes rapid improvement, and spontaneous improvement occurs even among patients with chronic low back pain. Placebo responses are as common and as powerful in this condition as in others. Thus, the use of randomized concurrent controls is essential if we are to know whether treatment results are better than natural history plus placebo effects.

Minimal Subject Attrition

Subjects who respond especially well or especially poorly may be more likely to drop out from a study than other subjects. If so, the results may be biased, so attrition must be minimized.

Blinding

Three parties with pre-existing biases may be involved in any research project: the patient, the therapist, and the person who assesses the outcomes. Efforts to blind all of these persons to treatment group assignments help to reduce potential bias, though blinding with regard to physical treatments is difficult. Nonetheless, it is usually possible at least to have a blind assessor measure study outcomes.

Equivalent Co-Interventions

Many treatments may be prescribed simultaneously in the management of back pain (e.g., medication, exercise, physical therapy, behavioral therapy), and patients often obtain treatments other than those prescribed by a single medical care provider. It is important to know whether such co-interventions were identified and were comparable among study groups.

Compliance

Clinical and research experience suggest that compliance with many physical treatments is difficult to

achieve, and is often worse than medication compliance (which in turn is often limited). Efforts to ensure and measure compliance are necessary to gauge efficacy of the intended therapy.

Contamination

Patients assigned to one treatment may seek out or inadvertently obtain the alternative treatment, becoming unintended "crossovers." This is especially a problem in long-term studies or for readily available treatments.

Statistical Power

If a study finds statistically significant differences between two treatments, then statistical power is not a problem. If no significant differences are found, it is essential to determine whether the sample size was adequate to detect clinically important differences.

Criteria for Applicability of Research Results

Adequate Demographic Description

It has been demonstrated that patient age, sex, educational level, employment status, compensation status, and source of recruitment all influence the likelihood of improvement. While many other features may be equally or more important, these are simple to ascertain and influence the generalizability of results.

Adequate Clinical Description

In many cases of back pain a firm diagnosis is impossible, but a careful clinical description of study subjects helps judge the applicability of results. Thus, the duration of pain, presence of sciatica, neurologic abnormalities, prior surgery, narcotic analgesic use, and other inclusion or exclusion criteria are essential in understanding to whom the results apply.

Adequate Description of the Intervention

The dose or intensity of treatment, frequency of treatments, duration of therapy, and description of techniques are necessary to reproduce or generalize the results.

Reporting All Relevant Outcomes

Death or cure are rare outcomes of back pain therapy, so other indicators are needed. Relevant outcomes should be considered from at least four categories: (1)

physiological (e.g., pain scales, range of motion, neurologic change); (2) functional (e.g., work status, activities of daily living, disability days); (3) costs, often estimated from charges or utilization of services; and (4) attitudes or perceptions, such as preferred therapy, satisfaction, or psychological test results. All of these may be clinically important, and concordance among different types of outcomes increases our confidence that findings are valid, generalizable, and clinically important.

In reviewing the literature on treatments for lumbar spine disorders, we have tried to consider each of these criteria, and to identify shortcomings. For interested readers or potential investigators, a more detailed and stringent list of research design criteria should be considered, and these are discussed elsewhere (20,34).

BARRIERS TO RESEARCH IN LOW BACK DISORDERS

There are a number of unique barriers to conducting valid therapeutic research among patients with low back problems. One of the most problematical is the uncertainty of diagnosis in most cases of low back pain. Even with the best medical evaluation, it has been estimated that up to 85% of patients with back pain will not have a definitive diagnosis of the underlying pathoanatomic cause (94). Indeed, there is substantial controversy concerning even the existence of many diagnoses, including trigger point syndromes, muscle spasm, and spinal instability (35,50,78). In the absence of clear cut diagnoses, it is important at least to provide detailed information concerning demographic and clinical features of the patients as described above. New classifications for patients with

low back pain, such as the one proposed by the Quebec Task Force on Spinal Disorders, should be useful in describing groups of patients and research subjects with somewhat homogeneous characteristics and prognoses (82) (Table 1).

Unlike most drug treatments, it is difficult to blind a clinical trial of physical treatments. Nonetheless, efforts to provide placebo treatments which resemble as nearly as possible the active treatment help to mask the identity of treatments (e.g., use of sham TENS as a control for true TENS; massage as a control for spinal manipulation; and traction with sub-therapeutic weight as a control for conventional traction). Furthermore, it should generally be possible to have someone assess patient outcomes who is truly blinded to the treatment assignment.

A third major problem is that there is little consistency as to the types of outcomes which are measured in most clinical studies. While it is important to record physiologic data and patient symptoms, actual patient behavior in the conduct of daily activities may be the most important outcome for patients and for society. There is a growing literature on the assessment of daily functioning among patients with back pain, and the newer measures appear to offer substantial advantages over some more traditional measures (23).

Dropouts and difficulty in long-term follow-up appear to be particularly common in trials of back pain therapy. This may occur because patients are substantially improved or because they are unhappy with lack of improvement. In either case, investigators must often make extraordinary efforts to find patients and may need to provide incentives for continued participation. Reasons for dropping out should always be identified.

TABLE 1. *Classification of activity-related spinal disorders (ref. 82)*

Classification	Symptoms	Duration of symptoms from onset	Working status at time of evaluation
1	Pain without radiation	a (<7 days)	
2	Pain + radiation to extremity, proximally	b (7 days–7 weeks)	W (working)
3	Pain + radiation to extremity, distally*	c (>7 weeks)	I (idle)
4	Pain + radiation to upper/lower limb neurologic signs		
5	Presumptive compression of a spinal nerve root on a simple roentgenogram (i.e., spinal instability or fracture)		
6	Compression of a spinal nerve root confirmed by Specific imaging techniques (i.e., computerized axial tomography, myelography, or magnetic resonance imaging) Other diagnostic techniques (e.g., electromyography, venography)		
7	Spinal stenosis		
8	Postsurgical status, 1–6 months after intervention		
9	Postsurgical status, >6 months after intervention 9.1 Asymptomatic 9.2 Symptomatic		
10	Chronic pain syndrome		W (working)
11	Other diagnoses		I (idle)

* Not applicable to the thoracic segment.

Finally, efficacy of a new treatment in the research setting does not necessarily mean a treatment will be effective in routine clinical practice. Effectiveness is a complex product of accurate diagnosis, efficacy of the treatment under ideal circumstances, physician skill in applying treatment, and patient compliance. A failure in any of these areas may render treatment ineffective, but the literature contains little information about any of these factors except efficacy.

RATIONALE FOR AND EFFICACY OF COMMON TREATMENTS

Bed Rest

Based on national surveys in the United States, rest is the most frequently used treatment for low back pain (27). Traditional recommendations for bed rest were vague, but periods of one to two weeks were typically discussed. There has been little evidence to support the efficacy of bed rest, and in some primary care settings, patients report missing an average of less than three days from their usual activities (84). While the direct costs of this treatment are small, the indirect costs in terms of lost time from work or usual activities may be substantial.

The traditional rationale for recommending bed rest was twofold: (1) many persons with mechanical back pain report symptomatic relief in the supine position, and this is especially true for persons who appear to have a herniated disc; and (2) intravital measurements demonstrate that intradiscal pressure is minimized in the supine position. Nonetheless, nearly 50% of patients with back pain report only minimal relief with bed rest (89), and intradiscal pressure rises to 75% of that in the standing position when patients merely roll to the side (75). Although intradiscal pressure may be important for persons who have a herniated disc, this condition probably accounts for only a small proportion of all cases of low back pain. For cases in which pain arises from paraspinal muscles, ligaments, facet joints, and other structures, a rationale for bed rest is less clear.

Only recently have randomized trials of bed rest been reported. The first of three randomized trials suggested that bed rest was superior to continued ambulation, but this study was conducted among young men in military training (95). The outcome assessments were not blinded, and both assessor and patient may have been aware of the investigators' hypothesis. The types of injuries experienced by vigorous young men in physically demanding circumstances may not be typical of those encountered in primary care. Certainly, these recruits were absent from their usual duties for a longer period than is generally reported in primary care populations. Finally, this study compared enforced bed rest with enforced ambulation, circumstances that do not reflect the

realities of civilian life. Most patients have the opportunity to combine both types of activity, adjusting activity and rest according to symptoms, demands, incentives, and advice.

It is not surprising that two subsequent trials in primary care medical practice reported different results than the military study. Our study of acute back pain in a walk-in clinic randomized 203 subjects to a recommendation of two days or seven days of bed rest (25). Patients with neuromotor deficits were excluded and follow-up was partially blinded. Pain resolution and return of function were equally prompt in the two treatment groups, but those given the shorter bed rest recommendation returned to work 45% sooner than those given the seven day recommendation (3.1 versus 5.6 days). A search for predictors of work absenteeism during the three month follow-up period identified only the bed rest recommendation as a significant correlate. Clinical variables such as self-rated pain severity, duration, number of prior episodes, spine flexion, or straight leg raising did not significantly predict work loss. Thus, it appeared that for patients with no neuromotor deficits, a two day bed rest recommendation was as effective as longer periods, and resulted in less restriction of usual activities.

A similar study was completed in a family practice clinic at which 270 patients were randomized to a recommendation of four days of bed rest versus none at all (40). Again, patients with neurologic deficits were excluded, and follow-up assessments were conducted by a blinded observer. Follow-up was conducted at regular intervals for an entire year, and there were no detectable differences in the pace or extent of pain resolution or return of function. Subjects randomized to receive no bed rest returned to their "usual activities" 42% faster than those in the bed rest group. These two trials suggested that brief if any bed rest is sufficient treatment for most patients with acute low back pain, and that while bed rest may provide some symptomatic relief, it does not alter the natural history of recovery.

Bed rest can certainly have a variety of important medical and social side effects. Table 2 lists some of the complications that are either documented or likely (13,56,74). It is important to prevent deconditioning even in persons who have herniated discs or other potential surgical problems. Thus, many experts recommend at least brief ambulation after three days of bed rest even

TABLE 2. *Side effects of bed rest*

Perception of severe illness: even myocardial infarction does not require a week of strict bed rest
Economic loss: absenteeism strongly related to bed rest recommendation
Muscle atrophy: 1.0%–1.5% per day
Cardiopulmonary deconditioning: 15% in 10 days
Acute complications: thromboembolism
Bone mineral loss, hypercalcemia, hypercalciuria

for patients with a herniated disc and neurologic impairments.

Patient compliance with bed rest is also problematical. In our trial, many potential candidates refused to participate because they were unwilling to observe any bed rest (25). Even among the subjects who enrolled, compliance with bed rest recommendations was poor. Among those randomized to receive the seven day recommendation, three-fourths reported fewer than seven days of bed rest. Furthermore, compliance with the supine position is difficult to achieve. Most patients given a prescription for bed rest will prop themselves up or sit to read or watch television. This raises intradiscal pressures higher than those in the standing position, subverting even the hypothetical physiological goals of bed rest (75). See Chapter 31 for discussion of the theoretical adverse effects of recumbency and disuse on spinal structures.

Exercise

There is persistent controversy about the best exercise programs for persons with low back pain. Various experts advocate flexion exercises, extension exercises, stretching regimens, and aerobic conditioning. Many treatment programs prescribe a combination, and although there is little agreement on specific regimens, there is a consensus that exercise plays a major role in the treatment of mechanical low back pain. As evidence against the efficacy of passive treatments (such as bed rest and traction) accumulates, there is a shift towards more active therapy, with involvement of the patient in various exercise programs.

Persons who are not aerobically fit tend to fatigue rapidly in performing repetitive tasks, and may therefore be more susceptible to back injuries. Aerobic exercise is often prescribed for patients with back pain with the rationale of improving muscular endurance, neuromotor control, coordination, mechanical efficiency, and, to some degree, strength of lower extremity and abdominal muscles. Additional benefits of aerobic exercise may include weight loss and favorable psychological effects, with reductions of anxiety and depression (77). See Chapter 31 for discussion of the theoretical beneficial effects of exercise on spinal structures.

To date there have been no published randomized trials of aerobic exercises among patients with low back pain. The most widely cited evidence for their benefit is a cohort study of Los Angeles firefighters, among whom higher levels of fitness predicted a lower risk of subsequent back problems. In this study, "fitness" was characterized by a combination of data from bicycle ergometry, muscle strength testing, and spine flexibility. Thus, the particular role of aerobic fitness in preventing back injury could not be isolated (10). In a more recent prospective cohort study in another industrial setting, aerobic fitness estimated from a submaximal treadmill exercise test had no predictive value with regard to subsequent back problems (4). These studies did not address the therapeutic use of aerobic exercise in patients with current back problems, and the role of aerobic fitness in treatment thus remains uncertain.

Nonetheless, aerobic exercise is often prescribed for the anticipated physiologic and psychologic benefits described above. The type of exercise is relatively unimportant, and walking, swimming, bicycling, and even jogging may be reasonable prescriptions. Because of the potential for raising intradiscal pressure, some authors caution against certain types of aerobic dance which require torsion and forward flexion, or exercise such as rowing (77).

Another program is based on stretching exercises, with the intention of improving the extensibility of muscles and other soft tissues to reestablish normal joint range of motion. In many cases, mobility becomes restricted in response to pain. Stretching exercises have been advocated for many years by Kraus, and recently popularized in the form of group instruction by the Young Mens Christian Association (YMCA) (53,54,55). The YMCA has reported that approximately 80% of persons with chronic back pain who enter their program report subjective improvement at the end of the six week training period (54,55). These observations are not controlled, however, and could conceivably be the result of natural history and placebo effects.

A very recent study tested a brief program adapted from that of the YMCA (28). Patients were randomly allocated to receive exercise plus local heat, or heat alone. There were 125 subjects with chronic low back pain who completed the trial, and the exercise group reported significantly greater improvement in pain severity, pain frequency, and self-rated activity level (Table 3). After the supervised instruction ended, however, compliance with the exercise regimen was poor, and group differences were lost after an additional two month follow-up. Thus, there is evidence for modest subjective improvements in pain with the stretching exercise regimen, but it appears that continuing efforts are necessary to maintain patient compliance.

Probably the best known of exercise regimens is the isometric flexion program popularized by Williams in the 1930s (96). The rationale of the flexion regimen was to widen intervertebral foramina and facet joints, reducing nerve compression; to stretch hip flexors and back extensors; to strengthen abdominal and gluteus muscles; and to reduce "posterior fixation" of the lumbosacral junction. Some have suggested that strengthening of the abdominal muscles could in effect develop a muscular "corset," reducing loads on the lumbar spine. A theoretical concern of this regimen is that certain flexion maneuvers result in substantial increases in intradiscal pressure, potentially aggravating bulging or herniated discs (75).

At least three randomized controlled trials of flexion exercises have been reported, but with conflicting results (Table 3). The trial by Kendall and Jenkins included patients with chronic pain and found the isometric flexion exercises to be superior to mobilizing exercises or extension exercises (52). The subsequent trial of Davies and his colleagues studied young adults with sub-acute pain and found that both an extension and a flexion exercise regimen were superior to no exercise at all (although results were not statistically significant) (18). The most recent trial examined middle-aged patients with acute back pain in a Canadian family practice. Subjects (n = 252) were randomized to receive isometric flexion exercises or no exercise and were followed for up to a year. No benefit for the exercise regimen could be demonstrated in functional recovery, range of motion, or pain severity. In some cases the trend was against the exercise regimen (40).

Recently, interest has turned to exercise regimens which emphasize extension principles. Perhaps the most widely publicized regimen is that of McKenzie, who advocates a complex program individualized according to the patient's symptoms (68). This program is more extensively described in Chapter 76, and emphasizes exercises that minimize or "centralize" radiating pain. One randomized trial of this program has been reported in a preliminary fashion, but a very high dropout rate compromised the certainty of results (29). Furthermore, the study has not been reported in sufficient detail to assess its methodologic adequacy. Nonetheless, the trial did purport to demonstrate an advantage of the McKenzie exercise regimen over traction or back school.

Danish investigators have reported their results with a much more intensive extension regimen which was not individualized according to patients' symptoms (64). In this program, patients performed three exercises with a

TABLE 3. *Methodologic details of randomized trials of exercise for low back pain*

Reference	Type of exercise	Patient description	Exercises adequately described or referred	Blind outcome assessment	Compliance reported?	Equal cointerventions	Result
Deyo (28)	stretching vs. no exercise	chronic pain	Yes	Yes	Yes	Yes	Exercise better than no exercise
Gilbert (40)	flexion vs. no exercise	acute pain	No	Yes	Yes	Yes	No significant benefit; trend against exercise
Kendall (52)	flexion vs. extension	chronic pain	Yes	Yes	No	Yes	Flexion better than extension or mobilizing exercises
Davies (18)	flexion vs. extension	sub-acute pain	Yes	Yes	No	Yes	No significant differences; trend favoring extension*
Manniche (64)	intensive extension regimen vs. mild extension regimen or mild combined regimen	chronic pain	Yes	Yes	No	Yes	Intensive extension regimen superior to others
Coxhead (15)	not specified	chronic sciatica, with or without back pain	No	No	No	Yes	No benefit*
White (93)	not specified	sub-acute or chronic (receiving workers' compensation)	No	No	No	No	No benefit*
Lidstrom (60)	2 combination regimens	back pain with sciatica, sub-acute or chronic	No	Yes	No	No	No benefit* of either regimen over no exercise

* Statistical power not reported.

large number of repetitions: (1) trunk lifting, performed by raising the unsupported trunk while lying prone on a couch, (2) leg lifting, performed with the trunk prone on a couch and the legs raised from a standing position to a horizontal position, and (3) a "pull to neck" with a weight pulley device drawn down behind the neck and shoulders. An intensive three month program of these exercises was superior to a milder version of the regimen or a less intensive combined flexion and extension program. The patients in this trial had chronic pain, but appeared to be highly functional, with 78% employed at the time of study entry. This regimen required almost two months before benefit became apparent, and the need for close supervision by a physical therapist was emphasized.

Table 3 lists three additional randomized trials of exercises for patients with low back pain, but these are difficult to interpret (15,60,93). The exercise regimens were not well described and statistical power was not considered.

Traction

The rationale for traction is to stretch the back, pulling vertebrae away from each other, and thereby potentially reducing protrusion of a bulging or herniated disc. It is generally advocated only for patients who have sciatica or a proven disc herniation. Physiologic studies have demonstrated that an applied weight of at least 25% of body weight is necessary to achieve distraction of the lumbar vertebrae, given the inertia and resistance of the body (83).

At least seven randomized clinical trials of conventional traction have been published, with striking consistency in their results. Table 4 summarizes these trials, none of which demonstrated any significant benefit for traction over the control treatment (15,60,65,66,79, 91,92). While these trials suffered from a variety of methodologic flaws (high attrition, unblinded assessments, and failure to consider statistical power), their

results are strikingly consistent. The only positive randomized trial we have identified (not shown in Table 4) is a study of an unconventional technique called "autotraction" in which the patient himself controls the tractive force (58). While this technique has been used in Sweden, it is not widely available in the United States, and there is at least one conflicting negative trial of this method (92). Furthermore, the patients studied by this method had sciatica as a significant symptom, rather than low back pain only.

A variety of devices have been marketed to apply the tractive force in novel ways, such as tilt tables, gravity inversion devices, and the "90-90 traction" method (14,39). No controlled trials of these devices were identified at the time of this review, and it is clear that gravity inversion has important ocular and cardiovascular side effects (33). These data clearly support the consensus view of the Quebec Task Force on Spinal Disorders which concluded that there was no scientific evidence to support the use of spinal traction despite its widespread application in practice (82).

Acupuncture

This treatment had its roots in ancient Chinese Taoist philosophy, without a scientifically acceptable rationale. Recent investigation suggests that acupuncture might act by principles of the "gate" theory of Melzack and Wall (71), which hypothesized that one type of sensory input (back pain) could be inhibited in the central nervous system (CNS) by another kind of input (in this case, needling). There also is evidence that acupuncture may stimulate production of endorphins as well as serotonin and acetylcholine within the CNS, enhancing analgesia. Unfortunately, acupuncture teaching and practice have often focused on the theory of stimulating traditional Chinese meridians (hypothetical lines of force that traverse the body from head to toe), the use of Chinese terminology, and extravagant claims for success in treating hepatitis, burns, hydrocephalus, and a host of other

TABLE 4. *Randomized controlled trials of conventional traction for sciatica or proven lumbar disc herniation*

Reference	N	Patient description	Control group	Blind outcome assessment	Results
Lindstrom (60)	62	sciatica	heat, rest	Yes	Negative
Weber (91)	86	herniated disc	sham traction[1]	No	Negative
Mathews (65)	27	sciatica	sham traction[1]	Yes	Negative
Coxhead (15)	292	sciatica	multiple treatments	No	Negative
Weber (92)[2]	215	herniated disc	sham traction[1]	Yes	Negative
Pal (79)	41	sciatica	sham traction[1]	Yes	Negative
Mathews (66)	143	sciatica	heat	Yes	Negative (except for women aged <45 years)

[1] Sham traction consisted of applying the traction apparatus with minimal weight (shown not to produce distraction of the vertebrae in radiographic studies).
[2] Used four different methods of traction.

TABLE 5. *Results of randomized trials of acupuncture therapy*

Control treatment	Reference	Included electrical stimulation	Results
Misplaced needling	Gaw (37)	?	Acupuncture equal to control
Misplaced needling	Godfrey (41)	No	Acupuncture equal to control[1]
Misplaced needling	Edelist (30)	Yes	Acupuncture equal to control[1]
Misplaced needling	Ghia (38)	Yes	Acupuncture equal to control[2]
Superficial lidocaine injection	Mendelson (72)	No	Acupuncture equal to control[1]
Sham TENS or subthreshold TENS	Lehmann (59)	Yes	Acupuncture superior to control
Sham TENs	MacDonald (63)	Yes	Acupuncture superior to control
Standard care	Gunn (43)	Yes	Acupuncture superior to control
Waiting list	Coan (12)	Yes	Acupuncture superior to control

[1] No significant group differences, but slight trend in favor of acupuncture.
[2] No significant group differences, but slight trend in favor of misplaced needling.

conditions (87). Claims for success in treating pain seem more circumspect and more plausible, even for those who are appropriately skeptical. Published studies have focused on chronic rather than acute pain.

Several randomized trials of acupuncture are summarized in Table 5 (12,30,37,38,41,43,59,63,72). All included only patients with chronic pain, although three of the studies included other problems in addition to low back pain (37,38,41). While the technique varied among studies, it was adequately described in most. Most studies employed an experienced acupuncturist, and many employed electrical needle stimulation as well as mechanical stimulation by pecking or twirling movements of the needles. In Godfrey's study (41), only 36% of the subjects had lumbosacral pain, but all or most of the subjects in the remaining studies had low back pain. Attrition was high in three studies, but their results are quite consistent with the others. Blinding was variable, and in one case an inventive scheme was developed to keep even the therapist blind as to whether he was providing acupuncture at appropriate or inappropriate sites (41). Despite the various design flaws identified, the results summarized in Table 5 are quite consistent. When compared against a treatment which involved no needling (sham TENS, standard physical and occupational therapy, or a waiting list) acupuncture appeared to offer a significant advantage. When compared to other needling techniques, however ("misplaced needling" is used to indicate placement at sites other than the prescribed Chinese meridians, or simply at tender areas), none of the studies showed a significant advantage for properly applied acupuncture. Since statistical power was generally not considered in these negative trials, it is important to examine any trends in the data suggesting a true effect which was "missed" due to small sample size. As Table 5 shows, however, one trial favored misplaced needling, one found virtually identical results for true and sham acupuncture, and three showed slight trends favoring true acupuncture. Thus, no consistent advantage is suggested, although a very small difference could have been missed in these trials.

Overall, these trials suggest that acupuncture is little more effective than placebo therapy which mimics active treatment. They strongly suggest that there is nothing special about the traditional Chinese meridians.

Transcutaneous Electrical Nerve Stimulation (TENS)

The use of TENS was originally based on the gate control theory of pain, which suggested that counterstimulation of the nervous system could modify pain perception (71). The theory first led to surgically implanted dorsal column stimulators, but the technique of TENS developed as a screening test for surgical candidates. The transcutaneous form of stimulation appeared to be effective itself (in uncontrolled observations), and TENS eventually became a widely accepted form of therapy. Later studies suggested that in certain stimulation modes, TENS could elevate spinal fluid endorphin levels, perhaps an additional mechanism for pain relief.

The early studies of TENS therapy were uncontrolled or used non-random allocation of research subjects to alternative treatments (61,62,81). Subsequent controlled trials suggested that TENS was superior to massage or equivalent to ice stimulation (69,70), but these trials suffered from small size, non-random allocation, unspecified dropout rates, and inadequate blinding. A small crossover comparison of TENS and acupuncture suggested that TENS was less effective than acupuncture, though differences did not achieve statistical significance with the sample size of 12. Perhaps the most widely cited evidence for the efficacy of TENS was a trial that employed conventional TENS in a crossover design, which, with perceptible stimulation, certainly precluded patient blinding. Furthermore, only a minority of patients had low back pain (88). Another randomized trial employed "sub-threshold" (imperceptible) TENS and reported no advantage over sham TENS. This was a small trial, however, and could be criticized because imperceptible stimulation may be ineffective (59). In a carefully blinded trial for arthritis pain, TENS was no more effective than sham TENS (57). A very recent trial was carefully blinded, avoided a crossover design, and used perceptible TENS in two different stimulation modes. There was no treatment benefit above sham TENS, and the trial was the largest randomized study of TENS for back pain reported to date (28). Thus, there remains no convincing evidence for the efficacy of TENS for chronic low back pain, and growing evidence against its efficacy. We have not reviewed its use in acute pain syndromes or conditions other than lumbar pain.

Corsets and Braces

Corsets and braces have been widely used for the purposes of restricting lumbosacral motion, providing abdominal support, and correcting posture. All of these potential benefits have been challenged, and some authors emphasize the potential for exacerbating disuse atrophy of important muscles (83). Only three randomized clinical trials of corset use have been identified, and failure to assess patient compliance or to blind observers confuses the interpretation of these studies (15,58,73). Perhaps the best designed study found that corsets were less effective than the use of "autotraction" (58). Thus, there is little scientific evidence to support the efficacy of spinal orthoses, and the Quebec Task Force on Spinal Disorders concluded that these devices are in common practice, but that there is no scientific evidence of their efficacy (82). There is some rationale, however, for the use of corsets and rigid braces in patients after spinal operations.

Biofeedback

Biofeedback has been advocated as a form of therapy for patients with chronic low back pain, based on the assumption that muscle tension or spasm may frequently produce pain. The concept of skeletal muscle spasm has been challenged (50), but the use of electromyographic (EMG) biofeedback to reduce muscle tension could nonetheless be appropriate.

Much of the early research on EMG biofeedback for low back pain consisted of uncontrolled case reports and case series. Only a small number of randomized controlled trials have been reported. Nouwen reported a small (n = 20) randomized trial of biofeedback in which the treatment was shown to produce a significant decrease in paraspinal EMG activity but no significant reduction in reported pain (76). A larger randomized trial similarly concluded that EMG biofeedback was no more effective than a placebo treatment or a waiting list (9). This was true for measures of pain, anxiety, depression, and paraspinal EMG. One trial purported to show an advantage to EMG biofeedback, but suffered from a high dropout rate (25%) and included both patients with low back pain and those with neck and shoulder pain (31).

The proportions of each type of patient were unclear and results were not separated for these two groups. Thus, the applicability of the results to patients with chronic low back pain remains uncertain. These studies support the conclusion of the Quebec Task Force on Spinal Disorders, that, like spinal orthoses, EMG biofeedback may be in common use, but there is no scientific evidence for its efficacy (82).

Drug Therapy

A variety of drugs are widely used in the treatment of low back pain. These include pure analgesics such as narcotic drugs and acetaminophen, anti-inflammatory drugs, the so-called muscle relaxants, and anti-depressant medications. Very few trials of pure analgesics for low back pain have been reported, and those which exist have important methodological flaws. Nonetheless, the general analgesic properties of medications such as codeine are well established, and clinical experience suggests that they are efficacious in the management of acute back pain syndromes. Because of their potential for abuse, and their lack of efficacy with chronic use, their use should be strictly time limited. That is, when these medications are used, patients should be instructed from the outset that they will not be used until "all the pain is gone," but rather for a fixed period of time, typically one week. There is wide agreement that narcotic analgesics are inappropriate in the management of chronic low back pain.

The nonsteroidal anti-inflammatory drugs (NSAIDs) have occasionally been studied specifically in the treatment of low back pain. Well designed trials suggest an advantage of several of these drugs over placebo in the management of acute low back pain. Drugs which have been specifically tested in this setting include naproxen sodium, diflunisal, and piroxicam, and it seems likely that most drugs in this category are efficacious (2,3,5,46). Unfortunately, most of these trials have not included an adequate description of their subjects, so that optimal selection of patients for this type of therapy remains unclear. Furthermore, these newer NSAIDs have not been shown to be superior to the less expensive aspirin, although gastrointestinal side effects are generally less frequent. The efficacy of these medications in the management of chronic (rather than acute) back pain syndromes remains unclear. Furthermore, side effects are relatively frequent, and the drugs should be used with appropriate caution. This is especially true for older patients, among whom reversable renal insufficiency and serious gastrointestinal bleeding may be most common (85) (see also Chapter 31).

The use of "muscle relaxant" drugs is predicated on the assumption that low back pain may frequently be a result of muscle spasm. As previously noted, the very concept of skeletal muscle spasm has been challenged

(50), but the possibility of increased muscle tone contributing to pain still seems reasonable. Nonetheless, the effects of muscle relaxant drugs in conventional oral doses may include minimal muscle relaxation, with sedation being the major effect. Unfortunately, these medications have often been tested in clinical trials where a variety of "muscle spasm" syndromes were tested together, including not only low back pain, but neck pain, and even extremity muscle pain (97). The overall results of such trials should be extrapolated to low back pain patients with caution for several reasons:

1. The clinical detection of muscle spasm appears not to be reproducible between expert physicians (90).
2. Anatomic, physiological, and psychological considerations may be different for low back pain as opposed to other pain syndromes.
3. Where results have been itemized according to clinical syndrome, results for low back pain are sometimes worse than for patients with other diagnoses.

Table 6 summarizes the results of muscle relaxant trials which have included only patients with low back pain (6,7,8,17,42,47,48). Unfortunately, most such trials have not provided an adequate clinical description of the study subjects so that, again, it is difficult to generalize the results in terms of patient selection. Nonetheless, it appears that at least some of these medications may have an advantage over placebos or pure sedatives. This has been particularly well demonstrated in the case of carisoprodol (8,47). Unfortunately, side effects appear to be quite common with all of these drugs (Table 6), and it remains unclear whether they add any clinical benefit to the use of nonsteroidal drugs alone. Because of the potential for habituation, it is probably important to strictly limit the use of these medications with a time schedule rather than according to patient symptoms. Like the use of narcotic analgesics, one week of use may be a generally appropriate guideline.

Tricyclic antidepressant medications are yet another class of medications most widely used for chronic pain syndromes for several reasons. First, it may be that prolonged somatic complaints such as low back pain are a marker for subclinical depression. Second, these drugs could have some inherent analgesic properties, as suggested in trials of tricyclic drugs for chronic neuritic pain. Further, many of these drugs are sedating, and may improve sleep among patients with night time pain. Table 7 summarizes several trials of anti-depressant drugs for chronic low back pain (1,44,49,80). Unfortunately, most of these trials suffer from a large dropout rate, possibly a consequence of medication side effects. The trial of Hameroff included only patients who were clinically depressed in addition to having chronic pain, and included both neck pain and low back pain (44). Thus, the applicability of the results to chronic low back pain alone is unclear. The only negative trial listed in Table 7 (that of Jenkins and colleagues) suffered not only from a high dropout rate, but also a relatively low dose of imipramine and a short trial duration (49). Perhaps the most persuasive of these studies is Alcoff's who studied only

TABLE 6. *Randomized trials of oral "muscle relaxant" drugs exclusively for low back pain*

Reference	N	Percent dropouts	Adequate patient description?	Side effects active drug (%)	Side effects placebo (%)	Results
Hindle (47)	48	10	No	0	0	Carisoprodol superior to placebo or butabarbitol
Boyles (8)	71	4	No	22 (C)	35 (D)	Carisoprodol superior to diazepam
Hingorani (48)	50	0?	No	40	16	Valium equal to placebo; statistical power not considered
Dapas (17)	200	32	No	68	30	Baclofen superior to placebo in severe group; overall results not reported
Berry (6)	112	14	Yes	41	21	Tizanidine equal to aspirin plus placebo in efficacy; Tizanidine group required less "rescue" aspirin
Berry (7)	105	10	Yes	45	31	Tizanidine plus ibuprofen superior to placebo plus ibuprofen
Gold (42)	60	0?	No (literally none)	25	5	Orphenadrine superior to phenobarbital or placebo at 48 hrs.; later results not reported

TABLE 7. *Randomized trials of tricyclic anti-depressant drugs for chronic low back pain*

Reference	Type and number of patients	Dropout rate	Adequate clinical description of subjects?	Results
Pheasant (80)	Chronic LBP n = 16	44%	Yes	Amitriptyline superior to placebo
Jenkins (49)	Chronic LBP n = 59	25%	No	Imipramine not significantly better than placebo
Alcoff (1)	Chronic or recurrent LBP n = 50	18%	Yes	Imipramine superior to placebo
Hameroff (44)	Chronic LBP or neck pain and clinically depressed n = 30	10%	No	Doxepin superior to placebo

patients with chronic or recurring low back pain (1). Except for the high dropout rate, this study was well designed, and showed an advantage of imipramine over placebo with regard to activity limitations and pain severity. Thus, there is suggestive, but still not definitive, evidence that tricyclic anti-depressants are efficacious in the management of chronic low back pain.

Manipulation

The types of manipulative therapy and their benefits (or lack thereof) will be discussed in Chapter 73.

THERAPEUTIC RECOMMENDATIONS

Based on the evidence presented here, several traditional treatments for low back pain may well be inefficacious. Although the data may not be conclusive, there appears to be growing evidence against the efficacy of conventional spinal traction for the treatment for sciatica or herniated discs, against the use of TENS for chronic low back pain, and against the use of corsets and biofeedback. The data concerning acupuncture are complex, but show that traditional acupuncture is not superior to misplaced needling, suggesting that needling alone may have important placebo or perhaps counterirritant effects. Acupuncture appears efficacious only when compared with non-invasive forms of therapy or no treatment at all. Furthermore, there is growing evidence against the efficacy of prolonged bed rest for even one to two weeks.

In contrast, there is growing evidence for the efficacy of several exercise regimens, as well as several types of drug therapy. Thus, based on incomplete but suggestive data, the following conservative treatment recommendations can be made. Note that the time frames used below to define acute, sub-acute, and chronic are Frymoyer's (35) and differ from those of the Quebec Task Force (82) (see Table 1).

General Considerations

Most patients have a strong desire for explanation of symptoms, and may need reassurance that most back problems are not disabling. Thus, it is important to explain the excellent prognosis for returning to work and usual activities, and to avoid using potentially frightening diagnostic terminology (e.g., ruptured disc, spine degeneration). Second, patients should be told that mild or moderate pain on activity will not cause permanent harm, and does not necessitate activity restriction. The advice to "let pain be your guide" appears to result in worse outcomes than specific time-limited prescriptions for medication and activity limitation (32). Third, there is growing epidemiologic evidence that general fitness measures such as weight reduction and smoking cessation may reduce the frequency and severity of back problems (24,36,45,51). Finally, patient compliance with therapy may be an important problem. The literature on patient compliance suggests that it is particularly difficult to modify patient lifestyle, as necessitated by prescriptions for exercise, smoking cessation, or weight reduction (86). The use of compliance-enhancing strategies may often be necessary, including the provision of both verbal and written instructions and frequent patient follow-up (86).

Acute Back Pain (Less than 6 Weeks)

Bed rest may not alter the natural history of recovery, but does provide transient symptomatic relief for many patients. Thus, it is often appropriate to prescribe brief bed rest, with two to three days sufficient for most patients. For the patient with a neurologic deficit related to a probable herniated disc, the bed rest recommendation may need to be longer and stricter, but there are no data to suggest its optimal duration.

The use of nonsteroidal anti-inflammatory drugs is appropriate, and muscle relaxant medications may also be beneficial. If the latter are used, their prescriptions should be strictly time-limited, typically to one week. There are few data to aid in the selection of patients most appropriate for muscle relaxant therapy.

Early ambulation should be encouraged for most patients. Even for those with disc herniations, it is often possible to begin brief ambulation after two or three days of bed rest. This helps to limit muscular and cardiovascular deconditioning, and loads on the intervertebral disc are only slightly higher than those in the side lying position. After acute pain has subsided, usually within two weeks, further aerobic conditioning is probably appropriate for most patients. The rationale is to improve endurance of the abdominal, lower extremity, and spine musculature, perhaps making subsequent strain less likely.

The specific choice of exercise is probably unimportant, and may include swimming, walking, bicycling, and even jogging for some patients. Major torsion or flexion forces on the spine should probably be avoided, so that rowing and certain types of aerobic dance may need to be individually evaluated. A minimum of three weekly exercise sessions of 20 minutes each appears necessary to result in cardiovascular conditioning.

Even for patients who may become surgical candidates, walking is highly appropriate. Mild exercise may help to avoid deconditioning, which impedes surgical recovery and subsequent rehabilitation. Patients whose pain persists beyond two weeks may be candidates for spinal manipulation, for which there is some evidence of efficacy, and which is discussed in Chapter 73.

Sub-Acute Back Pain (6 to 12 Weeks)

This may be a particularly important clinical group, because these patients have already demonstrated a worse-than-average clinical course, but have not yet become chronic pain patients. It may be that optimal management at this stage can help to prevent the emergence of chronic pain syndromes. Aerobic conditioning as for acute pain is probably appropriate, as well as stretching exercises such as those of the YMCA. At this stage, referral to a physical therapist or a structured group treatment program may be appropriate to provide closer supervision and better treatment adherence. If a highly individualized exercise regimen (such as that advocated by McKenzie) is to be used, this is an appropriate time for its initiation. Patients with radiating pain to the leg which "centralizes" on extension are probably the best candidates for this type of exercise. Extension exercises should be avoided if they aggravate the pain or if the patient is known to have spinal stenosis, spondylolisthesis, or moderate scoliosis.

The role of medications in this phase of treatment remains unclear. However, it is inadvisable to continue the use of narcotic analgesics or muscle relaxants at this stage.

Chronic Low Back Pain (Greater than 3 Months)

Certainly, the mere persistence of pain is not an indication for surgical intervention. Thus, the management of most such patients remains conservative. In this patient group, the prognosis becomes worse, and aggressive nonsurgical treatment appears to be important. There may often be important barriers to improvement that should be identified, including psychological problems, financial disincentives, and symptom amplification. For this group, referral to a formal pain management program may often be appropriate. Such programs often include "functional restoration" emphasizing both aerobic fitness and strengthening exercises (67). The recent work of Manniche and colleagues (64) suggests that some patients in this category will benefit from strenuous extension exercises. These clearly require specialized equipment and supervision by a physical therapist. The major goal of most structured pain treatment programs is the resumption of functioning, with pain relief as a secondary goal which often parallels functional restoration.

Pending further studies, it is reasonable to institute a trial of tricyclic anti-depressant therapy for these patients. Specific choice of anti-depressant agents is probably unimportant, and selection may be based on the profile of side effects and other properties which may be desirable (e.g., sedation or minimization of sedation). This is certainly appropriate for patients with clinical or questionnaire evidence of depression, but may also be helpful for those who are not overtly depressed.

FUTURE RESEARCH

Physicians who provide spine care should remain alert to emerging research results, and be critical in judging their validity and applicability. Major trials are currently underway for several exercise regimens, spinal manipulation, and other treatments. These could certainly modify or add to the recommendations described here. Aside from the need for more and better research on each of the modalities described here, there is a major need for compliance research which would help us to monitor and enhance patient compliance with often challenging recommendations.

ACKNOWLEDGMENTS

Preparation of this chapter was supported in part by the Northwest Health Services Research and Development Field Program, Seattle VA Medical Center, and by

Grant number HS 06344 from the U.S. National Center for Health Services Research and Technology Assessment.

REFERENCES

1. Alcoff J, Jones E, Rust P, Newman R (1982): Controlled trial of imipramine for chronic low back pain. *J Fam Pract* 14:841–846.
2. Amlie E, Weber H, Holme I (1987): Treatment of acute low-back pain with piroxicam: Results of a double-blind placebo-controlled trial. *Spine* 12:473–476.
3. Aoki T, Kuroki Y, Kageyama T, et al (1983): Multicentre double-blind comparison of piroxicam and indomethacin in the treatment of lumbar diseases. *Eur J Rheum Inflam* 6:247–252.
4. Battie MC, Bigos SJ, Fisher LD, Hansson TH, Nachemson AL, Spengler DM, Wortly MD, Zeh J (1989): A prospective study of the role of cardiovascular risk factors and fitness in industrial back pain complaints. *Spine* 14:141–147.
5. Berry H, Bloom B, Hamilton EB, et al (1982): Naproxen sodium, diflunisal, and placebo in the treatment of chronic back pain. *Ann Rheum Dis* 41:129–132.
6. Berry H, Hutchinson DR (1988): A multicentre placebo-controlled study in general practice to evaluate the efficacy and safety of tizanidine in acute low-back pain. *J Int Med Res* 16:75–82.
7. Berry H, Hutchinson DR (1988): Tizanidine and ibuprofen in acute low-back pain: Results of a double-blind multicentre study in general practice. *J Int Med Res* 16:83–91.
8. Boyles WF, Glassman JM, Soyka JP (1983): Management of acute musculoskeletal conditions: thoracolumbar strain or sprain. A double-blind evaluation comparing the efficacy and safety of carisoprodol with diazepam. *Todays Therapeutic Trends* 1(1):1.
8a. Brown BR Jr, Womble J (1978): see ref. 97.
9. Bush C, Ditto B (1985): A controlled evaluation of paraspinal EMF biofeedback in the treatment of chronic low back pain. *Health Psychol* 4:307–321.
10. Cady LD, Bischoff DP, O'Connell ER, Thomas PC, Allan JH (1979): Strength and fitness and subsequent back injuries in firefighters. *J Occup Med* 21:269–272.
11. Chalmers TC, Celano P, Sacks HS, Smith H Jr (1983): Bias in treatment assignment in controlled clinical trials. *N Engl J Med* 309:1358–1361.
12. Coan RM, Wong G, Ku SL, et al (1980): The acupuncture treatment of low back pain: A randomized controlled study. *Am J Chinese Med* 8:181–189.
13. Convertino V, Hung J, Goldwater D, DeBusk RF (1982): Cardiovascular responses to exercise in middle-aged men after 10 days of bedrest. *Circulation* 65:134–140.
14. Cottrell GW (1985): New, conservative, and exceptionally effective treatment for low back pain. *Comprehensive Therapy* 11(11):59–65.
15. Coxhead CE, Inskip H, Meade TW, et al (1981): Multicentre trial of physiotherapy in the management of sciatic symptoms. *Lancet* 1:1065–1068.
16. Currey HL, Greenwood RM, Lloyd GG, et al (1979): A prospective study of low back pain. *Rheumatol Rehabil* 18:94–104.
17. Dapas F, Hartman SF, Martinez L, et al (1985): Baclofen for the treatment of acute low-back syndrome: A double blind comparison with placebo. *Spine* 10:345–349.
18. Davies JE, Gibson T, Tester L (1979): The value of exercises in the treatment of low back pain. *Rheumatol Rehabil* 18:243–247.
19. Department of Clinical Epidemiology and Biostatistics, McMaster University Health Sciences Centre (1981): How to read clinical journals: V. To distinguish useful from useless or even harmful therapy. *Can Med Assoc J* 124:1156–1162.
20. DerSimonian R, Charette LJ, McPeek B, Mosteller F (1982): Reporting on methods in clinical trials. *N Engl J Med* 306:1332–1337.
21. Deyo RA (1982): Compliance with therapeutic regimens in arthritis: Issues, current status, and a future agenda. *Semin Arth Rheumat* 12:233–244.
22. Deyo RA (1983): Conservative therapy for low back pain: Distinguishing useful from useless therapy. *JAMA* 250:1057–1062.
23. Deyo RA (1988): Measuring the functional status of patients with low back pain. *Arch Phys Med Rehabil* 69:1044–1053.
24. Deyo RA, Bass JE (1989): Lifestyle and low-back pain: The influence of smoking and obesity. *Spine* 14:501–506.
25. Deyo RA, Diehl AK, Rosenthal M (1986): How many days of bed rest for acute low back pain? A randomized clinical trial. *N Engl J Med* 315:1064–1070.
26. Deyo RA, Diehl AK (1986): Patient satisfaction with medical care for low-back pain. *Spine* 11:28–30.
27. Deyo RA, Tsui-Wu Y-J (1987): Descriptive epidemiology of low-back pain and its related medical care in the United States. *Spine* 12:264–268.
28. Deyo RA, Walsh N, Martin D, Schoenfeld L, Ramamurthy S (1990): A controlled trial of transcutaneous electronic nerve stimulation (TENS) and exercise for chronic low back pain. *N Engl J Med* 322:1627–1634.
29. DiMaggio A, Mooney V (1987): The McKenzie program: Exercise effective against back pain. *J Musculoskel Med* December:63–74.
30. Edelist G, Gross AE, Langer F (1976): Treatment of low back pain with acupuncture. *Can Anesth Soc J* 23:303–306.
31. Flor H, Haag G, Turk DC, Koehler H (1983): Efficacy of EMG biofeedback, pseudotherapy, and conventional medical treatment for chronic rheumatic back pain. *Pain* 17:21–31.
32. Fordyce WE, Brockway JA, Bergman JA, Spengler D (1986): Acute back pain: A control-group comparison of behavioral vs. traditional management methods. *J Behav Med* 9:127–140.
33. Friberg TR, Weinreb RN (1985): Ocular manifestations of gravity inversion. *JAMA* 253:1755–1757.
34. Friedman LM, Furberg CD, DeMets DI (1983): *Fundamentals of clinical trials*. Boston: John Wright/PSG Inc.
35. Frymoyer JW (1988): Back pain and sciatica. *N Engl J Med* 318:291–300.
36. Frymoyer JW, Pope MH, Clements JH, et al (1983): Risk factors in low-back pain. An epidemiological survey. *Bone Joint Surg [Am]* 65:213–218.
37. Gaw AC, Chang LW, Shaw LC (1975): Efficacy of acupuncture on osteoarthritic pain. *N Engl J Med* 293:375–378.
38. Ghia JN, Mao W, Toomey TC, Gregg JM (1976): Acupuncture and chronic pain mechanisms. *Pain* 2:285–299.
39. Gianakopoulos G, Waylonis GW, Grant PA, et al (1985): Inversion devices: Their role in producing lumbar distraction. *Arch Phys Med Rehabil* 66:100–102.
40. Gilbert JR, Taylor DW, Hildebrand A, Evans C (1985): Clinical trial of common treatments for low back pain in family practice. *Br Med J* 291:791–794.
41. Godfrey CM, Morgan P (1978): A controlled trial of the theory of acupuncture in musculoskeletal pain. *J Rheumatol* 5:121–124.
42. Gold RH (1978): Orphenadrine citrate: Sedative or muscle relaxant? *Clin Therap* 1:451–453.
43. Gunn CC, Milbrandt WE, Little AS, Mason KE (1980): Dry needling of muscle motor points for chronic low-back pain: A randomized clinical trial with long-term follow-up. *Spine* 5:279–291.
44. Hameroff SR, Cork RC, Scherer K, Crago BR, Neuman C, Womble JR, Davis TP (1982): Doxepin effects on chronic pain, depression, and plasma opioids. *J Clin Psychiatry* 43:22–27.
45. Heliovaara M (1987): Body height, obesity, and risk of herniated lumbar intervertebral disc. *Spine* 12:469–472.
46. Hickey RF (1982): Chronic low back pain: A comparison of diflunisal with paracetamol. *NZ Med J* 95:312–314.
47. Hindle TH 3d (1972): Comparison of carisoprodol, butabarbital, and placebo in treatment of the low back syndrome. *Calif Med* 117:7–11.
48. Hingorani K (1966): Diazepam in backache: A double-blind controlled trial. *Ann Phys Med* 8:303–306.
49. Jenkins DG, Ebbutt AF, Evans CD (1976): Tofranil in the treatment of low back pain. *J Int Med Res* 4(Suppl 2):28–40.
50. Johnson EW (1989): The myth of skeletal muscle spasm [editorial]. *Am J Phys Med Rehabil* 68:1.
51. Kelsey JL, Githens PB, O'Connor T, et al (1984): Acute prolapsed lumbar intervertebral disc: An epidemiological study with special

reference to driving automobiles and cigarette smoking. *Spine* 9:608–613.

52. Kendall PH, Jenkins JM (1968): Exercises for backache: A double-blind controlled trial. *Physiotherapy* 54:154–157.

53. Kraus H (1965): *Backache, stress and tension: Cause, prevention, and treatment.* New York: Simon and Schuster.

54. Kraus H, Melleby H, Gaston SR (1977): Back pain correction and prevention. National voluntary organizational approach. *NY State J Med* 77:1335–1338.

55. Kraus H, Nagler W, Melleby A (1983): Evaluation of an exercise program for back pain. *Am Fam Phys* 28:153–158.

56. Krolner B, Toft B (1983): Vertebral bone loss: An unheeded side effect of therapeutic bed rest. *Clinical Science* 64:537–540.

57. Langley GB, Sheppeard H, Johnson M, Wigley RD (1984): The analgesic effects of transcutaneous electrical nerve stimulation and placebo in chronic pain patients: A double-blind non-crossover comparison. *Rheumatol Int* 4:119–123.

58. Larsson U, Choler U, Lidstrom A, et al (1980): Auto-traction for treatment of lumbago-sciatica: A multicentre controlled investigation. *Acta Orthop Scand* 51:791–798.

59. Lehmann TR, Russell DW, Spratt KF, et al (1986): Efficacy of electroacupuncture and TENS in the rehabilitation of chronic low back pain patients. *Pain* 26:277–290.

60. Lidstrom A, Zachrisson M (1970): Physical therapy on low back pain and sciatica: An attempt at evaluation. *Scand J Rehabil Med* 2:37–42.

61. Loeser JD, Black RG, Christman A (1975): Relief of pain by transcutaneous stimulation. *J Neurosurg* 42:308–314.

62. Long DM, Campbell JN, Gucer G (1979): Transcutaneous electrical nerve stimulation for relief of chronic pain. *Adv Pain Res Therap* 3:593–599.

63. MacDonald AJ, MacRae KD, Master BR, Rubin AP (1983): Superficial acupuncture in the relief of chronic low back pain: A placebo-controlled randomised trial. *Ann R Coll Surg Engl* 65:44–46.

64. Manniche C, Hesselsoe G, Bentzen L, Christensen I, Lundberg E (1988): Clinical trial of intensive muscle training for chronic low back pain. *Lancet* 2:1473–1476.

65. Mathews JA, Hickling J (1975): Lumbar traction: A double-blind controlled study for sciatica. *Rheumatol Rehabil* 14:222–225.

66. Mathews JA, Mills SB, Jenkins VM, et al (1987): Back pain and sciatica: Controlled trials of manipulation, traction, sclerosant and epidural injections. *Br J Rheum* 26:416–423.

67. Mayer TG, Gatchel RJ, Mayer H, Kishino ND, Keeley J, Mooney V (1987): A prospective two-year study of functional restoration in industrial low back injury: An objective assessment procedure. *JAMA* 258:1763–1767.

68. McKenzie RA (1979): Prophylaxis in recurrent low back pain. *NZ Med J* 89:22–23.

69. Melzack R, Jeans ME, Stratford JG, Monks RC (1980): Ice massage and transcutaneous electrical stimulation: Comparison of treatment for low-back pain. *Pain* 9:209–217.

70. Melzack R, Vetere P, Finch L (1983): Transcutaneous electrical nerve stimulation for low back pain. A comparison of TENS and massage for pain and range of motion. *Physical Therapy* 63:489–493.

71. Melzack R, Wall PD (1965): Pain mechanisms: A new theory. *Science* 150:971–979.

72. Mendelson G, Selwood TS, Kranz H, et al (1983): Acupuncture treatment of chronic back pain: A double-blind placebo-controlled trial. *Am J Med* 74:49–55.

73. Million R, Nilsen KH, Jayson MI, et al (1981): Evaluation of low back pain and assessment of lumbar corsets with and without back supports. *Ann Rheum Dis* 40:449–454.

74. Muller EA (1970): Influence of training and of inactivity on muscle strength. *Arch Phys Med Rehabil* 51:449–462.

75. Nachemson A (1976): The lumbar spine: An orthopaedic challenge. *Spine* 1:59–71.

76. Nouwen A (1983): EMG biofeedback used to reduce standing levels of paraspinal muscle tension in chronic low back pain. *Pain* 17:353–360.

77. Nutter P (1988): Aerobic exercise in the treatment and prevention of low back pain. *State Art Rev Occup Med* 3:137–145.

78. Osterweis M, Kleinman A, Mechanic D, eds. (1987): *Pain and disability: Clinical behavioral and public policy perspectives.* Washington, DC: National Academy Press.

79. Pal B, Mangion P, Hossain MA, Diffey BL (1986): A controlled trial of continuous lumbar traction in the treatment of back pain and sciatica. *Br J Rheum* 25:181–183.

80. Pheasant H, Bursk A, Goldfarb J, Azen SP, Weiss JN, Borelli L (1983): Amitriptyline and chronic low-back pain: A randomized double-blind crossover study. *Spine* 8:552–557.

81. Procacci P, Zoppi M, Maresca M, Francini F (1977): Hypoalgesia induced by transcutaneous electrical stimulation: A physiological and clinical investigation. *J Neurosurg Sci* 21:221–228.

82. Quebec Task Force on Spinal Disorders (1987): Scientific approach to the assessment and management of activity-related spinal disorders: A monograph for clinicians. Report of the Quebec Task Force on Spinal Disorders. *Spine* 12:S1–S59.

83. Quinet RJ, Hadler NM (1979): Diagnosis and treatment of backache. *Semin Arthritis Rheum* 8:261–287.

84. Rockey PH, Tompkins RK, Wood RW, Wolcott BW (1978): The usefulness of x-ray examinations in the evaluation of patients with back pain. *J Fam Pract* 7:455–465.

85. Roth SH (1988): Nonsteroidal anti-inflammatory drugs: Gastropathy, deaths, and medical practice. *Ann Intern Med* 109:353–354.

86. Sackett DL, Haynes RB, Tugwell P (1985): Compliance. In: *Clinical epidemiology: A basic science for clinical medicine.* Boston: Little, Brown.

87. Skrabanek P (1984): Acupuncture and the age of unreason. *Lancet* 1:1169–1171.

88. Thorsteinsson G, Stonnington HH, Stillwell GK, Elveback LR (1978): The placebo effect of transcutaneous electrical stimulation. *Pain* 5:31–41.

89. Waddell G (1987): 1987 Volvo award in clinical sciences. A new clinical model for the treatment of low-back pain. *Spine* 12:632–644.

90. Waddell G, Main CJ, Morris EW, et al (1982): Normality and reliability in the clinical assessment of backache. *Br Med J* 284:1519–1523.

91. Weber H (1973): Traction therapy in sciatica due to disc prolapse. *J Oslo City Hosp* 23:167–176.

92. Weber H, Ljunggren AE, Walker L (1984): Traction therapy in patients with herniated lumbar intervertebral discs. *J Oslo City Hosp* 34:61–70.

93. White AW (1966): Low back pain in men receiving workmen's compensation. *Can Med Assoc J* 95:50–56.

94. White AA 3d, Gordon SL (1982): Synopsis: Workshop on idiopathic low-back pain. *Spine* 7:141–149.

95. Wiesel SW, Cuckler JM, DeLuca F, et al (1980): Acute low-back pain: An objective analysis of conservative therapy. *Spine* 5:324–330.

96. Williams PC (1965): *The lumbosacral spine, emphasizing conservative management.* New York: McGraw Hill.

97. Brown BR Jr, Womble J (1978): Cyclobenzaprine in intractable pain syndromes with muscle spasm. *JAMA* 240:1151–1152.

The Adult Spine: Principles and Practice,
J. W. Frymoyer, Editor-in-Chief.
Raven Press, Ltd., New York © 1991.

CHAPTER 73

Spinal Manipulative Therapy in the Management of Low Back Pain

Scott Haldeman and Reed B. Phillips

DEFINITION AND HISTORY

Spinal manipulative therapy (SMT), also referred to as manipulation, manual therapy, or manual medicine, can be broadly defined as including all procedures where the hands are used to mobilize, adjust, manipulate, apply traction, massage, stimulate, or otherwise influence the spine and paraspinal tissues with the aim of influencing the patient's health. Some form of spinal manipula-

S. Haldeman, D.C., M.D., Ph.D., F.R.C.P.: Department of Neurology, University of California, Irvine; Consulting Neurologist, Santa Ana, California 92701.
R. B. Phillips, D.C., D.A.C.B.R., M.C.S.M., Ph.D.: Research Director, Los Angeles College of Chiropractic, Whittier, California 90609.

tion has been used by physicians since ancient times and has been referred to in the writings of such prominent authorities as Hippocrates (400 BC), Galen (130–120 BC), Avicenna (960–1037 AD), Ambrose Paré (1510–1590 AD), Percivall Pott (1715–1788), Sir James Paget (1844–1899) and many others (79,112).

Primitive forms of manipulation of the spine appear to have been available and widely used by almost every society in recorded history, from the ancient Roman, Greek, Japanese, and South American civilizations, through the Middle Ages including the folk medicines of India, Egypt, Bohemia, China, and Finland, to modern times (41,79,110,112). Throughout history, and in almost every society, some physician has evolved with the ability and skill to provide spinal manipulation as a service.

The past few years has seen a marked increase in the utilization of spinal manipulative therapy and its incorporation in the management of patients with low back pain. In 1976, it was estimated that 90 million patient visits, by 3.6% to 5% of the population, were made to chiropractors in the United States (20,52). By 1980, this estimate had increased to 120 million office visits per year (124). Over 50% of these visits to chiropractors were due to low back pain (7,123). Deyo (23) estimates that 30% of the low back pain population in the United States is seen by chiropractors.

There has been a rapid expansion of interest in SMT by medical physicians, physical therapists, and osteopaths. Increasing numbers of physicians are incorporating manipulation into their practices either by learning the technical skills themselves or by working more closely with other practitioners.

However, agreement on the effectiveness or role of manipulation in the management of patients with low back pain is lacking. Discussion on the topic has now moved from expression of strongly held opinions to one of academic debate as increasing amounts of research have been performed on the efficacy and methods of action. It is impossible for any physician who treats patients with low back pain to avoid discussion of the topic of spinal manipulation since a significant number of their patients will have received or will be considering this form of treatment. Understanding of the various theories, techniques of manipulation, research trials, indications and contraindications for manipulation is therefore becoming increasingly necessary for all clinicians who treat patients with low back pain.

CLINICAL EFFICACY

From 30% to 50% of all spinal manipulations administered each year are for the treatment of low back pain (7,96). Hence, the main thrust of clinical research into the effectiveness of SMT has been in the area of low back pain.

Reports from uncontrolled prospective and retrospective case studies have been difficult to interpret (53,91). The percentage of patients with low back pain who respond favorably to spinal manipulation varies from 51% in patients hospitalized for low back pain (15) to over 90% in patients seen in a private practitioner's office (5,34,108). The relative importance of the variation in manipulative skills and patient selection in explaining this difference is not clear (8,53).

An increased number of controlled clinical trials, which compare the results of manipulation to different forms of placebo treatments as well as many of the recognized conservative forms of treatments for low back pain, have been published. These trials have been summarized in Table 1 where the most optimistic results from the various papers have been quoted. In many cases, positive results were not seen on re-examination of patients after different periods of treatment (10,25,45); in other cases, positive results were seen to varying degrees (2,51,125). For specific criticism of this research one can refer to papers by Nachemson (93), Haldeman (53,55), Greenland et al. (49), Brunarski (8), and Ottenbacher and DiFabio (100).

In the mid 1970s, detuned ultrasound was used as a placebo in clinical trials testing the effectiveness of manipulation (3,44). Glover et al. (44) found manipulation to be significantly more effective than the placebo only in those patients who had their pain for less than seven days. This disappointing result may have been due to the fact that a relatively crude long lever manipulation was used. The results of Bergquist-Ullman and Larsson (3), on the other hand, showed significant improvement of more specific articulating and mobilization techniques over the placebo. The patients undergoing manipulation showed less pain after six weeks, less sick leave following treatment, and a *decreased* tendency to change their occupation. Manipulation combined with physiotherapy, however, was not found to be significantly more effective than a sophisticated and well organized back school.

The study by Coxhead et al. (18) suggests that combining treatments was more effective than utilizing a single treatment protocol. When manipulation, traction, exercise, and corsets were offered at the same time, the improvement rate increased from 69% for a single treatment protocol to 88%. Patients were also less likely to return for further treatment at a later date if they had received multiple treatment modalities.

When compared to bed rest and analgesia (19), analgesia alone (31), short wave therapy (106), heat, exercise, and massage (29), or mobilization (51), manipulation appears to be a significantly more effective method of treating low back pain. The only studies where the authors felt that there were no significant differences between the effectiveness of manipulation and the other conservative forms of treatment for low back pain were those by Doran and Newell (25) and by Godfrey et al. (45). However, a re-evaluation of the statistics from the Doran and Newell study has suggested that manipulation was indeed significantly more effective than the other treatment modalities after three weeks (49).

The studies at the University of California at Irvine (9,10,12,58) have helped to rule out the psychological effect of laying on of hands. By selecting patients who were unable to tell the difference between a manipulative thrust and simple massage, it was possible to demonstrate that there is something intrinsic to the manipulation which appeared to cause improvement of symptoms in patients with low back pain.

The positive effects of manipulation reported in these trials all appear to occur either immediately after the manipulation is given or within the first four to six weeks

TABLE 1. *Comparative and controlled trials on the effectiveness of manipulation in patients with low back pain (% improved)*

Reference	Time period	Manipulation	Analgesia and bed rest	Heat massage exercise	+ or − short wave	Physiotherapy	Back school	Massage	Corsets	Traction	Mobilization	Comments
Coyer and Curwen (19)	1 week	55%	27%									No stats
	6 weeks	88%	72%									No stats
Rasmussen (106)	2 weeks	92%			24%							p < 0.01
Evans et al. (31)	3 weeks	60%	18%									p < 0.05
Doran and Newell (25)	3 weeks	64%	49%			52%			49%			p < 0.05
	3 months	71%	56%			67%			68%			No stats
Glover et al. (44)	immediate	43%			12%							p < 0.05
	7 days	85%			70%							No stats
Sims-Williams et al. (113)	1 month	90%			73%							p < 0.1
Buerger (10)	immediate	83%						67%				p < 0.003
Bergquist-Ullman and Larsson (3)	1 year	40%			29%		36%					Without reference
Coxhead et al. (18)	4 weeks	53%		49%					50%	50%		Mean improvement
Hoehler et al. (58)	immediate	84%						68%				p < 0.05
	3 weeks	88%						68%				p < 0.05
Gibson et al. (1989)	2 weeks	12%			3%							No stats
	4 weeks	28%			28%							No stats
	12 weeks	42%			37%							No stats
Arkuszewski (2)	6 months	32%	12%									p < 0.05
Hadler et al. (51)	1 week	50%									10%	p < 0.025

Where different types of assessment or multiple assessments at different time periods were done, the most favorable results from manipulation are quoted. References should be checked for details.

of treatment. Attempts at evaluating the long term effects of a brief, two to four week treatment period using manipulation have not demonstrated any significant difference over controls at three or twelve months (3,18,58,113). However, no investigations have as yet been undertaken to determine the long-term effect of intermittent or regular manipulation, a protocol which is not uncommonly followed by certain practitioners of manipulation. Ottenbacher and DiFabio (100) did a meta-analysis on 57 studies on manipulation/mobilization. Their conclusions indicated that those studies which did not employ random assignment were more likely to support manipulation/mobilization. Furthermore, the use of manual therapy in conjunction with other therapies was more effective, especially when treatment effects were measured immediately following therapy.

Due to the psychosocial component of low back pain, subjective measures in the form of questionnaires and self-reporting data-gathering instruments are becoming

more accepted (see McDowell and Newell, ref. 88, for a complete review).

OBJECTIVE CHANGES FOLLOWING MANIPULATION

Attempts to document objective physical or radiographic changes following manipulation have been difficult. A number of research protocols have looked at range of motion as an objective measurement. Rasmussen (106) found significant improvement in the range of motion following manipulation when measuring the C7 to S1 difference in length on standing and forward flexion (for a review of the reliability issues associated with range of motion measures of the lumbar spine, see Liebenson and Phillips, ref. 76).

Fisk (37) demonstrated a statistical increase in straight leg raising in patients with back pain following manipulation when compared to manipulation in control subjects without pain. Bergquist-Ullman et al. (3) and Hoehler et al. (58) also demonstrated greater improvement in straight leg raising following manipulation compared with a placebo, as did Matthews et al. (85).

Roberts et al. (109) failed to show any roentgenographic changes in vertebral position following manipulation of the lumbar spine. Functional radiography is a common method used for evaluating spinal motion (27,68). Although changes in lumbar range of motion after manipulation have not been documented using x-rays, there are two reports of increased cervical range of motion following manipulation (59,62). Mathews and Yates (84) reported two patients where disc prolapses seen by epidurography were reduced by manipulation, but Wilson and Frederick (129) were unable to show changes in myelographic defects after manipulation under anesthesia. Similarly, Chrisman et al. (15) found that manipulation was much less effective in patients with myelographic evidence of disc herniation than in those with normal myelograms, and no change in myelographic appearance occurred after manipulation.

Attempts to look at muscle spasm before and after manipulation have been made by Grice (50) and by Diebert and England (24). Both of these papers reported changes in surface electromyographic activity in paraspinal muscles following manipulation. The number of patients studied and the recording methodology in these trials are open to criticism, thus further trials will be necessary to determine whether manipulation does have a positive effect on muscle spasm.

A 1984 paper by Terrett and Vernon (116) is of interest and has led to the suggestion that manipulation may influence cutaneous pain tolerance mechanisms. These authors report a 140% change in the level of paraspinal cutaneous pain tolerance following manipulation compared to controls. The possibility that this change in pain tolerance may be due to a release of endorphins has been suggested by Vernon et al. (122). They reported a small but statistically significant increase in serum beta endorphin levels in a small group of patients following spinal manipulation. The specificity and sensitivity of the techniques used for these determinations are not reported.

Other recent work has demonstrated quantifiable gait changes in low back pain patients treated by chiropractic manipulation (57). This work is in its early stages of development.

A THEORETICAL MODEL

Both practitioners and critics of manipulation have shown extreme ingenuity in the formulation of theories that might explain the clinical results from SMT. In the past, and to a lesser extent even today, practitioners of SMT can be separated into different schools (or professions) depending on adherence to a particular theory.

The major theories on which manipulation is based include the reduction of disc prolapse (21,82), the correction of posterior joint dysfunction (87), the mobilization of fixated or blocked vertebral joints (42,75,83,111), the reduction of nerve root compression (97,101), the normalization of reflex activity (60,72,80), and the relaxation of muscles (102). These theories have been the subject of debate at a number of conferences (11,46,54,73).

Increasing research into the pathology and physiology of back pain (39) has helped consolidate many of these theories into a model which is increasingly being used to explain the mechanism of action in manipulation. The model remains a generalized one, however, with many unexplained or untested components.

The model makes the assumption that spinal manipulation *influences* spinal motion. This is not an unreasonable assumption. Manipulation is primarily a force exerted against a movable spinal structure and is commonly associated with a click or pop to suggest that a joint has moved. As noted earlier, there is some evidence that manipulation does cause increased range of motion although this has not been firmly established. Spinal motion has been shown to have a beneficial effect on the nutrition and metabolism of the intervertebral disc (94) and restricted motion has been shown to be detrimental to peripheral synovial joints (1) and intervertebral discs (39). Spinal motion has been assumed to have beneficial effects on neurogenic reflexes (130) and may be responsible for relief of muscle spasm and other neurophysiological consequences related to its positive effects.

These considerations have led to the postulation of motion barriers that can be influenced by manipulation. The model is presented in Figure 1A. In this model, there are different ranges of motion for each spinal joint. The "active" range of motion is that motion which can be influenced by muscles. It is the range of motion in which exercise is performed and which is limited by the leverage capacity of muscles surrounding the joint. Beyond the active range of motion is the "passive" range of motion where stretching and mobilization techniques are utilized. The limit of this range of motion is the so called "physiologic barrier." Beyond that range is a smaller range of motion through which a joint can be moved without disrupting its ligaments. This so-called "paraphysiologic space" can be entered by a quick thrust in the direction of joint movement and results in the "pop" or "snap" that is a vacuum phenomenon in the joint and commonly occurs during the manipulation. The limit of this range is the so-called "anatomic barrier" and any attempt to exceed this limit will result in tearing of ligaments or bony collapse.

Restricted motion under this model can result in three ways (Figs. 1B–1D): First, the muscle may go into spasm or shorten due to contracture. The first of the three barriers is moved toward the neutral position. To restore

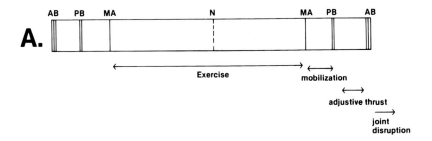

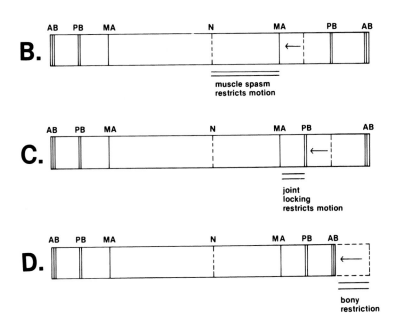

N = neutral position
MA = limit of muscle activity
PB = physiologic barrier
AB = anatomic barrier

FIG. 1. A conceptual model **(A–D)** for mobilization and manipulation.

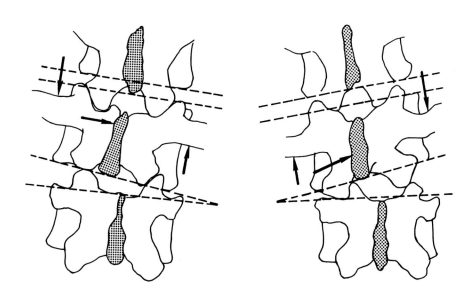

FIG. 2. The more classic method of "listing" vertebral position according to the direction of intervertebral disc wedging and the position of the spinous process in relation to the vertebral body. The arrows indicate the direction in which an adjustive thrust may be administered in each case.

motion one has to release the muscle spasm or stretch the shortened muscles. Second, the joint may lock on one side pulling the physiologic barrier toward the neutral point. This may or may not result in simultaneous movement of the anatomic barrier or the muscle activity barrier. Mechanisms for this restriction in motion include articular synovial pinching and disc herniation. To release this motion restriction it is necessary to give a manipulative thrust into the paraphysiologic space to stretch the ligaments and open the facets. Third, the bony structures may block movement through spur formation or deformity. Manipulation is not able to help in restoring motion in these cases.

INDICATIONS FOR MANIPULATION

The selection of patients who might benefit from SMT is difficult due to poor understanding of the pathogenesis of back pain and the unsophisticated techniques available to examine the spine. The breakdown of back pain into numerous different diagnostic categories has been somewhat controversial (92). However, studies on large groups of patients undergoing SMT have found differing results in patients diagnosed as having different symptom complexes or specifically diagnosed origins of their pain (66,69,103,108). This documentation has helped define those conditions most likely to respond to SMT (Table 2).

Uncomplicated Acute Low Back Pain (Quebec Classification Type 1)

This non-specific diagnostic category is used to include those patients with low back pain of recent onset in the absence of leg pain or radicular signs. It is this category of patients which Glover et al. (44) and Farrell and Twomey (33) found to be significantly more responsive following manipulation compared to a placebo treatment. The response was most obvious immediately after manipulation was given. The patients who responded to

TABLE 2. *Indications for manipulation in patients with low back pain*

Uncomplicated low back pain (lumbago)
Sciatica without neurological deficit
Uncomplicated chronic low back pain
Post-surgical chronic low back pain
Intervertebral disc degeneration, Type IV; bulging disc
Posterior facet syndrome
Sacroiliac syndrome
Sacroiliac strain
Piriformis syndrome
Psoas syndrome
Spondylolisthesis
Spinal stenosis: central stenosis and lateral entrapment

manipulation in the trial by Bergquist-Ullman and Larsson (3) had a median duration of symptoms of less than nine days prior to entering their trial. The trials by Buerger (9) and Rasmussen (106) were also on acute low back pain patients. Potter (103) noted that patients with acute back pain had the highest response rate compared to other groups of patients, with 93% of such patients either fully recovered or much improved following manipulation. Hadler (51) found manipulation to be more effective than mobilization in acute low back pain patients also.

Complicated Acute Low Back Pain (Quebec Classification Type 2 and 3)

These patients complain of low back pain of recent onset with either leg pain or neurological deficits. Leg pain or sciatica appears to respond very well to SMT (36,82,85). Both Potter (103) and Edwards (29) found that over 75% of patients with pain radiating into the buttock or down the leg recovered or improved considerably following spinal manipulation. Painful limited straight leg raising was one of the objective parameters shown to improve following spinal SMT in the blinded clinical trial by Buerger (9). When frank neurological deficit is present, many practitioners of manipulation become much more cautious (21,36). Most of the trials quoted earlier excluded patients with such deficits. Where patients with acute neurological deficit have been subjected to SMT, the results have been less rewarding (69,89,103,115).

Uncomplicated Chronic Low Back Pain

The only report that compares the results of SMT in patients with acute and chronic back pain is that by Potter (103). He concluded that chronic pain sufferers are less responsive to SMT but nevertheless reported an improvement in 71% of these patients. Ongley et al. (99) also found statistically significant treatment effects in the chronic low back pain patient utilizing manipulation in conjunction with injections compared to injections without manipulation. The results of SMT on patients referred to a university hospital for chronic back pain reported by Kirkaldy-Willis (66) varied greatly depending on the pathologic diagnosis, but in all cases over 65% of patients showed some degree of improvement. It should be remembered that this group of patients, by definition, were not recovering spontaneously.

Complicated Chronic Low Back Pain

The comments made about patients with acute low back pain complicated by leg pain or neurological deficit applies equally well to patients with chronic back pain. Potter (103) found that chronic leg pain improved in approximately 70% of patients treated with SMT, the number of successes dropping considerably when neurological signs were present. One interesting aspect of this study was the observation that previous back surgery did not significantly alter the results and therefore did not serve as a contraindication to manipulation. Kirkaldy-Willis and Cassidy (69) reported that patients with referred pain syndromes showed an improvement rate of 81% but if nerve compression signs and symptoms were present the improvement rate dropped to 48%.

Disc Degeneration and/or Herniation

The effect of spinal manipulation on intervertebral disc disease is controversial. Cyriax (21) and Maigne (82) think that the primary effect of manipulation is the reduction of nuclear protrusions in the disc. Mathews and Yates (84) claim to have demonstrated the reduction of disc prolapses by epidurography. On the other hand, Chrisman et al. (15) reported that manipulation in the patients with disc protrusion demonstrable by myelography was much less effective than in patients with normal myelograms. They were unable to demonstrate any reduction in positive myelogram findings following manipulation. Kirkaldy-Willis and Cassidy (66,69) were similarly unimpressed with the results of manipulation in patients with demonstrable lumbar disc herniation. Nonetheless, manipulation is being widely recommended for patients diagnosed as having intervertebral disc degeneration without frank herniation or neurological deficit (21,82,115,126).

The Posterior Facet Syndrome

Mennell (87), Lewit (75), and Gillett (42) are among the many practitioners of spinal manipulation who believe that the primary effect of manipulation is the mobilization of "fixated" or "blocked" posterior facet joints. In the differentiation of patients with chronic back pain by Kirkaldy-Willis (66), 72% of patients diagnosed as having posterior facet syndrome improved following SMT, a result he concluded was disappointing if the posterior facets were, in fact, the primary site of action of SMT. The later study by Kirkaldy-Willis and Cassidy (69) showed some improvement to 79% but noted that the presence of lumbar instability greatly reduced the effectiveness of SMT.

The Sacroiliac Syndromes

Some of the best results from spinal manipulation have been reported in patients where the diagnosis of sacroiliac syndrome has been made. Kirkaldy-Willis and Cassidy (66,69) and Riches (108) claim that over 90% of patients with this diagnosis show improvement in their back pain following manipulation. Many practitioners of manipulation (43,47,78) place a great deal of emphasis on the analysis of sacroiliac motion and position and choose their manipulation technique according to these findings. If one makes the diagnosis of sacroiliac syndrome, manipulation appears to be a very effective method of treatment. Sacroiliac and posterior joint syndromes have been reported to exist in combination in certain patients who respond well to manipulation (69).

The Muscle Syndromes

A variety of muscles have been implicated in the genesis of back pain including piriformis, psoas, quadratus lumborum, and the long paraspinal muscles (60,86,121). Specific manipulation techniques have been developed with the aim of stretching or manually massaging these muscles in an attempt to relax them (32). The importance of these muscle syndromes in the genesis of back pain remains speculative. However, if the diagnosis is made, we believe the treatment of choice is either manipulation or the injection of a local anesthetic.

Spondylolisthesis

Back pain associated with isthmic spondylolisthesis was found to improve through spinal manipulation in 85% of cases reviewed by Kirkaldy-Willis and Cassidy (66). These authors made it quite clear that no claim was being made that spinal manipulation influenced the degree of displacement of the lesion. Instead, they speculate that in most cases the spondylolisthesis was an incidental finding. Care was taken by these clinicians to avoid any direct force at the area of slippage. Manipulations were, instead, directed at the sacroiliac joint or the posterior joints above the level of slippage. The one point which appears to arise from this observation is that spondylolisthesis is in itself not a contraindication to nontraumatic specific short lever manipulation in skilled hands.

Spinal Stenosis

The results of manipulation in patients whose low back pain is diagnosed as being due to spinal stenosis are not good. Kirkaldy-Willis and Cassidy (66,69) and Potter (104) reported that a significant number of patients with either lateral spinal nerve entrapment or central spinal stenosis showed some improvement following manipulation. Very few of these patients became symptom free. Case reports on the beneficial effects of manipulation in patients with neurogenic claudication thought to be due to spinal stenosis have been presented by Henderson (56). Even in this report the relief these patients obtain from SMT was usually temporary.

CONTRAINDICATIONS TO MANIPULATION

Spinal manipulative therapy should not be considered a totally innocuous procedure. Although there are less than 100 reported cases where serious complications of manipulative therapy have occurred (70,77), these complications are often quite devastating. Extreme care should therefore be taken in the selection of patients and choice of manipulative techniques in order to minimize their occurrence.

By far the major portion of severe complications comes from injury to the cerebral circulation or spinal cord following cervical manipulation (4,70,117). Injuries from lumbar spine manipulation are much less common. The most frequently reported complication is the prolapse of a herniated intervertebral disc resulting in a cauda equina syndrome (61,107,115). These complications are probably due to the use of long lever, high force rotational manipulative techniques in the side lying position (70). The other painful complication of lumbar rotational or thoracic manipulation is spraining of the costovertebral or costochondral joints during rotation of the trunk. These painful incidents are again attributed to poor technique (70,82).

The contraindications for manipulation of the lumbar spine are listed in Table 3 and, for the most part, are based on common sense. They include the following.

TABLE 3. *Contraindications for high velocity manipulation techniques on the lumbar spine*

Unstable fractures
Severe osteoporosis
Multiple myeloma
Osteomyelitis
Primary bone tumors
Metastatic bone tumors
Paget's disease
Any progressive neurological deficit
Spinal cord tumors
Cauda equina compression
Central intervertebral disc herniations
Hypermobile joints
Rheumatoid arthritis
Inflammatory phase of ankylosing spondylitis
Psoriatic arthritis
Reiter's syndrome
Anticoagulant therapy
Congenital bleeding disorders
Acquired bleeding disorders
Inadequate physical and spinal examination
Poor manipulative skills

Under certain circumstances soft tissue non-force manipulation or mobilization procedures may still be possible.

Weakening of Bone Structure

Unstable fractures, severe osteoporosis, osteomyelitis, multiple myeloma, bony tumors, or any other disorder which results in weakened bone structure is the most obvious contraindication to spinal manipulation. Therefore, a patient who is being considered for manipulation should be carefully evaluated to exclude these conditions.

Severe or Progressive Neurological Deficits

There is some debate whether or not spinal manipulation should be applied to patients showing minor stable signs of radicular injury. Many practitioners of manipulation would not be inhibited from using light mobilization or traction maneuvers in such patients. Patients with signs of progressive neurological loss, acute cauda equina compression, or a spinal cord lesion, on the other hand, may require immediate surgical intervention and should not be subjected to any form of manipulation therapy.

Acute Inflammatory Joint Disease

The forceful manipulation of any joint that is acutely inflamed can be very painful. This is also true of the sacroiliac and posterior spinal articulations. For this reason, patients with such disorders as rheumatoid arthritis and the spondyloarthropathies should be carefully evaluated for any sign of acute inflammation of the spinal joints before manipulation is attempted. The ligamentous laxity and joint instability that can result from these disorders may also serve as contraindications to manipulation in the dormant stage of the arthritis, especially when this occurs in the cervical spine (70).

Bleeding Disorders

Manipulation of patients on anti-coagulant therapy can cause intraspinal hematoma formation (22). Therefore, patients who are on anti-coagulant therapy or who have a clotting abnormality, either inherited or acquired (e.g., liver disease), should not be subjected to any forceful manipulations.

Inadequate Examination or Manipulative Skills

Perhaps one of the greatest problems today in manipulation is the attempt by clinicians to apply these techniques without formal training. Reading a textbook or attending a weekend course does not convert an untrained clinician into a skilled practitioner of SMT. Many of the reported injuries following spinal manipulation can be attributed to inadequate examination to rule out contraindications or to the use of crude, long lever, high force techniques. In the same way, many of the disappointing results from manipulation which have been reported involved the use of primitive non-specific procedures. The expected results and number of complications are dependent on the ability of the clinician. Lack of examination and manipulative skills should therefore be considered a contraindication to SMT.

THE MANIPULABLE SPINAL LESION

One way of reviewing the principles on which spinal manipulation is based is to look at the clinical characteristics of the lesion to which the manipulation is applied. Despite the wide variation in the theorized mechanism of action of SMT, there is an amazing amount of agreement on the clinical nature of the manipulable spinal lesion. This lesion, also referred to as the subluxation, osteopathic lesion, vertebral fixation or blockage, spinal dysfunction, etc., has specific characteristics listed below and is determined primarily by manual palpation.

Over the past few years a number of studies have been performed to determine whether practitioners of manipulation can agree as to the nature and location of the manipulable lesion. An interesting observation was made at an international meeting on manipulation in 1984 (26). Clinicians from six countries were asked to localize the spinal lesion on patients without knowledge of clinical symptoms or the findings of other examiners. There was amazingly good agreement between these clinicians as to the level of the lesion, especially since there was considerable disagreement as to what constituted a manipulable lesion. Johnston (64) asked three to five examiners to examine a series of patients independently. He noted a high degree of inter-examiner agreement, which could not have been achieved by chance. Admittedly, the examiners required adhesive vertebral markers at different levels in order to achieve these results. McConnell et al. (81), on the other hand, showed a very low correlation in the findings of different osteopathic clinicians using their own techniques without any palpatory clues. Wiles (128) looked at the ability of pairs of examiners to agree on abnormalities in sacroiliac motion. Certain parameters of sacroiliac motion were palpated at a high level of correlation while others were not, and the degree of correlation seemed to relate to the degree of expertise and experience of the examining clinician.

Vertebral Malposition

Repeated studies on large groups of patients have shown that there is no relationship between vertebral malposition and low back pain (40,74,90). Nevertheless, many practitioners of manipulation continue to make fine radiographic measurements of vertebral positional relationships prior to manipulation. The prime reason for determining these relationships in practice is to determine the direction in which the manipulative thrust should be given, rather than the determination of the level of pathology. If the slope of the facets and the position of the vertebrae are known, a much smaller, less traumatic force can be given to correct the "manipulable lesion."

The so-called "listing" of the position of a vertebra is determined by measuring the direction in which the disc is wedged and noting the position of the spinous process in relation to its body (47,114). Figure 2 illustrates four of the classic spinal listings and demonstrates how such a listing might influence the direction in which a manipulation would be given. The significance and importance of these listings has yet to be evaluated. However, clinicians who take into account structural relationships of the vertebrae are convinced that they are capable of administering a more specific manipulation with greater ease and less trauma to the patient.

Abnormal Vertebral Motion

As already noted, the most widely held view on the primary effect of manipulation is that it increases the range of motion at a joint (83,87,115). The major criteria for the manipulable lesion by clinicians who adhere to this point of view are therefore "restriction," "fixation," or "blockage" of motion at a specific joint in the spine. The location and characteristics of the fixation must therefore be determined before a manipulation can be given. The primary technique for this evaluation is the palpation of motion in the various joints of the spine. Specific techniques for palpating motion in the sacroiliac joint and lumbar spine have been developed and are widely used.

There are multitudes of techniques for palpating motion at the sacroiliac joint (42,43,67,115). The following three-step procedure is one of the simpler methods.

Step 1

The examiner stands behind the patient and places his thumbs on the patient's posterior superior iliac spines gripping the iliac wings with his/her fingers. The patient is asked to elevate and flex his knee as high as possible. Normally this maneuver will cause the ilium on the side of the flexed leg to rotate posterior. The posterior superior iliac spine on that side will appear to dip inferior relative to the opposite side. Fixation of both sacroiliac joints will prevent movement of one ilium relative to the other and this motion will not be felt.

A

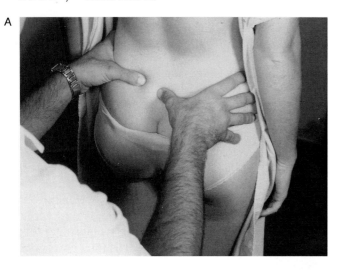

B

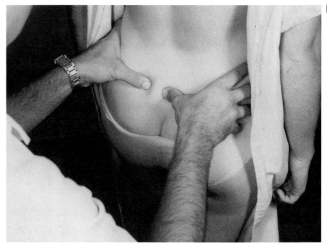

C

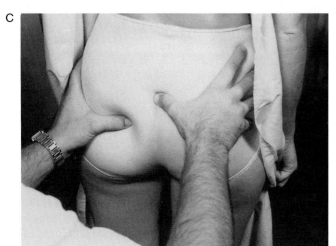

D

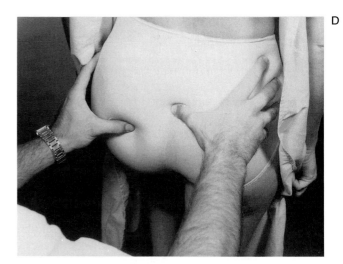

FIG. 3. Basic motion palpation tests for the sacroiliac joint. Test 1: One thumb is placed on the left posterior superior iliac spines (PSIS), the other on the second sacral tubercle (**A**). On elevation of the left leg, the PSIS on that side moves inferior (**B**). Test 2: One thumb is placed on the left ischium, the other is placed on the sacral apex (**C**). On elevation of the left leg, the ischium moves anterior and lateral (**D**).

Step 2

In the same position, the examiner palpates one posterior superior iliac spine with the thumb of one hand and palpates the second sacral tubercle with the thumb of the other hand (Fig. 3A). The patient is again asked to elevate the knee as high as possible on the side where the iliac spine is being palpated. With normal sacroiliac movement, the iliac spine will again be felt to dip posterior and inferior relative to the sacrum (Fig. 3B). Failure to perceive this movement is considered indicative of fixation of the upper portion of the sacroiliac joint on the side being palpated.

Step 3

The examiner can now attempt to palpate motion in the lower half of the sacroiliac joint by placing one

thumb on the ischium as close to the inferior aspect of the sacroiliac joint as possible (Fig. 3C). The thumb of the other hand is placed on the apex or tip of the sacrum. The patient once again elevates the knee as high as possible. The ischial contact point will normally be felt to move anterior, superior, and lateral relative to the sacral apex (Fig. 3D). Fixation of the inferior sacroiliac joint will prevent this movement.

Numerous variations of these palpation methods as well as techniques for determining movement of the sacroiliac joint during spinal flexion and lateral bending have been described.

The palpation of motion between segments of the lumbar spine is best perceived with the patient sitting (14,43,82). Each of the normal movements of lumbar spine may be palpated individually.

1. Flexion-extension motion can be perceived by palpating the interspinous space using the fingers or

A 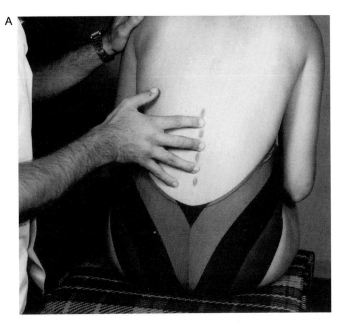 B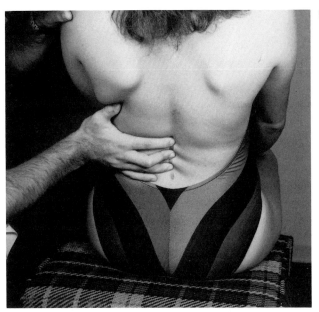

FIG. 4. A method for palpating flexion and extension movement in the lumbar spine. The fingertips are placed between the spinous processes, and the patient is moved into flexion and extension. **A:** Flexion palpation. **B:** Extension palpation.

hand. The examiner's non-palpating arm is used to grip the patient's shoulders and move the lumbar spine into flexion and extension. A smooth opening and closing of the interspinous spaces can be felt if normal motion is present (Fig. 4).

2. Lateral flexion motion is determined in a similar manner. The relative position of two adjacent spinous processes is determined by hooking the lower spinous process with one finger and pushing the upper spinous process with the other. The patient is passively assisted into lateral flexion by moving the patient's shoulders. Movement of the upper spinous process over the lower one can be perceived and absence of this movement is suggestive of a lateral bending fixation at that level.

3. In order to examine rotational movement, the examiner palpates two adjacent spinous processes and guides the patient's trunk into rotation. Movement of the superior spinous process over the inferior one can be perceived and should give the feeling of a step at the limit of rotation.

Lack of Joint Play

Springing of a joint and the determination of joint play and end feel is an integral part of the pre-manipulation spinal examination (82,87).

Neutral or static joint play is determined by springing each vertebra in the neutral position in both flexion/extension and rotation/lateral flexion directions. The patient is placed in the prone position with the abdomen supported. Lateral pressure is exerted over the spinous process from each side using the examiner's thumb. Counter pressure on the spinous process above or below with the thumb of the other hand can help localize the direction in which the vertebra is being stressed. Normally a pain-free spongy or "springy" movement can be perceived. Extreme tenderness with hard resistance to this pressure is considered an important indicator of a clinically significant manipulable lesion (82,87). Joint springing in the flexion/extension direction is accomplished by pressing over the transverse processes of the lumbar vertebrae unilaterally or bilaterally (Fig. 5).

The evaluation of "end play" or "end feel" is achieved through the same technique as that used for motion palpation. The vertebral joint being tested is placed at the limit of its passive range of motion and then stressed slightly beyond this limit (Fig. 6). A soft, springy, painless end feel at the limit of each motion should be palpable. The presence of pain or the feeling of solid resistance at the limit of motion is considered abnormal (42,82,87).

Palpable Soft Tissue Changes

On palpating the paraspinal tissues some clinicians believe it is possible to feel areas of subcutaneous tissue "thickening" or muscle contraction which are exquisitely tender. These "taut and tender fibers" or trigger points can be found in the long paraspinal muscles, shoulder girdle muscles (infraspinatus, supraspinatus, trapezius, rhomboids, levator scapulae), the pelvis (iliopsoas, piriformis, quadratus lumborum, glutei, tensor

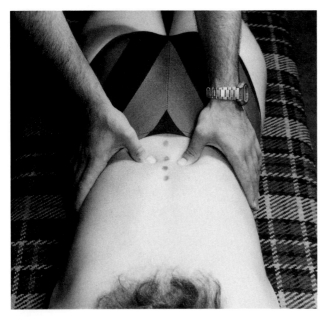

FIG. 5. The palpation of flexion and extension joint play in the neutral position by springing one segment of the lumbar spine.

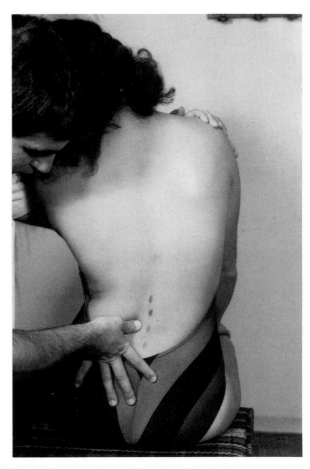

FIG. 6. The palpation of "end feel" in the lumbar spine on lateral flexion.

fascia lata), spinal ligaments (iliolumbar, anterior and posterior sacroiliac, interspinous, supraspinous, fascia lata), and bony prominences (posterior superior iliac spines, spinous processes, femoral trochanter). In the absence of a destructive lesion, these soft tissue changes are considered important indicators of the lesion which may respond to manipulation (82,87).

Muscle Contraction or Imbalance

One of the major goals of many manipulative procedures is to stretch or stimulate contracted muscles (86,115,121). The determination of muscular function is therefore an important part of the pre-manipulation spinal examination. The muscles which are most commonly evaluated for tender contraction in patients with low back pain include the piriformis, iliopsoas, quadratus lumborum, glutei, and erector spinae. The following examples will serve to illustrate how muscle imbalance is determined.

The so-called piriformis syndrome presents as back pain with or without leg pain, external rotation of the leg at rest (Fig. 7), limited internal rotation of the leg with the hip extended, and extreme tenderness on palpation of the muscle at its insertion above the acetabulum or over its belly on palpation through the rectum (67,86).

The iliopsoas muscle has been considered an important factor in causing abnormal hyperextension of the lumbar spine. The evaluation of this muscle is accomplished by observing the change in lumbar lordosis in standing and sitting, measuring the degree of hip exten-

sion and palpating for tenderness in the muscle as it passes over the pubic ramus to attach to the femur.

The role of the quadratus lumborum muscles in lateral flexion of the lumbar spine has been described and a possible role in some forms of scoliosis proposed (71,98). Since a number of manipulative techniques are aimed partly at stretching this muscle, it should be examined. This is done by observing any restriction in the lateral flexion of the lumbar spine and any tenderness on palpation over the muscle just lateral to the erector spinae muscles (120).

If the legs are determined radiographically to be of equal length and one leg is found to be higher than the other on lying prone or supine (Fig. 8), the short leg is considered to be due to elevation of the hip and pelvis on that side secondary to imbalance of the paraspinal muscles (120).

Painful limitation of straight leg raising which is not accompanied by motor, sensory, or reflex changes, is not aggravated by dorsiflexion of the foot, and has no bowstring sign, may be due to stretching of tight hamstring muscles or restricted movement in the hip or sacroiliac joints rather than sciatic nerve irritation. Buerger

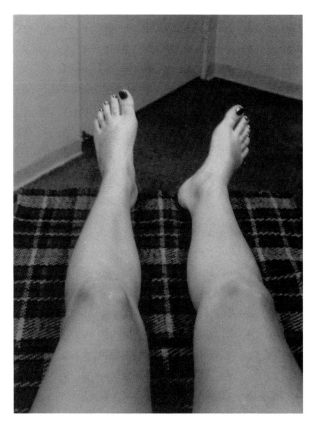

FIG. 7. The position of the legs in the supine position at rest in a patient with piriformis syndrome. Note the external rotation of the right leg thought to be caused by muscle imbalance.

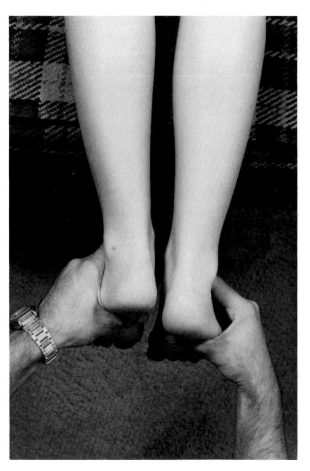

FIG. 8. Illustration of a functional short leg on the left in the absence of anatomical leg length deficiency. The shortening of the leg is thought to be secondary to paraspinal muscle imbalance.

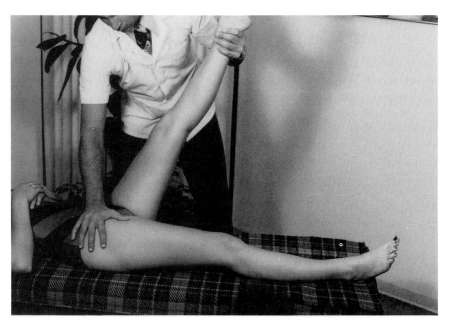

FIG. 9. The method for palpating pelvic tilt during straight leg raising.

(9) and Fisk (35) have shown that straight leg raising increases immediately after spinal manipulation when pelvis tilt is used as the end point for limited straight leg raising (Fig. 9). In the absence of sciatic nerve irritation, this maneuver first brings tension on the hip extensors followed by tilting of the pelvis and flattening of the lumbar lordosis.

MANIPULATIVE TECHNIQUES

The therapeutic goal of spinal manipulative therapy is to correct the manipulable lesion (subluxation, osteopathic lesion, somatic dysfunction, etc.), thereby presumably increasing motion in the hope that this, in turn, will benefit the patient. Since the exact mechanism of action of spinal manipulation and the nature of the lesion on which it has its effect are still theoretical, every manipulation must be considered a therapeutic trial. The effectiveness of any specific manipulative technique is therefore determined by its ability to correct the components of the manipulable lesion with the least amount of force and discomfort to the patient. The ideal manipulative procedure should take into account the structural relationship and facet orientation of the vertebrae being manipulated as well as any structural asymmetries. It should mobilize the areas of restricted or fixated joint movement, reduce painful or abnormal joint play and/or end feel, eliminate palpable soft tissue taut or tender fibers, and correct areas of muscle contraction or imbalance. These goals must be achieved without traumatizing the spinal or paraspinal tissues or causing pain.

There are a multitude of techniques which have been developed over the years to manipulate the spine. Each basic technique, in turn, has numerous variations and refinements. In the past there has been a tendency for practitioners of manipulation to form groups or factions under the leadership of a single teacher who has developed, perfected, and taught a particular system of techniques. Although this tendency is breaking down, there remain practitioners who practice exclusively those techniques as taught by Cyriax, while others practice techniques taught by Mennell, Lewit, Maigne, Paris, Kaltenbourn, Maitland, Palmer, Gonstead, DeJarnette, Toftness, Kimberly, Stoddard, Mitchell, etc. The relative effectiveness of one technique compared to another has yet to be evaluated, so the choice of manipulative technique continues to be based, to a large extent, on the skills a clinician has developed rather than on a rational understanding of the role of each separate manipulative procedure.

Although the adherents of many of these technique systems claim to have unique approaches to manipulation, the various techniques have much in common. It is possible to classify the majority of the spinal manipulative procedures into six subgroups. The remainder of the chapter will be devoted to a discussion of these six classes of manipulation. Examples have been chosen to illustrate the basic principles in each subgroup. It is impossible to describe every technique in detail. For further information, published textbooks and notes (see references) should be reviewed.

The Non-Specific Long Lever Manipulations

This class of manipulation includes all those procedures where a high velocity force is exerted on a part of the body some distance from the area where it is expected to have its beneficial effect. The long levers used for this type of manipulation include the leg, shoulder, pelvis, and thoracic spine. Although these manipulations have been widely used (17,21,44), they are generally considered to be the crudest and least effective of the manipulative techniques available. The long lever makes it very difficult, although not impossible, to make this type of manipulation specific to a particular segment. The force is exerted instead into a region of the spine. The segment which receives most of the mobilization is often the one which is already hypermobile rather than the vertebral level which is restricted. It is this type of manipulation which has been considered most likely to result in the herniation of degenerated intervertebral discs and damage to soft tissues.

The most commonly used long lever technique for the lumbar spine is the rotational manipulation described by Cyriax (21) and Coplans (17). The patient is placed in the lateral side lying position with the symptomatic side up. The hip and knee of the superior leg are flexed while the inferior leg is held in extension. The clinician stands in front of the patient and steadies the shoulder with his superior hand pushing it down to the table. With the other (inferior) hand, he contacts the pelvis or buttock and pulls the patient's pelvis toward him while letting the flexed leg hang over the side of the table (Fig. 10). The rotational slack is taken up with the inferior hand and a sharp controlled thrust is given to the pelvis or leg in the direction of rotation (downward and laterally).

There are a great number of variations to this technique:

1. It is possible to hook the foot of the patient's superior flexed leg into a popliteal fossa of the inferior leg. This allows the clinician to exert a force through the femur giving a long more powerful lever.

2. The patient can be placed in the supine position on the back with hips flexed and knees crossed. Both knees are twisted toward the clinician while the shoulders are kept flat on the table. The clinician holds the shoulders down with his superior hand while applying force through both legs at the knee. This forces rotation during lumbar side flexion.

3. A reversed long lever rotational manipulation can be

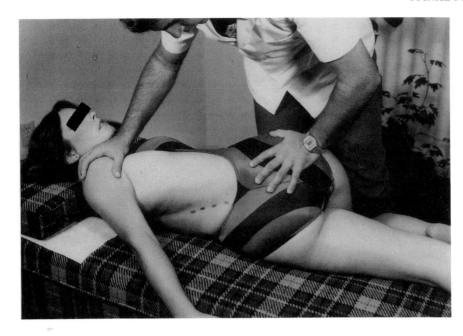

FIG. 10. The basic non-specific long lever rotational manipulation of the lumbar spine.

achieved by placing the patient in the side lying position with the clinician standing behind the patient. The thorax is rotated forward and the pelvis backward. The examiner forces the rotation by pressing simultaneously on the shoulder and pelvis.

The second group of non-specific manipulations are those that force extension of the lumbar spine. For most of these maneuvers the patient is asked to lie prone on the couch or table. The hands are placed either unilaterally or bilaterally alongside the spinous process. The patient is asked to relax, the slack in the lumbar spine is taken up, and a high velocity thrust forces the lumbar spine into extension. Considerably greater force can be exerted if one leg is elevated in extension and the other

used as a lever or simply held in maximum extension with one hand while the thrust is given with the other hand to the lumbar spine (Fig. 11).

It should be reiterated that these long lever manipulations are crude, non-specific, and potentially dangerous. Most experienced practitioners of manipulation seldom utilize them, and they are included here simply for completeness.

The Specific Short Lever High Velocity Spinal Adjustment

The manipulative procedure in widest usage by trained practitioners of SMT is the short lever high veloc-

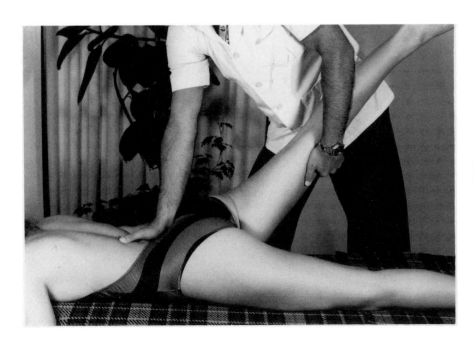

FIG. 11. The long lever extension manipulation of the lumbar spine.

ity thrust directed specifically at the manipulable lesion (subluxation, osteopathic lesion, etc.). In order to practice these techniques, it is essential that a clinician have some basic understanding of spinal mechanics, have the palpatory skills to diagnose the clinically significant manipulable lesion, and have developed, through experience, the ability to direct the adjustive thrust to one segment in a specific direction.

Once the clinically significant manipulable lesion has been found, the direction in which motion is lost has been determined, and the facet orientation and structural relationship between the vertebrae known, it is possible to work out a technique that will theoretically correct the lesion. The patient is placed in a position which will allow movement of the vertebra in the desired direction. Contact is taken with a relatively small portion of one hand (thumb, finger, pisiform). The spinal segments, either above or below the segment being manipulated, are locked by moving the spine to the limit of their passive range of motion (75,82). A high velocity, small amplitude thrust is then delivered through the contact arm and hand to the short vertebral lever (transverse process or spinous process) in the direction which will correct the segmental fixation.

Once again, it is impossible to list the numerous techniques and variations which have been developed to adjust the lumbar spine and sacroiliac joint. It is possible to perform such adjustments with the patient in the prone, supine, side lying, or sitting position and by using a variety of specially designed adjustment tables, blocks, and traction devices. The following four examples with variations will illustrate a few of the principles of lumbosacral adjusting.

Example 1

Adjustment of the sacroiliac joint is most frequently carried out with the patient in the side lying position (43,47). The side to be adjusted is placed up. The inferior leg is straight and the superior leg flexed. This brings the lumbar spine to its neutral position with the shoulders and hips vertically above each other. The inferior arm is drawn rostrally from under the patient with a minimum of spinal rotation and placed across the chest. The clinician's superior hand is placed on the patient's shoulder and pressure exerted rostrally with only that amount of spinal rotation and lateral flexion necessary to lock the spine down to the segment being manipulated. The pisiform eminence of the clinician's inferior hand is used to contact either the posterior superior iliac spine (for a flexion fixation of the sacroiliac joint) or the ischial tuberosity (for an extension fixation). The inferior leg is flexed to the point where resistance is felt in the sacroiliac joint (approximately 75 degrees for flexion fixations, 90 degrees for extension fixations). Traction is applied to the spine as the patient takes a deep breath and then slowly exhales and relaxes. A high velocity, low amplitude thrust is delivered through the clinician's inferior arm and hand while the superior arm simply stabilizes the trunk and spine. The direction of thrust is determined by the "listing" of the pelvis. For example, if the iliac spine is felt to have moved posterior and inferior, the thrust is rostral and anterior toward the patient's shoulder. If the superior ilium is felt to have rotated internally onto the sacrum, the direction of thrust is anterior toward the superior femur in an attempt to open the sacroiliac joint. The thrust on the ischium for an extension fixation is toward the patient's lower shoulder (43) (Fig. 12).

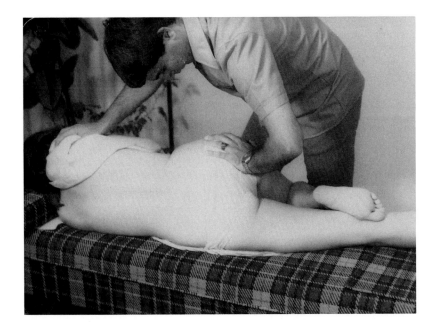

FIG. 12. The specific adjustment for an extension fixation of the sacroiliac joint.

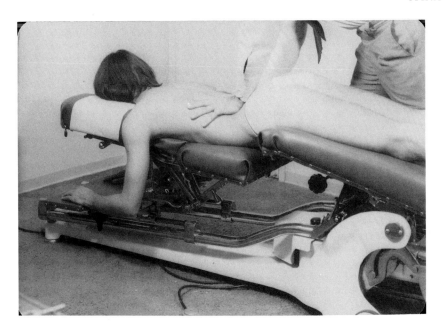

FIG. 13. The specific lumbar extension adjustment using a segmental table.

Manipulation of the lumbar spine can be carried out using a very similar technique. The patient is placed in the same position. The spine is locked down to the segment being manipulated through traction and slight rotation of the shoulder. The thrust is delivered to a transverse process or by hooking a spinous process.

With proper placement of the patient, it is seldom necessary to put weight on the femur or to maximally rotate the spine, thus reducing the chance of traumatizing the rib cage, hip joint, or intervertebral disc.

Example 2

The adjustment of the lumbar spine for an extension fixation can best be achieved with the patient prone

(47,48,114). A flat couch, however, does not allow for sufficient extension of the lumbar spine to achieve specific localization of the adjustive force. A number of adjusting tables have been developed to overcome this problem. The segmental table (Fig. 13) has a pelvic support that elevates and/or an abdominal support that drops away. This allows the pelvis to be locked while the lumbar spine is hanging in extension.

Another much less costly piece of equipment, the knee posture table, similarly allows for locking of the pelvis (on the femurs) with maximum extension of the lumbar spine. The position of the pelvis locking can be varied by changing the trunk femur angle for a perpendicular 90 degrees to 80 degrees or 100 degrees. This is achieved by moving the knees forward or backward. Contact is made

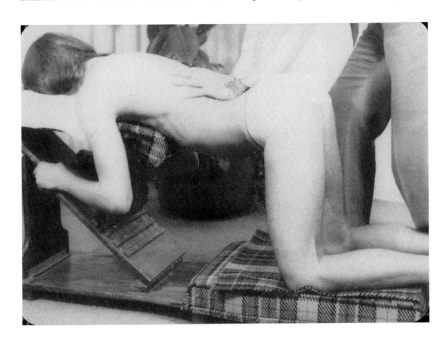

FIG. 14. The specific lumbar extension adjustment using the knee posture table.

over the transverse processes of the segment being adjusted either unilateral or bilateral (Fig. 14). The clinician may use either his thumbs or pisiform to make the contact. The use of the thenar or hypothenar eminences is less effective since it tends to dissipate the force over a number of segments thus reducing the specificity of the procedure.

The ability to deliver a very sharp, low amplitude thrust is necessary for this procedure. A single "thud" can often be heard and felt over the articulation being adjusted if the procedure is executed properly. Any excessive force or depth to the thrust can be painful. The decision as to whether the thrust should be given unilaterally or bilaterally and the exact direction for the thrust is dependent on the listing, the facet facings, and whether the fixation is unilateral or bilateral.

Example 3

Sitting rotary and lateral flexion manipulations can be quite specific. The clinician has the advantage of being able to maneuver the patient's spine in all three planes of motion prior to delivering the adjustive thrust (65,82). The main drawback is the inability to achieve segmental traction.

The patient straddles the edge of the adjusting table and clasps both hands across the chest on opposite shoulders or behind the neck. The clinician gains control of the trunk by grasping the shoulders or arms with one arm. The clinician's other hand is free to make contact in the lumbar spine. The patient can be maneuvered into flexion, extension, rotation, lateral bending, or any combination of these positions. The thrust is delivered to the transverse or spinous process of the lumbar segment being adjusted (Fig. 15). The position of the patient prior to giving the thrust and the direction of the thrust are once again dependent on the listing and the direction in which the segment is fixated. The thrust is an exaggerated movement of the trunk with localization being directed through the contact point in the lumbar spine.

Example 4

There are a wide variety of specific adjusting procedures that do not utilize a high velocity thrust. These techniques (along with mobilizing procedures) are particularly useful in the management of elderly patients where it may be advantageous not to use heavy force. Kimberly (65) describes a number of so-called "muscle energy" and "respiratory force" procedures. These procedures utilize the patient's own muscles to achieve the correction of a specific fixation. The basic principle of the techniques is to position the patient at the limit of a specific range of motion in the direction of the vertebral fixation. The segment being adjusted is held firm. When

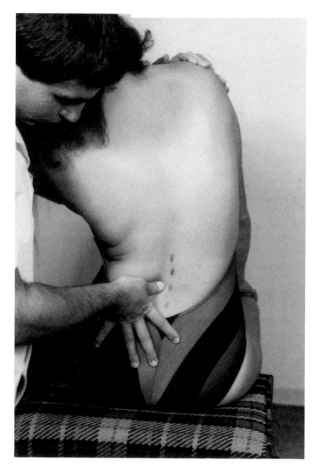

FIG. 15. The rotation-lateral flexion adjustment in the sitting position.

the patient relaxes, the slack created by the isometric contraction is taken up. In this way the passive range of motion of the segment which was held is increased. This process is repeated a number of times until movement is felt in the vertebra being adjusted. Muscle energy techniques have been developed in the sitting, prone, and supine positions for almost every direction of movement fixation. Patient positioning is very similar to that used for the high velocity, low amplitude thrust techniques. It is the use of the patient's own muscles rather than a dynamic thrust which is the distinguishing feature.

A simple example of this technique is that described by Kimberly (65) for a restricted or fixated sacroiliac joining where the posterior superior iliac crest is felt to have moved posterior and inferior (Fig. 16). The patient is placed prone with the clinician standing on the side opposite to that being adjusted. The clinician elevates the leg on the affected side with one hand and places the other hand on the iliac crest slightly above the posterior superior iliac spine. The leg is elevated in extension and pressure exerted on the iliac crest until the restrictive barrier at the limit of passive range of motion is engaged. The patient is then instructed to pull the leg downward

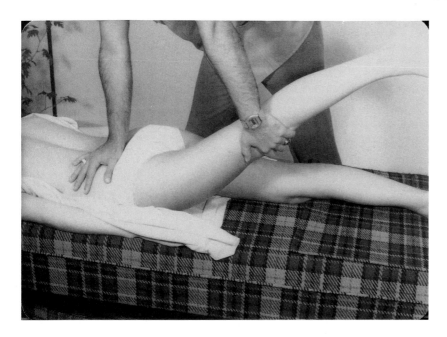

FIG. 16. An example of the muscle-energy adjustment. This adjustment is to correct a fixated sacroiliac joint with posterior-inferior misalignment of the ilium. The direction of the patient's muscle force is down toward the table.

toward the table against the resistance of the clinician's hand. The patient relaxes and the additional slack in the joint motion is taken up until the new restrictive barrier is engaged. The process is repeated two to three times until the fixation is corrected.

Vertebral Mobilization or Articulation

The procedures generally included under the term "mobilization" are those where a joint is forced beyond the limits of active muscle contraction and into the passive range of motion. There is no attempt to force the joint beyond its restrictive physiological barrier (16,83,95). These techniques are extremely valuable in patients with acutely painful joints or where there is some inherent danger to high velocity adjusting techniques (e.g., osteoporosis).

Four grades of mobilization are classically described (Fig. 17). A Grade I mobilization starts at the neutral position and has only very small excursion. A Grade II mobilization begins at the neutral position and has deeper excursion into the normal range of motion of the joint but does not attempt to reach the limit of passive motion. Grade III mobilizations begin approximately half way into the normal motion of the joint and carry through to the physiological barrier of the joint. A Grade IV mobilization has a short excursion at the limit of the passive motion of the joint.

Mobilization can be either specific to a single vertebral joint or non-specific to the entire spine or a large segment of the spine. It can be accomplished in flexion, extension, rotation, lateral flexion, or any combination of these movements. The positioning of the patient varies only slightly from that used in non-specific manipula-

tion and the specific spinal adjustment. It is the degree of movement and the lack of a thrust which distinguishes mobilization from these procedures.

In addition, mobilization can be performed in the neutral position by springing a joint in a specific direction. These neutral mobilizations are identical to the techniques used for determining neutral joint play. In this case, however, the goal is treatment rather than diagnosis. The springing of a joint is repeated a number of times, often with increasing depth (or grades of mobilization) until the full range of motion is achieved and is pain free. This may require repeated mobilizations over a number of days. Figure 18 illustrates specific rotation mobilization of a lumbar vertebra in the neutral position by lateral pressure over a spinous process. Figure 19 is an example of a technique for specific springing of the lumbar spine in extension.

Manual Traction or Muscle Stretching

The manual application of traction to the legs, arms, head, or trunk falls within the broad definition of spinal manipulative therapy. These techniques are non-specific for any one vertebral level or joint; the traction is applied to the entire spine. The major advantages over mechanical traction are that the clinician can monitor the amount of traction being given, change the direction of traction by altering the position of the leg or arm which is being pulled, and change the rhythm of intermittent traction.

There are two types of manual traction which have been described for the lumbar spine. The vertical traction technique (87,115) begins with the patient and clinician standing back to back. The patient grasps his own

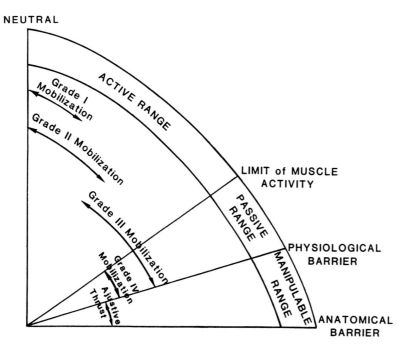

FIG. 17. An illustration of the relationship between the four grades of mobilization to the normal passive range of motion of a joint. The adjustment takes place between the physiological and anatomical limits of joint movement.

shoulders and the clinician reaches behind to grasp the patient's elbows. The clinician then bends forward, holding the patient's elbows rigid and lifts the patient from the ground. The patient is asked to flex his head, and the clinician, after taking up the ligamentous slack in the spine, gives the patient a sharp shake by lifting the patient suddenly higher. This causes straight extension of the spine. It is a clumsy maneuver but can be effective if vertebral traction and extension is required.

The application of traction to one or both legs has been used in an attempt to open the sacroiliac and posterior joints of the lumbar spine and to stretch the para-spinal muscles (6,43,83). This can take the form of sustained traction on the leg, a short tug on the leg, or a movement from the flexed leg position to the extended position followed by traction (Fig. 20). Bourdillon (6) recommends internal rotation of the leg prior to applying the leg tug.

The spray and stretch techniques developed by Travell (118,119) for the treatment of specific trigger points also fall under this heading. In this case, traction is applied to muscles rather than to a joint. Travell describes the myofascial trigger points as palpable tender firm bands of muscle which refer pain in a specific pattern often some

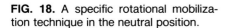

FIG. 18. A specific rotational mobilization technique in the neutral position.

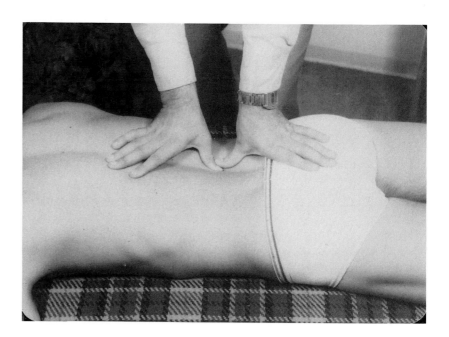

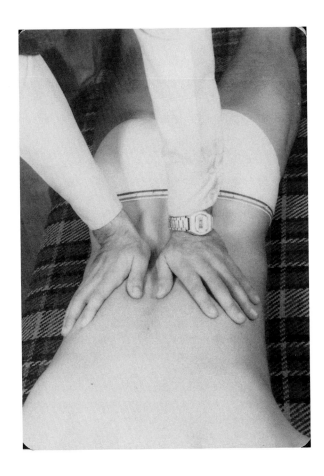

FIG. 19. An extension mobilization technique in the neutral position (springing of the lumbar spine).

distance from the trigger point. The trigger points which are considered important in low back and leg pain are those within the iliocostalis, gluteus medius, longissimus, multifidus, gluteus minimus, adductor longus, piriformis, and quadratus lumborum muscles. When a trigger point in a specific muscle is found in a patient with the appropriate pain pattern, the muscle should be stretched to determine the extent of motion restriction caused by the muscle contraction. While maintaining the muscle in the stretched position, the patient is asked to voluntarily relax the muscle and a stream of vapocoolant spray (fluoromethane) is directed at the muscle. The spray is applied in one direction from the trigger point toward its reference zone in slow even sweeps over

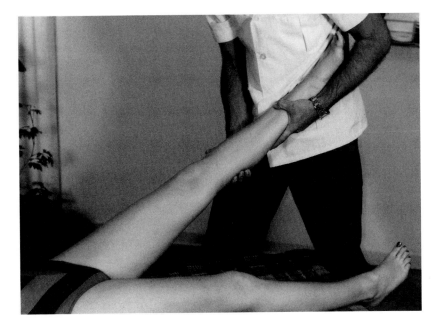

FIG. 20. An example of a traction manipulation using the leg. The force may be gradual, intermittent, or in the form of a sharp tug.

the skin. During the spraying, passive stretch is applied to the muscle with steady, gradually increasing force. The stretch is held at a tolerably painful point which does not result in any contraction or guarding of the muscle. The trigger point should disappear if the procedure is carried out properly. Figure 21 illustrates the technique for spray and stretch of the hamstring muscles.

More specific stretching techniques for specific spinal muscle groups have been published by Evjenth and Hamberg (32) where the patient is positioned in a manner which places specific muscles on stretch. The clinician then actively applies further force on the muscle levers to stretch it further.

Soft Tissue Massage

All forms of massage fall under the definition of manipulative therapy and are often referred to as manipulations (28,105). The massage techniques can be broken down into superficial stroking or effleurage, deep kneading or friction massage, and the hacking and clapping procedures.

Two types of massage deserve special mention in a discussion of low back pain. Connective tissue massage is a deep stroking massage which utilizes a twisting movement of the fingertips along specific planes of the back. The stroking is sufficiently deep as to cause discomfort to the patient and marked hyperemia of the skin. Claims of effective management of back pain have been made for this procedure (28,38).

Deep transverse friction massage is the specific focal application of massage across an injured tender muscle, tendon, or ligament (21). The theoretical basis of this procedure is to break down scar tissue and increase cir-

culation. The massage is given over a very small area and at right angles to the muscle or ligamentous fibers. Although this technique is usually recommended for known areas of soft tissue injury in the extremities, it is also being used to manipulate trigger points around the spine.

Point Pressure Manipulation

Many of the muscle syndromes considered to be associated with low back pain are said to respond to deep point pressure without any movement of the joint or massage of the muscle. The piriformis syndrome is the most commonly quoted example. The manipulative procedure recommended by Maxwell (86) and Edwards (30) utilizes constant heavy pressure over the piriformis muscle using the thumb or elbow for approximately 30 seconds or until spasm in the muscle is released. The easiest way to find the muscle is to have the patient in the lateral recumbent position with the affected side up. The tender contracted muscle can be felt just above the acetabulum when the patient's hip is flexed and adducted (Fig. 22).

There are a variety of practitioners of spinal manipulation who claim to be able to change symptoms, increase muscle strength, and influence health by exerting pressure over certain mapped points on the body. These procedures, which have been referred to under such titles as Rolfing, muscle balancing massage, acupressure, applied kinesiology, etc., recommend the application of deep point pressure over specific points on the body surface, often on an acupuncture meridian or over the same trigger points described by Travell (119). These procedures have as yet to be discussed in any peer-reviewed journal.

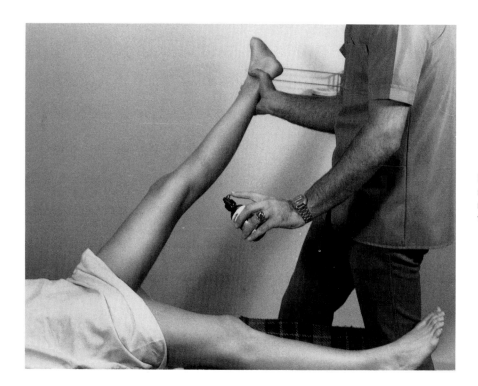

FIG. 21. An example of the spray and stretch manipulations. The hamstring muscles are stretched after applying vapocoolant spray.

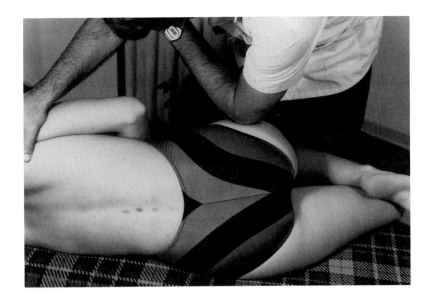

FIG. 22. An example of point pressure manipulation. In this case, the piriformis muscle is being manipulated.

They are often supported by unsubstantiated theories, and claims of success deserve mention only because of their popularity and repeated mention in the popular press.

CONCLUSION

Spinal manipulation over the past decade has moved from a procedure offered only by persons excluded from the mainstream of health care to one that is increasingly being seen as an alternative approach available to a physician who is treating patients with low back pain. Spinal manipulation is finally being subjected to scientific investigation. Its relative effectiveness compared with other treatments, and its effectiveness in different categories of patients with low back pain, are becoming increasingly evident. Both indications and contraindications are being more closely defined and some rational theory as to the mechanism of action of spinal manipulation is evolving. It remains, however, a procedure requiring both manual diagnostic and treatment skills which take time, interest, education, and experience to develop. There remain many valid criticisms of the theory and claims for spinal manipulation, and it will require considerably more research to determine its exact role in the management of low back pain. Despite these shortcomings, most physicians who treat back pain can develop a level of understanding of the treatment method to determine whether spinal manipulation is or is not a viable option for the management of their patients. As research in this area continues, the role of spinal manipulation in the treatment of low back pain can be expected to become clearer.

REFERENCES

1. Akeson WH, Amiel D, Woo S (1980): Immobility effects on synovial joints, the pathomechanics of joint contracture. *Biorheology* 17:95–110.

2. Arkuszewski Z (1986): The efficacy of manual treatment in low back pain: A clinical trial. *Manual Med* 2:68–71.
3. Bergquist-Ullman M, Larsson U (1977): Acute low back pain in industry. *Acta Orthopaed Scand* [Suppl] (170):1–117.
4. Blaine ES (1925): Manipulative (chiropractic) dislocations of the atlas. *JAMA* 85:1356–1359.
5. Bosshard R (1961): The treatment of acute lumbago and sciatica. *Ann Swiss Chiropractor's Assoc* 50–61.
6. Bourdillon JF (1970): *Spinal manipulation.* London: William Heineman Medical Books.
7. Breen AC (1977): Chiropractors and the treatment of back pain. *Rheumatol Rehabil* 16:46–53.
8. Brunarski DJ (1984): Clinical trials of spinal manipulation: A critical appraisal and review of the literature. *J Manipulative Physiol Ther* 7:243–249.
9. Buerger AA (1978): A clinical trial of rotational manipulation. *Pain Abstracts* 1:248. Second World Congress on Pain, International Association for the Study of Pain, Montreal, Canada.
10. Buerger AA (1979): A clinical trial of spinal manipulation. *Fed Proc* 38:1250.
11. Buerger AA, Tobis JS, eds. (1977): *Approaches to the validation of manipulative therapy.* Springfield: Charles C Thomas.
12. Buerger AA (1980): In the manipulation project. A controlled trial of rotational manipulation in low back pain. *Manuelle Medizin* 2:17–26.
13. Cassidy JD, Potter GE, Kirkaldy-Willis WH (1978): Manipulative management of back pain in patients with spondylolisthesis. *J Canad Chiropractic Assoc* 22(1):15–20.
14. Cassidy JD, Potter GE (1979): Motion examination of the lumbar spine. *J Manipulative Physiol Ther* 2:151–158.
15. Chrisman OD, Mittnacht A, Snook GA (1964): A study of the results following rotatory manipulation in the lumbar intervertebral-disc syndrome. *J Bone Joint Surg* [AM] 46:517–524.
16. Cookson JC (1979): Orthopedic manual therapy—An overview. Part II. The spine. *Physical Therapy* 59:259–267.
17. Coplans CW (1978): The conservative treatment of low back pain. In:Helfet AJ, Gruebel, Lee DM, eds. *Disorders of the lumbar spine.* Philadelphia: JB Lippincott.
18. Coxhead CE, Inskip H, Meade TW, North WR, Troup JD (1981): Multicentre trial of physiotherapy in the management of sciatic symptoms. *Lancet* 1:1065–1068.
19. Coyer AB, Curwen IHM (1955): Low back pain treated by manipulation: A controlled series. *Brit Med J* 1:705–707.
20. Croner CM (1976): *The nation's use of health resources, 1976 ed.* DHEW Publication No. (HRA) 77–1240.
21. Cyriax J (1971): *Textbook of orthopaedic medicine, vol 2, 8th ed.* London: Bailliere-Tindall.
22. Dabbert O, Freeman DG, Weis AJ (1970): Spinal meningeal hematoma, warfarin therapy and chiropractic adjustment. *JAMA* 214(11):2058.

23. Deyo RA, Tsui-Wu YJ (1987): Descriptive epidemiology of low-back pain and its related medical care in the United States. *Spine* 12(3):264–268.

24. Diebert PW, England RW (1972): Electromyographic studies. I: Consideration in the evaluation of osteopathic therapy. *J Am Osteopath Assoc* 72:221–223.

25. Doran DM, Newell DJ (1975): Manipulation in treatment of low back pain: A multicentre study. *Brit Med J* 2:161–164.

26. Dvorak J, Dvorak V, Schneider W (1985): *Manual medicine 1984.* Berlin:Springer Verlag.

27. Dvorak J, Froehlich D, Penning L, Baumgartner H, Panjabi MM (1988): Functional radiographic diagnosis of the cervical spine: Flexion/extension. *Spine* 13(7):748–755.

28. Ebner M (1978): Connective tissue massage. *Physiotherapy* 64:208–210.

29. Edwards BC (1969): Low back pain and pain resulting from lumbar spine conditions, a comparison of treatment results. *Austral J Physiotherapy* 15(3):104–110.

30. Edwards FO (1962): Pyriformis syndrome. *Academy of Applied Osteopathy Yearbook,* pp.39–41.

30a. England RW, Diebert PW (1972): see ref. 24.

31. Evans DP, Burke MS, Lloyd KN, Roberts EE, Roberts GM (1978): Lumbar spinal manipulation on trial. Part I. Clinical assessment. *Rheum Rehabil* 17:46–53.

32. Evjenth O, Hamberg J (1984) *Muscle stretching in manual therapy. A clinical manual, volume II, The spinal column and the TM joint.* Afta, Sweden: Alfta Rehab Forlag.

33. Farrell JP, Twomey LT (1982): Acute low back pain. Comparison of two conservative treatment approaches. *Med J Austral* 1:160–164.

34. Fisk JW (1971): Manipulation in general practice. *NZ Med J* 74:172–175.

35. Fisk JW (1975): The straight leg raising test: Its relevance to possible disc pathology. *NZ Med J* 81:557–560.

36. Fisk JW (1977): *A practical guide to management of the painful neck and back.* Springfield: Charles C Thomas.

37. Fisk JW (1979): A controlled trial of manipulation in a selected group of patients with low back pain favouring one side. *NZ Med J* 90:288–291.

38. Frazer FW (1978): Persistent post-sympathetic pain treated by connective tissue massage. *Physiotherapy* 64:211–212.

39. Frymoyer J, Gordon S (1989): *New perspective on low back pain.* Park Ridge: American Academy of Orthopedic Surgeons.

40. Frymoyer JW, Phillips RB, Newberg AH, MacPherson BV (1986): A comparative analysis of the interpretations of lumbar spinal radiographs by chiropractors and medical doctors. *Spine* 11:1020–1023.

41. Gibbons RW (1976): Chiropractic in America. The historical conflicts of cultism, and science. 10th annual history forum of Duquesne University.

41a. Gibson Grahame R, Harkness J, Woo P, Blagrave P, Hills R (1989): Controlled comparison of shortwave diathermy treatment with osteopathic treatment in non–specific low back pain. *Lancet* 1:1258–1260.

42. Gillett H, Liekens M (1973): *Belgian chiropractic research notes, 10th ed.* Brussels.

43. Gitelman R (1980): A chiropractic approach to biomechanical disorders of the lumbar spine and pelvis. In:Haldeman S, ed. *Modern developments in the principles and practice of chiropractic.* New York: Appleton-Century-Crofts.

44. Glover JR, Morris JG, Khosla T (1974): Back pain: A randomized clinical trial of rotational manipulation of the trunk. *Brit J Ind Med* 31:59–64.

45. Godfrey CM, Morgan PP, Schatzker J (1984): A randomized trial of manipulation for low-back pain in a medical setting. *Spine* 9:301–304.

46. Goldstein M, ed. (1975): The Research Status of Spinal Manipulative Therapy. NINCDS Monograph No. 15, DHEW Publication No. (NIH) Bethesda, 76–998.

47. Gonstead CS (1968): *Gonstead chiropractic science and art.* SCi-Chi Publications.

48. Grecco MA (1953): *Chiropractic technique illustrated.* New York: Jarl Publishing Co.

49. Greenland S, Reisbord LS, Haldeman S, Buerger AA (1980): Controlled clinical trials of manipulation: A review and proposal. *J Occup Med* 22:670–676.

50. Grice AA (1974): Muscle toning changes following manipulation. *J Can Chir Assoc* 19(4):29–31.

51. Hadler NM, Curtis P, Gillings AB, Stinnett S (1987): A benefit of spinal manipulation as adjunctive therapy for acute low-back pain: A stratified controlled trial. *Spine* 12(7):702–706.

52. Haldeman S (1975): Chiropractic: A dying cult or a growing profession? *Musings Quarterly* 1(3):53–57.

53. Haldeman S (1977): What is meant by manipulation? In:Buerger AA, Tobis JS, eds. *Approaches to the validation of manipulative therapy.* Springfield: Charles C Thomas, pp. 299–302.

54. Haldeman S, ed. (1980): *Modern developments in the principles and practice of chiropractic.* New York: Appleton-Century-Crofts.

55. Haldeman S (1983): Spinal manipulative therapy. A status report. *Clin Orthop* (179):62–70.

56. Henderson DJ (1979): Intermittent claudication with special reference to its neurogenic form as a diagnostic and management challenge. *J Canad Chiropractic Assoc* 23(1):9–19.

57. Herzog W, Nigg BM, Read LJ (1988): Quantifying the effects of spinal manipulations on gait using patients with low back pain. *J Manipulative Physiol Ther* 11(3):151–157.

58. Hoehler FK, Tobis JS, Buerger AA (1981): Spinal manipulation for low back pain. *JAMA* 245:1835–1838.

59. Hviid H (1971): The influence of chiropractic treatment on the rotary mobility of the cervical spine. A kinesiometric and statistical study. *Ann Swiss Chirop Assoc* 5:31–44.

60. Janda V (1985): Pain in the locomotor system—a broad approach. In: Glasgow E, Twomey L, Scull E, et al., eds. *Aspects of manipulative therapy, 2nd ed.* Melbourne: Churchill Livingstone, pp. 148–151.

61. Jennet WB (1956): A study of 25 cases of compression of the cauda equina by prolapse intervertebral discs. *J Neurol Neurosurg Psych* 19:109–116.

62. Jirout J (1972): The effect of mobilisation of the segmental blockade on the sagittal component of the reaction on lateroflexion of the cervical spine. *Neuroradiology* 3:210–215.

63. Johnston WL (1976): Interexaminer reliability in palpation. *J Am Osteopath Assoc* 76:286–287.

64. Johnston WL, Allan BR, Hendra JL, Neff DR, Rosen ME, Sills LD, Thomas SC (1983): Interexaminer study of palpation in detecting location of spinal segmental dysfunction. *J Am Osteopath Assoc* 82:839–845.

65. Kimberly PE (1979): *Outline of osteopathic manipulative procedures.* Kirksville: Kirksville College of Osteopathic Medicine.

66. Kirkaldy-Willis WH, Cassidy JD (1978): Effects of manipulation on chronic low back pain. Presented at a conference on manipulative medicine in the management of low back pain, sponsored by the University of Southern California and the North American Academy of Manipulative Medicine, October 1978.

67. Kirkaldy-Willis WH, Hill RJ (1979): A more precise diagnosis for low-back pain. *Spine* 4:102–109.

68. Kirkaldy-Willis WH, Farfan HF (1982): Instability of the lumbar spine. *Clin Orthop* (165):110–123.

69. Kirkaldy-Willis WH, Cassidy JD (1985): Spinal manipulation in the treatment of low back pain. *Can Fam Physician* 31:535–540.

70. Kleynhans AM (1980): Complications of and contraindications to spinal manipulative therapy. In: Haldeman S, ed. *Modern developments in the principles and practice of chiropractic.* New York: Appleton-Century-Crofts.

71. Knapp ME (1951): Function of the quadratus lumborum. *Arch Phys Med* 32:505–507.

72. Korr IM (1976): The spinal cord as organizer of disease processes: Some preliminary prospectives. *J Am Osteopath Assoc* 76:35–45.

73. Korr IM, ed. (1978): *The neurobiologic mechanisms in manipulative therapy.* New York: Plenum Press.

74. La Rocca H, Macnab I (1969): Value of pre-employment radiographic assessment of the lumbar spine. *Can Med Assoc J* 101:383–388.

75. Lewit D (1977): Manuelle Medizin. In: *Rahmen der Medizinischen Rehabilitation, 2 Auflage.* Leipzig: Johann Ambrosius.

76. Liebenson C, Phillips R (1989): The reliability of range of motion measurements for lumbar spine flexion: A review. *Chiropractic Technique* 1(3):69–78.

77. Livingston MC (1972): Spinal manipulation causing injury. *Brit Col Med J* 14:78–81.

78. Logan VF, Murray FM, eds. (1950): *Textbook of Logan basic methods.* St. Louis: LBM.

79. Lomax E (1975): Manipulative therapy: A historical perspective from ancient times to the modern era. In: Goldstein M, ed. *The research status of spinal manipulative therapy.* NINCDS Monograph No. 15, DHEW Publication No. (NIH) 76–998.

80. Lewit K (1985): *Manipulative therapy in the rehabilitation of the locomotor system.* London: Butterworths.

81. McConnell DG, Beal MC, Dinnar U (1980): Low agreement of findings in neuromusculoskeletal examinations by a group of osteopathic physicians using their own procedures. *J Am Osteopath Assoc* 79:441–450.

82. Maigne R (1972): *Orthopedic medicine. A new approach to vertebral manipulations,* translated by WT Liberson. Springfield: Charles C Thomas.

83. Maitland GD (1973): *Vertebral manipulation, 3rd ed.* London: Butterworths.

84. Mathews JA, Yates DA (1969): Reduction of lumbar disc prolapse by manipulation. *Brit Med J* 3:696–697.

85. Mathews JA, Mills SB, Jenkins VM, Grimes SM, Morkel MJ, Mathews W, Scott C, SiHampalam Y (1987): Back pain and sciatica: Controlled trials of manipulation, traction, sclerosant and epidural injections. *Brit J Rheumatol* 26:416–423.

86. Maxwell TD (1978): The piriformis muscle and its relation to the long legged scoatoc syndrome. *J Can Chirop Assoc* 22(2):1–56.

87. Mennell J (1960): *Back pain: Diagnosis and treatment using manipulative therapy.* Boston: Little, Brown.

88. McDowell I, Newell C (1987): *Measuring health. A guide to rating scales and questionnaires.* New York: Oxford University Press.

89. Morrison MC (1984): The best back to manipulate? *Ann Royal Coll Surg Engl* 66:52–53.

90. Nachemson A (1968): A long term follow-up study of non-treated scoliosis. *Acta Orthop Scand* 39:466–476.

91. Nachemson A (1975): A critical look at the treatment for low back pain. In: Goldstein M, ed. *The research status of spinal manipulative therapy.* NINCDS Monograph 15, DHEW Publication No. (NIH) 76:998.

92. Nachemson A (1976): The lumbar spine: An orthopedic challenge. *Spine* 1:59–71.

93. Nachemson A (1977): Pathophysiology and treatment of back pain: A critical look at the different types of treatment. In: Buerger AA, Tobis JS, eds. *Approaches to the validation of manipulative therapy.* Springfield: Charles C Thomas, pp. 42–57.

94. Nachemson A (1983): Work for all. For those with low back pain as well. *Clin Orthop* (179):77–85.

95. Nwuga VC (1976): *Manipulation of the spine.* Baltimore: Williams and Wilkins.

96. Nyiendo J, Phillips R, Meeker W, Kunsler G, Jansen R, Menon M (1989): A comparison of patients and patient complaints at six chiropractic college teaching clinics. *JMPT* 12(2):79–85.

97. Olmarker K, Rydevik B, Holm S, Bagge U (1989): Effects of experimental graded compression on blood flow in spinal nerve roots. A vital microscopic study on the procine cauda equina. *J Orthop Res* 7(6):817–823.

98. Olsen GA, Allan JH (1969): The lateral stability of the spine. *Clin Orthop* (65):143–156.

99. Ongley MJ, Klein RG, Dorman TA, Eek BC, Hubert LJ (1987): A new approach to the treatment of chronic low back pain. *Lancet* 2:143–146.

100. Ottenbacher K, DiFabio RP (1985): Efficiency of spinal manipulation/mobilization therapy: A meta-analysis. *Spine* 10(9):833–837.

101. Palmer DD (1910): *The science, art and philosophy of chiropractic.* Portland: Portland Printing House.

102. Perl ER (1975): Pain: Spinal and peripheral factors. In: Goldstein M, ed. *The research status of spinal manipulative therapy.* NINCDS Monograph No. 15, DHEW Publication No. (NIH) 76–998.

103. Potter GE (1977): A study of 744 cases of neck and back pain treated with spinal manipulation. *J Can Chiro Assoc* 21(4):154–156.

104. Potter GE (1979): Chiropractors [letter]. *Can Med Assoc J* 121:705–706.

105. Prosser E (1951): *Manual of massage and movements.* London.

106. Rasmussen GG (1977): Manipulation in low back pain: A randomized clinical trial. *Manuelle Medizin* 1:8–10.

107. Richard J (1967): Disk rupture with cauda equina syndrome after chiropractic adjustment. *NY State J Med* 67:2496–2498.

108. Riches EW (1930): End-results of manipulation of the back. *Lancet* 1:957–960.

109. Roberts GM, Roberts EE, Lloyd KN, Burke MS, Evans DP (1978): Lumbar spinal manipulation on trial. Part II. Radiological assessment. *Rheumatol Rehab* 17:54–59.

110. Schafer RC (1976): *Chiropractic health care, 2nd ed.* Des Moines: Foundation for Chiropractic Education and Research.

111. Schaefer R, Faye L (1989): *Motion palpation and chiropractic technic: Principles of dynamic chiropractic.* Huntington Beach: The Motion Palpation Institute.

112. Schiotz EH (1958): Vertebral manipulation therapy as seen from the viewpoint of medical history and in the light of primitive and popular medicine, osteopathy and chiropractic. *Tidsshr Nor* 78:359–372.

113. Sims-Williams H, Jayson MI, Young SM, Baddeley H, Collins E (1978): Controlled trial of mobilisation and manipulation for patients with low back pain in general practice. *Brit Med J* 2:1338–1340.

114. States AZ (1968): Spinal and pelvic technics. *Atlas of chiropractic technic, 2nd ed.* Lombard: National College of Chiropractic.

115. Stoddard A (1959): *Manual of osteopathic technique.* London: Hutchison.

116. Terrett AC, Vernon H (1984): Manipulation and pain tolerance. A controlled study of the effect of spinal manipulation on paraspinal cutaneous pain tolerance levels. *Am J Phys Med* 63:217–225.

117. Tissington-Tatlow WF, Bammer HG (1957): Syndrome of vertebral artery compression. *Neurology* 7:331–340.

118. Travell J (1957): Symposium on mechanism and management of pain syndromes. *Proc Rudolf Virchou Med Society* [Basel] 16:128–135.

119. Travell J (1976): Myofascial trigger points: Clinical view. *Advances in Pain Research and Therapy* 1:919–926.

120. Travell J (1978): The quadratus lumborum muscle. An overlooked cause of low back pain. Presented at a conference on manipulative medicine in the management of low back pain, sponsored by the University of Southern California and the North American Academy of Manipulative Medicine, Los Angeles, October 1978.

121. Travell J, Travell W (1946): Therapy of low back pain by manipulation and of referred pain in the lower extremity by procaine infiltration. *Arch Phys Med* 27:537–547.

122. Vernon HT, Dhami MSI, Arnett R (1985): Abstract. Canadian Foundation for Spinal Research symposium on low back pain, March 15–17, 1985, Vancouver.

123. Vear HJ (1972): A study into the complaints of patients seeking chiropractic care. *J Can Chirop Assoc* 16:9–13.

124. VonKuster T Jr (1980): *Chiropractic health care: A national study of the cost of education, service, utilization, number of practicing doctors of chiropractic and other key policy issues.* Washington: The Foundation for the Advancement of Chiropractic Tenets and Science.

125. Waagen G, Haldeman S, Cook G, Lopez D, DeBoer K (1986): Short term trial of chiropractic adjustments for the relief of chronic low back pain. *Manual Med* 2:63–67.

126. White AA, Panjabi MM (1979): *Clinical biomechanics of the spine.* Philadelphia: Lippincott.

127. Wiesel SW, Tsourmas N, Feffer HL, Citrin CM, Patronas N (1984): A study of computer-assisted tomography: 1. The incidence of positive CAT-scans in an asymptomatic group of patients. *Spine* 9:549–551.

128. Wiles MR (1980): Reproducibility and interexaminer correlation of motion palpation findings of the sacroiliac joints. *J Can Chirop Assoc* 24:59–69.

129. Wilson JN, Ilfeld FW (1952): Manipulation of the herniated intervertebral disc. *Am J Surg* 83:173–175.

130. Wyke BD (1976): The neurological aspects of back pain. In: *The lumbar spine and back pain.* M Jayson, ed. New York: Grune and Stratton, pp 189–256.

The Adult Spine: Principles and Practice,
J. W. Frymoyer, Editor-in-Chief.
Raven Press, Ltd., New York © 1991.

CHAPTER 74

Orthoses for Treatment of Low Back Disorders

Malcolm H. Pope

HISTORICAL OVERVIEW

Mankind has been bracing backs for millennia, though the devices used have undergone many revisions. Lumbosacral corsets have probably been in use at least since the Minoan period, around the year 2000 BC (20). Women have used corsets for almost as long to "improve" their figures. In the sixteenth century Vesalius condemned the practice because of adverse effects on the abdominal viscera. During the early twentieth century corsets became widely prescribed for back pain. Even electric corsets were advocated in the last portion of the nineteenth century. "Wilson's magnetic appliances cure 90% of cases; Cure without medicine; No cure no pay" (38).

Rigid braces date back to Paul of Aegina in 500 AD, who attempted to correct scoliosis by bandages and splints, and Ambroise Paré used a metal cuirass padded with rags. Sayre (57) popularized the use of plaster of paris casts. Paré's concept was improved by Lorenzo Heister in the eighteenth century and was called the

rior upright with a crossbar at the level of the shoulders. The concept has undergone many revisions since then (39), and today we have more than thirty different types of back supports available for the care of low back problems (3,50).

Back supports have enjoyed great acceptance by physicians. Less than 1% of 3,410 orthopedic surgeons responding to a survey stated that they never used support for low back pain sufferers (55). Usage has increased to the point where 250,000 corsets were prescribed in Britain in a one year period (3). Deyo and Tsui-Wu (15) found that 27% of low back patients use corsets or braces. Ahlgren and Hansen (1) showed that 75% of patients were still wearing corsets four years after they were prescribed. Some patients wear corsets for up to 20 years in the belief that they would not survive without them. Despite the risk of dependence, some patients are still provided with a spinal support as a placebo or because other measures have failed (29).

Such widespread use of corsets and braces suggests the need for a thorough understanding of their functions and applications in order to determine how, and under what conditions, to use them; what they can do and where they fall short; how they can help; and where, if misused or overused, they can cause problems.

M. H. Pope, Dr. Med. Sc., Ph.D.: McClure Center for Musculoskeletal Research, Vermont Rehabilitation Engineering Center, Department of Orthopaedics and Rehabilitation, University of Vermont, Burlington, Vermont 05405.

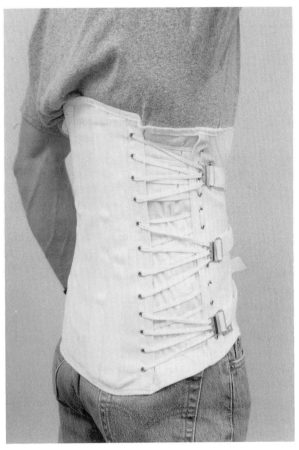

FIG. 1. The typical high laced corset brace.

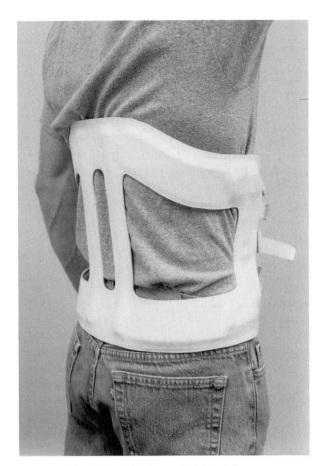

FIG. 2. The Knight or chair back brace.

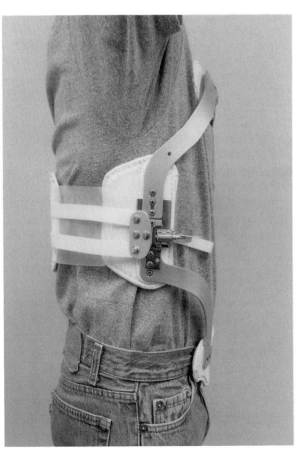

FIG. 3. The Jewett hyperextension brace.

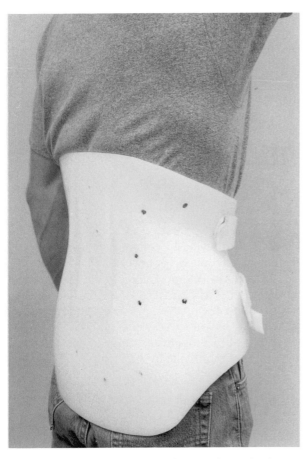

FIG. 4A. Low molded, anterior opening orthosis.

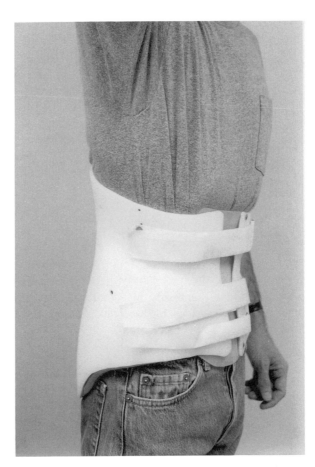

FIG. 4B. Low molded, anterior opening orthosis.

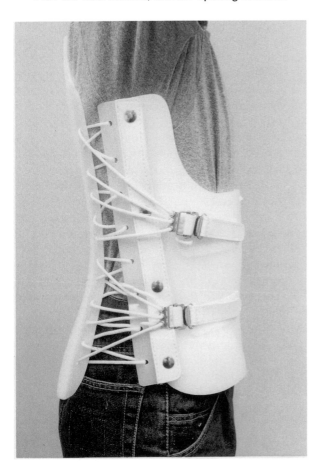

FIG. 5. Two-piece molded orthosis with adjustable side lacing.

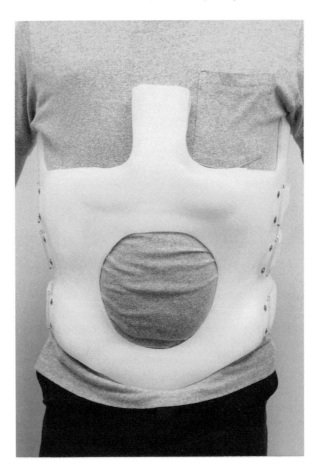

FIG. 6. Molded orthosis designed to increase hyperextension.

CLASSIFICATION OF ORTHOSES

A convenient classification system would include:

1. Trochanteric belts
2. Sacroiliac and lumbosacral belts
3. Corsets
4. Rigid braces
5. Hyperextension braces
6. Molded jackets.

Trochanteric Belts

The trochanteric belt goes around the pelvis between the trochanter and iliac crests. The belt, which is usually between 5 cm and 8 cm wide, buckles at the front. The belt is usually prescribed for sacroiliac joint pain and pelvic fractures.

Sacroiliac and Lumbosacral Belts

The so-called sacroiliac (SI) belt and lumbosacral belt are usually made of heavy cotton reinforced by light-weight stays. They differ in width with the sacroiliac belt of 10 cm to 15 cm wide and the lumbosacral belt of 20 cm to 30 cm wide. Pressure is applied by means of the adjustable laces on the side or back. The sacroiliac belt is meant to prevent SI motion by squeezing the joints together. Both belts are prescribed for low back pain.

Corsets

Corsets (Fig. 1) often extend over the buttocks and often have shoulder straps. Corsets have stays to provide rigidity and use laces at the back, side, or front. The shorter corsets are usually prescribed for low back pain whereas the longer corsets are used for problems in the mid-thoracic and lower thoracic spine.

Rigid Braces

The rigid brace is generally short with posterior uprights contoured to the dorsal spine and with pelvic and thoracic bands. Anterior pressure is applied by fabric and straps. Typical braces of this type are the Williams or Knight brace (Fig. 2). Both are usually prescribed for low back pain or segmental instability. The Knight brace (chair back type) has the function of immobilizing the lumbar spine in a neutral position. The Williams brace has no vertical uprights in the middle of the back and thus the low back can be pushed into flexion. The Raney flexion jacket, which reduces the lumbar lordosis and holds the patient in pelvic tilt, is popular amongst many clinicians.

Hyperextension Braces

The anterior hyperextension brace (Taylor or Jewett) employs an anterior rectangular metal frame to apply pressure over the pubis and upper sternum and counter pressure is applied at about the T10 level (Fig. 3). It is designed to prevent excessive flexion and is often used for anterior compression fractures.

Molded Jackets

These were previously constructed from plaster of paris but molded plastic is now more commonly used (Figs. 4A and 4B). Although the pressure is widely supported over the skin surfaces local abrasion can be a problem. Some such jackets are flexible and have anterior straps to provide access and support. These have been modified to provide greater flexibility in application (Fig. 5) or to provide hyperextension (Fig. 6).

CLINICAL UTILIZATION

Rationale

As noted above, braces and corsets come in many different types. Depending on the type chosen, braces may be designed to immobilize or support the spine in a neutral or upright, hyperextended, flexed, or sideways leaning position. Bracing of the lower back may be provided for low back pain, trauma (e.g., fractures), infections, muscular weakness, and, occasionally, metabolic bone disease such as osteoporosis. The majority of supports or braces, however, are prescribed for idiopathic LBP, prior to surgery or following the failure of surgery (45). Lucas (39) suggests that the objectives of spinal bracing are (a) control of pain, (b) protection from further injury, (c) assistance for muscle weakness, and (d) prevention and correction of deformity. Hipps (29) proposed that corsets and braces may promote a conditioned reflex and response reaction, which will develop tone and strength in weak abdominal muscles, improve patient posture, and decrease motion, thereby lessening pain. Million et al. (43) believed that the principal mechanism of symptom relief was by the restriction of motion. Bugge and Biering-Sörensen (7) have suggested that proprioceptive stimuli, local temperature elevation, and an increased feeling of safety in braces may help LBP sufferers.

By far the most common rationale, however, is that lumbar supports, including corsets and braces, compress the abdomen resulting in increased intra-abdominal pressure, which unloads the vertebral column itself (10,45,46). The topic of intra-abdominal pressure (IAP) is discussed further below.

Clinical Trials

Much opinion exists among clinicians regarding the use of corsets and braces. Mooney and Cairns (44) state that they use lumbosacral supports in about 5% of outpatient care programs as an aid in controlling the acute problem. They do not advocate their use in chronic low back pain. On the other hand, on the basis of a retrospective study, Alaranta and Hurri (2) suggest that a corset is reasonable therapy with patients with chronic LBP. A corset was found to be less expensive than other treatments. Likewise Amundsen and Weber (4) found that the use of a three point corset led to improved function in 53% of chronic LBP patients. However the numbers were small (20) and no control group was used. In an interesting study Coxhead et al. (11) found greater improvement in patients who used four different simultaneous treatment modalities (including corsets) compared to those who received fewer treatment modalities although this benefit was not sustained. Similarly, Larsson et al. (36) found that five simultaneous modalities worked better in the short run than either corset or bed rest alone. Noncomparative studies by Willner (64) support selected use of corsets.

Alaranta and Hurri (2) retrospectively studied 113 Finnish LBP patients. Thirty-seven percent of respondents claimed excellent or good relief from corsets. As shown in Table 1 males preferred low semi-rigid or elastic models and females preferred a high semi-rigid model. As shown in Table 2 the respondents had worn the corset quite recently.

Very few prospective trials have been reported. In a multicentered study, 456 British LBP patients were randomized into manipulation, corset, physical therapy, or analgesics (18). There was no difference between groups at 3 and 6 weeks and 3 months and 1 year. However, it was concluded that the corset alone was as effective as other treatments, less expensive than manipulation and physical therapy, and safer than drugs. Million et al. (43) found that a spinal support (metal stays) in a lumbosacral corset was important in relieving symptoms. These workers randomly allocated patients to a corset with or

TABLE 1. *Relation between subjective relief and type of corset according to sex*

| | Subjective relief | | | |
| | Excellent or good (%) | | Slight or negligible (%) | |
	Females	Males	Females	Males
Elastic (low)	7 (30)	7 (47)	16 (70)	8 (53)
Semi-rigid				
Low	5 (28)	5 (39)	13 (72)	8 (61)
High	16 (48)	2 (20)	17 (52)	8 (80)
Total	28 (38)	14 (37)	46 (62)	24 (63)

With permission from ref. 2

TABLE 2. *When did you last wear the corset?*

	Females (%)	Males (%)	All (%)
During the past week	32 (43)	13 (34)	45 (40)
2–4 weeks ago	13 (18)	9 (23)	22 (19)
1–2 months ago	10 (13)	4 (11)	14 (13)
3–4 months ago	8 (11)	6 (16)	14 (13)
6–9 months ago	3 (4)	2 (5)	5 (4)
9 months ago	8 (11)	4 (11)	12 (11)
Total	74 (100)	38 (100)	112 (100)

With permission from ref. 2.

without a support. Objective measures (SLR, lateral bend, flexion) did not differ between the groups but subjective measures did.

Haugh et al. (27) conducted a three week randomized controlled clinical trial of transcutaneous muscle stimulation (TMS) compared to lumbosacral corset on patients with non-specific semi-acute low back pain. An interesting feature of this study was that a heat sensitive compliance meter was sewn into the corset in an effort to measure and to improve compliance. Both treatment groups increased their muscle strength (assessed by maximum isometric extensor contractions) by similar amounts and increased their fatigue times by insignificant amounts. Neither group changed in extension flexibility, and the difference in flexion flexibility between the groups was not statistically significant. The only group difference that was of statistical significance (p < 0.05) was the greater reduction in pain for the TMS group.

It should be noted that the comprehensive Quebec Task Force Report (37) concludes that there is no documented evidence to suggest that braces reduce the period of disability. In addition, Flor and Turk (22) concluded that corsets and braces, although widely used, have no proven effect.

Perhaps, the most important consideration is the correct indication. For example Hipps (29) states that braces are more beneficial when (a) there is a localized area of spasm in an area of low back pain, (b) there is a limited range of movement in a certain part of the back, usually in a painful area, and (c) pain occurs or is aggravated by the movements of the spine.

The many hypotheses on mechanism of action of braces and corsets include:

1. Increased abdominal pressure may have an analgesic effect.
2. The lower margin of a corset may provide circumferential support around the pelvic ring.
3. There is an unloading effect on the trunk by support through thoracic musculoskeletal structures.
4. They insulate the skin and the increased warmth decreases pain sensation.
5. Increased pressure on the abdomen caused by the de-

vice results in hydraulic support for the painful back structures.

6. They physically limit the range of motion of the spine, thus decreasing stress to painful structures in the back.
7. Tactile stimulation from the device results in beneficial modification of muscle action with decreased stress on the back.

Negative Aspects

In spite of the wide clinical use of back supports, their use is not without drawbacks. There is a possible loss of muscle function and psychological addiction to the device (59). Quinet and Hadler (56) were also of the opinion that they are detrimental by leading to muscular atrophy. This is a concern voiced by many authors although neither of these effects has been proven. However, in most patients, it should be possible to eliminate use of a corset eventually, according to Kester (31).

MECHANICAL FUNCTION

Electromyography

Waters and Morris (62) found that while standing, both the chair back brace and a corset slightly decreased or did not change erector spinae EMG. An inflatable corset reduces electromyographic (EMG) activity particularly during heavy load. In slow or moderate walking no devices had any effect, but in fast walking the EMG activity was increased if a rigid brace was worn. It should be noted that Lumsden and Morris (40) found that a rigid brace actually increased intersegmental motion in rotation. Thus, the muscle activity may be an attempt to prevent the segmental rotation. Other work is equivocal: Grew and Deane (25) and Morris and Lucas (46) noted decreased EMG activity with corsets. Waters and Morris (62) and Nachemson et al. (49) found both increases and decreases depending on the task.

Intra-Discal Pressure (IDP)

Nachemson and Morris (48) used the method pioneered by Nachemson to measure the IDP under a variety of circumstances. Subjects who experienced pain during different activities were found to have increased IDP. This supports the view that these patients have greater muscle contraction due to the muscles splinting the spine. Likewise a valsalva (a voluntary increase in intra-abdominal pressure due to muscle contraction) actually increased IDP. Alternatively an inflatable corset decreased the IDP by 25%.

Intra-Abdominal Pressure (IAP)

Harman et al. (26) found that weight lifters who used a weight lifters' belt produced both a greater peak and faster rise in IAP than without the belt. The authors conclude that a lifting belt increases IAP and reduces disc pressure. The abdominal cavity, as well as the thoracic cavity, is pressurized to a greater extent when the spine is placed under increased load (5,13,19,34). This cavity pressure has long been conjectured to decrease spinal loading by introducing an extension moment across the lumbar spine which reduces the tension required in the posterior spinal muscles. Based upon controlled testing, however, Krag et al. (33) have shown that voluntary pressurization of the abdominal cavity causes the opposite effect, namely an *increase* of dorsal muscle activity.

Morris et al. (45) found that an inflatable corset increases the resting abdominal cavity pressure by about 10 to 15 mm Hg, but does not raise the peak pressures during a controlled lift. Grew and Deane (25) stated that the longer supports provide significant increases in pressure when the wearer is seated, and the corsets increased the pressure significantly when the wearer is walking. The same authors found that the patient group responded in a different manner than a control group in terms of spinal movement, but not in the developed IAP. Grew and Deane (25) concluded that over the period of treatment a patient becomes accustomed to the brace or corset. It was suggested that where the spine is lightly stressed, the support reduces the activity of the abdominal muscles. Under stressful activity the brace strengthens the wall and enables the wearer to increase the IAP.

Krag et al. (32) compared cloth lumbosacral corsets to Raney plastic jackets and no support in normal volunteers. They demonstrated that no significant effects were produced by either device, either for IAP or erector spinae EMG during isometric extension efforts. Finally Kumar and Godfrey (35) conducted a comparative evaluation of six commonly prescribed spinal supports. Volunteers were fitted with sacroiliac belt, lumbosacral corset, Harris, Macnab, Knight, and Taylor braces in turn and were asked to perform sagittal, lateral, and oblique lifts, and same level side to side weight transfers. The results show no significant difference in intra-abdominal pressure due to different spinal support in all activities studied. It was concluded that on the basis of the support through IAP there is no significant difference between the braces studied.

Motion

The efficacy of spinal braces in preventing intervertebral movements has been questioned by Norton and Brown (53). While gross movements are prevented, individual vertebral movements are sometimes increased.

These workers concluded that it seems highly unlikely that any device applied to the exterior of the body can effectively splint the lumbosacral region. Lumsden and Morris (40) found a modified chair back brace to be quite effective in restricting motion in standing whereas a corset was quite ineffective. In walking both the brace and the corset actually increased the axial rotation in the lumbar spine.

On the other hand Fidler and Plasmans (21) and Maier (41) on the basis of radiographic studies state that corsets and braces do, in fact, decrease motion. Grew and Deane (25) concluded that in order to reduce spinal movements by an appreciable amount, a rigid form of bracing is required, although a custom-fitted less rigid brace is better than a non-custom-fitted more rigid plastic shell. Corsets were said to provide little restriction of movement although the location of the stays can enable specific painful movements to be influenced. The shorter corsets restricted movement better than the longer ones.

Temperature

Dixon et al. (16) found that chronic LBP responds as well to the wearing of an insulated belt as to an ordinary corset, and suggested that the observed increase in the lumbar and thoracic skin temperature was the cause of symptom relief.

Likewise, similar findings were reported by Grew and Deane (25). These workers found that thicker or padded material over the lumbar skin can be used to raise its temperature by almost 2 degrees centigrade. However, the material must be held in contact with the skin. Apparently a rigid plastic jacket had a tendency to provide a cooling "funnel" which reduced its heating effectiveness.

BIOFEEDBACK

Another proposed mechanism of action is that tactile stimulation from the brace or corset results in behavioral modification of muscle action, therefore improved spinal support. EMG activity would presumably evidence this effect, but available reports are conflicting, and show EMG activity to be increased (30), decreased (9), or unchanged (42) in persons with low back pain. Two reviews, Dolce and Raczynski (17) and Nouwen (54) were equivocal.

It is accepted that low back pain is often caused by mechanical stress. Clinical observations indicate that positions of decreased stress such as lying down sometimes improve pain temporarily. However, prolonged bed rest does not appear to help in the long run (14), perhaps because of simultaneous muscle deconditioning.

As decreasing stress appears to improve LBP, stress reduction by an orthosis would presumably be desirable. Table 3 shows that even if compliance with feedback were perfect, neither tactile information from a corset, nor EMG signal, nor inclinometer signal provides adequate information about stress. The corset only provides information about flexion of the trunk, appropriate when standing but not when lying. Forward flexion either at the hips or in the trunk while standing provides a long lever arm for the force of gravity through the low back. With either movement, an inclinometer would be activated. When the trunk is partially flexed, EMG activity is increased, but with full flexion there is electrical silence (24). Holding an object while standing increases force and is countered by increased EMG activity (58,60) but would not activate an inclinometer. Force applied to the spine by the contraction of muscles in spasm (17) would be detected by EMG but not inclinometer.

Treatments involving EMG feedback have been reported both effective (23,50) and not effective (8) in treating low back pain. However, these reports focus on treatments applied for only one hour or less each day, in coordination with psychotherapy, rather than for longer treatment periods. Wolf et al. (65) and Nouwen (54) are the only two studies which involved longer periods of feedback: the latter showed no improvements, but the former, albeit dealing with only one patient, reported the treatment was superior. An inclinometer, a promising device for this application, has been used to monitor but not to treat persons with LBP (52). It has successfully improved head posture of children with cerebral palsy (66).

The feedback stimulus must be effective in changing behavior of the orthosis wearer. Feedback has been successfully used in ergonomics (11) applications. Wertsch

TABLE 3. *Feedback provided to decrease force on the spine*

	Ideal	EMG	Inclinometer	Corset
Standing trunk flexion	+	+	+	+
Standing hip flexion	+	+	+	−
Deceleration	+	+	+	−
Standing holding object	+	+	−	−
Back "spasm"	+	+	−	−
Trunk fully flexed	+	−	+	−
Lying trunk flexion	−	−	+	+

(63) reviewed substitution of tactile for visual sensation, described auditory and visual feedback to patients with insensate feet but pointed out that stimuli are often ignored. Szeto and Saunders (61) studied effectiveness of various feedback mechanisms. It is apparent that there is some possibility of a specially designed biofeedback orthosis having some potential for prevention of excessive forces or postural stresses.

FUTURE DIRECTIONS

Braces and corsets have been used for a very long time but it is only recently that clinical trials have been run to test their efficacy and experiments proposed to assess their mode of action. The clinical trials that have been published were often not prospective or were poorly controlled and with small numbers of subjects. Clearly priority needs to be placed in this area.

It is not clear that present braces or corsets reduce spine load or immobilize the spine. It is probable that biofeedback from the brace is an important positive aspect and further work should explore this issue.

ACKNOWLEDGMENT

We wish to acknowledge support from the National Institute of Disability and Rehabilitation Research through the Vermont Rehabilitation Engineering Center.

REFERENCES

1. Ahlgren SA, Hansen T (1978): The use of lumbosacral corsets prescribed for low back pain. *Prosthet Orthot Int* 2:101–104.
2. Alaranta H, Hurri H (1988): Compliance and subjective relief by corset treatment in chronic low back pain. *Scand J Rehab Med* 20:133–136.
3. American Academy of Orthopaedic Surgeons (1952): Braces, splints, show alterations. In: *Orthopaedic appliances atlas vol. 1*. Ann Arbor: Edwards.
4. Amundsen T, Weber H (1982): Korsettbehandling av kronisk rygg. *Tidsskr Nor Laegeforen* 102:1649–1651.
5. Bartelink DL (1957): Role of abdominal pressure in relieving pressure on lumbar intervertebral discs. *J Bone Joint Surg* [Br] 39:718–725.
6. Benn RT, Wood PH (1975): Pain in the back: An attempt to estimate the size of the problem. *Rheumatol Rehab* 14:121–128.
7. Bugge PM, Biering-Sörensen F (1987): Lumbar corset treatment. *Ugeskr Laeger* 149:577–579.
8. Bush C, Ditto B, Feuerstein M (1985): A controlled evaluation of paraspinal EMG biofeedback in the treatment of chronic low back pain. *Health Psychol* 4:307–321.
9. Collins GA, Cohen MJ, Naliboff BD, Schandler SL (1982): Comparative analysis of paraspinal and frontalis EMG, heart rate and skin conductance in chronic low back pain patients and normals to various postures and stress. *Scand J Rehab Med* 14:39–46.
10. Coplans CW (1978): Conservative treatment of low back pain. In: *Disorders of the lumbar spine*, AJ Helfet, LD Grubel, eds. Philadelphia: JB Lippincott.
11. Coxhead CE, Inskip H, Meade TW, North WR, Troup JD (1981): Multicentre trial of physiotherapy in the management of sciatic symptoms. *Lancet* 1:1065–1068.
12. Cushman WH, Little RH, Lucas RL, Pugsley RE, Stevens JA (1983): Equipment design. In: *Ergonomic design for people at work, vol. 1*. Belmont, CA: Eastman-Kodak Company, Human Factors Section, Lifetime Learning Publications.
13. Davis PR, Troup JDG (1964): Pressures in the trunk cavities when pulling, pushing and lifting. *Erg* 7:465–474.
14. Deyo RA, Diehl AK, Rosenthal M (1986): How many days of bed rest for acute low back pain? A randomized clinical trial. *New Engl J Med* 315(17):1064–1070.
15. Deyo RA, Tsui-Wu YJ (1987): Descriptive epidemiology of low-back pain and its related medical care in the United States. *Spine* 12(3):264–268.
16. Dixon ASJ, Owen-Smith BD, Harrison RA (1972): Cold sensitive, non specific, low back pain (a comparative trial of treatment). *Clin Trials J* 9:16–21.
17. Dolce JJ, Raczynski JM (1985): Neuromuscular activity and electromyography in painful backs: Psychological and biomechanical models in assessment and treatment. *Psychological Bulletin* 97(3):502–520.
18. Doran DM, Newell DJ (1975): Manipulation in treatment of low back pain: A multicentre study. *Br Med J* 2:161–164.
19. Eie N, Wehn P (1962): Measurements of the intra-abdominal pressure in relation to weight bearing of the lumbosacral spine. *J Oslo City Hosp* 12:205–217.
20. Evans A (1921): *The palace of Minos, vol. 1*. London: Macmillan, p. 503.
21. Fidler MW, Plasmans CM (1983): The effect of four types of support on the segmental mobility of the lumbosacral spine. *J Bone Joint Surg* [Am] 65(7):943–947.
22. Flor H, Turk DC (1984): Etiological theories and treatments for chronic back pain. I. Somatic models and interventions. *Pain* 19:105–121.
23. Flor H, Haag G, Turk DC (1986): Long-term efficacy of EMG biofeedback for chronic rheumatic back pain. *Pain* 27:195–202.
24. Floyd WF, Silver PHS (1955): The function of the erectores spinae muscles in certain movements and postures in man. *J Physiol* 129:184–203.
25. Grew ND, Deane G (1982): The physical effect of lumbar spinal supports. *Prosthet Orthot Int* 6:79–87.
26. Harman EA, Rosenstein RM, Frykman PN (1989): Effects of a belt on intraabdominal pressure during weight lifting. *Med Sci Sports Exerc* 21:186–190.
27. Haugh LD, Pope MH, Krag MH, MacDonald LP (1989): Treatment of semi-acute low back pain by transcutaneous muscle stimulation or lumbosacral corset: A randomized clinical trial. Presented at FCER meeting, Washington, DC, April 1989.
28. Hayne CR (1983): The case for spinal supports and education in back pain. *Practitioner* 277:1069.
29. Hipps HE (1967): Back braces: Types, functions and how to order and use them. *Medical Clin N Am* 51(5):1315–1343.
30. Janda U (1977): Muscle, central nervous motor regulation and a back problem. In: *The neurobiological mechanisms in manipulative therapy*, JM Korr, ed. New York: Plenum Press.
31. Kester NC (1969): Evaluation and medical management of low back pain. *Med Clin N Am* 53(3):525–540.
32. Krag MH, Byrne KB, Miller L, Haugh L, Pope MH (1987): Failure of intra-abdominal pressure to reduce spinal loads without and with lumbar orthoses. Proc Orthop Res Soc 33rd annual meeting, San Francisco, CA.
33. Krag MH, Gilbertson L, Pope MH (1985): Intra-abdominal and intra-thoracic pressure effects upon load bearing of the spine (Proc Orthop Res Soc 31st annual meeting, Las Vegas NV). *Orthop Trans* 9:358.
34. Kumar S, Davis PR (1973): Lumbar vertebral innervation and intra-abdominal pressure. *J Anat* 114:47–53.
35. Kumar S, Godfrey C (1986): Spinal braces and abdominal support. In: *Trends in ergonomics/human factors III*, Karwowski, ed. New York: Elsevier.
36. Larsson U, Choler U, Lidstrom A, Lind G, Nachemson A (1980): Autotraction for treatment of lumbago-sciatica. *Acta Orthop Scand* 51:791–798.
37. Le Blanc F, et al (1987): Scientific approach to the assessment and management of activity-related spinal disorders. A monograph for clinicians. Report of the Quebec Task Force on Spinal Disorders. *Spine* 12(7):S1–S59.
38. Lewis L, Smith HJ (1982): *Oscar Wilde discovers America*. New

York: Benjamin Blom, by arrangement with Harcourt, Brace and World.

39. Lucas DB (1969): Spinal bracing. In: *Orthotics,* S Licht, ed. Baltimore: Waverly Press, pp. 274–305.

40. Lumsden RM 2d, Morris JM (1968): An in vivo study of axial rotation and immobilization at the lumbosacral joint. *J Bone Joint Surg* [Am] 50:1591–1602.

41. Maier K (1962): Rontgenologischen Funktions Studien an der Lendenwirbet-saule bei Fivierung durch verbrauchliche korsette. *Z Orthop* 95:319–330.

42. Miller DJ (1985): Comparison of electromyographic activity in the lumbar paraspinal muscles of subjects with and without chronic low back pain. *Phys Ther* 65:1347–1354.

43. Million R, Nilsen KH, Jayson MI, Baker RD (1981): Evaluation of low back pain and assessment of lumbar corsets with and without back supports. *Ann Rheum Dis* 40:449–454.

44. Mooney V, Cairns D (1978): Management in the patient with chronic low back pain. *Orthop Clin N Am* 9(2):543–557.

45. Morris JM, Lucas DB, Bresler B (1961): Role of the trunk in stability of the spine. *J Bone Joint Surg* [Am] 43:327–351.

46. Morris JM, Lucas DB (1963): Physiological considerations in bracing of the spine. *Orthop Prosth Appl* 37:44.

47. Morris JM (1974): Low back bracing. *Clin Orthop* (102):126–132.

48. Nachemson A, Morris JM (1964): In vivo measurements of intradiscal pressure. *J Bone Joint Surg* [Am] 46:1077–1092.

49. Nachemson A, Schultz A, Andersson G (1983): Mechanical effectiveness studies of lumbar spine orthoses. *Scand J Rehab Med* (Suppl) 9:139–149.

50. Nattress LW, Litt BD (1962): Report 2: Survey to determine the state of services available to amputees and orthopedically disabled persons. Orthotic Services USA-1962. Washington, DC: American Orthotics and Prosthetics Association.

51. Nigl AJ, Fischer-Williams M (1980): Treatment of low back strain with electromyographic biofeedback and relaxation training. *Psychosomatics* 21:495–499.

52. Nordin M (1982): Methods for studying work load with special reference to the lumbar spine (thesis). Goteborg, Sweden.

53. Norton PL, Brown T (1957): The immobilizing efficiency of back braces; Their effect on the posture and motion of the lumbosacral spine. *J Bone Joint Surg* [Am] 39:111–139.

54. Nouwen A (1983): EMG biofeedback used to reduce standing levels of paraspinal muscle tension in chronic low back pain. *Pain* 17:353–360.

55. Perry J (1970): The use of external support in the treatment of low-back pain. *J Bone Joint Surg* [Am] 52(7):1440–1442.

56. Quinet RJ, Hadler NM (1979): Diagnosis and treatment of backache. *Sem Arthrit Rheum* 8:261–287.

57. Sayre LA (1877): *Spinal disease and spinal curvature.* London.

58. Schultz AB, Andersson GB, Haderspeck K, Ortengren R (1982): Analysis and measurement of lumbar trunk loads in tasks involving bends and twists. *J Biomech* 15:669–675.

59. Selby DK (1982): Conservative care of nonspecific low back pain. *Orthop Clin No Am* 13(3):427–437.

60. Seroussi RE, Pope MH (1987): The relationship between trunk muscle electromyography and moments in the sagittal and frontal planes. Proc Orthop Res Soc 33rd annual meeting, San Francisco, CA.

61. Szeto AY, Saunders FA (1982): Electrocutaneous stimulation for sensory communication in rehabilitation engineering. *IEEE Trans Biomed Eng* 29:300–308.

62. Waters RL, Morris JM (1970): Effect of spinal supports on the electrical activity of muscles of the trunk. *J Bone Joint Surg* [Am] 52:51–60.

63. Wertsch J (1985): Sensory substitution: State of the art and future technology. Milwaukee, WI: Proc Clement Zablocky VA Medical Center.

64. Willner S (1985): Effect of a rigid brace on back pain. *Acta Orthop Scand* 56:40–42.

65. Wolf SL, Nacht M, Kelly JL (1982): EMG feedback training during dynamic movement for low back pain patients. *Behav Therapy* 13:395–406.

66. Wooldridge CP, Russell G (1976): Head position training with the cerebral palsied child: Application of biofeedback techniques. *Arch Phys Med Rehab* 57:407–414.

Physical Therapy and Education

The Adult Spine: Principles and Practice,
J. W. Frymoyer, Editor-in-Chief.
Raven Press, Ltd., New York © 1991.

CHAPTER 75

The Physical Therapist Approach

Philip L. Witt

A comprehensive program of physical therapy is the cornerstone of modern treatment for adult spinal dysfunction in cases requiring non-surgical medical management. Also physical therapy plays a significant role in the recovery of patients whose conditions require surgical intervention. The focus of this chapter will be on physical therapy for non-surgical adult spinal dysfunction patients. Spinal dysfunction is defined as a functional incapacity regardless of the causation. This distinction between spinal dysfunction and pain is important. While the alleviation of back pain is certainly one of the goals of physical therapists, and the primary goal of patients, correction of or adaptation to the underlying dysfunction is of primary importance. The following discussion will be divided into two sections: Physical Therapy for Acute Spinal Symptoms and Physical Therapy for Chronic Spinal Dysfunction. General physical therapy goals and an overview of possible treatments will be addressed.

As in any rapidly developing clinical field, basic and applied research lags behind the development of treatment techniques (11). The profession of physical therapy is moving rapidly to close the gap. I will attempt to delineate techniques that have scientific or clinical support, or

that make common sense. Physical therapy is not alone in its attempts to develop and document sound treatments for spinal problems; nor does any profession have the definitive answer to spinal pain and dysfunction.

The basis for all physical therapy related to spinal dysfunction is a detailed history and physical examination. The majority of therapists follow a system of evaluation modeled after the work of Maitland (60).

The history covers topics such as, the area of the pain or stiffness; the behavior of symptoms such as symptom fluctuations, aggravators, relievers including rest, functional limitations; related questions (general health, weight loss, medications); and an account of present and prior episodes, current and previous treatment, contraindications, effect on the patient's life and on their goals. A part of the history identifies those conditions not amenable to physical therapy. The history permits the therapist to plan the objective exam, and to understand the effect that this problem has had on the life of the patient.

The objective exam is used to confirm clinical impressions garnered from the history, to localize pain causative structures, to set realistic short- and long-term goals, and to plan appropriate treatments to attain those goals. The exam includes the patient's posture, gait, willingness to move, deformity, swelling, and movement patterns; spinal movements within the physiological

P. L. Witt, Ph.D., P.T.: Division of Physical Therapy, University of North Carolina at Chapel Hill, Chapel Hill, North Carolina, 27599–7135.

range; passive movement tests which involve both accessory and physiological ranges; resistive tests; stress tests to reproduce symptoms; palpation to identify pain productive structures; special tests for specific anatomical structures; and a sensory and neurological examination.

Therapists attempt to reproduce the complaints of the patient through the objective examination. Great importance is placed on confirming subjective symptoms with objective signs. As emphasized throughout this text arthritic changes in spinal radiographs or a CT image of a herniated disc do not confirm that these are the cause of the pain or dysfunction in any given individual (93,94).

PHYSICAL THERAPY FOR ACUTE SPINAL SYMPTOMS

The major goals of therapists in the treatment of acute spinal dysfunction are: (a) alleviation of pain; (b) promotion of injured tissue healing; (c) relief of muscle spasm; (d) restoration of normal range of motion, spinal mechanics, and muscle function; (e) activity of daily living education; and (f) education to prevent future problems. Each goal should be addressed to achieve the best possible short- and long-term outcome. Although 90% of people with an acute back pain episode are pain free within approximately a month (25,79), the alleviation of the pain is not necessarily indicative of the resolution of the underlying problem (11). Correction of underlying dysfunction, which is usually related to biomechanics or fitness, is necessary for the prevention of future difficulties (8,13), including future disability (64).

Goal 1. Alleviate Pain

Pain relief can be attained by a variety of means dependent upon the source of the pain. Pain caused by what physical therapists term mechanical block (e.g., annular disc lesion or zygoapophyseal joint impingement) can sometimes be relieved by appropriately located and graded mobilization or manipulative maneuvers (26,27,33,47). There are numerous techniques for mobilization and manipulation but little evidence of the relative benefits of one versus the other (37,38,45,109). Therefore therapists usually choose those techniques best suited to their education, experience, and treatment philosophy.

Mobilization techniques are categorized according to the amount of movement being caused by the technique. Movements are graded on a scale of 1–5 (Fig. 1). Grades one and two primarily are used to relieve pain. Grades three through five are used on the premise they stretch muscles, ligaments, or joint capsules. Attention is also directed toward the treatment of pain presumed to be caused by muscle spasm through the application of a

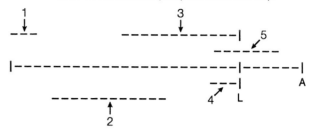

FIG. 1. Grades of movement (adapted from ref. 60).

L: Pathological limit of the joint.
A: Anatomic limit of the joint.
Grade 1: Small amplitude movement performed at the beginning of the range.
Grade 2: Large amplitude movement performed within the range but not reaching the end of the range.
Grade 3: Large amplitude movement performed up to the end of the available range.
Grade 4: Small amplitude movement performed at the limit of the available range.
Grade 5: Small amplitude, high velocity thrust beyond the currently available range.

combination of ice (1,6,57,112), electrical stimulation (58,74), gentle massage techniques (21,50), gentle active and passive movement therapy (92,106,111), and rest (24,110).

Pain arising from a disc herniation commonly is treated with positioning in trunk extension, postural corrections of lateral shifts, and rest (53,65,98). This approach will be discussed in detail in Chapter 76. As noted in that chapter the patient's pain induced compensatory posture is corrected and repositioning usually in extension is maintained which is hypothesized to decrease stress on the posterior vertebral structures and to allow migration of the nuclear material anteriorly (2,19,69, 70,72,99).

Pain thought to arise from other soft tissue sources (ligaments, fascia) is treated with rest, ice, positioning for comfort, gentle friction massage to prevent adhesions (20), and gradual active motion. Nerve root impingement pain and dural impingement pain are treated by first attempting to alleviate the mechanical derangement via treatments such as traction, positioning, and mobilization (42,61,95,96). This is followed by treatment for any compensatory muscle involvement, again including ice, massage, and gentle active movements.

People with acute pain from sources not amenable to physical therapy (tumors, vertebral fractures, kidney disease, gynecological disease) are referred to appropriate health care practitioners.

Goal 2. Promote Tissue Healing

Following the reduction of pain, promotion of healing is the next concern of the physical therapist. Injured structures that have a blood supply have the potential to heal (41,66). Treatment for acute back muscle strain and spinal ligament sprain is similar to the treatment for the same problems at any joint. Included in the regime are rest to reduce further trauma (24,110) and ice to limit the amount of edema (1,6). The physical therapist believes electrical stimulation will help control edema, and thereby promote healing (18,85,87,107).

Gentle movements and stretching may be instituted early in the recovery phase to maintain range of motion and to stimulate soft tissue nutrition (29,40,44,84, 88,103). Proper positioning is an important component of the program designed to enhance healing. Positioning is done according to the comfort of the patient, as well as based on the presumed pathology. The principal proponent of this technique is McKenzie (69,70,72,99). However, McKenzie and others emphasize that initial patient positioning is temporary. Eventually the patient must re-establish as much range of movement as possible in all directions (65).

Goal 3. Relieve Muscle Spasm

Muscle spasm has been implicated as a major cause of acute and chronic back pain (93,94), although, as pointed out in Chapter 16, underlying data in support of this concept are sparse. Many physical therapists believe acute muscle spasm may be the actual source of the pain and the decreased spinal mobility which may predispose the individual to injury of other tissues (15). On that premise, elimination of acute spasms is an important component of the treatment plan, particularly in the prevention of future long-term or recurrent back pain episodes. In fact, we believe untreated spasms may remain at a subclinical level, and are sufficient to predispose patients to future injury (65,79). Many techniques exist for achieving the relief of muscle spasms, most of which are based on clinical observation. However, rigorous clinical research has not documented the effectiveness of these techniques.

Ice that is applied directly over the area of acute muscle spasm has been shown to reduce the amount of spasm effectively (1,6,57,112). Gentle transverse friction massage has been advocated by Cyriax for the reduction of muscle spasm and the prevention of later adhesions (20). Slow, gentle massage and stretching techniques, commonly called myofascial release, are being used to reduce spasms and stretch fascia. Gentle movements designed to cause muscle to contract and relax are in common usage today as are low grade, oscillatory mobilization movements and stretching techniques (17,23, 35,77). Also, alleviation of underlying muscle spasms, accompanied by establishment of normal movement and education may help to reduce the number of recurrent back problems (12,51).

Goal 4. Restore Normal Range of Motion, Spinal Mechanics, and Muscle Function

Much of the diminished spinal range of motion observed in patients with acute back pain episodes will return with the elimination of pain and muscle spasm. People with recurrent back pain episodes may not be so fortunate. Most physical therapists advocate that any residual range of motion limitations be altered through high grade mobilizations and exercise to break range limiting adhesions and to stretch joint capsules (29,77). If the patient has a pre-existing limitation of motion, additional therapy may be needed. Muscle lengthening through a combination of stretching, followed by exercise in the lengthened range will be needed to stimulate the growth of new sarcomeres (4,32,34). Prolonged stretching of soft tissue will be needed to stimulate the laying down of longer collagen fibers (54,105). A combination of active and passive movement therapy (Proprioceptive Neuromuscular Facilitation, Feldenkrais, Trager Bodywork) may be used to promote pain free, coordinated spinal movements and to maintain the range of motion gained through stretching (91,102, 104,111). Many of the movement therapies have been developed outside of traditional medicine and have yet to be scientifically validated. I listed Feldenkrais' and Trager's work as examples because they are two forms of movement therapy that have had long clinical track usage, and make common sense.

Exercise is an important component of the complete care of any acute or chronic patient with spinal dysfunction. The better conditioned their muscles and cardiopulmonary systems are for the types of activities they will be performing, the easier and safer it will be for them to do their everyday activities (5,22). Specific therapeutic exercises for weak muscles may be prescribed (49,71). An important consideration, in addition to specific conditioning, is to regain muscle balance which is also thought to be affected and can prevent later reinjury (56,97).

General body conditioning is important as well. Injuries are more common when people are fatigued (5,46,75,80). The lower the person's overall fitness level, the more easily they become fatigued (3,5). Today, industry often wants to know if a patient is fit enough to return to work (63). While this is an extremely complicated question, physical therapists place increased reliance on computer-assisted back-evaluation devices to monitor objectively patient progress during treatment (52,55,62,80,101), and by establishing functional restoration programs to assess the ability of an individual to return safely to work (63).

Information obtained from the computerized back-evaluation systems is being used to predict if an individual is capable of performing a specific job. Even the best of these machines are not capable of a true simulation of "on the job" lifting. I do not believe their widespread application for this purpose is justified at this time (81,101).

Functional restoration (work-hardening) programs (see Chapter 13) have been developed to insure that a patient has become reconditioned for a particular task. Comprehensive programs involve an individual performing the same or similar job tasks required at their place of work, but in a controlled and monitored environment so that patient safety, muscle strength, endurance, and body mechanics can be evaluated and altered. Functional restoration systems can be quite simple or elaborate, utilizing computer-assisted multifunction stations (63,101). The most important component of the functional restoration programs is that patients are stressed sufficiently during the program to determine their future work status.

Goal 5. Educate Patients for Activities of Daily Living

In addition to the job task analysis and conditioning (mentioned previously), physical therapists help educate patients with correct body mechanics applicable to different daily requirements, methods of relaxation, and proper stretching techniques (50,67). Back schools in hospitals and industry have been developed to educate the public on how to protect their backs with a goal of lowering injury rates (7,9,39). This topic, its limitations, and use are discussed in Chapter 77.

Goal 6. Suggest Environmental Alterations

Physical therapists are concerned about the environmental conditions of the patient's home and workplace. Today, more therapists are working in the industrial setting making recommendations for job task assignments, workplace alterations, and scheduling changes to help relieve the stress of static positioning, repetitive motion, and muscle overload. Specially trained therapists are experienced at matching an ergonomic analysis of occupational environment with the realities of dealing with humans of differing physical characteristics.

PHYSICAL THERAPY FOR CHRONIC ADULT SPINAL DYSFUNCTION

Treatment of chronic spinal dysfunction is markedly different than the management of acute spinal pain. Treatment goals differ in that alleviating pain and promoting the healing of presumably injured tissue are not prime treatment objectives. Therefore, initial treatment for chronic dysfunction is fundamentally different. Although relief of pain should be one of the ultimate goals of therapy, I do not believe chronic pain can be ad-

dressed directly or rapidly and restoration of function is the first objective. This information must be given to the patients clearly because their primary goal most often is pain relief. Therapists must convince patients that their goals are not at odds with the patients'. Patient cooperation and participation are absolutely critical if a successful outcome is to be achieved.

Physical therapy goals for the treatment of chronic spinal dysfunction include: (a) improvement of spinal mobility and coordination of movement patterns, (b) gradual increase in both the quality and quantity of activities of daily living, (c) strength and endurance training, (d) relief of chronic muscle spasms, and (e) environmental alterations. Over time, all of these should cause some alleviation of pain; the reported pain is most likely caused by constant mechanical stressing of a variety of spinal structures by faulty biomechanics (43,78,86), poor conditioning (48), a physical manifestation of stress (82,93,94), self-perpetuating C-fiber input, sympathetic activation, or myofascial pain (30,31,83). Frequently, patients have undergone conscious and subconscious physical and psychological learning processes which promote decreased function and pain behavior (16,28,90,108). Treatments such as bed rest, ice, and other pain relieving modalities are of minimal value and conflict with the overall goal which is to get the individual active (63,73,111). Preparing patients both physically and psychologically for exercise programs and gradually rebuilding strength and endurance are critical steps in the process. In this context patients must take control over their own health, while the therapist's job is to encourage and develop an independent attitude while providing a treatment program for the patient. Once patients have seen progress is possible, they will be more willing and able to cooperate with the more physically challenging parts of the program.

The following discussion of the specific goals of treatment is designed to serve as a framework for the treatment of chronic spinal dysfunction. Little evidence exists to dictate one specific approach over another. While I personally have a preferred approach, I believe that any overall approach that the therapist knows well and is comfortable with can work if the program addresses the following goals.

Goal 1. Correct/Improve Spinal Mobility and Coordination of Movement Patterns

Establishing normal, or at least increasing, spinal mobility is important (65,77). Normal spinal biomechanics, as well as the normal functioning of muscles, is not possible if spinal segments have limited mobility. Force that is generated by muscles or externally applied to the spine cannot be dissipated properly if spinal segments have limited motion. The resultant stress may be directed to

areas not designed to absorb such stress, and secondarily cause sprain, strain, or degeneration (76).

Numerous techniques exist for establishing spinal mobility (11,65,77). Mobilization and manipulation techniques that are passive or self-mobilizing may be used (51). There are specific techniques designed to correct limited motions in very precise directions, and more general techniques designed to improve overall mobility. Appropriate use of both types of treatments may be needed to increase spinal mobility although following a specific technique or approach does not seem to influence the clinical outcome (37,38,45,109).

In conjunction with establishing spinal mobility is treatment designed to increase spinal coordination. While this area is just beginning to be studied for the spine (89), experience with other joints suggests that prolonged immobility and disuse can cause a loss in normal movement patterns (10,102). Movement techniques designed to facilitate coordination in people with generalized neurological problems appear to be effective with that population (10,14). Similar techniques could be applied to the chronic pain population. No matter what technique is used, patients must understand that it will be necessary to repeat the movements many times per day and over a prolonged period of time (111).

Goal 2. Increase Patients' Activities of Daily Living

Consistent with the main objective of increased movement, the therapist helps guide patients into gradually increasing their activities of daily living. People suffering from chronic spinal dysfunction tend to decrease their daily activity level because of pain. A gradual, controlled increase in activity will help patients make use of their new mobility and coordination.

Goal 3. Increase Patients' Strength and Endurance Training

Decreased general activity and spinal motion because of chronic pain will lead to a general decrease in muscle strength and endurance. Specific muscles critical to the control of spinal movement also may become deconditioned. Conversely the long-term success of treatment for this population will depend on gradual reconditioning. The two most common forms of exercise are weight lifting and swimming. Both are excellent with proper instruction on technique and progression. Other forms of exercise in use today are biking, rowing, stationary cross-country skiing, stair climbing, water aerobics, no impact or low impact land aerobics, and isokinetic or isodynamic exercise. Patients should be encouraged to take part in a variety of exercise programs rather than focusing only on a single exercise regime.

Goal 4. Relieve Chronic Muscle Spasm

Although the exact cause of most chronic pain remains unknown, I and others believe a major contributor may be chronic muscle spasm. While the spasm itself may not be painful (20), the resultant compensations in movement may cause pain and dysfunction. Unlike acute spasms which are thought to be caused by overactively contracting muscles, the pathophysiology of chronic spasms is unknown, nor do they respond to the same treatments. Ice application is not indicated but heat application may be beneficial presumably by increasing circulation to the area of spasm (36). Application of myofascial techniques including transverse friction massage combined with movement is reported to be successful (20).

Goal 5. Suggest Environmental Alterations

Environmental alterations are basically the same for chronic dysfunction patients as they are for the acute cases. However the extent of alterations may be greater. The same basic plan should be followed, i.e., altering the way patients use their environment and altering the environment. Changes in seating at home, work, and in the car may be needed. Information on appropriate bed mattresses should be provided. Physical changes at home and work should be suggested to allow the person to use better body mechanics. Work and activity schedules should be altered to allow patients to maximize their activity while minimizing the chance of reinjury.

Goal 6. Alleviate Pain

As previously mentioned, I do not believe there is much that can be done to directly address the pain component of chronic spinal dysfunction. As emphasized in this text, surgery is appropriate for a small minority of patients. Medication may help control some of the pain (30). Transcutaneous electrical nerve stimulation (TENS) also may be used for pain management but with no lasting benefits (59,68).

I believe it is better to have patients use their pain as a guide to activity level, rather than spend their time and money trying to mask the pain. The graded progression of a sound therapy program has as one of its goals reduction in pain as a result of the increased mobility, activity, and fitness level of the patient.

SUMMARY

This chapter was written as an introduction to physical therapy for the treatment of adult spinal dysfunction patients. We have some knowledge about what to do and why, but much remains to establish the scientific basis of our approach and treatment. Therapists cannot stop treating spine patients until the research is completed: utilizing currently available information and professional judgment, combined with logic, seems to provide effective treatment for many people suffering from acute and chronic spinal dysfunction.

Many chronic spinal dysfunction patients want and expect miracles. My greatest challenge as a physical therapist is to convince patients that the only miracle that will help is hard work, plenty of it, and mostly theirs (73).

REFERENCES

1. Abraham N (1974): Heat versus cold therapy for the treatment of muscle injuries. *Athletic Training* 9:4.
2. Adams MA, Dolan P, Hutton WC (1988): The lumbar spine in backward bending. *Spine* 13(9):1019–1026.
3. Adams TD, Yanowitz FG, Chandler S, Specht P, Lockwood R, Yeh MP (1986): A study to evaluate and promote total fitness among fire fighters. *J Sports Med Phys Fitness* 26:337–345.
4. Ashmore CR, Summers PJ (1981): Stretch-induced growth in chicken wing muscles: Myofibrillar proliferation. *Am J Physiol* 241:C93–C97.
5. Astrand P (1956): Human physical fitness with special reference to sex and age. *Physiolog Rev* 36(3):307–335.
6. Beirmane W (1955): Therapeutic use of cold. *JAMA* 157:189–192.
7. Bergquist-Ullman M, Larsson U (1977): Acute low back pain in industry. *Acta Orthop Scand* (170):1–117.
8. Biering-Sorenson F (1984): Physical measurements as risk indicators for low back trouble over a one year period. *Spine* 9:106–119.
9. Bigos SJ, Battie MC (1987): Acute care to prevent back disability: ten years of progress. *Clin Orthop* 221:121–130.
10. Bobath B (1979): *Adult hemiplegia: Evaluation and treatment.* 2nd. ed. London: William Heinemann Medical Books Limited.
11. Bourdillon JF, Day EA (1987): *Spinal manipulation,* 4th. ed. London: William Heinemann Medical Books, Chapter 1.
12. Buckle P, Stubbs D (1989): The contribution of ergonomics to the rehabilitation of back pain patients. *J Soc Occup Med* 39:56–60.
13. Cady LD, Bischoff DP, O'Connell ER, Thomas PC, Allan JH (1979): Strength and fitness and subsequent back injuries in fire-fighters. *J Occup Med* 21:269–272.
14. Carr J, Sheperd R, Gordon J, Gentle A, Held J (1987): *Movement science: Foundations for physical therapy in rehabilitation.* Rockville, Maryland: Aspen Publications.
15. Caillet R (1981): *Low back syndrome.* 3rd. ed. Philadelphia: F.A. Davis.
16. Carlsson AM (1986): Personality characteristics of patients with chronic pain in comparison with normal controls and depressed patients. *Pain* 25:373–382.
17. Codman E (1934): *The shoulder.* Boston: Thomas Todd.
18. Crisler GR (1953): Sprains and strains treated with ultrafaradic M-4 impulse generator. *J Fla Med Assoc* 40(1):32–34.
19. Cyriax J (1950): Treatment of lumbar disk lesions. *Br Med J* [Clin Res] 2:1434–1438.
20. Cyriax J (1982): *Textbook of orthopedic medicine, Volume one: Diagnosis of soft tissue lesions,* 8th. ed. London: Bailliere Tindall. pp. 16–17.
21. Danneskiold-Samsoe B, Christiansen E, Bach Andersen R (1986): Myofascial pain and the role of myoglobin. *Scand J Rheumatol* 15:174–178.
22. Darling RC (1947): The significance of physical fitness. *Arch Phys Med Rehabil* 28:140–145.
23. Deibert PW, England RW (1972): Electromyographic studies. 1. Consideration in the evaluation of osteopathic therapy. *J Am Osteopath Assoc* 72:221–223.
24. Deyo RA, Diehl AK, Rosenthal M (1986): How many days of bed rest for acute low back pain? *N Engl J Med* 315:1064–1070.
25. Dixon A StJ (1976): Diagnosis of low back pain. In: Jayson M, ed. *The lumbar spine and back pain.* New York: Grune and Stratton.
26. Doran DM, Newell DJ (1975): Manipulation in the treatment of low back pain: A multicentre study. *Br Med J* [Clin Res] 2:161–164.
27. Edwards B (1969): Low back pain and pain resulting from lumbar spine conditions: A comparison of results. *Aust J PT* 15:106.
28. Engel GL (1959): "Psychogenic" pain and the pain-prone patient. *AJM* 26:899–918.
29. Enneking WE, Horowitz M (1972): The intraarticular effects of immobilization on the human knee. *J Bone Joint Surg* [Am] 54:973–985.
30. Fields H (1987): *Pain.* New York: McGraw-Hill.
31. Fitzgerald M (1979): The spread of sensitization of polymodal nociceptors in rabbit from nearby injury and by antidromic nerve stimulation. *J Physiol* 297:207–216.
32. Goldberg AL, Etlinger JD, Goldspink DF, Jablecki C (1975): Mechanism of work-induced hypertrophy of skeletal muscle. *Med Sci Sports Exerc* 7:185–198.
33. Goldstein M, ed. (1975): *The research status of spinal manipulative therapy.* United States Dept of Health, Education, and Welfare.
34. Gollnick PD, Timson BF, Moore RL, Riedy M (1981): Muscular enlargement and number of fibers in skeletal muscles of rats. *J Appl Physiol* 50:936–943.
35. Grice A (1974): Muscle tonus changes following manipulation. *J Canad Chir Assoc* 19(4):29.
36. Griffin J, Karselis T (1978): *Physical agents for physical therapists.* Springfield, Illinois: Charles C Thomas.
37. Hadler NM, Curtis P, Gillings DB, Stinnett S (1987): A benefit of spinal manipulation as adjunctive therapy for acute low back pain: A stratified controlled trial. *Spine* 12:702–706.
38. Haldeman S (1983): Spinal manipulative therapy: A status report. *Clin Orthop* 179:62–70.
39. Hall H, Iceton JA (1983): Back school: An overview with specific reference to the Canadian Back Education Units. *Clin Orthop* 179:10–17.
40. Hendry NG (1958): The hydration of the nucleus pulposus and its relation to intervertebral disc derangement. *J Bone Joint Surg* [Br] 40:132–144.
41. Hettinga D (1979): Normal joint structures and their reaction to injury. *J Ortho Sports Phys Ther* 1:83–88.
42. Hood LB, Chrisman D (1968): Intermittent pelvic traction in the treatment of the ruptured intervertebral disk. *Phys Ther* 48:21–30.
43. Hult L (1954): Cervical, dorsal, and lumber spinal syndromes. *Acta Orthop Scand Suppl* 17:1–102.
44. Jarvinen M (1976): Healing of a crush injury in rat striated muscle. With special reference to treatment by early mobilization or immobilization. Thesis. Turku, Finland.
45. Jayson MI, Sims-Williams H, Young S, Baddeley H, Collins E (1981): Mobilization and manipulation for low back pain. *Spine* 6:409–416.
46. Jorgensen K, Nicolaisen T (1987): Trunk extensor endurance: Determination and relation to low back trouble. *Ergonomics* 30(2):259–267.
47. Kane RL, Olsen D, Leymaster C, et al (1974): Manipulating the patient. *Lancet* 1:1333.
48. Kelsey JL, White AA (1980): Epidemiology and impact of low back pain. *Spine* 5:133–142.
49. Kendall H, Kendall F, Boynton D (1952): *Posture and pain.* Baltimore: Williams and Wilkins.
50. Kessler R, Hertling D (1983): *Management of common musculoskeletal disorders: Physical therapy principles and methods.* Philadelphia: Harper and Row Publishers, pp. 208–209.
51. Klaber-Moffett JA, Chase SM, Portek I, Ennis JR (1986): A controlled prospective study to evaluate the effectiveness of a back school in the relief of chronic low back pain. *Spine* 11:120–122.
52. Klein R, Dorman T, Johnson C (1989): Proliferant injections for low back pain: Histologic changes of injectioned ligaments & objective measurements of lumbar spine mobility before and after treatment. *J Neurol Orthop Med Surg* 10(2):123–126.
53. Kopp JR, Alexander HA, Turocy RH, Levrini MG, Lichtman DM (1986): The use of lumbar extension in the evaluation and

treatment of patients with acute herniated nucleus pulposus. *Clin Orthop* 202:211–218.

54. LaBan MM (1962): Collagen tissue: Implications of its response to stress in vitro. *Arch Phys Med Rehab* 43:461–466.

55. Langrana NA, Lee CK (1984): Isokinetic evaluation of trunk muscles. *Spine* 9:171–175.

56. Larson CB (1961): Pathomechanics of backache. *Iowa Med* 51:643–650.

57. Lee JM, Warren MP, Mason SM (1978): Effects of ice on nerve conduction velocity. *Physiotherapy* 64:2–6.

58. Lee WJ, McGovern JP, Duvall EN (1950): Continuous tetanizing (low voltage) currents for relief of spasm. *Arch Phys Med Rehabil* 31:766–771.

59. Loeser JD, Black RG, Christman A (1975): Relief of pain by transcutaneous stimulation. *J Neurosurg* 42:308–314.

60. Maitland GD (1980): *Vertebral manipulation,* 4th. ed. London: Butterworth.

61. Mathews JA (1968): Dynamic discography; a study of lumbar traction. *Ann Phy Med* 9:275–279.

62. Mayer TG, Gatchel RJ, Kishino N, Keely J, Capra P, Mayer H, Barnett J, Mooney V (1985): Objective assessment of spine function following industrial injury: A prospective study with comparison group and one year follow up. *Spine* 10:482–493.

63. Mayer T, Gatchel R (1988): *Functional restoration for spinal disorders: A sports medicine approach.* Philadelphia: Lea & Febiger.

64. McGill CM (1968): Industrial back problems: A control program. *J Occup Med* 10:174–178.

65. McKenzie R (1981): *The lumbar spine: Mechanical diagnosis and therapy.* Upper Hill, New Zealand: Wright and Carman Limited.

66. Medoff R (1987): Soft tissue healing. *Sports Med* 3(2):67–70.

67. Meilman P (1979): Psychological aspects of chronic pain. *J Ortho Sports Phys Ther* 1:76–82.

68. Melzack R (1984): Acupuncture and related forms of folk medicine. In: Wall PD, Melzack R, eds. *Textbook Pain.* Edinburgh: Churchill-Livingstone. Chapter 3.

69. Nachemson A, Morris JM (1964): In vivo measurements of intradiscal pressure. *J Bone Joint Surg* [Am] 46:1077–1092.

70. Nachemson A (1966): The load on lumbar disks in different positions of the body. *Clin Orthop* 45:107–122.

71. Nachemson A, Lindh M (1969): Measurement of abdominal and back muscle strength with and without low back pain. *Scand J Rehab Med* 1:60–65.

72. Nachemson A (1975): Toward a better understanding of low back pain: a review of the mechanics of the lumbar disc. *Rheum and Rehab* 14:129–143.

73. Nachemson A (1983): Work for all: For those with low back pain as well. *Clin Orthop* 179:77–85.

74. Newman LB, Arieff AJ, Wasserman RR (1954): Present status in management of spasticity and spasm. *Arch Phys Med Rehabil* 35:427–436.

75. Nicolaisen T, Jorgensen K (1985): Trunk strength, back muscle endurance and low back trouble. *Scand J Rehabil Med* 17:121–127.

76. Nordin M, Frankel V (1989): *Basic biomechanics of the musculoskeletal system, 2nd ed.* Philadelphia: Lea & Febiger.

77. Paris SV (1983): Spinal manipulative therapy. *Clin Orthop* 179:55–61.

78. Paris S (1984): Functional anatomy of the lumbar spine. Thesis. Union Institute, Cincinnati, Ohio.

79. Paris S (1985): The role of the physical therapist in pain control programmes. *Clinics in Anaesthesiology* 3(1):155–167.

80. Parnianpour M (1988): The effect of fatiguing isoinertial trunk flexion and extension movement on patterns of movement and motor output. Thesis New York University, New York, New York.

81. Parnianpour M, Li F, Nordin M, Kahanovitz N (1989): A database of isoinertial trunk strength tests against three resistance levels in sagittal, frontal, and transverse planes in normal male subjects. *Spine* 14(4):409–411.

82. Parris W (1986): Chronic pain management: A logical approach. *J Tenn Med Assoc* 79:683–687.

83. Perl ER (1976): Sensitization of nociceptors and its relation to sensation. In: Bonica JJ, Albe-Fessard DG, eds. *Advances in pain research and therapy,* vol 1. New York: Raven Press, pp. 17–28.

84. Petrofsky JS, Phillips CA, Sawka MN, Hanpeter D, Stafford D (1981): Blood flow and metabolism during isometric contractions in cat skeletal muscle. *J Appl Physiol* 50:493–502.

85. Randall BF, Imig CJ, Hines HM (1953): Effect of electrical stimulation upon blood flow and temperature of skeletal muscle. *Am J Phys Med Rehabil* 32:22–26.

86. Rasch P, Burke R (1978): *Kinesiology and applied anatomy. The science of human movement.* Philadelphia: Lea & Febiger, pp. 210–241.

87. Reed BV (1988): Effect of high voltage pulsed electrical stimulation on microvascular permeability to plasma proteins: A possible mechanism in minimizing edema. *Phys Ther* 68(4):491–495.

88. Richardson D (1981): Blood flow response of human calf muscles to static contractions at various percentages of maximal voluntary contraction. *J Appl Physiol* 51:929–933.

89. Richter RR, VanSant AF, Newton RA (1989): Description of adult rolling movements and hypothesis of developmental sequences. *Phys Ther* 69:63–71.

90. Roy T, Trunks E (1982): *Psychosocial factors in rehabilitation.* Baltimore: Williams and Wilkins.

91. Rywerant Y (1983): *The feldonkrais method: Teaching by handling.* San Francisco: Harper and Row.

92. Saal JA, Saal JS (1989): Nonoperative treatment of herniated lumbar intervertebral disc with radiculopathy: An outcome study. *Spine* 14:431–437.

93. Sarno JE (1981): Etiology of neck and back pain: Autonomic myoneuralgia? *J Nerv Ment Dis* 169:55–59.

94. Sarno JE (1982): *Mind over back pain.* New York: Berkley Books.

95. Saunders HD (1981): Unilateral lumbar traction. *Phys Ther* 61:221–225.

96. Saunders HD (1983): The use of spinal traction in the treatment of neck and back conditions. *Clin Orthop* 179:31–38.

97. Schmidt G, Amundson L, Dostal W (1980): Muscle strength at the trunk. *J Orthop Sports Phys Ther* 1:165.

98. Schnebel BE, Watkins RG, Dillin W (1989): The role of spinal flexion and extension in changing nerve root compression in disc herniation. *Spine* 14(8):835–837.

99. Shah J, Hampson WG, Jayson MI (1978): The distribution of surface strain in the cadaveric lumbar spine. *J Bone Joint Surg* [Br] 60:246–251.

100. Shah J (1980): Structure, morphology and mechanics of the lumbar spine. In: Jayson M, ed. *The lumbar spine and low back pain.* London: Pitman Medical.

101. Smidt GL, Blanpied PR, White RW (1989): Exploration of mechanical and electromyographic responses of trunk muscles to high-intensity resistive exercise. *Spine* 14(8):815–830.

102. Sullivan P, Markos P, Minor M (1982): *An integrated approach to therapeutic exercise: Theory and application,* Reston, Virginia: Reston Publishing Company.

103. Sylven B (1951): On the biology of the nucleus pulposus. *Acta Orthop Scand* 20:275–279.

104. Trager M (1988): Moving with Milton Trager. *East West* 54–60.

105. Viidik A (1973): Functional properties of collagenous tissues. *Int Rev Connect Tissue Res* 6:127–215.

106. Waddell G (1987): 1987 Volvo Award in Clinical Sciences. A new clinical model for the treatment of low back pain. *Spine* 12:632–644.

107. Wakim KG (1953): Influence of frequency of muscle stimulation on circulation in the stimulated extremity. *Arch Phys Med* 34:291–295.

108. Watson D (1982): Neurotic tendencies among chronic pain patients: an MMPI item analysis. *Pain* 14:365–385.

109. Wells P, Frampton V, Bowsher D (1988): *Pain management in physical therapy.* Norwalk, Conn.: Appleton and Lange, pp. 214–216.

110. Wiesel SW, Cuckler JM, Deluca F, Jones F, Zeide MS, Rothman R (1980): Acute low back pain: An objective analysis of conservative therapy. *Spine* 5:324–330.

111. Witt PL (1986): Trager psychophysical integration; An additional tool in the treatment of chronic spinal pain and dysfunction. *Whirlpool* 9(2):24–26.

112. Wolf SL, Basmajian JV (1973): Intramuscular temperature changes deep to localized cutaneous cold stimulation. *Phys Ther* 53:1284–1288.

The Adult Spine: Principles and Practice,
J. W. Frymoyer, Editor-in-Chief.
Raven Press, Ltd., New York © 1991.

CHAPTER 76

Mechanical Assessment and Treatment of Spinal Pain

Ronald G. Donelson and Robin McKenzie

The patient with back and neck pain, with or without associated pain radiation from the midline, poses a diagnostic and therapeutic dilemma to the treating health care practitioner. These subjective complaints are frequently dismissed and the associated physical findings, such as limited motion, assumed to be non-specific and unreliable observations. Diagnostic imaging usually adds little new or useful information to guide treatment (40) (see also Chapter 71). As a result, the clinician is limited in his ability to formulate specific treatment.

The minimal significance attached to the history and physical in the majority of patients with spinal pain is strikingly in contrast to the relevance attached to these data in virtually all other joints. When the clinician evaluates a painful peripheral joint, the patient's history of pain relief and accentuation in response to motion, position, and activity is clearly helpful. At the completion of the history, a limited differential diagnosis usually is possible. The various structures suspected to be the source of pain are then tested in the physical examination by palpation and then by stressing the joint to its end-range of motion, actively and passively in all directions, while monitoring the pain response. In most patients with peripheral joint pathology, the examination limits the possibilities and the diagnostic imaging, if required, provides the confirmation of the clinical diagnosis.

We believe that the patient's history of pain and the systematized evaluation of motion have been underutilized in patients with spinal pain. Unlike the peripheral joint, spinal palpation usually gives little reliable information (10,26,34). However, the system of spinal evaluation developed by the senior author is useful; a thorough history of the patient's pain is elicited, followed by a systemized examination performed while the clinician monitors the patient's pain behavior.

A similar conclusion was reached by the Quebec Task Force on Activity-Related Spinal Disorders (40), which recommended that the majority of patients with spinal pain were best classified by their symptom location and by the presence or absence of neurologic deficits, rather than by pathoanatomic criteria. They concluded:

Of the numerous pathologic conditions of the spine, non-specific ailments of back pain in the lumbar, dorsal, and cervical regions, with or without radiation of pain, comprise the vast majority of problems found among workers. . . . The incidence in the general populations can only be greater.

    R. G. Donelson, M.D.: Department of Orthopedic Surgery, State University of New York, Health Science Center, Syracuse, New York 13202.
    R. McKenzie F.N.Z.S.P., Dip. M.T.: McKenzie Institute International, Waikanae, New Zealand.

They estimated that over 90% of spinal mechanical disorders fell into this non-specific category, and thus that only 10% of patients could be given a specific pathoanatomic diagnosis with our present technology and understanding.

We feel that a patient's QTF classification can be improved, often rapidly, by changing the patient's pain location and even occasionally reversing neurologic deficit. Additionally, specific patterns of pain behavior can be identified using these mechanical spinal test movements. We believe these pain patterns reflect the pathoanatomic cause, which most often is attributable to a specific spinal structure, the intervertebral disc. Additionally, we and others have found their diagnostic inferences usually permit the patient to self-correct the underlying painful disorder, often rapidly (8,20,24,25,30,31, 35,41). As a result, patients are educated and trained to treat their own painful spinal conditions. This self-reliance avoids dependency on pills, corsets, manual therapy, bed rest, and manipulation, none of which is of demonstrated long-term benefit. The treatment method we advocate also permits patients to apply their knowledge and techniques to prevent recurrences of back pain, or at least to terminate them more quickly.

In this chapter we will describe the system of spinal diagnosis and treatment developed by the senior author, the conceptual model of spinal pain that underlies it, and the clinical results achieved.

HISTORICAL PERSPECTIVE

The theory that the intervertebral disc content somehow shifts in the opposite direction of spinal bending was the result of a chance observation in 1956. A patient with a three-week history of low back and leg pain had been resistant to all treatment. On one visit, he inadvertently positioned himself in a prone, hyperextended position for 10 minutes (Fig. 1). Based on the then prevalent theories of spinal treatment, this "bizarre" position should have accentuated his symptoms. Instead, his leg, buttock, and most of his back pain was abolished completely. There was no other intervention to account for this dramatic improvement, which happened so rapidly that the position itself was thought to be responsible. The patient continued utilizing this position over the next several days. The peripheral leg pain never returned and the remaining central low back pain rapidly resolved. Thereafter the senior author began to evaluate the response of every patient with back and leg pain to the hyperextended position. Many responded similarly, including the rapid abolition of peripheral symptoms, and relief persisted. However, return to a flexed position often caused return of the peripheral symptoms. In other patients no response was observed and, in fact, some were worsened by spinal extension. Many of the patients who were worsened by extension responded to positioning in a lateral direction. Once the radiating pain centralized to the lumbar midline, extension for many was no longer painful and could be performed freely and fully.

Over the next six years, a large number of patients with low back and neck pain were studied, correlating intensity and location of symptoms with spinal movements, positions, and activities leading to a classification scheme. It was proposed that the different pain patterns present defined the likely causative mechanical disorder. It followed that these conditions would be most rapidly resolved if a corresponding and rectifying mechanical treatment method was utilized. Key to this system was the concept of centralization.

CENTRALIZATION

In a patient with asymmetrical low back or neck pain, with or without radiation into the extremities, the pri-

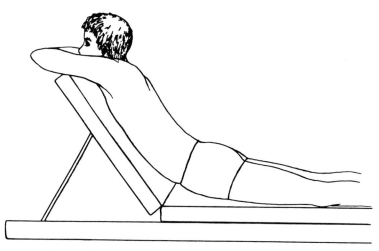

FIG. 1. Static end-range lumbar extension while prone.

mary purpose of the evaluation is to search for those movements or positions which transfer the perceived location of the pain toward the midline, a concept termed centralization. The senior author found in his clinical studies that centralization of asymmetric or radiating pain occurred in a great majority of patients, providing that all planes of spinal movements and combinations thereof were throughly explored. Once identified, this direction of exercise and movement could be utilized for initial treatment. When temporary avoidance of the movements in the direction which caused pain was employed, rapid recovery was commonplace in patients with acute pain. This concept of centralization became the cornerstone of the evaluation and treatment process. Based on these treatment observations, the authors' and others' clinical research has continued to accumulate information which supports this concept. For example, in our prospective, randomized clinical study (7), the assessment system in only the sagittal plane of spine movement was examined. The effects of loaded and unloaded lumbar end-range flexion and extension movements, both single and repeated, were studied in 145 symptomatic patients during a single session (7). Changes in pain location and intensity in this symptomatic group were documented with patients randomly assigned to 1 of 2 assessment protocols, differing only in the order with which the test movements were performed.

There were marked differences in pain intensity and location with the various movements; and each of the two assessment protocol groups demonstrated that these differences corresponded with the direction of test movement performed. The group mean with lumbar flexion increased both the central and most-distal pain intensity, as well as the distal location or extent of the radiating pain (peripheralization), although considerable variation was noted between patients. Extension on the other hand decreased both back and leg pain intensity and "centralized" the radiating pain. When the direction of movement that accentuated pain was ceased, the symptoms tended to subside when the spine was positioned in its "neutral" lordosis. At the conclusion of the relieving movements, the improvements were maintained. The differences in pain accentuation and reduction between the effects of these two directions of test movements was highly significant (p < .003).

Another study documented the assessment and treatment of 87 patients with low back pain and symptoms radiating into the buttock or leg (8). Centralization of the referred pain occurred in 76 (87%) patients during the first 48 hours of care, most commonly occurring during the first therapy assessment session. The later treatment of these patients followed our treatment guidelines: the direction of movement which induced centralization determined the direction of spinal bending exercise to be performed by the patient at home. At the same time, the patients were instructed to temporarily avoid bending or positioning the lumbar spine in the direction which aggravated symptoms. Most required extension movements and avoided flexion.

Treatment outcome for these patients was determined by an independent assessor. An excellent outcome required the patient to be pain-free and fully functional. If symptom relief was only partial, secondary criteria were considered, including the patients' satisfaction with their outcome, improvement in physical and neurologic examination, and return to work. A good result required improvement in all of the secondary criteria, a fair result was failure to achieve just one, and poor outcome was defined as no relief of symptoms.

Of the patients with symptoms for less than 4 weeks who experienced centralization of pain during their initial assessment, 91% had excellent treatment outcomes while another 7% were good (Table 1). Of those with symptoms for longer than 4 weeks, but less than 12 weeks, 77% of those whose pain centralized initially had excellent or good treatment results, while 81% of those with symptoms for greater than 12 weeks who centralized experienced excellent or good results with McKenzie treatment.

Six patients with symptoms for 4 weeks or less had referred pain which could not be centralized. Four patients (67%) were subsequently found to have significant lumbar disc herniation, including 3 who had extruded nuclear fragments and a 4th with internal disc disruption. All 4 have had excellent surgical results with a 4-year follow-up and were the only surgical patients in the study.

The centralization phenomenon occurs very commonly and is highly reliable in selecting effective treatment of the underlying disorder, particularly in patients

TABLE 1. *The occurrence or non-occurrence of centralization was correlated with treatment outcome in the three patient groups identified by their duration of symptoms at the time of evaluation*

Duration of symptoms (weeks)	Presence of centralization	Treatment outcome			
		Excellent	Good	Fair	Poor
0–4	Yes	43 (91%)	3 (7%)	0	1
0–4	No	0	1	1	4 (67%)
4–12	Yes	8 (62%)	2 (15%)	2	1
4–12	No	0	1	1	0
>12	Yes	8 (50%)	5 (31%)	2	1
>12	No	0	1	1	1

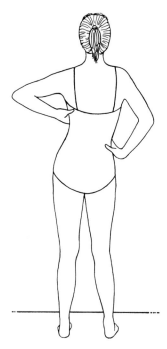

FIG. 2. One method of self-treatment in the spinal loaded position for correction of a lumbar lateral deformity.

with acute symptoms. It also has significant value as an outcome predictor of treatment success and seems to predict the presence of a lumbar disc herniation.

To consider the underlying mechanism responsible for this centralization phenomenon, several factors are quite apparent to those experienced in this evaluation technique. Centralization frequently occurs as a result of extension movements and at other times from laterally directed movements and only rarely with flexion.

For a movement to eventually centralize pain, it often must be performed repetitively. In fact, the initial movement will often aggravate or intensify the pain. Centralization also occurs much more rapidly if the initial movements are performed passively to end-range.

The rapid centralization or abolition of pain seems to mimic the rapid onset of the patient's symptoms. Of

note, these improvements usually remain, even after the conclusion of the centralizing movements, and the pain then tends not to return unless movement or positioning occurs in the opposite direction. This aggravating direction is typically the same movement which the patient reports caused the onset of the original pain (Figs. 2 and 3).

These characteristics of pain aggravation and relief are highly reminiscent of pain presentations in patients with "deranged peripheral joints," such as a displacement of the medial meniscus. The pain of a peripheral joint derangement rapidly commences at the time of displacement and is rapidly relieved with corrective end-range stresses. The pain also remains better thereafter unless the joint is returned to the original offending direction, which usually causes rapid return of the symptoms.

CENTRALIZATION PHENOMENON: THE CONCEPT OF ITS PATHOANATOMIC CAUSATION

The similarities between the onset of pain in internally deranged peripheral joints and the spine suggests that the nucleus pulposus may be the anatomic structure which displaces in the spine. The direction of displacement would account for the change in the location of symptoms. Such a mechanical causation seems most plausible to account for the rapid onset of symptoms and equally dramatic relief. Since this concept of nuclear displacement was proposed, biomechanical studies have demonstrated the normal nucleus moves posteriorly with flexion and anteriorly with extension (22,23,36,37,38). When the disc is degenerate, accelerated and quite dramatic displacements can occur, often suddenly (1,2,45). This concept of nuclear displacement also fits with Kirkaldy-Willis's observations of spinal degeneration (18,19), and particularly his view of spinal instability. This mechanical behavior of the nucleus has been used to form a conceptual framework and classification system of spinal pain presumed to be of mechanical origin.

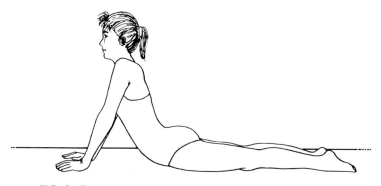

FIG. 3. End-range lumbar extension exercise while prone.

CLASSIFICATION OF SPINAL PAIN OF MECHANICAL ORIGIN

McKenzie has identified three syndromes based on pain aggravation and relief. Each syndrome has an analogy to tissue injury of peripheral joints. However, the spine does differ from peripheral joints in the centralization of radiating pain, which is thought to result from neuroanatomical relationships and the specific mechanical behavior of the intervertebral disc.

The syndromes are the basis for pathogenetic models which are useful for explaining symptoms and formulating rational treatment. They serve to educate practitioners and to provide patients with explanations for diagnosis and treatment. The patient must be an active participant in acute treatment and later in preventing or minimizing future episodes.

The Postural Syndrome

The postural syndrome represents a painful condition which occurs without any demonstrable underlying pathology. When normal tissues are placed in the position of prolonged or excessive stretch, pain is elicited which serves as a warning that damage may occur if the stress is not relieved. The pain almost immediately ceases when the position producing the tension is removed, since no damage has occurred. A good example of this phenomenon is the "hammerlock," a commonly used wrestling hold, which places the shoulder in a position of severe stretch. In this position the joint capsule and other periarticular structures are excessively stretched at the end-range of joint motion. The pain rapidly ceases when the joint is relieved of this position.

In elegant animal experiments involving both peripheral and spinal articulations, these excessive stretches are now identified to produce outbursts of electrical activity in the nerves supplying the joint being studied (9,11,12,13,21). Although direct measurements of electrical activity of nerves supplying the annulus fibrosus have not been made, biomechanical studies of the intervertebral disc in humans indicate that prolonged sitting, particularly in a vibrational environment, will cause significant increases in intradiscal pressure (29).

In the lumbar spine, this situation most commonly happens when we sit for a prolonged period in a slouched position, at the end range of flexion (Fig. 4). We believe the importance of maintaining normal lumbar lordosis cannot be overemphasized. The postural syndrome most commonly occurs in younger patients, who have been characterized as "hanging on their ligaments." The pain experienced is usually in or near the midline and does not radiate peripherally. Although the precise pain-producing structure cannot be specifically identified in the spine, the pain-producing position and the mechanical solution of shifting posture from the end-range are quite apparent. Since postural pain is experienced when the spine is left at the end-range for an extended time interval, examination of patients with these complaints typically reveals normal, pain free end-range movements in all directions (25).

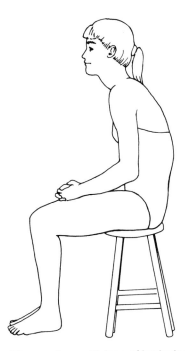

FIG. 4. Poor sitting posture with loss of lordosis in both lumbar and lower cervical regions.

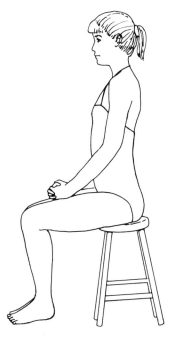

FIG. 5. Good sitting posture with lumbar and lower cervical lordosis present.

While patients with central pain from a pure postural syndrome, where no pathology seems to exist, are few in number, most other low back disorders have the stresses of poor posture superimposed upon them. Static loading of the spine in end-range flexion either precedes or perpetuates the underlying disorder, or both. Subsequent non-operative treatment trials without initially removing these aggravating postural stresses are commonly unsuccessful at resolving symptoms or preventing a progression of the underlying disorder.

Biomechanical studies strengthen this concept. In cadaver discs, the role of poor posture in predisposing the disc to failure was illustrated by Wilder (45) who exposed the discs to 1 hour of static flexion loading before applying stresses sufficient to produce posterior annular failures. The flexion pre-loaded discs were found to fail much earlier and with less applied force than those without prior flexion loading.

In a prospective, randomized, clinical study (25) of a population of low back pain patients with or without leg symptoms, correcting posture alone has been shown to be effective treatment. While these patients' symptoms were a result of undetermined pathology, significant improvement was observed over 48 hours with posture correction only (Fig. 5).

The Dysfunction Syndrome

Theoretically, continued exposure to end-range spinal flexion stresses can damage the annulus and other ligamentous structures which may then repair and heal. However, repetitive sub-clinical trauma, as well as the healing process, can result in contracture of these tissues, accompanied by loss of elasticity. The combination of pain, the underlying trauma, and healing events may over time cause a reduction in the joint's range of movement. End-range movements or positioning now places these shortened, nociceptor innervated structures on stretch, and produces premature end-range pain. Many of the events proposed in this conceptual model of dysfunction are similar to the pathologic events proposed by Kirkaldy-Willis (19) as the cause of his "dysfunction" stage of spinal degeneration. Similar to the postural syndrome, the pain of "dysfunction" is also experienced only at the end-range of spinal motions and most commonly is felt at or near the midline. If the shortened structure or scar tethers a nerve root, the pain might be experienced peripherally. The important physical findings are that pain is reported only when the shortened structure is placed on stretch at the end-range with loss of motion in this plane, the absence of mid-range pain, and the observation that repeated movements do not alter the intensity and location of the pain.

The Derangement Syndrome

The pain pattern of patients with the derangement syndrome is much different from that reported by patients with the postural and dysfunction syndromes. This pattern is present in the large majority of patients who seek treatment. It is also for this syndrome that the model of asymmetrical disc deterioration provides the most useful conceptual framework.

During the postural and dysfunctional phases, the nucleus is thought to be constrained by an intact annulus. In the derangement syndrome, significant damage to the annulus is proposed to have caused loss of constraint and, therefore, abnormal and asymmetric displacements are possible. As previously noted, this hypothesis is now supported by basic, biomechanical research (1,2,45). Depending on the location of annular stresses, the pain resulting from nucleur displacements may be midline or may lateralize (5,27,46). The patient reports a change in pain from being brief or positional, to one experienced in the mid-range of spinal motion. Initially the pain may resolve spontaneously and rapidly, particularly if the patient avoids the inciting spinal position.

In our sedentary society where prolonged lumbar flexion predominates (see Fig. 4), the continued stresses placed on the disc form the basis for episodes of recurrent pain, which often occur with increasing intensity. If the flexion lifestyle is temporarily abandoned, this progression can still be halted or reversed. Perhaps this is the strategy utilized instinctively by patients, which accounts for the high rate of "spontaneous" recovery and the favorable natural history of low back episodes.

If nuclear displacement progresses, the annulus deteriorates, further predisposing to an increase in pain intensity, in frequency of episodes, and in peripheralization of symptoms. Pathologic studies characterize this further damage to the annulus as the creation of actual fissures which become filled with displacing nuclear chemicals or actually sequestered nuclear fragments. In addition to mid-range spinal pain, movements may become obstructed in the direction of the displacement, similar to other peripheral deranged joints, thereby producing visible deformity. The directions of displacements and the resulting abnormal postures are as follows: kyphosis results when the nucleus displaces predominately in a posterior direction, scoliosis results when the direction is posterolateral or lateral, and fixed lordosis results with anterior displacement. It is this obstruction to curve reversal with bending that typifies this group of patients, and also forms the basis of a subclassification of the derangement syndrome.

With continued unidirectional stresses, nuclear displacement continues and may result in complete failure of the annulus (2). The pain typically now radiates distally into the extremity and neurologic deficits are common. This typical presentation of lumbar disc herniation

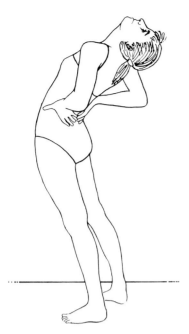

FIG. 6. Standing end-range lumbar extension.

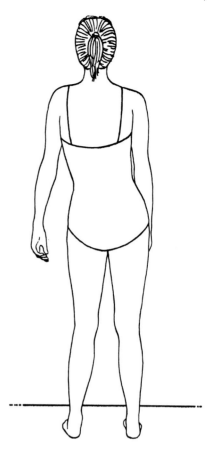

FIG. 7. Acute lateral lumbar deformity.

is no longer rapidly reversible, but symptoms can subside without surgical intervention (44).

The derangement category therefore includes those patients with or without acute spinal deformity, whose pain intensity and/or pain location change often quite rapidly, as the result of end-range bending movements or positioning. Pain location can be central or peripheralized, but usually can be rapidly centralized or abolished with repeated end-range movements and positioning (Fig. 6). As already noted, centralization of pain during the clinical evaluation is important to diagnosis, predicting the outcome of therapy, and determining the possible presence of extruded disc fragments (8). As the duration of constant and unrelieved symptoms lengthens, the more likely it becomes that the process will be irreversible.

Yet another important observation is whether test movements in all directions worsen or peripheralize the radiating symptoms or whether there is simply no or even just partial centralization obtained. In the first instance, the imaging studies usually reveal a large hernia-

tion or extrusion. In the second, however, lumbar CT or MRI often show no apparent external disc abnormality, but discography reveals internal disc pain and morphologic disruption.

Subcategories of Derangements

The subcategories of derangements are defined by the location of the pain and the presence or absence of acute spinal deformity. Based on pain location three subgroups are identified: the first has only central or symmetrical lumbar pain; the second has asymmetric pain which extends no further than the knees, and the third

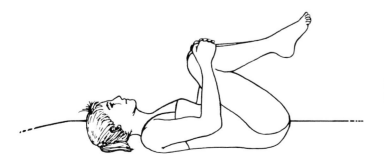

FIG. 8. Supine end-range lumbar flexion.

TABLE 2. *McKenzie mechanical syndromes*

	Postural	Dysfunction	Derangement*
Definition	End-range stress of normal structure	End-range stress of shortened structure (scarring, fibrosis, nerve root adherence)	Anatomic disruption and/or displacement within the motion segment
Findings with repeated movements	Full range of movement No pain during, or as a result of, movement (pain only with prolonged end-range stress)	Pain at limited end-range only No pain during motion No radiation (except nerve root adherence) *No centralization occurs* Does not progressively worsen or improve Pain stops shortly No rapid changes occur	Pain during movement (mid-range) Peripheralization occurs *Centralization occurs* Progressively worsens or improves Remains worse or better Rapid changes occur
Requirements of treatment	Requires posture correction Correction obtained only by patient	Requires remodeling Remodeling requires regular, frequent stretching, achieved only by patient	Requires reductive procedures Should be achieved only by patient whenever possible to educate for prevention of recurrences

* The Derangement category can be further broken down into subcategories according to the location of the patient's pain and the presence or absence of acute spinal deformity (see Table 3).

reports pain radiating below the knee. These subcategories (24) are virtually identical with the Quebec Task Force's diagnostic classifications reported in 1987 (40). Unlike the Quebec Task Force, we have subdivided each of these groups, characterized by pain location, into those patients with spinal deformity (Fig. 7), and those who have no deformity. As already noted, we believe this classification by deformity provides useful diagnostic information and guides treatment.

Mixed Syndromes

Although the delineation of syndromes is important, there are many patients who may present with the features of more than one, most commonly a derangement with a dysfunction. These combinations can be effectively analyzed and treated by a well-trained practitioner. For example, some patients have a significant loss of extension range due to a predominately flexed lifestyle, yet have had minimal or no symptoms. When displacement occurs, symptoms result. Although the treatment requires extension of the spine to centralize or abolish symptoms, the extension range is too limited by dysfunction to allow the position. In these patients, stretching must be performed initially to bring about sufficient extension range to allow centralization and pain relief (Fig. 8).

Tables 2 and 3 summarize the three principle syndromes and the subcategories of the derangement syndrome.

TABLE 3. *Derangement subcategories*

Derangement	Characteristics
1	Central or symmetrical pain No deformity
2	Central or symmetrical pain With or without radiation With kyphotic deformity
3	Unilateral or asymmetrical pain With or without proximal extremity pain (above elbow or knee) No deformity
4	Unilateral or asymmetrical pain With or without proximal extremity pain (above elbow or knee) With scoliosis (lateral) deformity
5	Unilateral or asymmetrical pain With or without proximal extremity pain (above elbow or knee) Extremity pain extending below the elbow or knee No deformity
6	Unilateral or asymmetrical pain With or without proximal extremity pain (above elbow or knee) Extremity pain extending below the elbow or knee With sciatic scoliotic deformity
7	Symmetrical or asymmetrical pain With or without proximal extremity pain (above elbow or knee) With deformity of accentuated cervical or lumbar lordosis

ASSESSMENT SYSTEM FOR SPINAL PAIN PATIENTS

A thorough history and physical examination that concentrates on the patient's symptoms is the foundation of any medical evaluation. In our assessment scheme, we place great emphasis on the range of spinal motion and postures which have produced pain acutely or in the past, and those spinal motions and postures which centralize that pain or abolish it. As already noted, we believe this protocol enables patients to be categorized according to the presumed pathology and provides the basis for treatment. This process is fully described elsewhere (24).

History

The patient's history should focus on items that relate to changes in location and intensity of pain. This analysis includes developing an understanding of the patient's home, work, and recreational requirements, which then determine the relevant static and dynamic forces which are being regularly applied to the patient's spine. One should inquire as to the precise location of the pain at onset and as the episode has continued. Typically, the initial central pain reported has only subsequently peripheralized. The intermittency or constancy of the symptoms, whether central and/or peripheral, and associated neurological complaints must also be carefully elicited. Pain which is intermittent or changes its location is easily treated. Pain which is truly constant is more difficult to treat and has a less certain prognosis, particularly when chronic. It is also important to differentiate pain characterized by recurrent episodes over many years from constant pain, because of the more favorable prognosis in those with recurring symptoms.

Examination

Although our examination includes all of the elements of the usual clinical evaluation of patients with back pain, it focuses particularly on the static and dynamic qualities of the patient's spine and relates these observations to pain location and intensity.

The patient's normal seating posture should be observed and the location and intensity of pain should be recorded. Frequently symptoms worsen while patients are seated during the interview in their "natural postures." Simple correction of the seating position at this point may have a noticeable impact, and many patients describe decreased pain intensity and may even centralize an asymmetric or peripheral pain. Similarly, the presence of an acute deformity is important information and is observed only in patients with a derangement. The deformity can frequently be abolished quickly and simultaneously during the examination process.

Repeated end-range spinal test movements of the involved region of the spine are the cornerstone of the examination and reveal important information when the location and intensity of the pain are monitored in response to these test movements. As the patient is systematically examined, the pain often will change in its location or even be abolished. It is most important that movements be taken to the end-range permitted by the patient in order to observe changes in pain patterns. Monitoring whether the pain occurs during the mid-range movements or only at the end-range is also important and helps differentiate the three major syndromes of spinal pain. Repeated spinal motions usually produce one of three changes in the patient's complaints: an increase in the intensity and/or peripheralization of symptoms, which implies displacements are increasing; a decrease in intensity and/or centralization of symptoms, which implies the displacement is being reduced; or no effect on symptoms. In the dysfunction syndrome, one will observe pain only at the end-range without mid-range pain, the pain will not increase or decrease in intensity with repetition, and the pain location does not change. Any change in location of pain would seem to indicate that a derangement exists.

Our examination routinely includes end-range test movements, into flexion, extension, and lateral bending (Figs. 2, 3, 6, 8), both in the standing or sitting weight-bearing posture, as well as non-weight-bearing positions during recumbency. The importance of repeating the movements cannot be overemphasized. Often the direction of movement that eventually centralizes or abolishes the pain increases pain on the first attempt. Conversely, the direction of spinal movement that has actually been aggravating the patient's problem often is not pain productive on the first attempt, but only worsens during repetition. Distinguishing the pain of derangement from dysfunction may require many repetitions in several different directions.

Even patients with acute severe pain can be helped dramatically if the principles of evaluating spinal movement are followed and taken slowly during the evaluation process. Patients with acute kyphotic or scoliotic deformities and intense pain often will have reduction of pain and elimination of deformity during their first clinic visit. Given the opportunity, patients in acute pain sometimes learn how to "reduce" the deformity and relieve their pain during the examination.

When the history is completed and an inventory taken of the effects of common positions, movements, and activities on the location and intensity of symptoms, we believe the patient's underlying pathology can then be surmised and treated specifically. In the majority of patients, this analysis relieves the practitioner of the need to obtain initial imaging studies, unless the problem is thought to warrant immediate surgery, such as the rare instances of cauda equina syndrome.

Treatment

Once the pain syndrome has been identified, "mechanical logic" forms the basis for appropriate treatment. The abolition of the patient's symptoms, especially when this occurs rapidly, would seem to confirm the accuracy of the analysis and dictates the choice for ongoing treatment.

Postural Syndrome

Patients with this condition need only to avoid the static loading produced by the end-range positioning to abolish and prevent their pain. Most often correction of sitting posture (Fig. 5) is required, although standing posture is relevant in some patients to the production of symptoms.

Dysfunction Syndrome

In this condition, the pain arises from adaptively shortened or contracted tissues, resulting in a premature restriction on the end-range of motion. For these patients frequent regular stretching of the painful tight structures over a 6 to 8 week interval is usually sufficient (Fig. 3). During treatment, lingering pain after the stretch implies the intensity of the stretch is excessive. As full range of movement is gradually restored, symptoms progressively resolve, and a pain-free, full range of movement results.

Derangement Syndrome

These patients are characterized by rapid onset of symptoms, rapid changes in pain location and intensity, deformities, and pain in the mid-range of motion. They require application of reductive postures and motions which will centralize and then abolish the pain. The patient can usually generate sufficient force, once the required direction for "reduction" is determined, thereby requiring the patient to assume increasing responsibility and independence for care. After pain has been abolished there are two additional phases of treatment. The "reduction" must be maintained allowing stabilization and eventually tissue healing to occur. This recovery is accomplished by adhering to the strategies learned in the initial evaluation and treatment. The final phase involves the recovery of motion in all directions, including the temporarily forbidden, previously "displacing" direction of movement. The appropriate determination of this phase is based upon cautious testing into the previously painful direction. Gradually the patient should be able to resume all functions.

In practice, any variance from these three phases during treatment usually recreates the patient's pain. The principles are similar to those of any other displacing injury. For example, in a Colles fracture reduction of the displacement fairly rapidly abolishes the pain. The maintenance of the reduction by cast or splint allows healing to continue. When the cast is removed, motion progresses until all normal motions are tolerated.

PREVENTION OF RECURRENT PAIN

The prevalence, incidence, recovery, and costs of low back pain are well documented in the literature (4,6,14,15,16,17,28,32,33,39). One of the major contributions to the cost and disability are recurrent episodes which occur in as many as 85% of patients (42). As noted by Valkenburg (42) and others (24), the severity and duration of each recurrence tend to increase, although the mechanical characteristics are usually similar to the previous episodes. These recurrences increase the risk for chronicity, disability, surgery, and costly rehabilitation. It is estimated that 85% of the costs of low back pain are spent on the 10% of patients with recurrent and chronically disabling symptoms (6).

Regardless of treatment, it is also natural for patients to associate their recovery with the treatment being used at the time of symptom resolution. When medications, braces, manipulation, and modalities are used, the patients will tend to seek the same treatments with the next recurrence and thus develop a dependency on an external system. We believe one of the major benefits of the system of diagnosis and treatment described here is that patients learn to self-treat mechanically and abolish their symptoms. With the initial treatment, they learn how to move their symptoms centrally or distally in a predictable fashion and then, as they recover, to abolish symptoms completely. They quickly learn the mechanics of their own pain disorder and with treatment are placed in the position to take control and resolve later episodes. Like other self-directed treatment programs, our approach places responsibility on patients for their own management and prevention.

Our goals for effective treatment, therefore, are measured by: the resolution of symptoms in more than 80% of patients within three months, and a hastened rate of functional recovery by the rapid abolition of symptoms. More importantly, we believe effective treatment should reduce the rate of recurrences and reduce or eliminate the disability of subsequent episodes utilizing patient self-treatment.

TREATMENT EFFICACY

Published studies refer to the system of diagnosis and treatment we have described here as the McKenzie approach and thus we will use this designation here. Much of the initial enthusiasm for this approach was based on clinical observation, rather than on rigorous scientific analyses. Subsequently, a number of studies have compared the use of the McKenzie approach with Williams flexion exercises (45a). In the earlier studies (30,31) all patients were acutely symptomatic, and in one study (30) all had confirmed disc lesions based on neurologic examination and myelography. Both studies demonstrated a significant benefit for the McKenzie approach with respect to the rate of pain reduction, restoration of spinal motion, increased straight leg raising comfort, and increased sitting capacity. The average number of treatments to achieve these results was significantly lower with the McKenzie approach than with the Williams flexion exercises. It is worth emphasizing that the Williams approach treats all patients essentially by the same protocol. In contrast, our system defines the treatment on the basis of the individualized mechanical needs of the patient, which are determined by the clinical assessment.

One of these studies (30) followed patients for two months and noted a reduction in the rate of recurrent episodes. This limited study suggests some capacity of the treatment to prevent further problems.

For many, correction of posture alone, with no other intervention, will significantly improve symptoms. In a prospective and controlled study, 210 patients with low back pain with or without referred pain were randomly assigned to either a lumbar kyphotic or lordotic group (25). Pain location and back and leg pain intensities were assessed during sitting over a 24- to 48-hour period under standardized clinical settings and general sitting environments.

When sitting with a lordotic posture, both back and leg pain intensity were significantly reduced and referred pain shifted toward the low back. This was in significant contrast to the group sitting with kyphotic posture who did not demonstrate these changes (p < .001).

Moreover, sitting in kyphosis appeared to be detrimental: of those patients with pain present above the knee, tested over a 10-minute standardized sitting trial, 5% of those sitting with a lordosis experienced pain that extended below the knee. In comparison, 22% sitting with a kyphosis developed pain below the knee.

This would indicate that centralization of pain, therefore, can occur and/or be enhanced by posture correction alone, even without the end-range positioning and exercises that are utilized during the complete McKenzie assessment and treatment process.

In another study, 136 symptomatic low back pain patients were randomly assigned to 1 of 3 treatment programs: established back school, 90/90 traction, or McKenzie (43). While patient attrition and unplanned crossovers to alternative treatments invalidated study results after the first week, the initial data were valid and noteworthy. Of those patients treated with the McKenzie approach, 97% had improved after 1 week. By contrast, only 50% improved with 90/90 traction and 38% with back school. The results of both of the latter treatments were similar to, or lower than, what might be expected with no treatment at all. As will be noted in Chapter 72, one of the confounding variables in this study was the therapist's enthusiasm for the McKenzie method, which resulted in unplanned treatment crossover.

A recent randomized study (41) has compared the McKenzie approach to a mini-back school program in treating acute low back pain in 100 patients representative of the working population. Fifty-four percent of the patients had pain radiating into the buttock, leg, or foot. Patient assessments were then made by an independent observer at 3 weeks, but by the unblinded investigator at 1 year. The average number of treatments in the patients receiving the McKenzie approach was 5.5, the median sick leave was 10 days, and 45% had first year relapses with a mean sick listing of 27 days. In comparison, the mini-back school program had an initial medical sick leave of 17.5 days and an 80% recurrence rate in the first year, with a mean sick listing of 40 days. The investigators concluded the McKenzie approach had efficacy in rate of symptom reduction, prevention of disability, and reduction of disability when symptoms did recur. It is of note that the 80% recurrence rate noted in the mini-back school approaches the 85% recurrence rate noted by Valkenburg (42).

Preliminary reports of a study in progress in England (35) indicate similar findings. Patients with symptoms for less than 3 weeks of low back pain, with or without referred symptoms, were randomly assigned to either McKenzie therapy or given a 28-day supply of Ketoprofen 200 mg. The study administrator was blinded as to the treatments assigned and patients were carefully protected from knowledge of the alternative treatment. At 6-month follow-up with a blinded assessor, patients treated with the McKenzie method are demonstrating a significant decrease in the degree of disability during recurrences. These long-term benefits suggest these patients can effectively deal with the early warning signs of a recurrence and minimize its progression and disability.

Although further clinical research is clearly needed, these data support the efficacy of the method we are advocating.

CONCLUSION

The approach we have described for treatment of spinal pain is often misunderstood. It does not treat all patients with extension as though it were the opposite of the Williams flexion exercises. It is also not based on the disc model of nuclear shifting in the direction opposite that of spinal bending. It is a much more complex discipline to practice than this brief description can convey.

The system is based primarily upon pain and its behavior, as well as the presence or absence of acute spinal deformity, as the only direct links the clinician has to deal with the unknown underlying pathology. Meanwhile, the large majority of acute and chronic patients can be effectively treated, and recurrences can be prevented or quickly resolved simply by monitoring the pain and its behavior during a comprehensive mechanical assessment which identifies and utilizes self-treatment to the fullest for a wide range of patients.

The impact of low back pain on our population and its high cost to our society strongly suggest that we cannot remain content with letting patients spontaneously recover while we dispense unproven, passive modalities. We also cannot justify performing invasive injection procedures, prescribing medications and bed rest, or applying manual therapy to a population of patients who can effectively treat themselves.

The success of the McKenzie system is dependent on the training and expertise of the physician and especially the therapist. Typically, two years of clinical experience with spine patients, coupled with appropriate education, is required by the therapist for effective evaluation and treatment of a wide range of spinal patients.

REFERENCES

1. Adams MA, Hutton WC (1982): Prolapsed intervertebral disc. A hyperflexion injury. *Spine* 7:184–191.
2. Adams MA, Hutton WC (1985): Gradual disc prolapse. *Spine* 10:524–531.
3. Deleted.
4. Biering-Sorensen F (1982): Low back trouble in a general population of 30-, 40-, 50-, and 60-year-old men and women: Study design, representativeness and basic results. *Dan Med Bull* 29:289–299.
5. Cloward RB (1959): Cervical diskography: A contribution to the etiology and mechanism of neck, shoulder and arm pain. *Annals of Surg* 150:1052–1064.
6. Deyo RA, Tsui-Wu YJ (1987): Descriptive epidemiology of low-back pain and its related medical care in the United States. *Spine* 12:264–268.
7. Donelson RG, Grant WD, Kamps C, Medcalf R (1990): Pain response to sagittal end-range spinal motion: A multi-centered, prospective, randomized trial. Presentation, North American Spine Society, Monterey, California.
8. Donelson R, Silva G, Murphy K (1990): The centralization phenomenon: Its usefulness in evaluating and treating referred pain. *Spine* 15:211–213.
9. Goel VK, Mjus GO (1986): Stress-strain characteristics of spinal ligaments. *Trans Orthop Res Soc* 11:370.
10. Gonnella C, Paris SV, Kutner M (1982): Reliability in evaluating passive intervertebral motion. *Phys Therapy* 62:436–444.
11. Grigg P, Hoffman AH (1982): Properties of Ruffini afferents revealed by stress analysis of isolated sections of cat knee capsule. *J Neurophysiol* 47:41–54.
12. Grigg A, Hoffman AH, Fogarty KE (1982): Properties of Golgi-Mazzoni afferents in cat knee joint capsule, as revealed by mechanical studies of isolated joint capsule. *J Neurophysiol* 47:31–40.
13. Grigg P, Schaible HG, Schmidt RF (1986): Mechanical sensitivity of group III and IV afferents from posterior articular nerve in normal and inflamed cat knee. *J Neurophysiol* 55:635–643.
14. Horal J (1969): The clinical appearance of low back disorders in the city of Gothenburg, Sweden. Comparisons of incapacitated probands with matched controls. *Acta Orthop Scand Suppl* 118:1–109.
15. Hult L (1954): Cervical, dorsal and lumbar spinal syndromes. *Acta Orthop Scand (Suppl)* 17:1–102.
16. Kellgren JH, Lawrence JS (1958): Osteo-arthrosis and disk degeneration in an urban population. *Ann Rheum Dis* 17:388–397.
17. Kelsey JL (1982): *Epidemiology of musculoskeletal disorders.* New York: Oxford University Press, pp. 145–167.
18. Kirkaldy-Willis WH, Farfan HF (1982): Instability of the lumbar spine. *Clin Orthop* 165:110.
19. Kirkaldy-Willis WH (1983): *Managing low back pain.* New York: Churchill Livingstone.
20. Kopp JR (1986): The use of lumbar extension in the evaluation and treatment of patients with acute herniated nucleus pulposus. A preliminary report. *Clin Orthop* 202:211–218.
21. Korkala O, Gronblad M, Liesi P, et al. (1985): Immunohistochemical demonstration of nociceptors in the ligamentous structures of the lumbar spine. *Spine* 10:156–157.
22. Krag MH, Seroussi RE, Wilder DG, Pope MH (1987): Internal displacement distribution from *in vitro* loading of human thoracic and lumbar spinal motion segments: Experimental results and theoretical predictions. *Spine* 12:1001–1007.
23. Kramer J (1981): *Intervertebral disk diseases.* Chicago: Year Book Medical Publishers.
24. McKenzie RA (1981): *The lumbar spine: Mechanical diagnosis and therapy.* Waikanae, New Zealand: Spinal Publications.
25. McKenzie RA, Williams M, Hawley J, Van Wijmen P, Reed R, Farry S, Jack M, Laslett M (1988): A comparison of the effects of two sitting postures on back and referred pain. *Abstracts of The International Society for the Study of the Lumbar Spine,* Miami, Florida. Accepted for publication in *Spine.*
26. Matyus TA, Bach TM (1985): The reliability of selected techniques in clinical arthrometrics. *Australian J Physiotherapy* 1:175.
27. Mooney V, Brown M, Modic M (1989): Intervertebral disc: Clinical perspectives. In: *New perspectives on low back pain,* JW Frymoyer, SL Gordon, eds. Park Ridge, Illinois: American Academy of Orthopaedic Surgeons.
28. Morris A (1985): Identifying workers at risk to back injury is not guesswork. *Occup Health Safety* 54:16–20.
29. Nachemson AL (1985): Advances in low-back pain. *Clin Orthop* 200:266–278.
30. Nwuga G, Nwuga V (1985): Relative therapeutic efficacy of the Williams and McKenzie protocols in back pain management. *Physiotherapy Practice* 1:99–105.
31. Ponte DJ (1984): A preliminary report on the use of the McKenzie protocol versus Williams protocol in the treatment of low back pain. *J Ortho Sports Phys Therapy* 6:130–134.
32. Pope MH (1983): Understanding and rehabilitation of low back disease. *Spinal Column* 1:9.
33. Pope MH, Frymoyer JW, Andersson G (1984): *Occupational low back pain.* New York: Praeger.
34. Potter NA, Rothstein JM (1985): Intertester reliability for selected clinical tests of the sacroiliac joint. *Phys Therapy* 65:1671–1675.
34a. Quebec Task Force on Spinal Disorders (1987): see ref. 40.
35. Roberts AP (1989): The conservative treatment of low back pain. Unpublished doctoral thesis, University of Nottingham, Nottingham, United Kingdom.
36. Schnebel BE, Simmons JW, Chowning J, Davidson R (1988): A digitizing technique for the study of movement of intradiscal dye in response to flexion and extension of the lumbar spine. *Spine* 13:309–312.
37. Seroussi RE, Krag MH, Muller DL, Pope MH (1989): Internal deformations of intact and denucleated human lumbar discs subjected to compression, flexion and extension loads. *J Orthop Res* 7:122–131.
38. Shah JS, Hampson WGJ, Jayson MI (1978): Distribution of surface strain in the cadaveric lumbar spine. *J Bone Joint Surg* [Br] 60:246–251.
39. Spengler DM, Bigos SJ, Martin NA (1986): Back injuries in industry: A retrospective study. I. Overview and cost analysis. *Spine* 11:241–245.
40. [Spitzer WO] (1987): Scientific approach to the assessment and management of activity-related spinal disorders. A monograph for clinicians. Report of the Quebec Task Force on Spinal Disorders. *Spine* 12:S1–S59.

41. Stankovich R (1990): Conservative treatment of acute low-back pain. A prospective randomized trial: McKenzie method of treatment versus patient education in "mini back school." *Spine* 15:120.

42. Valkenburg HA, Haanen HCM (1982): The epidemiology of low back pain. In: *American Academy of Orthopaedic Surgeons symposium on idiopathic low back pain,* AA White III, SL Gordon, eds. St. Louis: Mosby, pp. 9–22.

43. Vanharanta H, Videman T, Mooney V (1986): McKenzie exercises, back trac and back school in lumbar syndrome. Presented at annual meeting of the International Society for the Study of the Lumbar Spine, Dallas, Texas.

44. Weber H (1983): Lumbar disc herniation: A controlled prospective study with ten years of observation. *Spine* 8:131–140.

45. Wilder D, Pope MH, Frymoyer JW (1988): The biomechanics of lumbar disc herniation and the effects of overload and instability. *J Spinal Disorders* 1:16–32.

45a. Williams PC (1965): *The lumbosacral spine, emphasizing conservative management.* New York: Blakiston, pp. 80–93.

46. Wyke B (1976): Neurological aspects of low back pain. In: *The lumbar spine and back pain,* M Jayson, ed. New York: Grune and Stratton.

The Adult Spine: Principles and Practice,
J. W. Frymoyer, Editor-in-Chief.
Raven Press, Ltd., New York © 1991.

CHAPTER 77

Education

The Prevention and Treatment of Low Back Disorders

Margareta Nordin, Sherri Weiser, and Nachman Halpern

THE CONCEPT OF EDUCATION FOR LOW BACK DISORDERS

Until recently, much of the responsibility for personal health has been assigned to medical professionals. Today, the rising cost of health care, the increasing number of chronically ill individuals who must learn to manage their illnesses, and advancements in our knowledge of health and illness make it impractical for individuals to relinquish control of their health (51). Patient advocacy groups championing the patient's "right to know" have added to the demand for information about health and illness (14,80). Health education programs have proliferated in response to this demand.

Patient education programs have been successful in preventing and treating various chronic illnesses. This model has been applied to low back disorders as well. During the first half of the twentieth century, attempts to prevent back injuries were limited to on-the-job training in lifting techniques. More recently, the concept of back

education has broadened to include strength and fitness, ergonomics, physiology, personal lifestyle, and stress management (91).

The target of back education programs today includes the general population. The scope often goes beyond prevention to include treatment. Moreover, few education programs are limited to the presentation of information. Most are also concerned with changing attitudes, beliefs, and behavior in addition to imparting knowledge. The following is a description and review of low back education programs.

Who Needs To Be Educated?

Epidemiological data from numerous studies show that lifetime prevalence of back pain in the general population of industrialized countries is between 45% and 85% (19). In workers, absence due to back pain fluctuates between 30% and 50% depending on the nature of the work task. In the working population, the annual incidence of compensable back injury is about 2% (2).

Because most people afflicted with back pain are in the prime of their lives, back problems are more than a

  M. Nordin, R.P.T., Dr. Sci.; S. Weiser, Ph.D.; N. Halpern, M.A.: Hospital for Joint Diseases, Orthopaedic Institute, New York, New York, 10003.

health concern. Industry suffers considerable economic strain in terms of increased insurance premiums and decreased productivity. This underscores the need for back education programs that address the population at risk for back disorders as well as those already injured.

Much effort has gone into identifying those at high risk for back injury (5,12,16,31). Personal risk factors based on prospective studies include previous history of low back pain, age, and cigarette smoking. In women, childbearing history is a risk factor. Height, various indices of obesity, poor muscle strength, and impact aerobic exercise have also been reported as risk factors but the results of different studies are conflicting. Some risk variables for industrial back injury are recent job entry, amount of twisting and lifting, and job satisfaction (5,8,31,49,97).

While it is possible to target at-risk groups based on the findings described above, identifying a specific at-risk individual is more difficult. Even individuals who have every risk factor have only an increased probability of injuring their backs. Therefore, in the workplace pre-employment screening for potential back injury claimants presents legal and possibly ethical problems (38). A person may not be denied work because he or she is "at risk." In order to exclude a candidate, the employer must demonstrate that the person cannot fulfill the physical requirements of the job at the time of employment.

THE PREVENTION OF LOW BACK DISORDERS THROUGH EDUCATION

In the case of low back disorders, it is widely recognized that prevention is the ideal treatment but that it is often difficult to implement (58,72). Prevention programs are of three kinds: primary, secondary, and tertiary. Primary prevention aims at reducing the occurrence of low back pain before it occurs. Secondary prevention aims to reduce the severity and/or the recurrence of low back pain episodes. Tertiary prevention involves the reduction of disability and restoration of function in chronic low back pain patients. Each type of program will be discussed in turn.

Primary Prevention

Primary prevention programs for the population at large are uncommon for several reasons. As previously mentioned, accurate identification of at-risk individuals is difficult. Therefore, primary prevention programs have to address a substantial segment of the population. Given the magnitude of this task, funding for a public back injury prevention program is costly and difficult to justify. In addition, individuals who believe that the chance of becoming injured is remote may not be motivated to change their behaviors. Under these circum-

stances, intervention is fruitless. However, more focused primary prevention programs have begun to surface in the workplace, where back pain has taken a toll of about $6 billion each year in the United States (60,71,73, 102,103,108). Unlike traditional classes in proper lifting techniques, these programs include strength and fitness training, manual materials handling, personal lifestyle, stress management, and/or ergonomic principles. Each component will be discussed at length in the section entitled "Review of Back Education Program Content."

Several studies have assessed the value of a primary prevention program in industry. In two studies, there was a decrease in the number of reported back injuries and days lost following such a program (63,73). However, confounding factors made it difficult to credit the positive outcome to the back program alone.

In a 3-year prospective study by Versloot et al. (102) of 400 bus drivers in Holland, a significant decrease in absenteeism was achieved after a back injury prevention program was instituted. The average decrease in absenteeism was 6 days per employee per year. However, a similar study of 4,000 Swedish federal employees by Ljungberg and Sanne (60) did not support these findings. The conflicting results of these two studies may be attributed to system variables such as company support and the social security system, and program variables such as the use of model teachers and employee involvement. Further research is needed to clarify these questions.

Secondary Prevention

Secondary prevention programs are usually aimed at the patient with acute (less than one month) or sub-acute (one to three months) back pain. Back schools and management education training are two programs designed to reduce the severity and recurrence of back pain.

Back School

Back schools are taught in small groups of patients who suffer from acute or intermittent back problems. Delpech is generally believed to have initiated the "Back School" concept in the early part of the nineteenth century in Montpelier, France (77). Zachrisson-Forssell (110) is credited with developing the first formal back school in Stockholm in 1969. Since then back schools have enjoyed great proliferation internationally (35,56,63).

Back schools are based on the premise that educating patients about proper back care can prevent and reduce the severity of future back pain episodes. The patient is expected to adopt health-promoting behaviors and take responsibility for recovery. As such, back schools represent a divergence from more conventional passive treatment modalities.

The group format provides an economical way to transmit information and fosters a supportive atmosphere in which students exchange ideas freely. Classes generally consist of 4 to 12 patients who meet for 5 to 7 sessions of approximately one hour in length. The term "school" is used to encourage learning and retention of information (91).

Back schools are most frequently taught by physical therapists but have also been taught by other health care professionals. Topics covered include the causes of injury, physiology of the spine, fitness, posture, personal lifestyle, and the relationship between stress and pain (9,35,63).

It is difficult to gauge the effectiveness of back schools due to the variation in teaching methods and topics covered in different programs. An additional obstacle has been the lack of controlled studies, often difficult to achieve in clinical settings. Nonetheless, Bergquist-Ullman showed that back school is superior to passive treatment or no treatment (9). Her prospective controlled studies demonstrated that back schools effectively reduced the amount of lost work days in sub-acute low back pain (9) but had little effect on chronic back pain populations (56). Linton and Kamwendo, in a review of existing studies (59), also found conflicting results. These authors point out that the lack of positive results may have less to do with the content of back school than with the fact the students may not be retaining what they have learned (59). Efforts to assess knowledge and skills acquisition may be an important step in the evaluation of back schools.

Management Education

In industry, most prevention efforts have focused on the worker. It has become evident that the cooperation of management is a crucial component in the success of work-site health programs. Snook and White (91) point to the importance of training management in early detection and appropriate care of back disorders.

Management education includes the concept of creating a supportive environment where employees are encouraged to report new injuries, and then to manage them without work loss. Worker participation in on-site education programs also requires supervisor approval. Workers may participate more willingly if they are not penalized for lost work time.

Management may also be educated in the benefits of temporarily reassigning an injured worker to a less physically demanding job. In common practice, workers remain on disability leave until they are able to resume their normal responsibilities. However, statistics show that the likelihood of someone returning to work after 6 months of disability is slim (65,104). Remaining at work, even in a limited capacity, can help prevent chronic pain syndrome (72). Management can also learn ways of modifying the job to accommodate the worker (91). The benefits of these approaches may, in the long run, outweigh the costs (108).

Tertiary Prevention

It has been suggested that sub-acute pain becomes chronic as early as 6 to 7 weeks after onset (93). However, most pain centers classify pain as chronic after 3 months. At this point, the life of the patient may be seriously disrupted psychologically, socially, and financially. Education and training programs must take these factors into consideration in order to successfully rehabilitate the patient. Functional restoration programs and non-medical pain management are two treatment modalities for chronic pain in which patient education is an important component.

Functional Restoration

Perhaps the greatest challenge in treating chronic pain is getting the patient to go back to work. Functional restoration and some work hardening programs are distin-

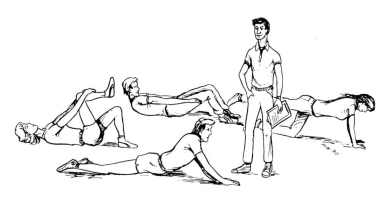

FIG. 1. Back school teaches principles of back care in a group setting.

guished by their aggressive approach to rehabilitation and their emphasis on returning the chronic pain patient to gainful employment. These programs utilize a behavioral paradigm in which the physical functioning criteria are set by the instructor rather than the patient, and accomplishment of goals is rewarded. Additionally, many of these programs simulate actual physical work tasks in order to prepare the patient to return to work after rehabilitation.

In 1985, Mayer et al. popularized a comprehensive functional restoration program for chronic low back pain patients (64). The program consisted of 54 hours of treatment per week for 3 weeks. It combined education, behavior training, physical fitness including endurance training, and work simulation. Objective functional capacity measurement techniques were used to guide the treatment program for pre- and post-evaluation.

Mayer et al. assessed the outcome of this program using a comparison group of patients who were unable to participate because they were denied insurance reimbursement (64). The study showed that 82% of the patients were reconditioned successfully and returned to work. In the no-treatment comparison group, only 40% of the patients returned to work. An identical functional restoration program was instituted at the New England Back Center with similar results (36) (see Chapter 13).

The return-to-work rates of these two programs are impressive. One must bear in mind, however, that the comparison groups in both studies were not randomly selected. Group differences may have been due to factors unrelated to the program. Also, due to the multidisciplinary nature of these programs, it is difficult to isolate the factors that contribute to success. Clinically controlled prospective studies, with and without the educational component, would be more informative in determining education's contribution to program success.

Non-Medical Pain Management

Pain of a chronic nature is rarely eliminated completely. Instead, chronic patients must learn how to reduce pain and come to terms with the pain that remains (92). Stress management techniques are used as a means of non-medical pain management, with pain identified as the main stressor one must learn to cope with.

Chronic pain patients are commonly characterized by disability disproportionate to their physical findings (95,104). Patients may remain sedentary due to fear of increased injury and pain or because of secondary gains associated with pain behaviors (28,54). Cognitive-behavioral techniques, where patients are rewarded for "well" behaviors, are taught to encourage return to pre-pain levels of functioning. These techniques also help to reassure the patient that normal activities will not exacerbate the injury (see Chapter 14).

REVIEW OF BACK EDUCATION PROGRAM CONTENT

Each of the topics covered in back injury prevention programs are based on current knowledge about the etiology and risk factors associated with lumbar spinal disorders. Although there is not total agreement, or scientific substantiation for all risk factors, the following are commonly included in designing curricula for education programs.

Manual Materials Handling

A number of handling techniques have been associated with back injury. The goal of manual materials handling training is to teach techniques that put less strain on the back. Occupational groups such as health care workers, construction laborers, garbage collectors, truck drivers, and machinists have a high risk of injury (43). These groups are prime targets for manual materials handling training.

Movements and postures associated with back injury comprise the content of most training programs. They are frequent lifting (25 times per day), twisting while lifting, heavy lifting (11.3 kg or more), static postures, forward bending and twisting of the trunk, and muscle fatigue (18,31,37,39,48,55,75,81,87). Of all these motions, perhaps the most deleterious is simultaneous twisting and forward bending of the trunk. Kelsey et al. (49) showed a sixfold increase in reported back injuries as a result of this movement.

Several studies have attempted to train workers in proper handling techniques (21,90,103). Manual materials handling education has, thus far, been unsuccessful in reducing injury rates. However, none of these studies attempted to assess the actual acquisition of new skills, or how the worker used the newly learned techniques on the job.

The inconsistent record of training programs also may be due to the fact that workers have only limited control of the way they handle materials. Some studies estimate that about 20% to 40% of all lifting motions can be attributed to individual worker technique (17,24,34). These studies suggest that avoiding twisting motions and maintaining the load close to the body (3) are the most important manual materials handling concepts to promote in order to reduce back injuries. Other motions require ergonomic solutions, such as workplace redesign.

Few studies have assessed manual materials handling education in terms of motor skills acquisition. Such studies are important because they indicate which skills can be effectively taught. Motion analysis showed that trainees can learn to get a good grip of an object, move smoothly and avoid jerky motions, hold a load close to the body, and extend the knees and hips while keeping

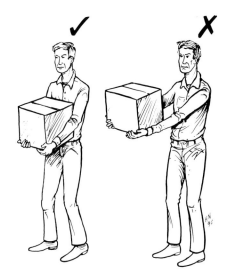

FIG. 2. The load should be kept close to the body.

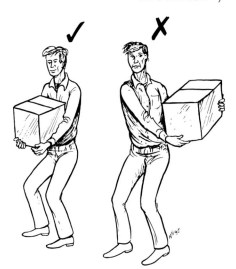

FIG. 3. Twisting while lifting should be avoided.

the trunk straight, particularly when handling heavy loads. The first two skills can be acquired in a 4 hour training program (17). The other skills require an intensive course of 35 hours (34). These findings limit the use of on-site training in industry.

The long-term retention of new skills is also important. Hultman et al. (41) have shown that subjects remember to keep their trunks straight after 3 months. Long-term retention is probably most sensitive to feedback and on-site reinforcement (17,21,41,96,103).

More research is needed to examine the effectiveness of manual materials handling training in reducing injury rates. Future studies should take into account the degree to which new motor skills have been acquired and retained, worker skill, and issues of compliance (52). In light of the estimate that 60% of reported back injuries could have been avoided by adopting safer moving techniques, manual materials handling training remains justifiable (34).

Strength and Fitness

Training in strength and fitness variably emphasizes musculoskeletal strength, cardiovascular fitness, aerobic capacity, endurance, and flexibility. While it is commonly believed that those in poor physical condition are prone to back injury, to date there is no scientific evidence to support this assertion (5,33,98). One study showed that firefighters who were fit were less likely to suffer back injuries over a four year period than their less fit coworkers (16). However, the failure of the investigators to control for such important baseline differences as age of subjects brings these findings into question.

In the largest prospective study to date, more than 3,000 employees underwent pre-employment testing (5).

After three years it was shown that those with poor general isometric strength were equally likely to report back pain as stronger workers. There was actually a trend for workers with greater strength to report increased back pain.

These studies used generic isometric strength and endurance, and cardiovascular fitness testing unrelated to specific work tasks, as measures of strength. Strength testing more closely related to physical requirements of the job may be more predictive of initial back pain episodes. This idea was brought to light in one study where testing was biomechanically designed to reflect job demands (50). However, too few back problems were reported to allow for an accurate data analysis. Prospective studies of dynamic strength are needed to uncover the relationship between strength and low back pain.

Flexibility has also been found to be a poor predictor of onset and severity of low back pain (5,12,98). Nonetheless, fitness programs have been shown to reduce overall absenteeism and medical costs in industry (16). People may also benefit psychologically from feeling fit. Therefore, until it is known for certain that fitness has no relationship to back pain, it may be prudent to include some strength and conditioning concepts in a back pain prevention program.

Personal Lifestyle

A person's lifestyle may be defined as eating habits, activity level, sleeping patterns, tobacco and alcohol consumptions, other substance use, and athletic pursuits. To the degree these factors are under an individual's control, they are important to emphasize in education programs. Eating habits have an effect on low back pain, insofar as obesity is a risk factor for back pain and its chronicity. Deyo (22) has reported that individuals in the fifth quintile of weight are at greater risk. He also noted taller people were at risk, but height is beyond the control of the individual.

Some of the issues in activity level have been discussed in the preceding section on "Strength and Fitness." Although the clinical data are inconclusive, there is a large body of basic information that demonstrates beneficial effects of aerobic activity on the metabolism and biomechanical integrity of muscles, ligaments, joints, and facets (30). This information lends credence to a clinical approach that stresses physical fitness not only in the prevention of back disease, but in overall health and well being.

As the antithesis of aerobic fitness, smoking appears to have a relationship to the incidence, severity, and resultant disability from low back disorders. Much of the clinical data is based on retrospective studies (31,97) and should therefore be viewed with some caution. Another study, also retrospective in design, showed a relationship of smoking to lumbar disc herniation (48). One prospective study found no relationship between smoking and onset of acute back pain (8), but in another study, however (5), smoking did have predictive value for future disability in a group of healthy subjects. The latter observation is consistent with cross-sectional epidemiologic surveys which show a significant interaction between smoking and disabling back complaints (84,85,101). In those same studies, alcohol consumption, drug use, poor eating habits, and sleep disturbances also were interrelated and predictors of disability. Thus, the question arises: is smoking a causal factor, or is it part of a broader set of psychosocial problems? Again the clinical data are unclear at this time, but basic disc research demonstrates a significant adverse effect of cigarette smoke and nicotine on intervertebral disc metabolism (see Chapter 31). Similarly, sleep disturbance has been related specifically to the clinical syndrome of fibromyositis. In fact, there is a school of thought suggesting that sleep disturbance is the primary event and back pain the outcome (see Chapter 35).

Lastly, some sports have been related to low back pain and even to sciatica. In particular, sports which involve twisting, such as golf, bowling, and tennis, have been associated with lumbar disc herniations (47). Other studies have suggested a relationship between mild non-disabling back pain and jogging and cross country skiing. A special example is the relationship between isthmic spondylolisthesis and gymnastics and American football.

The practical application of this knowledge in the prevention of back pain is limited. Certainly, no one would suggest a person give up sports to prevent back pain; conversely, a practical approach certainly would encourage both cessation of smoking and weight control.

Stress Management

There are a number of theories to explain the relationship between stress and pain. Muscle tension resulting from stress has been implicated as a causal factor in physiological theories (23,53,79,86). Psychological theories emphasize cognitive processes such as feelings of control and attitudes toward pain that moderate pain perception (11,32,46). Secondary gains which result from pain behaviors may also influence the subjective pain experience (28,54).

Several authors have associated stress with back disorders (76,107). The Bureau of National Affairs (15) has also claimed a relationship between stress and accidents. Work dissatisfaction was related to reports of back problems in several studies (5,13,42). In one investigation, work satisfaction was the best predictor of outcome among demographic and health status variables in patients suffering from back pain (5).

Palliative stress reduction strategies modify the stress response but do not directly alter the stressor. In relaxation training, the person is taught deep breathing and directed concentration, which reduces muscle tension (7,10). Cognitive coping strategies are based on the premise that maladaptive or negative thoughts result in stress-related feelings and behaviors (6,25,68). Such techniques encourage a shift in perspective so that the individual may feel more in control or perceive the pain differently.

A robust literature attests to the effectiveness of relaxation and cognitive coping strategies in reducing chronic pain (11,26,44,74,92,99,100). However, few studies address the use of these techniques for the prevention and treatment of acute back disorders (58). Those that do, suggest that early education in stress management may forestall chronicity (29,45).

Active coping strategies focus on the effective management of the environment as a means of attenuating the degree and the nature of stressors. Strategies include time management, goal setting, problem solving, social skills training, and assertion training. There is insufficient literature linking these techniques to control of low back problems, but pain management programs that include active coping skills have found them to be a useful complement to palliative coping strategies (32,36).

Stress Management in the Workplace

Work site stress management programs are increasing in popularity (27) and there is some evidence that they are successful in decreasing accidents (94). Often, the worker is chosen as the target for intervention. Identifying the workplace as the intervention site is an alternative approach and may result in innovations such as incentive programs, support groups, and modified workplace design. Since the worker and the work environment form an interactive system, it may be advisable to include elements of both approaches (67,76,88).

After reviewing a number of work site stress reduction programs, Pelletier and Lutz (76) identified several ingredients for success: Participation should be limited to "high risk" individuals who are motivated to learn. Classes should introduce a variety of stress management techniques, take place in a 4 to 8 week period, be of approximately 45 minutes in duration, and include 12 to 14 participants. Follow-up should include the reinforcement of skills as well as a method of program evaluation.

Ergonomic Principles

The ergonomic approach to injury control seeks to reduce the effect of biomechanical stress by eliminating the source of the hazard. The Proposed National Strategies for the Prevention of Leading Work-Related Diseases and Injuries (4) conclude that the ergonomic approach to workplace redesign may be the first choice for controlling musculoskeletal problems, with employee selection and training secondary (4). It has been estimated that almost half of all lifting motions are constrained by the design of the workstation. Therefore, it is not surprising that little improvement has been realized by training without the benefit of ergonomic changes in layout and object design (17,24,34).

Ergonomics education programs include the following topics: work physiology, anthropometrics/biomechanics, noise, job design, work organization, lifting, communication, and personnel issues. They are most effective in directing the trainees' attention away from management issues toward biomechanics and physiology as possible explanations for productivity problems (82). However, since the worker has limited control over ergonomic changes, it is best to educate management in

ergonomics (82). In fact, one long-term benefit of an ergonomic education program has been the growing number of ergonomic modifications initiated in organizations.

Several reports specify a reduction in low back pain as a result of ergonomic changes (78,89). Following an ergonomic education and workplace modifications program, Westgaard and Aaras (106) reported three results: a significant reduction of musculoskeletal-related sick leave, a reduction in labor turnover, and an increase in worker productivity. Other studies have supported these findings (78).

It may be concluded that education and training in ergonomic principles is of value. This may be particularly true for industries which require heavy and repetitive work. Little is known, however, about the efficacy of teaching ergonomic principles directly to employees. It is also not yet known whether these efforts directly affect back injuries (82).

ISSUES IN BACK EDUCATION AND TRAINING

Motivation and Learning

One of the most challenging aspects of health education is student motivation. Even the best program will fail if students are not interested in learning. The following section reviews some of the factors shown to facilitate learning and motivation in health education.

One approach to ensuring a high level of motivation has been to offer programs on a voluntary basis, excluding those with no desire to learn. Indeed, in most cases this is intuitively logical. However, there are two problems with this approach: One is that a person may volunteer for reasons having little to do with learning, such as the opportunity to be a part of a group or to get additional free time from work.

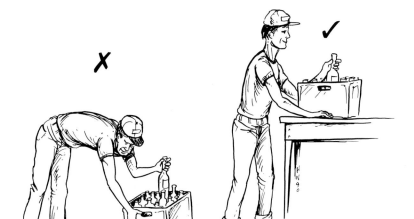

FIG. 4. Movements such as forward bending can be avoided by ergonomic workplace evaluations.

An additional problem is that voluntary programs may not attract those individuals who are most likely to benefit from education. Programs that identify at-risk individuals usually have a higher success rate than broadbased approaches (76). In addition, the likelihood of injury in certain jobs is so great that a mandatory training program may be justified. The advantages and disadvantages of a voluntary program must be considered with regard to these issues.

Regardless of the student's motivation level, certain principles of education and training have been shown to enhance learning. Students may learn best in group settings of 3 to 12 (80). Groups of this size permit the exchange of ideas and provide a supportive setting in which to learn. Patient education is also enhanced by the use of audio and visual aids (66,70) and the provision of relevant reading materials (66).

Programs that actively involve patients or students by emphasizing self-care and demonstrating treatments have been shown to be 1.5 to 3 times as successful as traditional education (80). Students are more likely to become involved in a topic that has relevance to them (109). The knowledge, beliefs, circumstances, and psychological status of the learner are important considerations in designing a program (69).

Studies have shown that patients' beliefs about their illness can differ substantially from those of health care providers (1,61). For example, one study showed that 50% of participants believed that their problem would become chronic (60). In addition, another investigation found that patients, even after being educated, gave anatomically incorrect descriptions of their back problem (1). The educator must be sensitive to erroneous beliefs and attempt to correct them before introducing new information.

Two crucial tools for keeping students motivated are frequent feedback on performance (62) and positive reinforcement. Reinforcement not only enhances the learning process but is shown to improve fine and gross motor skills (83), which are often required for back injury prevention.

Finally, health behaviors are deeply rooted and resistant to change. A successful education program must acknowledge the need for frequent and ongoing reinforcement. Principles of proper back care must be incorporated into lifestyle practices. Most current programs are of brief duration. Clearly, short-term education will not provide long-term solutions.

Program Content

Once the student is motivated to learn, another main issue in back education and training involves the transfer of information. Specifically, what information should be taught? In about 75% of all back injury cases, the cause of the problem is unknown. Therefore, most educators have used a trial and error approach to education, which reflects their basic beliefs about the etiology of back injury, as well as practical approaches to prevention.

Until more is known about how back pain develops, it is unlikely that one particular educational approach will be consistently effective. At this point, a multidisciplinary approach to back pain, particularly chronic pain, seems to be most reasonable, with one caveat. The importance of considering the individual characteristics and needs of the students cannot be underestimated. A successful educator will exercise sensitivity and flexibility in program content and emphasize the issues that are most appropriate to the students.

Furthermore, teaching methods are theoretically based and for the most part fail to emphasize the practical application of skills. The importance of practical information has been demonstrated in the success of functional restoration programs. Workplace intervention programs would be another example of this approach. More attention needs to be paid to translating information into the real life situation of the student.

Program Evaluation

Evaluations are a critical feature of any health education program and are done for several reasons. They allow the documentation of change, the justification of expense, and provide feedback about how to improve the program (40). Considering evaluation at the start-up phase of training also helps the instructor define course objectives.

Programs should be evaluated on parameters determined by program objectives. Outcomes are easier to assess when put in operational terms. Traditionally the goals of learning may be to increase understanding, change attitudes, change behavior, or reduce costs. Stated this way, it is unclear what quantifies a successful outcome. If, instead, the goal is to reduce absenteeism by, for example, 25%, the criteria for success can be clearly quantified.

Criteria for a successful program should be clearly decided on prior to the beginning of the course. Data can then be collected in such a way as to allow for before and after comparisons of these variables. It also helps to avoid post-hoc determinations of what defines a successful program.

Evaluation may be done using objective measures where certain behaviors or performances are quantified by observation. Subjective measures in a self-report format may also be used. Clearly, feelings and beliefs are more amenable to self-report, while knowledge and behavior are easier to observe. Since objective and subjective measures provide different information, it is best to use both (80).

Success criteria should, of course, be based on some meaningful quantity. The amount of change which makes the program worthwhile may be determined by a cost-benefit analysis. In general terms, costs may be quantified in terms of personnel, equipment, materials, and overhead. Benefits are considered the achievement of the course objectives. An education program may be considered successful when the benefits outweigh the costs.

A thorough discussion of program evaluation exceeds the scope of this chapter. A program evaluation done properly requires sophisticated knowledge and considerable skill. The reader is urged to consult reference material before undertaking an evaluation study (20).

SUMMARY AND CONCLUSIONS

Back education programs are an attempt to address the continuous rise in the prevalence and incidence of low back disorders. Back schools, training in manual materials handling, ergonomics, and stress management seem to be effective to a certain extent. Promising approaches such as functional restoration also depend heavily on education. To date, no one intervention provides a panacea.

The following points highlight the issues of importance to consider when developing a back education program: Educators should take a goal-oriented approach and, in light of the findings mentioned here, adopt realistic expectations for outcome. While a multidisciplinary approach to education is advisable, it is equally important to be flexible in terms of program content depending on the target population.

In industry, it is best to institute primary prevention programs to train the new employee. This way, the acquisition of poor working habits may be avoided. Ongoing prevention programs with frequent reinforcement must be implemented if a program is to succeed. Also, management must be educated about the importance of preventing and reducing the severity and recurrence of low back disorders.

Despite the paucity of conclusive findings in the area of back injury prevention education programs, it is too early to throw out the baby with the bathwater. As researchers and clinicians continue to elucidate the factors which result in a reduction in the severity and occurrence of back problems, better approaches to education and training will be developed.

The educational approach reflects a belief in the individual's ability to participate in his or her own health care and may be the strongest weapon we have in the battle against low back disorders. It may be concluded that, conceptually, back education represents a sound approach to the prevention and treatment of low back disorders. Future work should build upon existing attempts to translate these concepts into successful practical approaches.

ACKNOWLEDGMENTS

We are most grateful to Dr. M. L. Skovron and Dr. P. Brisson for their critical review of the manuscript. We also thank Joan Kahn for her time devoted to this project.

This project was supported by the HJD Research and Development Foundation.

REFERENCES

1. Adraschi C (1989): Personal communication.
2. Andersson G (1979): Low back pain in industry: Epidemiological aspects. *Scand J Rehabil Med* 11:163–168.
3. Andersson G, Ortengren R, Nachemson A (1976): Quantitative studies of back load in lifting. *Spine* 1:178–185.
4. Association of Schools of Public Health (ASPH) (1986): *Proposed national strategies for the prevention of leading work-related diseases and injuries,* Part 1, Washington D.C.: ASPH.
5. Battie M (1989): The reliability of physical factors as predictors of the occurrence of back pain reporters: A prospective study within industry. Doctoral dissertation, University of Gothenburg, Gothenburg, Sweden.
6. Beck A (1984): Cognitive approaches to stress. In: R Woolfolk, P Lehrer, eds. *Principles and practice of stress management.* New York: Guilford, pp. 255–305.
7. Benson H (1975): *The relaxation response.* New York: Avon.
8. Bergenudd H (1989): Talent occupation and locomotor discomfort. Thesis, Lund University, Malmo, Sweden.
9. Bergquist-Ullman M, Larsson U (1977): Acute low back pain in industry. *Acta Orthop Scand* (170):1–117.
10. Bernstein D, Given B (1984): Progressive relaxation: Abbreviated methods. In: R Woolfolk, P Lehrer, eds. *Principles and practice of stress management.* New York: Guilford, pp. 43–69.
11. Biedermann HJ, McGhie A, Monga TN, Shanks GL (1987): Perceived and actual control in EMG treatment of back pain. *Beh Res Therapy* 25:137–147.
12. Biering-Sorenson F (1984): Physical measurements as risk indicators for low-back trouble over a one-year period. *Spine* 9:106–119.
13. Bigos SJ, Spengler DM, Martin NA, Fisher L, Zeh J, Nachemson A (1986): Back injuries in industry: A retrospective study: II. Injury factors. *Spine* 11:246–251.
14. Bille D (1981): *Practical approaches to patient teaching.* Boston: Little, Brown.
15. Bureau of National Affairs (1984): *Personal policies forum survey* 132:3–11.
16. Cady LD, Bischoff DP, O'Connell ER, Thomas PC, Allen JH (1979): Letters to the editor: Authors' response. *J Occup Med* 21:720–725.
17. Chaffin D, Gallay LS, Woolley CB, Kuciemba SR (1986): An evaluation of the effect of a training program in worker lifting postures. *International Journal of Industrial Ergonomics* 1:127–136.
18. Chaffin DB, Park KS (1973): A longitudinal study of low-back pain as associated with occupational weight lifting factors. *American Industrial Hygiene Association Journal* 34:513–525.
19. Choler U, Larsson R, Nachemson A, Peterson LE (1985): Back pain: A trial of case management for patients with unspecific low back pain. Stockholm: SPRI Report 188 (in Swedish).
20. Cook T, Campbell D (1979): *Quasi-experimentation design and analysis issues for field setting.* Chicago: Rand McNally.
21. Dehlin O, Hedenrud B, Horal J (1976): Back symptoms in nursing aides in a geriatric hospital. *Scand J Rehab Med* 8:47–53.
22. Deyo RA, Tsui-Wu YJ (1987): Descriptive epidemiology of low-

back pain and its related medical care in the United States. *Spine* 12:264–268.

23. Dolce JJ, Raczynski JM (1985): Neuromuscular activity and electromyography in painful backs: Psychological and biomechanical models in assessment and treatment. *Psychological Bulletin* 97:502–520.

24. Drury CG (1985): Influence of restricted space on manual materials handling. *Ergonomics* 28:167–175.

25. Ellis A, Harper R (1975): *A new guide to rational living.* Los Angeles: Wilshire.

26. Fernandez E, Turk DC (1989): The utility of cognitive coping strategies for altering pain perception: A meta-analysis. *Pain* 38:123–135.

27. Fielding JE (1989). Work site stress management: National survey results. *J Occup Med* 31:990–995.

28. Fordyce WE (1988): Psychological factors in the failed back. *Int Disabil Stud* 10:29–31.

29. Fordyce WE, Brockway JA, Bergman JA, Spengler D (1986): Acute back pain: A control-group comparison of behavioral vs. traditional management methods. *J Behav Med* 9:127–140.

29a. Forssell MZ (1981): see ref. 110.

30. Frymoyer JW, Gordon S (1989): *New perspectives on low back pain.* Chicago: American Academy of Orthopaedic Surgeons.

31. Frymoyer JW, Pope MH, Clements JH, Wilder DG, MacPherson B, Askikaga T (1983). Risk factors in low back pain. *J Bone Joint Surg* [Am] 65:213–218.

32. Gottlieb H, Strite LC, Koller R, Madorsky A, Hockersmith V, Kleeman M, Wagner J (1977): Comprehensive rehabilitation of patients having chronic low back pain. *Arch Phys Med Rehab* 58:101–108.

33. Gyntelberg F (1974): One year incidence of low back pain among male residents of Copenhagen aged 40–59. *Danish Med Bull* 21:30–36.

34. Hale A, Mason I (1986): L'Evaluation du role d'urie formation kinetique dans la prevention des accidents de manutention. *Le Travail Humain* 49(3):195–208.

35. Hall H, Iceton JA (1983): Back school. An overview with specific reference to the Canadian Back Education Units. *Clin Orthop* (179):10–17.

36. Hazard RG, Fenwick JW, Kalisch SM, Redmond J, Reeves V, Reid S, Frymoyer J (1989). Functional restoration with behavioral support: A one-year prospective study of patients with chronic low-back pain. *Spine* 14:157–161.

37. Herrin GD, Jaraiedi M, Anderson CK (1986): Prediction of overexertion injuries using biomechanical and psychophysical models. *Am Ind Hyg Assoc J* 47:322–330.

38. Himmelstein JS, Andersson GB (1988): Low back pain: Risk evaluation and preplacement screening. *State Art Rev Occup Med* 3:255–269.

39. Holding D (1983): Fatigue. In: R Hockey, ed. *Stress and fatigue in human performance.* New York: John Wiley, pp. 145–165.

40. Holzemer W (1981): Evaluation of patient education programs. In: D Bille, ed. *Practical approaches to patient teaching.* Boston: Little, Brown, pp. 131–151.

41. Hultman G, Nordin M, Ortengren R (1984): The influence of a preventive educational program on trunk flexion in janitors. *Applied Ergonomics* 15:127–133.

42. Hurri H (1989): The Swedish back school in chronic low back pain II. *Scand J Rehab Med* 21:41–44.

43. Jensen R (1986): *Proceedings of the Human Factors Society, 30th Annual Meeting.* Santa Monica: The Human Factors Society.

44. Kabat-Zinn J, Lipworth L, Burney R (1985): The clinical use of mindfulness meditation for the self-regulation of chronic pain. *J Behav Med* 8:163–190.

45. Kamwendo K, Linton S (1986): Can pause-gymnastics prevent neck & shoulder pain. *Sjukgymnasten* 7:12–14.

46. Keefe FJ (1982): Behavioral assessment and treatment of chronic pain: Current status and future directions. *J Consult Clin Psychol* 50:896–911.

47. Kelsey JL (1975): An epidemiological study of acute herniated lumbar intervertebral discs. *Rheumatol Rehabil* 14:144–159.

48. Kelsey JL, Githens PB, O'Connor T, et al (1984): Acute prolapsed lumbar intervertebral disc: An epidemiologic study with special reference to driving automobiles and cigarette smoking. *Spine* 9:608–613.

49. Kelsey JL, Githens PB, White AA 3rd (1984): An epidemiologic study of lifting and twisting on the job and risk for acute prolapsed lumbar intervertebral disc. *J Orthop Res* 2:61–66.

50. Keyserling WM, Herrin GD, Chaffin DB, Armstrong TJ, and Foss ML (1980): Establishing an industrial strength testing program. *Am Ind Hyg Assoc J* 41:730–36.

51. Knowles J (1977): *Doing better and feeling worse: Health care in the United States.* New York: Norton, pp. 1–8.

52. Komaki J, Heinzmann AT, Lawson L (1980): The effect of training and feedback: Component analysis of a behavioral safety program. *J Applied Psychol* 65:261–270.

53. Kravitz E, Moore ME, Glaros A (1981): Paralumbar muscle activity in chronic low back pain. *Arch Phys Med Rehab* 62:172–176.

54. Kriegler JS, Ashenberg ZS (1987): Management of chronic low back pain: A comprehensive approach. *Semin Neurol* 7:303–312.

55. Lance BM, Chaffin DB (1971): The effect of prior muscle exertions on simple movements. *Human Factors* 13:355–361.

56. Lankhorst GJ, Van de Stadt RJ, Vogelaar TW, Van der Korst JK, Prevo AJH (1983): The effect of the Swedish Back School in chronic idiopathic low back pain. A prospective controlled study. *Scand J Rehab Med* 15:141–145.

57. Lindstrom I, Ohlund C, Eek C, Wallin L, Peterson L-E, Nachemson A (1989): Work return and low back pain disability: Results of a prospective randomized study in an industrial population [Abstract]. International Society for the Study of the Lumbar Spine (ISSLS), Kyoto, Japan.

58. Linton SJ (1987): Chronic pain: The case for prevention. *Beh Res Ther* 25:313–317.

59. Linton SJ, Kamwendo K (1987): Low back schools. A critical review. *Physical Therapy* 67:1375–1383.

60. Ljungberg P, Sanne H (1986): *Ryggbesvar.* Goteborg, Sweden: Statshalsan.

61. Lorig KR, Cox T, Cuevas Y, Kraines RG, Britton MC (1984): Converging and diverging beliefs about arthritis: Caucasian patients, Spanish speaking patients and physicians. *J Rheumatol* 11:76–79.

62. Marteniuk R (1986): Information processes in movement learning: Capacity and structural interference effects. *J Motor Behav* 18:55–75.

63. Mattmiller AW (1980): The California Back School. *Physiotherapy* 66:118–121.

64. Mayer TG, Gatchel RJ, Kishino N et al (1985): Objective assessment of spine function following industrial injury. A prospective study with comparison group and one-year follow-up. *Spine* 10:482–493.

65. McGill CM (1968): Industrial back problems: A control program. *J Occup Med* 10:174–178.

66. McKeachie W (1969): *Teaching tips: A guidebook for the beginning college teacher.* Lexington: D.C. Heath.

67. McLeroy K, Green L, Mullen K, Foshee V (1989): Can we reduce stress in American workers? A review of programs. *Advances* 6(1):16–19.

68. Meichenbaum D, Jarenko M (1983): *Stress reduction and prevention.* New York: Plenum.

69. Melvin J (1989): *Rheumatic diseases in adult and child: Occupational therapy and rehabilitation.* Philadelphia: Davis.

70. Moll JM (1986): Doctor-patient communication in rheumatology: Studies of visual and verbal perception using educational booklets and other graphic material. *Annals of the Rheumatic Diseases* 45:198–209.

71. Myers J, Riordan R, Mattmiller AW, Pelcher A, Levenson BS, White A (1981): Low back injury prevention at Southern Pacific Railroad: Five years experience with a back school model. International Society For The Study of The Lumbar Spine (ISSLS), Paris, France.

72. Nachemson A (1983): Work for all: For those with low back pain as well. *Clinical Orthop Rel Res* (179):77–85.

73. Nordin M, Frankel VH, Spengler DM (1981): A preventive back-care program for industry [Abstract]. International Society for the Study of the Lumbar Spine (ISSLS), Paris, France.

74. Ost LG (1987): Applied relaxation: Description of a coping technique and review of controlled studies. *Beh Res Therapy* 25:397–409.

75. Parnianpour M, Nordin M, Kahanovitz N, Frankel V (1988): The triaxial coupling of torque generation of trunk muscles dur-

ing isometric exertions and the effect of fatiguing isoinertial movements on the motor output and movement patterns. *Spine* 13:982–992.

76. Pelletier K, Lutz R (1989): Mindbody goes to work: A critical review of stress management programs in the workplace. *Advances* 6(1):28–34.

77. Peltier LF (1983): The "Back School" of Delpech in Montpellier. *Clinical Orthopaedics* (179):4–9.

78. Pope M (1987): Modification of work organization. *Ergonomics* 30(2):449–455.

79. Price JP, Clare MH, Ewerhardt FH (1948): Studies in low backache with persistent muscle spasm. *Arch Physical Med* 29:703–709.

80. Redmond BK (1988): *The process of patient education.* St. Louis: Mosby.

81. Riihimaki H (1985): Back pain and heavy physical work: A comparative study of concrete reinforcement workers and maintenance house painters. *Br J Industrial Med* 42:226–232.

82. Rohmert W, Laurig K (1977): Increasing awareness of ergonomics by in-company courses. A case study. *Applied Ergonomics* 8:19–21.

83. Rush D (1984): Peer behavior coaching soccer. *J Sport Psychol* 6:325–334.

84. Sandstrom J (1984): *Om Kroniska Landryggsbesvar.* Goteborg, Sweden: Goteborg Universitet.

85. Sandstrom J, Andersson GB, Wallerstedt S (1984): The role of alcohol abuse in working disability in patients with low back pain. *Scand J Rehab Med* 16:147–149.

86. Sargent M (1946): Psychosomatic backache. *New Engl J Med* 234:427–430.

87. Schultz A, Andersson GB, Ortengren R, Bjork R, Nordin M (1982): Analysis and quantitative myoelectric measurements of loads on the lumbar spine when holding weights in standing postures. *Spine* 7:390–397.

88. Seamonds B (1986): The concept and practice of stress management. In: S Wolf, ed. *Occupational stress.* Boston: PSG Publishing, pp. 153–163.

89. Simpson GC (1980): The economic justification for ergonomics. *Int'l J Ind Ergonomics* 2:157–163.

90. Snook SH, Campanelli RA, Hart JW (1978): A study of three preventive approaches to low back injury. *J Occup Med* 20:478–481.

91. Snook SH, White AH (1984): Education and training. In: MH Pope, JW Frymoyer, G Andersson, eds. *Occupational low back pain.* New York: Praeger, pp. 233–244.

92. Spinhoven P, Linssen AC (1989): Education and self-hypnosis in the management of low back pain: A component analysis. *Br J Clin Psychol* 28(pt 2):145–153.

93. [Spitzer WO, LeBlanc FE, DuPuis M] (1987): Scientific approach to the assessment and management of activity-related spinal disorders. Report of the Quebec Task Force on Spinal Disorders. *Spine* 12:S1–S59.

94. Steffy B, Jones J, Murphy L, Kunz L (1986): A demonstration of the impact of stress abatement programs on reducing employee's accidents and their costs. *Amer J Health Promotion* Fall:25–32.

95. Sternbach P (1978): *The psychology of pain.* New York: Raven.

96. Stubbs DA, Buckle PW, Hudson MP, Rivers PM, Worringham CJ (1983): Back pain in the nursing profession: I. Epidemiology and pilot methodology. *Ergonomics* 26(8):755–765.

97. Svensson HO, Andersson GB (1983): Low-back pain in forty to forty seven year old men: Work history and work environment factors. *Spine* 8:272–276.

98. Troup JDG, Foreman TK, Baster CE, Brown D (1987): The perception of back pain and the role of psychophysical tests of lifting capacity. *Spine* 12:645–657.

99. Turner JA (1982): Comparison of group progressive-relaxation training and cognitive-behavioral group therapy for chronic low back pain. *J Consulting Clin Psychol* 50:757–765.

100. Turner JA, Clancy S (1988): Comparison of operant behavioral and cognitive-behavioral group treatment for chronic low back pain. *J Consult Clin Psychol* 56:261–266.

101. Vallfors B (1985): Acute, subacute and chronic low back pain: Clinical symptoms, absenteeism and working environment. *Scand J Rehab Med* [Suppl] 11:1–98.

102. Versloot JM, Schilstra AJ, Tolen FJ, van Akkervehen PF (1988): Back school in industry, a prospective longitudinal controlled study (3 years) [Abstract]. International Society for the Study of the Lumbar Spine (ISSLS), Miami, Florida.

103. Videman T, Rauhala H, Asp S, Lindstrom K, Cedercruetz G, Kampoc M, Tola S, Troup JD (1989): Patient-handling skills, back injuries, and back pain. An intervention study in nursing. *Spine* 14:148–156.

104. Waddell G (1987): A new clinical model for treatment of low back pain. *Spine* 12:632–644.

105. Deleted.

106. Westgaard RH, Aaras A (1987): The effect of improved workplace design on the development of work related musculoskeletal illnesses. In: J Galer, ed. *Applied ergonomics handbook, 2nd ed.* London: Butterworths, pp. 185–196.

107. Wolf S (1986): Common and grave disorders identified with occupational stress. In: S Wolf, ed. *Occupational stress.* Boston: PSG Publishing, pp. 47–53.

108. Wood DJ (1987): Design and evaluation of a back injury prevention program within a geriatric hospital. *Spine* 12:77–82.

109. Woodruff A (1961): *Basic concepts of teaching.* Scranton: Chandler.

110. Forssell MZ (1981): The back school. *Spine* 6:104–106.

Congenital Abnormalities

The Adult Spine: Principles and Practice,
J. W. Frymoyer, Editor-in-Chief.
Raven Press, Ltd., New York © 1991.

CHAPTER 78

Classification, Non-Operative, and Operative Treatment of Spondylolisthesis

Leon J. Grobler and Leon L. Wiltse

Herbinaux (75), a Belgian obstetrician, noting a bony prominence of the sacrum that was obstructing labor, was probably the first person to recognize spondylolisthesis. The term spondylolisthesis was subsequently described by Kilian in 1854 (92) and is derived from the Greek words "spondylos" (meaning vertebra) and "olisthesis" (meaning to slip or slide). One year later,

L. J. Grobler, M.D.: Assistant Professor, Department of Orthopaedics, University of Vermont; Staff Orthopaedic Surgeon, Orthopaedics and Spinal Service, Medical Center Hospital of Vermont, Burlington, Vermont, 05405; Director of Surgical Services, Spine Institute of New England, Williston, Vermont, 05495.
L. L. Wiltse, M.D.: Clinical Professor, Department of Orthopaedic Surgery, University of California, Irvine, Irvine, California; Wiltse Spine Institute, Long Beach, California, 90806.

Robert (151) showed the lesion to be in the pars interarticularis, and Lambl (98) described spondylolysis as a defect of the pars interarticularis without vertebral slippage. Naugebauer (127) subsequently showed that forward displacement can occur by elongation of the pars interarticularis without an isthmic defect. Since that time, it has been recognized that spondylolisthesis constitutes a heterogeneous group of disorders that share the commonality of forward displacement of one vertebra on another.

CLASSIFICATION

The various classifications of spondylolisthesis have attempted to define specific lesions with respect to etiology and pathogenesis. None of these classifications includes retrolisthesis, which refers to a posterior translatory displacement of one vertebra on another, often accompanied by asymmetric posterior disc space collapse and facet subluxation. It is relevant to spondylolisthesis only because it is frequently seen at the level above the spondylolisthesis (Fig. 1). The term retrodisplacement is felt to be a more acceptable description than retrolisthesis, as "listhesis" refers to a downward or forward displacement. Laurent (100) suggested that it could be due to premature disc degeneration. Retrolisthesis (or retrodisplacement) occurred in 44% of L5-S1 spondylolisthesis cases reviewed by Henson (74).

Wiltse (214), Macnab (114), and Newman (129) individually attempted to create classifications, but later combined their concepts in what remains the most widely accepted classification (219) (Figs. 2A–2G):

Type I: Dysplastic spondylolisthesis
Type II: Isthmic spondylolisthesis
Type III: Degenerative spondylolisthesis
Type IV: Traumatic spondylolisthesis
Type V: Pathologic spondylolisthesis

Wiltse and Rothman (220) then suggested a common congenital component in the etiology of dysplastic and isthmic types of spondylolisthesis, and added to the original classification the post-surgical group.

Type I: Congenital or Dysplastic Spondylolisthesis. This subtype (Fig. 3A) is characterized by dysplasia of the upper sacrum and, more specifically, the facet joints. Wiltse and Rothman (220) conceptualized that this abnormality can lead to inability to resist shear stresses, and forward slippage follows. In some cases, increasing anterior shear abnormally stresses the pars interarticularis and leads to a thinned-out pars and eventually a pars stress fracture (115). The pars defect in these cases is a result of the slippage rather than the cause of it. However, in many cases the ring remains intact and, because it is intact, compresses the cauda equina rather soon. Eventually, the spinous process may come to rest on an S1 midline defect. This etiologic group most commonly starts in childhood and often presents with a listhetic crisis characterized by severe back pain, hamstring spasm, and possible neurological compromise.

Two subtypes are differentiated based on the predisposing congenital abnormality.

Subtype A. In this type (Fig. 3B), dysplastic articular processes are axially oriented, and there is often an accompanying spina bifida.

Subtype B. This type is characterized by articular processes that are sagittally oriented (Fig. 3C).

Type II: Isthmic Spondylolisthesis. Wiltse and Rothman (220) differentiate two subtypes.

Subtype A. Lytic type is due to a stress fracture of the pars interarticularis (Figs. 4A and 4B). It is uncertain if some patients have a congenitally weakened pars interarticularis (225). Clearly, some do not, and the lesion

arises de novo. O'Neill and Micheli (137) demonstrated healing of the pars defect in 90% of cases following a posterior intertransverse stabilization procedure only. Their findings support the theory that the lesion, being a stress fracture, if given enough time and adequate immobilization, will heal.

Subtype B. Here, the pars becomes elongated secondary to repeated cracking and healing of the stress fracture in the pars (Figs. 4C and 4D).

Type III: Degenerative Spondylolisthesis. This type (Fig. 2E) is due to long-standing intersegmental instability.

Type IV: Traumatic Spondylolisthesis. Wiltse and Rothman (220) emphasize that this lesion (Fig. 2F) is due to acute fractures in areas of the bony hook other than the pars interarticularis and is always due to major trauma.

Type V: Pathologic Spondylolisthesis. This lesion (Fig. 2G) is due to localized or generalized bone disease

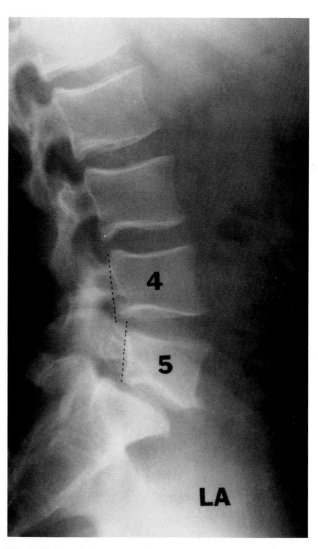

FIG. 1. Retrodisplacement above an L5-S1 spondylolisthesis in an adult patient presenting with low back pain.

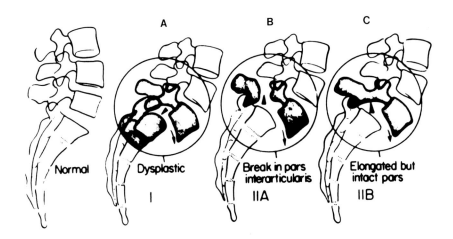

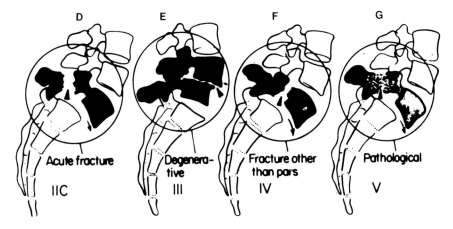

FIG. 2. The classification system proposed by Wiltse, Newman, & Macnab in 1976 (219) (Figure used with permission from ref. 22a).

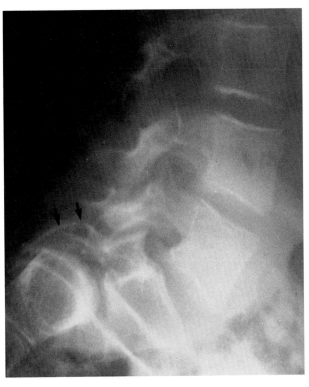

FIG. 3A: Congenital spondylolisthesis in a 14-year-old girl with an intact pars and hypoplastic superior sacral facet joint presenting with severe hamstring tightness. (Figs. 3B–3C follow.)

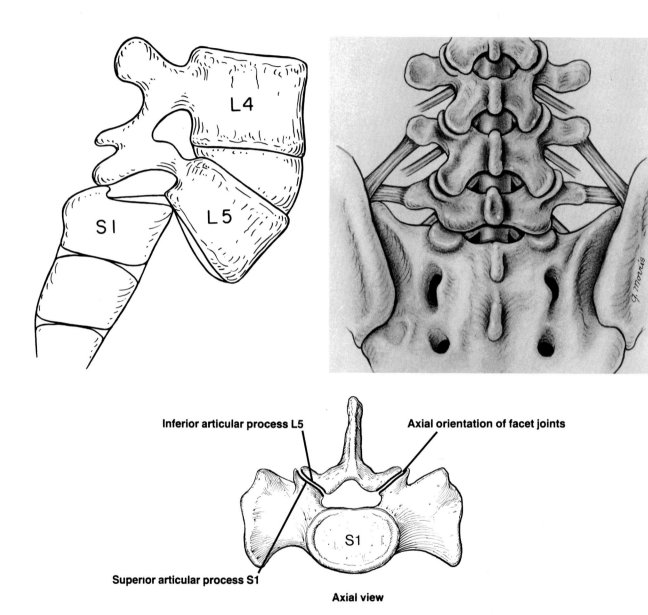

FIG. 3B: Clockwise from top left: lateral, posterior, and axial drawings showing the axial orientation of the facet joints.

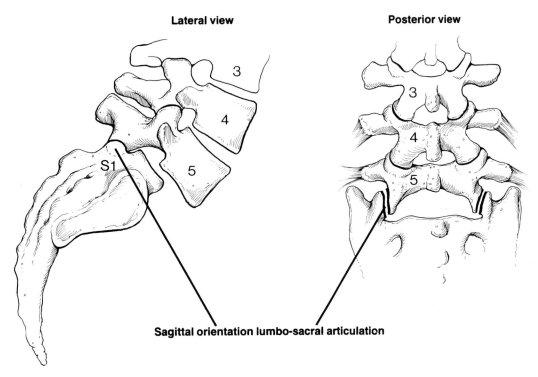

Lateral view

Posterior view

Sagittal orientation lumbo-sacral articulation

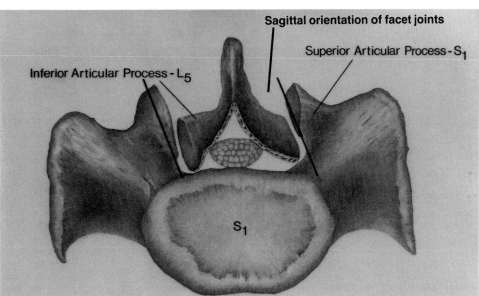

Sagittal orientation of facet joints

Superior Articular Process - S₁

Inferior Articular Process - L₅

S₁

FIG. 3C: Clockwise from top left: lateral, posterior, and axial drawings showing the sagittal orientation of the facet joints.

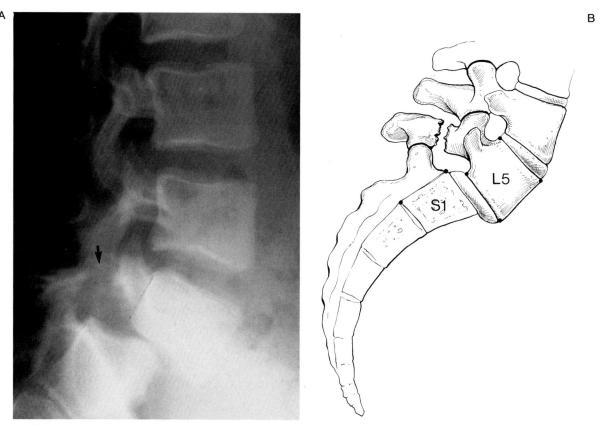

FIG. 4. A: Typical lytic isthmic spondylolisthesis (Subtype A) in a 16-year-old girl. **B:** Drawing outlines the pathology more clearly. (Figs. 4C–4D follow.)

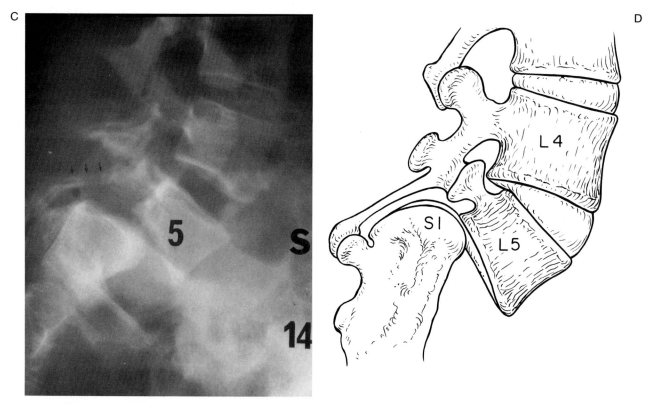

FIG. 4. *Continued* **C:** Intact but elongated pars in a 14-year-old girl with Grade III slip. **D:** Drawing illustrates the lesion.

and may present with an isthmic defect or elongated but intact pars.

Type VI: Post-Surgical Spondylolisthesis. This condition (102,210) is due to partial or complete loss of the posterior supporting structures and is secondary to a surgical procedure, ranging from overzealous decompression to post-surgical fracture of the neural arch.

Another classification has been proposed by Marchetti (116), who agrees with Wiltse (220) regarding a common congenital component in both the dysplastic and isthmic types, but suggests that the two subtypes are only different morphological expressions of the same etiologic process. He subsequently proposed the following classification based on etiological criteria only:

I. Developmental Spondylolisthesis. This category includes both congenital (dysplastic) and isthmic spondylolisthesis and consists of only two subgroups:
 A. Spondylolisthesis accompanied by lysis of the pars interarticularis.
 B. Spondylolisthesis accompanied by elongation of the pars interarticularis.
II. Acquired Spondylolisthesis
 A. Traumatic
  1. Acute fracture of the pars interarticularis: This type has a normal bony neural arch and follows sufficient and severe trauma such as a parachute injury (176), fall from height (181), or ejection from car (59). These injuries may affect other components of the neural arch, and the authors have never seen an isolated pars fracture, either unilateral or bilateral, without other parts of the vertebra being broken.
  2. Fatigue fracture of the pars interarticularis: Marchetti agrees with Wiltse (220) that repetitive stress at the isthmus can result in a stress fracture of the pars interarticularis in a patient with normal neural arch anatomy. Marchetti summarized his concept of traumatic spondylolisthesis as follows: "Either we are dealing with efficient trauma in a substantially normal bony structure and, therefore, to be included among acquired spondylolisthesis, or fractures in a congenitally dysplastic region, due to inefficient trauma under normal conditions, thereby classifiable under developmental types" (116).
 B. Iatrogenic
 C. Pathological
 D. Degenerative

Despite the evolving and controversial etiologic issues, we will use the Wiltse and Rothman classification. Our focus will be on the types of spondylolisthesis that commonly present in the adult. Because the clinical history and physical examination may not differentiate the various subtypes, radiologic criteria are most important. Before considering the clinical presentation and treatment, it is important to discuss the essential features of the radiographic evaluation, which form the basis for more of our current understanding of etiology, pathogenesis, prognosis, and an appropriate treatment regime.

RADIOGRAPHIC EVALUATION

Plain X-Rays

Large (14-inch × 17-inch) anteroposterior and lateral views are taken with the patient standing and should include the thoracolumbar and lumbosacral junctions. Midsagittal and spot lateral tomograms (Fig. 5A) are extremely helpful in outlining the bony contours so that accurate measurements can be made. If there is doubt, oblique views will show the pars sufficiently, especially if the tube is tilted slightly cranial to reduce the effects of the lumbar lordosis (Ferguson oblique view) (Figs. 5B and 5C).

Several x-ray measurements are made to determine the degree of slip. This is especially important in children with a progressing lesion, but rarely gives new information in the adult. Wiltse and Winter (223) published their guidelines for terminology and measurements in 1983, and with some modifications their approach is most widely used (Fig. 6). The essential information to be derived from these x-rays are:

1. Anterior displacement (slip, olisthesis, anterior translation) (Figs. 7A and 7B). Since Meyerding's classic description in 1932 (121), several methods have been described to measure the magnitude of forward displacement (21,117,120,128,195). Laurent and Einola (101) measured the anterior slip as a percentage of the width of the listhetic vertebral body. Although Lorenz and Bulo (108) found Meyerding's method the simplest and most reproducible, Taillard's method is most often used today (223). In this technique, the forward displacement of L5 is measured as a percentage of the maximum anteroposterior diameter of the first sacral vertebra. The method has a high inter- and intra-observer error, as reported by Danielson (33). Thus, consideration should also be given to the modified Boxall method, especially if research is being conducted (11). The amount of anterior displacement is expressed as a percentage obtained by dividing A by A'. It should be emphasized that it is not the absolute measurements but serial reproducible measurements by the same observer that are important and of clinical significance. Pizzutillo (146) also suggested using the so-called displacement index to evaluate displacement in cases in which landmarks are difficult to identify.
2. Sagittal rotation (slip angle) (Fig. 5A). This term describes the rotational relationship between the fifth

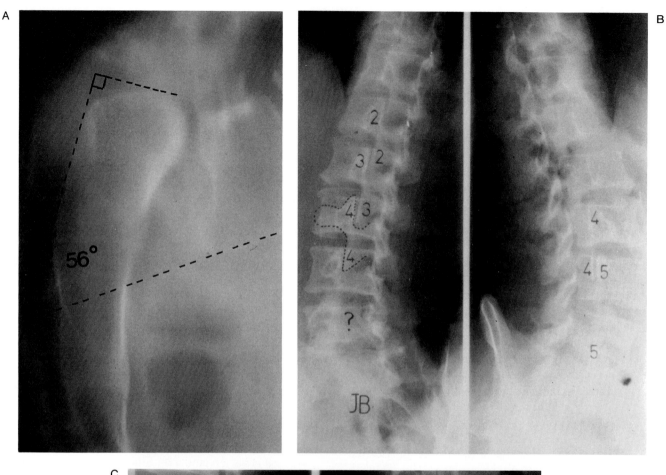

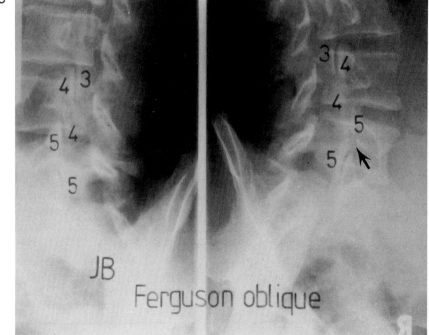

FIG. 5. Lateral tomogram **(A)** outlines bony landmarks for more accurate measurements. Standard oblique views **(B)** were unable to outline the L5 pars, but Ferguson oblique views **(C)** show pars defect clearly (see arrows).

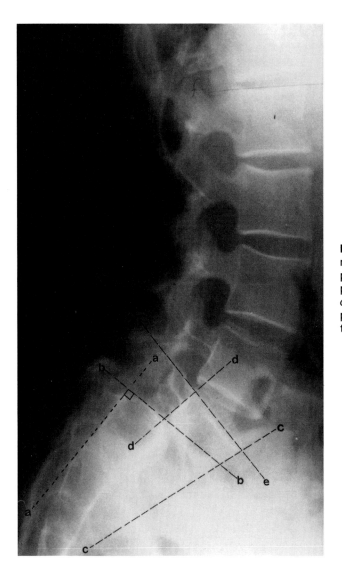

FIG. 6. The lines shown can be used to obtain and calculate measurements of clinical importance: *a-a:* Drawn along the posterior border of the first sacral vertebra. *b-b:* Drawn perpendicular to *a-a* intersecting upper border of the sacrum. *c-c:* Drawn parallel to the anterior border of L5. *d-d:* Drawn parallel to the posterior border of L5. *e-e:* Drawn parallel to the upper border of L5.

lumbar and first sacral vertebrae (sagittal rotation angle, or SRA). Because of frequent distortions of the upper sacral and lower fifth lumbar end plates, particularly on the congenital forms, measurements consist of the angle formed by intersection of a line along the posterior aspect of the body of S1 (a-a) and a line drawn along the anterior border of L5 (c-c). Several modifications can be used in selected cases (Figs. 8A–8C).

3. Sacro-horizontal angle (lumbosacral angle, Ferguson angle) (Fig. 9). The sacro-horizontal angle is the angle between a line drawn across the upper border of the first sacral vertebra and the horizontal. This measurement is more important in the young patient, but can be used to calculate the angle required to obtain an optimum angled anteroposterior view. Wiltse also used a modification of this angle in adults to decide what levels should be fused (220), as will be discussed later.

4. Lumbar lordosis and lumbosacral joint angle (Fig. 9). Lumbar lordosis is measured by calculating the curve formed by the intersection of lines drawn across the top of L1 and L5 (or S1), and measurement of the lumbosacral joint angle is shown. In the young patient with spondylolisthesis, increased lumbar lordosis is often found and is of secondary importance rather than etiologically significant.

5. Other measurements, including sacral inclination, the sacral horizontal angle, and the lumbosacral joint angle (Fig. 9).

Good quality supine oblique views are essential if spondylolysis is suspected but not proven. One must remember that up to 20% of pars defects may be unilateral (152,153,154,165). Oblique tomograms or 45-degree (can be varied from 20 degree-45 degree-60 degree; different degrees of obliquity often show defects better) oblique and 20-degree cranial tilt (Ferguson) views are important additional methods that can be used in difficult cases (Fig. 5C). Ferguson anteroposterior views (25 degrees caudocephalic) are essential to evaluate lumbosacral anomalies, including congenital anomalies (Figs.

A

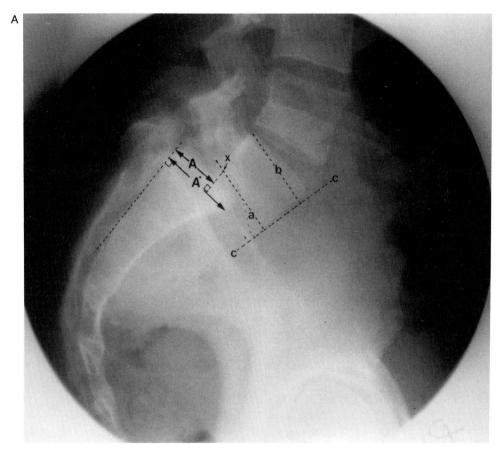

B

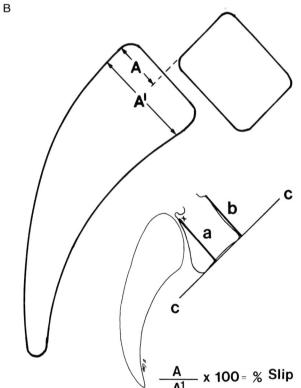

$$\frac{A}{A^1} \times 100 = \% \text{ Slip}$$

FIG. 7. A: Lateral x-ray (above) to calculate the percentage of slip by dividing A by A′. **B:** Determining the postero-inferior tip of L5 (marked x). Line b is drawn perpendicular to line a-c to the postero-superior tip of the body of L5. Line a is then drawn parallel to line b and is exactly the same length as line b. The point at which line a intersects the inferior border of L5 is point x, which is a constant in measuring percentage of slip.

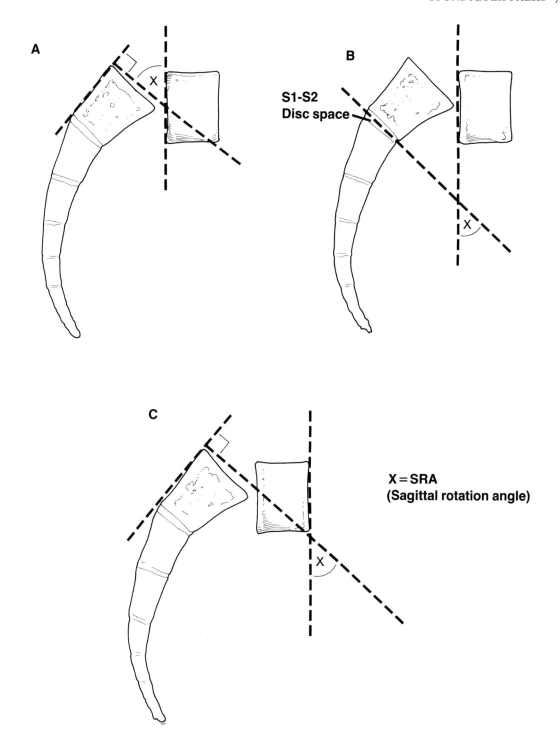

FIG. 8. Alternate methods **(A, B, and C)** to measure the slip angle (or SRA) if conventional landmarks are indistinct. Emphasis should be on serial and reproducible measurements.

10A and 10B), especially if accompanied by increased lumbosacral lordosis and in assessing the far out lateral syndrome (217). Supine flexion-extension views are used in evaluating both sagittal and translational mobility.

Radionuclide Scintigraphy (Technitium 99)

This technique is most sensitive for diagnosing suspected early stress fractures in the child and young athlete with relatively acute symptoms (25,139,144). A posi-

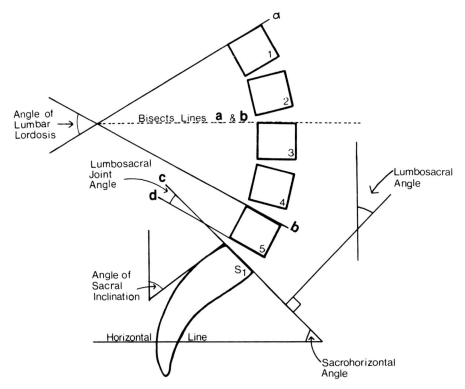

FIG. 9. Composite drawing showing the various angles in the normal lumbosacral spine (with permission from ref. 223).

tive scan is found in only 17% of patients with chronic pain who present with large and sclerotic pars defects (144). Thus, its usefulness is limited in patients with more chronic symptoms. Lowe (111), doing bone scintigraphy on military personnel with acute or a fairly recent history of low back pain and suspected fatigue fractures, found 43% had positive scintigrams. It was positive in only 13% with chronic low back pain, and none of the asymptomatic individuals had a positive scintigram.

An abnormal bone scan may be found in patients with an obvious unilateral defect on the contralateral side. This may be due to microfractures, reactive sclerosis (212), or healing of the original fracture accompanied by sclerotic stress changes in the contralateral pars due to incomplete healing or stress fractures (25,58,139,179, 191,193).

Bone scans are also extremely useful in athletes (112) who have had the diagnosis of stress fracture of the pars to evaluate healing and judge their return to high-level activities (82).

Computed Tomography

Not all patients with spondylolisthesis require additional imaging studies (65,161,162,196). Teplick found computed tomography to be more sensitive in the diagnosis of pars defects, especially in thin sclerotic lesions (196). Thus, CT may occasionally be useful in high-risk

athletes with negative bone scans and suspected fatigue fractures. Computed tomography can also be very helpful in diagnosing other causes of low back pain or in seeking the anatomical cause of radiculopathy in the adult with an established defect (118). It is essential that the CT sections be angled to cut as near as possible to right angles across the pars lesion. Computed tomography is often essential, and is the only method to differentiate congenital and isthmic spondylolisthesis in the adult.

Rothman feels strongly that by far the best way to determine spondylolisthesis (congenital or isthmic) is by CT evaluation. McAfee and Yuan found CT the most valuable method pre-operatively to visualize the "fibro-cartilaginous mass" often implicated in radiculopathies and its relation to the nerve root (118). To evaluate the possibility of foraminal impingement, para-sagittal reconstructions are also extremely useful (118). Nerve root infiltrations under CT guidance have also been found to be worthwhile in selected cases (90,91).

Magnetic Resonance Imaging

The primary finding on MRI (63,83,133) is the interruption of the cortical margins of the pars defect using sagittal images with short TR/TE or long TR/short TE pulse sequences (63). Grenier found MRI to be useful in patients with spondylolysis accompanied by spondylo-

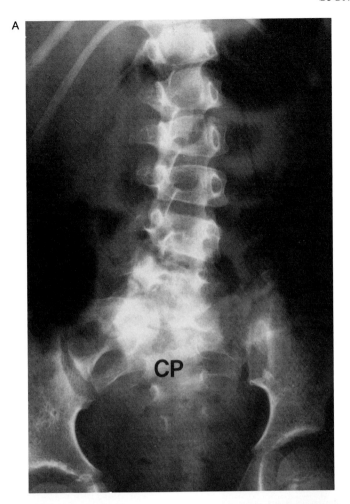

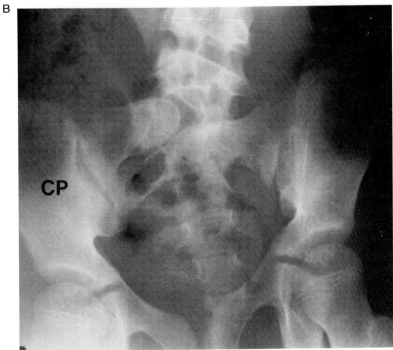

FIG. 10. Conventional **(A)** and cranial angled **(B)** view showing more detail of the lumbosacral junction.

listhesis. It was also useful in defining the causes of radiculopathy, including impingement of the nerve roots by the fibrocartilaginous tissue around the pars defect and foraminal stenosis, and exclusion of herniated nucleus pulposus at adjacent levels (161). One must appreciate that radiographic evidence of spondylolysis does not always reveal the true cause of the low back or leg pain, especially in the adult population.

CONGENITAL (DYSPLASTIC) SPONDYLOLISTHESIS

As already noted, this group is characterized by structural (congenital) anomalies of the lumbosacral junction (i.e., lowest lumbar vertebra and/or first sacral vertebra) and results in inadequate mechanical support to prevent forward slippage of L5.

Subtype A: Dysplastic Articular Processes in the Axial Plane

The axially oriented dysplastic articular processes may lead to the inability to resist forward thrust of L5 and spondylolisthesis may follow, frequently accompanied by spina bifida of the L5 and/or S1 lamina. The combination of axially oriented facet joints and spina bifida seems to predispose to spondylolisthesis. Due to the forward thrust of L5 on S1, the pars can elongate, come apart, or stay intact. If the pars interarticularis remains intact, neurologic symptoms usually occur only when the slippage exceeds 35% (224). If the pars elongates, it may be difficult to distinguish from Type IIB and axially oriented facets. CT scan studies will aid in differentiating these groups. If a pars defect occurs, it should be differentiated from Type IIA, although it will seldom change the treatment program. Zembo (225) reported on this condition occurring in facets, of which two were diagnosed at birth. It was found that the articular processes were horizontally oriented, resulting in a high-grade slip. Wynne-Davies and Scott (224) found that 11 of 12 patients with dysplastic spondylolisthesis had spina bifida occulta in the lumbosacral area. Dr. Wiltse feels that if a wide spina bifida of L5 or S1 is present, the olisthesis tends to appear earlier, slip is more severe, and is often accompanied by severe hamstring spasms. Fusion without decompression tends to improve back pain and/or neurological findings, including hamstring spasm.

Subtype B: Dysplastic Articular Processes in the Sagittal Plane

The sagittally oriented facet joints lead to forward slippage. This displacement can be accelerated by poorly developed posterior elements of L5 and/or S1. Because the neural arch is intact, high-grade slip seldom occurs, and the patients present with back and/or leg pain, hamstring spasm, and altered gait. In a few patients, Types IA and IB coexist.

Clinical Presentation

Dysplastic spondylolisthesis most often presents in the young child and adolescent, often as a listhetic crisis. When it presents in the adult, it is usually after the second decade. The treatment program is similar to that employed for the isthmic group and involves conservative treatment and, when necessary, decompression and/or stabilization. Usually when congenital spondylolisthesis presents in the adult, the deformity has an isthmic defect, but the radiologic characteristics of its congenital origin are present, e.g., hatchet-type vertebra and abnormally oriented facet joints L5-S1 detected only on CT scan evaluation.

The major types of spondylolisthesis presenting in the adult are isthmic and degenerative, which will form the major focus of the remainder of this section. For some strange reason, Type IB more commonly presents in adulthood.

ISTHMIC SPONDYLOLISTHESIS

The pars interarticularis is the connecting link between pedicle, transverse process, lamina, and the two articular facets acting as the pivotal center (Fig. 11A). The precise anatomic location of the pars lesion in relation to other anatomic structures is extremely important in understanding the pathogenesis, choosing the correct radiological diagnostic tests, and planning the appropriate surgical procedure.

The basic lesion consists of a stress or fatigue fracture of the pars interarticularis (5,103,222) and, therefore, forward slippage of L5 on S1 can occur with a normal relationship of the inferior lumbar to the superior sacral facets. As noted, two subtypes are identified and thought by some to be morphological expressions of the same disease (116,220).

Subtype A: Lytic Pars Defect

This subgroup (Figs. 11B and 11C) is described as a lytic lesion of the pars interarticularis following acute or repetitive fatigue stress (82). Severe trauma has been mentioned as a cause, but the most common mechanical cause is repetitive cyclic (flexion-extension) activity or a long-term repetitive positioning in lumbar lordosis (103) in a young athlete, accompanied by rotation. Hutton (79) found in vitro cyclic testing led to fatigue pars frac-

A

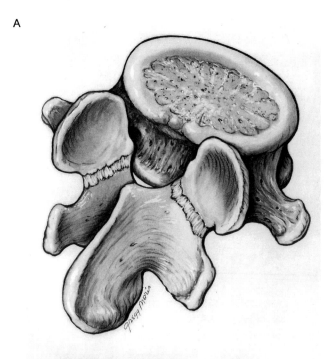

FIG. 11. Anatomical **(A)** and radiological **(B)** appearance of a lytic pars defect. Displacement **(C)** accompanied by normal relationship of facet joints.

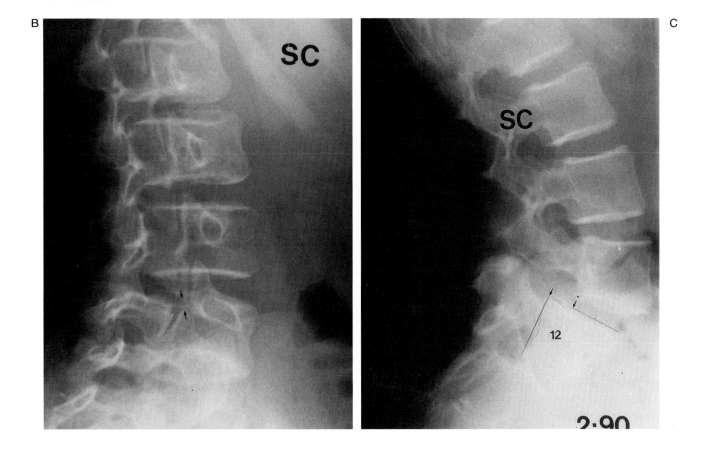

tures at relatively low cycles in the spinal column of a 14-year-old child subjected to these forms. The pars interarticularis is the pivot point where stress concentration is at its maximum, and Farfan (45) felt the possible mechanisms to be flexion overload, unbalanced shear forces, and forced flexion-extension. Both flexion (201) and/or extension (103,104,222) stress have been postulated as causative in the literature. Wiltse (213) found a distinct lesion of the pars interarticularis in an 8-month-old child. Borkow (9) described a case demonstrating a pars defect at age 4 months. Highest prevalence seems to occur at ages 5.5 to 7 years and during increased activity at ages 11 to 16. Wiltse postulates that children in the early age group already have the underlying predisposition (anatomical or dysplastic), and additional factors of increased activity at school and sitting for long periods in a lordotic posture set the stage for the lesion to occur. Occurrence is high in the adolescent and young adult, especially if involved in high-level sports activity relating to repetitive flexion/extension and rotation stress. Wiltse and Rothman (220) suggest that hypoplasia of the posterior arches of L5 and S1 predisposes to increased stress placed on the pars resulting in a stress fracture. This scenario may not be present in the young athlete. Letts emphasized the high incidence of stress fractures in high-level athletes and suggested that bone scans be done in the group that presented with back pain and no radiologically detectable isthmic lesion (103). A recent study by Wiltse and Rothman (220) also showed typical stress fractures in 6 young athletes who had previous radiographs showing normal bony anatomy, proving unquestionably that the etiology was a stress fracture. A high incidence of spina bifida was also found and correlates with previous reports on the isthmic group.

Subtype B: Elongation of the Pars Interarticularis

Elongation of the pars interarticularis can occur due to single or multiple healed stress fractures (Fig. 4C) that result in stretching of the pars interarticularis during the healing process. We agree with Marchetti that both subtypes represent the same basic etiologic mechanism.

The concept of a congenital component in the etiology of both the dysplastic and isthmic types was raised after CT scans showed hypoplasia of the superior articular processes of S1 occurring in some patients with both the isthmic and congenital groups (162). Congenital defects such as sacral spina bifida and hypoplasia of posterior sacral development were found in 94% of dysplastic and 32% of isthmic spondylolistheses (224). The hypoplasia of the facet joints could, therefore, be the underlying cause for slippage with initial intactness but eventual elongation, with resultant fracture of the pars found in the dysplastic type, or the stress or fatigue fracture of the pars in the isthmic type. In the latter situation, hypopla-

sia of the facet joints may lead to caudal displacement of the fulcrum of vertebral rotation, increased length of the lever arm, and resultant stress or fatigue fracture of the pars interarticularis. This compromises the posterior structures (by forward slippage with or without a pars defect), which resist the shear stress of the normal upright posture, and results in stress transferred to the intervertebral discs, leading to increased slip. Additional credence for a genetic causation is the familial incidence, which ranges from 27% to 69% (177,224), with the dysplastic form being more prevalent amongst first-degree relatives (33%). The familial incidence was found to be 40% in first-degree relatives over the age of 10 years (224).

Clinical Presentation

Prevalence. Isthmic spondylolisthesis occurs in the lumbar spine at the L5-S1 level in 82.1% of cases, L4-L5 level in 11.3%, L3-L4 level in 0.5%, L2-L3 level in 0.3%, and at other levels in 5.8% (153).

There seems to be a definite sex and racial difference, with black women (1.1%) having the lowest prevalence and white men (6.4%) the highest (73). Several reports state the increased prevalence of spondylolysis in certain population groups, e.g., Eskimos (185) and young sportsmen, ranging from 11% to 35% (160). The highest prevalence (36%) is found in weight lifters, and Rossi (160) found 50% of the Italian Olympic gymnastics team to have spondylolysis. Others at risk include college linemen in football (175), gymnasts (61,82,160), judoists (164,206), new army recruits (82,104), weight lifters (104), javelin throwers (160), pole vaulters (160), adolescents with thoracolumbar osteochondrosis (160), and loggers (104). Repetitive flexion (30), combined flexion-extension (48,97) and both forcible hyperextension and/or rotation (28) of the lumbar spine predispose the athlete to a pars stress fracture. Pars defects in gymnasts range widely, dependent on whether spondylolysis and/or spondylolisthesis is reviewed. The mechanism(s) could be explained by repetitive extension and/or rotation. It seems that by locking the L5-S1 facet joint in extension, rotational forces are directly transmitted to the pars interarticularis (Fig. 12). Fifty-one percent of O'Neill's (137) group relate their symptoms to competitive sports. An association is also found with idiopathic scoliosis, although the prevalence of 6.2% (51) is only minimally greater than in the population as a whole. This lesion seems to occur only in people with upright posture; no defects have been found in neuromuscular non-ambulators (157), but athetoid non-ambulating patients do have the defect with a greater prevalence of 9.8%, possibly due to a repetitive twisting motion. The defect is rare in animals, again indicating the importance of the upright posture (72,153).

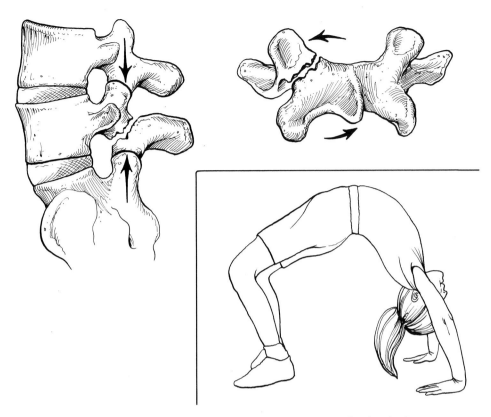

FIG. 12. Repetitive extension and rotation as a possible mechanism in the gymnast.

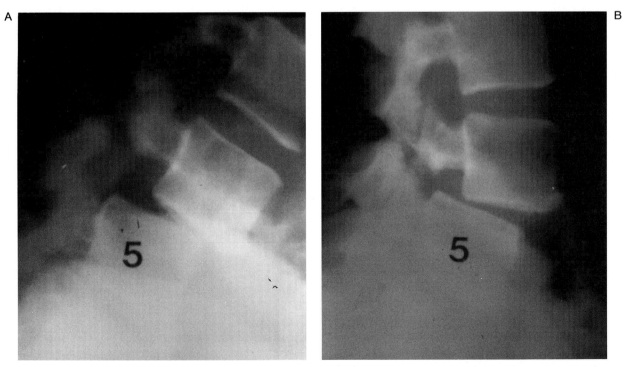

FIG. 13. Increased axial rotation on flexion **(A)** and extension **(B)** views indicating segmental instability.

Natural History

Wertzberger (209) emphasized the possible etiological factors that predispose to the progression of the slip. Although some authors feel that increased lordosis has etiologic significance, Sarasta (165) found that it was not a bad prognostic sign for further slippage. Few cases are reported before 5 years of age (163); most develop during the first year of school, and by age 7 the prevalence is 4% (54). A further 1.4% occur during adolescence, most appearing between 11 and 15 years (215). A few new cases even appear in early adulthood. Although the young patient is at risk for further slip, significant increase of slippage after adulthood is uncommon enough to be ignored as a clinical problem.

Marchetti (116) emphasized that the static forces that normally prevent slippage include the intervertebral disc, posterior ligamentous structures (i.e., anterior and posterior longitudinal ligamentous complex), the ilio-transverse ligaments, and the bony neural arch. Muscular action by reducing the lumbar lordosis (e.g., gluteals, hamstrings, and abdominals) may also play an important role. Degenerative changes in the adult tend to stabilize the spondylolytic process and do not seem to predispose to progressive slippage except in the degenerative form. More detailed discussions on spondylolisthesis in children and the risks for progression are discussed in Chapter 91.

In contrast to the L5-S1 isthmic lesion, there are indications that an isthmic lesion at the L4-L5 level may continue to be unstable in the third or fourth decade (Figs. 13A and 13B). This may be manifested by progressive slippage and increased symptoms (64), often necessitating surgical stabilization. The crucial role may be the stability given by the ilio-transverse ligament at the L5-S1 level and is presently being examined in our biomechanical laboratories.

PAIN IN SPONDYLOLISTHESIS

It seems appropriate to quote Ian Macnab's impression of the problem of low back pain as related to spondylolisthesis (115):

> The diagnosis is usually obscure or cannot be proven. Treatment perforce is empirical, and the results of treatment, in many instances, are unrewarding. Therefore, the demonstration on x-ray of a gross abnormality of this type is generally greeted with a sigh of relief: Here is a recognizable cause of backache; here is an easily understood and treated lesion. However, a word of caution must be interjected. Severe degrees of slip may be present in patients who engage in very vigorous activities and yet never suffer from backache.

Causes of Pain

Wiltse in 1976, and more recently Szypryt (194), observed (using MRI techniques) that in spondylolisthesis patients under age 25, the incidence of disc degeneration was equal to that in a control population, but in patients over 25 years, a statistically higher incidence of degeneration was found. The incidence of degeneration in the age group 25 to 45 years was found to be 70% (statistically significant). Farfan (45) stressed the role of torsion and shear forces on disc degeneration, and these stresses may well be accentuated in spondylolisthesis, resulting in accelerated degeneration. He also observed increased degenerative changes in the disc above the defect (Fig. 14A). We believe that the disc as the source of the pain can be evaluated by discography (Fig. 14B). Discography has been controversial (77), but more recent work by Weinstein (208) has clearly outlined the importance of this as a diagnostic test to exclude other causes for pain.

Macnab (115) reviewed patients who presented to his clinic with low back pain and found the prevalence of pars defect to be 7.6%, which does not differ substantially from the general population. Breakdown of these figures into three age groups revealed a higher prevalence in young people. These findings indicate that in patients under 25 years presenting with low back pain and radiologically proven isthmic spondylolisthesis, this lesion is most probably the cause of the symptoms (18.9%). Between 26 and 40 years, spondylolisthesis is often the cause of pain (7.6%), while over 40 years it is seldom the only cause of low back pain (5.2%). Disc degeneration in the adult is $2\frac{1}{2}$ times more common (69). Haraldsson and Willner (69) also found radiating pain to be present more often in the adult population (57% compared to 14%).

For example, Torgerson (198) found that 4.9% and Wiltse (222) found that 5% of low back pain patients had a demonstrable pars defect. Colonna (27) reported that over a 10-year period, in patients presenting with low back pain, only 50% of patients presenting a radiological pars defect had this as the cause of their symptoms (4,27,141). These symptomatic patients usually presented with low back pain following trauma, heavy lifting, and sudden rotation movements.

Therefore, it remains an enigma why symptoms so often develop only during adulthood if the lesion has most probably been present for many years. The precipitating factor in pain presentation trauma varies, and radiographs seldom show changes if compared to pre-injury films. Pre-employment radiographs, although controversial, give little new information, but legally may be very important to an employer. Work absence due to low back pain has been reported in 54% of adult patients with proven spondylolisthesis; 16% reported at least one month work loss each year (166).

In heavy laborers (2,119), the risk for low back pain is not increased if slippage is less than 10%, and there are no definitive studies regarding the 10% to 25% range. Above 25% slippage, the likelihood of low back pain has been found to be higher than in the general population and was also accompanied by earlier radiographic evidence of disc degeneration (165). However, no signifi-

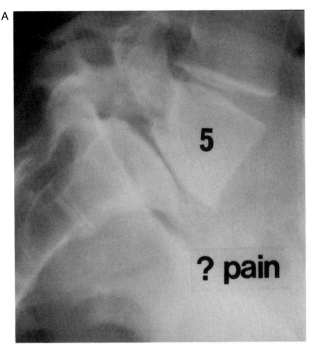 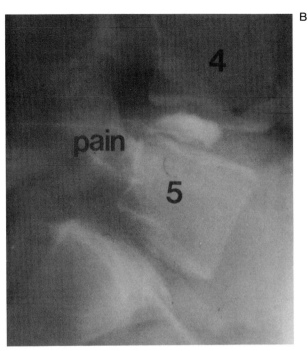

FIG. 14. The source of pain becomes a dilemma **(A)** in a case with two-level pathology and necessitates extreme care to make the correct decision. Despite the more obvious abnormality at the L5-S1 level **(B)**, discography reproduced this patient's pain at the L4-L5 level.

cant correlations exist between the severity of the symptoms and radiological findings (of disc space narrowing) in the adult. Severe radiological changes may accompany minimal symptoms, and minimal changes may be accompanied by severe pain complaints. It should be emphasized that there are clear differences in symptoms, radiographic findings, and results between young patients and adults (169). (Part of this dilemma is the lack of a basic understanding of the cause of pain.)

The pars, per se, has not been shown to be a pain-sensitive structure, and the mere existence of a lesion does not necessarily qualify it as the cause of symptoms. Wiltse (216) felt the cause of pain in spondylolisthesis to be (a) degeneration of a disc at the level of or adjacent to the pars defect, (b) nerve root impingement by fibrocartilaginous means, or (c) ligament tension due to loss of bony support. This observation emphasizes that spondylolysis should always be viewed as an incidental finding until proven otherwise, especially after the age of 40. However, symptomatic relief may temporarily follow local lidocaine injection, but why this occurs is uncertain. Other causes have, therefore, been sought.

Instability

Pearcy (140) found no instability at the level of the pars defect in undisplaced adult lesions, but Lowe (112) did find increased axial motion in Grade III and IV le-

sions, possibly due to weakening of the ligaments and discs. As already noted, progressive slip is rare in the adult, with the exception of L4-L5 lesions, which may represent an unstable lesion.

Other Causes of Pain

Macnab has noted that in the older adult, the disc at the level proximal to the spondylolisthesis may be the cause of pain rather than the pars defect itself. Macnab (115) advocated doing discograms at the level proximal to the slip in order to help determine whether the disc was a source of pain prior to fusion. Following radiological diagnosis of spondylolisthesis, the possibility of other extraspinal causes for back pain should be considered and excluded. The prevalence of Scheuermann's disease is higher in this population group, and the resultant hyperlordosis secondary to increased thoracolumbar kyphosis can be the cause of low back pain (135).

Radicular Pain

As noted, true radicular pain is found in 14% of patients with isthmic spondylolisthesis and its causation is more certain than low back pain. The radiculopathy may be caused by (a) disc prolapse that occurs above or below the pars defect or at the pars defect, (b) a fibrocartilaginous mass at the site of the pars defect, (c) stretching of the nerve, or (d) "far-out lateral syndrome" or other causes for peripheral neuritis (e.g., diabetes).

An extruded disc at the same level is relatively rare and was reported by Wiltse (218) in only 2 out of 50 cases; Briggs (17) found it in 1 out of 25 cases. A disc protrusion at an adjoining level is found more commonly and will obviously influence the treatment program.

The fibrocartilaginous mass formed at the proximal end of the pars defect can irritate and/or compress the L5 nerve root as it traverses around the L5 pedicle. The surgical technique employed in releasing this pressure is important and will be discussed in detail later. The S1 nerve root tends to be involved only if the slippage of L5 approaches 50% and is then due to impingement of the nerve between the distal end of the proximal stump and the body of S1.

Stretching of the nerve root as the proximal vertebra moves forward and pressure of the so-called corpotransverse ligament (115,199) has also been mentioned as a cause for radicular symptoms.

PRINCIPLES OF TREATMENT

Patient Education

Explaining the pathophysiology of the lesion to the patient in easily understandable terms will eliminate much of the anxiety and unknown factors, facilitate rational treatment, and improve the compliance to treatment goals. The goal in treating the adult patient, in contrast to the child, is pain control, not prevention of progression (12,216). This goal is most easily met in a patient with low-grade spondylolisthesis with mild symptoms. Work-related injuries often create additional anxiety and confusion for the patient, employer, and legal advisors. Realizing that spondylolisthesis is often a pre-existing lesion can facilitate early return to work and prevent chronic pain syndromes. Preventive measures to minimize twisting and rotational motions and emphasize posture and correct body mechanics in the workplace are important in general, as well as in the symptomatic patient. However, pre-employment x-rays are not a very useful strategy for primary prevention and were found not cost- or risk/benefit-effective. In France, pre-employment lumbar x-rays are obligatory for teachers of sports and physical activities (28).

Conservative Management

Exercise Program

Sinaki and Luttness (186) compared flexion and extension regimes in 48 patients with spondylolisthesis or Grade I isthmic spondylolisthesis followed over a 3-year period and reported better results using a flexion regime consisting of abdominal strengthening (isometric or isotonic), pelvic tilt, and chest-to-thigh exercises. Those results based on pain control, return to work, and recovery are summarized in Table 1. It is suggested that increased lumbar lordosis, which accompanies extension exercises, may lead to excessive stress on the pars, causing pain. The postural variation is also implicated as a causative factor in spondylolisthesis. By decreasing the lordotic posture, shear stress is thought by some to be minimized and lead to improvement in symptoms (50,62,80,82,157,222).

Bracing

Steiner and Micheli (190) described the use of the modified Boston brace in patients with symptomatic spondylolysis and spondylolisthesis (Grade I slip and less). They found 78% good or excellent results after a follow-up of 2.5 years. Braces were worn full time for 6 months, and activities consisted of a flexion exercise program and daily activities (including sports) within limits of pain. A distinct correlation was made between early brace treatment and osseous healing of a proven acute pars defect using clinical, radiological, and bone scan criteria. Age, delay in treatment, spina bifida, and activity on bone scan did not correlate with eventual results.

Other conservative modalities include bed rest, symptomatic medication, traction, manipulation, epidural injections, and facet joint infiltration, but none of these have been evaluated rigorously.

TABLE 1. *Data comparing results in flexion and extension exercise regimes in non-surgical treatment of spondylolisthesis*

Follow-up	Pain control		Return to work		Recovery*	
	FR	ER	FR	ER	FR	ER
3 months	73%	33%	68%	39%	58%	6%
3 years	81%	33%	76%	30%	62%	0%

FR = Flexion routine.
ER = Extension routine.
* Recovery based on rare episodes of mild pain, ability to perform normal job, and ability to perform leisure activities without restriction and not using brace.

Surgical Treatment

General

When pain becomes intractable, despite adequate conservative treatment for no less than 3 to 4 months, a surgical option should be considered. The pain at this time will usually influence the patient's quality of life, including work, sports, and other activities. However, as noted by Hanley in Chapter 91, a compensable cause for pain in patients with spondylolisthesis generally has a poor surgical outcome, and other non-operative options should be considered.

In a child with high-grade slip (beyond 50%) and below 10 years of age, surgery should be done if there is pain and any progressive slip. Surgery in a very young child should be resorted to with less delay than in an adult. Progressive slippage rarely occurs in the adult and, as already noted, isthmic spondylolisthesis is almost always a stable lesion, except at the L4-L5 level (64).

Neurological deficits, if present, often constitute a more certain surgical indication, depending on the extent of the nerve root compression, which as noted usually affects the L5 nerve root, secondary to the fibrocartilaginous mass, disc herniation, or foraminal stenosis.

How often conservative care fails and surgery is required is uncertain, although Monticelli found that in 15% of his cases conservative treatment failed and surgical treatment was needed (123). In preparing for an operation, a careful imaging evaluation should be done to clarify the causation of pain, including CT scan and/or MRI. As noted, we believe discography is an important adjunct.

Levels To Be Fused

After deciding that stabilization of the segment is indicated, an important question to be answered is how many levels need to be included. In the child and young adult, fusion of the L5-S1 unit is usually adequate, but in the adult population, the higher incidence of degenerative disc and facet disease at adjacent levels makes this decision more difficult.

We believe stabilization should include the L4-L5 level if that level is abnormal (concordant pain and disc degeneration) on discography, the L3-L4 level being normal. If both L4-L5 and L3-L4 levels are found to be abnormal, we would prefer to stabilize only the L5-S1 level. Wiltse proposed that inclusion of L4 should also be based on the degree of sagittal rotation of L5 on S1 (220). He suggested that if the "new" sacro-horizontal angle is less than 55 degrees, only the L5-S1 level be stabilized, and if it is more than 55 degrees, L4-L5 should also be included (provided the L3-L4 level is normal on discog-

raphy). Recent studies comparing results obtained by discography and MRI found high correlation (106). Hanley (68) suggested that L4-S1 fusion be done on all moderate (Grades I-II) spondylolisthesis cases, but we feel that more clinical data are needed to support this conclusion. We have not seen problems at the L4-L5 level after only L5-S1 fusion over a 10- to 15-year follow-up period.

Treatment Modalities

Posterior and Posterolateral Fusions: Grades I and II

There seems to be consensus of opinion that a one-level in situ fusion is the procedure of choice in Grades I and II symptomatic spondylolisthesis if the adjoining disc is found to be normal on discography (or MRI). We prefer to use the paraspinal approach (221) and posterolateral intertransverse and facet fusion (207) in all cases. Isometric exercises are started as soon as possible, and instructions are given regarding body mechanics. Accompanying decompression of the neural structures is done when indicated and will be discussed later. To summarize, we prefer not to automatically include the L4-L5 level, but to extend the fusion to L4 only if degenerative disc disease is found at the L4-L5 level on discography (L3-L4 must be normal), hypoplastic posterior elements (e.g., small transverse processes) are present, and the superior border of L5 is more than 55 degrees with the horizontal.

Results with in situ fusions vary from 94% union for one level to 84% for two-level fusions for this condition (216). Hanley (68) reported a non-union rate of 12% and excellent or good results in 60%. He also reported statistically significant unsatisfactory outcomes in males, those aged 30 to 50, smokers, cases in which pseudarthrosis developed, compensation cases, and patients who underwent a decompression for leg pain at the same time. Savini (168) reviewed posterolateral fusions in 20 patients and reported a fusion rate of 91.5% and good clinical results in 68%, showing a direct relationship between bony fusion and clinical outcome. Johnson et al. (85) reported an 80% likelihood of a good result with fusion in the presence of low back pain only. Haraldsson and Willner reviewed 45 patients after posterolateral in situ fusions by the same surgeon, finding indications for surgery in the younger group to be instability and in the adult to be nerve root compression and/or disc degeneration (69). In the group less than 20 years of age, 21 of 22 (95%) were completely free from symptoms, compared to 47 of 83 (57%) adult cases. The radiological fusion rate for both groups was 100% (69).

Kaneda (88) reported a 90.6% fusion rate in 53 patients using distraction instrumentation, but advised against using this method in greater than Grade II displacement because an increased slip angle was produced. Other methods of fixation include close loop sublaminar

A

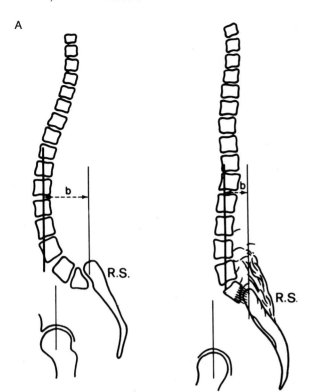

FIG. 15. A: Drawing shows improvement in the point of equilibrium after reduction and circumferential fusion in one of Savini's patients (with permission from ref. 3). **B:** A 12-year-old girl, presenting severe back pain and radicular symptoms necessitating a two-stage procedure consisting of posterior decompression-fusion and anterior strut grafting from L4 to S1. Note the improvement of the point of equilibrium. **C:** Excellent clinical and radiologic post-operative sagittal alignment.

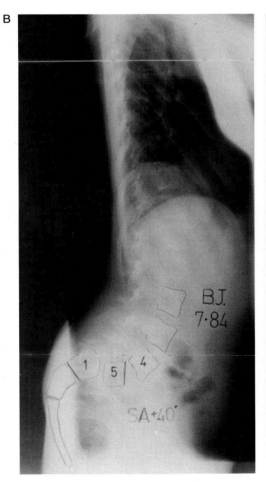

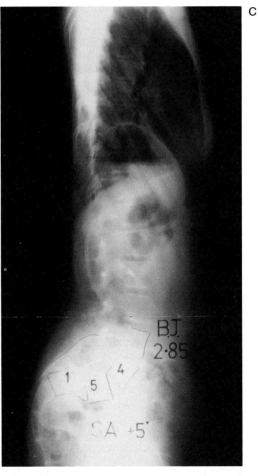

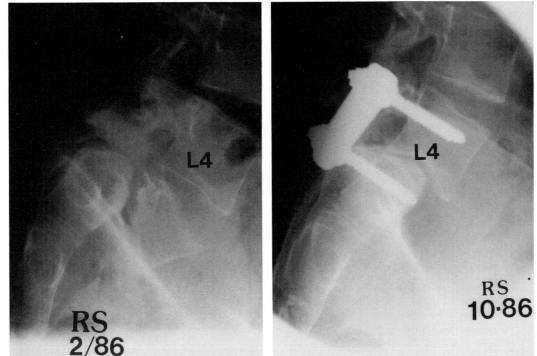

FIG. 16. Pre-operative **(A)** and post-operative **(B)** lateral x-rays of Grade V with spondylolisthesis after L5 vertebrectomy and restoration of sagittal contour (with permission from ref. 56).

fixation (53), Zielke apparatus (184), AO fixator (44), and numerous pedicular fixation devices, which are discussed in Chapter 92.

Posterior and Posterolateral Fusions: Grades III, IV, and V

Several studies are available on the surgical treatment for Grade III and IV spondylolisthesis in the adolescent, ranging from posterior fusion in situ (10,71,84,131, 143,172,187) to attempts at reduction using internal fixation devices (6,13,34,35,39,70,81,110,122,134,136, 169,171,182,188,189,226).

These procedures are extremely challenging and may lead to a high rate of complications (13,34,200). Although Schoenecker (170) reports neurodeficits in patients (all less than 18 years old) undergoing fusion in situ, most authors now agree that the indication for reduction of this deformity in the adult population is extremely rare, if not non-existent.

Reduction of severe spondylolisthesis is extremely controversial, and Ascani (3) attempted to predict the feasibility of reduction on biomechanical principles. He emphasized that in obtaining a reduction, an attempt should be made to restore the point of equilibrium (Figs. 15A–15C). Seitsalo (172) found that an increased lumbosacral kyphosis and subsequent compensatory hyperlordosis often led to increased back pain, even outside

the segment stabilized, and also noted increased S1 joint arthrosis. Gaines (56) suggests that for spondyloptosis (Grade V), spondylectomy in his experience is the procedure of choice (Fig. 16).

In some adult patients presenting with severe grade slips, the symptoms of back pain can be controlled by non-surgical methods. The patient with low-grade symptoms is treated conservatively and advised to restrict high-level performances, especially those requiring excessive lordosis (36). Harris and Weinstein (71) reported on 11 patients followed for an average of 17.8 years (range from 10 to 24 years) treated non-operatively and found that 55% had only mild symptoms and only one patient had to make significant changes in his life-style (work and recreational). For comparison, they studied 18 patients who underwent posterior surgical stabilization in situ with an average 23.6-year follow-up (range from 4 to 45 years) and found that 76% of the post-surgical cases had improved symptoms. This was compared with the 36% in the non-operative group (11 patients) who felt their symptoms were improved.

Seitsalo (172) reviewed 93 patients with slippage of more than 50% and found that pain after 13 to 18 years' follow-up correlated with the severity of the lumbosacral kyphosis. He suggested in selected cases that attempts to reduce the increased slip angle may be warranted. Surgical treatment is indicated if symptoms are not controlled by conventional conservative measures and significantly interfere with the patient's life-style, i.e., work, sports,

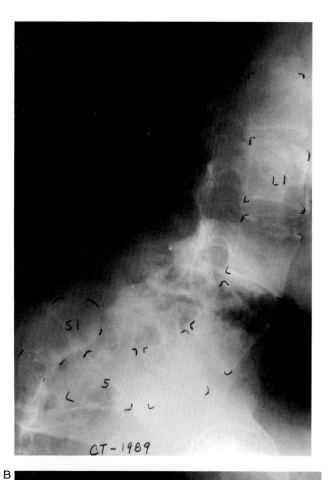

CT-1989

FIG. 17A: Pre-operative standing lateral radiograph **(left)** of a 22-year-old female with spondyloptosis and marked lumbar compensatory hyperlordosis. Prior attempts to obtain in situ fusion with C-D instrumentation were unsuccessful. She presented with progressive deformity, pain, mild radiculopathy, and concerns about deteriorating appearance (Figs. 17A–17E with permission from Dr. C. C. Edwards, ref. 39). (Figs. 17B-17C below.)

FIG. 17. *Continued.* **B:** Standing lateral radiograph one year following surgical correction. The deformity was reduced with the gradual application of distraction, posterior translation of the lumbar spine, and flexion of the sacrum using Edwards instrumentation. It was not necessary to resect the disc or perform an anterior release. There were no complications. **C:** AP radiograph at one year. It was necessary to instrument proximally to L3 only because prior surgery had disrupted the L3-L4 facets. At one year, the lateral fusion masses appear well consolidated. (Figs. 17D-17E follow.)

B

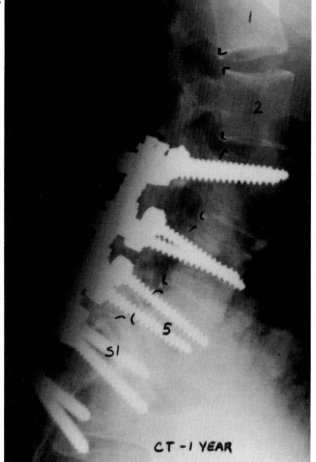

CT - 1 YEAR

C

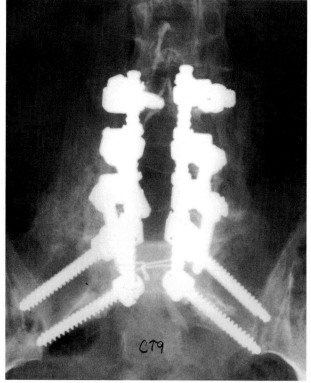

CT9

D

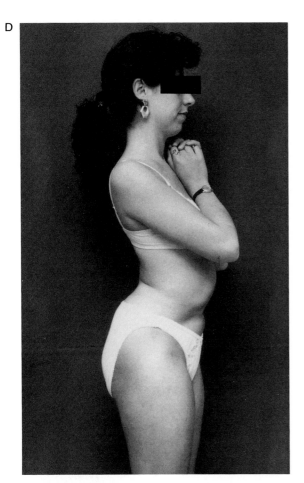

E

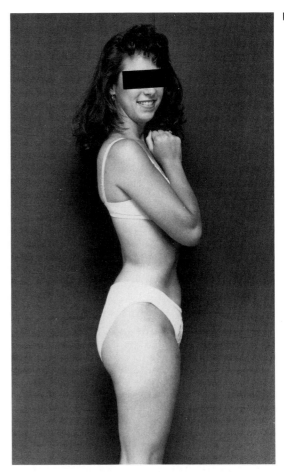

FIG. 17. *Continued.* Pre-operative clinical photograph **(D)** demonstrates anterior protrusion of the rib cage, loss of trunk height and waistline with ribs resting on iliac wings, pronounced compensatory thoracolumbar hyperlordosis, flank creases, and hip flexion contractures.

FIG. 17. *Continued.* Clinical photograph one year following surgical reconstruction **(E)** demonstrates normal sagittal alignment, restoration of trunk height and waistline, loss of flank and abdominal folds, and resolution of hip flexion contractures. The patient remains free of pain and without radiculopathy.

and recreational activities, or radiculopathy (including cauda equina symptoms) is present.

In adults who have Grade III or Grade IV spondylolisthesis presenting with radiculopathy, several procedures have been advocated, including posterior fusion in situ (71,84,143), removal of the posterior loose segment only (60), posterior decompression and fusion, reduction and posterior fusion, reduction and combined anterior and posterior fusion (6,11,34,136,183), and spondylectomy (37,56,57) combined with anterior and posterior fusion. In the presence of Grade III or IV slip and severe sciatica, Wiltse initially performed a posterior decompression followed by anterior arthrodesis one week later. Earlier, he had found excellent results in children (149) by performing only a posterior fusion; fusion rates exceeded 90% (125,154,202) using this technique. He then decided to follow these principles in the adult patient presenting with sciatica but no motor or cauda equina findings. In Grades III and IV, excellent results were found in 8 cases with an average slip of 82% (range from 66% to 118%) followed for 5.5 years. All patients had a solid fusion and returned to their previous employ-

ment. Only 1 of the 8 was a white-collar worker and none had work-related injuries.

Although Wiltse felt that posterolateral fusion was the procedure of choice, a high rate of non-union was reported (8,11,34,205) with this operation by others. For that reason, other approaches have been advocated. De-Wald reported on a combined anterior and posterior procedure in severe spondylolisthesis as the procedure of preference and felt that it was definitely indicated in failed posterior fusions. It should be emphasized that in a severe slip the posterior fusion mass is under tension and the anterior graft is biomechanically more sound being under compression. He suggested that attempts to reduce the slip should not be used in adults.

Smith and Bohlman (187) described 11 cases that were decompressed and stabilized using an anterior and posterior graft through a single posterior approach. They resected the posterior part of the first sacral vertebra as part of the decompressive procedure and stabilized the segment with a fibular graft, followed by transverse process fusion. All patients had Grade III or greater slip and

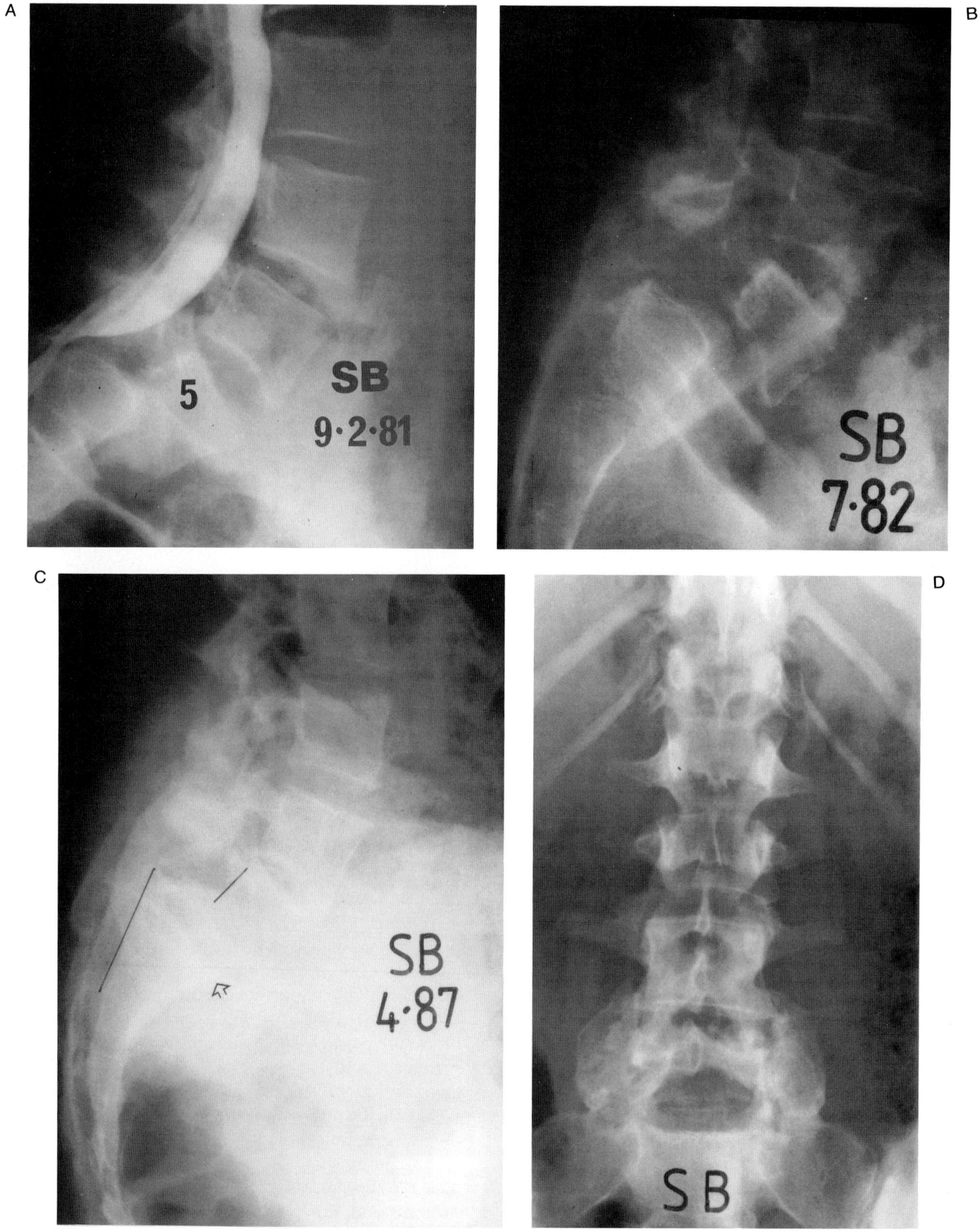

FIG. 18. A 16-year-old girl undergoing two-stage procedure. First stage **(A)**, posterior decompression-fusion L4-S1. Second stage **(B)**, anterior fibular strut graft. Good alignment and clinical result **(C and D)** after bony fusion was obtained.

all had severe neurological deficits. They reported excellent results, including recovery of bladder function. This technique is indicated only in selected cases.

Complication rates in the adult vary (11,15,34), but the overall consensus is that the risks of reduction in the adult in most cases outweigh the benefits (15,36,187). The mechanism of post-operative neurological compromise can vary from lengthening and traction to the cauda equina and proximal nerve root deficits (200) and soft tissue impingement by tense tissue and the corpotransverse ligament (36,199). The technical difficulties and special care needed in using pedicular fixation devices (36,39,109) also should be emphasized (Figs. 17A and 17B). Most authors feel that decompression of the neural elements is indicated if nerve compression, including motor deficit, intermittent claudication due to spinal stenosis, or cauda equina syndrome is present, although Peek (143) reports excellent results only stabilizing Grade III or IV slips even with minor neurological deficits.

In children with Grade III and IV slippage, reduction is not indicated if slip angle is small (empirically less than 55 degrees); if it is more than 55 degrees, reduction can be considered, but the high complication rate of 25% (95) must be acknowledged. The rate of major complications varies from 10% to 60% (11,13,172,182). Corrective procedures in children will not be discussed except to emphasize the high complication rate.

Anterior Interbody Fusion

Burns (22) did the first primary anterior interbody fusion for spondylolisthesis after Capener (23) suggested this approach in 1932. Van Rens et al. (205) felt this to be an excellent approach resulting in 21 out of 24 patients being pain free after 1 year and 20 out of 24 patients being pain free at 10 years' follow-up. He found that the best results were obtained in patients under the age of 30 in which an attempt was made to reduce the slip angle, suggesting that the deterioration and instability of adjoining levels were prevented. Selby advised that an anterior procedure is not optimal if the pathological process is posterior to the pedicles (174). Of practical concern is that the surface area for bony fusion becomes smaller as the slippage increases.

We do not advocate anterior fusion as a primary procedure and suggest it should be kept as a salvage procedure or as part of a two-stage procedure (Figs. 18A–18D). Boxall (11) also emphasized the high rate of progressive slippage after "solid" anterior fusion if displacement is more than 50% (10,11,32,138).

Others are not so pessimistic. Thomassen (197) reviewed his experiences with anterior interbody fusions done for spondylolisthesis and for disc degeneration and found the fusion rate to be very similar (85% and 84%,

respectively), but clinical improvement in low back pain was more substantial in spondylolisthesis (67% versus 54%); 73% of the spondylolisthesis group returned to work, compared to 50% of the degenerative group. A second-stage procedure that involved posterior transarticular screw fixation increased his fusion rate to 95% in the spondylolisthesis group and 93% in the degenerative group. Whitecloud (211) suggested combined anterior and posterior stabilization in the adult with high-grade slip, especially after wide decompression. Transvertebral pedicular strut graft gives adequate immediate stabilization and high fusion rate.

Posterior Lumbar Interbody Fusion

Hutter (78), using a modified Cloward technique, found that spondylolisthesis cases had 92% excellent or good results. By comparison, 85% of patients with primary discectomy and fusion had excellent or good results.

Several other authors emphasize the biomechanical advantages of the posterior lumbar interbody fusion (PLIF) procedure, advocating its use in spondylolisthesis (24,26,89,105,145). This procedure, although becoming more frequently used, has definite risks, including neurological damage and epidural scarring. If used, the operator should realize the technical pitfalls and risks involved. Wiltse feels that theoretically this procedure addresses the three criteria for ideal surgery in spondylolisthesis: It decompresses the neural components, it distracts the disc space, and it stabilizes the motion segment. But he emphasizes that pedicular fixation should be added to stabilize the motion segment. Recent laboratory work by McAfee (180) has shown, in contrast to previous suggestions, that PLIF alone increases instability. He suggests that if a PLIF is to be done, pedicular fixation be added.

Direct Repair of the Defect

In selected cases, direct repair of the pars defect has been advocated to ensure bony union of the defect without modifying the functional anatomy about the defect (7,19,20,126,132,142,204). Bradford (16) reported good and excellent results in 80% of his cases after successful fusion in 90%. Hambly (66) suggested its use in selected cases in which he combines fusion of the segment and the defect using intra- and intersegmental wiring. The advantage of this direct repair is the preservation of motion by not including the facet joint in the fusion. The use of a circlage wire around the transverse process bilaterally and the spinous process inferiorly, as described by Bradford (16), immobilizes the defect and a local bone graft is added (Figs. 19A–19F).

The weak link in such an approach seems to be the

A

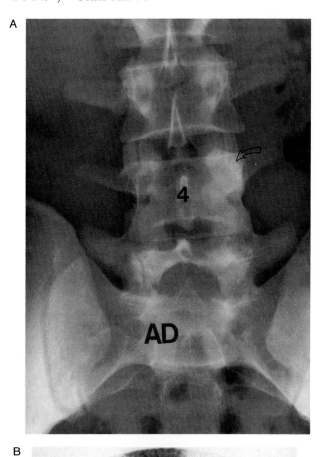

FIG. 19A: A 23-year-old high level athlete presenting with recent onset of low back and mostly right-sided hip pain. X-rays revealed sclerotic right L4 pedicle and bilateral pars defect seen on the oblique views. (Figs. 19B-19F follow.)

B

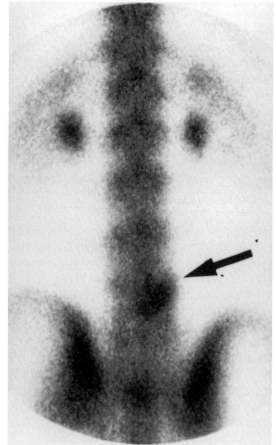

C

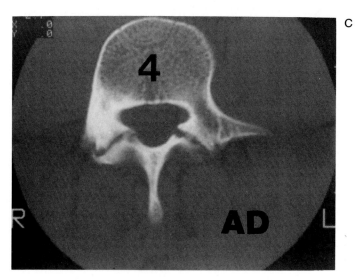

FIG. 19. *Continued.* Bone scan **(B)** shows increased uptake at that level and **(C)** confirmed sclerotic pars defect on the CT scan.

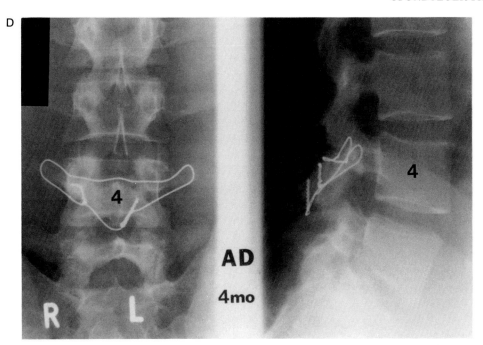

FIG. 19. *Continued.* Despite conservative treatment, this patient had continuous back pain with eventual decision for local repair of the pars defect at L4 by wiring procedure. Four months following surgery **(D)** good bone formation is evident.

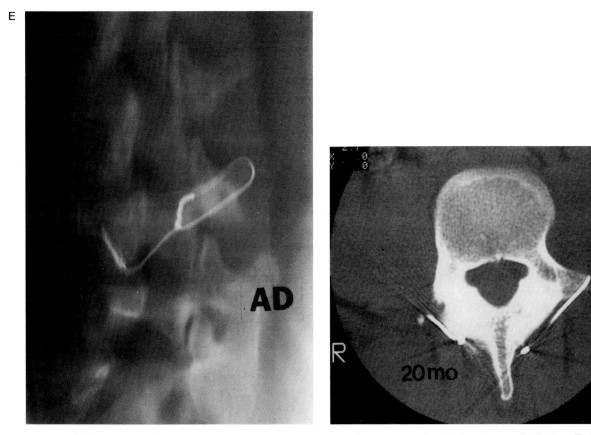

FIG. 19. *Continued.* CT scan and tomography at twenty months **(E and F)** show solid fusion. This patient had excellent relief of symptoms and returned to high level sports.

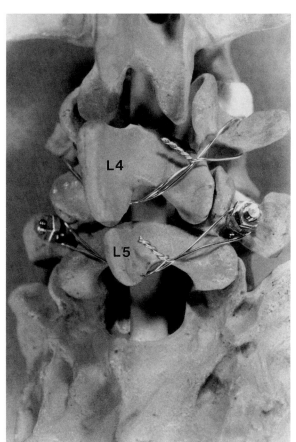

FIG. 20. Technique of pedicle screw-wiring shown on this model **(A)**. The L4 level was done using conventional wiring of the transverse processes **(B)**. Pedicle screw as fixation point was used at the L5 level.

transverse process, due to its inadequate bony strength, great variation in size, and difficulty in seating the wire around the strongest portion of the transverse process, especially L5. We feel that by using a pedicular screw as the anchoring point, this weak link can be eliminated and more effective decortication obtained without weakening the transverse process. This construct has been tested in the laboratory and found to be significantly more stable (Fig. 20). Esses and Kostuik (personal communication) obtained fusion in 10 out of 10 patients using a 4.5 mm malleolar screw, plus a graft in the defect. However, Morscher (124), after a number of screw breakages, has designed a hook plate that has distinct advantages (Fig. 21).

The suggested clinical indication for this procedure, therefore, is spondylolysis and minimal degrees of spondylolisthesis in the individual less than 30 years of age. However, a caveat is necessary.

We believe that normal discographic findings at the level of the defect are essential, as degenerative disc disease may be the primary cause for the persistence of pain and the poor clinical results that follow despite a solid pars repair. This could explain the discrepancy in Brad-

ford's findings where not all solidly fused patients had good clinical end results (16). For this reason, we feel that routine discography should be done at the level of the defect before considering local repair of the defect. Another useful diagnostic test is to see whether the infiltration of local anesthesia into the pars defect will relieve the pain. We also believe that the pedicle screw technique allows L5 defects to be repaired with ease.

Decompression Procedures

As previously discussed, compression of the lumbosacral nerve roots can occur due to different mechanisms, and each needs to be treated accordingly. Intraforaminal pressure can be due to the fibrocartilaginous mass or downward pressure of the pedicle. Extraforaminal pressure due to the corpotransverse ligament (199) can occur. Schoenecker (170) emphasized the tension on sacral roots due to pressure of the postero-superior border of the sacrum in isthmic spondylolisthesis and posterior arch of the fifth lumbar vertebra in dysplastic spondylolisthesis.

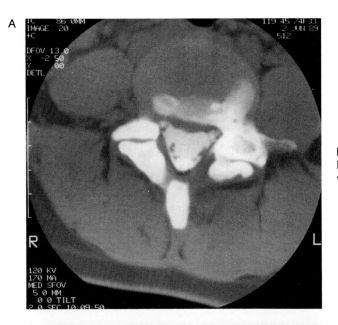

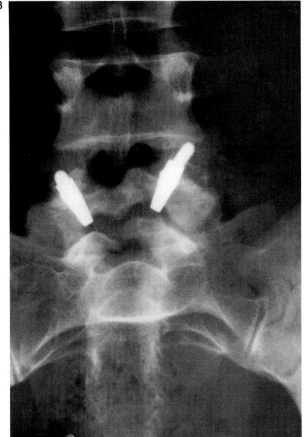

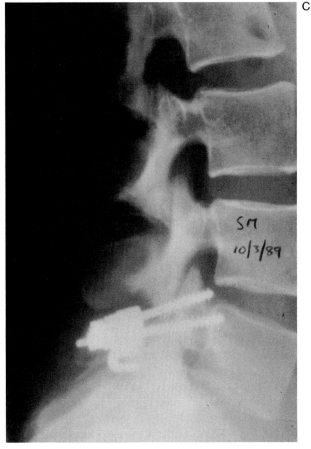

FIG. 21. A: CT scan demonstrates bilateral spondylolysis. Pain was relieved by infiltration with local anesthesia. **B:** AP view post-surgery. **C:** Lateral view. (Figs. 21D-21E follow.)

Fibrocartilaginous Mass

L5 radiculopathy can follow pressure due to the fibrocartilaginous proximal part of the pars defect and needs to be addressed in a distinct manner. Gill (60) advocated total resection of the loose neural arch, including the fibrocartilaginous mass, without a fusion procedure. He reported a satisfactory outcome in 75%. Further slippage following the Gill procedure without stabilization, especially in children, is often found. Lapras (99) reported a 68% good result, with 80% returning to pre-operative occupations following bilateral interlaminar decompression (including discectomy) without a stabilization procedure. Forty-four of his 45 patients were adults. It has

D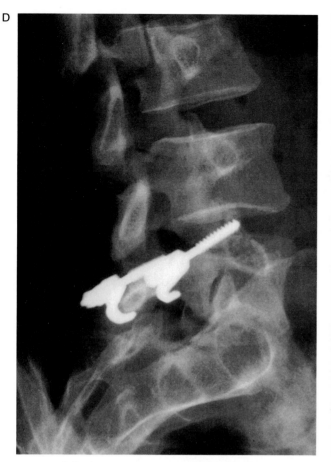

E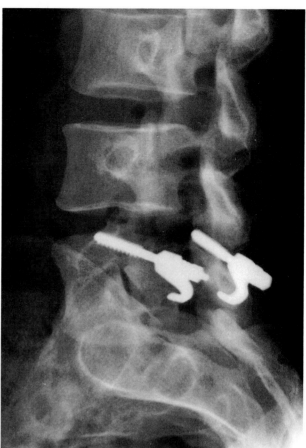

FIG. 21. *Continued.* Oblique views **(D and E)** demonstrate the spring loaded hook screw. The screw goes around the inferior aspect of the lamina. The screw bypasses the defect (healing is complete here). Bone graft is inserted into the defect at the time of surgery.

also been suggested that decompression of the L5 nerve root be done only on the symptomatic side accompanied by a stabilization procedure.

Technique of Decompression of the L5 Root (Figs. 22A–22C)

A routine midline incision is made and the spinous processes, laminae, facet joints, and transverse processes are exposed, depending on the levels to be fused (A). After identification of the L5 pars defect on the symptomatic side, the L4-L5 interlaminar space is isolated, the ligamentum flavum is excised, and the L5 nerve root is isolated at its origin. We emphasize the importance of identifying the nerve root proximal to the fibrocartilaginous mass before proceeding (B). The lamina and superior facet of the L5 vertebra are then removed with the L5 nerve root under direct vision. The L5 nerve root can now be freed as it traverses the inferior aspect of the pars on its way to the foramen around the pedicle (C). If necessary, part of the inferior portion of the pedicle may need to be removed to ensure that the nerve root is not stretched. The L5 nerve root can also be compromised

by a herniated nucleus pulposus at the same or proximal level.

Decompression of the L5 nerve root including discectomy is done in a routine fashion, as described in Chapter 84. Disc herniation at the level above may need only discectomy, especially if not accompanied by back pain (115,216).

Alar Transverse Process Impingement Syndrome (Far-Out Lateral Syndrome) (Fig. 23)

Wiltse (217) described this entity (see Fig. 23) whereby the L5 nerve root is compressed between the transverse process and the ala of the sacrum far laterally, secondary to degenerative scoliosis (Type I) or spondylolisthesis (Type II). This condition usually occurs in the middle-aged patient presenting with isthmic spondylolisthesis (slippage more than 20% to 30%). The common presentation is unilateral leg pain due to L5 nerve compression, which often does not respond to conservative measures. A CT scan usually shows the lateral canal to be stenotic only when there is more than 15% to 20% of slippage. Surgical decompression of the nerve often includes uni-

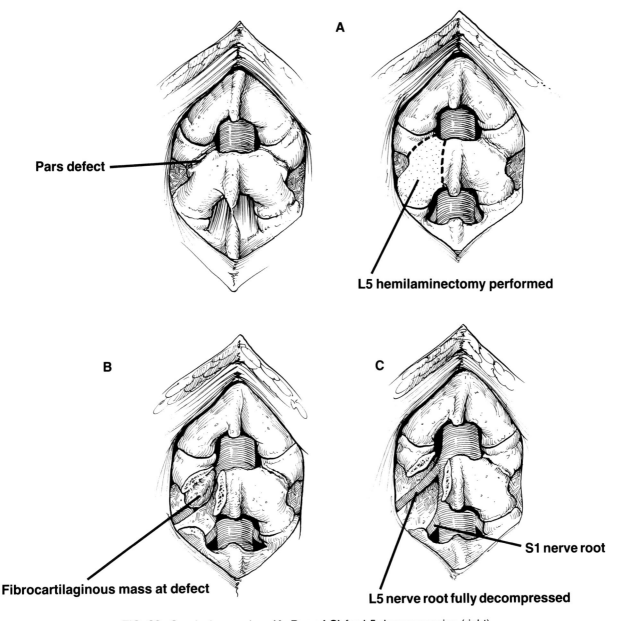

Pars defect

A

L5 hemilaminectomy performed

B

Fibrocartilaginous mass at defect

C

S1 nerve root

L5 nerve root fully decompressed

FIG. 22. Surgical procedure **(A, B, and C)** for L5 decompression (right).

lateral removal of the transverse process and lower part of the pedicle. Due to removal of a large bony component, contralateral fusion is indicated for most patients. More recently, pedicular fixation or posterior interbody fusion is suggested.

DEGENERATIVE SPONDYLOLISTHESIS

Degenerative spondylolisthesis (DS) is the forward slippage of one vertebra onto the next due to degenerative changes in the paravertebral joints and/or intervertebral discs at the same level, resulting in segmental instability. Junghanns (87), while reviewing Schmorl's collection of cadaveric spines, noticed forward slippage in specimens with an intact neural arch and suggested

the term "pseudospondylolisthesis." Macnab (113) emphasized that this was, in fact, a true displacement. He described the clinical entity in 22 patients and coined the term "spondylolisthesis with an intact arch." Newman and Stone (131) felt that this was not the only cause of spondylolisthesis in cases in which the arch was intact and suggested the term that is most widely accepted, namely, degenerative spondylolisthesis (DS).

Prevalence and Etiology

How often degenerative spondylolisthesis occurs is uncertain. In a radiographic survey in Holland, Valkenburg and Haanen (203) found that 10% of females over age 60 had a first- or second-degree slip. Farfan (46)

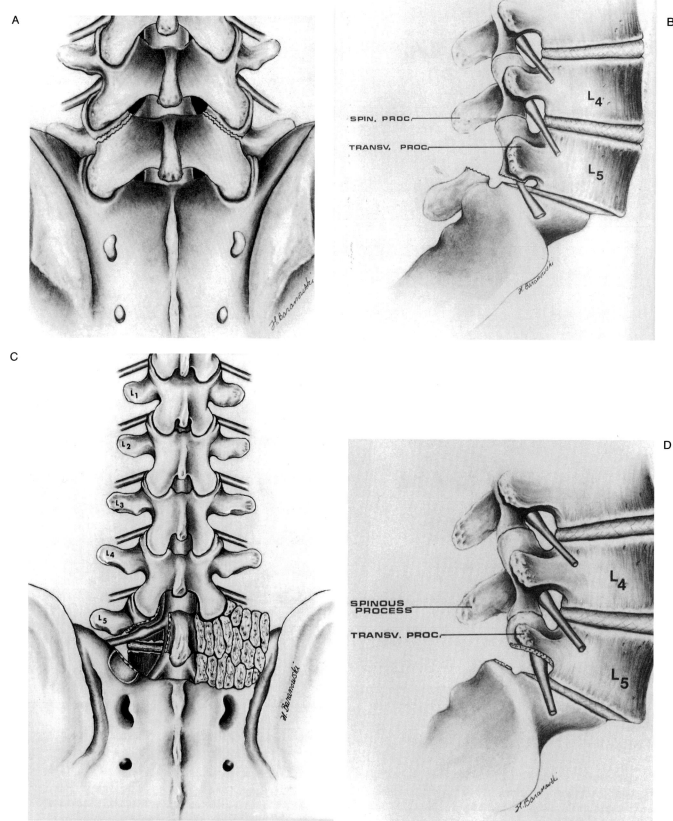

FIG. 23. Forward and inferior displacement of L5 vertebra on the sacrum can compress the L5 nerve against the ala(e) **(A and B)**. Decompression and fusion of the symptomatic side will usually solve the problem **(C and D)**, although an anterior fusion as a second stage was often indicated. (Figs. 23E-23F follow.)

E

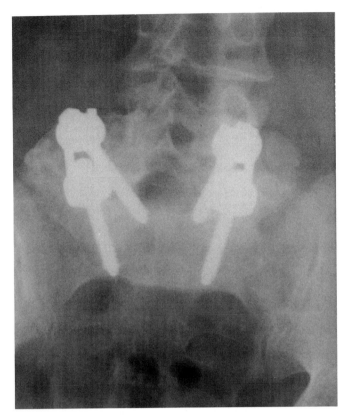

F

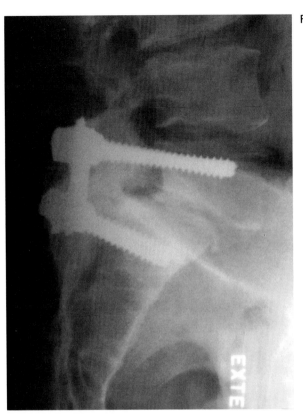

FIG. 23. *Continued.* More recently, one-level pedicle screw fixation has become the procedure of choice **(E and F).**

found the incidence to be 4.1% in autopsy specimens and emphasized that rotatory, in addition to forward, displacement be realized. The lesion occurs six times more often at the L4-L5 level; the L3-L4 level is the next most frequent level (155). It occurs five times more often in women, mostly in those over 40 years old (130,155). Sacralization of L5 is found four times more often than in the general population (155). Slippage seldom exceeds 25% to 30% (131,156), and the percentage of slippage in the adult seems to be proportional to the grade of disc degeneration up to a level where stabilization occurs.

Although the precise etiology of degenerative spondylolisthesis is unknown, the following factors to explain the predilection for L4-L5 involvement need discussion.

Progression of age-related disc degeneration, supra- and interspinous ligamentous aging (41), as well as deterioration of the facet joint cartilage may lead to shifting of the axis of rotation from the nucleus pulposus to a position near the facet joints, thereby placing more stress at this level (131,150) (Fig. 24).

Rosenberg (155), after reviewing the morphology of 20 skeletons and the radiographs of 200 patients, suggested that more stress was placed on the L4-L5 disc and facet joints, whereas the L5-S1 articulation is distinctly more stable for the following reasons:

1. The L5-S1 articulation, being in the coronal plane, is more stable than the sagittal placement of the L4-L5 facet joint, which predisposes the L4-L5 articulation to anterior displacement (1,167).
2. The fifth lumbar vertebra is stabilized by a large L5 transverse process, which supports strong muscular and ligamentous (ilio-lumbar) attachments (1). In contrast, the L4 transverse process is smaller, less strong, and supports fewer ligamentous attachments (52).
3. A decreased lumbosacral angle or increased lumbar lordosis increases the shear stress at the L4-L5 level, particularly when there is a block-shaped L5 lumbar vertebra.

There is also a high prevalence of L5 sacralization, resulting in more rotational and shear stress placed on the L4-L5 level. Disc resorption at L5-S1 results in a more stable level at the expense of more stress on the L4-L5 level. Additional predisposing factors leading to a hypermobile L4-L5 level can result from a low-lying iliac crest. The high placement of the L4 vertebra is measured by the intercrestal line (47). Farfan found this group of patients placed more stress on the L4-L5 level. Normally, the intercrestal line is situated at or above the

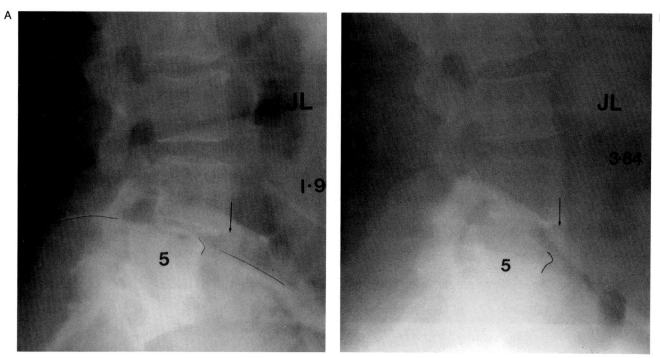

FIG. 24. A 64-year-old female presenting with symptomatic L4-L5 degenerative spondylolisthesis **(A)** and her x-rays showing minimal displacement 6 years before this presentation **(B)**.

lowermost one quarter of L4, but in a group of degenerative spondylolisthesis patients it was found to be at or below this level. This situation would reduce the protection given to L4 by soft tissue structures between the iliac crests, predisposing to slippage. In addition, females have more general mobility of their spines.

The pathophysiology can thus be explained by degenerative changes initially developing in the inferior facet of L4, followed by osteophyte formation, segmental instability, and increased forward and rotational translational slippage. This translational motion is usually halted by the superior facet of L5 and, if the joint is sagittally orientated, by the superior aspect of the L5 vertebra. This forward motion of L4 on L5, the hypertrophic joints of L4-L5, and the rotational component play significant roles in spinal and/or nerve root outlet stenosis. This translational and rotational force also results in compression and/or traction forces on the neural elements (nerve roots and/or cauda equina). The disc degeneration usually precedes paravertebral facet arthrosis, leading to increased slip and segmental spinal stenosis (40,42,43).

Signs and Symptoms

Patients present primarily with low back pain secondary to facet arthrosis in 80% of cases (158) and characteristics similar to symptomatic spinal degeneration, in general. Progression can lead to leg pain varying from sciatica to intermittent claudication resulting from cen-

tral spinal stenosis. Compression of the neural elements occurs at the level of the degenerative facet joints, with resultant local spinal stenosis and lateral recess stenosis most often involving the L5 nerve root, but frequently involving L4. The clinical presentation can be surprisingly benign, despite the radiographic appearance and minimal objective clinical findings, e.g., good range of motion and negative compression and tension signs (43). The amount of radiological slippage does not seem to correlate with clinical findings (156). As in many forms of spinal stenosis, the symptoms are often aggravated by a lordotic and improved by flexion stance. The clinical presentations can, therefore, be as follows:

1. The patient may have back pain with or without leg pain. Brown and Lockwood (18) found that 5.6% of patients presenting to their clinic with low back pain showed evidence of DS. They also found low back pain and proximal leg pain in 78% of their cases. Trauma, as a presenting factor, was found in only 14%.

2. The patient may present with predominantly leg pain. Tension signs are often absent, even in the sciatic type. Back pain may or may not be present. This presentation accounts for 42% of cases. The exiting L5 nerve root can be compressed by an L4-L5 disc protrusion at the same level, hypertrophy and direct pressure on the L5 nerve root by the hypertrophic superior facet of L5, or the guillotine-like pressure of the inferior articular process against the superior aspect of the L5 body.

3. The patient may have intermittent claudication characterized by calf pain brought on by walking, typical

of spinal stenosis. This presentation constituted 80% of Epstein's cases (43), but in other series was the primary presentation in 42%. Severe cauda equina compression with paresis/paralysis or bladder symptoms was found to be rare. Exuberant bone formation at the facet joint, capsular thickening, hypertrophy of the ligamentum flavum, and excess fluid in the capsule all contribute to the local spinal stenosis seen on myelography. The finding of hourglass constriction coincides with the typical history of intermittent claudication. Claudication of vascular origin must be excluded by clinical assessment and other definite tests, e.g., Doppler evaluation, if needed. Accompanying osteoarthritis of the hips is found in 11% to 17% (155) and may make differential diagnosis difficult. Reynolds found EMG changes in 41%, of which 80% involved the root below the slip, that is, L5 (147).

Radiological Findings

Routine anteroposterior, lateral, and oblique views clearly reveal the degenerative change at the L4-L5 level. In contrast to isthmic spondylolisthesis, spina bifida is seldom found (1). The lumbosacral spine is also found to be less lordotic (increased lumbosacral angle) (155). Both standing lateral and supine flexion-extension lateral views will reveal the presence of spondylolisthesis and help measure the degree of instability. However, the amount of slippage does not seem to correlate with the severity of the symptoms. Forward displacement has been found not to exceed 33% and has been measured to progress approximately 2 mm every 4 years (49). Dye-enhanced CT scan supplies the most information regarding both the bony and soft tissue components of the pathology. Magnetic resonance imaging is supplementary to plain films or CT scan and is becoming more widely used. Parasagittal reconstructions of the foraminae will often clearly outline the bony impingement of the nerve root, usually L5, in the foramen.

Conservative Treatment

Pain is the major presenting symptom, and conservative treatment benefits many patients. Modalities available include exercise programs, bracing, non-steroidal

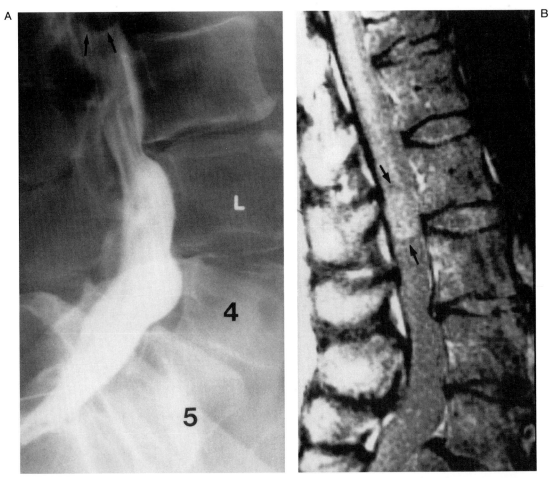

FIG. 25. A 63-year-old male presenting with degenerative spondylolisthesis of L4-L5 and on myelography **(A)** noting a filling defect at level of L1-L2, more clearly outlined by MRI **(B)**. Excision of this benign neurogenic tumor alleviated this patient's pain.

A

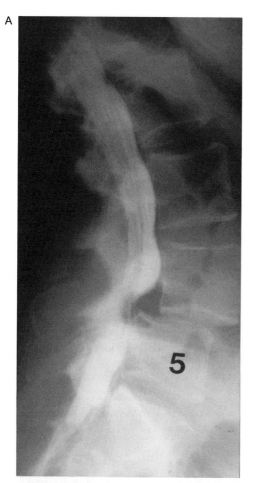

B

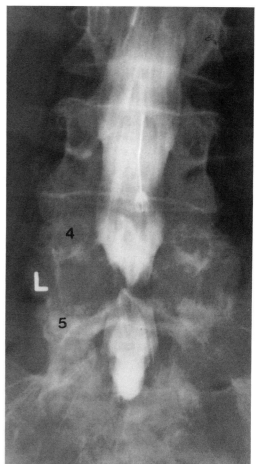

C

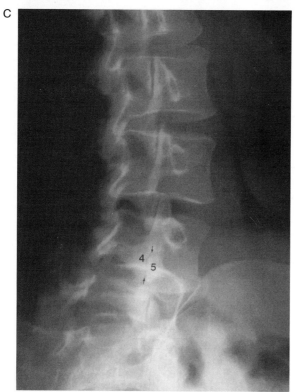

FIG. 26. This 46-year-old woman presented with typical spinal claudication and this L4-L5 Grade II degenerative spondylolisthesis. The myelographic appearance on both lateral (A) and AP (B) view. The localized L4-L5 degenerative facet joint disease is clear (C). (Figs. 26D-26F follow.)

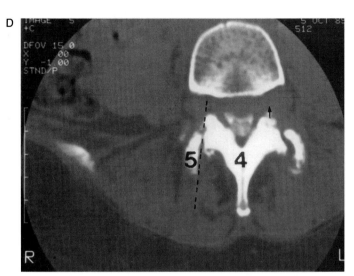

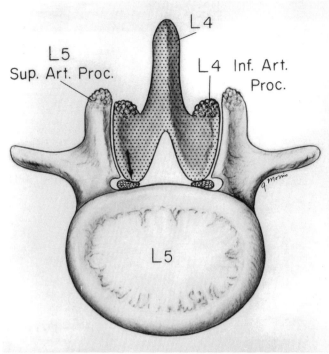

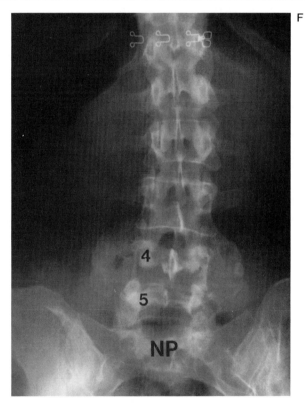

FIG. 26. *Continued.* Computed tomography **(D)** shows the sagittal orientation of the facet joint with a forward displacement of the posterior arch of L4 with narrowing of the canal as well as L5 nerve root compromise as outlined on the schematic drawing **(E)**. With a one-level decompression and stabilization, she was asymptomatic and back to her normal activities at the time of recent follow-up **(F)**.

anti-inflammatory drugs and pain medication, facet joint infiltrations, and epidural blocks. These patients have medical problems of concern in 40% of cases (18), which require careful evaluation. Other causes of back and/or leg pain should always be excluded in this group of patients (Fig. 25). In many patients, low back pain often responds well to conservative treatment. Stenotic symptoms or radiculopathy are the most common indication for surgery, rather than low back pain alone.

Surgical Treatment

Surgical treatment following unsuccessful conservative treatment is reported to be necessary in 10% to 15%

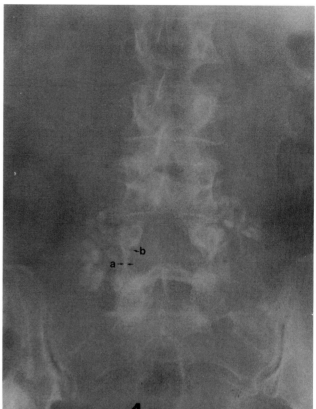

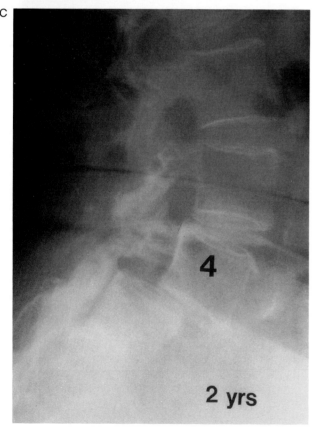

FIG. 27. A 68-year-old woman presenting with L4-L5 degenerative spondylolisthesis and myelographic defect at this level **(A)**. At the time of surgery, she had minimal displacement lying prone. Bony posterior decompression and one-level fusion was done using allograft. Four months following surgery the allograft is shown with minimal incorporation and indications of a pars fracture most probably due to over-zealous decompression **(B)**. At two years she was asymptomatic but showed progressive forward displacement and stabilization procedure was planned **(C)**.

of patients (130,155). Patients presenting with neurological involvement tend to do consistently better than those with only low back pain (14). Surgical decompression for the right indication has a high rate of success and can be offered even to the very elderly (Fig. 26). The primary goal is to adequately decompress the neural structures while not destabilizing the functional spinal segment. Preparation for surgery must be comprehensive and should include evaluation by an internist, cessation of drugs such as salicylates, if possible, to prevent excess bleeding, and a thorough discussion of options and possible complications with patient and family, making sure their expectations are realistic. With proper selection, careful evaluation, and experienced anesthesiologists, both operative blood loss and operative complications can be minimized. In high medical risk cases, epidural anesthesia can be very effective and save both time and blood loss. In this group of patients, positioning during surgery is very important and should be planned carefully to avoid pressure sores and venous hypertension. Degenerative spondylolisthesis is often part of a generalized degenerative condition and, therefore, cervical arthrosis and a decreased range of motion in other joints should alert the operating room staff in the positioning of the patient.

In deciding on a surgical plan, the importance of adequate decompression is widely accepted, but the extent of decompression and especially the necessity for routine fusion is still very controversial.

Fusion Alone. In the young patient, single-level segmental instability due to facet arthrosis can lead to degenerative spondylolisthesis. In the absence of neurological involvement, a single-level stabilization procedure can be done with good results. We recommend a posterolateral fusion supplemented, if warranted, by internal fixation.

Decompression Alone. Most surgeons agree that adequate decompression at the site of the degenerative spondylolisthesis is the procedure of choice for patients with neurological compromise, differing only on their interpretation of "adequate" measures for decompression without compromising stability, as well as when primary fusion is indicated. Wide decompression has been advocated by some authors as being necessary for adequate decompression, but increases the risk of increased slippage and/or symptoms (Fig. 27).

Rosomoff (158) emphasized that wide laminectomy and partial facetectomy were not sufficient and advocated total laminectomy and total facetectomy for adequate decompression, a view not shared by many surgeons now. He felt that progression of the slip was part of the natural disease process and reported that this was not a problem in his patients. Others do not agree; however, Dall and Rowe (31) did find results similar to Rosomoff's. In a retrospective analysis, they obtained distinctly better results when total facetectomy was compared to wide foraminotomies with preservation of the facet joints (relief of pain in 83% of cases compared to 36%). Post-operative slippage was found to be minimal and usually occurred within the first year.

In contrast, Lombardi and Wiltse (107), reporting on 6 cases done prior to 1976, found only 33% good or excellent results when the articular processes were removed, and subsequently abandoned this approach.

Rosenberg (155) also reported residual symptoms of instability if the entire articular process was excised. Today total laminectomy and facetectomy are rarely indicated because of clinical results that often result from progressive slippage (31,107,158,159).

At the other extreme, localized decompression of the nerves (168) (uni- or bilateral) is not universally followed by satisfactory results (155). However, several studies have shown that adequate decompression and subsequent good clinical results can be obtained by partial laminectomy and partial medial facetectomy (43,107,130,148).

The following surgical approach has been found by the authors to produce adequate decompression (Figs. 28A–28E). Adequate midline exposure localizes the hypertrophic L4-L5 facet joints, confirmed by intra-operative radiographs. After the L4-L5 interspinous ligament is excised, the lamina of L4 is removed as shown, depending on the extent of compression (Fig. 28A). Partial laminectomies at L3 and/or L5 depend on the pre-operative images and clinical presentation (Fig. 28B). Care should be taken to preserve the pars interarticularis of L4 and the maximum portion of the L4-L5 facet joints. The usual primary site of neural compromise is the hypertrophied and subluxed facet joints compressing the neural elements against the superior aspect of the L5 vertebral body. The medial bony components of the facet joints are removed and the thickened ligamentum flavum and capsule isolated and excised, carefully retracting the neural structures medial, noting that the epidural fat is usually absent. The medial, anterior, and caudal portions of the inferior facet of L4 are next removed to expose the superior articular process of L5. This bony prominence is then excised flush with the medial border of the L5 pedicle. Isolating the pedicle (P) will localize the path of the L5 nerve root for adequate visualization and total decompression. A major point of pressure is found to be between the hypertrophic inferior articular process (of L4) and the posterior superior rim of L5 (Fig. 28D) and careful, but adequate, decompression is needed. The pedicle of L4 is also isolated and subsequent decompression is thus obtained from pedicle to pedicle. The upper part of the L5 lamina is removed until adequate decompression of the L5 root and cauda is obtained. Care must be taken in removing the ligamentum flavum, as it can adhere to the dura, creating a risk of

A

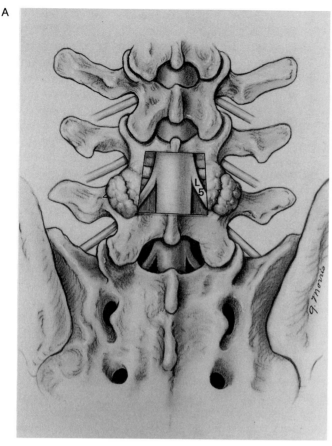

FIG. 28. Series **(A-E)** demonstrating the surgical procedure for adequate decompression and one-level intertransverse fusion (if indicated) for L4–L5 degenerative spondylolisthesis.

B

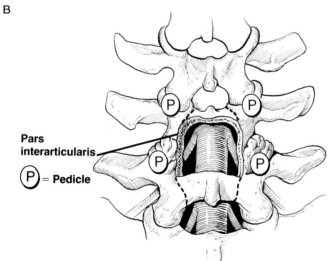

Pars
interarticularis

Ⓟ = Pedicle

C

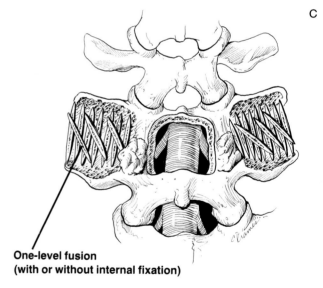

One-level fusion
(with or without internal fixation)

dural tear. By decompressing from pedicle to pedicle in all directions, adequate portions of the facet joints and pars interarticularis of L4 are usually preserved. The identical procedure is done bilaterally if clinically indicated. Before closure, the exposed dura is covered with Gelfoam or fat grafts. Depending on the patient's age, stability, and radiographic appearance, we prefer to add a one-level intertransverse fusion with or without internal fixation (Fig. 28C). However, this view is controver-

sial. When the entire facet joint or pars interarticularis of L4 is removed, fusion is always necessary.

The extent of decompression with removal of the articular processes at that level alone is shown schematically in Figures 28D and 28E. Midline posterior decompression alone was reported by Lombardi and Wiltse (107) as giving only 33% good to excellent results and led to a 10% increase in slip within the first year. However, the slip did not seem to influence the end results. Fitzgerald

D

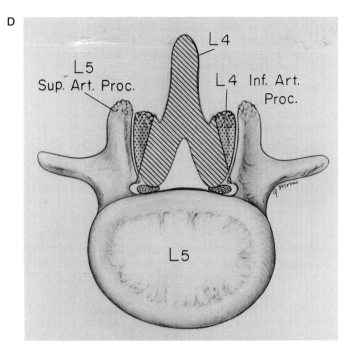

E

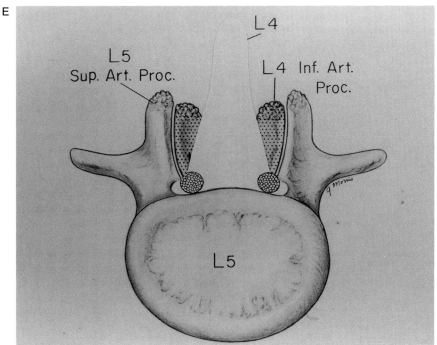

and Newman (52) used a similar midline approach and felt that fusion was indicated only in the younger, more active patients. Brown and Lockwood (18) reported 12% progressive slip following wide decompression without fusion.

Rosenberg (156) was more selective and advised that stabilization should be done only in cases with progressive slippage and pain. Increase in slip (as much as 15%) was seen in 5 out of 30 patients, occurring mostly in the first year (31,102,107). Increased slippage was reported, mostly following extensive resections including facet joints (18). Although no correlation was found comparing increased slippage and clinical outcome (31,76, 86,107,148), less optimal results were found after total facetectomy, often associated with progressive post-operative slippage (86,107,148).

Reynolds and Wiltse (148) reported 78% good or excellent results despite increased slippage in cases in which articular processes were resected. They suggested that fusion be reserved for patients younger than 60 years if they are in good health.

Epstein (43) emphasized that adequate decompres-

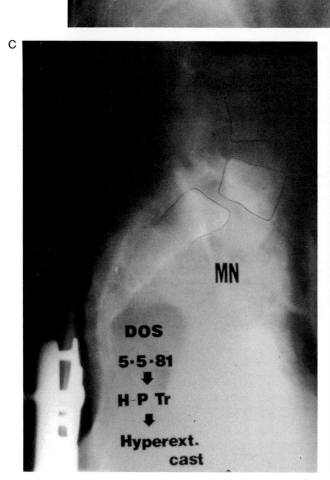

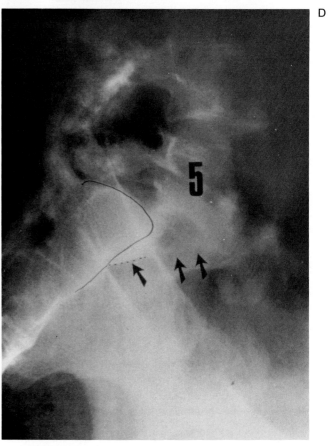

FIG. 29. This 25-year-old male was involved in a direct injury working in a timber yard. X-rays shortly after injury **(A)** show a pars defect and, two weeks later, lateral view shows Grade IV spondylolisthesis **(B)**. Posterior decompression, halo-pelvic traction, and anterior fibular strut grafting **(C)** followed. Eight months later, the patient had solid bony fusion with no pain **(D)**.

sion must include total laminectomy of L4 and L5, unroofing the lateral recesses wide and adding foraminotomies. Failure in his group of patients was associated with inadequate decompression, long history of disability, peripheral neuropathy, diabetes mellitus, hyperlordosis, obesity, and depression, rather than increased slippage. Others have more strongly advocated fusion.

Recently Herron and Trippi (76) reported excellent results following decompression without stabilization in 24 patients. They found an average improvement in back pain of 84% and in leg pain of 92%. Pre-operative flexion-extension radiographs showed less than 2 mm translation in all cases and an average post-operative slip of 8 mm (no case greater than 4 mm compared to pre-operative status). They emphasized preservation of pars interarticularis of L4 and as much of facet joints as needed.

Shenkin and Hash (178) reported that in 59 patients undergoing decompression without fusion, 10% revealed further slippage, and this number increased to 15% in three-level decompressions. Comparing Herron's (compression alone) and Lombardi's (compression alone and compression and fusion) groups of patients, no statistical difference was evident in the outcome.

Lombardi (107), reporting on decompression with medial facetectomies and foraminotomies preserving the maximum amount of facet joint and pars, found good or excellent results in 80%. After combining this approach with a one-level intertransverse fusion, the results were improved to 90%. Although this is not a statistically valid study, it suggests a rationale for fusion. Likewise, Feffer (49), in a preliminary study, found in a small group of patients that fusion did improve their clinical results when compared to those with no fusion.

Hanley (67) and others (55) emphasized that this condition is not only a translation deformity, but includes a rotational element. For this reason, neural compromise can be caused by both direct pressure due to bone and ligamentous hypertrophy and traction due to the rotational component. Hanley felt that fusion in situ does not address the rotational component and suggested Harrington distraction instrumentation for correction, but pointed out that excessive distraction will aggravate the translational deformity. Selby also felt that a Luque rectangular instrumentation was beneficial for reduction of translational deformity, although its effect on torsional correction was unclear (173). With the advent of

A

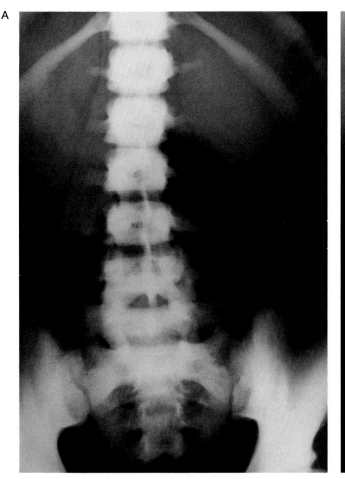

B

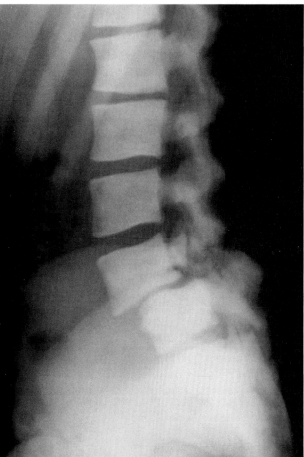

FIG. 30. This 36-year-old male presents with low back pain. The radiographs **(A and B)** show typical marble bone disease and the presence of pathological spondylolisthesis with an isthmic defect. He has responded to conservative treatment.

pedicular fixation, further reports are awaited, as both the translational and rotatory deformities can be corrected and held stable by most pedicular fixation systems.

The criteria for fusion today are variable. Wiltse (216) reported that posterolateral fusion was desirable in patients less than 65 years of age. However, he now feels that fusion is indicated in most patients, and age is not a contraindication. Patients with large disc heights have the greatest risk of post-operative slip, and this radiographic finding is used as an indication. If disc removal is required with decompression, a fusion is warranted.

In summary, it is felt that adequate decompression is essential and that stabilization procedures, at least at this time, are controversial. The following guidelines should be considered:

1. The patient's general medical status should be considered and fusion avoided, if possible, in elderly patients with major medical illness.
2. Iatrogenic instability due to extensive decompression necessitates stabilization in most patients. Fracture of the pars, usually bilaterally, will occur fairly frequently after wide midline decompression in these osteoporotic patients, and this may be as often as one in ten.
3. A patient less than 60 to 65 years old who is active and healthy more often qualifies for stabilization.
4. A patient with a large disc space or a patient who requires disc excision is a prime candidate for stabilization.

TRAUMATIC SPONDYLOLISTHESIS

Acute fractures of the pars interarticularis are rare and always due to severe trauma in a previously normal anatomical structure (29,38,93,94,96,192,220).

This form of spondylolisthesis (Fig. 29) and its place in the classification has not been clear, even following Wiltse, Newman, and Macnab's classification. These authors stated that this type is secondary to an acute injury affecting other parts of the neural arch, including the pedicle but excluding the pars. Sufficient trauma occurring in normal structures with no underlying developmental abnormalities would be classified by Marchetti (116) as an acquired form. In some cases, this may be difficult to differentiate from true lumbosacral dislocations. The authors have never seen a case in which bilateral pars fractures occurred with no other fractures in the vertebra.

PATHOLOGICAL SPONDYLOLISTHESIS

In this group, the bony strength is insufficient to resist forward motion of the proximal vertebra on the one below (Fig. 30).

Subtype A

In this type, a generalized skeletal disease leads to lysis or elongation of the bony components. The causations reported include Albers-Schoenberg, arthrogryposis, syphilitic disease, Von Recklinghausen's disease, osteochondroplasia, Larsen syndrome, Marfan syndrome, and osteomalacia (115).

Subtype B

This condition is due to localized bone destruction secondary to tumor and infection. It represents a rare complication that may be very difficult to manage because of the associated anterior column destruction.

POST-SURGICAL SPONDYLOLISTHESIS

The incidence of this form is rising and needs to be emphasized. As previously noted, the most common etiology is extensive decompression with sacrifice of the facets. A less common form is observed following midline posterior fusion and is termed "spondylolysis aquisita." The proposed etiology for the latter is devascularization of the neural arch, inadvertent fracture at the time of decortication, or weakening of the neural arch due to decortication with secondary fatigue fracture (see Chapter 98). Today, this condition is rare, as midline fusion has been abandoned by most surgeons in favor of other fusion techniques.

REFERENCES

1. Albrook D (1957): Movements of the lumbar spinal column. *J Bone Joint Surg* [Br] 39:339–345.
2. Apel DM, Lorenz MA, Zindrick MR (1989): Symptomatic spondylolisthesis in adults four decades later. *Spine* 14:345–348.
3. Ascani E, Salsano V, Montanaro A, Vicini M (1986): The surgical treatment of severe cases of spondylolisthesis: Critical considerations. In: *Progress in spinal pathology: Spondylolisthesis II.* Bologna, Italy: Italian Scoliosis Research Group.
4. Bailey W (1947): Observations on the etiology and frequency of spondylolisthesis and its precursors. *Radiology* 48:107–112.
5. Baker DR, McHolick W (1956): Spondylolisthesis and spondylolisthesis in children. *J Bone Joint Surg* [Am] 38:933–934.
6. Balderston RA, Bradford DS (1985): Technique for achievement and maintenance of reduction for severe spondylolisthesis using spinous process traction wiring and external fixation of pelvis. *Spine* 10:376–382.
7. Beckers L (1986): Buck's operation for treatment of spondylolysis and spondylolisthesis. *Acta Orthop Belg* 52:819–823.
8. Bohlman HH, Cook SS (1982): One-stage decompression and posterolateral and interbody fusion for lumbosacral spondyloptosis through a posterior approach. Report of two cases. *J Bone Joint Surg* [Am] 64:415–418.
9. Borkow SE, Kleiger B (1971): Spondylolisthesis in the newborn. A case report. *Clin Orthop* (81):73–76.
10. Bosworth DM, Fielding JW, Demarest L, Bonaquist M (1955): Spondylolisthesis: A critical review of a consecutive series of cases treated by arthrodesis. *J Bone Joint Surg* [Am] 37:767–786.
11. Boxall D, Bradford DS, Winter RB, Moe JH (1979): Management of severe spondylolisthesis in children and adolescents. *J Bone Joint Surg* [Am] 61:479–495.

12. Bradford DS (1978): Spondylolysis and spondylolisthesis. In: Chou SN, and Seljeskog L, eds. *Spinal deformities and neurological dysfunction.* New York: Raven Press, pp. 175–200.

13. Bradford DS (1979): Treatment of severe spondylolisthesis: A combined approach for reduction and stabilization. *Spine* 4:423–429.

14. Bradford DS (1983): Management of spondylolysis and spondylolisthesis. *Instr Course Lect, Am Acad Orthop Surg.* St. Louis: C.V. Mosby, 32:151–162.

15. Bradford DS, Gotfried Y (1987): Staged salvage reconstruction of grade IV and V spondylolisthesis. *J Bone Joint Surg* [Am] 69:191–202.

16. Bradford DS, Iza J (1985): Repair of the defect in spondylolysis or minimal degrees of spondylolisthesis by segmental wire fixation and bone grafting. *Spine* 10:673–679.

17. Briggs H (1949): Discussion of intervertebral foramen constriction. *JAMA* 140:476.

18. Brown MD, Lockwood JM (1983): Degenerative spondylolisthesis. *Instr Course Lect, Am Acad Orthop Surg.* St. Louis: C.V. Mosby, 32:162–169.

19. Buck JE (1970): Direct repair of the defect in spondylolisthesis. *J Bone Joint Surg* [Br] 52:432–437.

20. Buck JE (1979): Direct repair of the defect in spondylolysis. *J Bone Joint Surg* [Am] 61:479.

21. Burkhardt E (1940): Spondylolisthesis. *Schweiz Med Wochensch* 70:1093.

22. Burns BH (1933): An operation for spondylolisthesis. *Lancet* 1:1233.

22a. Camins M, O'Leary P, eds. (1987): *The lumbar spine.* New York: Raven Press, p. 258.

23. Capener N (1932): Spondylolisthesis. *Brit J Surg* 19:374–386.

24. Cloward RB (1953): The treatment of ruptured lumbar intervertebral discs by vertebral body fusion: Indications, techniques, after care. *J Neurosurg* 10:154–168.

25. Collier BD, Johnson RP, Carrera GF, et al. (1985): Painful spondylolysis or spondylolisthesis studied by radiography and single-photon emission computed tomography. *Radiology* 154:207–211.

26. Collis JS (1985): Total disc replacement: A modified posterior lumbar interbody fusion. *Clin Orthop* (193):64–67.

27. Colonna PC (1954): Spondylolisthesis. Analysis of two hundred one cases. *JAMA* 154:398–402.

28. Commandre FA, Taillan B, Gagnerie F, Zakarian H, Lescourgues M, Fourre JM (1988): Spondylolysis and spondylolisthesis in young athletes: 28 cases. *J Sports Med Phys Fitness* 28:104–107.

29. Cope R (1988): Acute traumatic spondylolysis. Report of a case and review of the literature. *Clin Orthop* (230):162–165.

30. Cyron BM, Hutton WC (1979): Variations in the amount and distribution of cortical bone across the partes interarticularis of L5. A predisposing factor in spondylolysis? *Spine* 4:163–167.

31. Dall BE, Rowe DE (1985): Degenerative spondylolisthesis. Its surgical management. *Spine* 10:668–672.

32. Dandy DJ, Shannon MJ (1971): Lumbosacral subluxation (Group 1 spondylolisthesis). *J Bone Joint Surg* [Br] 53:578–595.

33. Danielson B, Frennered K, Selvik G, Irstam L (1989): Roentgenologic assessment of spondylolisthesis. *Acta Radiologica* 30:65–68.

34. DeWald RL, Faut MM, Taddonio RF, Neuwirth MG (1981): Severe lumbosacral spondylolisthesis in adolescents and children: Reduction and staged circumferential fusion. *J Bone Joint Surg* [Am] 63:619–626.

35. Dick W (1984): Innere fixation von Brust- und lenden-wirbel-frakturen. *Aktuelle Probleme in chirurgie und orthopaedie 28.* Bern, Switzerland: Verlag Hans Huber.

36. Dick WT, Schnebel B (1988): Severe spondylolisthesis. Reduction and internal fixation. *Clin Orthop* (232):70–79.

37. Dimar JR, Hoffman G (1986): Grade 4 spondylolisthesis: Two stage therapeutic approach of anterior vertebrectomy and anterior-posterior fusion. *Orthop Rev* 15:504–509.

38. Edvardsen P (1983): Traumatic lumbar spondylolisthesis: Anterior fusion by means of a fibular graft. *Injury* 14:366–369.

39. Edwards C (1990): Prospective evaluation of a new method for complete reduction of L5-S1 spondylolisthesis using corrective forces alone. Presented at the American Academy of Orthopaedic Surgeons, New Orleans, LA. To be published in *Orthopaedic Transactions* 14(3).

40. Ehni G (1975): Effects of certain degenerative diseases of the spine, especially spondylolysis and disc protrusion on the neural contents particularly in the lumbar region: Historical account. *Mayo Clin Proc* 50:327–338.

41. Epstein JA, Epstein BS, Lavine L (1962): Nerve root compression associated with narrowing of the lumbar spinal canal. *J Neurol Neurosurg Psychiat* 25:165–176.

42. Epstein JA, Epstein BS, Lavine LS, Carras R, Rosenthal AD, Sumner P (1973): Lumbar nerve root compression at the intervertebral foramina caused by arthritis of the posterior facets. *J Neurosurg* 39:362–369.

43. Epstein NE, Epstein JA, Carras R, et al. (1983): Degenerative spondylolisthesis with an intact neural arch: A review of 60 cases with an analysis of clinical findings and the development of surgical management. *Neurosurgery* 13:555–561.

44. Esses SI (1989): The AO spinal internal fixator. *Spine* 14:373–378.

45. Farfan HF (1973): *Mechanical disorders of the low back.* Philadelphia: Lea and Febiger.

46. Farfan HF (1980): The pathological anatomy of degenerative spondylolisthesis: A cadaver study. *Spine* 5:412–418.

47. Farfan HF, Kirkaldy-Willis WH (1981): The present status of spinal fusion in the treatment of lumbar intervertebral joint disorders. *Clin Orthop* (158):198–214.

48. Farfan HF, Osteria V, Lamy C (1976): The mechanical etiology of spondylolysis and spondylolisthesis. *Clin Orthop* (117):40–55.

49. Feffer HL, Wiesel SW, Cuckler JM, Rothman RH (1985): Degenerative spondylolisthesis: To fuse or not to fuse. *Spine* 10:287–289.

50. Ferguson RJ, McMaster JH, Stanitski CL (1975): Low back pain in college football linemen. *J of Sports Med* 2:63–69.

51. Fisk JR, Moe JH, Winter RB (1978): Scoliosis, spondylolysis, and spondylolisthesis. Their relationship as reviewed in 539 patients. *Spine* 3:234–245.

52. Fitzgerald JA, Newman PH (1976): Degenerative spondylolisthesis. *J Bone Joint Surg* [Br] 58:184–192.

53. Flatley TJ, Derderian H (1985): Closed loop instrumentation of the lumbar spine. *Clin Orthop* (196):273–278.

54. Frederickson BE, Baker D, McHolick WJ, Yuan MA, Lubicky JP (1984): The natural history of spondylolysis and spondylolisthesis. *J Bone Joint Surg* [Am] 66:699–707.

55. Frymoyer JW, Selby DK (1985): Segmental instability: Rationale for treatment. *Spine* 10:280–286.

56. Gaines RW (1990): Treatment of spondyloptosis with L5 vertebrectomy and reduction of L4 onto the sacrum. To be published.

57. Gaines RW, Nichols WK (1985): Treatment of spondyloptosis by two-stage L5 vertebrectomy and reduction of L4 onto the S1. *Spine* 10:680–686.

58. Gelfand MJ, Strife JL, Kereiakes JG (1981): Radionuclide bone imaging in spondylolysis of the lumbar spine in children. *Radiology* 140:191–195.

59. Gerard Y (1962): Spondylolisthesis de la cinquieme lombaire d'origine traumatique. *Mem Acad Chir Paris* 88:57–62.

60. Gill GC, Manning JC, White HL (1955): Surgical treatment of spondylolisthesis without spine fusion. *J Bone Joint Surg* [Am] 37:493–520.

61. Goldberg MJ (1980): Gymnastic injuries. *Orthop Clin No America* 11:717–726.

62. Gramse RR, Sinaki M, Ilstrup DM (1980): Lumbar spondylolisthesis: A rational approach to conservative treatment. *Mayo Clin Proc* 55(11):681–686.

63. Grenier N, Kressel HY, Schiebler ML, Grossman RI (1989): Isthmic spondylolysis of the lumbar spine: MR imaging at 1.5 T. *Radiology* 170:489–493.

64. Grobler LJ, Haugh LD, Wiltse L, Frymoyer JW (1989): L4-5 isthmic spondylolisthesis: Clinical and radiological review in 52 cases. Presented at the Fourth Annual Meeting of the North American Spine Society, Quebec City, Canada, June/July.

65. Grogan JP, Hemminghytt S, Williams AL, Carrera GF, Haughton VM (1982): Spondylolysis studied by computed tomography. *Radiology* 145:737–742.

66. Hambley M, Lee CK, Gutteling E, Zimmerman MC, et al.

(1989): Tension band wiring—Bone grafting for spondylolysis and spondylolisthesis. A clinical and biomechanical study. *Spine* 14:455–460.

67. Hanley EN (1986): Decompression and distraction-derotation arthrodesis for degenerative spondylolisthesis. *Spine* 11:269–276.

68. Hanley EN Jr, Levy JA (1989): Surgical treatment of isthmic lumbosacral spondylolisthesis. Analysis of variables influencing results. *Spine* 14:48–50.

69. Haraldsson S, Willner S (1983): A comparative study of spondylolisthesis in operations on adolescents and adults. *Arch Orthop and Trauma Surg* 101(2):101–105.

70. Harrington PR, Tullos HS (1971): Spondylolisthesis in children. Observations and surgical treatment. *Clin Orthop* (79):75–84.

71. Harris IE, Weinstein SL (1987): Long-term follow-up of patients with grade-II and IV spondylolisthesis. Treatment with and without posterior fusion. *J Bone Joint Surg* [Am] 69:960–969.

72. Hasbe K (1913): Die wirbelsaule der Japaner. *Z Morph Anthrop* 15:259–380.

73. Hensinger RN (1983): Spondylolysis and spondylolisthesis in children. *Instr Course Lect, Am Acad Orthop Surg*. St. Louis: C.V. Mosby, 32:132–151.

74. Henson J, McCall IW, O'Brien JP (1987): Disc damage above a spondylolisthesis. *Br J Radiol* 60:69–72.

75. Herbinaux G (1782): *Traite sur diverse accouchemens laborieux et sur les polypes de la matrice*. Bruxelles: De Boubers.

76. Herron LD, Trippi AC (1989): L4-5 degenerative spondylolisthesis. The results of treatment by decompressive laminectomy without fusion. *Spine* 14:534–538.

77. Holt EP Jr (1968): The question of lumbar discography. *J Bone Joint Surg* [Am] 50:720–726.

78. Hutter CG (1983): Posterior intervertebral body fusion. A 25-year study. *Con Orthop* 179:86–96.

79. Hutton WC, Cyron BM (1978): Spondylolysis: The role of the posterior elements in resisting the intervertebral compressive force. *Acta Orthop Scand* 49:604–609.

80. Hutton WC, Scott JRR, Cyron BM (1977): Is spondylolisthesis a fatigue fracture? *Spine* 2:202–209.

81. Inoue S, Ozaki K (1972): Anterior fusion for spondylolysis and spondylolisthesis. *Saigai-Igaku* 15:919–934.

82. Jackson DW (1979): Low back pain in young athletes: Evaluation of stress reaction and discogenic problems. *Am J Sports Med* 7:364–366.

83. Johnson DW, Farnum GN, Latchaw RE, Erba SM (1989): MR imaging of the pars interarticularis. *Am J Radiol* 152(2):327–332.

84. Johnson JR, Kirwan EO (1983): The long-term results of fusion in situ for severe spondylolisthesis. *J Bone Joint Surg* [Br] 65:43–46.

85. Johnson LP, Nasca RJ, Dunham WK (1988): Surgical management of isthmic spondylolisthesis. *Spine* 13:93–97.

86. Johnsson KE, Willner S, Johnsson K (1986): Post-operative instability after decompression for lumbar spinal stenosis. *Spine* 11:107–110.

87. Junghanns H (1930): Spondylolisthesen ohne spalt in zwischengelenkstueck. *Arch fuer Orthopaedische Unfallchir* 29:118–127.

88. Kaneda K, Kazama H, Satoh S, Fujiya M (1986): Follow-up study of medial facetectomies and posterolateral fusion in isthmic spondylolisthesis. 53 cases followed for 18–89 months. *Clin Orthop* 203:159–167.

89. Keim HA (1977): Indications for spine fusions and techniques. *Clin Neurosurg* 25:266–275.

90. Kikuchi S, Hasue M (1988): Combined contrast studies in lumbar spine diseases. Myelography (peridurography) and nerve root infiltration. *Spine* 13:1327–1331.

91. Kikuchi S, Hasue M, Nishiyama K, Ito T (1984): Anatomic and clinical studies of radicular symptoms. *Spine* 9:23–30.

92. Kilian JF (1854): *Schilderungen neuer backenformen und ihrer verhalten im leben*. Mannheim: Bassermann and Mathy.

93. Kleinberg S, Burman MS (1942): Spondylolisthesis: Report of three cases in adults with forward displacement of the vertebrae below the level of the laminar defect. *J Bone Joint Surg* 24:899–906.

94. Klinghoffer L, Murdock MG (1982): Spondylolysis following trauma. A case report and review of the literature. *Clin Orthop* (166):72–74.

95. Kostuik JP (1978) Morbidity Committee statistics. Presented at Scoliosis Research Society.

96. Krenz J, Troup JDC (1973): The structure of the pars interarticularis of the lower lumbar vertebrae and its relation to the etiology of spondylolysis. *J Bone Joint Surg* [Br] 55:735–741.

97. Lafferty JF, Winter WG, Gambaro SA (1977): Fatigue characteristics of posterior elements of vertebrae. *J Bone Joint Surg* [Am] 59:154–158.

98. Lambl DL (1855): Zehn thesen ueber spondylolisthesis. *Zbl Gynak Urol* 9:250.

99. Lapras C, Pierluca P, Pernot P, Mottollese C (1984): Treatment of spondylolisthesis (stage I-II) by neurosurgical decompression without either osteosynthesis or reduction. *Neurochirurgie* 30(3):147–152.

100. Laurent LE (1958): Spondylolisthesis. *Acta Orthop Scand* (Suppl) 35.

101. Laurent LE, Einola S (1961): Spondylolisthesis in children and adolescents. *Acta Orthop Scand* 31:45.

102. Lee CK (1983): Lumbar spinal instability (olisthesis) after extensive posterior spinal decompression. *Spine* 8:429–433.

103. Letts M, Smallman T, Afanasiev R, Gouw G (1986): Fracture of the pars interarticularis in adolescent athletes: A clinical biomechanical analysis. *J Ped Orthop* 6:40–46.

104. Libson E, Bloom RA, Dinari G (1982): Symptomatic and asymptomatic spondylolysis and spondylolisthesis in young adults. *Int Orthop* 6:259–261.

105. Lin PM (1982): *Posterior lumbar interbody fusion*. Springfield: Charles C Thomas.

106. Linson MA, Crowe CH (1990): Comparison of magnetic resonance imaging and lumbar discography in the diagnosis of disc degeneration. *Clin Orthop* (250):160–163.

107. Lombardi JS, Wiltse LL, Reynolds J, Widell EH, Spencer C (1985): Treatment of degenerative spondylolisthesis. *Spine* 10:821–827.

108. Lorenz R, Bulo W (1982): Schweregradeinteilung der spondylolisthesis. Anwendbarkeit und wert verschiedener messverfahren. *Rontgenblaetter* 35:275–276.

109. Louis R (1988): Pars interarticularis reconstruction using plates and screws with grafting without arthrodesis. *Rev Chir Orthop* 74(6):549–557.

110. Louis R, Maresca C (1977): Stabilisation chirurgicale avec reduction des spondylolyses et des spondylolisthesis. *Int Orthop* 1:215–225.

111. Lowe J, Schachner E, Hirschberg E, Shapiro Y, Libson E (1984): Significance of bone scintigraphy in symptomatic spondylolysis. *Spine* 9:653–655.

112. Lowe RW, Hayes TD, Kaye J, Bagg RJ, Luekens CA (1976): Standing roentgenograms in spondylolisthesis. *Clin Orthop* (117):80–84.

113. Macnab I (1950): Spondylolisthesis with an intact neural arch: The so-called pseudo-spondylolisthesis. *J Bone Joint Surg* 32:325.

114. Macnab I (1975): Paper presented at the meeting of the International Society for the Study of the Lumbar Spine, London.

115. Macnab I (1990): *Backache, 2nd ed*. Baltimore: Williams and Wilkins, pp. 84–103.

116. Marchetti PG, Bartolozzi P (1986): Spondylolisthesis: Classification and etiopathogenesis. In: *Progress in spinal pathology: Spondylolisthesis II*. Bologna, Italy: Italian Scoliosis Research Group.

117. Marique P (1951): Le spondylolisthesis. *Acta Chir Belg Suppl* 3:3–89.

118. McAfee PC, Yuan HA (1982): Computed tomography in spondylolisthesis. *Clin Orthop* (166):62–71.

119. McCarroll JR, Miller JM, Ritter MA (1980): Lumbar spondylolysis and spondylolisthesis in college football players. *Am J Sports Med* 14:484–486.

120. Meschan I (1945): Spondylolisthesis. A commentary on etiology, and an improved method of roentgenographic mensuration and detection of instability. *Amer J Roentgenol* 53:230–243.

121. Meyerding HW (1932): Spondylolisthesis. *Surg Gynecol Obstet* 54:371–377.

122. Michel CR (1971): Reduction et fixation des spondylolisthesis et des spondyloptoses. *Rev Chir Orthop* 57 (Suppl I):148–157.

123. Monticelli G, Costanzo G (1986): Spondylolysis and spondylo-

listhesis: Treatment. In: *Progress in spinal pathology: Spondylolisthesis II.* Bologna, Italy: Italian Scoliosis Research Group.

124. Morscher E, Gerber B, Fasel J (1984): Surgical treatment of spondylolisthesis by bone grafting and direct stabilization of spondylolysis by means of a hook screw. *Arch Orthop Trauma Surg* 103(3):175–178.

125. Nachemson A (1976): Repair of the spondylolisthetic defect and intertransverse fusion for young patients. *Clin Orthop* (117):101–105.

126. Nachemson A, Wiltse LL (1976): Editorial: Spondylolisthesis. *Clin Orthop* (117):2–3.

127. Naugebauer F (1881): Die entstehung der spondylolisthesis. *Centralab fur Gynak* 5:260–261.

128. Newman PH (1965): A clinical syndrome associated with severe lumbosacral subluxation. *J Bone Joint Surg* [Br] 47:472–481.

129. Newman PH (1975): Classification of spondylolisthesis. Presented at the Meeting of the International Society for the Study of the Lumbar Spine, London.

130. Newman PH (1976): Surgical treatment for spondylolisthesis in the adult. *Clin Orthop* (117):106–111.

131. Newman PH, Stone KH (1963): The etiology of spondylolisthesis with a special investigation. *J Bone Joint Surg* [Br] 45:39–59.

132. Nicol RO, Scott JH (1986): Lytic spondylolysis. Repair by wiring. *Spine* 11:1027–1030.

133. Norman D (1987): The spine. In: Brant-Zawadzki M, Norman D, eds. *Magnetic resonance of central nervous system.* New York: Raven Press, pp. 289–328.

134. O'Brien JP, Mehdian H, Jaffray D (1988): Reduction of severe lumbosacral spondylolisthesis: A report of 22 cases with follow-up from 4–12 years. Abstracts of meeting in Miami, April. Toronto: Int. Soc. for the Study of the Lumbar Spine 25.

135. Ogilvie JW, Sherman J (1987): Spondylolysis in Scheuerman's disease. *Spine* 12:251–253.

136. Ohki I, Inoue S, Murata T, Mikanagi K, Shibuya K (1980): Reduction and fusion of severe spondylolisthesis using halo-pelvic traction with wire reduction device. *Int Orthop* 4:107–113.

137. O'Neill DB, Micheli LJ (1989): Post-operative radiographic evidence for fatigue fracture as the etiology in spondylolysis. *Spine* 14:1342–1355.

138. Osterman K, Lindholm TS, Laurent LE (1976): Late results of removal of the loose posterior element (Gill's operation) in the treatment of lytic lumbar spondylolisthesis. *Clin Orthop* (117):121–128.

139. Papanicolaou N, Wilkinson RH, Emans JB, Treves S, Micheli LJ (1985): Bone scintigraphy and radiography in young athletes with low back pain. *Am J Rad* 145:1039–1044.

140. Pearcy M, Shepherd J (1985): Is there instability in spondylolisthesis? *Spine* 10:175–177.

141. Pease CN, Najat H (1967): Spondylolisthesis in children. Special reference to the lumbosacral joint and treatment by fusion. *Clin Orthop* (52):187–198.

142. Pedersen AK, Hagen R (1988): Spondylolysis and spondylolisthesis. Treatment by internal fixation and bone grafting of the defect. *J Bone Joint Surg* [Am] 70:15–24.

143. Peek RD, Wiltse LL, Reynolds JB, Thomas JC, Guyer DW, Widell EH (1989): In situ arthrodesis without decompression for Grade III or IV isthmic spondylolisthesis in adults who have severe sciatica. *J Bone Joint Surg* [Am] 71:62–68.

144. Pennell RG, Maurer AH, Bonakdarpour A (1985): Stress injuries of the pars interarticularis: radiologic classification and indications for scintigraphy. *Am J Rad* 145:763–766.

145. Perrin G, Goutelle A, Fischer G, Monib H (1984): Lumbosciatica caused by spondylolisthesis. Results of the surgical treatment by facetolaminectomy and interbody arthrodesis by the posterior approach in a series of 66 cases. *Neurochirurgie* 30(6):387–393.

146. Pizzutillo PD, Mirenda W, MacEwan GD (1986): Posterolateral fusion for spondylolisthesis in adolescents. *J Pediat Orthop* 6:311–316.

147. Reynolds J (1987): Spondylolisthesis. In: White AH, Rothman RH, Ray CD, eds. *Lumbar spine surgery: Techniques and complications.* St. Louis: C.V. Mosby, pp. 279–285.

148. Reynolds JB, Wiltse LL (1979): Surgical treatment of degenerative spondylolisthesis. Abstract. *Spine* 4:148–149.

149. Reynolds JB, Wiltse LL (1988): The surgical treatment of high grade spondylolisthesis in children by in situ fusion. Presented at the meeting of the North American Spine Society, Colorado Springs, Colorado, July.

150. Rissanen PM (1964): Comparison of pathological changes in intervertebral disc and interspinous ligaments of the lower part of the lumbar spine in the light of autopsy findings. *Acta Orthop Scand* 34:54–65.

151. Robert K (1855): Eine eigentuemliche angeborene lordose, wahrscheinlich bedingt durch eine verschiebung des koerpers des letzen lindenwirbels auf die vordere flaeche des ersten kreuzeinwirbels. *Monat Geburtkunde Frauenkrank* 5:891–894.

152. Roche MB (1950): Healing of bilateral fracture of the pars interarticularis of a lumbar neural arch. *J Bone Joint Surg* [Am] 32:428–429.

153. Roche MB, Rowe GG (1951): Incidence of separate neural arch and coincident bone variations. *Anat Rel* 109:233–252.

154. Rombold C (1966): Treatment of spondylolisthesis by posterolateral fusion, resection of the pars interarticularis, and prompt mobilization of the patient. *J Bone Joint Surg* [Am] 48:1282–1300.

155. Rosenberg NJ (1975): Degenerative spondylolisthesis: Predisposing factors. *J Bone Joint Surg* [Am] 57:467–474.

156. Rosenberg NJ (1976): Degenerative spondylolisthesis: Surgical treatment. *Clin Orthop* (117):112–120.

157. Rosenberg NJ, Bargar WL, Friedman B (1981): The incidence of spondylolysis and spondylolisthesis in nonambulatory patients. *Spine* 6:35–38.

158. Rosomoff HL (1980): Lumbar spondylolisthesis: Etiology of radiculopathy and role of the neurosurgeon. *Clin Neurosurg* 27:577–590.

159. Rosomoff HL (1981): Neural arch resection for lumbar spinal stenosis. *Clin Orthop* (154):83–89.

160. Rossi F (1978): Spondylolysis, spondylolisthesis, and sports. *J Sports Med and Physical Fitness* 18:317–340.

161. Rothman SLG, Glenn WV Jr (1983): Spondylolysis and spondylolisthesis. In: Newton TH, Potts DG, eds. *Computed tomography of the spine and the spinal cord.* San Anselmo: Clavadel, pp. 267–280.

162. Rothman SLG, Glenn WV Jr (1984): Spondylolysis and spondylolisthesis. In: Post JD, ed. *CT of the lumbar spine.* Baltimore: William & Wilkins, pp. 591–615.

163. Rowe CG, Roche MB (1953): The etiology of separate neural arch. *J Bone Joint Surg* [Am] 35:102–110.

164. Rubens-Duval A, et al. (1960): Le rachis des ceintures noires de judo. *Rev du Rheumatisme* 27(7):233–241.

165. Sarasta H (1984): Prognostic radiologic aspects of spondylolisthesis. *Acta Radiol* 25:427–432.

166. Sarasta H (1987): Long-term clinical and radiological follow-up of spondylolysis and spondylolisthesis. *J Pediat Orthop* 7:631–638.

167. Sato K, Wakamatsu E, Yoshizumi A, Watanabe N, Irei O (1989): The configuration of the laminas and facet joints in degenerative spondylolisthesis. A clinicoradiologic study. *Spine* 14:1265–1271.

168. Savini R, Cervellati S, Draghetti M, Palmisani M, Ponzo L (1986): The surgical treatment of spondylolisthesis in the adult. In: *Progress in spinal pathology, vol II.* Bologna, Italy: Italian Scoliosis Research Group.

169. Scaglietti O, Frontino G, Bartolozzi P (1976): Technique of anatomical reduction of lumbar spondylolisthesis and its surgical stabilization. *Clin Orthop* (117):165–175.

170. Schoenecker PL, Cole HO, Herring JA, Capelli AM, Bradford DS (1990): Cauda equina syndrome after in situ arthrodesis for severe spondylolisthesis at the lumbosacral junction. *J Bone Joint Surg* [Am] 72:369–377.

171. Schollner D (1975): Ein neues verfahren zur reposition und fixation bei spondylolisthesis. *Orthop Praxis* 11:270–274.

172. Seitsalo S, Oesterman K, Hyvarinen H, Schlenzka D, Poussa M (1990): Severe spondylolisthesis in children and adolescents. *J Bone Joint Surg* [Br] 72:259–265.

173. Selby DK (1983): When to operate and what to operate upon. *Orthop Clin North Am* 14:577–588.

174. Selby DK, Henderson RJ, Blumenthal S, Dossett D (1987): Ante-

rior lumbar fusion. In: White AH, Rothman RH, Ray CD, eds. *Lumbar spine surgery.* St. Louis: C.V. Mosby.

175. Semon RL, Spengler D (1981): Significance of lumbar spondylolysis in college football players. *Spine* 6:172–174.

176. Serre H (1956): Spondylolyse traumatique vraie. Fracture isolee des isthmes de L5 anterieurement normaux. *Rev Rheum* 23:44.

177. Shahriaree H, Sajadi K, Rooholamini SA (1979): A family with spondylolisthesis. *J Bone Joint Surg* [Am] 61:1256–1258.

178. Shenkin HA, Hash CJ (1979): Spondylolisthesis after multiple bilateral laminectomies and facetectomies for lumbar spondylolysis: Follow-up review. *J Neurosurg* 50:45–47.

179. Sherman FC, Wilkinson RH, Hall JE (1977): Reactive sclerosis of a pedicle and spondylolysis in the lumbar spine. *J Bone Joint Surg* [Am] 59:49–54.

180. Shirado O, Zdeblick T, Ward KE, McAfee PC (1990): Biomechanical evaluation of posterior spinal stabilization methods for lumbosacral isthmic spondylolisthesis. Presented at the 1990 Am. Acad. for Ortho. Surgeons, New Orleans.

181. Sicard A, Leca A (1960): Les spondylolisthesis traumatiques. *Presse Med* 31:1207.

182. Sijbrandij S (1981): A new technique for the reduction and stabilization of severe spondylolisthesis. *J Bone Joint Surg* [Br] 63:266–271.

183. Sijbrandij S (1983): Reduction and stabilization of severe spondylolisthesis. *J Bone Joint Surg* [Br] 65:40–42.

184. Simmons EH, Capicotto WN (1988): Posterior transpedicular Zielke instrumentation of the lumbar spine. *Clin Orthop* (236):180–191.

185. Simper LB (1986): Spondylolysis in eskimo skeletons. *Acta Orthop Scand* 57:78–80.

186. Sinaki M, Luttness MP, Ilstrup DM, Chu CP, Gramse RR (1989): Lumbar spondylolisthesis: Retrospective comparison and three-year follow-up of two conservative treatment programs. *Arch Phys Med Rehabil* 70(8):594–598.

187. Smith MD, Bohlman HH (1990): Spondylolisthesis treated by a single-stage operation combining decompression with in situ posterolateral and anterior fusion. *J Bone Joint Surg* [Am] 72:415–421.

188. Snijder JG, Seroo JM, Snijder CJ, Schijvens AW (1976): Therapy of spondylolisthesis by repositioning and fixation of the olisthetic vertebra. *Clin Orthop* (117):149–156.

189. Steffee AD, Sitkowski DJ (1988): Reduction and stabilization of grade IV spondylolisthesis. *Clin Orthop* (227):82–89.

190. Steiner ME, Micheli LJ (1985): Treatment of symptomatic spondylolysis and spondylolisthesis with the modified Boston brace. *Spine* 10:937–943.

191. Sty JR, Starshak RJ, Babbit DP (1980): Bone scintigraphy: The sclerotic pedicle (Wilkinson syndrome). *Clin Nucl Med* 5:558.

192. Sullivan CR, Bickell WH (1960): The problem of traumatic spondylolisthesis: A report of three cases. *Am J Surg* 100:698–708.

193. Swee RG, McLeod RA, Beabout JW (1979): Osteoid osteoma. Detection, diagnosis, and localization. *Radiology* 130:117–123.

194. Szypryt EP, Twining P, Mulholland RC, Worthington BS (1989): The prevalence of disc degeneration associated with neural arch defects of the lumbar spine assessed by magnetic resonance imaging. *Spine* 14:977–981.

195. Taillard W (1955): Le spondylolisthesis chez l'enfant et l'adolescent. *Acta Orthop Scand* 24:115.

196. Teplick JG, Laffey PA, Berman A, Haskin ME (1986): Diagnosis and evaluation of spondylolisthesis and/or spondylolysis on axial CT. *AJNR* 7:479–491.

197. Thomassen E (1985): Intercorporal lumbar spondylodesis. 312 patients followed for 2–20 years. *Acta Orthop Scand* 56:287–293.

198. Torgerson WR, Dotter WE (1976): Comparative roentgenographic study of the asymptomatic and symptomatic lumbar spine. *J Bone Joint Surg* [Am] 58:850–853.

199. Transfeldt EE, Bradford DS, Robinson D, Heithoff K (1987): The cause of neurologic deficit in acute spondylolisthesis (listhetic crisis) and in reduction of grades III-IV spondylolisthesis. *Orthop Trans* 11:112.

200. Transfeldt EE, Dendrinos GK, Bradford DS (1989): Paresis of proximal lumbar roots after reduction of L5-S1 spondylolisthesis. *Spine* 14:884–887.

201. Troup JD (1976): Mechanical factors in spondylolisthesis and spondylolysis. *Clin Orthop* (117):59–67.

202. Turner RH, Bianco AJ Jr (1971): Spondylolysis and spondylolisthesis in children and teenagers. *J Bone Joint Surg* [Am] 53:1298–1306.

203. Valkenburg HA, Haanen HCM (1982): The epidemiology of low back pain. In: White AA, Gordon SL, eds. *Proc Am Assoc Orthop Surg Symposium on Low Back Pain.* pp. 9–22.

204. van der Werf GJ, Tonino AJ, Zeegers WS (1985): Direct repair of lumbar spondylolysis. *Acta Orthop Scand* 56(3):378–379.

205. van Rens TJ, van Horn JR (1982): Long-term results in lumbosacral interbody fusion for spondylolisthesis. *Acta Orthop Scand* 53(3):378–379.

206. Villiaumey J, Brondani JC (1972): Etude radiologique de la colonne vertebrale de jeunes ceintures noires. 5eme Conference des Maladies Rhum, Aix le Bains, France.

207. Watkins MB (1953): Posterolateral fusion of the lumbar and lumbosacral spine. *J Bone Joint Surg* [Am] 35:1014–1018.

208. Weinstein JN, Walsh TR, Spratt KF, Lehman TR, Aprill C, Sayet H (1990): Lumbar discography: A control prospective study of normal volunteers to determine the false/positive rate. Presented at the Annual Meeting of the Am. Acad. of Orthop. Surgeons, New Orleans.

209. Wertzberger KL, Peterson HA (1980): Acquired spondylolysis and spondylolisthesis in the young child. *Spine* 5:437–442.

210. White AH, Wiltse LL (1975): Spondylolisthesis after extensive lumbar laminectomy. *J Bone Joint Surg* [Am] (Proceedings) 58:727–728.

211. Whitecloud TS 3rd, Butler JC (1988): Anterior lumbar fusion utilizing transvertebral fibular graft. *Spine* 13:370–374.

212. Wilkinson RH, Hall JE (1974): The sclerotic pedicle: Tumor or pseudotumor? *Radiology* 111:683–688.

213. Wiltse LL (1962): Etiology of spondylolisthesis. *J Bone Joint Surg* [Am] 44:539–560.

214. Wiltse LL (1969): Spondylolisthesis: Classification and etiology. *Symposium of the Spine, Am Acad Orthop Surg.* St. Louis: C.V. Mosby, p. 143.

215. Wiltse LL (1975): Paper read at the Meeting of the International Society for the Study of the Lumbar Spine. London.

216. Wiltse LL (1977): Spondylolisthesis and its treatment: Conservative treatment; fusion, with and without reduction. In: Ruge D, Wiltse LL, eds. *Spinal disorders: Diagnosis and treatment.* Philadelphia: Lea & Febiger, pp. 193 ff.

217. Wiltse LL, Guyer RD, Spencer CW, Glenn WV, Porter IS (1984): Alar transverse process impingement of the L5 spinal nerve: The far-out syndrome. *Spine* 9:31–41.

218. Wiltse LL, Hutchinson RH (1964): Surgical treatment of spondylolisthesis. *Clin Orthop* (35):116–135.

219. Wiltse LL, Newman PH, Macnab I (1976): Classification of spondylolysis and spondylolisthesis. *Clin Orthop* (117):23–29.

220. Wiltse LL, Rothman LG (1989): Spondylolisthesis: Classification, diagnosis, and natural history. *Seminars in Spine Surgery* 1(2):78–94.

221. Wiltse LL, Spencer CW (1988): New uses and refinements of the paraspinal approach to the lumbar spine. *Spine* 13:696–706.

222. Wiltse LL, Widell EH Jr, Jackson DW (1975): Fatigue fracture: The basic lesion in isthmic spondylolisthesis. *J Bone Joint Surg* [Am] 57:17–22.

223. Wiltse LL, Winter RB (1983): Terminology and measurement of spondylolisthesis. *J Bone Joint Surg* [Am] 65:768–772.

224. Wynne-Davies R, Scott JHS (1979): Inheritance and spondylolisthesis. A radiographic family survey. *J Bone Joint Surg* [Br] 61:301–305.

225. Zembo MM, Roberts JM, Burke SW, King AG, Nadell J (1986): Congenital spondylolisthesis. Presented at Scoliosis Research Society Meeting 21st Annual Meeting, Bermuda, Sept.

226. Zielke K, Strempel AV (1986): Posterior lateral distraction spondylodosis using twofold sacral bar. *Clin Orthop* (203):151–158.

The Adult Spine: Principles and Practice,
J. W. Frymoyer, Editor-in-Chief.
Raven Press, Ltd., New York © 1991.

CHAPTER 79

Congenital Neurological Disorders of the Lumbar Spine Presenting in the Adult

Luis Schut, Leslie N. Sutton, and Anne–Christine Duhaime

GENERAL CONSIDERATIONS

Approximately 40% of all congenital malformations have some involvement of the cranial or spinal elements and this group of congenital anomalies is collectively referred to as the dysraphic state. While the majority of these lesions are obvious at birth, there are a large number of patients who are not diagnosed in the neonatal stage but rather present later on in life with disorders that are congenital in nature. This chapter will outline the various types of spinal dysraphism, particularly those that may present in a delayed fashion, discuss the anatomy and pathology of each, and consider various medical and surgical treatments as well as the clinical outcome that can be expected.

Spinal dysraphism (11) is a general term used to describe congenital malformations involving abnormal closure and development of the neural tube and neighboring structures as well as the posterior midline anat-

L. Schut, M.D., L. N. Sutton, M.D., A. C. Duhaime, M.D.: Children's Hospital of Philadelphia, University of Pennsylvania School of Medicine, Department of Neurosurgery, Philadelphia, Pennsylvania 19104.

omy. The classical spina bifida aperta has occurred when the skin is open or sealed only by a very thin layer of tissue. The most benign form of spina bifida aperta is the meningocele, which is a cystic lesion consisting only of an outpouching of meninges filled with spinal fluid. By definition, the patient should be neurologically intact and the major immediate risk to the patient is spinal fluid leakage with subsequent meningitis. Surgical repair of this lesion should be performed shortly after birth and this does not present a challenge to the neurosurgeon.

A more complex lesion of the spina bifida aperta type is myelomeningocele, and in this entity there is an open neural plate lacking a central canal. The area is surrounded by rudimentary dura and leptomeninges and the patient will have anywhere from moderate to severe neurological deficit very frequently accompanied by clinically significant hydrocephalus requiring shunting (65%) and Arnold Chiari malformation (95%). These lesions are obvious at birth and if surgical repair is undertaken the patient will most likely survive the neonatal period. However, additional problems may become manifest later on in childhood or adult life, such as tethering of the spinal cord, severe scoliosis, and signs and symptoms referable to the Arnold Chiari malformation.

The delayed spinal problems will be discussed in more detail later on.

Another type of spina bifida aperta is myeloschisis, which is a large open placode without meninges and may include most of the spinal canal. There is severe neurological deficit and the majority of these children do not survive. An unusual form of open spinal dysraphism is that in which there are areas of meningeal herniation which are very small or form at a later stage of fetal life and then undergo secondary atrophy. They are referred to as meningocele manque or atretic meningocele and there is usually a small redundant area of scarred skin which leads internally to an atrophic sac. Fibrous bands of tissue can be followed to the dura and to the spinal cord and they may contain non-functional nerve roots. The spinal cord and/or the nerve roots can be attached by way of adhesions and essentially represent an intrauterine healing of a small myelomeningocele. They are of importance to us because they can produce a later onset of symptoms due to tethering of the spinal cord.

In contraposition to the cases of spina bifida aperta, patients with an occult spinal dysraphism do not have an obvious lesion at birth (15). In this group of developmental abnormalities there is an intact skin covering and patients may have either a congenital, progressive, or potential neurological deficit. In contrast to spina bifida aperta, these defects are three times more commonly seen in females than in males and are rarely associated with Arnold Chiari malformation or hydrocephalus. The recognition of this group of disorders is important because correction with prophylactic surgery can halt the progression of neurological damage (14).

In the differential diagnosis of congenital spinal dysraphic lesions presenting later in life are those that produce symptoms via tethering of the spinal cord, including thickened filum terminale, tethered myelomeningocele, and diastematomyelia. Congenital dermal sinus tracts may present with tethering or infection. Epidermoid and dermoid tumors, neuroenteric cysts, anterior sacral meningoceles, lipomas, and lipomyelomeningoceles produce symptoms from compression or traction. The clinical presentations of the various forms of occult spinal dysraphism are relatively similar.

OCCULT SPINAL DYSRAPHISM: SIGNS AND SYMPTOMS

Cutaneous Manifestations

Cutaneous malformations occur in over 80% of all cases of occult spinal dysraphism and may present singly or in combination. The most frequent are subcutaneous lipomas, telangiectasias, hemangiomas, areas of abnormal pigmentation, atrophic skin, and accessory appendages (Fig. 1). The most striking of all is hypertricosis, which is a hairy patch that always occurs in the midline. While these patches may be small in size, more commonly they are wide and sometimes they get to be so prominent that the parents or patient shave the area. It is to be noted that the appearance and location of the cutaneous lesion predicts neither the type of underlying anomaly nor the exact intraspinal level at which it occurs.

Neurological Examination

By the time of the patient's presentation to the examining physician there is usually some muscular weakness and gait disturbance, sometimes accompanied by

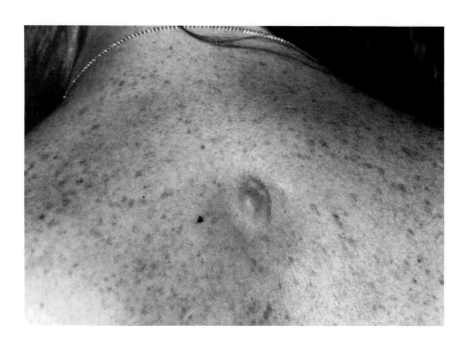

FIG. 1. Skin tag in neuroenteric cyst.

marked atrophy or asymmetry of the lower extremities. These findings are usually a combination of neurological and orthopedic abnormalities which are known collectively as the neuromusculoskeletal syndrome. More than 60% of these patients will be seen with a combination of foot and ankle deformity, short legs, muscle weakness and atrophy, changes in the distal reflexes with loss or hyperactivity of the reflex, sensory loss that may be patchy, trophic changes of the skin, pathological reflexes, and spasticity. The examination will commonly show both upper and lower motor neuron changes due to involvement of the anterior horn cells and roots along with the effects of tethering of the spinal cord itself; these signs are often asymmetric. The particular symptom that precipitates the visit to the physician is frequently the onset of pain, which may be localized to the area in question or may radiate in a nerve root distribution. This pain is accompanied by a stiff back and exacerbated by motion of the spine.

Finally, scoliosis and other forms of spinal curvature may be present with or without other features of the neuromusculoskeletal syndrome in up to 12% of the patients. This will be much higher in some forms of occult spinal dysraphism, such as in diastematomyelia where it approaches 70%–95%. Left curves and painful or rapidly progressive scoliosis increase the odds of a neurogenic cause. Obviously, this should be taken into consideration when evaluating patients with idiopathic scoliosis.

Unilateral or bilateral deformity of the foot of the cavus varus variant with hammer toes or clawed toes is also a frequent finding, particularly in cases of leptomyelolipoma.

Urological Examination

Bladder function is disturbed in more than 30% of these patients. Incontinence of the neurogenic type is usually seen. This may be accompanied by perianal sensory loss and decreased rectal tone, particularly if lower motor neuronal involvement is present. This will be accompanied by frequent urinary tract infections, which may be the only presenting symptom. Urodynamic testing may disclose bladder dysfunction even before symptoms become apparent.

RADIOLOGICAL INVESTIGATIONS

Plain X-Rays

Plain x-rays of the spine will usually show some anomalies that are not pathognomonic of any one of these disorders. The most common finding will be spina bifida occulta, which is the occurrence of failure of formation of the spinous processes and laminas of one or more vertebral segments with or without neurological deficit.

Generally this is an incidental finding on plain x-rays and can be found in as many as 17% of all adults with a higher frequency in younger children. It is most frequently found at S1 with L5 being the second most common segment involved (Fig. 2). Other findings on plain x-ray of the spine may include hemivertebrae, failure of fusions, bony spurs, butterfly vertebrae or other anomalies of the vertebral bodies, hemisacral anomalies such as the scimitar sacrum, and abnormal widening of the spinal canal. All of these may be accompanied by scoliosis or other abnormal curvatures of the spine.

Myelography

Until recently, myelography was the diagnostic test of choice to determine the presence or absence of spinal cord and nerve root involvement. However, this has been almost totally replaced by CT scan and, much more recently, by MR images of the spine.

In our clinical practice, myelography is only performed if there is a discrepancy between the neurological examination and findings on MRI or if for any reason it is necessary to confirm the suspected diagnosis.

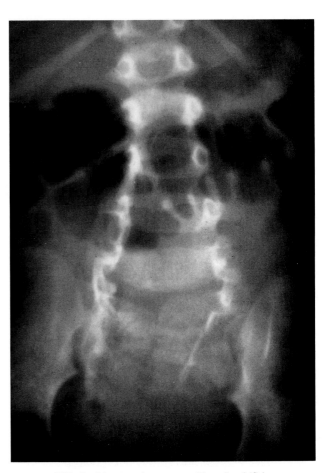

FIG. 2. Abnormal sacrum with spina bifida.

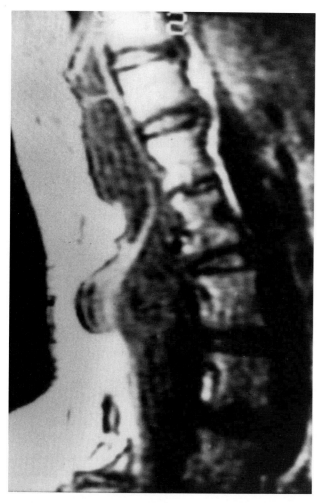

FIG. 3. Combined lesion, tethered cord, and hydrosyringomyelia.

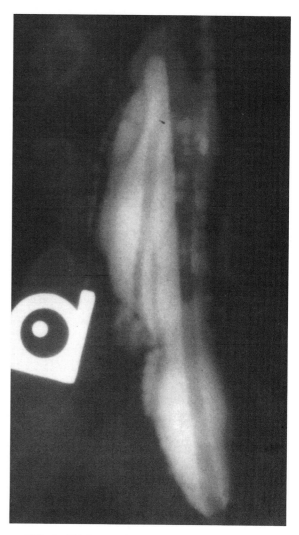

FIG. 4. Thickened filum terminale tethered cord.

Ultrasonography

Ultrasonography has been proven useful only in very small infants and, obviously, if there is a very large spina bifida. Tethering of the spinal cord can sometimes be seen by ultrasonography and attempts have been made to try to correlate the absence of pulsation on real-time ultrasonography with the development of retethering.

CT Scan

CT scan done following injection of intrathecal metrizamide is capable of demonstrating all of these anomalies with startling clarity. Of great help is sagittal reconstruction of the spinal canal which will allow the examining physician to demonstrate not only the type of anomaly but the anatomic localization.

MRI

MR imaging has almost completely replaced all of the above diagnostic tests in our clinical practice (2). With the obvious advantages of being non-invasive and with-out risk of radiation, it has become the tool of choice for the diagnosis of occult spinal dysraphism. It provides clear demonstration of soft tissue anomalies including the spinal cord and nerve roots. The major drawback is that MRI does not show the bony anatomy as well as other studies. However, this is of secondary importance and can be easily complemented with CT scan or plain x-rays.

One of the unexpected benefits of MRI examination of the spine is the demonstration of combined lesions occurring in spinal dysraphism (Fig. 3). It will be found with relatively high frequency that the lesion for which the patient is being studied is only one of several that will be seen on examination.

DIFFERENTIAL DIAGNOSIS IN OCCULT SPINAL DYSRAPHISM

Tethered Spinal Cord and Thickened Filum Terminale

This refers to a form of occult spinal dysraphism in which an association of a low-lying conus with a short

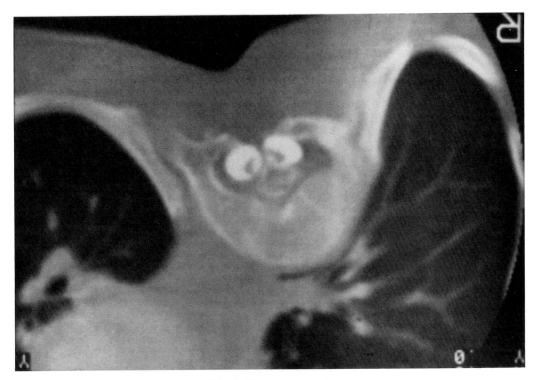

FIG. 5. Diastematomyelia.

thickened filum terminale is found. The filum may terminate at the caudal portion of the thecal sac or may attach more proximally to the posterior aspect of the dura mater (Fig. 4). Sometimes the syndrome is seen in association with the cutaneous manifestations of myelomeningocele manque or atretic myelomeningocele previously described. Some cutaneous manifestation is found in almost half of the cases and low back or leg pain is a prominent feature of the syndrome. In addition, the patients may manifest all or part of the orthopedic and neural syndrome as well as the urological disturbances of neurogenic bladder.

On further investigation, the patient usually will be noticed to have a spina bifida but this is not pathognomonic. MRI will demonstrate the low position of the conus medullaris below the level of L2 (7) and with relatively high frequency will be able to demonstrate the thickened filum terminale and its insertion into the posterior aspect of the dural canal. If myelography is performed, images should be obtained not only in the commonly used prone position but also the patient should be turned supine, since this will be the only way the thickened posterior filum terminale will be seen in a number of cases.

Surgical correction of the problem is straightforward, requiring laminectomy or laminotomy over the lowermost segment of the lumbar spine and upper sacral levels (10). The dura is opened in the midline and the filum terminale is identified. The filum is usually more than 2 mm in diameter, easily recognizable by its insertion in the posterior dura and its different color from the nerve roots. It is sectioned after coagulation close to the dura since it does have a very large vascular supply that has to be occluded prior to sectioning. While it is rare to see the filum terminale ascend rapidly after dissection, by measuring markers placed on the proximal portion it has been reported to have ascended as much as 2 cm in some cases.

The complaint of pain is quickly relieved and retethering of this particular form would be exceptional. Neurologic deficits usually remain static, but occasionally may improve after surgery.

Diastematomyelia

Diastematomyelia (9) is a primary developmental malformation leading to the division of the spinal cord into two halves (Fig. 5). This can be accompanied by either spina bifida occulta or aperta and the cleft may be partial or complete. As noted above, the term refers exclusively to the defect in the spinal cord and not to the bony or cartilaginous spur that may traverse the defect. This entity is to be distinguished from true diplomyelia in which there are two complete spinal cords, each having anterior and posterior horns and its own set of nerve roots. The existence of true diplomyelia has been questioned by many authors and in some cases may be considered an extreme form of diastematomyelia.

More than one level can be involved in diastematomyelia and it is often accompanied by all the manifestations of occult spinal dysraphism at the same or other levels of the spine. The most common location for the cleft is at the lower thoracic or upper lumbar regions, but it can occur at any level.

Patients with diastematomyelia may present with scoliosis, neurogenic bladder, back pain, gait disturbance, muscular atrophy, or deformity of the foot and calf. The pain may be related to physical exercise and progression of the disorder sometimes leads to loss of sphincter control and spastic paraparesis. The physiopathology of the progression of the symptomatology (17) is related to the normal movement of the spinal cord with activity, especially with hyperflexion which is prevented by the presence of a septum. This may lead to spinal cord damage not only via a direct pressure phenomenon but also by traction interfering with the vascular supply to the cord. The condition may sometimes appear to be of no clinical significance in a patient with normal neurological function, but it is not rare to see a patient who has been considered to be stable deteriorate later on in life following a relatively minor injury to the back or surgery such as correction of scoliosis or other procedures requiring spinal manipulation. The variety of diastematomyelia that is most clinically significant is the one in which a bony, fibrous, or cartilaginous septum is found with a sleeve of dura intervening between the two hemicords.

Virtually all of these patients will have significant spinal deformity with scoliosis which is accompanied by other vertebral anomalies such as hemivertebrae and spina bifida.

On radiological examination only about half of the plain x-rays of the spine will reveal the septum which, as mentioned before, usually lies between T12 and L4. The diagnostic procedures of choice at the present time are metrizamide-enhanced CT scan and MRI; the latter may be difficult to interpret because of the presence of curvature of the spine. Nevertheless, on MRI studies the two halves of the cord can be clearly seen and the relationship of the septum to the cleft can be identified. Special attention should be given to investigating the whole of the spinal cord since secondary malformations, such as thickened filum terminale with tethering of the spinal cord distally, are frequently present. An acquired Arnold Chiari type of malformation may also be seen.

Absolute indications for surgical removal (13) of the septum include progression of neurological deficit and as a preliminary prophylactic operation prior to scoliosis surgery. Prophylactic surgery should also be considered if there is radiological evidence that the septum is actually encroaching on the lowermost portion of the cleft

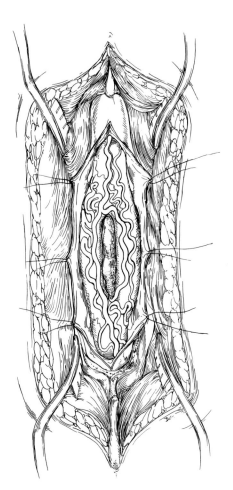

FIG. 6. Diastematomyelia, surgical view.

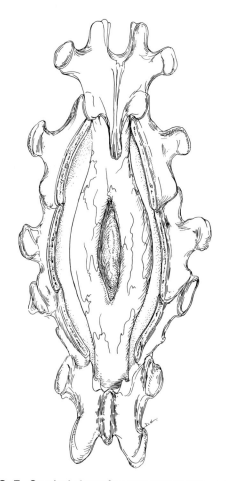

FIG. 7. Surgical view after removal of bony spur.

and/or if the patient is subject to repeated trauma to the spinal canal.

The surgical procedure involves laminectomy above and below the site of the septum (Fig. 6). This is followed by the removal of the septum and the dural cuff that surrounds it using fine rongeurs and the high-speed drill under magnification (Fig. 7). The septum is removed until it is flush with the anterior aspect of the spinal canal. It is usually not necessary or possible to close the anterior dura, but the posterior dura opening should be closed in a watertight fashion using a dural patch when necessary. If a thickened filum terminale is present, which is relatively common, a secondary laminectomy or laminotomy may be necessary to detach it from the spinal dura.

Neuroenteric Cysts

The same embryological abnormality that produces diastematomyelia can theoretically result in herniated ectoderm, which can differentiate into a neuroenteric cyst (8). Specifically, if the notocord is split and herniation of the yolk sac or primitive intestinal cavity occurs along with migration of mesenchymal elements through the neural plate, such an anomaly would result. Neuroenteric cysts are masses in the intramedullary or intradural extramedullary space, most commonly occurring in the ventral thoracic spinal canal, which may cause spinal cord compression. The posterior elements of the vertebrae are usually intact, but cases have been reported where the neuroenteric cyst has herniated through the ectoderm and these are visible on the back of the patient. Radiological examination will reveal a mass either in the posterior mediastinum or posterior mesenteric region with a second cystic component in the spinal canal. These rare entities require surgical removal of the mass which consists of drainage of the cyst and removal of the cyst wall.

Congenital Dermal Sinus Tract

This anomaly consists of an epithelium-lined tract extending from the skin to various depths toward the spinal canal and spinal cord (12). The tract may end anywhere between the skin and the central canal and it may

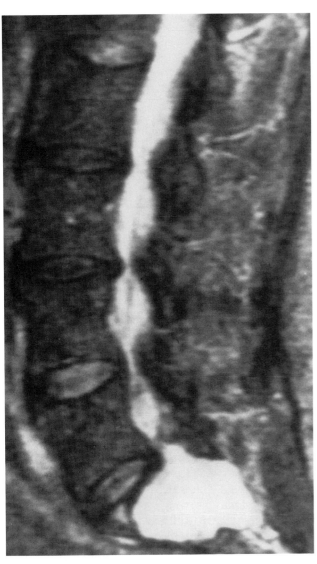

FIG. 8. MRI of anterior sacral meningocele.

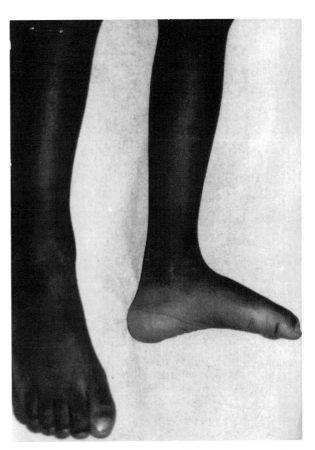

FIG. 9. Orthopedic manifestations of spinal lipoma. Left foot and leg show atrophy and early clawing.

include cysts such as dermoid or epidermoid tumors, or even teratomas. Dermal sinus tracts are sometimes associated with other types of dysraphic states and are most commonly found in the lumbosacral region. They can, however, occur anywhere in the midline, including the scalp. These may present later on in life as infections, including meningitis and intradural or extradural abscess, or as mass lesions compressing the spinal cord or the cauda equina. Plain films may demonstrate the spina bifida occulta but may also be normal (5). MRI will usually clearly demonstrate the tract and will disclose the presence or absence of intraspinal extension, tumors, and related anomalies.

Surgical treatment involves careful dissection of the tract following it cephalad from the skin defect. The surgeon should be prepared to continue the exploration intraspinally and this may necessitate a laminectomy at several levels followed by an intradural exploration of the tract if it is found to be entering the spinal canal. The authors have been surprised sometimes by finding a very large unsuspected intradural tumor which may extend for several segments and require far more complicated operation than was originally anticipated.

Anterior Sacral Meningocele

This is an uncommon form of spina bifida, usually found in an asymptomatic adult. Anterior meningoceles (1) are very uncommonly associated with posterior fusion defects and frequently have no accompanying neurological deficit or cutaneous manifestations (Fig. 8). The sacs herniate anteriorly through a defect in the sacral or lower lumbar spine producing an intrapelvic mass. This will produce pressure on the bladder or rectum and is often exacerbated or brought to the attention of the clinician with the increased intrapelvic congestion of pregnancy, explaining why these problems are usually found in females (16). The symptoms may include constipation, dysmenorrhea, and dysparunia due to pressure on the lumbosacral plexus. Radiologically, the spinal defect will be relatively easily seen on plain films with large portions of the sacrum missing, and CT scan or MRI will demonstrate the large pelvic cyst and bony defect.

The surgical correction involves a posterior approach in which the dural pedicle that connects the sac to the spinal canal is isolated and closed. Sometimes this can become a major surgical challenge since there will be occasional cases of nerve roots actually entering the sac and exiting through an independent dural cuff. This will require individual dural closures around each of the nerve roots prior to the plication and obliteration of the sac itself. Transabdominal or transpelvic procedures are far more dangerous and carry great risk of injury to the nerve roots and the possibility of the introduction of infection and secondary fistulas. Anterior meningoceles

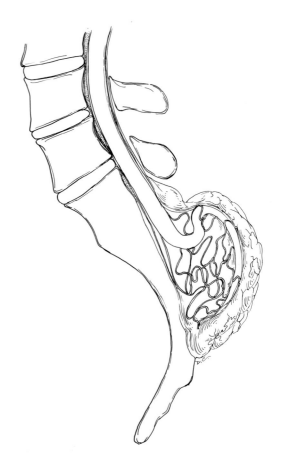

FIG. 10. Spinal lipoma.

rarely can occur at other levels, and in these cases are usually associated with neurofibromatosis.

Spinal Lipomas

By far the most common cause of an adult patient presenting with late onset of symptoms related to occult spinal dysraphism will be found in those harboring so-called spinal lipomas. This disorder has also been called lipomyelomeningocele or lipoma of the cauda equina. Actually, the true anatomic-pathological appearance of this family of anomalies is quite different from what these terms imply, since very seldom will there be herniation of neural elements outside the canal, and the problem is far more complicated than a simple lipoma occurring in the canal. Instead, the anomaly consists of a lipomatous mass which enters the spinal canal and attaches itself not to the nerve roots or to the cauda equina but to the spinal cord, which is itself anomalous in that it extends well into the lumbosacral level of the canal.

The patient with this anomaly presents with the previously-described syndrome (3), either urological, or-

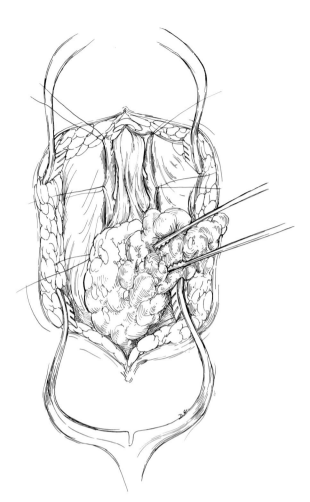

FIG. 11. Spinal lipoma, view at surgery.

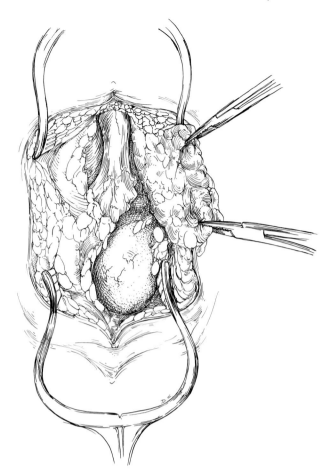

FIG. 12. Surgical repair of spinal lipoma.

thopedic, or neurological in nature or with a combination of these manifestations (Fig. 9). The late onset of symptomatology may be due to traction on the spinal cord or, more likely, compression of the conus medullaris or cauda equina by an increased mass of the lipoma with mechanical distortion and ischemia that will be progressive. While the lipomatous mass itself is a hamartoma and does not increase its number of cells through the life of the patient, the mass can increase in volume by increasing the fat content of each individual cell.

Pathologically, we can describe three types of spinal lipomas (6). The first and simplest are those fibrolipomas of the filum terminale that are attached only to the filum in the intrathecal or extrathecal area and are extremely easy to remove surgically. Unfortunately, they constitute the minority of clinical cases. The second type is the fibrolipoma of the dura mater in which the mass attaches to the coverings of the spinal canal but not to the neural structures. Again, this is a relatively unusual presentation. By far the most common presentation, and one that presents the most challenge to the operating surgeon, is that of leptomyelolipoma in which the fatty mass in the subcutaneous tissue penetrates through a de-

fect in the lumbar fascia through the bony spine and dura to insert into the spinal cord itself, usually at the level of the conus medullaris. The lipoma may insert at either the caudal aspect of the conus, with a relatively well defined interface between lipoma and neural elements, or it may insert into the dorsal aspect of the spinal cord with neural elements ventral to the fatty mass. This latter situation again produces confusion in the interpretation of the radiological studies and at the time of surgery, since at first glance it appears that the nerve roots are actually coming through the fatty tissue. In our experience, this is not the case and there is an interface between fat and neural tissue that can be found with careful investigation.

The radiological investigation of choice at the present time is MRI of the spine which will demonstrate not only the subcutaneous lipoma but the site of its entrance into the spinal canal, the amount of fatty tissue within the canal, and the site of its attachment to the spinal cord. MRI will also help the surgeon in planning his approach to the release of the lipoma since it will define the number of segments above the entrance of the canal that need to be investigated to find the interface with the neural tissue and will give an idea of the nature of attachment of the lipoma to the spinal cord. Other useful techniques include CT scan with or without metrizamide and ultrasonography, particularly in the young patient.

The goals of surgery are to untether the spinal cord (4) from the lipoma and from the thickened filum terminale if this is present. Also, by decreasing the mass of the lipoma, direct compression of the spinal cord will be relieved (Figs. 10, 11, and 12). At the time of surgery, somatosensory evoked potentials are useful in determining the amount of lipoma removal that is safe. Magnification and laser are useful in detaching the lipoma from the spinal cord without interfering with neural function.

It is of utmost importance to close the dura mater in a watertight fashion, since one of the major complications in this operation is CSF leakage. The spinal canal must be reconstructed with sufficient room for the neural elements to move within the canal and to prevent retethering by allowing CSF to cover all of the neural elements. If necessary, a dural graft is employed to provide a sufficiently capacious dural sac to effect these surgical goals.

LATE ONSET OF SYMPTOMS IN PATIENTS WITH PREVIOUSLY REPAIRED MYELOMENINGOCELE

The most common cause of delayed deterioration in a patient with myelomeningocele is that of retethering of the spinal cord at the site of previous surgery. Symptoms and signs of this phenomenon include back or leg pain, increasing motor or sensory deficit, a change in the bladder or bowel pattern, progressive orthopedic deformity of the lower extremities, increasing spasticity, or progressive scoliosis. As most patients with myelomeningocele will have anatomic and radiographic tethering of the placode, and because of the difficulty in differentiating progressive orthopedic changes from those due to a static neurogenic imbalance, the role of surgical untethering in these cases has remained somewhat controversial. Nonetheless, there are clearly some patients in whom progressive symptoms appear to stabilize and occasionally improve after the cord is untethered and the spinal canal is reconstructed.

The surgical procedure involves identifying the normal spinal cord above the level of the placode and disconnecting the placode from adherent scar tissue. The canal is then reconstructed with care taken to allow for an adequate CSF space around the terminal cord. The actual spinal level of the neural elements does not usually change as a result of surgery, but improvement is thought to be due to lessening of the chronic ischemic and traction injury to which the cord is subjected during movement.

It should be noted that in cases in which scoliosis surgery has been performed without untethering of the cord, impaction of the hindbrain at the level of the

Chiari malformation has been reported. For this reason, untethering of the cord at the time of a major scoliosis procedure is recommended.

The Chiari malformation itself can cause symptoms later in life. These can include occipital headaches, progressive lower cranial nerve dysfunction including voice changes and chronic aspiration, weakness and numbness of the upper extremities, and progressive myelopathy. Several surgical procedures have been recommended including bony decompression alone, dural opening, and plugging of the obex, but in each the goal is to reduce the mechanical compression at the level of the cervicomedullary junction. It should be noted that hydrocephalus may exacerbate symptoms referable to the Chiari malformation, so shunt function should always be tested prior to planning posterior fossa decompression. In some cases, maximizing shunt function will obviate the need for posterior fossa surgery.

Another problem that can develop in these patients is syringomyelia. This may occur at any level and, in fact, may extend into the brain stem as syringobulbia. Presentation is usually with motor and sensory changes and sometimes pain referable to the level of the syrinx. As syringomyelia often occurs in association with the Chiari malformation, surgical correction may include an approach to both problems with posterior fossa decompression and wicking or shunting of the syrinx cavity. Sometimes a terminal syrinx will occur near the site of a tethered cord and these two problems may be approached at the same operation as well. For large symptomatic syrinxes we prefer a syringopleural shunt as the negative intrathoracic pressure promotes drainage of the low-pressure syrinx cavity.

It is not uncommon for a patient with myelomeningocele to lose functional abilities very gradually, without ever presenting with a specific acute complaint. While it may sometimes be difficult to pinpoint which anatomic abnormality in these complicated patients is contributing to which aspect of the functional decline, careful clinical and radiographic follow-up and appropriate intervention may prevent the deterioration that is too often seen in these patients as they reach adolescence and adulthood.

REFERENCES

1. Amacher AL, Drake CG, McLachlin AD (1968): Anterior sacral meningocele. *Surg Gyn Obstet* 126:986–994.
2. Brophy JD, Sutton LN, Zimmerman RA, et al (1989): Magnetic resonance imaging of lipomyelomeningocele and tethered cord. *Neurosurg* 25(3):336–340.
3. Bruce DA, Schut L (1979): Spinal lipomas of infancy and childhood. *Childs Brain* 5:192–203.
4. Chapman PH (1982): Congenital intraspinal lipomas: Anatomic considerations and surgical treatment. *Childs Brain* 9:37–47.
5. Cheek WR, Laurent JP (1986): Dermal sinus tracts. In: *Concepts in pediatric neurosurgery, vol. 6.* New York: Karger, pp. 63–75.
6. Emery JL, Lendon RG (1969): Lipomas of the cauda equina and

other fatty tumours related to neurospinal dysraphism. *Dev Med Child Neurol* [Suppl] 20:62–70.

7. Fitz CR, Harwood-Nash DC (1975): The tethered conus. *Am J Roentgenol* 125:515–523.

8. French BN (1982): Midline fusion defects and defects of formation. In: Youmanns JR, ed. *Neurological surgery, 2nd ed.* Philadelphia: Saunders, pp. 1346–1350.

9. Guthkelch AN, Jones RA, Zierski J (1971). Diastematomyelia. *Dev Med Child Neurol* [Suppl] 13(25):137–138.

10. Hoffman HJ, Hendrick EB, Humphreys RP (1976): The tethered spinal cord: Its protean manifestations, diagnosis and surgical correction. *Childs Brain* 2:145–155.

11. James CC, Lassman LP (1960): Spinal dysraphism. *Arch Dis Child* 35:315–327.

12. Matson DD, Jerva MJ (1966): Recurrent meningitis associated with congenital lumbosacral dermal sinus tract. *J Neurosurg* 25:288–297.

13. Meacham WF (1967): Surgical treatment of diastematomyelia. *J Neurosurg* 27:78–85.

14. Pang D, Wilberger JE Jr (1982): Tethered cord syndrome in adults. *J Neurosurg* 57:32–47.

15. Schut L, Pizzi F, Bruce DA (1977): Occult spinal dysraphism. In: McLaurin RL, ed. *Myelomeningocele.* New York: Grune & Stratton, pp. 349–368.

16. Villarejo F, Scavone C, Blazquez MG, et al (1983): Anterior sacral meningocele: Review of the literature. *Surg Neurol* 19:57–71.

17. Yamada S, Zinke DE, Sanders D (1981): Pathophysiology of "tethered cord syndrome." *J Neurosurg* 54:494–503.

Degenerative Conditions of the Spine
Diagnosis and Treatment

The Adult Spine: Principles and Practice,
J. W. Frymoyer, Editor-in-Chief.
Raven Press, Ltd., New York © 1991.

CHAPTER 80

Radiculopathies: Lumbar Disc Herniation and Recess Stenosis

Patient Selection, Predictors of Success and Failure, and Non-Surgical Treatment Options

John W. Frymoyer

The basic objective for any musculoskeletal operation is to relieve pain, reduce deformity, and improve function. In the lumbar spine, the general methods available to achieve these goals are decompression and/or stabilization. The basic principles of lumbar fusion were developed by Hibbs and Albee in 1911 (1,28), but the real impetus for modern lumbar spinal surgery was Mixter and Barr's 1934 description (48) of the clinical syndrome and surgical treatment of lumbar intervertebral disc her-

J. W. Frymoyer, M.D.: Professor of Orthopaedics, Director, McClure Musculoskeletal Research Center, Department of Orthopaedics and Rehabilitation, University of Vermont, Burlington, Vermont, 05405.

niation. Fifty years later one of the first patients operated on by those surgeons was reevaluated (16). As part of the case report, a quote from Dr. Mixter was presented:

> Newton is of particular historic interest because he represents the first case where the lumbar intervertebral disk was recognized as the cause of symptoms. . . . As such he is the man who started the whole mess.

Clearly, Mixter was expressing his concern about the over-utilization and complications of surgical disc excision in the management of low back pain and sciatica.

In this chapter, the general indications for operative treatment of lumbar spine diseases are reviewed. This is from the perspectives of epidemiology, the determinants of success and failure, and the alternatives for non-operative treatment. The basic message is: Successful lumbar spine surgery requires an unequivocal, pathologic causation, where clinical symptoms and signs are congruous with carefully selected imaging studies in a patient who is not unduly influenced by psychosocial circumstances, or whose surgical outcome will produce better results than the "natural history" of the disease process itself. Violation of this principle is the dominant cause of failure, rather than failure to choose the right operation from the wide menu of decompression and stabilization procedures currently available to the spinal surgeon.

EPIDEMIOLOGY OF LUMBAR SPINE SURGERY

The reported lifetime incidence of lumbar spine surgery varies from country to country and ranges from 1% to 3%. The lower incidence figures are reported from Scandinavia and Great Britain, while the highest annual rates are recorded in the United States. Pokras and associates (51) report that 69.5 Americans/100,000 population undergo a lumbar disc excision each year. Another calculation estimates the annual incidence of disc excision to be 71/100,000 with an additional 31/100,000 patients who have spinal stabilization (15,53). By comparison, the annual rate of disc excision in Finland is 41/100,000 while in the United Kingdom the figure for disc excision and fusion is 10/100,000. However, these figures reveal only part of the issue; Kane (35) has estimated as much as a ten-fold regional variation across the United States in the annual incidence of lumbar spine surgery. Furthermore, there is some evidence that the surgical treatment of the lumbar spine is increasing as shown in Figure 1 (53).

How can we explain as much as a ten-fold variation between countries, and a far greater difference between some parts of the United States and European countries? Epidemiologic data demonstrate no significant difference in the incidence and point prevalence of sciatica and low back pain between countries or regions of the United States. Although occupational factors are related

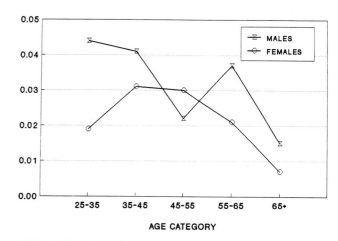

FIG. 2. Data have been analyzed from the NHANES II survey, a national survey of non-institutionalized and non-military United States adult population. The percentage of population in a given age category who have undergone lumbar surgery is shown. For example, the prevalence of surgery in males age 25 to 35 is 4.4%, while in females over age 65 the prevalence is 1.5% (Cats-Baril W, Frymoyer JW, unpublished data).

to an increased risk of sciatica or severe low back pain, national and regional differences in occupation are unlikely to explain such large variations.

Greater insight into the likely causation is derived from Wennberg's studies of regional variations in the utilization of surgical procedures (64). He reports elective operations such as carpal tunnel decompression, hysterectomy, prostatectomy, and tonsillectomy have as much as ten-fold regional variations in their use. The common factors of these procedures are that they are elective, they are used for the relief of non-life threatening conditions, and there is no clear medical consensus for their indications. In comparison, the rate of operation remains constant between regions when there is clear consensus about the indications and benefits of surgery. A good example of the latter is the operative management of a fractured hip in the elderly, where surgical rates are quite uniform. Wennberg (64) has concluded that the major determinant for operative intervention is based on the surgeon's personal preference and regionally accepted standards of care, rather than variations in disease incidence. This would seem to be the most likely reason for the differences in lumbar surgery, a perspective supported by newer analyses of lumbar decompression in the state of Maine (36).

There is also some evidence that the choice for surgical intervention relates to other demographic and occupational determinants, rather than to strict medical indications. We have analyzed the NHANES (7) (National Health and Nutrition Examination Survey), which represents a United States population-based survey, representative of the non-institutionalized, non-military population of this country (11). Figures 2, 3, and 4 present data

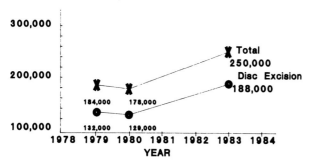

FIG. 1. The rate of lumbar spinal surgery is given including total lumbar operations, as well as operations specifically for lumbar disc herniation (adapted with permission from ref. 53).

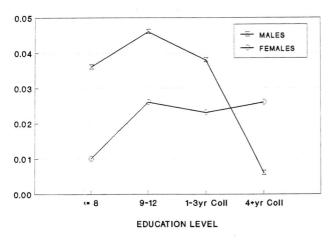

FIG. 3. The prevalence rate of lumbar spinal surgery is stratified for males and females as a function of educational level. Note the highest rates are in the mid-range of educational background (Cats-Baril W, Frymoyer JW, unpublished data).

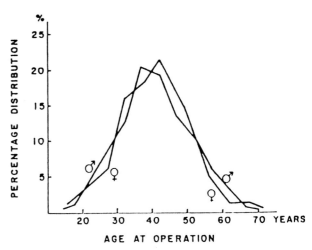

FIG. 5. The age of lumbar spinal surgery for males and females is depicted. Note this figure is derived from a study of patients undergoing surgery and indicates the peak years are in the early part of the fifth decade of life (with permission from ref. 55).

for this population sample and demonstrate the wide variation in the prevalence of lumbar spinal surgery as a function of education, income level, and age. Some of these differences are partially explained by the epidemiology and natural history of spinal disease. For example, the age relationships observed are the result of the age at which lumbar disc herniation most commonly occurs. Spangfort (55) has meticulously reviewed over 10,000 lumbar disc excisions culled from the world's literature. His results (Fig. 5) demonstrate that peak prevalence of the operation is at age 42 for both men and women. In addition, there may be other interactions that indirectly explain some of the variation seen in Figures 2, 3, and 4. For example, heavy occupation, lower income, and less education would be expected to interact and be covariates.

Based on all of these data, it appears that lumbar surgical prevalence and incidence are highly variable. This suggests that many factors participate in the operative decision, independent of the patient's symptoms or disease process.

THE MEASURE OF SUCCESS AND FAILURE IN LUMBAR SPINAL SURGERY

There are three broad measures of success and failure: How well did the patient fare after the operation? What were the requirements for further operation or treatment of complications? And how would the patient have fared if the surgery had not been performed? In a society that is concerned about health care costs, it is likely the cost-benefit ratio will be imposed in the future as another significant measure of success.

HOW WELL DO PATIENTS FARE AFTER LUMBAR SURGERY?

The goal of lumbar spinal operations is usually to relieve pain and improve function, rather than to reduce deformity, with the exception of the subset of adult patients with significant post-traumatic, developmental, or acquired postural deformities. If the objectives of pain relief and improved function are met, the operation should be termed successful. However, it is surprising how often functional criteria are not included as part of published reviews of lumbar surgery and how much the measure of function influences the surgical result. To determine the effects of outcome criteria on surgical results, a comparison was made of patients who had undergone lumbar disc excision and lumbar disc excision

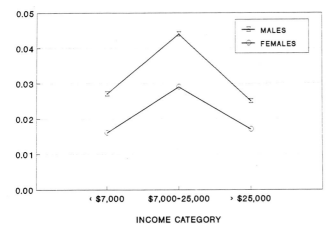

FIG. 4. The prevalence rate of lumbar spinal surgery is stratified for males and females as a function of family income level. The highest rates are in those with incomes of $7,000 to $25,000 (Cats-Baril W, Frymoyer JW, unpublished data).

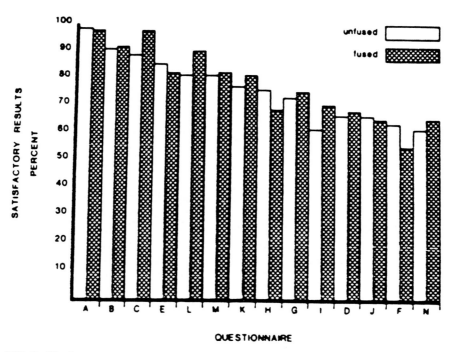

FIG. 6. The long-term results from discectomy with or without fusion in 207 patients have been manipulated by utilizing 14 published criteria for success or failure. Note the wide variation in results that occurs simply as a function of questionnaire format (with permission from ref. 31).

combined with fusion 10 or more years after the operation (31). As part of this analysis, a questionnaire was designed which included 14 previously published outcome measures for lumbar disc operations. Thus, a comparison was being made of the same patient group, where only the criteria for success were varied. Figures 6 and 7 present these results. It is apparent there are statistically significant differences in surgical results, produced solely by the measures used to classify "satisfactory" and "unsatisfactory" outcomes. The best results were obtained with those outcome measures based on patient satisfaction, less favorable results were based on reduced pain, and the least favorable results included functional criteria, usually determined by return to work. Thus, using various outcome measures can effectuate significantly different interpretation of surgical results.

COMPLICATIONS AND NEED FOR FURTHER SURGERY

Another measure of success or failure is the need for subsequent surgery or the prevalence of operative complications, which may produce symptoms of greater severity or morbidity than the original condition. The need for further surgery following lumbar disc excision ranges from 5% to 15% (14). It is uncertain whether these different failure rates represent variations in surgical technique, different surveillance methods, or different duration of follow-up evaluation. Moreover, the sources of failure are somewhat different in the various published operative follow-up studies (14). Some studies indicate the dominant need for re-operation is the failure to recog-

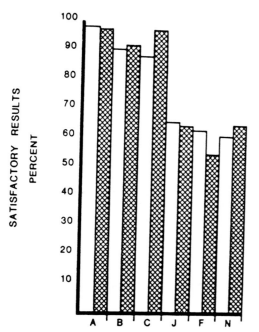

FIG. 7. The highest and lowest outcome measures are compared for the questionnaire survey depicted in Figure 6. Note that when these extremes are compared, a significant difference occurs (p = 0.01) (with permission from ref. 31).

nize lateral nerve root canal stenosis (5), or the failure to identify a co-existent instability (21). Others report the dominant source of failure is recurrent disc herniation, or that symptoms result from ongoing spinal degeneration (14).

The other significant causes of operative failure are true perioperative complications. Again, there is wide variation in the reported prevalence of these complications, which will be discussed in detail in Chapters 89 and 98.

NATURAL HISTORY OF SCIATICA: RESULTS OF NON-OPERATIVE TREATMENT

The third issue is how the patient would have fared if surgery had not been performed. Since most published operative reports do not include a non-surgical control or comparison group, this question is unanswerable for many of the pathologic conditions which serve as the broad operative indications for lumbar spine surgery. Colonna (8) made the first attempt to introduce a comparison group into the analysis of surgical results of lumbar disc excision. He retrospectively studied a small sample of patients with clinical symptoms, signs, and myelograms confirmatory of lumbar disc herniation. At an average follow-up interval of 2.7 years (range 1–8 years), 60% of the surgically treated group were pain free, and all but 13% were satisfied with their care. In the comparison (non-surgical) group, 29% were pain free and 32% were dissatisfied with their care. He concluded surgical intervention favorably influenced the natural history of lumbar disc herniation. A more comprehensive retrospective review was undertaken by Hakelius

(23), whose study included 166 patients who underwent surgery and 417 patients who were treated non-operatively. Figure 8 demonstrates the return to work and shows a slower rate initially in the operatively treated group, but an improved functional recovery 6 months later. He conducted a longer-term analysis of these patients with an average observation interval of 7 years, 4 months (range 3 to 13 years). There appeared to be little difference between the treatment and comparison group with respect to muscle paresis and sensory losses. In the non-operated comparison group, 77% had no motor symptoms and only 6% had significant complaints. However, physicial examination revealed 16% of the comparison group had continued objective evidence of what Hakelius termed "more extensive paresis" and 39% had continued evidence of great toe paresis. Similarly, sensory symptoms were identified in only 6%, while 72% had no sensory complaints. These figures were not significantly different from the surgically treated cohort. Recurrent sciatica occurred in 12% of the operated and comparison group; the occurrence of later disability was also similar.

A longer term retrospective comparison of surgically and non-surgically treated American World War II veterans was conducted by Nashold and Hrubec (49). From a cohort of 4,872 individuals treated from 1944 to 1945, they were able to identify a representative subset of 1,123 patients treated for sciatica, of which 395 had disc excision. Seventy percent of the patients were available 20 years later. During the 20-year interval, almost 50% of the surgically and non-surgically treated patients had changed jobs because of back problems. An equivalent degree of "disability" by clinical examination was identified in both groups. A second operation was required in

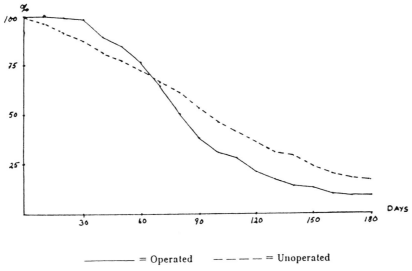

FIG. 8. The recovery from an acute episode of sciatica due to lumbar disc herniation, treated with or without surgery, is depicted. The outcome criterion used in this study was return to work (with permission from ref. 23).

TABLE 1. *Treatment after randomization—One year assessment (N = 126)*

Result	Conservative treatment			Operation		
	Remained in original group[1]	Operation	Total[2]	Operated as planned[1]	Not operated	Total[2]
Good	16	8	24	39	0	39
Fair	24	4	28	15	1	16
Poor	9	4	13	5	0	5
Bad	0	1	1	0	0	0
Total	49	17	66	59	1	60

Table shows the assessment of the results of conservative and operative treatment of patients with myelographically proven lumbar disc herniation one year after the randomization (with permission from ref. 62).
[1] Remained in original group/operated as planned: Chi-square for trend (1 d.f.) = 10.16, p = 0.0015.
[2] Total randomized material: Chi-square for trend in proportions, equidistant scoring of groups (1 d.f.) = 10.24, p = 0.0015.

14.7% of the surgically treated patients, and 13.9% of the non-surgically treated cohorts. They concluded that surgical intervention had little long-term impact. The major criticism of this study is the comparison of veterans to the civilian population.

These retrospective analyses have been followed by Weber's (62) classic prospective controlled study. He analyzed patients presenting with unequivocal clinical symptoms and signs of sciatica due to lumbar disc herniation confirmed by myelographic evaluation. Prior to the initial randomization, patients with severe muscle paresis, who were not improving with conservative management, were excluded from the study. Of the 280 patients presenting to him, 67 (25%) had significant muscle weakness or unrelenting pain and were surgically treated. Another 87 patients showed continuous improvement during the hospitalization and elected ongoing conservative treatment. The remaining 126 patients were randomized to the conservative treatment group, which was 6 weeks of physiotherapy and education, or to conventional disc excision without fusion. The follow-up interval has been extended to 10 years. These data are presented in Tables 1 and 2. The overall conclusion reached from this study is that surgical decompression of a herniated lumbar disc has the beneficial effect of earlier relief of sciatica and the initial period of disability. After 4 years, surgery does not influence the results with respect to recurrent symptoms or disability. Restoration of muscle weakness was similar in both groups; 20 patients at 4 years, and 5 patients at 10 years had residual weakness. Thirty-five percent of both patient groups had residual numbness at the final, 10-year evaluation.

The conclusion reached by these studies is that surgical intervention reduces the period of symptoms of disability in the patients with appropriate indications for surgery. In turn, the key element for success is patient selection, which must be analyzed with respect to the pathologic condition being treated, the operation chosen to treat that pathology, and the patient characteristics, the most important of which are psychosocial function and workers' compensation. In short, the "natural history" of a disease should be the standard by which surgical success is judged. Only when we know that we can improve upon the natural history can we be certain of our surgical indications.

INDICATIONS BASED ON PATHOLOGY

Intervertebral disc herniation is the most common indication for lumbar surgery; three-quarters of all pres-

TABLE 2. *Treatment results in randomized group—Ten years assessment*

Result	Conservative treatment			Operation		
	Remained in original group[1]	Operation	Total[2]	Operated as planned[1]	Not operated	Total[2]
Good	27	10	37	34	1	35
Fair	18	7	25	16	0	16
Poor	4	0	4	4	0	4
Bad	0	0	0	0	0	0
Total	49	17	66	54	1	55
Died	0	0	0	3	0	3
Not examined	0	0	0	2	0	2
Total	49	17	66	59	1	60

Table shows the assessment of the results of conservative and operative treatment of patients with myelographically proven lumbar disc herniation ten years after the randomization (with permission from ref. 62).
[1] Remained in original group/operated as planned: Chi-square for trend (1 d.f.) = 2.56.
[2] Total randomized material: Chi-square for trend (1 d.f.) = 1.76.

ently performed lumbar spine operations are for this condition (53). There is also the greatest knowledge regarding positive and adverse selection factors in the treatment of lumbar disc herniae. There is little debate about the absolute indications for lumbar disc excision when the patient presents with a cauda equina syndrome. This condition affects 0.24% to 2% of patients with a known lumbar disc herniation and is viewed as a surgical emergency (39,55). From 5% to 20% of these patients will present with significant and progressive muscle paresis or unrelenting severe pain (23,24,62). Although Hakelius and Hindmarsh (24) showed delays up to 3 months had a minimal effect on the ultimate recovery of strength, most surgeons advocate earlier surgery when it is apparent improvement is not occurring. Thus, 5% to 20% of patients present with reasonably unequivocal indications for their operation.

The majority of patients with lumbar disc herniation, however, have as their dominant complaints pain and varying degrees of functional limitation, rather than significant neuromuscular dysfunction. The earliest attempts to analyze the predictors of success in this later group of patients with lumbar disc herniation was performed by Hirsch and Nachemson (29) and Spangfort (55). Hirsch and Nachemson evaluated the predictive value of the pre-operative clinical symptoms and signs and myelographic imaging. Their results are presented in Tables 3 and 4 and demonstrate that the more certain the diagnosis of disc herniation, the greater the probability of success. Spangfort reached essentially the same conclusion in his studies. Further analyses indicate the following factors are important determinants of success.

Clinical History

The patient has an unequivocal history of sciatica, defined as pain radiating in the distribution of a lumbar dermatome, below the level of the knee, accompanied by one or more neuromuscular complaints such as weakness or sensory loss. A dominant complaint of low back pain or atypical sciatica are poor indications.

TABLE 3. *Outcome of lumbar disc surgery as a function of intraoperative findings*

Operative findings	Unimproved or poor
Prolapses	4% (8/179)
Root adhesions	27% (4/15)
Negative	32% (12/38)

Table compares surgical success rate as a function of operative findings. Note that far superior results are obtained when unequivocal surgical findings of disc prolapse are present and a high percentage of poor results occurs when findings are negative or equivocal (with permission from ref. 29).

TABLE 4. *Predictive value of the pre-operative physical findings to the operative finding of disc prolapse*

	Number of patients	Incidence of prolapses
Neurologically positive, Lasègue negative	20	55%
Neurologically positive, Lasègue positive	155	86%
Neurologically positive, Lasègue positive	43	66%
Neurologically negative, Lasègue negative	14	43%

Table demonstrates the importance of pre-operative findings in predicting the likelihood of disc prolapse (with permission from ref. 29).

Clinical Signs

The patient has unequivocal physical signs, of which nerve root tension signs are the most predictive. A straight leg raising test (SLR) is less confirmatory of lumbar disc herniation as the angle necessary to produce sciatica increases. Below a level of 30 degrees, the SLR is highly predictive, above 50 degrees its diagnostic significance is reduced (54,59). The reproduction of pain in the symptomatic extremity upon elevation of the well extremity (a contralateral SLR) is highly specific for herniation (54). Among other physical signs, the hierarchy of predictive value is in order of decreasing importance (reflex asymmetry, motor weakness, sensory loss). In combination, physical signs are accurate in predicting the presence of a disc herniation in 75% of patients presenting with sciatica, but are less predictive of the precise level of the herniation (24).

Imaging Studies

The issues regarding imaging sensitivity, specificity, and predictive value have been presented in other chapters. A summary of this information is presented in Table 5. Asymptomatic "volunteer" populations also demonstrate 30% to 40% significant pathology, including disc herniations when they are subjected to myelogra-

TABLE 5. *Diagnostic sensitivity and specificity of commonly used imaging studies compared for the evaluation of lumbar disc herniation*

Diagnostic test	Sensitivity	Specificity
CT scanning	0.92	0.88
Metrizamide myelography	0.90	0.87
Iophendylate myelography	0.80	0.90
Discography	0.83	0.78
Epidural venography	0.87	0.70
Electromyography	0.92	0.38

With permission from ref. 32.

phy, CT scans, and magnetic resonance imaging (3,39,65). The fundamental conclusion is that imaging studies are only as predictive as they confirm the clinical signs and symptoms. The decision for operative intervention should be based primarily on the basis of history and physical examination. Imaging studies are primarily confirmatory and to exclude other causes of sciatica (i.e., tumor).

INDICATIONS FOR SPECIFIC OPERATIONS IN LUMBAR DISC HERNIATION

A wide menu of operative approaches can be used to treat lumbar disc herniation. The basic question is "Does the choice of operation influence the results obtained?" Because there are no controlled prospective studies comparing surgical alternatives, comparison of results for the treatment of the same condition is not possible.

The so-called "gold standard" in the surgical management of lumbar disc herniation is the intralaminal approach with minimum sacrifice of bone structures as presented by Spengler in Chapter 84. The treatment alternatives include chemonucleolysis with chymopapain, percutaneous discectomy, and microdiscectomy.

Nordby will present the comparative results for chymopapain in Chapter 81. The conclusion is that the results for chymopapain are slightly less predictable than surgical excision. Low back pain is a significant problem in 20% to 30% of patients treated by chymopapain for intervals up to 6 weeks. There are a small number of catastrophic neurologic and allergic complications which can be avoided by proper technique and pre-operative treatment. In the longer term, the results of chymopapain and surgery appear similar. Weinstein and associates performed a 10-year follow-up survey of patients undergoing the two alternative treatments. Although there were significant selection biases in the two cohorts, the results appeared similar based upon elegant functional and clinical criteria. In conclusion chymopapain remains a viable treatment option for surgeons who use the technique regularly and for younger patients with contained lumbar discs and no element of spinal stenosis. A more interesting question is whether or not there are benefits to the regained disc space height that follows chymopapain. It has been shown in experimental animals (22) and in human studies that chymopapain produces an initial reduction of disc space height followed by restoration. In comparison, patients who have undergone lumbar disc excision virtually always demonstrate disc space narrowing that persists (18).

Percutaneous discectomy is evolving, but at present there are insufficient data to assess its long-term results. Mooney in Chapter 82 addresses the basic issue of how removal of 4 to 6 grams of nuclear material can influence radiculopathy, particularly when the later CT and MRI studies show little or no change in the geometry and size of the protrusion. This suggests that radicular pain may largely be the consequence of other biochemical or neurologic mediators, rather than dominantly a result of the size of the compressive lesion. Non-controlled and short-term comparisons of the results of percutaneous discectomy and standard surgical decompression suggest the results are less predictable with the percutaneous technique. The notion that the hole of entry of the cutting tool will provide a future escape for recurrent herniations is unlikely, based upon in vitro biomechanical studies (44). The technique appears contraindicated when a sequestered fragment is associated with the radiculopathy; this possibility is best determined by MRI. Percutaneous discectomy is a viable alternative in patients with non-sequestered lumbar disc lesions, and in the short-term has less predictable results, which are less favorable than routine discectomy. Offsetting this disadvantage should be the shorter duration of treatment and recovery.

Microdiscectomy (see Chapter 83) has many advocates who emphasize the major benefit is stronger illumination of the operative field and less morbidity because of the smaller incision. Additional benefits cited are reduced scarring and more rapid recovery (67). Detractors of this technique cite an increased risk of missing significant pathology, operating at the wrong level, a higher rate of recurrence, and a higher infection rate. Presently, there is little information to prove the additive benefits or risks, other than that return-to-work rate and duration of hospitalization appear similar when this technique is compared to the traditional surgical techniques (46). Moreover, the technique advocated by McCulloch in Chapter 83 has a significant learning curve and is not a technique for the occasional spinal surgeon. His technique is also very different from the use of the microscope after standard surgical incision and intralaminal exposure.

Regardless of the technique used, there appears to be little benefit to attempting to remove more than the obviously sequestered fragments. The notion one can totally excise the disc is unfounded. Even under controlled laboratory circumstances no more than 30% of the nucleus is routinely removed (6).

The other issue is the use of fusion as an adjunct to lumbar disc excision. Mixter and Barr (48) believed disc herniation was the manifestation of a structural weakness, where continued deterioration would inevitably follow. They logically surmised correction of the structural weakness would reduce that risk. Subsequently, the benefits of the "combined operation" have been debated ad nauseum. The data suggest minimal added benefit for fusion in the surgical management of patients who have monoradiculopathy due to lumbar disc herniation, with respect to future back pain or need for further operation.

There is no doubt recurrent disc herniations under a sound spinal fusion are rare (17,18), but this positive effect does not reduce the need for further operation. The major source of short-term failure is pseudarthrosis, although the presence of this defect in spinal radiographs does not necessarily predict clinical failure (18). In the longer term, patients with fusion are at greater risk for symptoms due to changes at the intervertebral level adjacent to their fusion, including the development of spinal stenosis, with or without degenerative instability. However, the radiographic appearance of instability and stenosis occurs far more often than symptoms. Lehmann and associates (43) analyzed patients 20 or more years following their fusion and observed radiographic evidence of instability and stenosis in 40%, but few had clinical symptoms. Similarly, flexion-extension radiographic evaluation of patients who underwent L4-S1 fusions an average of 13.7 years previously (range 10 to 20 years) showed 20% fulfilled Knutsson's (38) criteria for instability, but only 5% were symptomatic (18). More distressing has been the observation that the relief of low back pain was equivalent whether or not fusion was performed, and that the results of repeat operations were less satisfactory when the first operation had included a fusion (17,19).

OTHER FACTORS THAT INFLUENCE RESULTS AND PATIENT SELECTION

Age

There is little compelling information to suggest age as a major determinant in the success of lumbar disc excision, although it influences the level of the herniation (55).

Sex

The older literature suggested females have less favorable outcomes, particularly when the operation is performed at an older age. Other surveys show little difference (17). However, there is no doubt that a female with a lumbar disc herniation is less likely to be hospitalized or treated surgically than her male counterpart, but the reasons for this difference are unclear (37,55,58).

Level of Spinal Pathology

The results for L4-L5 disc excision are variously reported to be less favorable than L5-S1, although this finding is by no means uniform. One explanation given is that the L4-L5 level is at greater risk for instability (21). There is little question that the radiographic criterion of instability, i.e., a positive Knutsson's sign, is found commonly when L4-L5 disc excision has been performed previously and the female is selectively at risk (18). However, the radiographic finding is minimally associated with any increased risk of low back pain or recurrent sciatica and the issue is debatable.

Adjunctive Treatments

Basic animal research demonstrates that interpositional free-fat grafts (40,42,47,69) prevent later epidural scarring, but clinical investigations have not yet rigorously proven the efficacy of this treatment method. However, one additional factor does appear to be of major importance when fusion is part of the surgical procedure: Brown (4) has shown that L4 to sacrum, posterolateral fusion is 90% in non-smokers, while radiographic evidence of successful fusion is only 60% in smokers.

INDICATIONS BASED ON NON-MEDICAL FACTORS

Up to this point, this chapter has focused on the organic pathology, indications for operations based on that pathology, physical complications that follow, and the alternative operations available for disc excision. However, this perspective does not account for perhaps the most important sources of failure in lumbar spinal surgery, which result from non-organic, socioeconomic, and psychological variables. An analysis of patients presenting to rehabilitation units and/or as candidates for surgery following previous spine operations reveals organic pathology does not account for the majority of failures. This view is supported by the following general observations:

1. Analysis of long-term follow-up data indicate over one-half of these patients with surgical failures do not have a pathological basis for their continued symptoms (13,19). Even with extensive studies few will have an indication for further surgery. For example, only 13% of patients undergoing metrizamide-enhanced CT scan had surgically correctable pathology (52).
2. Analyses of patients with failed surgery demonstrate a high proportion of non-organic factors (2,20,26,27, 57,66).

The non-physical factors that predict failure include:

Perception of Fault

There is ample evidence that a claim for workers' compensation and third party payment negatively affects surgical treatment in lumbar disc disease. In fact, the workers' compensation cohort has less favorable re-

TABLE 6. *Costs of successful cases compared with unsuccessful cases*

	No. cases	Compensation costs ($) (average/claim)	Medical costs ($) (average/claim)	Total claim costs ($) (average/claim)
Group I chemonucleolysis				
Successful	17	11,254	9,319	20,573
Unsuccessful	44	23,138	18,603	41,741
Group II surgical discectomy				
Successful	26	14,266	13,741	28,007
Unsuccessful	18	17,209	13,125	30,334

Table shows the costs for treating patients who had a successful outcome versus an unsuccessful outcome for chymopapain and standard lumbar disc excision. The costs in each category are further broken down into the compensation costs and the medical costs (with permission from ref. 50).

sults from non-surgical treatment of all types (33,57,68) as well as an increased risk of complications following diagnostic tests such as myelography (25). A prospective comparison of workers' compensation versus "private pay" patients showed the results following simple disc excision were significantly less favorable in the compensation group. In particular, a blue collar worker with compensation had the least favorable surgical outcome (34). Today, it is common to stratify the sample into the compensation and non-compensation populations. Similarly, analyses of patients entering rehabilitation programs reveal a disproportionate number of the clients are receiving workers' compensation or benefits from other entitlement programs. Of interest is the observation that these entitlement programs have less impact when the follow-up survey is extended beyond the period of compensation payment (19). The cynical perspective suggests that claim settlement removes the incentive to remain symptomatic and disabled. This perspective is partially supported when surgical results are analyzed in patients with entitlement benefits that are not time-limited. In Nashold and Hrubec's study of veterans (49), poorer results were observed in the patients who were receiving continued disability payments. A less cynical perspective would conclude these were the more severely affected patients and continued disability was the inevitable outcome.

The economic impact of this problem is significant. Norton (50) has analyzed all workers' compensation pa-

tients who had lumbar spinal surgery over a one-year interval in the state of Oregon. Tables 6 and 7 present his data. The ultimate economic indicator he used was the cost per successful case, which was $110,000 for chymopapain, and $60,000 per successful laminectomy.

PSYCHOLOGICAL FACTORS

The objective analysis of psychological factors as they affect treatment outcome has been heavily based on the Minnesota Multiphasic Personality Inventory (MMPI). The Hy (Hysteria), Hs (Somatization), and D (Depression) scales have been the usual focus for the analysis of treatment failures. These scales also correlate with other psychologic test instruments, such as the pain drawing and non-organic physical signs reported by Waddell (60). Wiltse and Rocchio (68) found patients undergoing chemonucleolysis had significantly poorer results when the Hy and Hs scales were elevated, independent of the objective physical signs and myelographic findings. Similar results have been obtained in patients treated by lumbar disc excision and spinal fusion (26,27,33,57). Somewhat conflicting data have been obtained by Weber (62) from his randomized prospective survey of Norwegians. He found patients with psychological dysfunction who were randomized to the surgically treated group fared better than the patients randomized to the non-surgical treatment cohort, providing the clinical signs and myelogram were unequivocal.

TABLE 7. *Costs of cases meeting AAOS–AANS criteria compared with cases not meeting AAOS–AANS criteria*

	Group I chemonucleolysis		
	Compensation costs ($) (average/claim)	Medical costs ($) (average/claim)	Combined costs ($) (average/claim)
Criteria met			
Satisfactory results (9)	10,370	9,800	20,170
Unsatisfactory results (15)	17,458	13,736	31,194
All cases (24)	14,800	12,260	27,060
Criteria not met			
Satisfactory results (8)	10,413	9,241	19,654
Unsatisfactory results (29)	26,581	20,994	47,575
All cases (37)	23,085	18,453	41,538

Table shows the costs for treating patients and the outcomes are compared for patients who fulfilled the AAOS–AANS criteria for chymopapain injection and those who did not (with permission from ref. 50).

TABLE 8. *Rating scale for predicting surgical success*

Category	Maximum points allowed for category	Points assigned to parameters
I. *Neurologic signs*	25	
A. Weakness, consistent		
Associated with positive EMG		25
EMG normal		10
B. Atrophy (>2 cm)		10
C. Reflex absent or asymmetric		
Patient ≤ 50 years of age (add 5 points if EMG positive)		20
Patient > 50 years (add 15 points if EMG positive)		10
D. No clinical signs; EMG positive		15
II. *Sciatic tension signs*	25	
A. Crossed straight leg raising positive		20
B. Pelvic list		15
C. Dysrhythmia of lumbar paraspinal muscles with motion		15
D. Ipsilateral straight leg raising positive		5
III. *Personality factors (MMPI scores)*	25	
A. Normal (includes depression)		25
B. Abnormal (impulsive/schizophrenic)		10
C. Elevated hysteria (>1 SD, <2 SD)		10
D. Conversion reaction or hysteria (>2 SD)		0
IV. *Lumbar myelography*	25	
A. Positive and correlates with clinical findings		25
B. Equivocal nerve root asymmetry		10
C. Positive, but does not correlate with clinical findings (excludes spinal stenosis)		0
D. Normal		0
Total	100	

Table shows a patient evaluation form with a rating scale for the prediction of surgical success. A score of 100 would be the best possible and would predict a high degree of successful outcome, whereas lower scores predict less likelihood of success.
Abbreviations: EMG, electromyogram.

As a subset of this problem, substance abuse also is a major issue and confounds surgical and non-surgical treatment. This topic has been carefully analyzed by Loeser in Chapter 14, and the presence of substance abuse serves as an important contraindication to surgery, unless the indications are obvious based upon pathology.

IMPACT OF NON-ORGANIC FACTORS ON INDICATIONS FOR LUMBAR SPINAL SURGERY

Although worker's compensation and psychologic factors clearly influence surgical outcomes, there are important and complex interactions between organic pathology and the other non-organic factors. Spengler (56), Herron (27), and Hurme (33) have created indication checklists and algorithms which provide a means for the clinician to predict the chance of success (see Table 8).

NON-SURGICAL ALTERNATIVES FOR TREATMENT

As the individual surgeon attempts to define indications for surgical treatment, it is equally important to define the alternatives for non-surgical treatment. In Chapter 72, Deyo gives a comprehensive review of conservative management and alternatives and thus only a summary is presented here.

Bed rest remains the treatment of choice but, based on clinical and biologic research, the duration of treatment should be restricted. For patients with back pain the optimal duration is as short as two days. For patients with sciatica the information is less certain, but seven days appears optimal (10). For the patient with sciatica not relieved by bed rest, additional efficacious treatment includes autotraction (41) and exercise (see Chapter 76), although aerobic programs appear more appropriate than flexion exercises when the underlying pathology is a lumbar disc herniation. The role of epidural steroids is more controversial, with some studies indicating a beneficial effect (12), while others indicate no effect with a risk of significant complications (9). The latter conclusion has been criticized because the duration of post-injection observation was limited to two days. Given the favorable natural history of both low back pain and sciatica as presented here and in other chapters, the majority of patients can resume function, and pain can be adequately managed with non-operative treatment. In the patient population with the predictably poorest outcomes, i.e., those with psychologic dysfunction, workers' compensation, and poorly defined pathologic causation for their symptoms, the comprehensive rehabilitation programs advocated by Mayer (45) and reported in Chapter 13 by Hazard have success rates exceeding surgical intervention by functional criteria.

SUMMARY AND CONCLUSIONS

The indication for any operation is that the surgeon believes there is a reasonable probability of relieving the patient's pain and improving function over the natural history of the disease process. Except for a very small subset of patients with severe or progressing neurologic dysfunction or life-threatening pathology, the majority of patients with low back pain and sciatica present with only relative indications. Thus, for the majority of patients the selection of an operative or non-operative approach is based on the relative probability of success or failure. The success of lumbar surgery in these patients ultimately is based on the unequivocal demonstration of pathology, amenable to surgical treatment, the selection of patients whose psychosocial circumstances give them a reasonable probability of successful outcome, and the performance of the operation best suited to the pathology. Most critical to success is the pathology; patient selection is next most important; and selection of a particular operation is least important, particularly when lumbar disc herniation is being treated. In today's society, success must be measured not only by relief of pain, but by the patient's return to work, except in the elderly. In this subgroup of elderly, outcome will eventually be measured by "cost-benefit" ratios.

Based on these premises, a predictable success rate is obtained when the patient presents with the unequivocal symptoms, signs, and confirmatory imaging studies of lumbar disc herniation; when the patient does not believe the herniation was the result of a work-related, compensable "injury," and when psychologic testing reveals minimal dysfunction. Conversely, a low rate of success is predictable when the signs and symptoms are uncertain and the imaging studies are equivocal; when the patients believe their symptoms are work related; and when the operative findings reveal minimal pathology.

Although the surgical technique may influence the results by a factor of 10%, the other non-surgical issues will influence the results far more significantly. "Surgical checklists" and algorithms are effective aids to the treating physician in predicting the probability of success or failure and thus are an important means for determining surgical indication.

Although this chapter focuses primarily on lumbar disc herniation, the evidence strongly indicates the same principles are important in determining the indications for surgical treatment of other pathologic conditions affecting the lumbar spine.

REFERENCES

1. Albee FH (1911): Transplantation of a portion of the tibia into spine for Pott's disease. *JAMA* 57:885.
2. Beals RK, Hickman NW (1972): Industrial injuries of the back and extremities: Comprehensive evaluation—an aid in prognosis and management: A study of one hundred and eighty patients. *J Bone Joint Surg* [Am] 54:1593–1611.
3. Boden SD, Davis DO, Dina TS, Patronas NJ, Wiesel S (1989): The incidence of abnormal lumbar spine MRI scans in asymptomatic patients: A prospective and blinded investigation. Presented at the meeting of the International Society for Study of the Lumbar Spine, Kyoto, Japan.
4. Brown CW, Orme TJ, Richardson HD (1986): The rate of pseudarthrosis (surgical nonunion) in patients who are smokers and patients who are nonsmokers: A comparison study. *Spine* 11:942–943.
5. Burton C (1981): The role of spine fusion: Question 4. *Spine* 6:291.
6. Capanna AH, Williams RW, Austin DC, Darmody WR, Thomas LM (1981): Lumbar discectomy—percentage of disc removal and detection of anterior annulus perforation. *Spine* 6:610–614.
7. Cats-Baril WL, Frymoyer JW (1989): Demographic predictors of low back pain, low back pain disability and back surgery: Analysis of the NCHS data base. Presented at International Society for the Study of the Lumbar Spine meeting, Kobe, Japan.
8. Colonna PC, Friedenberg ZB (1949): The disc syndrome. Results of conservative care of patients with positive myelograms. *J Bone Joint Surg* [Am] 31:614–618.
9. Cuckler JM, Bernini PA, Wiesel SW, Booth RE Jr, Rothman RH, Pickens GT (1985): The use of epidural steroids in the treatment of lumbar radicular pain: A prospective, randomized, double-blind study. *J Bone Joint Surg* [Am] 67:63–66.
10. Deyo RA, Diehl AK, Rosenthal M (1986): How many days of bed rest for acute low back pain? A randomized clinical trial. *N Engl J Med* 315:1064–1070.
11. Deyo RA, Tsui-Wu YJ (1987): Descriptive epidemiology of low-back pain and its related medical care in the United States. *Spine* 12:264–268.
12. Dilke TF, Burry HC, Grahame R (1973): Extradural corticosteroid injection in management of lumbar nerve root compression. *Br Med J* 2:635–637.
13. Finnegan WI, Fenlin JM, Marvel JP, Nardini RJ, Rothman RH (1979): Results of surgical intervention in the symptomatic multiply-operated back patient. Analysis of 67 cases followed for 3–7 years. *J Bone Joint Surg* [Am] 61:1077–1082.
14. Frymoyer JW (1981): The role of spine fusion. Question 3. *Spine* 6:284–290.
15. Frymoyer JW (1989): Are we performing too much spinal surgery? *The Iowa Orthopaedic Journal* 9:32–36 (Department of Orthopaedics, University of Iowa).
16. Frymoyer JW, Donaghy RM (1985): The ruptured intervertebral disc: Follow-up report on the first case fifty years after recognition of the syndrome and its surgical significance. *J Bone Joint Surg* [Am] 67:1113–1116.
17. Frymoyer JW, Hanley E, Howe J, Kuhlmann D, Matteri R (1978):

Disc excision and spine fusion in the management of lumbar disc disease: A minimum ten-year followup. *Spine* 3:1–6.

18. Frymoyer JW, Hanley EN Jr, Howe J, Kuhlmann D, Matteri RE (1979): A comparison of radiographic findings in fusion and non-fusion patients ten or more years following lumbar disc surgery. *Spine* 4:435–440.

19. Frymoyer JW, Matteri RE, Hanley EN, Kuhlmann D, Howe J (1978): Failed lumbar disc surgery requiring second operation. A long-term follow-up study. *Spine* 3:7–11.

20. Frymoyer JW, Rosen JC, Clements J, Pope MH (1985): Psychologic factors in low-back-pain disability. *Clin Orthop* (195):178–184.

21. Goldner JL (1981): The role of spine fusion: Question 6. *Spine* 6:293–303.

22. Gotfried Y, Bradford DS, Oegema TR Jr (1986): Facet joint changes after chemonucleolysis-induced disc space narrowing. *Spine* 11:944–950.

23. Hakelius A (1970): Prognosis in sciatica: A clinical follow-up of surgical and non-surgical treatment. *Acta Orthop Scand (Suppl)* 129:1–76.

24. Hakelius A, Hindmarsh J (1972): The comparative reliability of preoperative diagnostic methods in lumbar disc surgery. *Acta Orthop Scand* 43:234–238.

25. Herkowitz HN, Romeyn RL, Rothman RH (1983): The Indications for Metrizamide Myelography. *J Bone Joint Surg* 65A:1144–1149.

26. Herron LD, Turner J (1985): Patient selection for lumbar laminectomy and discectomy with a revised objective rating system. *Clin Orthop* (199):145–152.

27. Herron LD, Turner J, Clancy S, Weiner P (1986): The differential utility of the Minnesota Multiphasic Personality Inventory. A predictor of outcome in lumbar laminectomy for disc herniation versus spinal stenosis. *Spine* 11:847–350.

28. Hibbs RH (1911): An operation for progressive spinal deformities. *NY J Med* 93:1013.

29. Hirsch C, Nachemson A (1963): The reliability of lumbar disk surgery. *Clin Orthop* (29):189–194.

30. Hitselberger WE, Witten RM (1968): Abnormal myelograms in asymptomatic patients. *J Neurosurg* 28:204–206.

31. Howe J, Frymoyer JW (1985): The effects of questionnaire design on the determination of end results in lumbar spinal surgery. *Spine* 10:804–805.

32. Hudgins WR (1983): Computer-aided diagnosis of lumbar disc herniation. *Spine* 8:604.

33. Hurme M, Alaranta H (1987): Factors predicting the result of surgery of lumbar intervertebral disc herniation. *Spine* 12:933–938.

34. Kahanovitz N (1990): Personal communication.

35. Kane WL: Personal communication.

36. Keller RB, Soule DM, Wennberg JE, Hanley DF (in press): Dealing with geographic variations in hospital use: The experience of the Maine Medical Assessment Program's orthopaedic study group. *J Bone Joint Surg*.

37. Kelsey JL (1982): *Epidemiology of musculoskeletal disorders,* New York: Oxford University Press, pp. 145–167.

38. Knutsson F (1944): The instability associated with disk degeneration in the lumbar spine. *Acta Radiol* 25:593–609.

39. Kostuik JP, Harrington I, Alexander D, Rand W, Evans D (1986): Cauda equina syndrome and lumbar disc herniation. *J Bone Joint Surg* [Am] 68:386–391.

40. LaRocca H, Macnab I (1974): The laminectomy membrane. Studies in its evolution, characteristics, effects and prophylaxis in dogs. *J Bone Joint Surg* [Br] 56:545–550.

41. Larsson U, Choler U, Lidstrom A, et al (1980): Auto-traction for treatment of lumbago-sciatica: A multicentre controlled investigation. *Act Orthop Scand* 51:791–798.

42. Lee CK, Alexander H (1984): Prevention of postlaminectomy scar formation. *Spine* 9:305–312.

43. Lehmann TR, Spratt KF, Tozzi JE, Weinstein JN, Reinarz SJ, El-Khoury GY (1987): Long-term follow-up of lower lumbar fusion patients. *Spine* 12:97–104.

44. Markolf KL (1972): Deformation of the thoracolumbar intervertebral joints in response to external loads. *J Bone Joint Surg* [Am] 54:511–533.

45. Mayer TG, Gatchel RJ, Kishino N, et al. (1985): Objective assessment of spine function following industrial injury: A prospective study with comparison group and one-year follow-up. *Spine* 10:482–493.

46. McCulloch J, Kahanovitz N (1987): Surgical discectomy and microdiscectomy chemonucleolysis. A clinical and cost effect study. Presented at the International Society for Study of the Lumbar Spine, Rome.

47. Mikawa Y, Hamagami H, Shikata J, Higashi S, Yamamuro T, Hyon S-H, Ikada Y (1986): An experimental study on prevention of postlaminectomy scar formation by the use of new materials. *Spine* 11:843–846.

48. Mixter WJ, Barr JS (1934): Rupture of the intervertebral disc with involvement of the spinal canal. *N Engl J Med* 211:210–215.

49. Nashold BS, Hrubec Z (1971): *Lumbar disc disease: A twenty-year clinical follow-up study.* St. Louis: Mosby.

50. Norton WL (1986): Chemonucleolysis versus surgical discectomy: Comparison of costs and results in workers' compensation claimants. *Spine* 11:440–443.

51. Pokras R, Graves EF, Dennison CF (1982): *Surgical operations in short-stay hospitals: United States, 1978,* Series 13, No. 61. Hyattsville, Maryland: DHEW Publication (PHS) 82-1722.

52. Pyhtinen J, Lahde S, Tanska EL, Laitinen J (1983): Computed tomography after lumbar myelography in lower back and extremity pain syndromes. *Diag Imag* 52:19–22.

53. Rutkow IM (1986): Orthopaedic operations in the United States, 1979 through 1983. *J Bone Joint Surg* [Am] 68:716–719.

54. Scham SM, Taylor TK (1971): Tension signs in lumbar disc prolapse. *Clin Orthop* (75):195–204.

55. Spangfort EV (1972): The lumbar disc herniation: A computer-aided analysis of 2,504 operations. *Acta Orthop Scand (Suppl).* 142:1–95.

56. Spengler DM, Freeman CW (1979): Patient selection for lumbar discectomy. An objective approach. *Spine* 4:129–134.

57. Spengler DM, Freeman C, Westbrook R, Miller JW (1980): Low-back pain following multiple lumbar spine procedures: Failure of initial selections. *Spine* 5:356–360.

58. Thomas M, Grant N, Mashall J, et al. (1983): Surgical treatment of low backache and sciatica. *Lancet* 2:1437–1439.

59. Troup JD (1981): Straight-leg-raising (SLR) and the qualifying tests for increased root tension: their predictive value after back and sciatic pain. *Spine* 6:526–527.

60. Waddell G, McCulloch JA, Kummel E, Venner RM (1980): Non-organic physical signs in low-back pain. *Spine* 5:117–125.

61. Weber H (1978): Lumbar disc herniation: A prospective study of prognostic factors including a controlled trial. Part II. *J Oslo City Hosp* 28:89–113.

62. Weber H (1983): 1982 Volvo Award in Clinical Science. Lumbar Disc Herniation. A controlled, prospective study with ten years of observation. *Spine* 8:131–140.

63. Weinstein J, Spratt KF, Lehmann T, McNeill T, Hejna W (1986): Lumbar disc herniation: A comparison of the results of chemonucleolysis and open discectomy after ten years. *J Bone Joint Surg* [Am] 68:43–54.

64. Wennberg J, Gittelsohn A (1973): Small area variations in health care delivery. *Science* 182:1102–1108.

65. Wiesel SW, Tsourmas N, Feffer HL, Citrin CM, Patronas M (1984): A study of computer-assisted tomography. I. The incidence of positive CAT scans in an asymptomatic group of patients. *Spine* 9:549–551.

66. Wilfling FJ, Klonoff H, Kokan P (1973): Psychological, demographic and orthopaedic factors associated with prediction of outcome of spinal fusion. *Clin Orthop* (90):153–160.

67. Williams RW (1986): Microlumbar discectomy. A 12-year statistical review. *Spine* 11:851–852.

68. Wiltse LL and Rocchio PD (1975): Preoperative psychological tests as predictors of success of chemonucleolysis in the treatment of the low-back syndrome. *J Bone Joint Surg* [Am] 57:478–483.

69. Yong-Hing K, Reilly J, de Korompay V, Kirkaldy-Willis WH (1980): Prevention of nerve root adhesions after laminectomy. *Spine* 5:59–64.

The Adult Spine: Principles and Practice,
J. W. Frymoyer, Editor-in-Chief.
Raven Press, Ltd., New York © 1991.

CHAPTER 81

Chemonucleolysis

Eugene J. Nordby

The clinical use of chymopapain when first reported in 1963 was given an ambivalent greeting. Some hailed it as the greatest advance in treatment of a herniated disc since Mixter and Barr's report of 1934 (42); others decried it as simply a placebo effect or as a toxic substance too dangerous to pursue. After more than 25 years of research, double blind trials, FDA approval, and extensive clinical use, the differing views persist, and each has its vocal and literary advocates. Although I am convinced of its safety and efficacy when the drug is properly used, a balanced view of its indications and complications is the aim of this chapter. Although Lyman Smith coined the term "chemonucleolysis" to describe the treatment of intervertebral disc lesions by the intradiscal injection of the enzyme chymopapain, others have expanded its use to include collagenase (8,13,60).

HISTORY

Eugene Jansen and Arnold Balls isolated chymopapain in 1941 from crude papain derived from the latex of the fruit of Carica papaya (30). Papaya latex contains three enzymes in addition to chymopapain: protease, lysozyme, and papain. While seeking an enzyme that would reduce circulating protein in blood, Lewis Thomas in 1956 injected rabbits intravenously with crude papain and noticed that their ears drooped. Forty-eight hours later the erect position was resumed, pointing to a reversible action on the chondral intracellular substance of the ears. The injection also softened the trachea, but had no apparent effect on other tissues (72).

Intrigued by Thomas's article, Lyman Smith postulated a possible therapeutic use in chondroplastic tumors. Although chymopapain had no effect on tumors, Smith found that intradiscal injection in rabbits discretely removed the nucleus pulposus, but left the annulus largely intact (61).

Other proteolytic enzymes were also investigated and found to have a similar effect on disc tissue, but toxicologic studies revealed chymopapain to be the least toxic and to have the most specific action on chondromucoprotein (26).

Animal experiments were then expanded to the normal discs of mice, dogs, cats, and monkeys, and then to dachshunds, an achondroplastic breed with herniated discs (57). Eighty-six percent of these dogs made a lasting

E. J. Nordby, M.D.: Department of Orthopaedics, University of Wisconsin Medical School, Madison, Wisconsin, 53705.

TABLE 1. *Double-blind trials of chymopapain*

	Schwetsenau et al. (57a)	Fraser (25a)	Javid et al. (31)	Dabezies et al. (17)
Year	1975	1981	1981	1987
Patients	104	60	108	159
Chymopapain success	58%	80%	82%	71%
Placebo success	49%	57%	41%	45%
Dosage	1 ml/4 mg	2 ml/8 mg	2 ml/8 mg	2 ml/8 mg
Formula	Discase	Discase	Chymodiactin	Discase
Placebo	CEI	Saline	Saline	CEI

recovery from nerve root compression, and no deleterious effects were observed.

Subsequently, Smith sold the patent for chymopapain to Baxter-Travenol Laboratories for $1. They then formulated Discase, a trademarked combination of chymopapain, cysteine sodium sulfite, and EDTA in lyophilized form containing 10,000 units per vial. Smith injected the first patient in 1963 and some 75 investigators in the United States and Canada eventually injected about 17,000 patients in the Phase III trial, which ended in July 1975.

In 1974, extensive one-day instructional courses were presented by the American Academy of Orthopaedic Surgeons to 1,600 orthopedists in anticipation of the drug's release. Soon thereafter, the FDA authorized a randomized double blind study of Discase. This study was inconclusive and resulted in the withdrawal of the NDA by Baxter in 1975.

With the popularity of chemonucleolysis still high in the United States, many patients were referred to Canada for chymopapain (Discase). Investigational use of chymopapain also continued in Australia and England. A Yugoslavian product (Lekopain) was widely used in the Eastern Bloc countries and to a lesser extent in France and Italy with favorable results. In an attempt to bypass the FDA, legislation was passed in Indiana, Illinois, and Texas to allow use of chymopapain within each state, but only in Texas was the product developed and used as "Chemolase."

Baxter-Travenol then began a blind study of chymopapain versus CEI (Cysteine-Edetate-iothalamate) or saline control, which allowed patients to have a laminectomy in the United States or go to Canada for chymopapain, if they had a placebo failure. Significant difficulty was encountered in accumulating adequate numbers of trial participants, and the results were finally published in 1988. One hundred seventy-three participants at 25 locations reported 71% success with Discase as compared to 45% with CEI (17). Saline was dropped from the randomization scheme and, therefore, this control was absent.

In 1979, Smith Laboratories developed a new formula of chymopapain and established a double blind protocol. This drug, termed Chymodiactin, was formulated by (a) omitting one protein fraction of the three present in Discase, since it is not proteolytic, and (b) retaining only cysteine to stabilize the chymopapain in the sulphydryl form. Tests showed Chymodiactin to be proteolytic for the nucleus pulposus and to have a long-term stability at room temperature, unlike Discase, which required refrigeration and lost potency over a brief time interval. After reconstitution Chymodiactin retained full activity for two hours at room temperature (64).

A randomized double blind study was authorized by the FDA in 1981 in seven centers and included cooperating orthopedic surgeons and neurosurgeons. The meticulously performed study enrolled 108 patients by July 1, 1981, and the final results of a six-month follow-up

TABLE 2. *Illinois study of efficacy: Patient self-evaluation*

	3 weeks	6 weeks	3 months	6 months
Excellent	107 (7.2%)	249 (17.2%)	475 (34.1%)	683 (48.7%)
Good	811 (54.7%)	876 (60.3%)	685 (49.2%)	543 (38.7%)
Fair	340 (22.9%)	189 (13.0%)	129 (9.3%)	58 (4.1%)
Poor	163 (11.0%)	81 (5.6%)	51 (3.7%)	39 (2.8%)
Failure (includes patients requiring surgery)	62 (4.2%)	57 (3.9%)	51 (3.7%)	79 (5.6%)
Total	1,483	1,452	1,391	1,402

With permission from ref. 41.
Excellent = Normal activity and no pain.
Good = Able to work with some limitation of activity, and some pain occasionally needing mild pain killer.
Fair = Unable to work except at very light work, and frequent pain needing a strong pain killer.
Poor = Much limitation of activity, high degree of pain, very minor improvement.
Failure = Severe pain and limitation, no improvement.

TABLE 3. *Illinois study of efficacy: Physician evaluation*

	3 weeks	6 weeks	3 months	6 months
Excellent	103 (7.0%)	326 (22.4%)	584 (42.0%)	843 (62.1%)
Good	816 (55.0%)	819 (56.4%)	611 (44.0%)	363 (26.8%)
Fair	432 (29.1%)	211 (14.5%)	106 (7.6%)	54 (4.0%)
Poor	89 (6.0%)	57 (3.9%)	36 (2.6%)	22 (1.6%)
Failure (includes patients requiring surgery)	43 (2.9%)	40 (2.8%)	52 (3.7%)	75 (5.5%)
Total	1,483	1,453	1,389	1,357

With permission from ref. 41.

Excellent = Requires no analgesics for back pain, is able to return to previous or comparable employment, and is able to participate in desired recreational activities.

Good = Requires non-narcotic analgesics, is able to return to work, is limited in stressful activities, and does no heavy lifting.

Fair = Requires regular non-narcotic analgesics with occasional narcotics, must do only light work, and is relieved sufficiently not to wish further surgery.

Poor = Somewhat improved, but not happy with result and requires other major intervention.

Failure = No better in any manner or may be worse.

showed composite successful results on 82% of those receiving Chymodiactin and 41% of those who received placebos. No major complications were reported (31). Table 1 summarizes the results of these double blind trials.

A second open study in Illinois was designed to allow a two-level injection and treatment of compensation cases, if not over six months in duration. Thirty-seven doctors, only twelve of whom had been previous investigators, performed the Chymodiactin injections in 1,498 patients after a one-day course of training was arranged for them, their pharmacists, and their nurses. The success rate in this open trial was approximately 90% (Tables 2 and 3) (41).

Complications among those 1,498 patients included four cases of anaphylactic shock, two of whom died, and one case of acute transverse myelitis 21 days after a successful injection. In spite of extensive study, a causal relationship between chemonucleolysis and acute transverse myelitis was not established (20).

The successful outcome of the double blind study and the Illinois open trial with Chymodiactin resulted in FDA approval for clinical use of the enzyme on November 10, 1982 (23).

In mid-1982, the Executive Committee of the American Association of Neurological Surgeons (AANS) and the American Academy of Orthopaedic Surgeons (AAOS) formed a joint committee on chymopapain to develop and offer a course on intradiscal therapy. Over a four-month period, 6,214 doctors attended the instructional courses given by a volunteer faculty of 99 prior investigators and patterned after the 1974 course and the Illinois trial instructional day. This effort was complemented by full sets of educational materials that were provided to each residency program in neurosurgery and orthopedic surgery. Baxter Laboratories' Discase was approved by the FDA on January 18, 1984. Despite this

major educational effort, a very high usage was encountered, followed by reports of hemiparesis and paraplegia resulting from intrathecal injection. Ultimately, this resulted in both manufacturers discontinuing the product and selling their rights to a larger company, in part because of product liability suits.

BIOCHEMISTRY AND TOXICOLOGY

The currently manufactured chymopapain differs from the original formulation as follows: One protein electrophoretic peak has been removed; the disodium edetate has been omitted, since no heavy metals should be present in the purified product; and sodium bisulfite has been omitted as a stabilizer, since it was never shown to have this property (Fig. 1). The current formulation is stable without use of refrigeration for up to three years (64). The proteolytic enzyme chymopapain acts by hydrolysis to split the peptide bonds of proteoglycan molecules. This liberation of the polysaccharide (glucosaminoglycans) (GAG) side chains results in loss of their capacity to bind water molecules, which then diffuse out of the cartilaginous matrix of the disc and reduce intradiscal pressure. The activity of chymopapain is limited and must act quickly at the injection site to obtain a therapeutic effect because of diffusion, dilution, and inactivation by Alpha-2-macroglobulin, a general inhibitor of proteolytic enzymes present in all tissue fluids and sera (63).

After diffusion from the disc, the enzyme remaining bound to the proteoglycan (GAG) and its fragments pass into the circulation and are excreted in the urine. Chymopapain is further deactivated by cathepsins and the production of specific antibodies within seven days.

Chymopapain degrades the nucleus pulposus but leaves the annulus fibrosus essentially intact because of

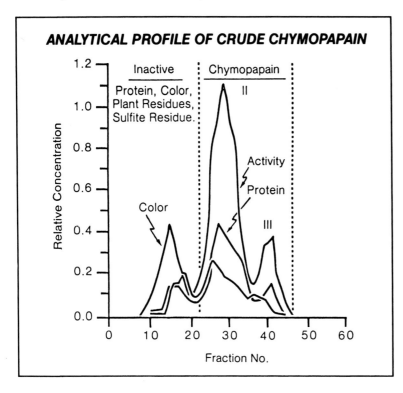

FIG. 1. Analytical profile of chymopapain showing the inactive components separable by column chromatography which are removed in chymodiactin and present in Discase (with permission from ref. 64).

the largely collagenous composition of that structure. This allows narrowing of the disc space, but in younger tissue reconstitution occurs within a year, indicating that the chondrocyte-mediated synthesis of nuclear proteins is not irrevocably impaired (5). The phenomenon is dose related.

Table 4 outlines chymopapain toxicology. Most toxic effects of chymopapain injection result from the proteolysis of glucosamino-glycan in the capillary wall. Large doses can cause lethal systemic hemorrhage, which is most commonly intrathecal. The resultant compressive effects of the bleeding can cause paraplegia or death. This catastrophic complication can be prevented in experimental animals by venting the dura either by needle or opening a flap, thus decompressing the dura. If the animal recovers, no residual arachnoiditis is identified. Vessels other than capillaries have a fibrous cover that prevents chymopapain from having any effect on them (Table 5).

TABLE 4. *Chymopapain toxicology*

1. Mechanism: Proteolysis of capillaries, GAG structure
2. Lethality: Systemic—from petechial hemorrhage, clots
   Intrathecal—from CSF pressure increase
3. Does not affect: Sensory or motor nerves
   (5 mg [2,500 units] per kg) Dura mater
                               Collagen
                               Heart rate, blood pressure
                               Clotting factors

Limited by serum inhibition

With permission from ref. 64.

TABLE 5. *Intrathecal toxicity*

Mechanism:
Capillary rupture → CSF pressure increase via petechial hemorrhage
Cisternal tap controls pressure and prevents death

With permission from ref. 64.

The enzyme does not directly affect sensory and motor nerves, or dura mater. Thus, chymopapain is not neurotoxic. Spinal nerves are not affected by epidural application of chymopapain because of their fibrous covering and the likely counteraction of Alpha-2-macroglobulin (27,77). Experiments showing axonal death or intraneural fibrosis are all secondary to interference with the capillary microcirculation exposed to the enzyme. In dogs, there is no measurable effect on heart rate, blood pressure, or clotting factors (Table 6).

TABLE 6. *No effect from chymopapain injection*

Sciatic nerve (frog, rabbit) threshold voltage
Sensory nerve (corneal, intradermal)
Dura mater (doses up to 8× human)
  Dogs, 5 mg (2,500 units) per kg
  Heart rate, blood pressure, carotid occlusion reflex, clotting factors.
Maximum human dose:
0.36 mg (143 units) per kg

With permission from ref. 64.

The other major complication attributable to the use of chymopapain is the potential for anaphylactic reaction, similar to all foreign proteins. Although it is much less antigenic than animal serum, about 1% of the world's population has potential for reaction to chymopapain because of prior exposure to the antigen. The chymopapain protein, although quite pure, is cross reactive to commercial sources of papain such as meat tenderizers, papaya fruit, beer, toothpaste, digestive aids, cosmetics, contact lens washing solutions, laboratory reagents, and some treated leathers (69).

Sensitivity to chymopapain can be detected prior to injection by skin testing or direct measurement of the patient's antibodies (IgE) by tests such as the RAST (Radioallergo Sorbent Test) or FAST (Fluorescent Allergo Sorbent Test). Although all procedures can detect sensitivity to chymopapain, there has been little formal evaluation of the skin test, and anaphylaxis has been reported following epidermal injection (35).

INDICATIONS FOR USE OF CHYMOPAPAIN

Patient Selection

In spite of the technical advances in imaging, the keystone to selection of a proper candidate for chymopapain injection is a documented history of sciatica and a competent physical examination of the lumbar spine, which denotes lumbar disc herniation. The myelogram, discogram, CT scan, MRI imaging, and EMG are only confirmatory to examination.

Stated simply, chymopapain is indicated in the treatment of unremitting sciatica due to a proven herniated nucleus pulposus that has not responded to adequate conservative measures in a patient considered amenable to discectomy. Additionally, McCulloch and Macnab have found that those patients having two symptoms, two signs, and one diagnostic investigation positive for a herniated nucleus pulposus are more likely to respond to chemonucleolysis using chymopapain. Using this "rule of five," symptoms should include sciatic leg pain dominant over back pain; specific neurological symptoms such as paresthesia in the leg or foot; signs such as straight leg raising limited to 50% of normal with or without crossover pain and with or without a positive bow-string sign and at least two neurologic abnormalities, such as reflex alterations, wasting, weakness, or sensory loss; and a confirmatory positive water-soluble myelogram, CT scan, or MRI (37,38). Of course, many of these patients will recover with conservative treatment. Since the action of chymopapain is to change the water-binding properties of the nucleus mucoprotein, it is obvious that only a problem of discogenic origin can respond to injection with chymopapain and that other causes of sciatica, such as lateral recess stenosis, will not benefit.

In cases of sciatica, it is difficult to establish when a specific period of conservative treatment has been adequate because some patients will have increasing pain or progressive neurological changes requiring intervention earlier than in a situation in which unrelenting pain is the major complaint. Of course, profound acute or progressive neurological changes, particularly the cauda equina syndrome, are a contraindication to the use of chymopapain, and adequate neural decompression is the treatment of choice (46).

Age is also a consideration in patient selection. Those over age 60 may have sufficient degeneration to have depleted the mucoprotein in the nucleus pulposus. This decision must be individualized because patients in their early eighties have demonstrated relatively normal hydrated discs by MRI studies and theoretically could respond to that drug.

Specific recommendations for the use of chymopapain in those under 20 years of age have been lacking because of a paucity of studies in that age group. Sutton has reported performing chemonucleolysis on 24 patients under the age of 19 and found the results to be 96% satisfactory comparable to an age-matched cohort previously subjected to open discectomy. The surgery group had a higher recurrence rate of 25% as compared to 8% in those treated by chymopapain (66,68). Lorenz and McCulloch (36) treated 55 adolescents between the ages of 13 and 19 with 44 considered successful (80%) and 11 failed. The failures all had laminectomies that revealed sequestrated discs in 4, adhesions about the nerve root in 2, segmental instability in 1, a foraminal stenosis in 1, and no cause found in 1; 2 operative reports were unobtainable. Of the discectomies, 4 had good results, 5 fair, and 2 got no relief.

In 10 patients, ages 13 to 19, I have found only one who did not have a satisfactory result (48). That patient required discectomy and was found to have a persistent herniated portion of the disc in the epidural area giving nerve root compression while the intradiscal material was absent. I believe this failure was a result of too little enzyme being injected to dissolve the nucleus. From this experience, I believe that the increased amount of mucoprotein present in a young disc requires more chymopapain to neutralize it than would a more mature disc. Others do not agree. Recent research indicates that chymopapain does not have a dose-response relationship, but rather acts in an "all or nothing" fashion (33).

CONTRAINDICATIONS TO USE OF CHYMOPAPAIN

The major specific contraindications to the use of chymopapain include allergy to papain or papaya. A second injection of chymopapain is generally believed to be contraindicated in that the initial exposure may have sensitized the individual. This belief has been challenged by Sutton in a series of 33 re-injections where he has done prior serum testing (Chymofast test) to determine the IgE titer and had found reaction in only 9%. The last 12 patients in his series were pre-treated with H_1 and H_2 blockers, and there were no allergic reactions (67).

As already noted, progressive significant neurological change such as cauda equina syndrome is a specific contraindication because the response to chymopapain is time dependent, and it is essential to have prompt relief of neural pressure. Visual identification is also desirable from a medico-legal perspective (49).

Pregnancy is a contraindication. No series of pregnant women have been studied.

The most absolute and obvious contraindication to injection of a disc with chymopapain is the finding of a normal disc by discography or MRI. Other relative contraindications to the use of chemonucleolysis include spinal stenosis, since a bony impingement cannot be ameliorated by chymopapain; severe spondylolisthesis; and old infection of the disc or vertebrae, since it is possible to rekindle present latent infections. Radiographic evidence of osteoarthritis may obstruct needle insertion and may also be a relative contraindication to the procedure. Unsuccessful prior open discectomy at a symptomatic level is likely to prejudice a successful outcome of a chymopapain injection because of the presence of fibrosis. Emotional instability and the complicating factor of a medico-legal action are also obvious relative contraindications to any definitive back treatment and have been associated with poor results. Likewise, psychologic disturbances have been associated with less successful results (78).

In addition to these specific contraindications, relative contraindications include diabetes mellitus, depending on its severity and control, and the presence of neuropathy. Patients with workers' compensation have significantly poorer results, not necessarily because of the etiology of the problem but probably because of the frequently cited lack of motivation among such patients to admit to a successful outcome. Communication or language barrier can also be a problem in explaining the procedure so that there can be an understanding of the expectations and possible complications, and the resultant increased risk of medico-legal action (78).

Lastly, it is worth re-emphasizing the important role of the history and physical examination. In these days, CT and MRI examinations often appear to take the place of a well-conducted history and physical. The images should have clinically correlated definitive changes to be pertinent. Too often one sees a radiologist's reading of a "possible small defect which may represent a herniating nucleus pulposus" become a "probable herniating disc" in the next office note and a "definitive

TABLE 7. *Contraindications to chymopapain injection*

Absolute
1. Allergy to chymopapain
2. Cauda equina syndrome–bowel or bladder paresis
3. Pregnancy
4. Normal discogram

Relative
1. Diabetes with peripheral neuropathy
2. Spinal stenosis
3. Spondylolisthesis–severe
4. Old infection of the disc or vertebrae
5. Osteoarthritic spur as source of nerve root pressure
6. Extensive osteoarthritis to prevent needle insertion
7. Repeat injection of chymopapain
8. Allergy to iodine-containing compounds
9. Unsuccessful surgery at symptomatic level
10. Emotional instability
11. Medico-legal cases
12. Language barrier

With permission from ref. 46.

herniated disc" in the following note, which forms the basis for a definitive procedure, usually without relief of the patient's symptoms. These contraindications are summarized in Table 7.

TECHNIQUE

To accomplish chemonucleolysis it is necessary in a sterile manner to place a needle through the skin of the back and end in the central nucleus pulposus of the intervertebral disc while avoiding obstructing bones, spinal nerve, and a vulnerable thecal sac. Very errant placement may actually injure abdominal contents. To place such a needle comfortably and accurately, it is essential to be able to think three dimensionally while having only two-dimensional images. From long observation, it is doubtful that such stereognostic ability can be taught; one must be born to it. However, specially designed mannequins are available to teach the basic skill with which the operator must be comfortable before proceeding further.

To minimize the potential anaphylactic reaction that currently occurs in about 0.3% of patients (down from 1% earlier), it is helpful to premedicate with histamine 1 and histamine 2 receptor blockers 24 hours before injection (50). This does not prevent anaphylactic reaction but ameliorates the reaction so that treatment is more effective. Oral diphenhydramine 50 mg four times daily serves as an H_1 blocker, and oral cimetidine 300 mg or Ranitidine hydrochloride 150 mg four times a day represent H_2 blockers (51). Since steroids are thought to stabilize cell membranes and thus reduce the release of chemical mediation for anaphylaxis, some doctors use methylprednisolone sodium succinate 250 mg IV one hour prior to the procedure. However, no statistical evidence supports this position. Hydration is most important, and oral or intravenous hydration prior to injection is essential.

At the same time, it is important to avoid medications known to promote release of histamine such as Urecholine, dextran, beta blockers, long-acting curare, and morphine.

Anesthesia

Anesthesia may be general or local. If a general anesthetic is employed, the halogens should be avoided, since they may sensitize cardiac tissue to epinephrine and lead to cardiac arrhythmia. General anesthesia has the advantage of allowing intubation in case of laryngospasm in anaphylaxis, but the use of succinylcholine or a tracheostomy can accommodate this complication in patients with local anesthesia. At the present time there is no statistically valid difference in the occurrence of anaphylaxis as related to anesthesia (50).

Local analgesia has the advantage of allowing patients to respond to impending anaphylaxis and avoids post general anesthesia morbidity. It also allows appreciation of a nerve root being touched by a needle and, thus, can prevent nerve trauma; the risk of intrathecal injection is reduced. This technique is generally the preferred one.

An emergency tray must be present to be ready to treat anaphylaxis, whatever the anesthesia.

Procedure

The procedure of injection may be performed in a surgical suite or in a special procedure room of an x-ray department so long as the necessary equipment, anesthesia, emergency cart, and trained personnel are available in a clean environment.

Positioning

Positioning the patient on a table that has a built-in fluoroscope or allows the use of a C-arm fluoroscope is most important to present bony landmarks to guide successful placement of the needle. The prone or lateral decubitus position is satisfactory so long as the patient can be properly positioned and stabilized to allow a lateral approach to the intervertebral space (58).

In the lateral position (Fig. 2) with the left side down, with a pad or cushion under the left hip and the knees and hips flexed, it is possible to maintain a stable position with four-inch adhesive straps. Overlap of the vertebral bony margins of the intervertebral disc space often obscures the clear view of needle placement. This can be overcome by tilting the fluoroscopic or x-ray machine head to optimize the angulation of the x-ray beam. This maneuver will open up the view of the disc space and make placement easier (Figs. 3 and 4). Radiation exposure of the patient in the usual well-conducted procedure is equivalent to that of a five-view lumbosacral spine series.

Needle Placement

After sterile skin preparation, as for any surgical procedure, the area is draped and the iliac crest and spinous processes identified. The level to be injected is determined with the fluoroscope and an 18-gauge needle 6 inches in length is placed 8 to 10 cm superior to the spinous processes and directed at about a 45° angle toward the disc space (Fig. 5). The needle is advanced in 1 to 2 cm increments in a "stop and go and look" fashion to allow a change in course if it is not properly directed (Fig. 6). The progress is viewed in the AP and lateral projections of the fluoroscope, which must be of suffi-

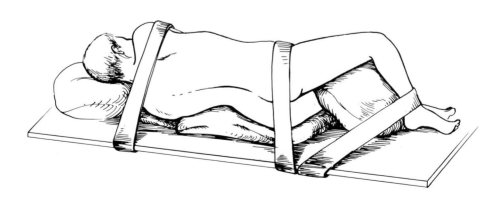

FIG. 2. Left lateral decubitus position. The spine is held perpendicular by adhesive straps. An inflatable pillow is under the left flank and the hips are acutely flexed.

A

B

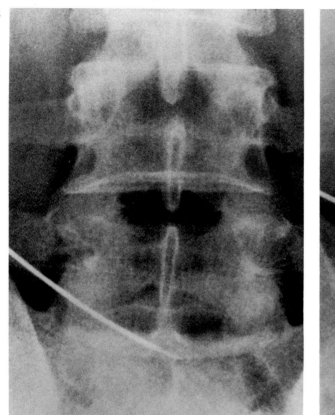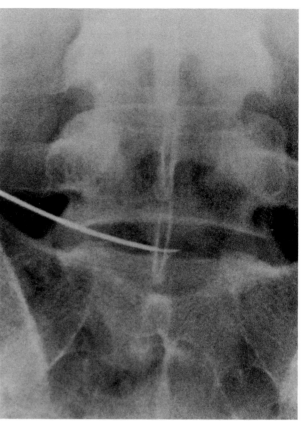

FIG. 3. AP radiogram with beam perpendicular (**A**) shows a distinct L4–L5 interspace but an indistinct image at L5–S1. AP radiogram with craniocaudal angulation of the x-ray beam (**B**) "opens up" the L5–S1 interspace (with permission from ref. 58).

FIG. 4. On the left, the L5–S1 interspace appears narrowed because of superimposition of the posterior lip of S1 on the anterior lip of the adjacent L5 surface. On the right, by angulation of the x-ray beam, the overlapping of the intervertebral margins disappears to give a clear view of the L5–S1 interspace (with permission from ref. 58).

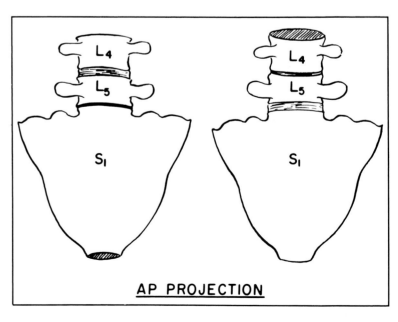

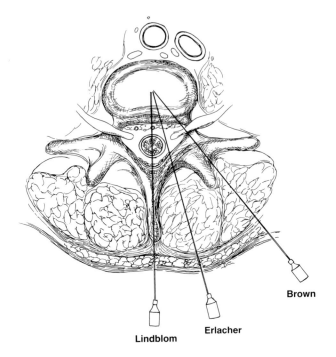

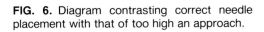

FIG. 5. Comparative needle placements in lumbar discography showing the posterior approach midline of Lindblom, the posterolateral approach of Erlacher, and the 45-degree lateral approach of J. Brown.

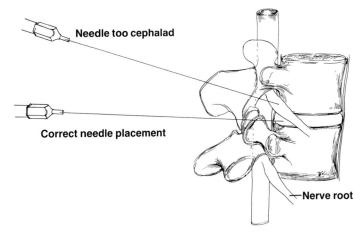

FIG. 6. Diagram contrasting correct needle placement with that of too high an approach.

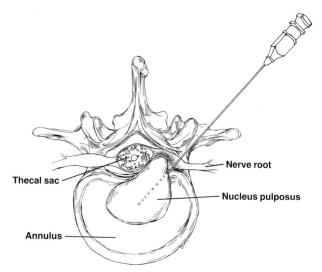

FIG. 7. Proper needle placement seen in axial view by the lateral approach.

Thecal sac

Annulus

Nerve root

Nucleus pulposus

cient strength and quality to give a clear view of the area. The L3–L4 and L4–L5 levels can be reached in this manner, and the needle tip should be at the center of the disc upon completion (Fig. 7).

For needle placement at the L5–S1 interspace it is necessary to avoid the iliac crest. To do this, the needle is started about 1 cm distal to placement for the L4–L5 level, angled 45° with the trunk and, in addition, about 30° caudally, again viewing the progress of the needle tip toward the intervertebral space placement in the nucleus pulposus.

Various needle systems may be used. The 18-gauge 6-inch spinal-type needle with obturator is most commonly used. A variation is to bend the distal 1.5 cm of the 18-gauge needle away from the bevel and, by rotation, maneuver about bony obstructions and change directions (14). A double needle technique is popular among others; an 18-gauge needle is used as a sleeve to approach the disc space and a 22-gauge needle at least 2 inches longer is placed through the first needle to enter the disc (Fig. 8). This 22-gauge needle may also be bent at the tip to aid maneuverability (71). In performing radiographically controlled needle placement it is important that attending personnel use proper protection. The surgeon, scrub nurse, anesthesiologist, and others remaining in the room during fluoroscopy or the taking of x-rays should wear lead aprons. Protective gloves and avoiding exposure of the hands of the operator also diminish exposure to radiation.

Needle Placement Confirmation

In early clinical trials, discography was used routinely to confirm needle placement and the presence of disc

degeneration (Fig. 9). Originally it was thought that intradiscal injection of a radio-opaque fluid might have some inhibitory effect on chymopapain, possibly by neutralizing its enzymatic activity. Naylor et al. measured enzyme activity by absorption spectrometry and found that Hypaque, Conray, and Urografin actually enhanced chymopapain action (43), but metrizamide had a slight inhibitory action. Animal experiments later showed that a mixture of contrast material and chymopapain was more toxic than either substance alone when intrathecal injection occurred (29). If discography is performed, the water-soluble non-ionizing contrast agents are probably the least irritative (Figs. 10, 11, and 12), and if epidural dye leakage occurs, this serves as no contraindication to injection.

Another means to confirm needle placement is discometry. As originally promulgated by McCulloch, this technique can be used by determining relative resistance in injecting water instead of radio contrast material (39). Injection of water into a nucleus pulposus or a leaking disc will give less resistance than an annular injection. A normal adult disc may hold up to 2 cc of fluid with considerable resistance.

As an additional safety precaution, advancement of the needle beyond the annulus without the stylet in place may be done to test for an intrathecal injection, which should produce a back flow of cerebrospinal fluid. Such a finding, of course, means that a change in needle position is essential before injection, and some people will abort the procedure if CSF is observed.

Drug Reconstitution and Injection Technique

Once a needle is properly placed, the chymopapain should be reconstituted with sterile water and drawn into separate syringes for testing and injection to avoid deac-

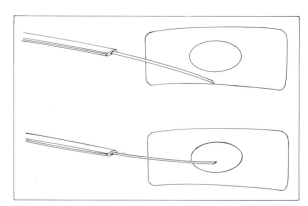

FIG. 8. Double needle technique showing correction of position of the 22 gauge inner needle by withdrawal, rotation, and reinsertion (with permission from ref. 71).

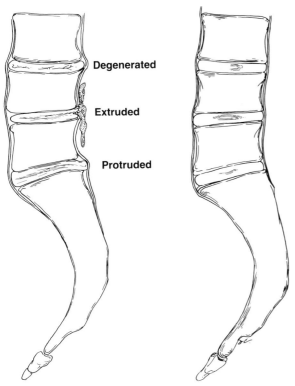

FIG. 9. Disc patterns in discography; abnormal on left and normal on right.

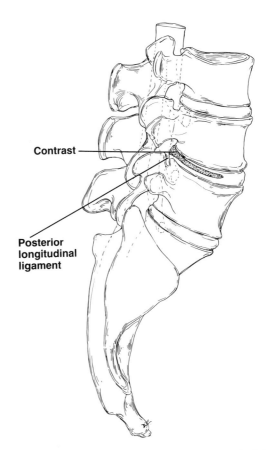

Contrast

Posterior
longitudinal
ligament

FIG. 10. Lateral discogram showing contrast material contained but elevating posterior longitudinal ligament.

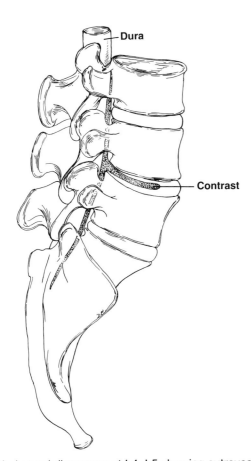

Dura

Contrast

FIG. 11. Lateral discogram at L4–L5 showing extravasation of radio-opaque material in the epidural space. This is not a contraindication to injecting chymopapain.

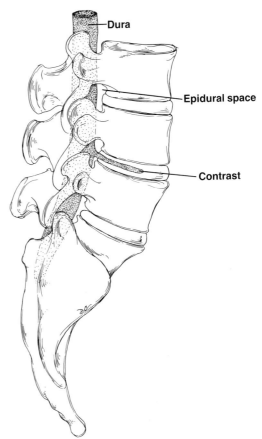

Dura

Epidural space

Contrast

FIG. 12. Lateral discogram at L4–L5 showing intrathecal flow of radio-opaque material from a congenital connection of the interspace and thecal sac to produce a myelogram. This is a contraindication to injecting chymopapain.

tivation of the enzyme by any reflux. Alcohol used on the vial stopper should evaporate before a needle is inserted, since alcohol contamination will neutralize chymopapain (14,73,74). The average dosage with Chymodiactin has been 1.5 cc total (3,000 units), using 0.3 cc as a test dose to determine any sensitivity. After 10 minutes the remaining 1.2 cc may be injected if there is no reaction. Recent studies suggest that as little as 1,000 units (0.5 cc) may be sufficient and seems to reduce much of the post-operative muscle spasm and back pain. However, it is well to place the 1,000 units in 2 cc volume for dispersion (33).

The enzyme should be injected slowly and with the least force possible to avoid unnecessary intradiscal pressure or theoretically the production of a cauda equina syndrome by sudden disc extrusion.

The stylet of the needle is replaced and the needle withdrawn. Since 95% of allergic reactions, such as anaphylactic shock, occur within 15 minutes, observation in surgery should be continued for this time before transporting to the recovery area.

Post-Chymopapain Aftercare

Although some have treated chemonucleolysis patients as outpatients, a day or two post-operative care allows instruction to be given in getting out of bed without straining the back, gradual ambulation as tolerated, and patient education. Any movement that is painful should be avoided. Sitting is often poorly tolerated and should initially be avoided.

While the sciatica or radiated leg pain is often promptly relieved after chemonucleolysis, back pain following the procedure is so frequent (20% to 40%) that many surgeons do not consider it a complication. A lesser number will have severe pain and spasms. Both groups of patients may be treated with ice packs, heat pads, analgesics, muscle relaxants, or the temporary use of a corset-type support.

Walking and side-stroke swimming are excellent convalescent measures that can be started almost immediately and then gradually increased in duration and intensity.

Ordinarily, the patient can return to light or sedentary work in two to four weeks and, with proper reconditioning, heavy work in six to twelve weeks, depending on the pre-injection condition of the muscles and the relief of symptoms.

COSTS OF TREATMENT

Estimates of the relative costs of chemonucleolysis and laminectomy in the treatment of lumbar intervertebral disc herniations find no general agreement, probably because of the many variables present. Post-opera-

tive complications, failed procedure, recurrence of a herniated nucleus pulposus, surgeon's fees, hospital charges, and loss of patient's income all have been considered in various studies. When only hospital charges are compared, there is ample evidence that the cost of chemonucleolysis is less than that of laminectomy. Rameriz and Javid have shown that the average hospital charges for chemonucleolysis are 23% less than those for open surgery (53). McCulloch reported a similar result (40). Reports from France and Australia also confirm this finding (3,28). Length of stay is, of course, the major factor in the lesser hospital charges for chemonucleolysis.

COMPLICATIONS

Tables 8 and 9 summarize the incidence of complications.

Immunological

The most common serious complication of chymopapain is an allergic response, in particular anaphylactic shock. This complication was reported in about 1% of patients; the use of IgE serum sensitivities and skin testing has currently reduced this incidence to about 0.3%. There continues to be a predilection of females over males of about 10 to 1 and of black females over Caucasian females of 3 to 1 (0.7% as compared to 2.0%). The post-marketing survey of the Boots (USA) Company, Inc., for 1987–88 shows an overall rate of anaphylaxis of 0.18% (50). A similar study in Europe by Bouillet placed the rate of anaphylaxis at 0.2% (4). The use of H_1 and H_2 blocking agents, while not shown to influence the incidence of anaphylaxis, has made any reaction more amenable to treatment. If anaphylaxis occurs, the current drug of choice for treatment is epinephrine (0.5 to 1.0 ml of a 1:10,000 dilution) intravenously or intermuscularly. Epinephrine is approximately 200 times the strength of ephedrine. One hundred percent oxygen by inhalation and intravenous infusion of colloids and crystalloids in

TABLE 8. *Comparative complications*

Neurological dysfunction post-operatively	
Laminectomy	0.29%
Chemonucleolysis	0.05%
Infection post-operatively	
Laminectomy	0.31%
Chemonucleolysis	0.07%
Death post-operatively	
Laminectomy	0.05%
Chemonucleolysis	0.02%

TABLE 9. *Complications*

Anaphylaxis	0.3%
Vascular	
Cerebral aneurysm or AVM	4
Intrathecal injection	17
Cerebral accident	5
Subarachnoid hemorrhage	3
Post anti-coagulant	2
Pheochromocytoma	1
Etiology unknown	4
Neurological	
Acute transverse myelitis	6
Cauda equina syndrome	3
Guillain-Barré syndrome	1
Etiology unknown	8
Seizures	4

volume of several liters are important to combat the hypovolemic shock present. Elevation of the lower extremities with the patient supine also will help to increase venous return to the heart and insure cardiac output. Dopamine may be useful if sustained adrenergic drugs are required. Dopamine hydrochloride in doses of as much as 5 microgram per kg/min increases cardiac output and reduces peripheral resistance as well as improving renal blood flow. Two hundred milligrams of Dopamine are dissolved in 250 ml of 5% dextrose and water for intravenous administration.

Less dangerous allergic reactions include a rash or urticaria, which ordinarily respond to antihistamines or steroid ointments, and serum sickness, which may require oral or injectable steroids.

Vascular

The only vascular effect attributable to chymopapain per se is capillary bleeding. In therapeutic dosage the only likely place to observe this effect is by intrathecal injection where the pia and arachnoid capillaries are at risk (26). The amount of bleeding incurred will depend on the dosage of chymopapain, the additional presence of radiocontrast material (which will make it more toxic), and the titer of cystatin C and kininogen present in the cerebrospinal fluid. The latter substances are antiproteases naturally occurring and on an average will neutralize 1.3 to 2.6 mg of chymopapain (10).

Vascular complications included thirty-five reported incidents of central nervous system hemorrhage. Eighteen were indirect or incidental. Included in the group were four cerebral aneurysms and cerebrovascular malformations; five cerebral accidents; four etiology unknown; three subarachnoid hemorrhages, of which two occurred in anticoagulated patients; and one pheochromocytoma (52). These vascular events were incidental to the procedure and were thought to be due to causes other than chymopapain. Seventeen of the thirty-five incidents involved intrathecal injection, and the complications are most likely attributable to the enzyme's action, as described below (Fig. 13).

Neurological

There were eighteen patients with paraplegia or paraparesis from causes other than central nervous system

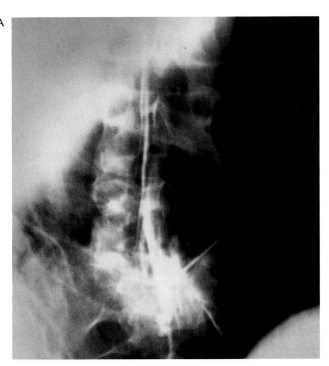
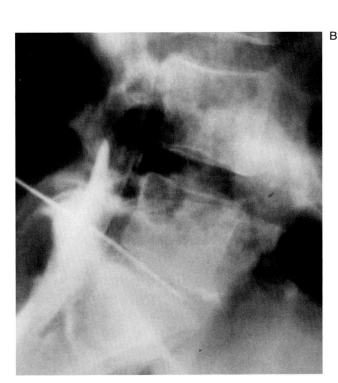

FIG. 13. A and **B:** Intrathecal injection.

hemorrhage (52). Six of these eighteen patients had the diagnosis of acute transverse myelitis (ATM) with onset two to five weeks post injection. A recent study of these cases indicates that two and probably a third case fit the criteria of ATM while of the other three, one involved a likely intrathecal injection, one was multiple sclerosis, and one a cauda equina syndrome 30 minutes following a subsequent laminectomy. The relationship of chymopapain to ATM, if any, has not been determined in spite of extensive study—which is not surprising, since very little is known about the etiology of ATM. Three of the six patients have shown improvement over time. Of the remaining twelve patients with neurologic complications, three people with extruded fragments developed a cauda equina syndrome. They recovered with treatment, but one has a slight extensor hallucis longus weakness and one remains impotent. One patient had a Guillain-Barré syndrome with complete recovery. In eight patients the etiology of neurologic involvement is unknown: one paraplegia, mid-thoracic transverse myelopathy; one paraparesis after two weeks, probably related to drug abuse; and six transient paraparesis, five who made a complete recovery within four days and one with a four-year history of episodes of mild weakness, who improved.

Four patients sustained seizures, none attributable to chymopapain; two probably as a complication of contrast material and two were epileptics.

Since April 15, 1984, there have been about 60,000 injections of chymopapain and no new cases of ATM have been reported. The last reported paraplegia secondary to intrathecal injection was in April 1987 (52).

A comparison of neurological dysfunction post-operatively with laminectomy shows a 0.05% overall rate of neurological defect with chemonucleolysis, while that reported in a survey of community hospitals in the United States in 1980 for laminectomy is 0.29%, or six times as frequent (54). The incidence of infection from laminectomy in 1980 was 0.31%, or four times the overall rate for chemonucleolysis, which is reported to be 0.07% (54). These comparisons are shown in Table 8.

A compilation of complications in the investigational period prior to FDA release of chymopapain in 1982 for the United States is well-documented by Watts and is of similar distribution (75).

Mortality

The post-marketing surveillance covering the first 105,000 patients revealed 9 deaths in the 35 patients already discussed who had central nervous system hemorrhages. Four of the nine deaths were unrelated to the procedure, such as ruptured cerebral aneurysm and cardiovascular malfunction; in three the etiology was unknown. There was one cerebral infarct—probably secondary to intrathecal injection—and one subarachnoid hemorrhage in a patient whose three siblings and father had died of cerebrovascular accidents.

A total of six deaths were secondary to anaphylaxis, four reported since November 1982 and two reported in the original Illinois clinical trial.

Three cardiovascular deaths with known underlying severe disease were unrelated to chymopapain. Additional cases of death include two following infection, one from meningitis and the other from generalized septicemia. One known alcoholic died of a hepatic coma, and another patient of pulmonary embolism (52).

These deaths from all causes not necessarily due to chymopapain occur at an incidence of 0.02%, as compared to 0.05% for laminectomy in 1980 in the United States, or 2½ times greater (54).

LONG-TERM FAILURES

Failure following a technically well-performed chemonucleolysis is largely due to a sequestrated fragment of nucleus pulposus that is either surrounded by fibrous tissue or isolated by healing of the tear in the posterior longitudinal ligament. Perineural fibrosis secondary to the inflammatory reaction caused by disc protrusion is another source of failure. Chymopapain has no influence on fibrosis (44).

Other causes of failure following chemonucleolysis include residual disc protrusion, spinal stenosis, facet hypertrophy, nerve root entrapment, bone spur formation, and acute cauda equina compression due to forcible injection (44).

If failure of chymopapain injection occurs, there is no impediment to performance of discectomy. No abnormality is found at surgery in the epidural space, dura, or about the nerve roots due to chymopapain (9,11,19,56).

RESULTS OF CLINICAL TRIALS

In a series of 1,344 patients injected 8 to 13 years previously, 739 were evaluated by questionnaire. Overall evaluation showed a satisfactory result (25% to 100% relief) in 76%. Of the satisfactory results, 51% were excellent (85% to 100% relief), 16% were good (50% to 85% relief) and 9% were fair (25% to 50% relief) (48). Of the 24% unsatisfactory results, 7% had no relief and no further treatment, 13% had a subsequent laminectomy with 63% of them achieving a satisfactory result, and 4% had a fusion post injection with 58% having a satisfactory recovery (48). This study also addressed the results of chymopapain in patients who had been treated by prior surgery. Of 739 patients surveyed in a long-term follow-up,

119 (16%) had had a laminectomy prior to injection with chymopapain. A successful outcome was noted in 55%, 24% of them excellent. In contrast, there were 526 not heard from in the survey who had previously shown a 72% success rate, but only 1% of them excellent (48).

When patients with prior surgery, midline discs, and spondylolisthesis were eliminated from the analysis to form a category of "ideal patients," there was a satisfactory result in 82%, 60% of which were excellent, further emphasizing the importance of patient selection in the outcome of the procedure (48).

A Texas trial using Chemolase reported the collective post-marketing clinical experience of 21 orthopedic surgeons and neurosurgeons with 919 patients accumulated from 1980 to 1982. Of these patients, 408 were evaluated. The success rates were 93% at one month, 92% at three months, and 93% at six months. Significantly poorer results were found in Hispanics, blue-collar workers, and patients covered by workers' compensation insurance. Adverse reactions were noted in 5% of cases; 1.1% had anaphylaxis (59).

A compilation of long-term results by 13 authors was made to include 3,130 patients whose follow-up ranged from 7 to 20 years. Overall satisfactory results in this large group were 77%, varying from 71% to 93% (47). In comparison, a review of the literature of patients treated by laminectomy reported a composite of success in 77% (53). Thus the success of the procedure is deemed comparable, although admittedly these studies are neither controlled nor randomized.

Others such as Crawshaw et al. (16) and Ejeskar, Nachemson, et al. (21) have reported much less favorable results. In England, satisfactory results were found in 48%, while in Sweden the figure was 53%. With laminectomy, satisfactory results occurred in 89% in England and 64% in Sweden. Unfortunately, both of these studies done at about the same time used Discase from the same drug supplier. In that time period two batches of Discase were recalled by that supplier because of lack of potency. Therefore, it is possible that both of those studies suffered from use of noneffective chymopapain (45).

A prospective comparison of chemonucleolysis and surgical discectomy in 100 closely supervised military personnel found after one year that 78% of the chymopapain-treated patients had a satisfactory outcome, compared to 80% of the discectomy patients. Seventy-eight percent of the chymopapain group and 79% of the discectomy group returned to full military duty. Although this study shows comparable results with chemonucleolysis and discectomy when careful patient selection is practiced, the conclusion drawn by the investigators was that chemonucleolysis should be utilized prior to discectomy whenever appropriate (1). Similar comparable results were found in a ten-year follow-up analysis of 156 patients who had either chemonucleolysis or discectomy. No significant difference was found in the two

groups (76), using elegant outcome criteria. Again, the authors noted that these were not randomized or controlled.

Perhaps the most significant finding in the long-term follow-up studies is that there have been no late complications reported. The concern that spinal stenosis would result from disc space narrowing has not been observed.

USES OF CHYMOPAPAIN IN OTHER CONDITIONS

When the first cervical injection was done by Joseph Brown in 1964, the patient had initial relief and then developed a Brown-Sequard syndrome later proved to be due to a fatal malignant hemangioendothelioma. Nevertheless, this resulted in cervical injections being prohibited. Recently, a small series was reported from Spain with 100% success that gives cause for further investigation in this area of the spine. Since only the "soft disc" herniation will respond to chemonucleolysis, exacting diagnosis will be necessary to be able to recommend intradiscal therapy (12) for these patients.

An intriguing use of chymopapain has been in the proposal stage for some time, but definitive studies have not been forthcoming. Animal experiments have shown that the mobility of the motion segment is increased by surgical or enzymatic removal of the nucleus pulposus (62). If the intervertebral disc at the apex of a scoliotic curve and one on both sides were injected, it is postulated that closed reduction of the curve and cast or jacket maintenance might simplify the treatment of juvenile and adolescent scoliosis. Such an effect has been obtained in the past by surgical discectomy but has not been popular because of the extensive nature of the surgery (55). Injection of the discs might overcome this objection.

Investigational work is under way to determine the probability that chymopapain blocks the chemical mediators that cause irritation to the nerve root from a herniated disc. The proposed action of chymopapain is to disrupt the formation of prostaglandins.

Lastly, work on developing a purer form of chymopapain continues. Removal of impurities and nonessential protein substances is being accomplished. Animal studies have demonstrated its lytic effect on the nucleus pulposus.

OTHER INTRADISCAL INJECTABLES

Collagenase

Sussman presented collagenase in 1948 as an enzyme that would digest the collagen of a herniated disc to relieve the symptoms of nerve root compression (65). In 1980, Bromley and associates reported further studies conducted on dogs and monkeys with a more purified collagenase called Nucleolysin (Advance Biofactures Corp., Lynbrook, NJ). A wide range of safety was demonstrated in all tissues except for intrathecal injection. No allergenicity was found in guinea pig studies (7). An initial series of 52 patients had 78% successful results with no systemic or local toxic effects. Failures were found to be secondary to disc extrusion (6).

There continues to be work done on collagenase. Animal experiments and Phase III human investigation was stopped in 1984 after operative findings in Germany revealed involvement of end plates, bone, ligaments, and epidural fat (2). It was determined that the collagenase used in the German studies was of greater potency than recommended, and similar findings were not identified in the United States (24). Lack of allergic reactions to collagenase has been a major benefit, but the pain relief experienced even in successful cases often takes three to six weeks to develop (8).

Chu presented 252 patients with herniated discs treated by epidural injection of low doses of collagenase. Although three to eight weeks were usually required for relief, he reported 77% satisfactory results. About 50% of the cases not responding to the initial injection were re-injected with "relief in the majority" and without allergic response. He favors epidural rather than intradiscal injection because it does not cause disc space narrowing and possible later stenosis. Unlike with chymopapain, narrowing of the disc space that follows injection of collagenase is irreversible (13).

Aprotinin

Based on the osmotic system of the intervertebral disc, Aprotinin (Transylol-Bayer A. G., Leverkusen) has been utilized for its pressure-reducing effect. Aprotinin contains an alkaline polypeptide with a molecular weight of 6,512, and even intrathecal administration has not resulted in any appreciable damage. Experiments have shown significant reduction in intradiscal pressure in human intervertebral specimens. A series of 212 patients received intradiscal injection of Aprotinin, transdurally in the midline without anesthesia. Spinal headache occurred in 11% of patients. Sixty-seven patients (32%) later had discectomy because of no improvement. A two-year follow-up showed 57% of patients without their previous symptoms. The cases that failed and underwent surgery showed that discs with nuclear protrusion beyond the annulus did not respond to this treatment (34).

A French study of 140 patients injected with Iniprol (Aprotinin, Choay Laboratories) found 61% good results and 39% "medium or bad results." It concluded that Aprotinin was non-neurotoxic, weakly antigenetic, low in cost, and did not cause articular changes or arachnoiditis, but its efficacy was about 10% less than that of chy-

mopapain. The study also concluded that it is applicable to fewer patients with disc problems and appeared to have a "proinfectuous effect." In another series of 125 cases there was a 5% infection rate. A more complete study is said to be underway (15).

Chondroitinase

Chondroitinase ABC (CABC) is a product of the bacterium proteus vulgaris and is a highly specific disaccharidase with potential desirable enzymatic action on the nucleus pulposus. The effect of various concentrations of CABC injected into rabbit intervertebral discs has been compared with alternative levels injected with chymopapain, sterile water, or needled only. Examination showed the chymopapain and Chondroitinase injected discs had narrowing by radiologic examination and degradation of the nucleus pulposus by gross and microscopic evaluation. Histological review indicated dose-related and time-dependent morphological histochemical changes in the disc matrix. A "halo effect" was found that has not been previously noted in enzymatic treatment of the intervertebral disc. Additional studies are underway with this enzyme (22).

Cathepsins

Additional studies have been made on naturally occurring proteolytic enzymes produced by the human body —the cathepsins. Cathepsin G, obtained from human neutrophil leukocytes, chymotrypsin purified from human pancreatic juice, and Cathepsin B purified from human liver have been compared with chymopapain using rabbit intervertebral discs as the experimental model. All enzymes removed the nucleus pulposus, with Cathepsin G and chymotrypsin as effective as chymopapain. Cathepsin B was about half as effective as the others. Further study is under way. One proposed benefit is that an enzyme of human derivation should be less antigenic than a foreign protein (18).

SUMMARY

Chymopapain injection is a safe procedure when performed properly and is effective in relieving radiculitis caused by a herniating nucleus pulposus and appears to give results similar to those for discectomy. Much of the controversy and poor results reported result from poor patient selection or technical error.

Chymopapain causes capillary bleeding intrathecally and may interrupt the microcirculation of nerve tissue, but is not itself neurotoxic. It also does not cause fibrosis or arachnoiditis.

Because it is a foreign protein, chymopapain is allergenic

and can cause anaphylaxis, which can be ameliorated or modified by pre-injection of H_1 and H_2 blocking agents.

The incidence of death, infection, and neurological complications is significantly less with chemonucleolysis than with laminectomy.

Cost comparisons show a 23% saving in hospital charges with chemonucleolysis as compared to laminectomy.

Work continues in the search for improved chemonucleolytic enzymes of increased safety and effectiveness.

REFERENCES

1. Alexander AH, Burkus JK, Mitchell JB, Ayers WV (1989): Chymopapain chemonucleolysis versus surgical discectomy in a military population. *Clin Orthop* (244):158–165.
2. Artigas J, Brock M, Mayer HM (1984): Complications following chemonucleolysis with collagenase. *J Neurosurg* 61:679–685.
3. Bochu M, Demiaus C, Vignon E (1986): The cost of chemonucleolysis. A preliminary study. In: Bonneville J-F, ed. *Focus on chemonucleolysis.* Berlin, Heidelberg: Springer-Verlag, pp. 123–125.
4. Bouillet R (1987): Complications de la nucléolyse discale par la chymopapain. *Acta Orthop Belgica* 53:250–260.
5. Bradford DS, Oegema TR Jr, Cooper KM, Wakando K, Chad EY (1984): Chymopapain, chemonucleolysis, and nucleus pulposus regeneration. A biological and biochemical study. *Spine* 9:135–147.
6. Bromley JW, Gomez JG (1983): Lumbar intervertebral discolysis with collagenase. *Spine* 8:322–324.
7. Bromley JW, Hirst JW, Osman M, Steinlauf P, Gennace RE, Stern H (1980): Collagenase. An experimental study of intervertebral disc dissolution. *Spine* 5:126–132.
8. Brown M (1983): *Intradiscal therapy: Chymopapain or collagenase.* Chicago: Year Book Medical Publishers, pp. 120–127.
9. Burkus JK, Alexander AH, Mitchell JB (1988): Evaluation and treatment of chemonucleolysis failures. *Orthopedics* 11:1677–1682.
10. Buttle DJ, Abrahamson M, Barrett AJ (1986): The biochemistry of the action of chymopapain in relief of sciatica. *Spine* 11:688–694.
11. Carruthers CC, Kousaie KN (1982): Surgical treatment after chemonucleolysis failure. *Clin Orthop* (165):173–175.
12. Castresana FG, Herrero CV (1989): Cervical chemonucleolysis. Presentation of three cases. Early results. International Intradiscal Therapy Society meeting, Orlando, Florida, March 10.
13. Chu KH (1987): Collagenase chemonucleolysis via epidural injection. *Clin Orthop* (215):99–104.
14. Chung BU (1985): Bent-tip single needle technique. In: Brown JE, Nordby EJ, Smith L, eds. *Chemonucleolysis.* Thorofare, New Jersey: Slack, pp. 143–165.
15. Clarisse J, Lesoin F, Pruvo JP, Courtecuisse P, Krivosic I, Gozet G, Deramond H, Viaud C (1986): Nucleolysis using Aprotinin injection: A study of 140 cases. In: Bonneville J-F, ed. *Focus on chemonucleolysis.* Berlin, Heidelberg: Springer-Verlag, pp. 147–151.
16. Crawshaw C, Frazer AM, Merriam WF, Mulholland RC, Webb JK (1984): A comparison of surgery and chemonucleolysis in the treatment of sciatica: A prospective randomized trial. *Spine* 9:195–198.
17. Dabezies EJ, Langford K, Morris J, Shields CB, Wilkinson HA (1988): Safety and efficacy of chymopapain (Discase) in the treatment of sciatica due to a herniated nucleus pulposus. Results of a randomized double-blind study. *Spine* 13:561–565.
18. Dando PM, Morton DB, Buttle DJ, Barrett AJ (1988): Quantitative assessment of human proteinases as agents for chemonucleolysis. *Spine* 13:188–192.
19. Deburge A, Rocolle J, Benoist M (1985): Surgical findings and results of surgery after failure of chemonucleolysis. *Spine* 10:812–815.
20. Eguro H (1983): Transverse myelitis following chemonucleolysis: Report of a case. *J Bone Joint Surg* [Am] 65:1328–1330.
21. Ejeskar A, Nachemson A, Herberts P, Lysell E, Andersson G, Irstam L, Peterson LE (1983): Surgery versus chemonucleolysis for herniated lumbar discs: A prospective study with random assignment. *Clin Orthop* (174):236–242.
22. Eyrell JC, Brown M (1988): The effects of chondroitinase ABC on rabbit intervertebral disc. Presented at the international Intradiscal Therapy Society meeting, Fort Lauderdale, Florida, March 12.
23. FDA Drug Bulletin (1982): Chymopapain approved. 12:17–18.
24. Fisher RG (1985): Complications of chymopapain chemonucleolysis. (letter). *J Neurosurg* 62:621–622.
25. Flanagan N, Smith L (1986): Clinical studies of chemonucleolysis patients with ten- to twenty-year follow-up evaluation. *Clin Orthop* (206):15–17.
25a. Fraser RD (1984): Chymopapain for the treatment of intervertebral disc herniation. The final report of a double–blind study. *Spine* 8:815–818.
26. Garvin PJ, Jennings RB, Smith L, Gesler RM (1965): Chymopapain: A pharmacologic and toxicologic evaluation in experimental animals. *Clin Orthop* (41):204–223.
27. Gesler RM (1969): Pharmacologic properties of chymopapain. *Clin Orthop* (67):47–51.
28. Goldstein G, Gross PF (1985): The treatment of herniated disc in Australia. Costs and benefits of intradiscal injection of chymopapain and surgery. *Aust Family Phys* 14:1179–1190.
29. International Research and Development Corp., Manawan, Michigan (1985): Study of chymopapain and various contrast dyes in the subarachnoid space in baboons. Report to Smith Laboratories.
30. Jansen EF, Balls AK (1941): Chymopapain: A new crystalline proteinase from papaya latex. *J Biol Chem* 137:459–460.
31. Javid MJ, Nordby EJ, Ford LT, Hejna WJ, Whisler WW, Burton C, Millett DK, Wiltse LL, Widell EH, Boyd RJ, Newton SE, Thisted R (1983): Safety and efficacy of chymopapain (Chymodiactin) in herniated nucleus pulposus with sciatica. Results of a randomized, double-blind study. *JAMA* 249:2489–2494.
32. Kiester PD (1989): Research Department. Boots (USA) Company, Inc., Lincolnshire, Illinois.
33. Kiester PD, Anderson GBJ, McNeill TW, Williams J (1989): Is the effect of chymopapain on disc proteoglycans dose related? North American Spine Society paper, Quebec City, Canada, June 30.
34. Kraemer J, Laturnus H (1982): Lumbar intradiscal instillation with aprotinin. *Spine* 7:73–74.
35. Lockey RF, Benedict LM, Turkeltaub PC (1987): Fatalities from immunotherapy (IT) and skin testing (ST). *J Aller Clin Immunol* 79:660–677.
36. Lorenz M, McCulloch J (1985): Chemonucleolysis for herniated nucleus pulposus in adolescents. *J Bone Joint Surg* [Am] 67:1402–1404.
37. McCulloch JA (1977): Chemonucleolysis. *J Bone Joint Surg* [Br] 59:45–52.
38. McCulloch JA (1980): Chemonucleolysis. Experience with 2,000 cases. *Clin Orthop* (146):128–135.
39. McCulloch JA (1983): Discometry. In: McCulloch JA, Macnab I. *Sciatica and chymopapain.* Baltimore: Waverly Press.
40. McCulloch JA (1985): Costs: Surgery vs chemonucleolysis. In: *Alternatives in Spinal Surgery* 2:3–4.
41. McDermott DJ (1985): Clinical trial results. In: Brown JE, Nordby EJ, Smith L, eds. *Chemonucleolysis.* Thorofare, New Jersey: Slack, pp. 61–70.
42. Mixter WJ, Barr JS (1934): Rupture of the intervertebral disc with involvement of the spinal canal. *N Engl J Med* 211:210–215.
43. Naylor A, Earland C, Robinson J (1983): The effect of diagnostic radiopaque fluids used in discography on chymopapain activity. *Spine* 8:875–879.
44. Nordby EJ (1983): Chymopapain in intradiscal therapy. *J Bone Joint Surg* [Am] 65:1350–1353.
45. Nordby EJ (1985): A comparison of discectomy and chemonucleolysis. *Clin Orthop* (200):279–283.
46. Nordby EJ (1985): Diagnosis and patient selection. In: Brown JE, Nordby EJ, Smith L, eds. *Chemonucleolysis.* Thorofare, New Jersey: Slack, pp. 45–60.

47. Nordby EJ (1986): Editorial comment. Long-term results in chemonucleolysis. *Clin Orthop* (206):2–3.
48. Nordby EJ (1986): Eight- to 13-year follow-up evaluation of chemonucleolysis patients. *Clin Orthop* (206):18–23.
49. Nordby EJ, Lucas GL (1973): A comparative analysis of lumbar disk disease treated by laminectomy or chemonucleolysis. *Clin Orthop* (90):119–129.
50. Periodic adverse drug experience to the FDA on Chymodiactin (1987): The Boots (USA) Company, Inc., Lincolnshire, Illinois.
51. Philbin DM, Moss J, Akins CW, Rosow CE, Kono K, Schneider RC, VerLee TR, Savarese JJ (1981): The use of H_1 and H_2 histamine antagonists with morphine anaesthesia: A double-blind study. *Anesthesiology* 55:292–296.
52. Post marketing survey (1982–1986): Smith Laboratories, Northbrook, Illinois.
53. Rameriz LF, Javid MJ (1985): Cost effectiveness of chemonucleolysis versus laminectomy in the treatment of herniated nucleus pulposus. *Spine* 10:363–367.
54. Rameriz LF, Thisted R (1989): Complications and demographic characteristics of patients undergoing lumbar discectomy in community hospital. *Neurosurg* 25:226–231.
55. Roaf R (1960): Vertebral growth and its mechanical control. *J Bone Joint Surg* [Br] 42:40–59.
56. Roggendorf W, Brock M, Gorge HH, et al. (1984): Morphological alterations of the degenerated lumbar disc following chemonucleolysis with chymopapain. *J Neurosurg* 60:518–522.
57. Saunders WC (1964): Treatment of the canine intervertebral disc syndrome with chymopapain. *J Am Vet Med Assoc* 145:893.
57a. Schwetsenau PR, Ramirez A, Johnston J, et al (1976): Double-blind evaluation of intradiscal chymopapain for herniated lumbar discs: Early results. *J Neurosurg* 45:622–627.
58. Shields CB, Arpin EJ (1985): Prone position chemonucleolysis. In: Brown JE, Nordby EJ, Smith L, eds. *Chemonucleolysis.* Thorofare, New Jersey: Slack, pp. 119–127.
59. Simmons JW, Stavinoha WB, Knodel LC (1984): Update and review of chemonucleolysis. *Clin Orthop* (183):51–60.
60. Smith L (1969): Chemonucleolysis. *Clin Orthop* (67):72–80.
61. Smith L, Garvin PJ, Jennings RB, Gesler RM (1963): Enzyme dissolution of the nucleus pulposus. *Nature* 198:1311–1312.
62. Spencer DL, Miller JAA, Bertolini JE (1984): The effect of intervertebral disc narrowing on the contact force between the nerve root and a simulated disc protrusion. *Spine* 9:422–426.
63. Stern IJ (1969): Biochemistry of chymopapain. *Clin Orthop* (67):42–46.
64. Stern IJ (1985): The biochemistry and toxicology of chymopapain. In: Brown JE, Nordby EJ, Smith L, eds. *Chemonucleolysis.* Thorofare, New Jersey: Slack, pp. 11–28.
65. Sussman BJ (1968): Intervertebral discolysis with collagenase. *J Natl Med Assoc* 60:184–187.
66. Sutton CJ Jr (1985): Current concepts in chemonucleolysis. International Congress and Symposium Series. Royal Society of Medicine, London 72:205–211.
67. Sutton CJ Jr (1986): Repeat chemonucleolysis. *Clin Orthop* (206):45–49.
68. Sutton CJ Jr (1988): Chemonucleolysis in the management of herniated lumbar discs in the adolescent. International Intradiscal Therapy Society meeting, Fort Lauderdale, Florida, March 10.
69. Tarlo SM, Shaik W, Bell B, et al. (1978): Papain-induced allergic reactions. *Clin Allergy* 8:207–215.
70. Taylor TK (1971): Intervertebral disc prolapse in children and adolescents. *J Bone Joint Surg* [Br] 53:357.
71. Thomas JC, Wiltse LL (1985): The double needle technique using local anesthesia. In: Brown JE, Nordby EJ, Smith L, eds. *Chemonucleolysis.* Thorofare, New Jersey: Slack, pp. 129–142.
72. Thomas L (1956): Reversible collapse of rabbit ears after intravenous papain and prevention of recovery by cortisone. *J Exp Med* 104:245–252.
73. Trosier O, Gozian E, Durey A, Rodineau J, Goundt-Halbout MC, Pelleroy B (1980): Traitment des lombo-sciatiques per injectio intradiscal d'enzymes proteolytiques (nucleolyse) 80 observations. *Nouvelle Presse Medicale* 19:227.
74. Ventrile CT, Kozlov BA (1978): Papain therapy in the treatment of lumbar osteochondroses. Symposium Lek. Published in Ljubliana, Yugoslavia.
75. Watts C (1977): Complications of chemonucleolysis for lumbar disc disease. *Neurosurg* 1:2–5.
76. Weinstein JN, Lehmann TR, Hejna W, McNeill T, Spratt K (1986): Chemonucleolysis versus open discectomy. A ten year follow-up study. *Clin Orthop* (206):50–55.
77. Wiltse LL (1977): Letter to the editor. *Spine* 2:237.
78. Wiltse LL, Rocchio PD (1975): Preoperative psychological tests as predictors of success of chemonucleolysis in the treatment of the low-back syndrome. *J Bone Joint Surg* [Am] 57:478–483.

The Adult Spine: Principles and Practice,
J. W. Frymoyer, Editor-in-Chief.
Raven Press, Ltd., New York © 1991.

CHAPTER 82

Percutaneous and Suction Discectomy

Vert Mooney

Although it would seem we have good understanding of the role of the herniated nucleus as the major source of sciatica, this is not necessarily the case. We still do not understand why imaging studies demonstrate a significant herniated disc in 20% to 30% of the population who are asymptomatic. We do not know why after successful discectomy the CT scan 6 weeks later shows an unchanged annular profile in the majority of cases (28). We have long thought the disc herniation was a fragment of nuclear tissue from deep within the disc protruding into the spinal canal. Now based on collagen typing, this fragment seems to be repair tissue and not the nucleus (24). Our understanding of the disc as a source of sciatica is constantly being challenged. With that challenge, newer promising treatments such as percutaneous discectomy are developing.

THE CONCEPT OF THE HERNIATED NUCLEUS AS A CAUSE OF PAIN: HISTORIC BACKGROUND

The presence of sciatica was known to ancient physicians but anatomic source was unclear. By 1864, Lasegue (23) described the clinical findings in sciatica, but attributed it to neuritis. Surgical excision of disc material to relieve sciatic pain and impairment was first reported by Oppenheim (32) in 1909. The source of this lesion

was thought to be a neoplasm defined as a enchondroma rather than disc tissue. The fact that disc material could displace into the spinal canal was demonstrated by Middleton and Teacher in 1911 (26) from autopsies. These displacements followed violent events and seem to have little relationship to the common clinical picture we see today. The concept of compression of a nerve root by soft tissue with the creation of subsequent pain and physical deficit was introduced by Elsberg in 1915 (9a). The abnormality he described, however, was the soft tissue of "ligamentum subflavum" which was compressing the nerve root. He did demonstrate that upon removal of this soft tissue the pain was relieved. He also recognized that the change in the soft tissue near the nerve root could create sciatic pain and suggested that perhaps these events would develop on the posterior margins of the vertebral disc. Finally, in 1929, Dandy operated on two patients with cartilaginous masses pressing on the nerve roots, which he thought was the cause of their sciatica (6). He described detached fragments of cartilage from an intervertebral disc and noted the absence of inflammation and the presence of cartilaginous cells. A drawing from his paper shows a clear understanding that the loose cartilage emerged from the intervertebral disc. Because the pre-operative diagnosis had been malignancy, his approach was transdural. The cauda equina syndrome in one of his two patients gradually resolved. He surmised that the lesion was not an enchondroma and termed it a "simulated tumor."

After observing the same clinical presentations and operative findings, Mixter and Barr (27) proposed the

V. Mooney, M.D.: Professor of Orthopaedic Surgery, California College of Medicine, University of California, Irvine Medical Center, Orange, California, 92668.

concept of the lesion of lumbar disc herniation. Comparison of the histologic findings in their patients to the autopsy findings of Schmorl documented the origin of the material was from the intervertebral disc. Surprisingly, they reported that the herniated disc was only somewhat more common than tumors, outnumbering them three to one. Because of continuing question of tumor and the poor radiographic localization then available, wide laminectomies and transdural approach was their advocated method of exploration. Mixter and Barr did create one conceptual milestone which was misleading. They insisted that a disc-lesion be defined as a rupture rather than a herniation, even though they pointed out that most of their cases seemed to be unrelated to major trauma. Rupture implicates a single traumatic event, whereas hernia suggests a progressive lesion with successive overload. This concept to a certain extent continues to cloud our understanding of the pathophysiology of the disc lesion, as well as medical-legal issues of causality. It is nonetheless on the basis of this primary work that the concept of disc prolapse seemed secure. In the words of Macnab, the "dynasty of the disc" emerged as the major explanation for lumbago and sciatica. This simplistic view seemed to answer the important clinical questions. Little attention seemed to be focused on why it happened.

PATHOLOGICAL MECHANISMS UNDERLYING THE CLINICAL SYNDROME OF LUMBAR DISC HERNIATION

Over the decades, the clinical picture became clear. As noted by Mixter and Barr, the majority of patients did not have a single major traumatic event sufficient to have created the problem. The concept then emerged that tears in the annulus could occur and nuclear material could creep into the crevices. Peripheral tears of the annulus were noted in biomechanical and cadaver studies (10), and also were observed in discographic studies (15). That peripheral tear could occur independent of full thickness radial tears in the annulus was emphasized by Parke (33). He pointed out that significant trauma, which produces radial tears in the laboratory, is not necessarily the initiating lesion of the degenerating disc which later becomes a herniation. Support for this concept is derived from studies in sheep demonstrating that a surgically created peripheral laceration of the annulus results in herniation many months later (43a).

Yet another important aspect in the pathophysiology of the deteriorating disc is whether migrating nuclear material is the inciting cause or the result of a deteriorating annulus. CT discography, using water soluble contrast media, shows that a cleft in the annulus is filled by migrating nuclear material. Did increased pressure force create the environment that allowed this nuclear mate-

rial to tear the inner fibers of the annulus, and thus create a stress riser which eventually eroded more peripheral annular fibers to emerge as hernia? Or is the nuclear material a passive agent, which merely flows into a void space in the annular cleft? In identifying the role of the percutaneous discectomy, this capacity of nuclear flow seems to have important implications. Basic biomechanical research also supports this concept.

For example, cyclic events are associated with tears of the annulus, initiated at the inner portion of the disc, which progress radially to the periphery. Adams and Hutton (2) showed that cyclic flexion injury to the disc would eventually create a posterior prolapse in young, well hydrated discs. Later, Krag (20) demonstrated potential for a nuclear flow within the intervertebral disc. Using cyclic flexion, he could show that metal pellets would gradually move posterior in the non-degenerate disc. Thus, these cadaver studies seem to document the potential for material to "flow from one position to another." None of these studies have been done in a living individual and, thus, the reality of nuclear flow has not been demonstrated. However, the question can be asked, "If the material can flow peripherally, is it possible for the material to flow back toward the center—if the space is evacuated?" It is this conceptual model which provides a justification to remove the material in an alternative way to the posterior approach. Moreover, the posterior approach has the liability to destroy some supporting structures of the posterior elements, as well as scar, when the nerve root is surgically exposed. It has been pointed out that it is no longer necessary to totally evacuate the disc to achieve a successful nerve root decompression (40).

Why not avoid the problems created by the posterior approach completely? Historically an answer to this question emerged in the 1940s. Lane and Moore (22) did anterior discectomies for herniated disc disease with moderate success. Due to the morbidity of this approach, it never became popular in the United States. In contrast, anterior treatment for the herniated disc became much more acceptable in Japan. In 1958, Suzuki (41) reported remarkably successful outcomes in his first 30 patients. This success continued and by 1984 a much larger series of cases of anterior disc excision and bone graft replacement was summarized by Inoue (17). In this review of 350 patients followed over 10 years, a spectacular 97% of patients reported they had excellent results for relief of sciatica and 72% reported relief of associated back pain. From a scientific and clinical perspective, these studies had significant limitations. Prolonged bed rest after the surgery was necessary and some complications and morbidity are inherent with the anterior approach. Because fusion was part of the procedure, was stabilization the basis for long-term success? The second part of the question was answered by Nakano (29), who used an abdominal approach and then did a 5 mm perforation in the anterior longitudinal ligament with direct exposure and removal of disc material by standard forceps. No fusion was done. At 5-year follow-up, 95% of his patients were satisfied and had gone back to their original jobs. Only 4% had to have repeat operations. Nakano's clinical experience points out that for the majority of patients with herniated discs, decompression can be achieved by an indirect route. The anterior surgical approaches also appeared to have the potential to remove trapped posterior fragments which are partially extruded into the spinal canal. When asked how much disc material should be removed, Nakano indicated that it was wise to wait after disc material had been removed initially because small pieces would often migrate anteriorly associated with decompression of more central tissue. This clinical observation seems to confirm the potential for anterior migration of nuclear material following creation of a new space more centrally.

CLINICAL EXPERIENCE WITH ATTEMPTS TO ACHIEVE NUCLEAR FLOW

All of the evidence suggests that decompression of the herniated disc by an indirect approach depends upon the potential for nuclear migration or flow. Does this happen in the clinical setting? To date only one study has tried to objectively identify displacement of nuclear material (43). Males suffering with back pain who had CT-discogram before and after flexion and extension exercises demonstrated no changes in radiographic appearances. Variations in the discographic appearance pre- and post-exercise were no greater than could be accounted for by measurement technique. Thus, change in the location of nuclear material could not be proven. However, the exercise regimen proposed by McKenzie (Chapter 76) and the clinical results suggest nuclear displacement and replacement may occur.

A study by Kopp (19) focused at repetitive extension exercises. This study evaluated results when extension exercises were applied to a group with clinical diagnosis of lumbar disc disease who had already had 6 weeks of bed rest and who had leg pain worse than back pain. Sixty percent improved following cyclic extension exercises as advocated by McKenzie. Those who improved were able to achieve full range of extension. Of those who did not improve, 93% could not achieve full extension range and later required surgical treatment. The common surgical finding in these patients was an extrusion of nuclear material. In a later study, Donelson (8) could demonstrate that extension exercises would relocate the pain in most patients. Only 4 of the 80 patients he studied had a poor outcome. Of those patients who could not achieve relocation of pain, 3 required disc removal for complete disc prolapse. These exercise programs seem to focus on relocating displaced nucleus

with the assumption that motion to the disc has the potential for nuclear flow.

If decompression of the disc is the therapeutic goal for the symptomatic herniated disc, what other maneuvers are available? Certainly a time tested maneuver has been bed rest. It should be noted that experimental studies have shown that a total amount of rehydration in the disc will occur within two hours of recumbency (42). It takes about 8 to 10 hours, however, for the fluid within the disc to finally be squeezed out to the baseline state. Thus, prolonged bed rest can offer no advantage to improved hydration of the disc. Further attempts to decompress the disc have been made using traction. Certainly bed traction when compared with other maneuvers had not been demonstrated to be more favorable (35). Other types of traction have been described, such as 90/90 traction (21), gravity traction (5), inversion traction (38), and auto traction. None of these methods have been shown to be of benefit compared to other passive maneuvers (44) or compared to one another.

Another maneuver that might be expected to affect the status of nuclear material is manipulation. Certainly chiropractors and osteopaths for years have provided successful paramedical treatments for a large number of back pain sufferers, but to date no one has ever identified the physiologic event associated with chiropractic manipulation. It is possible, however, that nuclear material could be "rearranged" by these maneuvers, but to date no researcher has investigated the effects of manipulation on herniated discs, despite research directed to this objective (4,11,43a).

Although the combined clinical and scientific information is by no means complete, it forms a plausible basis for treatment by percutaneous discectomy.

HISTORY OF PERCUTANEOUS DISCECTOMY

The concept that chemical removal of nuclear material internally could affect peripheral nerve root irritation was demonstrated clinically first by Lyman Smith (39) with the introduction of chymopapain and supported by a number of subsequent clinical studies (see Chapter 81). Unfortunately complications such as death, significant neurologic deficit, and allergic reaction marred the effective clinical application of this drug in many surgeons' hands.

In 1975 Hijikata (14) published a report on a series of patients who had been successfully treated by a percutaneous discectomy approach. He used specially designed instruments placed through a 5 mm cannula and inserted against the lateral annulus. A circular incision was made in the annulus, and the nuclear material was grasped with a modified pituitary forceps. The success rate was about 80% in the patients presented.

Kambin began to use a percutaneous posterior lateral

discectomy in 1973. Initially he combined a laminectomy with a dorsolateral evacuation of the nucleus using Craig-type instruments. These kinds of instruments had previously been used for bone biopsies and were not particularly suited to the needs of disc evacuation. Better instruments were designed by Jacobson, a neurosurgeon in Miami. He used a direct lateral approach with fluoroscopic guidance. Due to the size of the surgical approach, general anesthesia was used. A 1 inch incision was made over the iliac crest, a speculum was passed through this and then a #40 chest tube was passed to the annulus. The annulus was incised and the disc was removed by the special instruments. Jacobson recommended careful pre- and intraoperative radiographs to avoid lacerating the intestines. He had experience with over 300 patients. Unfortunately, despite his warning, several complications of bowel and peripheral nerve injury occurred. Anatomic variations also were observed and the lateral approach was abandoned because of the unacceptably high level of morbidity which occurred (12). Using the posterolateral approach, however, Kambin persisted with his experience and this forms the basis for the approach used today.

PATIENT SELECTION FOR PERCUTANEOUS DISCECTOMY

Selection of a proper patient for percutaneous discectomy must be based on the demonstration of a structural abnormality creating nerve root irritation that is potentially reversible by decompression of nuclear material. If extruded nuclear material can be demonstrated, or if lateral recess syndrome exists, decompression of the nucleus internally will be of no benefit. The starting point in the evaluation therefore must be based on an appropriate clinical history and physical examination. If the irritated nerve root is the source of pain, leg pain must be expected as the most significant part of the complaint. Ideally, the leg pain is unilateral and more severe than the back pain. However, central disc herniations can occur. In these patients, bilateral leg pain with or without significant back pain can be the clinical presentation.

When identifying the patient's pain, the relationship of the pain to posture and activity is valuable information. Pain that increases with prolonged standing or sitting, but can be relieved by recumbency, suggests the possibility that percutaneous discectomy might be effective. The pain that is constant no matter what posture is tried and unrelated to time suggests the source of the nerve root irritation is fixed and also suggests a trapped disc fragment or extruded disc. The patient is less likely to be a good candidate for the procedure and will more likely require a posterior procedure.

The physical examination must also demonstrate nerve root irritation and the straight leg raising test must confirm that sciatica is present. If straight leg raising of the asymptomatic leg reproduces pain down the symptomatic leg, this finding usually suggests a large herniating disc. In this case, imaging studies should be carefully reviewed because a disc fragment that is too large or extruded may be present. These patients are not candidates for the percutaneous procedure. Careful neurologic examination is also necessary to detect sensory motor or reflex changes suggested by a pain drawing characteristic of a radiculopathy. Motor weakness is often better defined by history of weakness than by specific testing.

Once a history and physical are done, imaging studies are required, of which the most appropriate is the MRI. Because this imaging study has the ability to outline the contour of the annulus, as well as relative water content, more information can be identified concerning the extruded disc. The MRI should demonstrate three elements: (1) an asymmetric protrusion of the lumbar intervertebral disc; (2) a posterior displacement adjacent to the spinal nerve root; and (3) a lack of symmetry relative to the epidural fat. In the older age group, a CT scan also is warranted due to greater sensitivity of this test to identify foraminal intrusion and nerve root entrapment.

Important additional information is the definition of an extruded fragment. Is the disc herniation outside of the annulus and trapped by the posterior longitudinal ligament? It appears that an extruded fragment will contain more water and thus appear lighter on the T2-weighted image (25). A contained herniation in the T2-weighted image has the same dark coloration as the degenerated disc. This is a valuable definition as to whether the patient is a candidate for surgical laminectomy or a percutaneous discectomy. In this regard, the CT discogram is valuable to identify the connection between the internal nuclear material and that at the periphery. It has been noted by Edwards that a non-staining herniation by CT discography has only a 50% good result by chymopapain injection. Probably it would be even worse by percutaneous discectomy, although this study has not been accomplished (9) (Fig. 1). The size of the protrusion is also valuable information. If a herniation is 50% or greater than the anterior posterior diameter of the thecal sac, there is probably a greater than 90% chance that this is an extruded fragment and the patient is not a good candidate for percutaneous discectomy (13). Similar results have been found for chemonucleolysis (34). The size of the spinal canal also is an important consideration. A herniation in a smaller trefoil spinal canal is more significant than a small herniation in a very large canal.

Two other areas of definition are important. One is to clarify to what degree the pain problem is secondary to instability and associated nerve root entrapment as opposed to only a herniation. Standing lateral x-rays are often very helpful and compared to recumbent lateral may show a difference in relative position of the vertebral bodies, which suggests instability. This condition is not appropriate for percutaneous discectomy. A patient

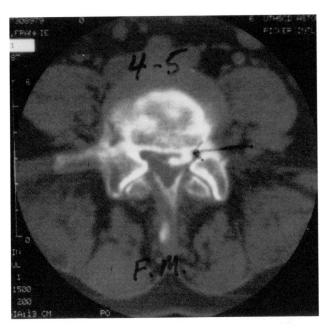

FIG. 1. CT discogram of L4-L5 disc, which demonstrates a subligamentous herniation. This patient had corresponding neural deficits as well as reproduction of pain on the occasion of discography, not ideal for percutaneous discection.

with a very narrowed disc space also is an unlikely candidate for percutaneous discectomy, because of technical problems that will be encountered.

Another emerging use of percutaneous discectomy is the patient with recurrent herniation after successful surgery. One of the most significant problems is the definition between a recurrent disc at a site of previous surgery or pain associated with residual scar. There are two ways in which it can be determined if recurrent disc on scan is an offender. First, the CT discogram will clearly identify the presence of nuclear material relative to scar. This is also an excellent way of determining whether there is connection of the internal nucleus with the periphery disc protrusion. If recurrent disc and connections to the nucleus are present, percutaneous discectomy is an ideal approach because the potential for additional scarring within the spinal canal is avoided. A second maneuver, which recently has emerged as a means by which scan can be differentiated from disc material, is the use of gadolinium. Diffusion of this contrast material into vascularized tissues allows distinction of vascularized scar from non-vascularized tissues such as the disc. In the post-surgical patient, of course, this is a very important consideration and at least one of these two tests should be done to clarify before percutaneous discectomy is considered.

TECHNIQUE

Percutaneous Discectomy

Similar instrumentation had been used for several years by ophthalmologists to remove the vitreous humor of the eye with a special sucking-cutting instrument. The basic tool had originally been directed toward neurosurgical use for removal of brain tumors, but never became successful. Onik (31) noted the ability of this tool to remove the fibro-gelatinous material typical of the vitreous humor of the eye. With appropriate redesign and re-engineering, a cutting device was produced which could pass down a 2 mm cannula. Also due to the reciprocal design of the cutting tool, flexibility was available in the probe and, thus, approach to the L5-S1 level could be accomplished. The first cases using the suction technique were done in association with Dr. James Morris of San Francisco in 1984. First report of this method of disc removal was in 1985 (30) (Figs. 2 and 3). The alternative approach is that of Kambin (18).

In all percutaneous procedures, positioning is very important. Confirmatory location of the area of interest must be accomplished fluoroscopically before the procedure is begun. The AP view must demonstrate the spinous processes to be in the middle of the vertebral body and, thus, a true view without rotation. The lateral view must demonstrate the endplates of the appropriate disc space to be parallel and to be in the middle of the screen. Of course confirmatory localization is necessary to assure the appropriate disc space is being approached. Thus, it is often necessary to count the disc space from below. It is often useful to place a small water bag under the patient's waist if the lateral decubitus position is chosen. This tends to avoid a sag of the lumbar spine in the mid lumbar area and to allow the lumbar spine to be parallel to the floor.

Kambin Approach

In the Kambin approach, the patient lies prone and is lightly sedated. A site 8 to 9 cm lateral to the mid line is chosen and a long 18 gauge needle is inserted into the annulus. Obviously the correct positioning of the needle is a necessary step. An attempt is made to insert the needle parallel to the vertebral endplates and into the center of the disc as visualized in the anteroposterior and lateral x-ray positions. The techniques of this approach are identical to that for chymopapain as described in Chapter 81 (Fig. 4A). Following appropriate position of the needle, a small diameter Kirschner wire is introduced through the needle. Following that, a cannulated blunt trocar with an external diameter of 4 mm and a length of 19 cm is passed over the K-wire and directed towards the annulus. The cannulated trocar allows insertion of various instruments while avoiding injury to surrounding soft tissues. The guide wire is removed before insertion of the instruments. Once radiographic confirmation is achieved, a larger cannula is passed over the original one with an external diameter of 6 mm, internal diameter of 4.9 mm, and a length of 16 cm. A small cutting instrument with an external diameter of 2.5 mm centered on the hollow tube and fitted snugly

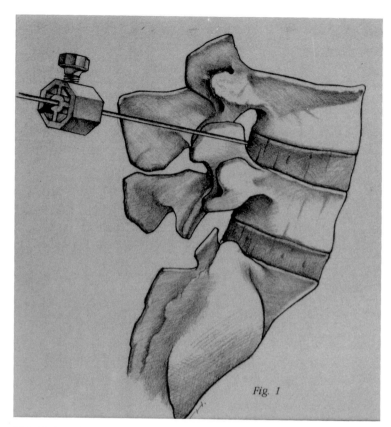

FIG. 2. Localization of the trochar at the L4-L5 level from the posterior lateral approach.

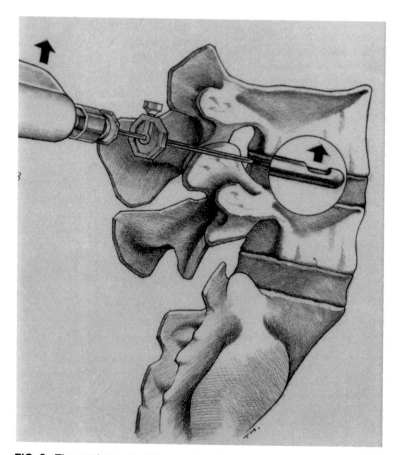

FIG. 3. The cutting port of the suction discectomy nucleotome. Reciprocal slicing by a small guillotine knife inside of the tube creates 1 mm chunks of tissue which are flushed away. The localization of the cutting port can be determined by the orientation of the nucleotome handle.

A

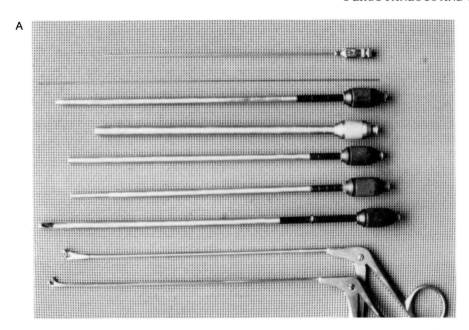

FIG. 4. A: The Kambin instruments. The enlarging cannulas are evident. In addition, the positioning cannula to allow location of the special rongeurs is noted. (Figs. 4B–4C follow.)

B

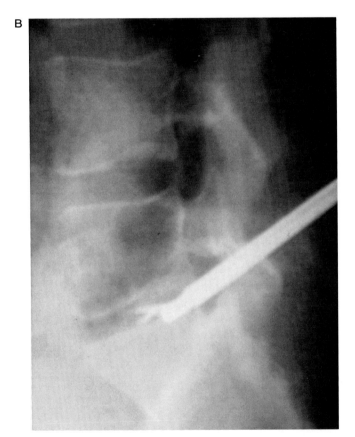

C

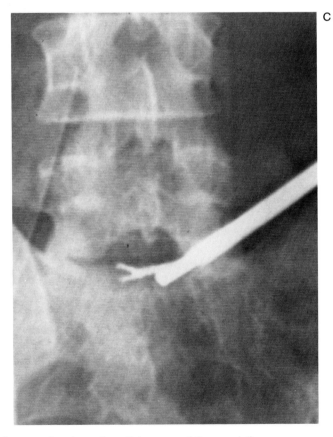

FIG. 4. B and C: Use of the positioning cannula to allow greater circumferential access of the specially designed forceps. The angulation allows removal of additional material and access to the L5-S1 level.

inside the sheath is used to cut a hole in the annulus. This is followed by a larger cutter with an external diameter of 4 mm, which is used to enlarge the annular fenestration (Figs. 4B and 4C). Now with the annulus windowed and soft tissues protected, and a sufficiently large cannula in place, straight and curved forceps are introduced through the sheath into the disc space. These forceps are specially designed for this purpose and may be angulated slightly to remove additional material. Further evacuation is aided by aspiration with a 50 cc lure-lock syringe fitted to the cutting instrument or the forceps deflector. The procedure under these circumstances is continued until no more material can be evacuated.

Suction Discectomy

The technique advocated is similar to that described by Kambin and also similar to that advocated for chymopapain injection and discography. Although the positioning can be done either prone or lateral, most surgeons are more comfortable with a lateral decubitus position, while most radiologists seem to be more comfortable with a prone position which requires a special table. When the prone position is used, flexion of the hips is of benefit to reduce lumbar lordosis and, thus, allow a larger entry zone posteriorly. This posture can be accomplished easily in the lateral decubitus position with the patient merely bending the hips.

In contrast to the Kambin procedure, the procedure using the suction nucleotome is initiated with an 18 gauge, 25 cm long hubless stainless steel trocar. This is inserted obliquely toward the posterior margin of the intervertebral disc from a site which has been identified earlier using the fluoroscope. The fluoroscope allows the appropriate level to be identified, and the posterolateral approach about 10 cm from the mid line is chosen. Local anesthesia is necessary and the patient is merely sedated. The trocar is passed slowly to the area of interest with confirmatory fluoroscopic views as necessary. Once the trocar is in the appropriate position, a 2.8 mm cannula with an internal blunt-ended, tapered dilator is placed over the hubless trocar. When the cannula and dilator are in the correct position, the dilator is removed. The dilator extends past the cannula 2 mm so that once the dilator is removed the cannula moves forward slightly and is pressed up against the annulus. A 2 mm open-ended, circular cutting tool is placed through the cannula, over the guide wire, to cut the hole in the annulus. Fluoroscopic confirmation is necessary if sensation of abutment on the annulus is not available. A few rotations of the cutting trocar are necessary, then the cannula can be passed through the hole in the annulus. It should be passed only a few millimeters. It is now appropriate to remove the trocar and pass the nucleotome into the disc space (Fig. 5).

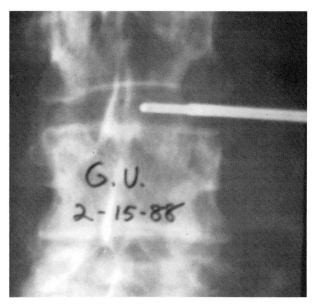

FIG. 5. Proper location of the nucleotome should be as near as possible to the center of the disc. Suction discectomy is occurring here at the L3-L4 level.

The nucleotome is 20 cm long with a rounded tip and closed in with a single port. It functions according to the same principle as the guillotine instruments used in arthroscopic surgical procedures. The reciprocating action of the cutting tool has a 2 mm travel. Aspiration occurs concurrent with the cutting and is pneumatically driven; this allows flexibility of the instrument. The material is suspended in saline, which has reached the port by flowing distally between the inner cannula and the walls of the outer tube. This slurry is aspirated through the inner cannula into a collection bottle. The inner cannula reciprocates at approximately 180 cycles per minute permitting rapid cutting and aspiration of disc material. The negative pressure is about 600 mm of mercury. The disc material is removed until none is easily obtained and usually requires 20 to 30 minutes to accomplish. This particular instrument does not allow as large a circumference of potential evacuation as the Kambin tool. The amount of disc material that can be removed is questionable and will be discussed later.

In both the percutaneous and suction techniques, the L5-S1 approach is more difficult due to the height of the iliac crest and, in fact, was originally thought to be a relative contraindication. However, this disc space can now be approached by proper positioning and special instruments (Fig. 6). In general, the procedure at L5-S1 is often easier in women due to their wider pelvis and, thus, a less steep angle necessary for the approach of the L5-S1 level. Positioning can be helped at L5-S1 in several ways.

First, slight angulation of the pelvis inferiorly is feasible if the superior leg is adducted. This can be accomplished in the lateral decubitus position by flexing the

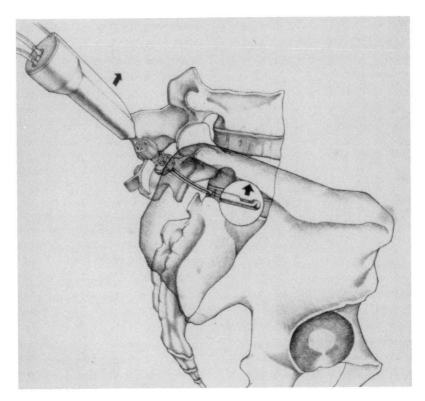

FIG. 6. The nucleotome is inserted into the L5-S1 disc space. The flexible shaft of the nucleotome allows access to the disc space lying below the iliac crest.

inferior hip, but allowing the superior hip to be extended. The weight of the leg will slightly tilt the pelvis.

Secondly, radiographic control is most important in appropriate instrument placement at the L5-S1 area. Romy (36) described an oblique approach, which may facilitate entry. The basic strategy is to find the path to the disc with the central x-ray beam along which the trocar can then be aimed. The key to this approach is positioning of the fluoroscopic unit so that the endplates are parallel, and in the oblique position the superior articular facet of the first sacral segment is posterior to the entry site while the iliac crest is anterior. This leaves a small triangle with the inferior endplate of L5 making the third line as seen under fluoroscope. In these circumstances one can use a needle holder and place the trocar down the line of the fluoroscopic beam. If the angle is correct, the needle appears as a single dot over the path to the disc. As the needle or trocar deviates from the appropriate line, more of the metal is seen.

Thirdly, in that the trocar should approach the L5-S1 disc space in a parallel manner, the entry area of the skin should be that area just superior to the iliac crest which allows the trocar to be parallel to the L5-S1 interspace as it enters the skin and skims over the top of the iliac crest. Local anesthetic may be necessary at the iliac crest. Trial and error efforts may be necessary before the final position is achieved. Sometimes the angle is so steep that the trocar cannot enter the annulus and remain straight.

Under these circumstances the curved cannula supplied by the manufacturer can be brought over the trocar and by bending the trocar slightly, entry into the disc space can be achieved. Once the cannula is in place, the procedure is the same as for the other levels. The curved cannula is 15 cm long and 3.5 mm in diameter. The curve has a 24 cm radius. Because the curved cannula is somewhat larger than the basic cannula, initial introduction of the straight cannula is helpful to serve as a dilator for soft tissues before the insertion of the curved cannula. The curved cannula has a teflon sleeve internally so that the nucleotome and other instruments can more easily pass within it. This curved cannula also has the benefit that it allows rotation and, thus, a greater area of disc may be removed than at other levels.

This approach does have problems in that most portable C-arms have such a narrow distance between image intensifier and x-ray tube that positioning may abut against the table. For this reason, before initial application to a patient, trial with cadavers or mannequins should be accomplished using the equipment anticipated to be used in the hospital setting.

RESULTS

Evaluation of results should be made in the context of the selection procedure and the criteria for success. The original investigators for this procedure decided to evaluate results purely on the basis of success or failure. Success was identified as follows: (1) moderate to complete pain relief, (2) no narcotic medications, (3) a return to pre-injury functional status, and (4) satisfaction by the patient with the procedure. Failure of any of these criteria resulted in the patient being classed as a failure. In the selection process, patients were identified as those who fulfilled strict criteria for inclusion in the original protocol and those who were not in the protocol. The protocol utilized was essentially the same as previously used for patients selected for chemonucleolysis. To qualify as a candidate in the protocol, the patient had to have leg pain worse than back pain, evidence of nerve root tension, imaging studies which correlated with the clinical picture, and failure of spontaneous healing or conservative treatment for at least 6 weeks. Those patients who did not meet all of the criteria identified above, but still were considered by the clinicians to be candidates for the procedure, were identified as being out of protocol. The early results of the 17 original investigators are presented in Table 1. One third of the patients operated upon were out of protocol. As a group, the patients were equally distributed to males and females. The average age was 41. The average period of pre-operative care was 11.5 months and the minimal period of follow-up evaluation was 12 months. The success of those patients meeting protocol criteria was about 75% as noted in Table 2. The success rate was about 50% for those patients who had treatment, but were not in the strict protocol as is seen in Table 3. Sex or age seemed to make no difference in success or failure.

All the reports from this procedure have not been excellent of course. The most disappointing results were reported by Kahanovitz et al. at the 1989 meeting of the International Society for the Study of the Lumbar Spine at Kyoto, Japan, May 15–19, 1989. At this meeting it was reported that only 55% of the 39 patients in a multicenter series had a good result as defined by not needing additional surgery. At that same meeting, investigators from other parts of the world gave reports as well, as is reflected by Table 4. Although different criteria were used for success and failure in these reports, most of the experience was over a 70% success rate (1).

The sources of failure were interesting and there seemed to be little difference between those in protocol and those out of protocol. Table 5 demonstrates the sources of failure for out of protocol while Table 6 demonstrates the same information for the patients in protocol. Certainly the presence of a free fragment was the most common source of failure, followed by spinal stenosis which was a significant factor in those patients out of protocol. Incomplete decompression apparently due to technical factors was the most common source of failure for those in protocol.

With growing experience, better selection criteria, and greater experience with the procedure, some improvement in results can be expected. To date, Davis has the largest experience with this procedure. He has recently prepared a report on 518 consecutive patients (7), which showed a higher success rate with greater experience. In those patients receiving no compensation, an 87% success rate was defined at 6 months follow-up (Table 7). Davis also demonstrates an interesting aspect of the percutaneous discectomy. There were 44 cases who presented as failures from previous laminectomies, but who had a pain-free interval before recurrence of pain. In these individuals with apparent recurrent disc herniation, there was a 91% success rate (Table 8). In his series, there were 36 patients over the age of 36; the older patients had less significant success rate and 30% failure rate.

Others have compared the results of chymopapain and percutaneous discectomy procedures (37). Schweigel noted a 14-year experience with 3,000 cases of chymopapain and a 2.5-year experience with 300 cases of percutaneous discectomy. His success rate was 78% for the percutaneous procedure, nearly exactly the same as his success rate using chymopapain. In reporting his results, Schweigel has identified some of the technical problems with this procedure. He noted that in two of his early failures, he had entered the side opposite to the symptoms. Following failure of the procedure, he repeated the procedure entering on the side of the symptoms and had a good result. He, thus, notes that it is necessary to be more precise in instrument placement than in the case of chymopapain. He also emphasizes the importance of placing the nucleotome central and posterior to be as close as possible to the herniated material. However, there was little relationship between amount of disc material removed and success or failure. He also noted another aspect of percutaneous discectomy which is of interest. A relatively small number of patients were significantly symptomatic with a central herniation, which generally caused pain in both legs. Fifty-five of his 300 cases had this condition and achieved an 82% success rate.

None of the reports indicate significant back pain following the procedure. Although it was common to note disc space collapse following chymopapain, this radiographic finding has not been noted following percutaneous discectomy.

How often is this procedure performed relative to other procedures available for disc herniations? Two surgeons, Maroon and Day, have focused on that question. Both indicate that about 20% of their patients had discectomies performed by the percutaneous approach (3). This would suggest very strict adherence to patient selection criteria.

The most heartening aspect of this procedure, however, is its safety. In the 495 patients reported by the original investigators there was one disc space infection

TABLE 1. *Protocol*

	N	%
(I) In	327	66.1
(O) Out	168	33.9
Total	495	100.0

TABLE 2. *In protocol success/failure*

	N	%
(S) Success	246	75.2
(F) Failure	81	24.8
Total	327	100.0

TABLE 3. *Out protocol success/failure*

	N	%
(S) Success	83	49.4
(F) Failure	85	50.6
Total	168	100.0

TABLE 4. *ISSLS percutaneous reports 1989 (ref. 1)*

Series	Success	Author
30	83%	Ooi, Japan
49	65%	Cho, Korea
137	74%	Cotta, Germany
150	72%	Hijikata, Japan
39	55%	Kahanovitz, United States

TABLE 5. *Findings at secondary procedure in patients out of protocol*

Free fragment	41
Spinal stenosis	16
Incomplete decompression	6
Pending surgery	22
Total	85

TABLE 6. *Findings at secondary procedure in patients in protocol*

Free fragment	30
Spinal stenosis	6
Bulging disc	7
Vertebral fracture	1
Incomplete decompression	16
Pending surgery	21
Total	81

TABLE 7. *Davis results: Patients at 6 months follow-up or greater (ref. 7)*

Overall	
Number of cases	518
Successful	439 (85%)
Failures	79 (15%)

Non-compensated cases	
Number of cases	427
Successful	371 (87%)
Failures	56 (13%)

Compensated cases	
Number of cases	91
Successful	68 (74%)
Failures	23 (26%)

TABLE 8. *Previous laminectomies*

Number of cases	44
Successful	40 (91%)
Failures	4 (9%)

and one psoas hematoma. There was no nerve damage or major vascular damage. All other investigators to date report an excellent safety record. It is estimated that the incidence of infection for this procedure probably is about the same as for discography which is probably about 1 in 1,000. To this date no major vascular or neural damage has been reported. However, it must be remembered that a similar safety record was reported for chymopapain, only to be followed by significant complications when its use became more widespread.

Obviously, a procedure such as this which is relatively so simple and might even be considered innocuous has a great risk for overutilization. This is a procedure which generally can be done on an outpatient basis and for which patients can be assured that their risks are significantly less than for standard surgical approaches. No long-term damage to the disc or supporting structures has ever been reported. Even in those patients who are not held in the strict protocol of radiculopathy, secondary to herniated discs, a 50% success rate has been reported (see Table 3). In these out of protocol patients, what is accomplished? Indeed in those successful results in protocol, what really has happened? At this point in time we really don't know. There does not seem to be a very great relationship between the amount of nuclear material removed and success of procedure. Perhaps the benefit of the procedure is by mechanism of disc decompression in a structure which, for various reasons, has increased pressure. It seems unlikely that the actual protrusion is significantly reduced; repeat CT scans days or a week after the procedure show little anatomic change. However, repeat discography accomplished two weeks after the procedure does not reveal leaking of contrast externally.

Probably the correct answer to the question "What is the place of percutaneous discectomy?" is not yet available. Only by careful follow-up and evaluation of pre- and post-operative findings will the answers become clear. This procedure, however, does present exciting opportunities for further investigation and evaluation. By easy access to the disc of the symptomatic individual, a greater understanding of the pathophysiology of this lesion will emerge and wider applications will be forthcoming. Indeed, the procedure has been used for biopsy and evacuation of disc space infections. Perhaps because of the ease of access, this procedure at some time in the future will be used for the instillation of therapeutic agents within the disc. The history of its use is still quite short and there is much to be learned in the future.

REFERENCES

1. *Abstracts* (1989): International Society for the Study of the Lumbar Spine. Kyoto: Japan, pp. 39, 42, 60, 67, 84.
2. Adams MA, Hutton WC (1982): Prolapsed intervertebral disc: A hyperflexion injury. *Spine* 7:184–191.
3. Blum RS (1988): Technology marches on, or does it? Chemonucleolysis, percutaneous nucleotomy and imaging procedures: A review. Presented at the California Society of Industrial Medicine in Surgery, Carmel, California, July 14–17.
4. Breen AC (1977): Chiropractors and the treatment of back pain. *Rheum Rehab* 16:46–53.
5. Burton CV (1986): The gravity lumbar reduction therapy program. *J Musculoskel Med* 3:12.
6. Dandy WE (1929): Loose cartilage from intervertebral disk simulating tumor of the spinal cord. *Arch Surg* 19:660–672.
7. Davis WG, Onik G, Helms C (accepted for publication): Automated percutaneous discectomy. *Spine.*
8. Donelson R (1986): Centralization phenomenon. Its usefulness in evaluating and treating sciatica. *Orthop Trans* 10:533.
9. Edwards W, et al (1987): CT discography: Prognostic value in selection of patients for chemonucleolysis. *Spine* 12:792–795.
9a. Elsberg CA (1915): Pain and other sensory disturbances in diseases of the spinal cord and their surgical treatment. *Am J Med Sci* (ns) 149:337–339.
10. Farfan HF, Cossette JW, Robertson GH, Wells RV, Kraus H (1970): The effects of torsion on the lumbar intervertebral joints: The role of torsion in the production of disc degeneration. *J Bone Joint Surg* [Am] 52:468–497.
11. Farrell JP, Twomey LT (1982): Acute low back pain: Comparison of two conservative treatment approaches. *Med J Australia* 1:160–164.
12. Friedman WA (1983): Percutaneous discectomy: An alternative to chemonucleolysis? *Neurosurgery* 13:542–547.
13. Fries JW, Abodeely DA, Vijungco JG, et al (1982): Computed tomography of herniated and extruded nucleus pulposus. *J Comput Assist Tomogr* 6:874–887.
14. Hijikata S, Yamagishi M, Nakayama T, et al (1975): Percutaneous discectomy: A new treatment method for lumbar disc herniation. *J Toden Hosp* 5:5.
15. Hirsch C (1948): An attempt to diagnose the level of disc lesion clinically by disc puncture. *Acta Orthop Scand* 18:132.
16. See Vernon-Roberts, et al, ref. 43a.
17. Inoue S, Watanabe T, Hirose A, et al (1984): Anterior discectomy and interbody fusion for lumbar disc herniation: A review of 350 cases. *Clin Orthop* (183):22–31.
17a. International Society for the Study of the Lumbar Spine (1989): see ref. 1.
18. Kambin P, Sampson S (1986): Posterolateral percutaneous suction-excision of herniated lumbar intervertebral discs. *Clin Orthop* (207):37–43.
19. Kopp JR, Alexander AH, Turocy RH, et al (1986): The use of lumbar extension in the evaluation and treatment of patients with acute herniated nucleus pulposus. *Clin Orthop* (202):211–218.
20. Krag MH, Seroussi RE, Wilder DG (1987): Thoracic and lumbar internal displacement distribution from an in vitro loading of human spinal motion segments: Experimental results and theoretical predictions. *Spine* 12:1001–1007.
21. Lancourt JE (1986): Traction techniques for low back pain. *J Musculoskel Med* 3:44.
22. Lane JD Jr, Moore ES Jr (1948): Transperitoneal approach to the intervertebral disc in the lumbar area. *Ann Surg* 127:537–551.
23. Lasegue C (1864): Considerations sur la sciatique. *Arch Gen Med* (S6) 4:55.
24. Lipson SJ (1988): Metaplastic proliferative fibrocartilage as an alternative concept to herniated intervertebral disc. *Spine* 13:1055–1060.
25. Masaryk TJ, Ross JS, Modic MT, et al (1988): High-resolution MR imaging of sequestered lumbar intervertebral discs. *Ann J Neuroradiol* 9:351–358.
26. Middleton GS, Teacher JH (1911): Injury of the spinal cord due to rupture of an intervertebral disc during muscular effort. *Glasgow Med J* 76:1–6.
27. Mixter WJ, Barr JS (1934): Rupture of the intervertebral disc with involvement of the spinal canal. *New Engl J Med* 211:210–215.
28. Montaldi S, Fankhauser H, Schnyder B, de Tribolet N (1988): Computed tomography of the post operative intervertebral disc and lumbar spinal canal: Investigation of 25 patients after successful operation for lumbar disc herniation. *Neurosurgery* 22:1014–1022.

29. Nakano N, Nakano T (1986): Long-term results of anterior exterior peritoneal lumbar discectomy. *Orthop Trans* 10:537.

30. Onik G, Helms C, Ginsburg L, Hoaglund F, Morris J (1985): Percutaneous lumbar discectomy using a new aspiration probe. *Am J Neuroradiol* 6:290.

31. Onik GM, Morris J, Helms C, et al (1987): Automated percutaneous discectomy: Initial patient experience. *Radiology* 162:129.

32. Oppenheim H, Krause F (1909): Veber Ein Klemmung bzw. Strangulation der cauda equina. *Deutsche Med Wchnschr* 35:697.

33. Park WM, McCall MB, O'Brien JP, Webb JK (1979): Fissuring of the posterior annulus fibrosus in the lumbar spine. *Br J Radiol* 52:382–387.

34. Postacchini F, Lami R, Massobrio M (1987): Chemonucleolysis versus surgery in lumbar disc herniations: Correlation of results to preoperative clinical pattern and size of the herniation. *Spine* 12:87–96.

35. Quinet RJ, Hadler NM (1979): Diagnosis and treatment of backache. *Sem Arth Rheum* 8:261–287.

36. Romy M (1985): Chemonucleolysis technique: New oblique approach requires no measurements. *J Neurol Orthop Med Surg* 6:47.

37. Schweigel J (1988): Compression of chymopapain and percutaneous discectomy. In: *Automated percutaneous lumbar discectomy*, G Onik, CA Helms, eds. San Francisco: Radiology Research and Education Foundation, pp. 85–92.

38. Sheffield FJ (1964): Adaptation of tilt table for lumbar traction. *Arch Phys Med Rehab* 45:469–472.

39. Smith L (1964): Enzyme dissolution of the nucleus pulposus in humans. *JAMA* 187:137–140.

40. Spengler DM (1982): Lumbar discectomy: Results with limited disc excision and selective foraminotomy. *Spine* 7:604–607.

41. Suzuki J (1958): Anterior body fusion for lumbar disc herniation. *Japanese Orthopaedic Association* 32:948.

42. Urban JP, Holm S, Maroudas A, et al (1982): Nutrition of the intervertebral disc: Effect of fluid flow on solute transport. *Clin Orthop* (170):296–302.

43. Vanharanta H, Ohnmeiss MS, Rashbaum R, et al (1988): Effect of repeated trunk extension and flexion movements as seen by CT discography. *Orthop Trans* 12:650.

43a. Vernon-Roberts B, Osti OL, Fraser RD (1990): A sheep model of disc degeneration initiated by a peripheral annulus tear. *Abstracts.* International Society for the Study of the Lumbar Spine, June 13–17, 1990, Boston, p. 21.

44. Weber H (1983): Lumbar disc herniation: A controlled, prospective study with ten years of observation. *Spine* 8:131–140.

The Adult Spine: Principles and Practice,
J. W. Frymoyer, Editor-in-Chief.
Raven Press, Ltd., New York © 1991.

CHAPTER 83

Microdiscectomy

John A. McCulloch

A successfully completed surgical procedure followed by a poor result quickly leads to the realization that the ultimate outcomes are far more dependent on patient selection than surgical technique. Obviously, a poorly done operation carries with it a greater risk of failure. But given competent surgical expertise, there is little apparent difference in outcome between a microsurgical discectomy and standard laminectomy/discectomy. Why, then, should a modification of a well-accepted technique be promoted?

Progress in medicine is founded on obvious principles and flourishes in the milieu of dialogue between supporters and critics. If a new idea or technique can stand

rigorous critique, the essence of science, it survives. It doesn't take a lot of criticism to make a bad idea go away. It is in this setting that more surgeons are advancing the idea of microsurgery for lumbar disc disease. The advocates of microdiscectomy believe there are many advantages to using the microscope over loupes and also believe their approach enhances wound healing.

ADVANTAGES OF USING THE MICROSCOPE

I believe there are significant advantages to the use of the microscope:

1. The microscope offers greater degrees of magnification than possible with loupes. With loupes, a surgeon may work for a limited period of time at 3 to 4 times magnification. As the loupe magnification increases, the

J. A. McCulloch, M.D.: Professor of Orthopaedics, Northeastern Ohio Universities, College of Medicine, Rootstown, and 75 Arch Street, Suite 501, Akron, Ohio, 44304.

length of time a surgeon can work is decreased because it is more difficult to fix the line of vision for extended periods of time. Further, as loupe magnification increases, the surgeon becomes momentarily disoriented on looking up from the field.

2. The optics of the microscope compress the dimensions needed for 3-dimensional visualization (stereopsis) of the operative field (Fig. 1).

3. The illuminating system of the microscope has two advantages: (a) it is very intense (40,000 footcandles), and (b) it is directly along the line of vision (Fig. 2). These optical/illuminating advantages enhance the ability to see the nerve root and encroachment pathology, to cauterize epidural veins safely, to distinguish between scar tissue and nerve root in re-operations, and, finally, to allow the assistant to see as well as the operating surgeon, making the microscope a powerful teaching instrument in a training program.

4. A hidden benefit of the microscope is the more disciplined thinking it forces on the surgeon. The moment a surgical incision is limited, the more imperative it becomes for the surgeon to know exactly where to position the incision and exactly what is to be found at the time of exposure. This forces him to look more critically at the patient and the imaging investigation. No longer can the surgeon seek and find; the pathology to be found and its exact location must be precisely localized before the limited skin incision is made. Sophisticated imaging modalities are essential. In this context the microscope can be viewed as merely a tool that gets the surgeon to the scene of the pathology.

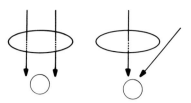

FIG. 2. Coaxial vs paraxial illumination. With paraxial illumination (loupes and headlight) (right), a wider incision is needed to get the light into the depth of the wound.

WOUND HEALING

The second broad set of advantages, I believe, relates to wound healing. Some surgeons would say that the length of the incision is not important because wounds heal side-to-side, not end-to-end. Admittedly, skin incisions heal side-to-side and the length of the skin incision is not important, except for cosmesis. The major issues are the wound hematoma and the magnitude of peridural scar (Fig. 3) (19). Larocca and Macnab (14), in developing their hypothesis for laminectomy membrane, observed: "The fibrous response was always more marked when a wide operative exposure was employed." Unfortunately, this observation was not enlarged upon because the thrust of their research was to show the value of a Gelfoam membrane, used to separate the exposed dura and nerve roots from the erector spinae muscles.

It is also important to emphasize the less muscle dissection that occurs, the less potential dead space there is for hematoma. When a limited wound incision is made, there is a reduced requirement for healing by secondary intention and, in the end, less scar (Fig. 4).

Figure 5 demonstrates the advancing front of wound healing that encircles the dead space hematoma that fills a paraspinal incision. There is such an organized mass of cells and events involved in wound healing that the healing wound can be considered a "temporary organ unto itself" (19). This process of wound healing is affected by local factors such as the amount of tissue damage made at the time of the incision, the number of sutures inserted, and the presence or absence of other necrotic debris and infection. In the end, this healed wound is represented by scar.

A further disadvantage is the denervation that occurs in larger paraspinal incisions. This was documented by Macnab et al. (16) in a clinical study of 113 patients, showing some measure of denervation of the paravertebral muscles on EMG in 96% of the cases. Denervation was shown to persist for many years following surgery, and reinnervation was only partial.

A final argument in support of the smallest possible wound is the observation in repeat spine surgery that the best place to look for normal structures, such as unscarred dura, is behind normal bone or ligamentum flavum. Thus, if a spine exposure can be accomplished with

A

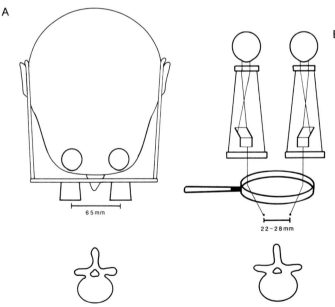

65 mm

22–28 mm

FIG. 1. Stereopsis (3-dimensional) visualization requires at least 65 mm for interpupillary distance with loupes (**A**). Through the optics of the microscope, this distance is compressed to 22–28 mm (**B**), meaning a much smaller incision is needed to maintain 3-D vision in the depth of the wound.

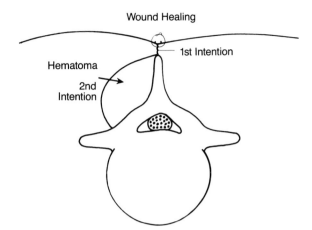

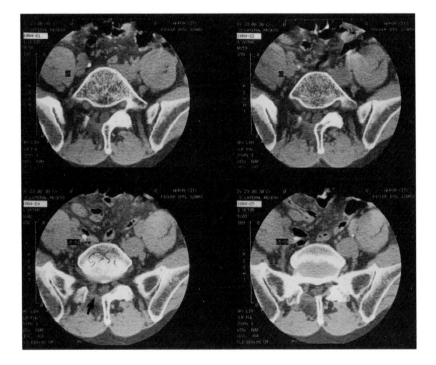

FIG. 3. Skin is expected to heal by primary intention, but if dead space is left behind by a longer paraspinal incision, it will fill with hematoma and heal by secondary intention (scar). Dead space is reduced when the smallest possible invasion (microsurgery) is used.

FIG. 4. A post-operative microdiscectomy on CT. Note the laminectomy membrane and very little scar around the dura and root (right L5-S1) (arrow).

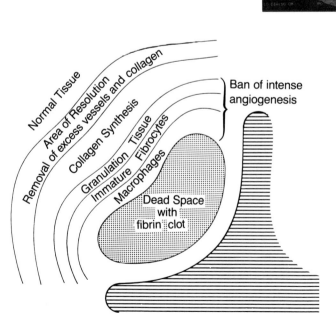

FIG. 5. The module of wound healing—a complicated, multifaceted "organ unto itself."

maintenance of as much normal anatomy as possible, such as bone or ligamentum flavum, then the ultimate scar tissue formation around the dura and nerve roots will be reduced. One of the advantages of microsurgery is that the surgical exercise can be accomplished with limited removal of ligamentum flavum and lamina.

Finally, I believe one of the major benefits is early mobilization. Kahonovich et al. (12) compared a group of patients who had standard laminectomy to a group of patients who had a microsurgical exposure. In terms of surgical outcome, the results of the two groups were identical except for post-operative morbidity and length of stay in hospital. The patients who underwent a microsurgical approach had a much reduced post-operative morbidity and a much shorter hospital stay. A patient who can get out of bed the same day as the surgical procedure and be home the next day has tremendous advantage over a patient who has a more painful wound and requires longer bedrest and hospitalization. The general benefits of early mobilization include a reduced incidence of pulmonary and vascular complications (such as atelectasis and thrombophlebitis). Such early mobilization also affects the basic physiology of wound healing.

The three basic molecular steps in local wound healing outlined by Peacock in 1967 (19) are: intracellular synthesis of tropocollagen molecules; extracellular assembly of fibrils and fibers; and formation of ground substance. A fundamentally important property of the healing wound is its tensile strength, which is directly related to collagen formation and orientation. Salter and co-workers (24) have shown that when wounds healed with continuous passive motion (CPM) are compared to immobilized wounds, the former wounds healed better both qualitatively and quantitatively. These investigators postulated that the tension of CPM enhanced the formation and alignment of collagen.

These advantages were seen by Halstead in 1913 who stated: "I believe that the tendency will always be in the direction of exercising greater care and refinement in operating, and that the surgeon will develop increasingly a respect for tissues; a sense which recoils from inflicting, unnecessarily, insult to structures concerned in the process of repair." This historic observation on his part is becoming more important as more and more surgery is being done through limited exposures.

INDICATIONS FOR MICROSURGERY

Indications for Surgery in Herniated Nucleus Pulposus (HNP)

One only has to review the natural history of lumbar disc disease to realize that spinal surgeons play a palliative role in the management of this problem in the majority of patients as shown by Weber (25) and Hakelius (10)

TABLE 1. *Weber's results (1983)*

	Non-surgical results	Surgical results
1 year	60% better	92% better
4 years	No statistical difference between the two groups	
10 years	No difference between 4-year and 10-year follow-up	

(Table 1). From these and other studies on the natural history of sciatica due to a disc herniation, one can only conclude that sciatica usually is a transient, self-limiting condition. Satisfactory resolution over time is likely to occur, regardless of the method of treatment intervention, be it surgery or conservative treatment. If one is proposing surgical intervention, then it is essential to prove that surgery carries with it a high rate of initial success with limited risk to the patient and the least expense possible to the payers for the service.

In this light, the indications for microsurgical discectomy are no different from the indications for any discectomy. They include:

Bladder and Bowel Involvement. The acute massive disc herniation that causes bladder and bowel paralysis is usually a sequestered disc that requires immediate surgical excision for the best prognosis. I have yet to encounter a disc herniation that was too large to be removed through a microsurgical wound.

Increasing Neurological Deficit. If, in spite of conservative treatment, the weakness or sensory loss appears to be increasing on repeated examination, discectomy is indicated.

Significant Neurological Deficit with Significant and Persisting Straight-Leg-Raising Reduction. This is a relative indication supported by the work of Weber and Hakelius.

Failure of Conservative Treatment. This is the most common reason for surgical intervention (3), a topic discussed in Chapter 80.

Recurrent Episodes of Sciatica. Conservative treatment can also fail in that the patient experiences recurrences of the sciatic syndrome. Table 2 outlines the use of "recurrences of sciatica" as an indication for surgical intervention.

TABLE 2. *Recurrent sciatica: indications for surgery*

First episode	90% of patients will get better and stay better
Second episode	90% of patients will get better, but 50% of the patients will have a recurrence of symptoms—consider surgery
Third episode	90% of the patients will get better but almost all will have recurrent episodes of sciatica —propose surgery

This condition is to be distinguished from recurrent HNP (disc herniation recurring after previous surgery).

DISADVANTAGES OF MICROSURGERY

Knowing the limitations of a technique is the key to avoiding problems and maximizing its potential. Microsurgery has inherent disadvantages that will lead to complications if not understood and overcome.

Limited Field of Vision

The diameter of the field of vision in microsurgery is less than 50 mm. If that field is not centered over the pathology, fragments of disc and bony encroachment will be missed. Recently, manufacturers have introduced new microscopes that increase the area of the visual field (Fig. 6).

Limited Field of Work

A 1-inch skin incision is commonly mentioned in microsurgical articles. Actually, the incision is usually 1 to 1½ inches, especially if the patient is large or obese. Assuming a 1½ inch skin incision, the area for instrumentation is even less than the potential field of vision. This limited operating field requires special instrumentation (straight instruments of small diameter), manipulated precisely, to avoid errors and damage to important neurological structures. Failure to accept this limitation has led those learning the technique to have an increased incidence of dural tears and root damage. There are occasions when the surgical exercise will be occurring near the edge of the microscope field. At this point, it is important to stop and reposition the microscope so that the working area is centered. Once the limited field of work is acknowledged and instrumentation is adapted, problems will be significantly reduced.

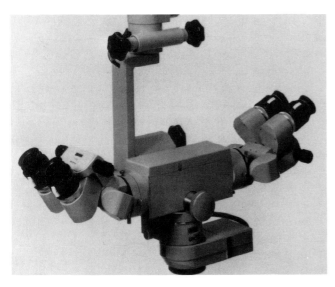

FIG. 6. The new Zeiss MD microscope that has increased the size of the operative field.

Bleeding

A small amount of bleeding into a limited operative field interferes with visualization and completion of the surgical exercise. The difference between 25 ml of blood loss and 100 ml of blood loss under the microscope is significant. Every effort in pre-operative preparation (e.g., taking the patient off anti-inflammatory medication), intra-operative patient positioning on the operating room table, and meticulous hemeostasis have to be considered to avoid this disadvantage.

Infection

Wilson and Harbaugh (30,31) have reported an increased rate of disc space infection following microsurgery. This increase is most likely because of the presence of the microscope directly over the wound. Although the microscope is sterilely draped, there are exposed parts of the microscope (eyepieces) that have the potential to contaminate the wound. As well, the limited operating space between the microscope and the wound introduces another element of potential break in proper surgical technique that can result in wound contamination.

PRINCIPLES OF THE MICROSCOPE

Before embarking on microdiscectomy, the operator needs to select the instrument which will work for him and understand the function of its component parts.

The Microscope Head and Optics

The operating microscope is a combination of binocular field glasses and a magnifying glass (Fig. 7). Interposed between the binocular and the magnifying glass is a magnifying chamber that allows for increasing or decreasing the size of the image (Fig. 8). The microscope, as constructed, is a series of lenses and prisms that allow for transformation of an image to the retina. Optical deficiencies, such as reflections and glare, have to be factored out of the system to improve image quality. This has resulted in an instrument of very complicated design that is impossible to explain in this brief chapter. There are excellent works (13) that explain the microscope in more detail, but this section will serve as a very basic summary of the microscope assembly important for lumbar disc surgery.

Objective Lens (The Magnifying Glass)

Objective lenses with focal length ranging from 150 to 400 mm are available in 25-mm increments. The focal length of an objective lens is a close approximation of the

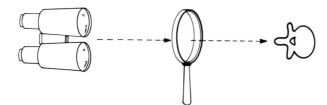

FIG. 7. The microscope, simply stated, is a pair of binoculars, looking through a magnifying glass.

distance between the lens and the point of anatomy that is in focus (Fig. 9).

For spine surgery, it is usual that a 300-, 350-, or 400-mm lens is used. The surgeon must try the various lenses to choose the most comfortable position relative to standing at the microscope and operating on the patient. As well, there must be a comfortable distance between the bottom of the microscope and the depth of the wound in which to manipulate instruments. The author's personal preference is a 350-mm lens.

The Binocular Assembly

The binocular assembly consists of two components (Fig. 10): the binocular tube and the eyepieces. The image formed by the objective lens is, in turn, magnified by the binocular assembly.

The function of the binocular tubes is to take the image of the objective, which is translated in infinity, and converge it to something that can be viewed by the human eye. With the addition of eyepieces, the optical system in the binocular assembly becomes convergent.

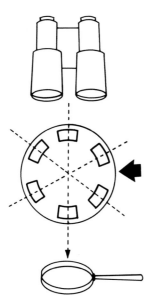

FIG. 8. A magnifying chamber (arrow) allows for greater or lesser magnification during the procedure, as called for by the surgeon.

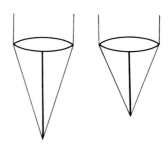

FIG. 9. The focal length of the objective lens determines the distance between the bottom of the microscope and the field in focus.

Binocular tubes can be straight or inclined. The most popular model today is the tiltable binocular tube that allows for individual adjustment of the angle of the binocular tube. This is most helpful when the surgeon and the assistant are of different heights.

Eyepieces

Another portion of the magnification equation for the microscope is added by the eyepieces. The convergent system in the binocular tube produces an intermediate-sized image, which is magnified by the eyepieces for viewing by the human eye. Eyepieces for the Zeiss microscope are measured by 10×, 12.5×, 16×, and 20×. For the Wild microscope, the eyepieces are 10×, 15×, and 20×. The eyepieces on each of these microscopes are adjustable, with 8 diopters to correct for visual acuity problems. It is possible to wear eyeglasses when using the binocular-tube-eyepiece assembly by folding back the rubber cups on the eyepieces. The use of eyeglasses is recommended when correction for astigmatism is necessary. If the use of eyeglasses is required only for myopia or hyperopia, then it is possible to operate without eyeglasses, using the diopter adjustments on the eyepieces to achieve focus.

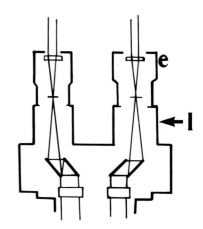

FIG. 10. The binocular tube has eyepieces (e) and length (l) that effect the final degree of magnification.

Interpupillary Distance

Interpupillary distance varies from surgeon to surgeon. The eyepieces must be adjusted for interpupillary distance so that the two images are fused and stereoscopic or 3-dimensional appreciation of the image occurs.

Magnification Chamber

The final piece of the microscope that determines the size of the image structures is the magnification chamber, as depicted in Figure 8. It is a Galilean telescopic system that allows for alteration in the magnification setup between the binocular assembly and the objective lens. The actual magnification factor achieved with the chamber can be 0.4×, 0.6×, 1.0×, 1.6×, or 2.5×. The magnification chamber can be (a) a turret drum setup that clicks in at the above-listed magnification factors, or (b) a zoom magnifying chamber. The zoom system is a mechanized chamber controlled by a foot pedal or dial on the microscope that gives a continuous magnification range from 0.5 to 2.5, using a single optical system.

Common Optics for Lumbar Disc Surgery

The magnification formula governing any microscope is:

$$Mag = \frac{Binocular\ tube\ length}{Objective\ focal\ distance}$$
$$\times\ Eyepieces \times Mag\ Chamber$$
$$MT = Fb/Fo \times Me \times Mc$$

For a Zeiss microscope, the equation would be:

$$MT = \frac{170}{350} \times 12.5 \times 1.0 = 6.07$$

Using the 1.6 magnification setting, the formula would change to:

$$MT = \frac{170}{350} \times 12.5 \times 1.6 = 9.7$$

Illumination Strength

As magnification increases, the amount of illumination decreases. However, the change in brightness is not enough to interfere with surgery.

Illumination Systems

An advantage of the illuminating system of the microscope is the coaxial path of the observation and illumination beams (Fig. 2).

The ideal illumination system provides enough brightness to the light so that the anatomy can be clearly seen. It should also be economical and consistent. In addition, when the source fails (burned-out bulb), it should be easily replaced. A constant problem with all lighting sources in the microscope is the generation of heat. Obviously, the least amount of heat generation is the most desirable.

The choices for illuminating the microscope are as follows:

Incandescent (tungsten coil) light. This is the oldest and cheapest source of light in the operating microscope. Either (a) 6-volt, 30-watt, or (b) 6-volt, 50-watt bulbs have been used, with the higher wattage used when documentation equipment is attached to the microscope. In the early microscopes, the bulb was close to the microscope head and the heat generated was significant.

Halogen (tungsten coil) bulb. The halogen bulb is the most popular choice for illumination today. It is a more sensitive light than the incandescent bulb, with a greater blue spectrum. This results in the surgical site appearing whiter and brighter. The standard halogen bulb used is 12 volts, 100 watts. This produces light with a brightness of 160,000 lux or 14,860 foot-candles.

The metal vapor lamp. This system forms the basis of the Superlux-40 by Zeiss, which produces over 40,000 footcandle power.

Light Transfer Systems

Light is transferred through the microscope in one of two ways:

Prisms and filters. If an incandescent bulb is used close to the microscopic head, then its light source is transferred through the objective with a series of prisms and filters, as depicted in Figure 11.

Fiberoptics. A more popular choice is fiberoptics (Fig. 12). This allows for placement of the light source at a distance from the microscope head, making it easier to control heat and easier to change bulbs when they burn

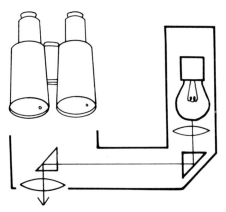

FIG. 11. A light source close to the microscope has to be reflected into the wound via prisms.

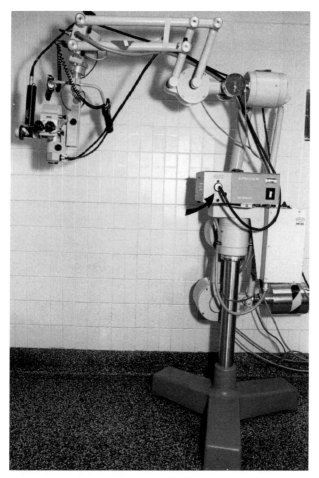

FIG. 12. A more popular choice that generates less heat within the microscope is a distant light source carried into the microscope via a fiberoptic cable (arrow).

out during the procedure. The disadvantages of fiberoptic systems are that (a) they are expensive, and (b) with continuing use and bending of the fiberoptic cable, the glass fiberoptic cables break, reducing the light.

The author's present setup is a Superlux-40 (Zeiss) light source powered by a 12-volt, 100-watt halogen bulb with the light carried to the microscope by a fiberoptic cable (Fig. 12).

TECHNIQUE OF MICROSURGERY FOR HERNIATED NUCLEUS PULPOSUS

The frame and position most universally used is shown in Fig. 13. The patient is stable in the kneeling position and is not hyperflexed at the hips and knees. The abdomen is free, thereby relieving pressure on the abdominal venous system and in turn decreasing venous backflow through Batson's plexus into the spinal canal. In this position it is easy to obtain an intra-operative lateral x-ray of the lumbosacral spine, which is usually desirable.

Identification of Level and Side

The level of surgical intervention should be marked before prepping and draping (Fig. 14). In most cases, the side of entry is predetermined by the symptoms. On occasion, a midline disc herniation may be approached from either side but preferably from the most symptomatic side.

Skin Incision and Exposure of Interlaminar Space

The skin incision, $\frac{1}{2}$ to $\frac{3}{4}$ of an inch on either side of the marking line, is made beside the spinous processes rather than in the midline. Blunt dissection is used to expose the lumbodorsal fascia, which, in turn, is opened in a curvilinear fashion (Fig. 15). The skin opening and fascial incision are designed to do the least amount of damage to the interspinous-supraspinous ligament complex. The subperiosteal muscle dissection and elevation is confined to the interlaminar level being exposed.

Entry to the Spinal Canal

Inspect the interlaminar interval, and decide which type of entry to the epidural space will be used. The alternatives are:

Transligamentous entry. Crossing the ligamentum flavum to enter the spinal canal is the simplest, most direct route to the pathology. If the interlaminar interval is narrowed by degenerative changes, then other routes are necessary.

Removal of a portion of the cephalad lamina. This is a popular neurosurgical approach, whereby the inferior portion of the proximal lamina is removed before removing the ligamentum flavum. There are many times when a microsurgical disc excision can be accomplished without removing any lamina, which is why most microsurgeons prefer the transligamentous approach.

Detachment of the distal insertion of the ligamentum flavum from the caudal lamina. At the base of the inferior facet usually lies a fatpad which is directly posterior to the base of the superior facet (Fig. 16). In difficult openings, such as in patients who had had previous surgery (26), this is a safe haven. The facet fatpad is usually easy to find and will lead the microsurgeon out of trouble more often than not. From there, exposure can proceed along the inferior border of the cephalad lamina or the superior edge of the caudad lamina (Fig. 16).

Across the pars interarticularis, removing the inferior facet. This is a very aggressive method of entry which is sometimes used for decompression of a foraminal stenosis or removal of a foraminal disc. This approach increases the risk of instability of the segment.

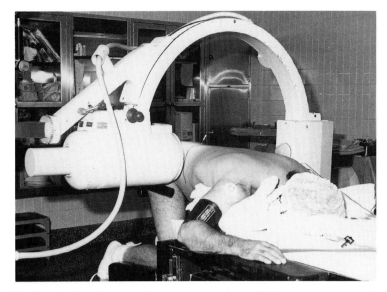

FIG. 13. The kneeling position, taking pressure off the abdomen and allowing blood to flow from the epidural veins, through Batson's plexus, into the vena cava. (Note the image intensifier and needle in position to mark the disc space level.)

Extent of Interlaminar Exposure Relative to Pathology

With pre-operative knowledge of the location of the pathology in the spinal canal, a plan of cephalad-caudad laminar excision can be followed. For example:

1. A third-story HNP in the L5 segment requires removal of some of the cephalad and caudad laminar edges during an L4-L5 exposure (Figs. 17, 18, 19).
2. A second-story HNP in the L4 segment requires removal of at least half the cephalad lamina (Fig. 20).

The Lateral Edge of the Nerve Root

Once in the spinal canal, finding the lateral edge of the nerve root, using blunt dissection, is the single most important step to take. After defining the lateral border of the nerve root and retracting the root medially, it is possible to become more aggressive with the Kerrison to achieve the cephalad or caudad laminar excision necessary to deal with the pathology.

If the lateral edge of the nerve root cannot be found, the following are important considerations:

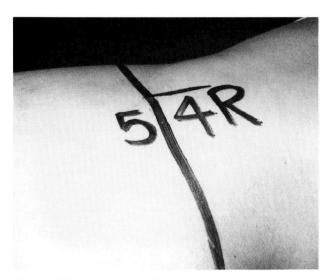

FIG. 14. The limited surgical incision requires exact pre-operative marking.

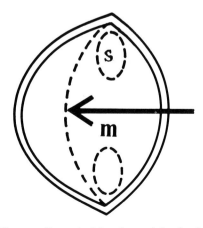

FIG. 15. The curvilinear incision through lumbodorsal fascia and erector spinae fascia (arrow) (s = spinous process; m = midline supraspinous ligament area) that spares the interspinous/supraspinous ligament complex.

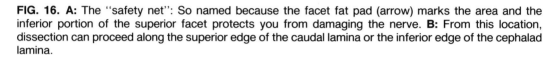

FIG. 16. A: The "safety net": So named because the facet fat pad (arrow) marks the area and the inferior portion of the superior facet protects you from damaging the nerve. **B:** From this location, dissection can proceed along the superior edge of the caudal lamina or the inferior edge of the cephalad lamina.

1. An axillary disc is displacing the root laterally;
2. There is osteophytic lipping of the medial edge of the superior facet, which is obstructing the view and will require removal;
3. Adhesions are present; or
4. There is an anomalous root.

It is a good basic rule not to use sharp tools in the spinal canal until the lateral border of the nerve root has been located.

If trouble is encountered in finding the lateral edge of the nerve root or if there are concerns there is any root lateral to the root, it is important to remember the following basic rule:

Nerve roots are intimately related to pedicles (Fig. 17): If a nerve root cannot be found, find a pedicle and the root will be immediately beside it. If the nerve root is isolated, check that the medial bony wall of the pedicle is lateral to a probe, as proof that no other nerve tissue is lateral. Before retracting the nerve root, the lateral border must be clearly defined as described above. There should be no adhesions tethering it. Microsurgery is a two-handed procedure; one hand holds and manipulates the root and the other hand operates. For this reason, it is best for the surgeon to hold the root retractor, which allows proper positioning and retraction necessary to complete the operation.

Dealing With Canal Pathology

The object of the surgical exercise is to leave a freely mobile nerve root. This requires removal of the obvious portion of ruptured disc and also includes a diligent

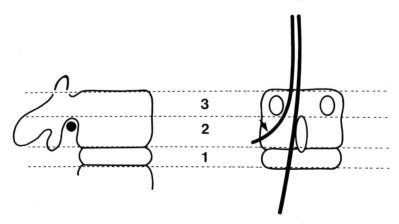

FIG. 17. For the purposes of a microsurgical exploration, each lumbar anatomical segment is divided into 3 levels or stories: 1st story: disc level; 2nd story: foraminal level; 3rd story: pedicle level. The exiting nerve root (arrow) passes beside and beneath the pedicle and is numbered by that pedicle.

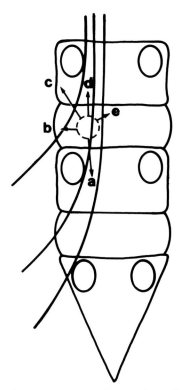

FIG. 18. Disc fragments may migrate down into the third story of the level below (a), laterally into the first story (b), or up into the second story of the same segment (c and d).

search of the canal, along with probing of the foramen, for residual discal or bony pathology. In the end, the patient must be left with a freely mobile nerve root.

Removing Intradiscal Tissue

How much disc to remove from within the discal cavity is an unresolved issue. Removal of as much disc as possible implies curettage of the interspace, including removal of the endplates. Critics of this approach point out the following:

1. It is not possible to remove all intradiscal material in this manner, no matter how long the surgeon works.
2. This aggressive approach increases the risk of damage to visceral structures, anterior to the disc space.
3. The incidence of chronic back pain produced by conditions such as sterile discitis and instability is increased.
4. Although there are some articles in the literature to suggest that this extensive intradiscal debridement decreases the recurrent HNP rate, there are other articles refuting the position. In the end, the only reasonable prospective controlled study is Spengler's (23), which suggests that limited disc excision is all that is necessary.

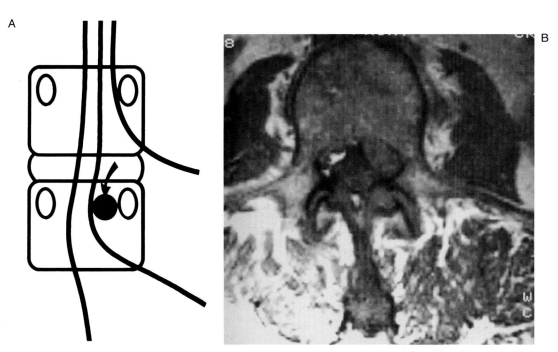

FIG. 19. A and B: A third story (pedicle) HNP (herniated nucleus pulposus) from the disc space above (arrow).

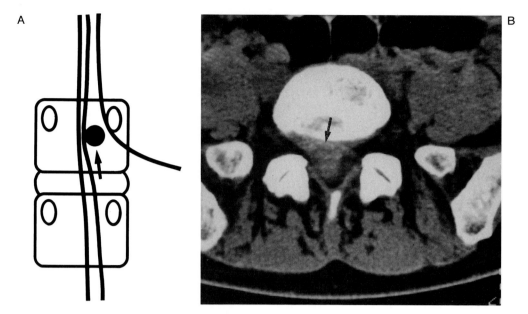

FIG. 20. A and B: A second-story disc herniation.

The advantages of limited disc removal are less trauma to endplates and less dissection; less nerve root manipulation; the low infection rate is prevalently lower; reduced risk of damage to structures anterior to disc space (vessel perforation); and less disc space settling occurring post-operatively.

THE FORAMINAL DISC HERNIATION

The technique just described uses the interlaminar window, with which we are all familiar (Fig. 21). When a disc herniation migrates laterally into the foramen (Fig. 22), there is another window of opportunity into the spinal canal—the intertransverse window (Fig. 21).

Foraminal disc herniations occur in approximately 3%–10% of all disc herniations (1). They migrate superiorly and laterally to lie in Macnab's "hidden zone" (Fig. 22B). There, they irritate and compress the exiting nerve root (Fig. 23). An attempt to remove this disc herniation through the standard interlaminar window results, more often than not, in loss of a facet joint, possibly destabilizing the level (Fig. 24).

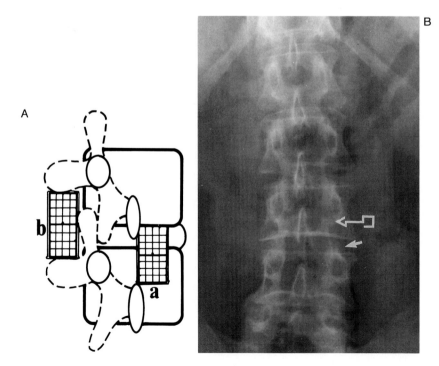

FIG. 21. A: There are two windows of opportunity into the spinal canal: (a) the interlaminar window, and (b) the intertransverse window. **B:** Note the location of the lateral border of the pars (arrow) and the extent of the disc space lateral to this point (smaller arrow) at all levels except L5.

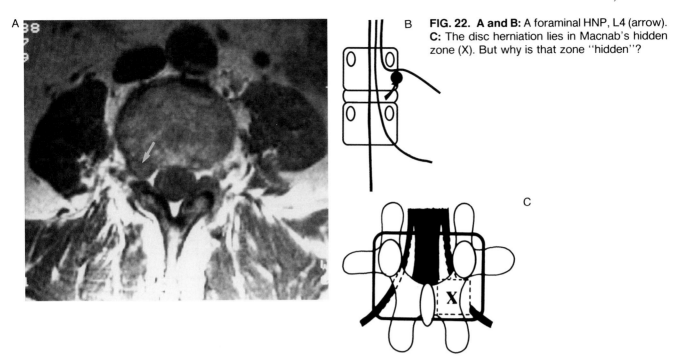

FIG. 22. **A and B:** A foraminal HNP, L4 (arrow). **C:** The disc herniation lies in Macnab's hidden zone (X). But why is that zone "hidden"?

Clinical Presentation

Most foraminal disc herniations occur at the L4-L5 and L3-L4 levels, affecting the L4 and L3 roots respectively. They tend to occur in older patients (average age 50) who have a wide disc space rather than degenerative and narrowed disc spaces. The onset is usually sudden and the usual presentation is severe anterior thigh pain, interfering with all functions except sitting. Sleep patterns are grossly disrupted because the positive femoral stretch test does not allow the patient to lie on the back

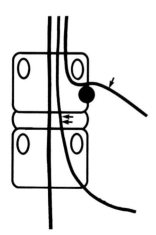

FIG. 23. A foraminal disc compresses the exiting nerve root (single arrow) and not the traversing root (double arrows).

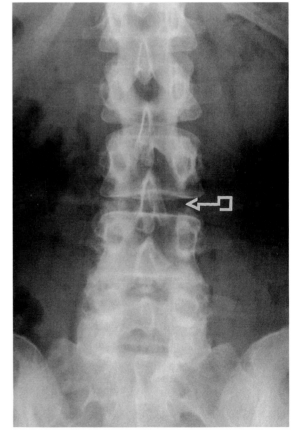

FIG. 24. An interlaminar approach to an L3 disc herniation which resulted in loss of a facet joint (arrow).

A

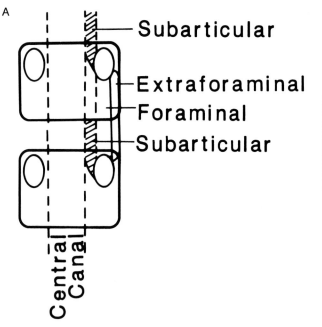

Subarticular

Extraforaminal

Foraminal

Subarticular

Central Canal

B

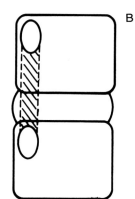

FIG. 25. A: The three regions of the lateral zone: (1) the subarticular, (2) the foraminal, and (3) the extraforaminal. B: The boundaries of the foraminal zone (pedicle-to-pedicle and pedicle-to-pedicle).

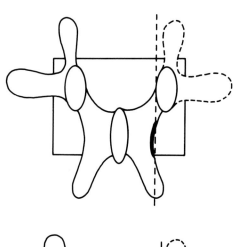

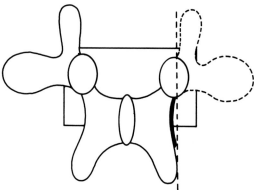

FIG. 26. The key to understanding the boundaries of the foramen, noting that the lateral border of the pars is on the same sagittal plane as the medial border of the pedicle. Another way of understanding this concept is to note that there is no bony roof to the foramen; the posterior boundary is the intertransverse ligament. This applies to all lumbar levels except L5, shown at the bottom.

or in the prone position with the thigh extended. Neurological examination, especially the sensory examination, will usually give a clue as to what root is involved. The very positive femoral stretch test together with the fairly negative SLR test will alert the examiner to the possibility of a higher lumbar disc lesion.

Often, these disc ruptures do not respond to conservative care, or the pain is so severe that the patient is not prepared to accept too long a conservative treatment program.

Operative Technique

The lateral zone can be divided into three regions (Fig. 25). Foraminal disc herniations lie in the foramen or extraforaminally. The key to understanding the boundaries of the foramen is depicted in Fig. 26. The foramen has no bony roof and the best way to approach the region for a full view of the pathology without sacrificing the facet joint is through the intertransverse window. The method chosen is the paraspinal approach (35) (Fig. 27). The results using this technique will be reported later.

RESULTS

Two hundred twenty-three patients who had a microdiscectomy or microdecompression have been followed by the author. The diagnoses have included 185 herniated nucleus pulposus, 24 lateral zone stenosis, and 14 combining the two. There were 154 males and 69 females. The average age was 46 years (15–85 years). The

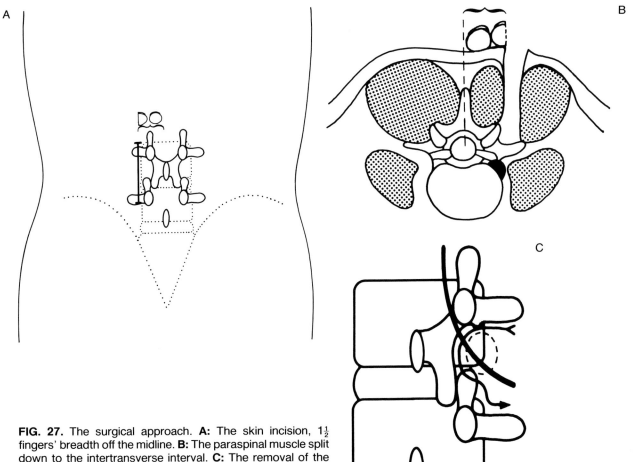

FIG. 27. The surgical approach. **A:** The skin incision, $1\frac{1}{2}$ fingers' breadth off the midline. **B:** The paraspinal muscle split down to the intertransverse interval. **C:** The removal of the intertransverse ligament to identify the nerve root and the disc fragment.

TABLE 3. *Functional grade*

	Grade	Rating	Description
Satisfactory:	I	Excellent	Complete relief of symptoms, back to normal
	II	Good	Mild discomfort, able to participate in all activities; do not require medications or bracing
Unsatisfactory:	III	Fair	Better than pre-operative state, significant limitations of activities and/or requiring medications and/or bracing
	IV	Poor	No better than pre-operative status, unable to return to work

TABLE 4. *Previous lumbar spine procedures (Group I)*

Diagnosis	Total	Primary cases	Previous discolysis	Previous laminectomy
HNP	185	119 (64.3%)	58 (31.4%)	8 (4.3%)
LZS*	24	15 (62.5%)	7 (29.2%)	2 (8.3%)
HNP and LZS	14	9 (64.3%)	5 (35.7%)	0
	223	143 (64.1%)	70 (31.4%)	10 (4.5%)

* Lateral zone stenosis (subarticular and foraminal)

TABLE 5. *Compensation cases (Group I)*

Diagnosis	Total cases	Compensation cases
HNP	185	41 (22.2%)
LZS*	24	2 (08.3%)
HNP and LZS	14	4 (28.6%)
	223	47

* Lateral zone stenosis

TABLE 6. *Level of surgery (Group I)*

Level	Number	Frequency
L1-L2	1	0.4%
L3-L4	16	7.2%
L4-L5	106	47.5%
L5-S1	94	42.2%
2 levels	6	2.7%
	223	100.0%

TABLE 7. Results (Group I)

Grade I	Excellent	108	48.4% ⎫	
Grade II	Good	61	27.4% ⎬	75.8%
Grade III	Fair	17	7.6% ⎫	
Grade IV	Poor	37	16.6% ⎬	24.2%
		223	100%	

average follow-up was 19 months (10–28 months). Eighty patients had undergone previous procedures prior to their microsurgical intervention. Seventy of these 80 patients had failures of previous chymopapain treatment, while the remaining 10 had undergone previous laminectomy (Table 4). There were 47 patients with pending compensation cases in this group (Table 5). Table 6 shows the distribution of the affected segments.

The clinical evaluation of results was made using a modification of Spangfort's criteria (Table 3): Those with Grade I and II classification were considered satisfactory. Those with Grade III or IV classification were considered unsatisfactory. On this functional grading scale, any patients who had limitations in their activity level or had not returned to work were deemed failures. Some patients with an unsatisfactory result were working with continuing symptoms but were not seeking further care. Other patients were relieved of leg pain but were not working, and they were also classified as an unsatisfactory result.

Average blood loss was 166 ml. The average post-operative hospitalization lasted 2.3 days. The result of surgery was rated "excellent" in 108 patients (48.4%), "good" in 61 patients (27.4%), "fair" in 17 patients (7.6%), and "poor" in 37 patients (16.6%) (Table 7). Satisfactory and unsatisfactory results were further analyzed by diagnosis and presence or absence of previous surgery (Tables 8–10).

In patients with pending compensation cases, 31 (66%) obtained a satisfactory result, while 16 (34%) obtained an unsatisfactory result. In patients without compensation pending, 138 (79%) obtained a satisfactory result, while 38 (21%) had an unsatisfactory result.

One hundred eighty-nine patients worked prior to their operative procedure. Of the 34 patients who were not employed, 21 were retired, 11 were housewives, and 2 were students. One hundred seventy-one (90.5%) of the 189 patients returned to their previous work at an average 2.2 months post-operatively. Eighteen patients (9.5%) were unable to return to work because of continu-

ing back or leg symptoms. Thirty-five (74.4%) patients with compensation cases pending returned to work at an average 3.2 months post-operatively, while 136 patients (95.7%) without compensation cases pending returned to work at an average 1.6 months post-operatively.

The 10.8% complication rate in Group I patients seems very high (Table 11). It is important to emphasize that 223 patients in this group represent my first cases of microsurgical intervention. Obviously, there was a learning curve involved, and most of these complications—specifically the dural tears—occurred early in the microsurgical experience. The six dural tears were all considered minor punctures, except for one which required repair. The other five "tears" were not repaired, and none of the six tears led to further complications.

All 6 cases of wrong-level explorations were discovered intraoperatively, and the correct level was subsequently exposed. Five of the 6 cases were one level too high, which is the most common wrong-level error in microsurgery. They occurred most commonly in the obese patient and in the patient with hyperlordosis in the kneeling position. The basic rule to obey in order to avoid wrong-level explorations is as follows: Know beforehand exactly what pathology is to be encountered. When that pathology is not encountered on operative exposure, one must be immediately suspicious of wrong-level exploration. If there is any reason for doubt, it is essential to obtain an intraoperative x-ray to verify the operative level exposed.

Those patients with minor superficial infections were recorded and easily treated. Of more concern is an almost 1% disc-space infection rate, which is unacceptably high, although not different from that reported by Spangfort (22). The likely reason for this is manipulation of the microscope, which has nonsterile exposed eyepieces over the wound. Some of these patients received prophylactic antibiotics and some did not, but there was no consistent relationship between prophylactic antibiotics and the presence or absence of infection. A review of the literature reveals a range of disc-space infection rates. Spangfort's (22) large and comprehensive series reports a rate of 2%. Goald (8) (0% in 477 patients) and Williams (27) (0% in 530 patients) deal only with pathology within the canal and do not invade the disc space in the limited fashion used in this series. Eberling et al. (6), after reviewing a number of articles, concluded that the infection rate is the same for microsurgery and standard laminectomy/discectomy. Dauch (5) concluded that the

TABLE 8. Results in patients by diagnosis (Group I)

	HNP	LZS*	HNP and LZS	Total
Satisfactory	146 (78.9%)	12 (50%)	11 (78.6%)	169 (75.8%)
Unsatisfactory	39 (21.1%)	12 (50%)	3 (21.4%)	54 (24.2%)
	185 (100%)	24 (100%)	14 (100%)	223 (100%)

* Lateral zone stenosis (subarticular and foraminal)

TABLE 9. *Results in patients without previous surgery (Group I)*

	HNP	LZS*	HNP and LZS	Total
Satisfactory	100 (84%)	8 (53.3%)	8 (88.9%)	116 (81.1%)
Unsatisfactory	19 (16%)	7 (46.7%)	1 (11.1%)	27 (18.9%)

* Lateral zone stenosis (subarticular and foraminal)

TABLE 11. *Complications (Group I)*

Dural tear (minor)	6	(2.70%)
Wrong level exploration*	6	(2.70%)
Hemorrhage requiring transfusion	3	(1.35%)
Superficial wound infection	2	(0.90%)
Disc space infection	2	(0.90%)
Increase neuro deficit	2	(0.90%)
Hematoma	1	(0.45%)
Gastritis	1	(0.45%)
Urinary retention	1	(0.45%)

* Recognized during surgery

infection rate for standard laminectomy/discectomy (2.8%) was much higher than that for microsurgery (0.4%).

Two patients had an increase in their neurological deficits (increased weakness) which was considered minor but definite. Both of these patients recovered and had no residual problems.

Miscellaneous complications of wound hematoma, gastritis, and urinary retention were also recorded. The low incidence of urinary retention is the result of ambulation of patients on the day of (or on the day after) microsurgical intervention. Although a complication rate of 10.8% seems unusually high, these were considered minor complications with minimal effect on the hospital stay and no effect on the ultimate result.

Results in Patients with Foraminal Lesions

Using the interlaminar approach in 22 patients, 10 facet joints were sacrificed (Table 12). Since switching to the paraspinal approach, 6 patients, as reported in Table 13, and a further 23 patients, have had the disc rupture removed through a paraspinal approach without loss of a facet joint.

LONG TERM FOLLOW-UP OF MICRODISCECTOMY

In a recent publication, Williams (29), Young (34), Yasargil (2), and Caspar (4) have reported their long term results. Williams had the longest follow-up at 15 years with a 98.8% successful outcome defined as a pa-tient who is economically productive (if he or she desires), physically comfortable without addictive medication, and free of sciatic pain. Of this group, 14.8% required re-operation to reach the "surgical cure" rate, leaving him with an overall success rate on initial surgery of 85.2%. Unfortunately, an "estimated" 30% of his patients were lost to follow-up, which detracts significantly from the validity of the analysis. Twenty-three patients of 989 followed (2.3%) experienced minor complications such as wound infection (8), transfusion (4), and wound dehiscence (11).

Young reported on 481 patients followed from 6 months to 54 months post-operatively. Although not clearly stated, it would appear that he had an 86% success rate without a clear-cut definition of success or failure outlined.

Yasargil reported on 236 patients 1 month to 10 years post-operatively with an 87.3% excellent result. His complication rate was low (8.5%) and all were minor.

Caspar reported 299 patients but excluded his first year's experience with the technique. The patients averaged 44 years of age and there was a male/female ratio of 3:2. The follow-up in the microdiscectomy group was not less than 2 years and averaged 2.8 years, revealing a 92.7% success rate (93.7% return-to-work rate). His complication rate was 12.9% but he reported no serious, permanent complications.

The author's results for the foraminal disc herniations are outlined in Tables 12 and 13. Abdullah (1) and Postacchini (20) have reported similar results, although they both recommended the more difficult interlaminar win-

TABLE 10. *Results in patients with previous surgery (Group I)*

	HNP	LZS*	HNP and LZS	Total
Satisfactory	46 (69.7%)	4 (44.4%)	3 (60%)	53 (66.3%)
Unsatisfactory	20 (30.3%)	5 (55.6%)	2 (40%)	27 (33.7%)

* Lateral zone stenosis (subarticular and foraminal)

TABLE 12. *Foraminal HNP: Follow-up*

Patients	28
M:F ratio	3:2
Average age	57 years
Side	L = R
Level	L4 = 14
	L3 = 11
	L2 = 2
	L5 = 1

TABLE 13. *Foraminal HNP: Results*

Interlaminar Approach = 22 (loss of facet joint in 10)
Paraspinal Approach = 6 (loss of facet joint in 0)
Success 23/28 = 82%
Failure 5/28 = 18%

dow. Each publication described facet joint loss in limited detail.

The problem with all these results, including the author's, is that they represent uncontrolled retrospective analyses. Although it might be possible to conclude that microsurgery delivers results equivalent to standard laminectomy/discectomy, there is no support for the conclusion sometimes expressed that microsurgery delivers superior results to standard laminectomy/discectomy.

CONCLUSION

Obviously, microsurgical intervention for lumbar disc disease is a controversial subject. To some, it represents a gimmick. To others, it implies the advancement of surgery to different technical levels that use the combination of magnification and illumination to facilitate and limit operative exposure (9,11,15,18,27,28,32). This series and other reports leave no doubt about the decreased length of hospitalization following microsurgical intervention and, thus, the decreased cost of caring for patients. This decreased utilization cost, along with preliminary results comparable to those of standard laminectomy/discectomy, offers an advantage for microsurgical intervention. A hidden advantage of microsurgical intervention is the necessity for an extremely accurate pre-operative diagnosis before the surgical exposure is undertaken. Microsurgery is not seek-and-find surgery, and thus it is imperative that an accurate diagnosis be made in regard to the level of pathology, the nature of pathology, and the extent of pathology before a microsurgical procedure is undertaken. The increased infection rate in this series and in Wilson's (30,31) series is critical to resolve and probably centers around the presence of a partially nonsterile instrument over the operative field. Wrong-level surgical intervention is a constant problem for microsurgeons.

In spite of these initial setbacks in microsurgical experiences, the procedure has become simply one of the many options available to the patient population with varied spine problems.

REFERENCES

1. Abdullah AF, Wolber PG, Warfield JR, Gunadi IK (1988): Surgical management of extreme lateral lumbar disc herniations: Review of 138 cases. *Neurosurg* 22:648–653.
2. Abernathey CD, Yasargil MG (1990): Results of microsurgery. In: *Microsurgery of the Lumbar Spine,* RW Williams, JA McCulloch, PH Young, eds. Rockville: Aspen, pp. 223–226.
3. Bell GR, Rothman RH (1984): The conservative treatment of sciatica. *Spine* 9:54–56.
4. Caspar W (1990): Results of microsurgery. In: *Microsurgery of the Lumbar Spine,* RW Williams, JA McCulloch, PH Young, eds. Rockville: Aspen, pp. 227–231.
5. Dauch WA (1986): Infection of the intervertebral space following conventional and microsurgical operation on the herniated lumbar intervertebral disc. *Acta Neurochir* (Wien) 82:43–49.
6. Ebeling U, Reichenberg W, Reulen HJ (1986): Results of microsurgical lumbar discectomy. *Acta Neurochir* (Wien) 81:45–52.
7. Feldman R, McCulloch JA (submitted for publication): Microsurgery for lumbar root encroachment.
8. Goald HJ (1980): Microlumbar discectomy: Follow-up of 477 patients. *J Microsurg* 2:95–100.
9. Goald HJ (1986): A new microsurgical reoperation for failed lumbar disc surgery. *J Microsurg* 7:63–66.
10. Hakelius A (1970): Prognosis in sciatica: A clinical follow-up of surgical and non-surgical treatment. *Acta Orthop Scand* [Suppl] 129:1–76.
11. Hudgins WR (1983): The role of microdiscectomy. *Orthop Clin North Am* 14:589–603.
12. Kahanovitz N, Viola K, McCulloch J (1989): Limited surgical discectomy and microdiscectomy: A clinical comparison. *Spine* 14:79–81.
13. Lang WH, Muchel F (1981): *Zeiss microscopes for microsurgery.* Berlin: Springer-Verlag.
14. LaRocca H, Macnab I (1974): The laminectomy membrane. *J Bone Joint Surg* [Br] 56:545–550.
15. Loew F (1986): Different operative possibilities for treatment of lumbar disc herniations. *Neurosurg Rev* 9:109–111.
16. Macnab I, Cuthbert H, Godfrey C (1977): The incidence of denervation of the sacro-spinales muscles following spinal surgery. *Spine* 2:294–298.
17. Mandel RJ, Brown MD, McCollough NC 3d., et al. (1981): Hypotensive anesthesia and autotransfusion in spinal surgery. *Clin Orthop* (154):27–33.
18. Merli GA, Angiari P, Tonelli L (1984): Three years experience with microsurgical technique in treatment of protruded lumbar disc. *J Neurosurg Sci* 28:25–31.
19. Peacock EE Jr (1967): Dynamic aspects of collagen biology, I. synthesis and assembly. *J Surg Res* 7:433–445.
20. Postacchini F, Montanaro A (1979): Extreme lateral herniations of lumbar disks. *Clin Orthop* (138):222–227.
21. Sachdev VP (1986): Microsurgical lumbar discectomy: A personal series of 300 patients with at least 1 year of follow-up. *Microsurg* 7:55–62.
22. Spangfort EV (1972): The lumbar disc herniation: A computer-aided analysis of 2,504 operations. *Acta Orthop Scand* [Suppl] 142:1–95.
23. Spengler DM (1982): Lumbar discectomy. Results with limited disc excision and selective foraminotomy. *Spine* 7:604–607.
24. Van Royen BJ, O'Driscoll SW, Dhert WJ, Salter RB (1986): A comparison of the effects of immobilization and continuous passive motion on surgical wound healing in mature rabbits. *Plast Reconstr Surg* 78:360–368.
25. Weber H (1983): Lumbar disc herniation: A controlled, prospective study with 10 years of observation. *Spine* 8:131–140.
26. Weir BK, Jacobs GA (1980): Reoperation rate following lumbar discectomy. An analysis of 662 lumbar discectomies. *Spine* 5:366–370.
27. Williams RW (1978): Microlumbar discectomy: A conservative surgical approach to the virgin herniated lumbar disc. *Spine* 3:175–182.
28. Williams RW (1986): Microlumbar discectomy: A 12-year statistical review. *Spine* 11:851–852.
29. Williams RW (1990): Results of microsurgery. In: *Microsurgery of the Lumbar Spine,* RW Williams, JA McCulloch, PH Young, eds. Rockville: Aspen, pp. 211–214.
30. Wilson DH, Harbaugh R (1981): Microsurgical and standard removal of the protruded lumbar disc: A comparative study. *Neurosurgery* 8:422–427.
31. Wilson DH, Kenning J (1979): Microsurgical lumbar discectomy: Preliminary report of 83 consecutive cases. *Neurosurgery* 4:137–140.

32. Yasargil MG (1977): Microsurgical operation of herniated lumbar disc. *Adv in Neurosurg* 4:81.
33. Yong-Hing K, Reilly J, DeKorompay V, Kirkaldy-Willis WH (1980): Prevention of nerve root adhesions after laminectomy. *Spine* 5:59–64.
34. Young PH (1990): Results of microsurgery. In: *Microsurgery of the Lumbar Spine,* RW Williams, JA McCulloch, PH Young, eds. Rockville: Aspen, pp. 215–222.
35. Zindrick MR, Wiltse LL, Rauschning W (1987): Disc herniations lateral to the intervertebral foramen. In: *Lumbar Spine Surgery,* AH White, RH Rothman, CD Ray, eds. St. Louis: Mosby, pp. 195–207.

The Adult Spine: Principles and Practice,
J. W. Frymoyer, Editor-in-Chief.
Raven Press, Ltd., New York © 1991.

CHAPTER 84

Lumbar Discectomy

Indications and Technique

Dan M. Spengler and John W. Frymoyer

INDICATIONS

Many patients present to orthopedists for evaluation of low back pain and/or sciatica (10). Based on Weber's studies (25) and the natural history of sciatica, 80% or more of these patients can be managed by non-operative treatment. Patients who do not respond to non-operative treatment and who, in addition, have objective findings consistent with lumbar disc herniation may be considered for elective discectomy (10,19). Results from lumbar discectomy vary from 46% to 90% excellent outcomes (21). This variation largely can be attributed to pre-operative selection criteria (22). In addition to improved selection criteria, the technique for lumbar discectomy has been enhanced over the past several years (8,20). This procedure has, in the past, been referred to as lumbar laminectomy, which in our opinion does not represent an appropriate descriptive term. Lumbar laminectomy suggests a much more complete and potentially destabilizing exposure of the neural elements, which is indicated in patients who have significant central lumbar spinal stenosis, lateral recess stenosis, or are undergoing a revision of a failed prior operation.

Patients who present with evidence of significant pro-gressive neurologic deficit, particularly cauda equina symptoms, should be rapidly evaluated and undergo prompt surgery should the pre-operative evaluation confirm a disc herniation. The majority of patients, however, who present to a doctor's office with low back complaints have symptoms which alter the perceived quality of life for the individual rather than cause significant neurologic loss. Objective criteria should be used to evaluate these individuals to determine the likelihood of response from lumbar discectomy (21,23). If patients are carefully selected by such objective criteria, the rate of success from lumbar discectomy should exceed 85% (19,21). If the surgeon observes a lower success rate among his patients, the indications for surgery should be carefully reviewed. Although newer approaches to manage patients who suffer from lumbar disc herniation are always worth consideration, at present no controlled studies have been published to support many of the newer strategies being discussed. Since the natural history of patients who suffer from low back pain with sciatica is one of progressive improvement, an invasive therapy should be considered successful only if a control group of comparable subjects has also been included (19). Indications for lumbar discectomy are straightforward and can be easily quantified pre-operatively (21,23). Major categories that must be assessed prior to surgical intervention include neurologic signs, sciatic tension signs, psychologic factors, and imaging studies (21,23). Since the vast majority of lumbar disc herniations involve nerve roots L4, L5, and/or S1, neurological manifestations for each of these nerve roots will be reviewed.

D. M. Spengler, M.D.: Professor and Chairman, Department of Orthopaedics and Rehabilitation, Vanderbilt University Medical Center, Nashville, Tennessee, 37232.
J. W. Frymoyer, M.D.: Professor of Orthopaedics, Director, McClure Musculoskeletal Research Center, Department of Orthopaedics and Rehabilitation, University of Vermont, Burlington, Vermont, 05405.

In a patient who has an L4 nerve root dysfunction, decreased sensation to pin prick may be observed over the medial aspect of the leg in the saphenous nerve distribution. The knee reflex may also be diminished or absent. In addition, quadriceps weakness may be observed. A positive femoral stretch test is the confirmatory tension sign.

In a patient who has an L5 radiculopathy, sensory changes are typically noted in the dorsal webspace between the great toe and the second toe. Although no reflex changes are usually observed, a reflex that is variably present, the posterior tibial, may be elicited in a few patients (3). Motor weakness is usually present in the extensor hallucis longus, extensor digitorum communis, and/or tibialis anterior. And in addition, the peroneal muscles may also be weak.

In a patient with an S1 radiculopathy, the sensory disturbance is noted over the lateral border of the foot. The ankle reflex exhibited may be diminished to absent. Pushoff weakness may be observed when the patient attempts to hop on the symptomatic extremity because of weakness of the gastrocsoleus muscles. However, this is rare (18). Weakness of the extensor hallucis longus is a more common finding (7).

In addition, progressive neural deficits should be clarified. It is important to determine clinically significant worsening of motor weakness in essential motor groups from insignificant paresis which occurs in muscles of less functional importance. Thus, an increase in weakness of the extensor hallucis longus from four-fifths to three-fifths would not be considered significant. However, a similar change in the triceps surae group or in the tibialis anterior muscle would be significant. The latter group of patients require more rapid evaluation and treatment.

In both the L5 and S1 radiculopathy, a positive straight leg raising test is the confirmatory nerve root tension sign. These sciatic tension signs are observed in most patients who have a lumbar disc herniation. However, the typical sciatic tension response is less dramatic in the elderly patient than in the adolescent or young adult (18).

These nerve root tension signs include the classical ipsilateral straight leg raising, well leg raising, dysrhythmia with flexion to the lumbar spine, and/or listing of the pelvis to one side. The traditional ipsilateral straight leg raising test can often be misinterpreted by the unsophisticated examiner as emphasized in Chapters 15 and 71. Distracting tests should be used to ensure that a patient has true sciatic tension. For example, if a patient can straighten both knees to 180 degrees in the sitting position, yet complains bitterly of pain with 10 degrees of straight leg raising in the supine position, no evidence for sciatic tension exists. In this instance, considerable evidence would exist for symptom amplification.

Over-interpretation of sciatic tension signs clearly contributes to unwarranted surgical procedures. Conversely, when a well straight leg raising test is performed and produces pain on the contralateral affect leg, the probability is high that a disc herniation exists. Dysrhythmia with forward flexion is a less specific but useful tension sign. This finding is present when the paraspinous muscles contract eccentrically during an attempt to flex. Its value is because these asymmetric contractions cannot be simulated by a patient who amplifies his symptoms and is, therefore, an objective confirmatory sign. However, the direction of the list is not a sensitive or specific sign of the location of the disc herniation.

These clinical symptoms and signs define the usual presentation of a patient with lumbar disc herniation. As shown in Chapter 71, the usual neurologic presentation of an L5–S1 herniation is an S1 radiculopathy, while the L4–L5 herniation typically involves the L5 root. However, there are a number of important variations in the classic picture which alter the clinical presentation and operative approach.

First, and most importantly, is the cauda equina syndrome, secondary to a massive central disc herniation which constitutes a surgical emergency. To reemphasize this syndrome, the symptoms which should alert the physician to this problem include any or all of the following: (a) numbness in the perineum or bilateral lower extremity numbness, (b) lower extremity weakness which is usually symmetrical, and (c) difficulty with urination. All of these neurologic symptoms may be accompanied by significant low back pain which often radiates into both extremities. The confirmatory physical findings may include: (a) decreased perception to pin prick in the perineum and lower extremities, usually in a symmetrical distribution but early in the evolution of the syndrome; (b) asymmetrical distributions, (c) decreased motor strength in all muscle groups innervated by nerve roots distal to the lesion; and (d) decreased to absent anal sphincter tone and absent anal wink (11).

A rarer subset of patients who may present with a cauda equina has as the pathology an intra-dural herniation. This has been reported in one of 300 patients operated upon by Dandy (2), 2 of 753 cases reported by Peyser and Harari (15), and was estimated by Graves (6) to occur in 0.13% of operated disc lesions. These reports, as well as isolated case studies (9,12,17) support a view that the presentation is usually that of a cauda equina syndrome which often is misinterpreted to be intra-dural tumor.

The other presentations relate to the differing locations of the disc or nerve roots, which may alter the classic relationship between disc level and nerve root. These include the far lateral disc, a disc fragment within the foramina, and disc lesions in association with segmentation abnormalities or conjoint nerve roots. The far lateral disc (see Chapter 71) typically affects the nerve root one or more levels higher than the classic paracaudal or pararhizal lesion. Thus, an L5–S1 far lateral disc affects the L5 rather than the S1 root and occasionally will affect the L4 root. Similarly, a lesion solely within the foramina will affect the exiting nerve root and place the nerve root deficit one level higher than the usual presentation. These lesions can be suspected particularly in a younger patient who has a clinical presentation of L4 nerve involvement since true L3–L4 herniations are fairly rare in this age group (18).

In patients with segmentation abnormalities, similar discrepancies may be noted which may lead to operating upon the wrong level. A conjoint nerve root may also alter the clinical presentation, but its greater importance is the difficulty which it poses in decompression. Lastly, a disc herniation can occur and be symptomatic at more than one level. In the earlier literature, this was thought to be a common occurrence and affect as many as 10% of patients (14). With newer imaging techniques this seems a gross overestimate, and the real prevalence is probably closer to 1%. However, in the case of far lateral herniations, one study indicated two-level lesions occur in 15% of these patients (1). All of these variations should be anticipated from careful pre-operative imaging studies, particularly MRI or CT scan, particularly when the latter technique is myelographically enhanced.

OTHER PRE-OPERATIVE EVALUATION TECHNIQUES

Psychological factors can be assessed using a number of criteria. The pain drawing correlates well with more formal personality tests (16,19). The pre-operative Minnesota Multiphasic Personality Inventory (MMPI) represents an excellent instrument to predict outcome in patients who suffer from lumbar disc herniations (21,23). In our studies, patients who have significant psychological problems do less well following elective lumbar discectomy procedures in spite of the fact that a disc herniation is confirmed.

Imaging studies are necessary to reaffirm the clinical impression of a disc herniation, but should not be used as the dominant criterion for patient selection. The lumbar myelogram with a CT scan following injection of the contrast material in my view is the most accurate study. Magnetic resonance imaging is also being used more frequently to evaluate the spinal canal, and some proponents report it is now the imaging method of choice. The MRI is quite sensitive, and hence, careful correlation with clinical signs and symptoms must be undertaken to prevent overinterpretation. In our opinion, the CT scan

TABLE 1. *Objective patient evaluation form (OPES)*

Category	Maximum points allowed for category	Point assignments
I. Neurologic signs	25	
A. Weakness consistent with level of lesion		
Associated with positive EMG		25
Associated with normal EMG		10
B. Atrophy (>2 cm)		10
C. Reflex absent or asymmetric		
Patient ≤ 50 years of age (add 5 points if EMG positive)		20
Patient > 50 years of age (add 15 points if EMG positive)		10
D. No clinical signs; EMG positive		15
II. Sciatic tension signs	25	
A. Positive crossed straight leg raising[a]		20
B. Pelvic list		15
C. Dysrhythmia of lumbar paraspinal muscles during back motion		15
D. Positive ipsilateral straight leg raising[b]		5
III. Personality factors (MMPI scores)	25	
A. Normal (includes depression)		25
B. Abnormal (impulsive/schizophrenic)		10
C. Elevated hysteria or hypochondriasis scales or both (>1 SD, <2 SD)		10
D. Conversion reaction or hysteria (>2 SD)		0
IV. Lumbar myelography/CT scan	25	
A. Positive and correlates with clinical findings		25
B. Equivocal nerve root asymmetry		10
C. Positive, but does not correlate with clinical findings		0
D. Normal		0
Total	100	

With permission from ref. 23.
[a] Positive when straight leg raising on asymptomatic side. Causes pain to be perceived by patient in symptomatic buttock, thigh, or leg.
[b] Standard straight leg raising test.

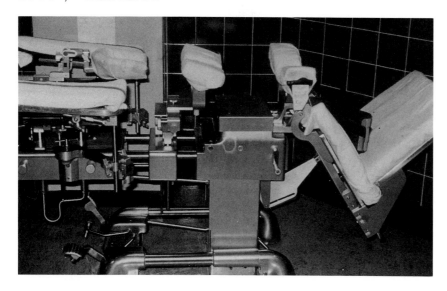

FIG. 1. Roger Anderson (Tower) table. Key feature is that abdominal viscera hang free.

alone has not been helpful as the sole pre-operative imaging study to recommend discectomy (26).

Despite the specificity of many of the clinical symptoms, signs and imaging studies, we often obtain an electromyogram to quantify pre-operative electrical abnormalities. However, nearly 20% of patients with disc herniations will not exhibit any electrical signs of abnormality (21,23). Nevertheless, if positive findings are identified, the clinician is reassured that a radiculopathy is present.

Once a patient has been thoroughly assessed, an Objective Patient Evaluation Form (OPES) score is generated (Table 1). Lumbar discectomy is recommended to those individuals who have failed a course of non-operative treatment (usually 2 to 8 weeks) and who have an OPES score of 50 or greater (21,23). Patients who have less than 50 points on the OPES are unlikely to improve following discectomy and, hence, are generally more appropriately managed by non-operative treatment. While the pre-operative MMPI represents the best predictor for outcome, the pre-operative imaging studies represent the most effective pre-operative predictor for surgical findings. In a well-selected series, post-operative results should approach 90% good outcomes. Recurrence rates should approximate 2% within the first 12 months following surgery (19).

SURGICAL TECHNIQUE (SPENGLER)

Once the patient has been evaluated, lumbar discectomy can be recommended should the patient's quality of life be adversely affected and the above criteria met. Patients who undergo elective lumbar discectomy should receive intravenous antibiotics in the operating room prior to beginning the surgery. Once the patient has been anesthetized, careful positioning is essential. I use the Roger Anderson (Tower) table (Fig. 1). After the patient has been positioned on this table, blood loss is lessened because of the decreased venous pressure on Batson's plexus. Careful attention to detail is essential during positioning. The surgeon must carefully inspect the eyes, ulnar nerves, genitalia in males, and breasts in females to assure that excessive pressure does not exist. Once the patient has been positioned, the lower back is prepped with an antiseptic solution. I recommend the use of loupe magnification (×2.5) plus a fiberoptic headlight (Fig. 2). Loupe magnification facilitates the exposure and improves tissue handling. Higher magnifications can be used but are not necessary. Once the patient has been properly draped, a vertical midline incision is made overlying the interlaminar space of choice (Fig. 3). The well-centered incision is approximately 6 cm in length. Dissection is carried through the skin and subcutaneous tissue to the level of the lumbar fascia. Hemostasis is obtained and self-retaining retractors inserted. The lumbar fascia is opened directly over the spinous processes of the motion segment of interest. Thus, if the L4–L5 interspace is being approached, the incision using electrocautery occurs directly on top of the spinous process of L4, then of L5. A continuation between L4 and L5 is then extended using cautery, and dissection is carried down to the laminae. I always expose the lamina on both the left and right sides, but others only expose one side. This bilateral exposure facilitates dissection and visualization. In addition, a midline entry into the canal is assured which, in my opinion, lessens the likelihood of nerve root injury. However, others expose only the side of involvement. Once the lamina has been exposed, a towel clip is placed on the spinous processes and a lateral intra-operative radiograph obtained (Fig. 4). Radiographic localization is important to minimize wrong-level procedures. Once the appropriate level has been verified, the interlaminar space is exposed. A larger, self-retaining retractor is inserted, and a Penfield 1 elevator used to gently dissect the ligamentum flavum from the

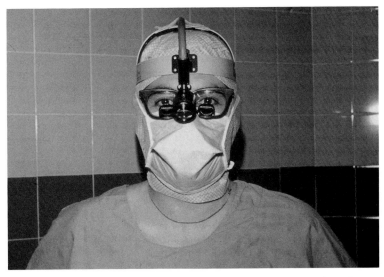

FIG. 2. Loupe magnification (2.5×) and a fiberoptic headlight enhance visualization.

anterior surface of the lamina from the midline toward the side of the herniation (Fig. 5). The 45 degree angled Kerrison rongeur is used to enhance visualization in the midline (Fig. 6). The raphe of the ligamentum flavum is identified. With the use of a Penfield 4 elevator, followed by a Penfield 3, the midline of the flavum is exposed. A no. 15 blade on a long-handled scalpel is used to divide the flavum using the Penfield to protect the underlying dura (Fig. 7). The ligamentum flavum is excised from the side of the herniation using upbiting rongeurs and/or curets (Fig. 8). Once the flavum has been excised, attention is turned laterally to the lateral reflection of the flavum. This tissue is carefully removed to expose the dural

sac and nerve root (Fig. 9). A midline entry into the epidural space lessens the likelihood for neural injury. Once the dura and nerve root are fully visualized, a Penfield 4 and a freer are used to gently mobilize the nerve root and dura. Care must be taken during this portion of dissection to handle the nerve root gently. In my experience, approximately one-third of patients who undergo surgery for a herniated lumbar disc also have a degree of lateral recess stenosis. Proper pre-operative planning through a careful assessment of the CT scan will usually identify these patients prior to the procedure. Once the lateral recess stenosis is recognized by the decrease in

Text continues on page 1794.

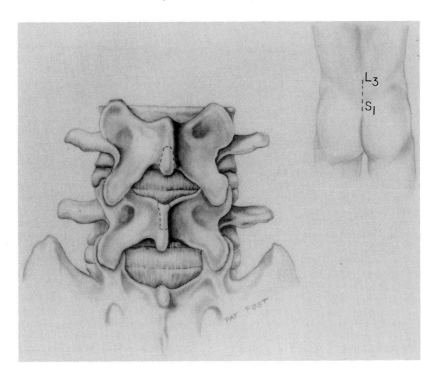

FIG. 3. Initial incision is made overlying interlaminar space of choice.

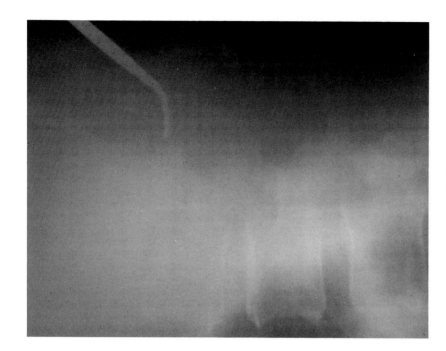

FIG. 4. Radiographic localization lessens likelihood for wrong-level procedure.

FIG. 5. Penfield 1 initiating dissection of the ligamentum flavum from the anterior lamina.

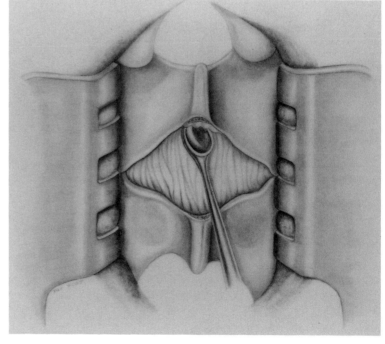

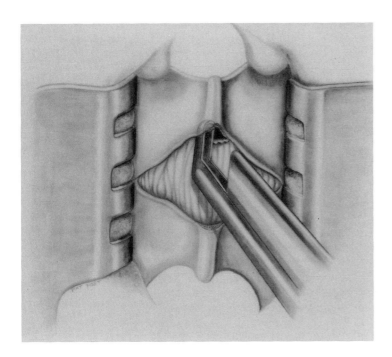

FIG. 6. Rongeur (45 degree) is used in the midline to expose raphe of the flavum.

FIG. 7. Ligamentum flavum is divided using a 15 blade protected by a Penfield 3 elevator.

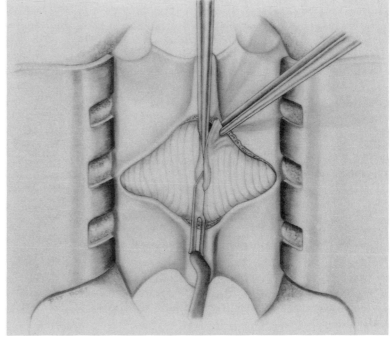

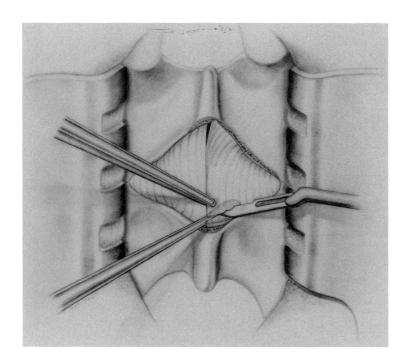

FIG. 8. Ligamentum flavum can be removed by sharp technique curets, or by angled upbiting rongeurs.

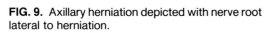

FIG. 9. Axillary herniation depicted with nerve root lateral to herniation.

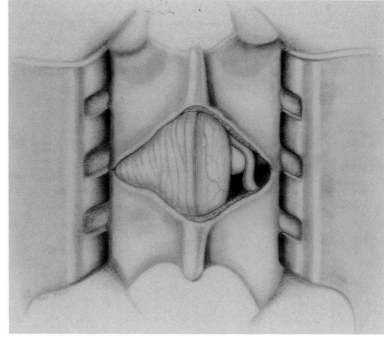

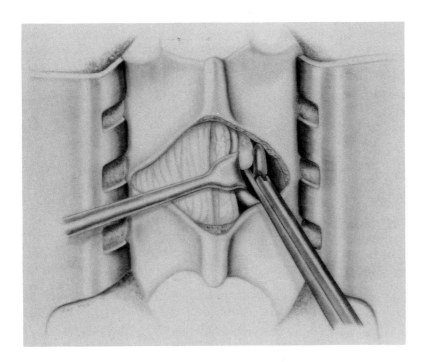

FIG. 10. Nerve root retracted medially to facilitate disc removal.

FIG. 11. If nerve root displaces easily 1 cm, decompression has been adequate.

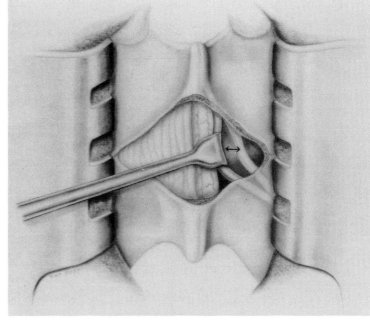

normal nerve root mobility (<1 cm), the upbiting Kerrison rongeurs will be required to enlarge the recess and the neural foramina to completely free the nerve root. Although by definition a portion of the zygoapophyseal joint is resected in this situation, the amount of joint removed is usually insufficient to warrant a stabilization procedure. Failure to recognize lateral recess stenosis is certainly a cause for failed lumbar spine surgery. Usually the nerve root can be easily displaced medially to expose the disc herniation. Once the disc herniation has been observed, pituitary rongeurs are used to remove the offending extrusion (Fig. 10). A Love nerve root retractor protects the nerve root from injury. If necessary, the initial incision into the annulus should be in the direction of the nerve root, so that in the event of a root entry the likelihood for major damage will be lessened. I perform a limited discectomy and make no attempt to remove the entire intervertebral disc. This technique has no higher recurrence rate (19) than the more formal and complete discectomy procedures advocated by others. In addition, a recent study by Balderston et al. has shown that patients who have limited discectomy are less likely to complain of low back pain on follow-up. Once the disc has been removed with pituitary rongeurs, the nerve root is mobilized to ensure that at least 1 cm of medial displacement is possible (Fig. 11). When this objective has been reached, the wound is irrigated and an interposition membrane of gel foam is put in place. The wound is then closed in layers over a drain. Blood loss seldom exceeds 150 cc.

UNUSUAL DISC HERNIATIONS

The standard surgical approach may be altered when the type or site of disc herniation is unusual.

Surgical Approach

Cauda Equina Syndrome

When cauda equina syndrome is present, the recommended approach of bilateral exposure becomes essential. In these instances the dura should be exposed by removal of the ligamentum flavum on both sides. As this is done great care should be taken not to enter the dura which frequently is pushed dorsally under the ligament. A wide approach is necessary into the lateral recesses, which may necessitate removing a portion of the superior articular facet to insure that the nerve roots are adequately visualized. On occasion it may be necessary to de-bulk the disc from the side opposite the major portion of the disc fragment to avoid traction on the already injured nerve root. It is also essential to be certain that the entire bulk of the free fragment has been removed which may necessitate a generous laminectomy.

Intradural Disc Herniation

It is rare that an intradural disc herniation can be removed by the usual methods. Dural adhesions are commonly reported (12,14), which may be the result of an inflammatory reaction. Also, these lesions are thought to be more common when there has been a previous operation at that level and, thus, fibrous tissue and adhesions are more apt to be present (12). Thus, a wide bony decompression has been advocated, accompanied by transdural excision (9). Following the removal of the fragment, the posterior but not the anterior dura is repaired.

Far Lateral and Intra-Foraminal Discs

These lesions (Fig. 12) cannot be easily removed through the usual approach previously outlined. Although taking down the entire facet is one alternative advocated by some (4,24), an alternative approach is extra-foraminal as advocated by Wiltse (28). The proponents (4) of going from the midline through the facets suggest instability is not a subsequent problem, and believe the nerve root can more easily be identified. Furthermore, they believe the surgeon can have greater confidence of complete decompression. However, many do not share this view.

The Wiltse (27,28) approach and the details of anatomic dissection are detailed in Chapters 82 and 83. Here we will present the principles. The incision is 3 to 5 cm from the midline, followed by blunt dissection of the paraspinal muscles. At this point, radiographs are taken and the transverse processes cleared of soft tissues. The intertransverse ligaments and fascia are entered using knife or curet, followed by removal of those structures between the transverse process. The nerve is identified and is usually 2 to 4 mm anterior to the fascia and is directed at a 45 degree angle (Fig. 13). The nerve is followed medially and the disc identified. If a free fragment is present this is removed. If only a bulge is present, the annulus is incised and easily identifiable fragments removed (Fig. 14).

If the lesion is intra-foraminal, a portion of the facet may be taken down laterally to expose the nerve root canal, although McCulloch points out the usual anatomic location of these lesions makes this rarely necessary. In fact, as will be shown in Chapter 83 it is more likely a portion of the lateral pars interarticularis will be sacrificed to achieve adequate exposure.

Closure in both instances is routine, with the use of a free fat graft to cover the nerve.

Conjoint Nerve Roots

The key element in dealing with conjoint nerve root and disc herniation is the pre-operative recognition of

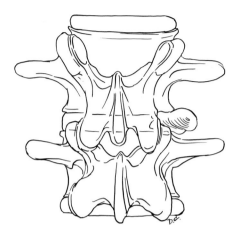

FIG. 12. Far lateral disc lesion. Note the relationship to transverse processes.

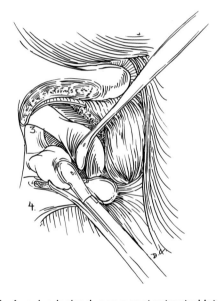

FIG. 14. Annulus incised, nerve root retracted laterally, disc removed with pituitary rongeur.

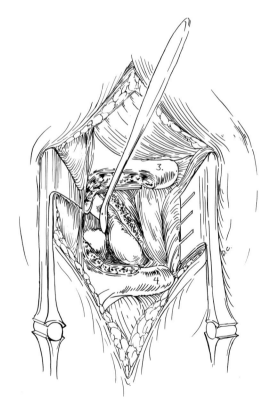

FIG. 13. Nerve identified and retracted at a 45 degree angle.

the lesion. The details of the imaging techniques used and their interpretation are given in Chapters 20, 22, and 23. From the perspective of the surgical approach, the key principle is a wide exposure, including, if necessary, sacrifice of a portion of the superior articular facet and significant laminectomy. It is essential to see all aspects of the nerve root back to its axilla and into the lateral gutter, before any attempt is made at retraction.

Segmental Abnormalities

The only importance of this abnormality in lumbar disc excision is the greater need for intra-operative radiographs to be certain that the level is correct.

Surgical Results

The surgical results vary by the pathologic condition being treated.

Cauda Equina Syndrome

The outcome of a cauda equina lesion is time-dependent. Traditionally, a "grace period" of 6 hours has been identified as optimum to insure neurologic discovery. However, Kostuik (11) found longer time intervals may be compatible with neurologic recovery, but still advocated it was prudent to perform the surgery as soon as feasible. Even with prompt recognition and adequate decompression, the neurologic outcome is not assured. Similarly, if the lesion is intra-dural, the outcome is variable, and because of the inflammatory reaction produced, may be followed by focal arachnoiditis.

Far Lateral and Intra-Foraminal Lesion

The results are variable using the transfacetal approach. McCulloch (see Chapter 83) found unsatisfactory results, whereas with the extra-foraminal approach the results were markedly improved. Faust (5) (see Chapter 80) had 14 good and excellent results in 15 patients treated by the extra-foraminal approach using neurologic and pain relief criteria. Epstein (4) indicates results are generally good with the transfacetal approach and segmental instability is not a later problem.

Conjoint Root

There is consensus that surgical results with conjoint roots are poorer overall, with an increased risk of neurologic residual.

COMPLICATIONS/PITFALLS

Proper localization of the intervertebral disc level is essential to lessen the likelihood of a wrong-level procedure. Counting mobile spinous processes is not as accurate and should not represent the sole method to localize spinal level. Gentle technique is required during the exposure and manipulation of the dura and nerve roots to lessen neural injury. The exposure must be adequate, which implies that the lateral extension of the exposure must be fully developed. The surgeon must be especially careful in the event an axillary disc herniation is identified so that the laterally displaced nerve root is not injured. All of the potential hidden zones for disc herniation should be inspected and the nerve root mobilized to ensure at least 1 cm of mobility (13). Nerve root foramina can be probed using a Penfield 3 elevator to ensure that no lateral disc herniation is present. We seldom use electrocautery within the vertebral canal since we believe nerve root injury can occur through electrical stimulation. We are also concerned about increased scar formation with the use of electrocautery within the canal. We obtain hemostasis by using small squares of thrombin-soaked gel foam with cottonoids.

As with any surgical procedure, a list of potential complications that might occur would be exhaustive. Certainly, injuries to the iliac arteries and veins, visceral injuries to virtually any structure from the appendix to the ureter have been reported in association with a lumbar discectomy procedure. Errors in diagnosis may also occur so that a patient may have symptoms suggestive of a lumbar disc herniation which in fact may be related to other problems such as referred pain from such intra-abdominal pathological processes as an aneurysm or a malignancy. By developing a thorough diagnostic assessment and judicious intra-operative technique, these extraordinary complications will be minimized.

POST-OPERATIVE CARE

Once the surgical procedure has been performed, the patient is placed in a lumbosacral binder for 1 month. Patients generally like the binder since abdominal support is provided. Thirty days following discectomy, patients begin an aggressive trunk strengthening program involving both flexion and extension. Progress can be monitored by the use of a multi-axis dynamometer. Motivated patients with high physical demands on the job are released for full duty approximately 4 months following surgery. Patients who have office-type jobs may be released to work within the first 10 days. In the event that a patient does not respond to lumbar discectomy, a thorough re-evaluation should be undertaken to exclude the multiple possible causes for low back symptoms. In addition, the surgeon should carefully reaffirm that the proper intervertebral disc level was addressed at the time of surgery. Although difficult to interpret in the first days to weeks following surgery, imaging studies should be repeated. Imaging studies often do not change substantially, even in those individuals who have extruded disc herniations and marked clinical improvement. Additional studies could be useful to provide further data.

We believe that lumbar discectomy represents a safe, predictable procedure to manage patients who suffer from lumbar disc herniation. Complications are few. Results are excellent.

REFERENCES

1. Abdullah AF, Wolber PG, Warfield JR, Gunadi IK (1988): Surgical management of extreme lateral lumbar disc herniations: Review of 138 cases. *Neurosurgery* 22:648–653.
2. Dandy WE (1942): Serious complications of ruptured intervertebral disks. *JAMA* 119:474–477.
3. Donaghy RM (1946): The posterior tibial reflex. A reflex of some value in the localization of the protruded intervertebral disc in the lumbar region. *J Neurosurg* 3:457–459.
4. Epstein JA (1989): Discussion on extreme lateral lumbar disc herniation. *J Spinal Dis* 2:138.
5. Faust SE (1990): Personal communication.
6. Graves VB, Finney HL, Mailander J (1986): Intradural lumbar disk herniation. *AJNR* 7:495–497.
7. Hakelius A, Hindmarsh J (1972): The comparative reliability of preoperative diagnostic methods in lumbar disc surgery. *Acta Orthop Scand* 43:234–238.
8. Holmes HE, Rothman RH (1979): Technique of lumbar laminectomy. *American Academy of Orthopaedic Surgeons Instructional Course Lectures* 28:200–207.
9. Jenkins LE, Bowman M, Cotler HB, Gildenberg PL (1989): Intradural herniation of a lumbar intervertebral disc. *J Spinal Dis* 2:196–200.
10. Kane W (1980): Incidence of lumbar discectomy. Presented at the 6th Annual Meeting of the International Society for the Study of the Lumbar Spine, New Orleans, Louisiana.
11. Kostuik JP, Harrington I, Alexander D, Rand W, Evans D (1986): Cauda equina syndrome and lumbar disc herniation. *J Bone Joint Surg* [Am] 68:386–391.
12. Lee Shih-Tseng, Fairholm D (1983): Intradural rupture of lumbar intervertebral disc. *Canad J Neurol Sci* 10:192–194.
13. Macnab I, Dall D (1971): The blood supply of the lumbar spine and its application to the technique of intertransverse lumbar fusion. *J Bone Joint Surg* [Br] 53:629–638.
14. O'Connell JE (1951): Protrusions of the lumbar intervertebral discs. A clinical review based on five hundred cases treated by excision of the protrusion. *J Bone Joint Surg* [Br] 33:8–30.
15. Peyser E, Harari A (1977): Intradural rupture of lumbar intervertebral disk: Report of two cases with review of the literature. *Surg Neurol* 8:95–98.
16. Ransford AO, Cairns D, Mooney V (1976): The pain drawing as an aid to the psychological evaluation of patients with low-back pain. *Spine* 1:127–134.
17. Smith RV (1981): Intradural disc rupture. *J Neurosurg* 55:117–120.
18. Spangfort EV (1972): The lumbar disc herniation: A computer-aided analysis of 2,504 operations. *Acta Orthop Scand (Suppl)* 142:1–95.
19. Spengler DM (1982): *Low back pain.* New York: Grune and Stratton.
20. Spengler DM (1988): Lumbar discectomy. In: *Operative Orthopaedics. Vol 3.* Philadelphia: Lippincott, pp. 2055–2064.
21. Spengler DM, Freeman CW (1979): Patient selection for lumbar discectomy. *Spine* 4:129–134.
22. Spengler DM, Freeman C, Westbrook R, Miller JW (1980): Low-back pain following multiple lumbar spine procedures. *Spine* 5:356–360.
23. Spengler DM, Ouellette E, Battie M, Zeh J (1990): Elective discectomy for herniation of a lumbar disc. *J Bone Joint Surg* [Am] 72:230–237.
24. Tarlov ET (1989): Discussion on extreme lateral lumbar disc herniation. *J Spinal Dis* 2:137–138.
25. Weber H (1983): Lumbar disc herniation: A controlled, prospective study with ten years of observation. *Spine* 8:131–140.
26. Wiesel SW, Tsourmas N, Feffer HL, et al. (1984): A study of computer-assisted tomography. *Spine* 9:549–551.
27. Wiltse LL (1987): In: Watkins RG, Collis JC, eds. *Lumbar discectomy and laminectomy.* Rockville, Maryland: Aspen.
28. Wiltse LL (1989): Discussion on extreme lateral lumbar disc herniation. *J Spinal Dis* 2:134–137.

Claudication

The Adult Spine: Principles and Practice,
J. W. Frymoyer, Editor-in-Chief.
Raven Press, Ltd., New York © 1991.

CHAPTER 85

Spinal Stenosis

Development of the Lesion, Clinical Classification, and Presentation

J. Desmond O'Duffy

HISTORICAL BACKGROUND

An early description of lumbar stenosis and its surgical treatment was in 1893 by W. A. Lane (18) of Guy's Hospital, London. His patient had a well-defined cauda equina syndrome and complained of difficult gait and "weakness of her back and insecurity of her legs." Lane was able to diagnose coexistent spondylolisthesis intra-operatively, even ruling out spondylolysis, without the use of x-ray.

> From the great density of the spinous process and lamina I concluded at once that there was no carious focus in the vicinity. On attempting to remove the lamina of the fifth lumbar vertebra, after cutting off its very prominent, largely developed and dense spinous process, it was found to be placed in the upper part of the sacral canal quite in front of its normal position. It was removed piecemeal with great difficulty. When the dura matral sheath of the cauda equina of the right side was seen to have been so severely compressed as not to expand then the bone pressing on it was removed (18).

Early descriptions of neurogenic claudication and its relief by forward flexion were in 1889 (38) and 1911 (1).

J. D. O'Duffy, M.B.: Department of Rheumatology, Mayo Clinic, Rochester, Minnesota, 55905.

Hypertrophic changes in the lumbar spine were stressed in the early reports. The concept of "congenital stricture of the spinal canal" was later proposed by Sarpyener (39). However, his series of 12 children contained examples of both upper and lower neuron disease. Verbiest, a Dutch surgeon, has championed the contribution of congenital narrowing (47), although a countryman of his, Van Gelderen (46), had earlier proposed that a hypertrophied ligamentum flavum might be responsible. Nevertheless, Verbiest defined the clinical syndrome and, using Lipiodol as contrast agent, confirmed the spinal obstruction. Although Macnab drew attention to "spondylolisthesis with an intact neural arch" he did not mention myelography or describe the neurogenic claudication which some of his patients may, in hindsight, be presumed to have had (21). Kirkaldy-Willis reviewed the subject of lumbar stenosis in 1974 (17). The relative merits of congenital narrowing versus hypertrophic changes are still debated. In my opinion, those who espouse the latter make a stronger case.

The concept of cervical disc protrusion was proposed by Stookey in 1928 (41) and enlarged on in 1948 by Brain (5). These authors did not clearly define cervical myelopathy from cervical disc disease. Later Pallis, Jones, and Spillane associated a myelopathy with cervical osteophytes and subluxation (30). Their descriptions have been enlarged upon subsequently by the British neu-rologists Lees (19) and Nurick (28,29).

LUMBAR STENOSIS

Definition

There are no widely accepted diagnostic criteria for lumbar stenosis. Most authors have described a set of stereotyped symptoms in patients with myelographic ob-struction. Uden stated, "The definition and classifica-tion of spinal stenosis are arbitrary and artificial" (44). Most would agree with Epstein that there is "an incongru-ity between the capacity and the contents of the lumbar spinal canal [that] may give rise to compression of the roots of the cauda equina" (12). Since the antero-poste-rior (A-P) diameter of the canal varies in symptomatic patients from 10 to 15 mm, overlapping generously with asymptomatic individuals, there can be no definition based on arbitrarily defined intra-spinal diameters (27,44). The cardinal symptom of lumbar stenosis is neurogenic claudication (3,4,13,17,33,47,51). This is an intermittent pain and/or paresthesia in the legs brought on by walking and standing, and relieved by sitting or lying down. Confirmation of the diagnosis requires my-elographic evidence of obstruction to distal flow of ra-dio-contrast material and, when indicated, compression of the caudal sac at laminectomy.

Development of the Lesion

A role for the disc in promoting canal stenosis has been proposed (24,27). Its contribution, however, has been questioned (9), and even cast in some doubt (32). Frequently, there is neither radiologic evidence of disc space degeneration nor computerized tomography (CT) nor myelographic evidence of disc protrusion.

Congenital narrowing of the canal has long been pro-posed (3,9,26,27,47). Developmentally, the lumbar canal reaches its full internal diameters in childhood. With growth it is the bony structures, not the lumen, that enlarge. The lumbar canal is normally narrowest at the level of L3 and L4 and indeed stenosis is most common at these sites. Before CT scanning, the normal A-P diame-ter was generally regarded to be 12 to 15 mm when mea-sured radiologically or intra-operatively (27).

Using dynamic CT-myelographic techniques, Pen-ning and Wilmink (32) evaluated internal diameter and cross sectional area of the caudal sac in 12 patients with myelographically proven lumbar stenosis and in con-trols. All measurements were done in flexion and exten-sion and were corrected for radiologic enlargement of 35%. There was no significant difference between bony sagittal or interpedicular diameters between the two groups. However, a discrepancy in the area within the dura was significant; 105 mm³ (range 70–138) in ste-notics versus 145 mm³ (range 86–230) in controls. It was proposed that the key to stenosis was the enlarging apophyseal joints. By a series of reconstructed diagrams the authors showed that the canal opens up in flexion, especially anteriorly, and reduces in extension. This ob-servation can explain the clinical relief afforded by flex-ion as the lateral recesses at the anterolateral angles of the canal carrying the emerging nerve roots obtain the larg-est bonus of area increase during flexion.

Table 1 lists contributing factors to lumbar stenosis. Figure 1 is a diagram of normal and pathologic lumbar vertebrae. Vertebra B is taken to represent the situation in congenital canal stenosis (or achondroplasia) but ver-tebra C with hypertrophic changes is the lesion most commonly encountered. The hypertrophy of the apophyseal joints narrows the space between the disc an-teriorly and the superior articular facets laterally (32). This pincer movement can be guessed at on lumbar CT when the normal epidural fat is reduced. The normal symmetric bulging of the disc in extension may make a minor contribution and in some patients with the classic syndrome of neurogenic claudication an unexpected disc protrusion coexists (9,13,32,51).

Gross features of canal stenosis are thickened laminae, facet hypertrophy, thickened ligamentum flavum, and narrow lateral recesses (27,33,51). At times, cysts from the apophyseal joints contribute. Does the ligamentum flavum contribute to stenosis? Some authors have re-ported that it may be 7 to 8 mm thick instead of the usual 4 mm or less (17,51), but at times the ligament has a normal thickness (51). Rauschning holds that the liga-ment thickness is more apparent than real, i.e., due to volume redistribution in a shortened spinal canal (36). In degenerative joint disease, the lesions are loss of carti-lage, increased bone formation, joint effusion, and liga-mentous hypertrophy. I propose that canal stenosis is entirely due to osteoarthritis. Whether stenotics have an excess of osteoarthritis elsewhere has not been prospec-tively studied. There probably is an association with hip degenerative joint disease (4).

Achondroplasts have reduced canal volume, develop facet joint disease, and commonly are found to have ei-ther lumbar stenosis or cervical myelopathy or both (35). Paget's disease of bone may produce the syndrome and symptoms may respond either to calcitonin or to surgi-cal decompression (48). Post-spinal fusion stenosis, al-though important, is not discussed here.

Metabolic diseases have seldom been incriminated. Calcium pyrophosphate crystals were found in four pa-tients' lumbar disc at re-laminectomy (11). Since none had typical chondrocalcinosis elsewhere, the significance of this finding is unknown. Diffuse intervertebral skele-tal hyperostosis (Forestier's disease) that produces bony bridging at multiple anterior vertebral junctions was re-ported in association with lumbar stenosis, but the main

A

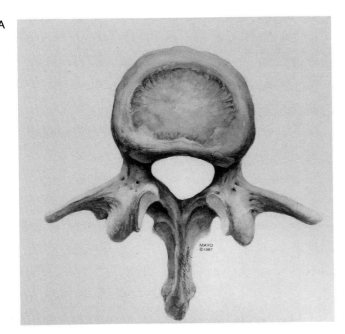

FIG. 1. A: Normal lumbar canal.

B

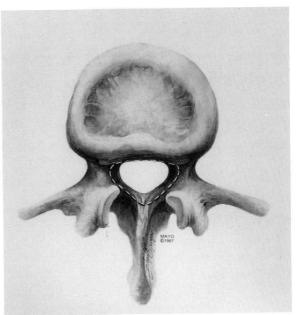

FIG. 1. B: Congenital narrowing of lumbar canal.

C

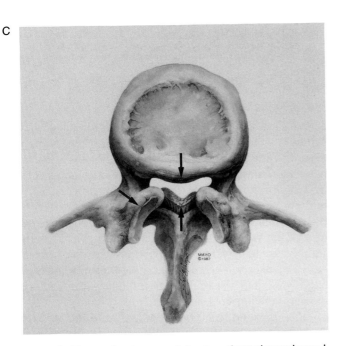

FIG. 1. C: Narrow lumbar canal due to enlarged apophyseal joints, ligamentum flavum, and prominent vertebral bossing (with permission from ref. 30a, Floyd Hosmer, artist).

TABLE 1. *Contributing factors to lumbar stenosis*

A. Degenerative
Lumbar spondylosis (common)
Diffuse intervertebral skeletal hyperostosis
B. Paget's disease of the bone
C. Congenital narrowing
D. Achondroplasia
E. Post-fusion narrowing
F. Fluorosis

operative finding was a 10 mm thick uncalcified ligamentum flavum as in lumbar spondylosis (16).

Ischemia of nerve roots has been proposed by Blau and Logue (3) and by Naylor (27). However, despite successful surgery in their patients, no ischemia was proven. Since the dura is not normally opened to allow nerve root inspection during laminectomy, it has not been possible to prove ischemia. However, since the pain persists while standing still, it is unlikely that ischemia is present. One of our patients died within 12 hours of three-level laminectomy. Autopsy examination of the excised cauda equina revealed segmental compression of the nerve roots with demyelination corresponding to the compressions of the roots at regular intervals (13). These demyelinated zones corresponded to the myelographic blocks. There was no evidence of ischemia.

TABLE 2. *Symptoms of lumbar stenosis in 68 patients*

	Symptom	Prevalence (%)
Description	Pseudoclaudication	94
	Standing leg discomfort	94
	⎧ Pain	93
	⎨ Numbness	63
	⎩ Weakness	43
	Bilateral	69
	Accompanied by back pain	65
Site	⎧ Whole limb	78
	⎨ Above knee only	15
	⎩ Below knee only	7
	Radicular pain only	6

With permission from ref. 13.

Clinical Presentation

Most patients are men. As the symptoms are difficult to correlate and signs are scarce or absent the patients have often been misdiagnosed. Typical misdiagnoses are psychoneurosis (17), osteoarthritis of the hip (4), and trochanteric bursitis. The cardinal symptom is pseudo-claudication (Table 2). This "neurogenic" claudication is usually bilateral and is reported as pain or weakness in the muscles of the thighs and calves provoked by both standing and walking, and relieved within minutes by sitting or lying down (3,13,17,33,47,51). Patients often report an accompanying numbness that may be described as a "rubbery" sensation or as "pins and needles" (3). Typically, the symptoms involve both lower extremities (13). Whereas other cauda equina diseases produce sphincteric disturbances, stenosis seldom does (3). Sparing of the lower roots can be understood when one considers their central protected position in the lumbar canal. That they may at times be involved is evidenced by a patient who could only urinate when sitting (51).

If patients persist in walking they notice that their legs get weak and they may fall (13,17,33). All the symptoms reduce when the patient adopts a flexed position (Fig. 2). Patients achieve this by leaning on shopping carts, church pews, forward on lawn-mowers, or against walls. Patients avoid lines at supermarkets or shopping in malls and, when forced to stand for long, will shift weight from one foot to the other. One patient when questioned about her walking and standing limits responded "one block and one hymn!" In advanced cases, patients adopt a simian posture and, even in recumbency, can assume a flexed or fetal position.

In true vascular claudication, by contrast, muscle pain is cramping, has no paresthetic quality, and is provoked by walking and relieved by standing. Whereas cycling provokes vascular claudication, it is well tolerated by stenotics as they are not weight-bearing and are in a flexed posture.

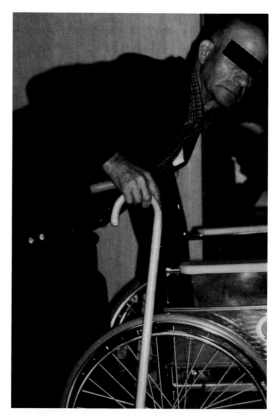

FIG. 2. Patient leaning on a wheelchair to get relief from neurogenic leg pain (with permission from ref. 30a).

Patients usually have no singular history of lumbar pains in early life and, unless spinal instability coexists, have surprisingly little back pain. Patients know their walking limits, often less than 100 meters. When asked to show where the pain is, a standing patient will describe the radicular symptoms with a sweeping downward motion of the two hands pointing from buttocks to heels. Valsalva maneuver will not provoke symptoms, whereas in discogenic sciatica it does. Low back pain, when present, is mild and has a mechanical quality (13,33,51). In the series of Hall, et al., at Mayo Clinic (13) less than 20% of patients could recall pre-existing discogenic sciatica. This may be normal for a middle-aged cohort.

Signs of stenosis are shown in Table 3. Few physical findings are present (6,13). The patient may be in a wheelchair or using a cane. If patients are observed standing or walking, they are soon seen to adopt a flexed

TABLE 3. *Neurologic signs of lumbar stenosis*

Reduced or absent ankle reflex	43%
Knee reflex decreased or absent	18%
Objective weakness	37%
Positive straight leg raising test	10%
Electromyogram abnormal	92%

With permission from ref. 13.

TABLE 4. *Differential diagnosis of lumbar stenosis*

Vascular claudication–atherosclerotic
Osteoarthritis of hip or knees
Lumbar disc protrusion

Unrecognized neurologic disease ⎰ Intraspinal tumor
⎱ Arteriovenous malformation
Peripheral neuropathy

posture. Reduced pedal pulses were noted in 9% of our series (13). In the same group of 68 patients, deep tendon reflexes were reduced at the ankles in 43% and at the quadriceps in 18%. The symptoms are shown in Table 2. Objective weakness was detected in 37%. Coexisting upper motor neuron lesions may at times occur since cervical myelopathies can coexist (13).

Decreased range of lumbar motion, although usually reported, is of little value in the diagnosis (13). The straight leg raising test of Lasegue is usually negative. Weakness, when present, is usually mild, can be unilateral or bilateral, and is usually in muscles innervated by L5 and S1 roots. This weakness can be evoked by attempts to walk on the heels or forefeet. When patients stand up for a few minutes they will seek a flexed posture as in leaning on the examining table. Walking non-stop for a few minutes will induce symptoms. At times the deep tendon reflexes, when rechecked after exertion, may disappear or be reduced (3).

The differential diagnosis of lumbar stenosis is shown in Table 4.

Diagnostic Tests

Electromyography, in the hands of an expert, reveals one or more radiculopathies in 92% of patients (13). The most typical pattern is bilateral multiple radiculopathies with evidence of paraspinal muscle involvement. At times paraspinal denervation may not be elicited. The chronic neurogenic changes include increase in motor unit amplitude, and fibrillation potentials.

Radiographs of the lumbar spine show degenerative disc disease in 70% of this elderly patient population and osteoarthritis of the facet joints in 62% (13). If A-P views of the lumbar spine show the apophyseal joints, this is a clue that can favor stenosis, as it suggests that the canal is sharply pitched like an A-frame roof and therefore not commodious. A degenerative spondylolisthesis, most often of grade I of L4 on L5, was seen in 35% of our series. This is the most reliable radiologic sign. Patients may have one or more degenerative lumbar discs, i.e., spondylosis. The spondylolisthesis is a late phase of osteoarthritis of the facet joints.

CT scans are commonly overinterpreted as evidence of lumbar stenosis. CT was predicted to become the leading diagnostic test (7,14,23) because it can reveal the lateral recesses and the reduction of epidural fat. Advanced CT machines provide high resolution. However, when CTs were read "blindly" in asymptomatic patients there were abnormal results in 35%. Moreover, up to 9% of asymptomatic "normal" controls were thought to have spinal stenosis (49). In another study of patients surgi-

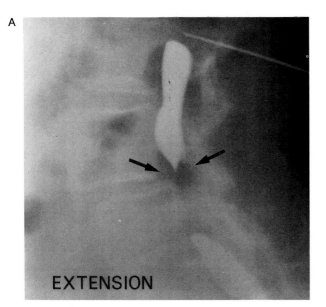
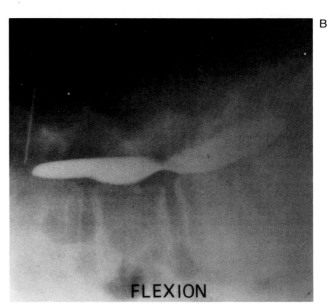

FIG. 3. Myelogram in lumbar stenosis. **A:** In extension: hour-glass deformity at L4-L5. Note grade I slip of L4 on L5. **B:** After flexion, radiocontrast passes below the block (with permission from ref. 13).

cally proven to have spinal stenosis, CT was diagnostically inferior to metrizamide myelography (2).

Besides false-positive results, the other difficulties with CT are time consumption, technical difficulty, and false-negative results (13,43,45). Window width differences can cause variation of measurements. Since the normal diameters of the lumbar canal vary between ethnic groups as well as between individuals, one cannot interpret diameters as absolute guidelines (10,34). In our series, 9% of patients had myelographic stenosis only at L1 or L2 or both, an area that is missed on conventional CT. Moreover, CT interpretation can miss a stenosis even within the area of viewing (13). At present, CT is best deferred until myelography and then used as an ancillary test. CT enables the radiologist to view foramens at and below the level of blocks, sites that are missed in lateral recess stenosis (24).

Myelography is the gold standard in diagnosis (9,13,34,47). It is essential when laminectomy is considered. The contrast material, usually injected with the patient in extension at L1 or L2, is blocked to caudal flow either completely or subtotally (13,17,47). Usually 10 to 15 ml contrast is needed (33,51), enough to fill the caudal subarachnoid space. Many neurosurgeons insist on tilting the table so that contrast can be allowed to flow cephalad. Otherwise, unsuspected high lesions are missed. Whereas pantopaque was formerly used (33,51), it is now preferable to use agents such as Iopamidol in order to prevent arachnoiditis (22,40). Flexion of the spine may allow blocked contrast material to flow distally (Fig. 3) thereby revealing if there are other blocks (9,44).

Selection of patients for surgery depends on the severity of pain, presence or absence of serious concomitant disease, and a realistic expectation that good to excellent operative results may not exceed 75% (13). Of approximately 1,000 lumbar stenotics seen at Mayo Clinic annually, it is estimated that no more than 200 are operated.

CERVICAL CANAL STENOSIS

Although cervical spondylosis or disc degeneration is common and affects most people over 50, spondylotic cervical myelopathy is uncommon. Stenosis in the cervical spine is less common than lumbar stenosis, but the two coexist so frequently, it is important to outline the symptoms of cervical disease (see Chapter 55).

The early descriptions of both cervical disc protrusion and spondylotic myelopathy had overlapping features (41,50). One early report described "extradural ventral chondromas" as tumors pressing on the cervical cord (41) and another discussed the relative merits of disc protrusion versus a degenerative or neoplastic process in causing myelopathy (5).

Development of the Lesion

As the cervical cord A-P diameter averages 10 mm and the internal spine diameter at C4 averages 17.7 mm, there is a large safety margin. The cervical discs, especially C5-C6 and C6-C7, degenerate in middle life showing signs of central dehydration (37). Spondylotic bars develop at the posterior margins of the vertebral bodies just above and below the disc. The "chondroma" described by Stookey (41) is a posterior bony exostosis and degenerated annulus fibrosus. This boss in front in combination with a hypertrophied ligamentum flavum and laminae behind compress the cord (8,28,29,37). Subluxations of vertebrae can occur (28,29). The end result of the multi-level compression is an indented cervical cord (Fig. 5) as with lumbar stenosis. Ischemia of the cord is not a likely contributor (8). A limited classification of cervical canal stenosis is shown in Table 5.

The corticospinal tracts are demyelinated below the level of compression whereas the ascending spinothalamic tracts are demyelinated above it (50). The cord may be deeply indented by spondylotic bars at several levels (Fig. 4). Cervical nerve roots can be compressed as the bars extend into the foramens. The nerve roots show compression of their dural sleeves (42).

The debate over the contribution of congenitally narrow canal versus spondylotic changes parallels that for lumbar stenosis. Thus, the putative culprits incriminated again are internal osteophytes, subluxations, ligament hypertrophy, and ischemia (28,29,37). Arguing against a constitutional narrowing are the findings by Nurick (28,29) of nearly equivalent internal spinal diameters in stenotics and controls. As deduced radiologically, the mean minimum A-P diameter of stenotic cervical spines in myelopathic patients was 14.6 mm, whereas in controls it was 16.2 mm.

Clinical Presentation

Patients are usually 45 to 65 years old (19,28,29), with a 60 to 40 male to female ratio. Few patients with cervical spondylosis, even when followed for six years or more, develop myelopathy (19). Patients with myelopathy usually present with a disorder of gait and often have a history of cervical radiculopathy. Neck pain is often

TABLE 5. *Non-malignant causes of cervical stenosis with myelopathy*

Acquired	Cervical spondylosis
	Paget's disease, gout
	Fluorosis (ref. 25)
Congenital	Multiple hereditary exostoses (ref. 15)
	Maroteaux-Lamy syndrome
	Achondroplasia (ref. 35)

A 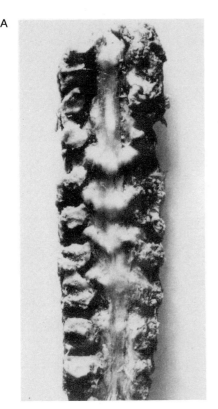 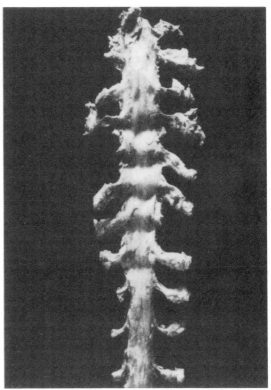 B

FIG. 4. A: Interior view of cervical canal showing transverse bars corresponding to **B,** indentations on stenotic cervical cord in same patient (with permission from ref. 50).

absent, and this adds to the difficulty in diagnosis. Spastic paraparesis is the most common syndrome (20) (Table 6). Depending on the site of the lesion, the upper extremities may have upper or lower motor neuron lesions or both (19,37,50). Babinski responses and increased knee and ankle jerks are expected, unless there is coexistent peripheral neuropathy or lumbar stenosis. In this case, leg reflexes may also be reduced. Involvement of spinothalamic tracts is usually revealed by a vague sensory level, and radicular involvement can give severe paresthesiae and hypesthesia in the hands. Posterior column involvement is detected by reduced vibratory or joint sense in the lower extremities.

Weakness and wasting of hand muscles, at times with fasciculations, may occur (5). Cord compression at C6 is suspected when a patient presents with hyperactive triceps tendon jerks and absent biceps reflexes. Symmetry is not necessary as Brown-Sequard lesions can be mimicked (5). Sphincter disturbances are seen in half the patients (20,37).

A sudden worsening of all symptoms and signs may be produced by neck trauma (19), but the course of spondylotic myelopathy is usually indolent. In a careful, mostly prospective study, the natural history of cervical spondylotic myelopathy was observed (19). All patients had extensor plantar responses. Episodes of worsening preceded referral and they occurred at infrequent intervals over a period of 2 to 30 years. Of 51 controls, patients having spondylosis without myelopathy, none developed myelopathy during long observation. These authors recommended a conservative approach to the myelopathy (19).

TABLE 6. *Symptoms and signs of myelopathy caused by spondylotic cervical myelopathy in 32 patients*

Type	Percent
Motor	
Hyper-reflexia	87
Babinski sign	54
Spastic gait	54
Sphincter disturbance	49
Arm weakness	31
Paraparesis	21
Quadriparesis	10
Brown-Sequard	10
Hand atrophy	13
Fasciculation	13
Sensory	
Vague sensory level	41
Proprioceptive loss	39
Cervical dermatome sensory loss	33
Pain	
Radicular, arm	41
Cervical pain	26

With permission from ref. 20.

Radiologic Diagnosis

Cervical spine roentgenograms (Fig. 5A) reveal disc space degeneration at C5-C6 and C6-C7, and foraminal encroachment seen on oblique views is due to Luschka joint exostoses. CT reveals spondylosis (Fig. 5B) but does not prove myelopathy. In a study by Penning (31), CT when combined with myelography predicted that concentric compression of the cord in a narrowed canal would cause symptoms when the cord cross-sectional area was reduced to about 60 mm², i.e., by 30% from normal (31). Conventional myelography reveals obstruction to caudal contrast flow in neck extension (31). It may be supplemented with CT (Fig. 5B). If there is no block, then post-myelogram CT is probably unnecessary (31).

Magnetic resonance imaging (MRI) can, when clinical findings are strongly suggestive, supplant myelography

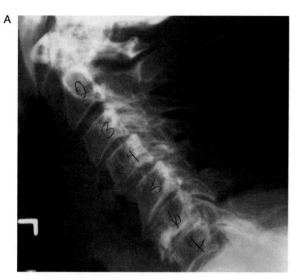

FIG. 5. A: Disc degeneration at C5-C6 and C6-C7, and subluxation at C3-C4.

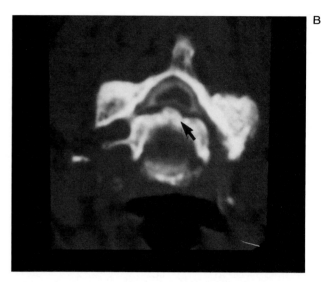

FIG. 5. B: Spondylotic bar seen in CT-metrizamide myelogram protruding posteriorly compressing cord at C5-C6.

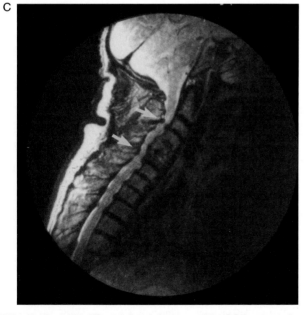

FIG. 5. C: MRI T2-weighted image with CSF appearing white, showing multi-level stenoses, worst at C3-C4 and C6-C7 (with permission from ref. 30a).

TABLE 7. *Differential diagnosis of cervical spondylotic myelopathy*

Cervical cord tumor
Syringomyelia
Cervical disc herniation
Arteriovenous malformation
Multiple sclerosis
Amyotrophic lateral sclerosis
Sub-acute combined degeneration
Neurosyphilis
Rheumatoid arthritis with subluxation

(22). The cervical canal on sagittal T2-weighted images shows multi-level stenosis (Fig. 5C). Moreover, MRI can rule out mimics, including intraspinal tumors and arteriovenous malformations. Cervical scoliosis makes MRI difficult to interpret. As with lumbar stenosis, the cerebrospinal fluid protein below the level of block is usually elevated. Cisternal myelography may be needed either when a block is not overcome by flexion or is multi-level, e.g., from C3-C6.

The differential diagnosis of cervical spondylotic myelopathy is shown in Table 7.

ACKNOWLEDGMENT

The author is deeply appreciative of the expert assistance provided by Mrs. Leisa Leisen in the preparation of this manuscript.

REFERENCES

1. Bailey P, Casamajor L (1911): Osteoarthritis of the spine as a cause of compression of the spinal cord and its roots: With reports of 5 cases. *J Nerv Ment Dis* 38:588–609.
2. Bell GR, Rothman RH, Booth RE, et al (1984): A study of computer-assisted tomography. Comparison of metrizamide myelography and computed tomography in the diagnosis of herniated lumbar disc and spinal stenosis. *Spine* 9:552–556.
3. Blau JN, Logue V (1961): Intermittent claudication of the cauda equina. *Lancet* 1:1081–1086.
4. Bohl WR, Steffee AD (1979): Lumbar spinal stenosis: A cause of continued pain and disability in patients after total hip arthroplasty. *Spine* 4(2):168–173.
5. Brain WR, Knight GC, Bull JW (1948): Discussion on rupture of the intervertebral disc in the cervical region. *Proc Roy Soc Med* 41:509–516.
6. Ciric I, Mikhael MA (1985): Lumbar spinal-lateral recess stenosis. *Neurologic Clinics* 3:417–423.
7. Dorwart RH, Volger JB 3d, Helms CA (1983): Spinal stenosis. *Radiol Clin North Am* 21:301–325.
8. Dunsker SB (1980): Cervical spondylotic myelopathy: Pathogenesis and pathophysiology. In: *Seminars in neurological surgery. Cervical spondylosis,* S Dunsker, ed. New York: Raven Press, pp 119–134.
9. Ehni G (1969): Significance of the small lumbar spinal canal: Cauda equina compression syndromes due to spondylosis. 1. Introduction. *J Neurosurg* 31:490–494.
10. Eisenstein S (1983): Lumbar vertebral canal morphometry for computerized tomography in spinal stenosis. *Spine* 8:187–191.
11. Ellman MH, Vazques LT, Brown NL, et al (1981): Calcium pyrophosphate dihydrate deposition in lumbar disc fibrocartilage. *J Rheum* 8(6):955–958.
12. Epstein JA, Epstein BS, Lavine L (1962): Nerve root compression associated with narrowing of the lumbar spinal canal. *J Neurol Neurosurg Psychiatry* 25:165–176.
13. Hall S, Bartleson JD, Onofrio BM, et al (1985): Lumbar spinal stenosis. Clinical features, diagnostic procedures and results of surgical treatment in 68 patients. *Ann Int Med* 103(2):271–275.
14. Hammerschlag SB, Wolpert SM, Carter BL (1976): Computed tomography of the spinal canal. *Radiology* 121:361–367.
15. Johnston CE 2d, Sklar F (1988): Multiple hereditary exostoses with spinal cord compression. *Orthoped* 11(8):1213–1216.
16. Karpman RR, Weinstein PR, Gall EP, et al (1982): Lumbar spinal stenosis in a patient with diffuse idiopathic skeletal hypertrophy syndrome. *Spine* 7(6):598–603.
17. Kirkaldy-Willis WH, Paine KW, Cauchoix J, et al (1974): Lumbar spinal stenosis. *Clin Orthop* (99):30–50.
18. Lane WA (1893): Case of spondylolisthesis associated with progressive paraplegia; laminectomy. *Lancet* 1:991.
19. Lees F, Turner JW (1963): Natural history and prognosis of cervical spondylosis. *Br Med J* 2:1607–1610.
20. Lunsford LD, Bissonette DJ, Zarub DS (1980): Anterior surgery for cervical disc disease. Part 2: Treatment of cervical spondylotic myelopathy in 32 cases. *J Neurosurg* 53:12–19.
21. Macnab I (1950): Spondylolisthesis with an intact neural arch: The so-called pseudo-spondylolisthesis. *J Bone Joint Surg* [B] 32(3):325–333.
22. Masaryk TJ, Modic MT, Geisinger MA, et al (1986): Cervical myelopathy: A comparison of magnetic resonance and myelography. *J Comp Assist Tomogr* 10(2):184–194.
23. McAfee PC, Ullrich CG, Yuan HA, et al (1981): Computed tomography in degenerative spinal stenosis. *Clin Orthop Related Res* 161:221–234.
24. McIvor GW, Kirkaldy-Willis WH (1976): Pathological and myelographic changes in the major types of lumbar spinal stenosis. *Clin Orthop* (115):72–76.
25. Misra UK, Nag D, Husain M, Ray PK, et al (1988): Endemic fluorosis presenting as cervical cord compression. *Arch Environ Health* 43(1):18–21.
26. Nasca RJ (1987): Surgical management of lumbar spinal stenosis. *Spine* 12:809–816.
27. Naylor A (1979): Factors in the development of the spinal stenosis syndrome. *J Bone Joint Surg* [B] 61(3):306–309.
28. Nurick S (1972): The pathogenesis of the spinal cord disorder associated with cervical spondylosis. *Brain* 95:87–100.
29. Nurick S (1972): The natural history and the results of surgical treatment of the spinal cord disorder associated with cervical spondylosis. *Brain* 95:101–108.
30a. O'Duffy JD (1989): Spinal stenosis. In: *Arthritis and allied conditions: A textbook of rheumatology, 11th ed.,* DJ McCarty, ed. Philadelphia: Lea and Febiger, pp. 1464–1472.
30. Pallis C, Jones AM, Spillane JD (1954): Cervical spondylosis. *Brain* 77:274–289.
31. Penning L, Wilmink JT, Van Woerden HH, et al (1986): CT myelographic findings in degenerative disorders of the cervical spine: Clinical significance. *AJR* 146:793–801.
32. Penning L, Wilmink JT (1987): Posture-dependent bilateral compression of L4 or L5 nerve roots in facet hypertrophy. A dynamic CT-myelographic study. *Spine* 12:488–500.
33. Pennal GF, Schatzker J (1971): Stenosis of the lumbar spinal canal. *Clin Neurosurg* 18:86–105.
34. Postacchini F, Ripani M, Carpano S (1983): Morphometry of the lumbar vertebrae: An anatomic study in two caucasoid ethnic groups. *Clin Orthop* (172):296–303.
35. Pyeritz RE, Sack GH, Udvarhelyi GB (1980): Cervical and lumbar laminectomy for spinal stenosis in achondroplasia. *Johns Hopkins Medical Journal* 146:203–206.
36. Rauschning W (1987): Normal and pathologic anatomy of the lumbar root canals. *Spine* 12:1008–1019.
37. Rowland LP (1984): Cervical spondylosis. In: *Merritt's textbook of neurology, 7th ed.,* LP Rowland, ed. Philadelphia: Lea & Febiger, pp. 310–312.
38. Sachs B, Fraenkel J (1900): Progressive ankylotic rigidity of the spine (spondylose rhizomelique). *J Nerv Ment Dis* 27:1–15.
39. Sarpyener MA (1945): Congenital stricture of the spinal canal. *J Bone Joint Surg* 27:70–79.
40. Sortland O, Magnaes B, Haug T (1977): Functional myelography with metrizamide in the diagnosis of lumbar spinal stenosis. *Acta Radiologica* [Suppl] 355:42–54.
41. Stookey B (1928): Compression of the spinal cord due to ventral extradural cervical chondromas. *Arch Neurol Psychiatry* 20:275–291.
42. Taylor AR (1953): Mechanism and treatment of spinal-cord disorders associated with cervical spondylosis. *Lancet* 1:717–720.
43. Thijssen HO, Keyser A, Horstink MW, et al (1979): Morphology of the cervical spinal cord in computed myelography. *Neuroradiol* 18(2):57–62.
44. Uden A, Johnsson KE, Jonsson K, et al (1985): Myelography in

the elderly and the diagnosis of spinal stenosis. *Spine* 10(2):171–174.

45. Ullrich CG, Binet EF, Sanecki MG, et al (1980): Quantitative assessment of the lumbar spinal canal by computed tomography *Radiology* 134:137–143.

46. Van Gelderen C (1948): Ein orthotisches (lordotisches) kaudasyndrom. *Acta Psychiatr Neurol* 23:57–68.

47. Verbiest H (1954): A radicular syndrome from developmental narrowing of the lumbar vertebral canal. *J Bone Joint Surg* [B] 36(2):230–237.

48. Weisz GM (1986): Lumbar canal stenosis in Paget's disease. *Clin Orthop Related Res* (206):223–227.

49. Wiesel SW, Tsourmas N, Feffer HL, et al (1984): A study of computer-assisted tomography. I. The incidence of positive CAT scans in an asymptomatic group of patients. *Spine* 9:549–551.

50. Wilkinson M (1971): *Cervical spondylosis: Its early diagnosis and treatment, 2nd ed.,* M Wilkinson, ed. Philadelphia: W.B. Saunders, pp 49–55.

51. Yamada H, Oya M, Okada T, et al (1972): Intermittent cauda equina compression due to narrow spinal canal. *J Neurosurg* 37:83–88.

The Adult Spine: Principles and Practice,
J. W. Frymoyer, Editor-in-Chief.
Raven Press, Ltd., New York © 1991.

CHAPTER 86

Lumbar Decompression for Spinal Stenosis

Surgical Indications and Technique

Dan M. Spengler

Lumbar spinal stenosis is a common clinical syndrome, which affects a significant number of individuals usually associated with advancing age (1,3,5,9). Although spinal stenosis can be identified in any age group, the most common type, degenerative stenosis, generally occurs in patients beyond the fifth decade (9). Lumbar spinal stenosis refers to the resultant clinical syndrome which occurs as the volume of the lumbar spinal canal is diminished from any cause (3,8). Several theories exist as to the cause for symptoms seen in patients who have diminished spinal canals. Direct pressure occurs, but by itself is insufficient to cause symptoms. Pressure plus inflammatory changes in surrounding tissues could explain symptoms. Evidence also exists that symptoms are the result of a decrease in arterial supply to the nerve roots. Venous engorgement of the epidural veins also occurs and may contribute to increasing symptoms by further diminishing the volume of the spinal canal (3,8,9). Studies have shown that the clinical syndrome of lumbar spinal stenosis is more commonly associated with patients who have an AP diameter of the dural sac of less than 10 mm (3). This value can be measured from CT scans following myelography. The measurements are most accurate at L4-L5 and above, since the dural sac normally tapers at L5-S1. Several anatomical structures contribute to a diminishment in size of the spinal canal, including the zy-goapophyseal joints, ligamentum flavum, intervertebral disc, and synovial tissue (8).

SURGICAL INDICATIONS

Degenerative stenosis occurs in an elderly patient population. Age alone, however, does not represent a contraindication to surgery. Consultation with a vascular surgeon or internist or both is often essential to ensure that there is not significant vascular disease, and to clarify pre-operative risk factors. The critical indicator for surgery revolves around the patient's own perception of his or her quality of life. This variable is different for everyone, but forms a major criterion for consideration of surgical intervention (9).

Patients with lumbar spinal stenosis usually complain of pain in the back, buttocks, lower extremities, or any combination (5,9). Patients may also complain of numbness, burning, weakness, in combination or separately. Walking exacerbates symptoms, which can often be relieved by sitting or lying down (pseudoclaudication). Some patients, particularly females, report changes in urinary function, such as increased frequency or nocturia. A recent onset of incontinence in a female with other symptoms of spinal stenosis indicates viscerogenic dysfunction unless otherwise disproven. These symptoms are generally insidious in onset, although on occasion a patient may present with an acute symptom of incontinence. Some individuals develop symptoms when a previously compromised spinal canal is further

D. M. Spengler, M.D.: Professor and Chairman, Department of Orthopaedics and Rehabilitation, Vanderbilt University Medical Center, Nashville, Tennessee, 37232.

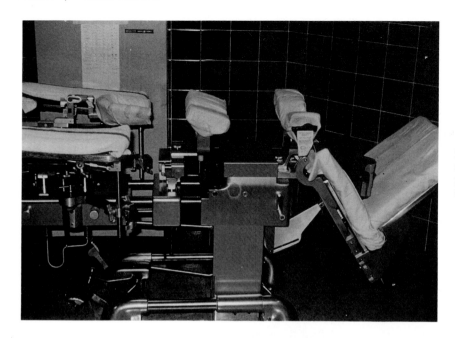

FIG. 1. Roger Anderson (Tower) table used to position patient so as to minimize pressure on abdominal content (see text on pages 1815–1818).

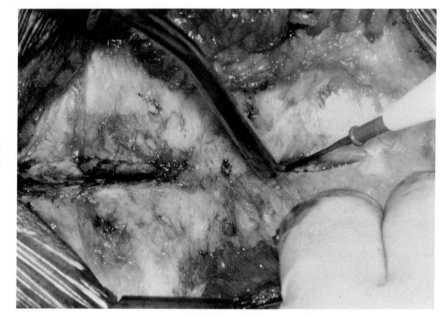

FIG. 2. Incisions with electrocautery over spinous processes to lessen bleeding.

compromised by an intervertebral disc protrusion. Other patients with stenosis complain of increasing pain in the evening, and are often awakened at night. Even though these symptoms are often associated with malignancy, spinal stenosis can also represent the source of symptoms.

Although most patients with lumbar stenosis have significant subjective complaints, the physical examination usually reveals few findings (9). A methodical, thorough examination is required to exclude other causes for low back symptoms, such as referred pain from an abdominal aneurysm or from a neoplasm. The most common physical findings in patients who have lumbar stenosis include pain with extension of the lumbar spine, weak-

ness of the extensor hallucis longus, and sensory changes that follow specific dermatomes. Sciatic tension signs are infrequent and when present usually indicate a component of lateral recess stenosis. A careful examination of the hip joints must be included, since many patients with osteoarthritis of the hip will complain of pain in the buttock, groin, and/or lower back. Often, patients in this age group may in fact have both lumbar spinal stenosis and osteoarthritis of the hip. These patients form a subset of individuals who are particularly difficult to manage. Comprehensive assessment is necessary. In some patients, surgical management for both conditions becomes necessary.

Imaging studies form the key method to confirm the

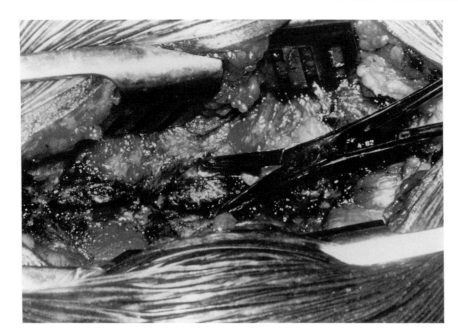

FIG. 3. Towel clip prior to radiograph to identify appropriate vertebral level precisely.

FIG. 4. Raytech sponges assist to control bleeding during dissection.

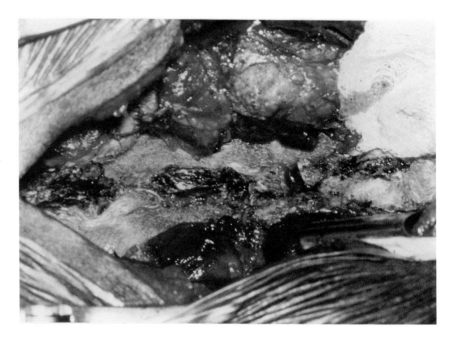

diagnosis of lumbar stenosis. Plain radiographs of the lumbar spine are indicated to exclude other pathological processes. Although the diagnosis of lumbar spinal stenosis can be suspected on the basis of plain radiographs, additional studies are mandatory prior to surgical intervention. Since the majority of patients with degenerative stenosis are elderly, there is a higher likelihood that these patients may have a neoplasm. Because of this possibility, a bone scan is an important diagnostic test.

I believe lumbar myelography followed by CT scanning provides the single best study to reaffirm the diagnosis of spinal stenosis and to provide critical information concerning pre-operative planning (2,3). This study permits the dural sac to be precisely measured. The ex-

tent of the decompression can also be planned from the studies. In the event of a complete block or a high grade stenosis, the computed tomographic scans must be studied distal to the block to determine the length of the surgical decompression (6). Finally, the myelogram permits evaluation of the conus medullaris to exclude an intraspinal tumor.

Magnetic resonance imaging is rapidly evolving as a popular method to assess patients with spinal disorders (see Chapter 23). Despite this current enthusiasm I recommend surgery in patients with lumbar stenosis only after I have reviewed the myelogram-CT scan.

Other studies are often warranted prior to performing surgery on the patient with symptoms suggestive of spi-

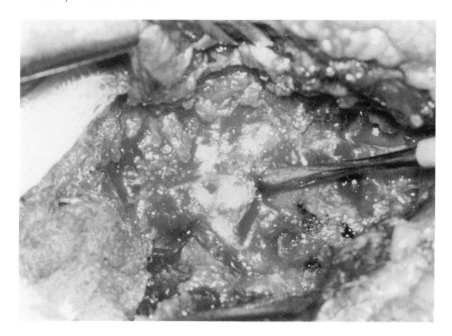

FIG. 5. Freer or Penfield 1 elevator used to initiate stripping of ligamentum flavum from anterior lamina.

FIG. 6. Angled (45°) rongeur used to expose midline raphe of the ligamentum flavum.

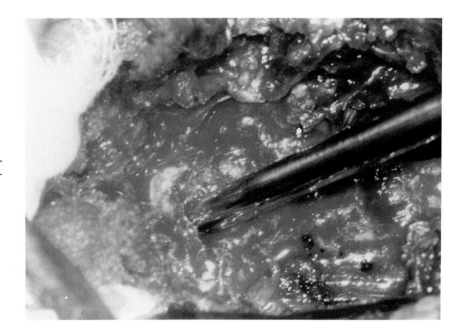

nal stenosis. Electrodiagnostic studies are useful to document the extent of neural involvement and to aid in pre-operative planning. Approximately 80% of patients who have lumbar spinal stenosis demonstrate changes on electromyographic examination (9). Certainly, the absence of electromyographic changes does not exclude the diagnosis of spinal stenosis, but the presence of electrical changes in selected nerve roots often assists the surgeon with pre-operative planning to ensure that these nerve roots are carefully inspected at the time of intervention. Somatosensory or motor evoked potentials used pre- and inter-operatively are currently undergoing assessment in the surgical treatment of spinal stenosis and appear to hold great promise (see Chapter 26).

The main psychological factor that should not be overlooked in the elderly patient is depression (10). Disincentives to improvement, such as wage-replacement benefits and litigation, must always be considered, but these are seldom involved in patients who are more than 65 years of age. Primary depression, which is not uncommon in this age group, can, however, result in a confusing differential diagnosis. Most patients who have true depression have some somatic complaints, and prompt recognition and early treatment of the underlying depression may result in marked diminution of such symptoms (10). On the other hand, patients who have a chronically painful condition do not always exhibit depression, and fewer than 20% of patients who have had a stroke or who have cancer are clinically depressed (7).

Based on all of these considerations, the indications

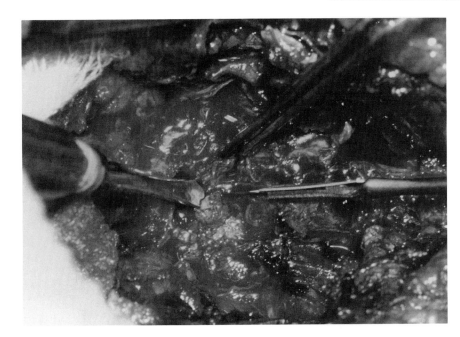

FIG. 7. Sharp division of the ligamentum flavum in the midline using a Penfield 3 to protect underlying dura.

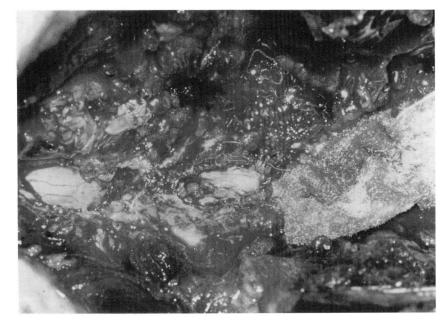

FIG. 8. Laminotomies above and below maximum stenosis have been completed.

for decompression are (1) actual or impending cauda equina syndrome; (2) increasing peripheral neurologic abnormality, particularly weakness; and (3) increasing or unrelenting claudication, which interferes with the patient's quality of life.

SURGICAL TECHNIQUE

After the institution of anesthesia of choice and after the administration of an intravenous antibiotic, the patient is placed in the prone position. I use the Roger Anderson (Tower) table (Fig. 1). This table allows proper positioning to ensure that the abdominal viscera hang free without pressure. The hips are flexed approximately

40 degrees, and the patient is suspended from the thorax and both iliac crests by padded supports. If, however, spinal fusion is to be contemplated as an addition to decompression, the patient should be positioned with the hip joints hyperextended to prevent the development of a flat back (loss of lumbar lordosis). This is especially true if internal fixation is to be used as an adjunct to fusion. Care must be taken during positioning so that there is no pressure on the eyes. As in lumbar disc surgery, I recommend the use of a fiberoptic headlight and loupe (2.5×) magnification. Following positioning, skin preparation, and surgical draping, a straight incision is made from the spinous process of L2 to the spinous process of S1. For purposes of this description, I assume a

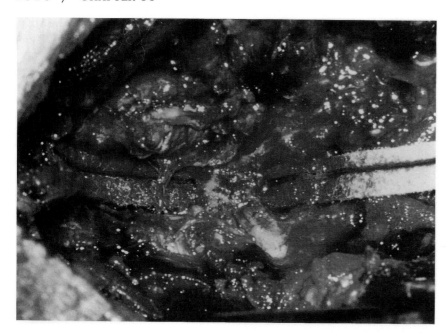

FIG. 9. Cottonoid underneath lamina protects dura.

FIG. 10. Maximum stenosis level is saved for last.

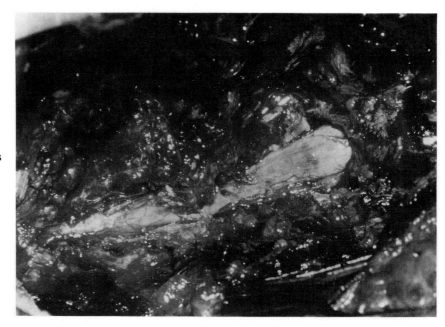

decompression from L3 to S1. If lesser decompression is necessary, the incision may be shortened accordingly.

Dissection proceeds to the thoracolumbar fascia; self-retaining retractors are placed after meticulous hemostasis has been achieved with cautery. Spinous processes are identified and an incision with electrocautery is made directly over the middle of each of the spinous processes (Fig. 2). Pickups provide tension to dissect around the spinous processes so as not to enter the paraspinous muscle envelope. Subperiosteal dissection is more effective and less bleeding is encountered. I use electrocautery for this portion of the dissection. Once all of the spinous processes have been delineated, dissection continues so

as to connect the incision from process to process. A towel clip is attached to one or two spinous processes and a lateral intra-operative radiograph is taken to accurately localize level (Fig. 3). Cobb elevators are used to strip the paraspinous muscles from the spinous processes and lamina. Dissection is continued laterally to the zygoapophyseal joints.

In patients with lumbar spinal stenosis, this portion of the dissection is more difficult than in other patients. The lamina are more vertical and the zygoapophyseal joints are enlarged, so that elegant stripping becomes difficult. Raytech sponges are packed into the wound on one side while the opposite side undergoes similar exposure (Fig. 4). Large Cobb elevators are used in sequence until the lamina and zygoapophyseal joints are exposed throughout the area for decompression. Once this phase of the dissection has been completed, large self-retaining retractors are positioned to clearly expose all of the posterior elements. The interlaminar spaces are cleared using rongeurs, elevators, and/or curettes. The inferior portion of the L3 spinous process and all of the intervening spinous processes are then removed. If the major stenotic segment is L4-L5, attention would first be turned to the L3-L4 interspace followed by the L5-S1 interspace. I recommend that the most stenotic motion segment be approached last after the dura has been exposed at the more normal levels to minimize dural tears. The midline of the L5-S1 interlaminar space is identified, and a Penfield 1 or a Freer elevator used to separate the ligamentum flavum from the lamina (Fig. 5). A 45 degree angled rongeur is used to further expose the ligamentum flavum in the midline to identify the midline raphe (Fig. 6). A Penfield 4 elevator is used to free the undersurface of the ligament. A Penfield 3 elevator is inserted underneath the ligamentum flavum (Fig. 7). Once the Penfield 3 elevator is in place, a #15 blade on a long-handled knife divides the flavum in the midline to the next lamina. Curettes or upbiting rongeurs can be used to more completely excise the ligamentum flavum. Once a laminotomy has been completed below the level of maximum stenosis, a similar approach is repeated above the level of maximum stenosis (Fig. 8). Cottonoids are used to protect the dura. Once the laminotomies have been performed above and below the block, dissection proceeds from cephalad and caudad toward the area of maximal stenosis.

In patients with spinal stenosis, the dura is usually adherent to the undersurface of the lamina as well as to the undersurface of the ligamentum flavum. Dural lacerations can be minimized with this technique. I pass a cottonoid under each lamina to protect the dura during the dissection (Fig. 9). Upbiting rongeurs are used to divide the lamina in the midline. Thus, a central midline decompression is created from L3 to S1. Once the midline dura has been exposed in its entirety, the surgeon should continue the decompression in the posterolateral gutter on the side of the spine opposite the surgeon. Forty-five degree angled rongeurs are used. A Penfield 1 elevator and cottonoids assist to protect the neural elements. Hemostasis is obtained by gentle packing with sterile, absorbable gelatin sponges and cottonoids. Cautery should be minimized within the spinal canal, since additional scar tissue may be generated. On occasion, however, bipolar cautery is essential to achieve proper hemostasis. The area of high-grade stenosis is decompressed last using extreme care (Fig. 10). Once the posterolateral gutter has been completed on one side with appropriate foraminotomies for any nerve roots that do not move 1 cm medially easily, the surgeon moves to the opposite side of

the table and performs a similar dissection on the opposite side. Foraminotomy, if felt to be necessary, may be accomplished by a number of different methods dependent upon the degree of stenosis. If mild, simple undercutting of the foramina with a 45 degree angled antral punch may suffice. If major, it may be necessary to remove most or all of the pars interarticularis. If the latter is done, particularly if bilateral, then a fusion should generally be added.

If the pedicle is a major factor resulting in "kinking" of the nerve root as described by Macnab (7a), then the use of a small sharp osteotome to remove the inferior aspect of the pedicle as the root rounds the pedicle will help to decrease the angular deformity of the nerve root. All freshly exposed bone areas should be overcoated with bone wax to decrease post-operative bleeding.

If the nerve root(s) are compromised by the overlying facets, undercutting of the facet may suffice to decrease neural compression. It may be necessary to remove the medial half of the superior facet or all of the facet. In a lateral recess stenosis, the overhanging superior facet may often need to be undercut or removed. We have found that this is most easily accomplished with the use of a small sharp osteotome which allows the bone to break away without fully penetrating the osseous projection and avoids damage to the underlying neural structures. The bone fragments can then safely be removed with a forceps. Once this dissection has been completed, the dura should be pulsatile and the nerve roots free and mobile. Intra-operative ultrasound may now be used to

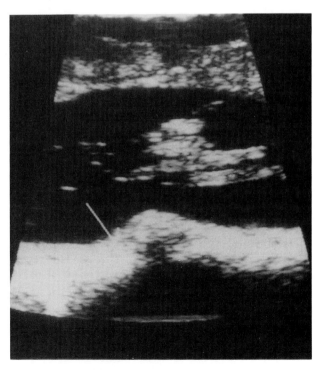

FIG. 11. Intra-operative ultrasound demonstrating anterior disc prominence in sagittal view.

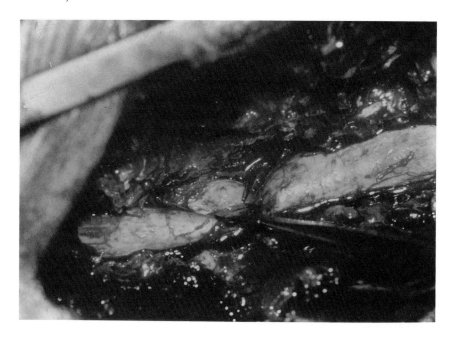

FIG. 12. Following retraction of dura to midline, large disc herniation is exposed.

FIG. 13. Surgery has been completed. Dura is pulsatile; nerve roots are free.

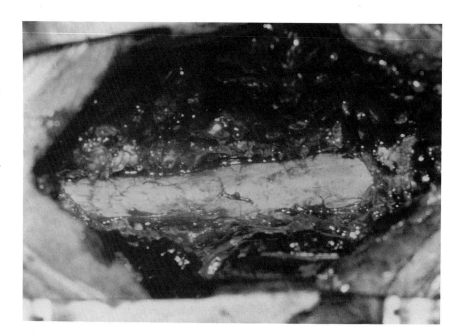

assess the anterior structures (Fig. 11). With or without ultrasound, careful inspection must be performed anteriorly to identify any evidence for disc herniation (Fig. 12). Assuming there is no evidence for any anterior decompression, surgery is now complete (Fig. 13). Hemostasis is obtained and an interposition membrane of fat and/or sterile, absorbable gelatin sponge is placed. The wound is then irrigated and closed in layers over a drain.

Controversy exists as to the necessity of adding a fusion in the presence of decompression for spinal stenosis. It is definitely indicated where decompression for a degenerative spondylolisthesis is done in conjunction with discotomy (these issues will be discussed in Chapters 78 and 90). Recent reports have shown that anterior slip following decompression for degenerative spondylolisthesis is significantly decreased with the addition of fusion, particularly with internal fixation (see Chapter 78). It has been shown that the destruction of a unilateral facet enhances instability as does removal of greater than 50% of both facets. Since spinal stenosis generally occurs in the more elderly person, where the viscoelastic properties of the spine are decreased, fusion is probably not indicated in the presence of significant disc narrowing. If the disc spaces remain reasonably open, the addition of fusion in the presence of facet destruction should be considered.

SPECIFIC COMPLICATIONS

In a recent literature review (also see Chapter 89), patients who undergo decompression of the lumbar spine for the treatment of acquired degenerative stenosis were shown to have good outcomes approximately 85% of the time (5,9). Patients who do not improve following decompression should be reassessed to exclude another cause for the symptom complex. Complications which can occur following this decompression are numerous. Wound infection, thrombophlebitis, urinary tract infection, and/or pulmonary complications may develop. Unique local complications include technical problems, such as dural lacerations with or without injury to the neural structures. Although neural complications are infrequent, dural lacerations occur more commonly due to the thin dura typical in patients with spinal stenosis. Patients must also be followed closely to recognize a postoperative cauda equina syndrome. If neurologic progression is observed following surgery, repeat myelography and/or prompt return to surgery appears to be the most appropriate method to deal with this complication. Bleeding can also be encountered, especially since most patients with stenosis have engorged epidural veins. Control of bleeding has not been a common problem in my practice. I have always been able to obtain hemostasis by the use of thrombin-soaked pledgets and cottonoids.

POST-SURGICAL MANAGEMENT

After surgery, the drain is removed within 24 to 48 hours. The patient is provided with an abdominal binder and mobilized the day following surgery. Certain frail, elderly patients require additional time prior to being mobilized, but the sooner the patient is mobilized, the better. Patients are usually discharged approximately 7 days following surgery. Active strengthening exercises are provided approximately 6 weeks following surgery. The extent and scope of the rehabilitation plan varies with each individual patient. For those individuals who desire maximum rehabilitation, strengthening using fitness machines is recommended to increase both abdominal and extensor muscle tone. In addition, an aerobic exercise program is outlined and implemented. This program will also vary with the interests of the patient, but can include walking, swimming, bicycling, and jogging. Patients are evaluated with standing lateral radiographs to ensure that no progressive slip or abnormality in spinal alignment develops. I do not perform a routine fusion procedure for a patient with lumbar stenosis who has a normally aligned lumbar spine. If a patient has a degenerative spondylolisthesis, I recommend posterolateral stabilization with the selective use of pedicle implant systems to further stabilize the spine.

REFERENCES

1. Arnoldi CC, Brodsky AE, Cauchoix J, Crock HV, Dommisse GF, Edgar MA, Gargano FP, Jacobson RE, Kirkaldy-Sheldon J, Tile M, Urist R, Wilson WE, Wiltse LL (1976): Lumbar spinal stenosis and nerve root entrapment syndromes: Definition and classification. *Clin Orthop* (115):4–5.
2. Bell GR, Rothman RH, Booth RE, Cuckler JM, Garfin S, Herkowitz H, Simeone FA, Dolinskas C, Han SS (1984): A study of computer-assisted tomography. II. Comparison of metrizamide myelography and computed tomography in the diagnosis of herniated lumbar disc and spinal stenosis. *Spine* 9:552–556.
3. Bolender N-F, Schonstrom NS, Spengler DM (1985): Role of computed tomography and myelography in the diagnosis of central spinal stenosis. *J Bone Joint Surg* [Am] 67:240–246.
4. Eismont FJ, Green BA, Berkowitz BM, Montalvo BM, Quencer RM, Brown MJ (1984): The role of intraoperative ultrasonography in the treatment of thoracic and lumbar spine fractures. *Spine* 9:782–787.
5. Hall S, Bartleson JD, Onofrio BM, Baker HL Jr, Okazaki H, O'Duffy JD (1985): Lumbar spinal stenosis. Clinical features, diagnostic procedures, and results of surgical treatment in 68 patients. *Ann Intern Med* 103:271–275.
6. Herkowitz HN, Garfin SR, Bell GR, et al (1987): The use of computerized tomography in evaluating non-visualized vertebral levels caudad to a complete block on a lumbar myelogram. *J Bone Joint Surg* [Am] 69:218–224.
7. Katon WJ (1985): Prevalence of depression in chronic disease. Presented at the Symposium on Depression and Chronic Disease, sponsored by Roerig, Division of Pfizer Pharmaceuticals, San Diego, California, April 19, 1985.
7a. Macnab I (1977): *Backache.* Baltimore: Williams and Wilkins, p. 212.
8. Schonstrom NS, Bolender N-F, Spengler DM (1985): The pathomorphology of spinal stenosis as seen on CT scans of the lumbar spine. *Spine* 10:806–811.
9. Spengler DM (1987): Degenerative stenosis of the lumbar spine. *J Bone Joint Surg* [Am] 69:305–308.
10. Ward NG (1986): Tricyclic antidepressants for chronic low-back pain. *Spine* 11:661–665.

The Adult Spine: Principles and Practice,
J. W. Frymoyer, Editor-in-Chief.
Raven Press, Ltd., New York © 1991.

CHAPTER 87

Microsurgical Spinal Laminotomies

John A. McCulloch

The merging of the technologies of magnetic resonance imaging (MRI) with the magnification and illumination characteristics of the microscope has dramatically changed the surgical treatment of spinal canal stenosis (SCS) (13). The use of the microscope to limit the surgical exposure in SCS is made possible by MRI pinpointing the soft tissue and bony stenotic lesion. The surgical procedure that has evolved has been variously named the intersegmental resculpturing or laminoplasty procedure, or simply a laminotomy (2). The advantage of considering this limited surgical approach lies in the fact that it is possible to save all the important soft tissue and bony stabilizing structures, yet at the same time remove the pathology encroaching on the cauda equina.

Before describing the technical approach, it is necessary to outline the limited types of spinal stenotic lesions that are amenable to a microsurgical operation. The classification of spinal stenosis has been outlined in Chapter 85. Acquired spinal stenosis is described as a lesion developing in mobile segments as part of the aging process. Abnormal motion, usually secondary to disc degeneration, results in osteophyte formation, ligamentum infolding or hypertrophy, facet hypertrophy, and/or annular bulging. In turn, these changes encroach upon neural structures and reduce the space available to the cauda equina and nerve roots.

J. A. McCulloch, M.D.: Professor of Orthopaedics, Northeastern Ohio Universities, College of Medicine, Rootstown, and 75 Arch Street, Suite 501, Akron, Ohio, 44304.

The classic symptom of spinal stenosis is limitation of walking distance due to leg symptoms, which may cause leg pain, to feelings of heaviness, fatigue, aching, numbness, and/or unsteadiness. The common denominator is that these symptoms limit the walking distance and cause the patient to "limp or be lame," hence the term claudication. Since the claudication has its pathological origin in the cauda equina, rather than the vascular tree, the symptom complex associated with spinal stenosis has become known as neurogenic claudication. This symptom complex is so prevalent that it forms the foundation of the definition of spinal canal stenosis:

Claudicant limitation of leg function in the presence of a stenotic spinal canal lesion on x-ray imaging, and in the absence of vascular impairment to the lower extremities.

CLASSIFICATION

The standard classification of SCS (1) was outlined in Chapter 85. This etiological classification and the term spinal stenosis are used by most authors to describe canal and "lateral recess" stenosis. This arbitrary division of spinal stenosis into lateral zone stenosis (LZS) and spinal canal stenosis (SCS) helps in understanding the two conditions but, at best, is an artificial separation that often does not stand the test of clinical medicine when a patient presents with stenosis involving both anatomical regions. The focus of this chapter is canal stenosis.

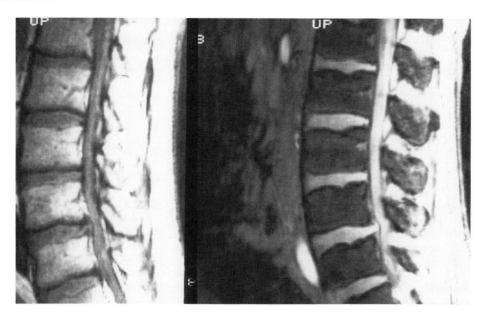

FIG. 1. Congenital SCS. The entire canal, all three stories (see Fig. 5) of each segment and multiple segments are narrowed in this sagittal MRI. A small disc protrusion is present at L4-L5, which tipped this patient into symptoms.

Purely congenital spinal stenosis is uncommon and a disease affecting multiple spinal segments (Fig. 1). It is not an entity that can be dealt with by a limited laminotomy procedure. The three most common forms of spinal stenosis, two of which lend themselves to one procedure, are acquired degenerative conditions:

Spinal canal stenosis (SCS) due to a degenerative spondylolisthesis (Fig. 2) is the most common form (4,9). Because of the forward and/or lateral translation (slip) of one vertebral segment on the next, a vertebral segmental instability is implied for which many surgeons would propose a combined decompression and stabilization procedure. This author is in agreement with that position and such a wide operative exposure cannot possibly be done through a limited microsurgical laminoplasty.

The next two conditions are approachable through limited surgical intervention with the microscope: Spinal canal stenosis (SCS) due to degenerative changes in the soft tissue and joints of the lumbar spine without a degenerative spondylolisthesis (Fig. 3) (6), and lateral zone stenosis (LZS) due to degenerative changes in the subarticular, foraminal, and extraforaminal regions of the lateral zone (Fig. 4).

PATHOANATOMY OF SPINAL CANAL STENOSIS

The surgical anatomy of the structural lesion in SCS is the key to understanding the limited surgical procedure to relieve the cauda equina stenosis. Each vertebral segment can be divided into three layers (Fig. 5). (For want

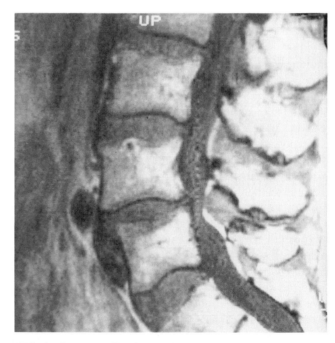

FIG. 2. Sagittal MRI (T1-weighted) showing a degenerative spondylolisthesis, L4-L5, with SCS. Note the buckling of the ligamentum flavum stenosing the canal largely in the "first story."

of better terminology, the author has designated these three layers as the three stories in a house.) On reviewing Figure 3, one can see that the stenotic lesion is largely confined to the first story of the anatomical segment with some extension into the third story of the anatomical segment below and some extension above into the sec-

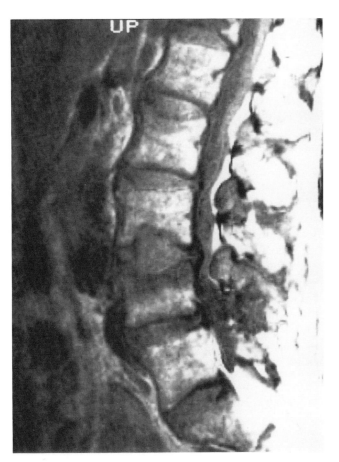

FIG. 3. Sagittal MRI (T1-weighted) showing SCS in multiple segments without a degenerative spondylolisthesis (slip). There is a very early slip, L4 on L5, but the stenotic levels are at L2-L3 and L3-L4.

ond story of the same anatomical segment. Figures 6 and 7 show a predominant "first story" lesion due to degenerative changes in the facet joints, disc space, and ligamentum flavum. These degenerative changes are in the form of hypertrophy and unfolding of the ligamentum flavum, annular bulging of the degenerating and collapsing disc, and osteophyte formation at the edges of the vertebral bodies or lips of the facet joints (12). Of the three, infolding of the ligamentum flavum is the major lesion. Note again that the major location of stenosis in Figures 3, 6, and 7 occurs predominantly in the first story of each segment, extending somewhat down into the third story of the segment below, and even less so up into the second story of the same segment. Between the midpoints of the pedicles and at the junction of the third and second stories there is virtually no stenosis (Figs. 3, 6, and 7).

Linking a series of segments together and being aware that canal stenosis is always most prominent in the first story, one can appreciate that the constriction of canal stenosis occurs between the take-off of nerve roots. Thus, canal stenosis at the disc space level of L4-L5 (first story

of L4) is a constricting ring between the take-off of the fourth root above and the fifth lumbar nerve root below (Fig. 12). Because the ligamentum flavum is such an important contributor to stenosis, some detail of its anatomy and degeneration are important to understanding the operative approach.

THE LIGAMENTUM FLAVUM

The ligamenta flava are paired structures that connect adjacent lamina (Fig. 8). The ligamentum flavum's elastin/collagen content and its attachment to the lamina make it a unique structure.

Elastin/Collagen Content

The elastic content of the ligamentum flavum is approximately 80% versus a collagen content of 20%. This high elastic content gives the ligament a yellow appearance, hence the name yellow ligament. It is probably a passive structure, acting much like a rubberband when lumbar vertebrae flex and extend. During flexion, the ligamentum flavum stretches but does not inhibit that motion. On return to neutral and extension, it returns to its resting, but still taut, position without buckling. With aging, the ligamentum flavum loses its elastic properties, becomes more collagenous in nature, and, as a result, permanently buckles or folds into the spinal canal as seen in Figures 3, 6, and 7.

Attachment of Ligamentum Flavum

The paired ligamenta flava are separated by a midline cleft (Fig. 8). Laterally, they extend to the anterior aspect of the facet joint, blending with the anterior capsule of the facet joint (Fig. 9). The important attachments are to the cephalad and caudal lamina. Note that the insertion

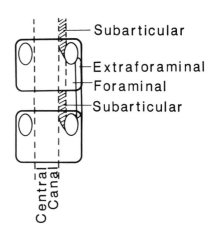

FIG. 4. The lateral zone divided into its three regions.

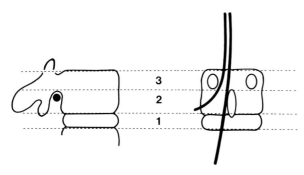

FIG. 5. The three "stories" in each anatomical segment. First story: the disc. Second story: the foramen. Third story: the pedicle.

of the proximal edge of the ligamentum is into the anterior surface of the midportion of the cephalad lamina. Its distal edge inserts along the superior border of the caudad lamina. Total unilateral excision of the ligamentum flavum requires removal of the inferior half of the cephalad lamina, the superior edge of the caudal lamina, and the medial margin of the facet joint (Fig. 11). In completing this limited excision, the stenosis of the canal can be alleviated. Further, this limited interlaminar approach is facilitated by the microscope.

Segments Involved in Spinal Canal Stenosis

Most often, SCS is a multisegmental disease or presents at a "slip" or "listhetic" level, which precludes a

microsurgical approach. Less than one-third of SCS patients will have unisegmental involvement at a non-slip level and be possible candidates for microsurgical approach. Although it is theoretically possible to use this microsurgical approach at two stenotic levels, its use in multisegmental decompressions is tedious and inadvisable. Multilevel cases are probably best handled with loupes. The single level most frequently affected is L4-L5 and the level least affected is L5-S1.

INVESTIGATION

Investigation of a patient with SCS can be difficult. Because of the age group affected, it is important to rule out other conditions, such as infection, tumors, and other non-mechanical causes of back pain. A high percentage of these patients may also have vascular disease, and it is necessary to establish that aortoiliac or femoral arterial insufficiency is not the dominant cause for their symptoms. Neurological symptoms require consideration of all possible causes, including generalized neurological disorders unrelated to the spine.

Radiological Investigation

Plain x-ray films of most patients with low back pain are routinely ordered but yield little information about a patient with SCS. Their greatest use is to rule out other conditions, such as tumors or infection. Radiographs do reveal the degenerative changes within the disc space and

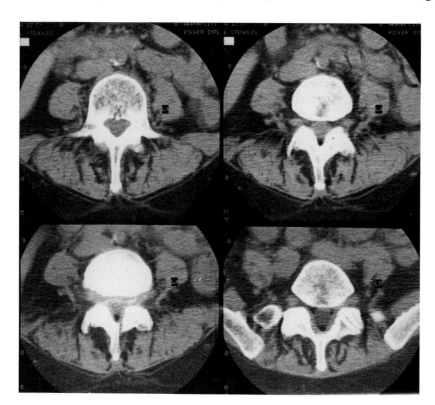

FIG. 6. Axial CT scans showing stenosis of cauda equina (bottom left). Above and below this "napkin ring" is a patent canal.

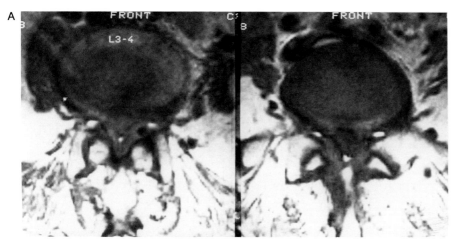

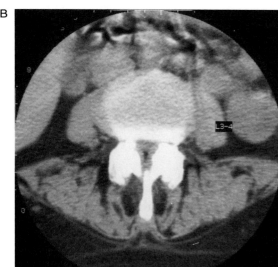

FIG. 7. A: Axial MRI (T1-weighted) showing the same napkin ring stenosis, L3-L4. B: Axial CT showing vertebral body and facet joint lipping contributing to the stenotic lesion.

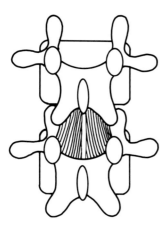

FIG. 8. The ligamenta flava are paired interlaminar structures separated by a midline cleft.

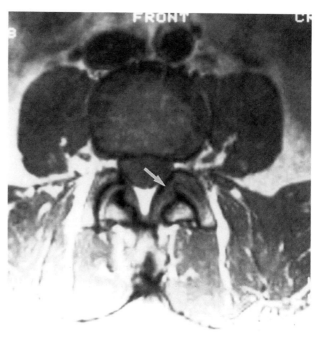

FIG. 9. The lateral portion of the ligamentum flavum blends with and becomes part of the anterior portion of the facet joint capsule (arrow).

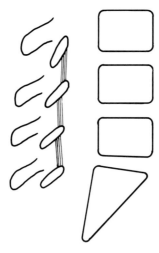

FIG. 10. A lateral schematic showing the attachment of the ligamentum flavum to the anterior aspect of the cephalad lamina and to the posterior edge of the caudal lamina.

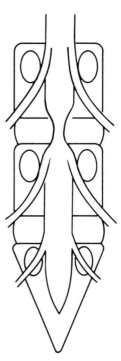

FIG. 12. The napkin ring stenotic lesion in the first story of L4, stenosing the canal between the L4 and L5 roots.

the facet joints, along with osteophytic formation. Vertebral body translation, which affects the ultimate surgical decision, is also obvious on plain x-ray films.

Many investigators have attempted to define SCS by using plain x-ray measurements of the spinal canal. These have routinely failed. Until recently, myelography has been the gold standard for the investigation of a patient with SCS, most often in conjunction with CT. Some authors have advocated the use of standing flexion and extension myelographic films, but they yield little information that cannot be obtained with mandatory investigation by MRI or CT-myelography. More recently, MRI has had a major influence on the diagnosis of SCS and is used as the only pre-operative investigative imaging procedure (other than plain x-rays) by many sur-

geons. The exception to this statement is the patient with degenerative scoliosis and spinal stenosis who still needs a CT-myelogram. These imaging modalities are all pre-operative tools that simply document a structural lesion which must fit perfectly with the clinical presentation.

The contraindications for microsurgical intervention are multiple level disease and/or a slip level. One level or, at most, two level SCS without a slip level may be approached with a microsurgical operation.

MICROSURGICAL LAMINOPLASTY FOR SPINAL CANAL STENOSIS

The principles that must be adhered to when considering a limited microsurgical procedure for SCS are:

1. The disease must be confined to one or, at the most, two segments.
2. If the decompression is going to be confined to the central canal, the surgeon must not leave behind encroachment in the lateral zone that may be causing symptoms.
3. Through a limited microsurgical approach, the soft tissue and bony encroachment of the cauda equina must be completely removed.
4. The limited surgical approach must spare the other important soft tissue and bony supporting structures of the segment, i.e., the interspinous/supraspinous ligament complex, the facet joints (except for their me-

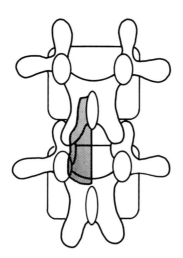

FIG. 11. A schematic showing that excision of the ligamentum flavum requires removal of the inferior half of the cephalad lamina, the superior edge of the caudal lamina, and the medial edge of the facet joint.

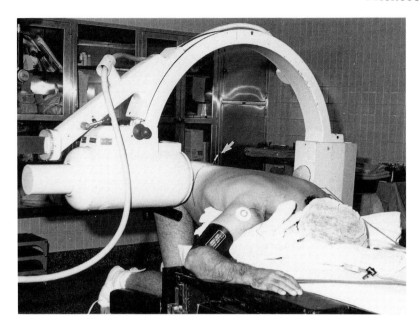

FIG. 13. In the kneeling position, under general anesthesia, an image intensifier is used for localization of the segment to be decompressed. A needle (arrow) marks the inferior edge of the vertebral segment to be decompressed.

dial edges), and the annulus/posterior longitudinal ligament complex, in an attempt to maintain as much stability as possible.

Although the primary goal is to relieve the patient's leg symptoms that limit walking ability, one must not lose sight of the mechanical back pain that is present. It is important to explain to patients prior to surgical intervention that although significant relief of leg pain often occurs, it may not be complete and some back pain will almost certainly remain. It is unusual that these residual *back* symptoms will restrict activities any more than they did pre-operatively.

Operative Procedure

It is usual that a patient with unisegmental SCS will show radiological evidence of bilateral disease. However, given the limited mortality associated with the procedure, it is my practice in these circumstances to perform a bilateral decompression. For example, in a decompression at L4-L5, the following steps are taken to complete a bilateral interlaminar decompression or laminoplasty from one side.

The procedure is best done with the patient in the kneeling position, starting with image intensifier localization of the segment to be decompressed (Fig. 13). The bilateral decompression should be done from the *most symptomatic side.* Assuming the most symptomatic side is the left, the skin and fascial incision for L4-L5 are shown in Figure 14. Subperiosteal muscle dissection is

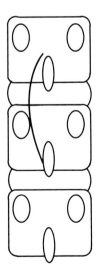

FIG. 14. A unilateral incision is made in the lumbodorsal fascia to save the supraspinous/interspinous ligament complex during decompression of each side.

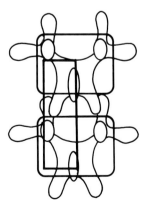

FIG. 15. The extent of the exposure reveals all of the lamina above and the upper half of the lamina below the interspace to be decompressed.

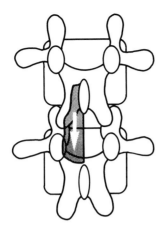

FIG. 16. Working proximal-to-distal, the inferior half of the cephalad lamina is removed and the interspace is decompressed proximal-to-distal.

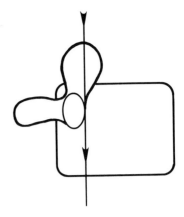

FIG. 17. The medial edge of the superior facet is removed laterally as far as the medial edge of the pedicle.

carried out, such that the entire lamina of L4 and the upper half of the lamina of L5, as well as the interlaminar space of L4-L5, are visible (Fig. 15).

Because of the interlaminar narrowing and shingling of SCS, it is rarely possible to directly cross the ligamentum flavum to gain entry to the epidural space. In this situation, one of two approaches is used:

1. Removal of the inferior half of the cephalad lamina up to the origin of the ligamentum flavum. The ligamentum flavum is then removed proximal-to-distal (Fig. 16).
2. Identification of the distal attachment of the ligamentum flavum from the caudal lamina and then peeling it off the superior edge of the caudal lamina. The ligamentum flavum is then removed distal-to-proximal.

Regardless of the method used, the entire ligamentum flavum must be removed, as well as the medial edges of the inferior facet of L4 and the superior facet of L5. The medial edge of the superior facet is removed laterally as far as the medial edge of the pedicle (Fig. 17).

This results in a complete decompression of the first story, the adjacent portions of the second story above, and the third story below. Removal of the medial edge of the superior facet also decompresses the subarticular zone (Fig. 17), but the foraminal and extraforaminal zones are not decompressed with this approach. When the decompression is finished, the supraspinal/interspinous ligament complex is intact, the facet joints are intact, and the disc space is undisturbed. There are rare occasions when a ruptured lumbar disc is associated with SCS and requires removal, but the routine opening of the disc space at the time of a SCS decompression is to be discouraged as this may result in irreversible progressive instability.

Once the unilateral laminoplasty has been completed, the decompression of the opposite side is started. The most anterior fibers of the interspinous ligament are removed. The bony masses that form the confluences of the spinous processes and the two laminae are then removed. And finally, the bulk of the opposite ligamentum flavum is then removed, a procedure best accomplished by tilting the operating table away from the surgeon and angling the microscope across the spinal canal (Figs. 18 and 19). During this portion of the laminoplasty it is essential to retract the cauda equina. Eventually, the laminar attachments of the ligamentum flavum and the lamina itself are excised to complete the interlaminar decompression. The opposite side laminoplasty is not considered complete until the roots above and below the constrictive lesion are seen along with the far edge of the dural sheath and its adjacent disc space.

If a second level laminoplasty is necessary, a similar procedure, as above, is carried out. The usual setting is for an L3-L4 decompression to accompany an L4-L5 interlaminar decompression. In this situation, a two-level, bilateral laminoplasty can be accomplished through a unilateral approach, using a 2 to 3 inch incision, sacrificing only ligamentum flavum, lamina, and medial edges of the facet joints causing the stenosis, while saving the supraspinous/interspinous ligament complexes, preserving the integrity of the facet joints, and not violating the disc. The resulting post-operative stability allows for early post-operative ambulation and, most often, a hospital discharge in 2 to 3 days.

RESULTS

Prior to mid-1988, the author was not using the microsurgical laminoplasty for spinal canal stenosis. A review of 72 standard, non-microsurgical spinal canal ste-

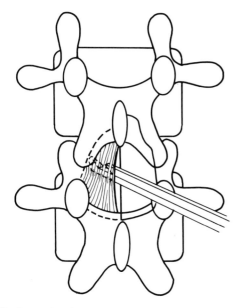

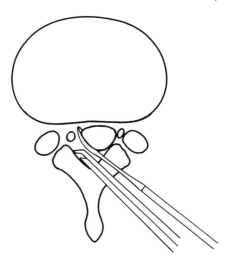

FIG. 19. Retracting the dura to the operating side.

FIG. 18. Operating from one side and retracting the dura to the operating side, the opposite ligamentum flavum can be decompressed. This is facilitated by angling the microscope across to the opposite side.

nosis surgeries (minimum 1-year follow-up, maximum 4-year follow-up) revealed that 21 were decompressions alone and 51 were decompressions and fusions. Of the 21 non-surgical decompressions, there were four failures due to continuing leg symptoms thought to be due to inadequate decompression. Ten decompressions were single level and eleven were multilevel, with L4-L5 the most common level decompressed and L5-S1 the least common level decompressed. No significant complications occurred.

With the increased use of MRI, especially sagittal sections, it became evident that the main lesion in acquired spinal canal stenosis occurred in the first story of the anatomic segment (Figs. 3, 6, and 7). This led to the introduction of the microsurgical decompression of the offending level of the anatomical segment through a bilateral midline exposure in 1988 (10). By early 1989, it became evident that when completing the second decompression on one side, the prior contralateral decompression could be seen through the ipsilateral operating side. Personal communication with Young (14) led to the next step in evolution: the bilateral interlaminar decompression laminoplasty through a unilateral interlaminar portal (Figs. 18 and 19). Since 1989, this technique has been used with no complications, except for one post-operative phlebitis, and good initial results. Obviously, acceptable scientific follow-up is not yet available.

The concept of a limited laminotomy for the treatment of spinal canal stenosis has been published by Aryanpur and Ducker (3), describing a 90% successful out-

come in 32 patients with "focal lateral recess stenosis." Although this is a different group from midline spinal canal stenosis as reported in this chapter, the concept of limited surgical intervention for one variety of spinal stenosis has proven useful in their hands with no complications reported.

COMPLICATIONS

The specific perils of operating with the microscope have been covered in Chapter 83 on microsurgery for lumbar disc disease. The added complications in bilateral laminotomies through a unilateral portal include inadequate decompression of the opposite side and dural tears from inadequate retraction at the time of Kerrison use on the opposite side.

CONCLUSION

SCS is a relentlessly progressive narrowing of the lumbar spinal canal that insidiously decreases the space available for the cauda equina. The resulting symptoms are quite disabling, yet patients present little clinical evidence of nerve root involvement. The diagnosis is often elusive until the patient undergoes myelographic and/or CT investigation. MRI is playing an increasing role in the diagnosis of canal stenosis.

For patients with unisegmental disease or two-level involvement without a slip level, a laminoplasty or resculpturing procedure represents a very limited surgical procedure that in its early development offers good results (Figs. 20 and 21) (2,14). It is this author's opinion that this approach is facilitated by the microscope, so much so that a bilateral laminoplasty can be completed through a unilateral interlaminar window.

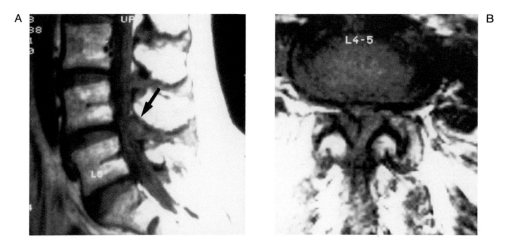

FIG. 20. A: Pre-operative sagittal MRI (T1-weighted) showing stenotic lesion, L4-L5 (arrow). **B:** Pre-operative axial MRI (T1-weighted) showing stenosis.

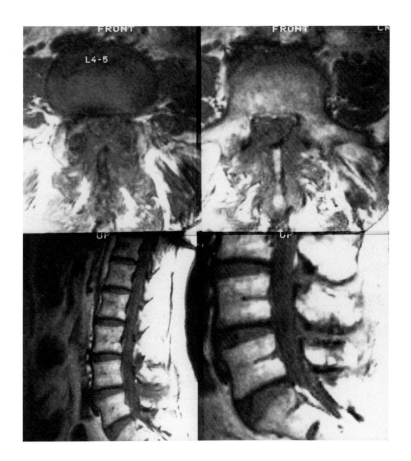

FIG. 21. MRI 6 months post-operative. Top row: Axial image (T1-weighted) showing decompressed spinal canal. Bottom row: Sagittal image (T1-weighted) showing decompressed spinal canal. This procedure was done through a bilateral approach, since abandoned for the bilateral decompression through a unilateral interlaminar window.

ACKNOWLEDGMENT

The author would like to thank Dr. Paul Young, neurosurgeon, St. Louis University, St. Louis, Missouri, for showing him the bilateral decompression of SCS through the unilateral interlaminar portal.

REFERENCES

1. Arnoldi CC, Brodsky AE, Cauchoix J, et al (1976): Lumbar spinal stenosis and nerve root entrapment syndromes: Definition and classification. *Clin Orthop* (115):4–5.
2. Aryanpur J, Ducker T (1988): Multilevel lumbar laminotomies for focal spinal stenosis: Case report. *Neurosurgery* 23:111–115.
3. Aryanpur J, Ducker T (1990): Multilevel lumbar laminotomies: An alternative to laminectomy in the treatment of lumbar stenosis. *Neurosurgery* 26:429–433.
4. Epstein NE, Epstein JA, Carras R, Lavine LS (1983): Degenerative spondylolisthesis with an intact neural arch: A review of 60 cases with an analysis of clinical findings and the development of surgical management. *Neurosurgery* 13:555–561.
5. Epstein JA, Epstein BS, Lavine LS (1962): Nerve root compression associated with narrowing of the lumbar spinal canal. *J Neurol Neurosurg Psychiatry* 25:165–176.
6. Johnsson K (1987): *Lumbar spinal stenosis: A clinical, radiological and neuro-physiological investigation.* Special publication of Dept. Of Orthopaedics, Malmo General Hospital, Lund University, Malmo, Sweden.
7. Kirkaldy-Willis WH, Wedge JH, Yong-Hing K, Reilly J (1978): Pathology and pathogenesis of lumbar spondylosis and stenosis. *Spine* 3:319–328.
8. Lin P (1981): Internal decompression for multiple levels of lumbar stenosis: A technical note. *Neurosurgery* 11:546–549.
9. Macnab I (1950): Spondylolisthesis with an intact neural arch—The so-called pseudospondylolisthesis. *J Bone Joint Surg* [Br] 32:325–333.
10. McCulloch JA (1990): Microsurgery for spinal canal stenosis: The resculpturing or laminoplasty procedure. In: *Microsurgery of the lumbar spine,* RW Williams, P Young, JA McCulloch, eds. Rockville: Aspen, pp. 199–210.
11. Schonstrom HSR, Bolender NF, Spengler DM (1985): The pathomorphology of spinal stenosis as seen on CT scans of the lumbar spines. *Spine* 10:806–811.
12. Verbiest H (1975): Pathomorphologic aspects of developmental lumbar stenosis. *Orthop Clin North Amer* 6:177–196.
13. Williams RW (1978): Microlumbar discectomy: A conservative surgical approach to the virgin herniated lumbar disc. *Spine* 3:175–182.
14. Young S, Veerapen R, O'Laoire SA (1988): Relief of lumbar canal stenosis using multilevel subarticular fenestrations as an alternative to wide laminectomy. *Neurosurgery* 23:628–633.

The Adult Spine: Principles and Practice,
J. W. Frymoyer, Editor-in-Chief.
Raven Press, Ltd., New York © 1991.

CHAPTER 88

Laminoplasty of the Thoracic and Lumbar Spine

John P. Kostuik

The purpose of a laminoplasty is to decompress the contents of the spinal canal and at the same time maintain stability and preservation of the posterior bony ligamentous complex. This technique in the cervical spine is a well-established approach to complex cervical disease, as described by Hirabayashi (2) and Matsuzaki (8). However, thoracic and lumbar spine laminoplasty is relatively uncommon.

ALTERNATIVE APPROACHES TO SPINAL STENOSIS

The indications for a laminoplasty are similar to those for laminectomy involving more than one level. A laminoplasty is usually performed for decompression of spinal stenosis. Stenosis can involve the entire neural canal and may affect both the anterior and posterior transverse diameters (Figs. 1 and 2). Frequently the lateral recesses are involved, as demonstrated on CT scan, and can be either generalized or isolated. In posterior decompression techniques for both the thoracic and the lumbar spine, the choice of operative approach is individualized. The objective is to decompress the lumbar canal and all involved lateral recesses. Three localized areas of lateral recess stenosis are usually caused by bony hypertrophy

on the deeper aspect of the articular processes as described by Macnab (6). When pathology requires only a unilateral single or two-level approach, a simple posterior decompressive procedure can be done with preservation of the facets, usually without compromising spinal stability. Similarly, if the stenosis is bilateral but isolated to one level, then a simple laminectomy usually can be done. However, if the problem requires multiple-level decompression with potential sacrifice of facets, then laminoplasty may be indicated.

In the usual posterior decompression for spinal stenosis without preservation of the posterior elements, the surgical technique involves three stages. First is the coronal plane resection of the spinous processes; second is the sagittal plane resection of the lamina; and third is the oblique plane resection of the deep surface of the facet joints, which usually allows these joints to be preserved (Fig. 3). However, if there is a pre-existing instability such as in degenerative spondylolisthesis or if the facet joints are markedly hypertrophied, then a bilateral resection is often required, resulting in compromised stability. This liability becomes even greater when radical resection is done for multilevel stenosis.

Rosomoff (10) has stated that neural arch resection for lumbar spinal stenosis is the ideal method for decompression. He described a technique in which complete resection of the posterior elements was done, including removal of the articulations, and radical decompression was accomplished by excising the pars interarticularis. He stated that this single procedure alleviated the majority of, if not all, problems of neural encroachment resulting from spinal stenosis. He recorded only one patient

J. P. Kostuik, M.D., F.R.C.S.(C): Professor of Orthopaedics, University of Toronto, Toronto, Ontario; and Head, Combined Division of Orthopaedic Surgery, Toronto General/ Mount Sinai Hospitals; Chief, Dewar Spinal Unit, The Toronto Hospital, Toronto, Ontario, Canada M5G 2C4.

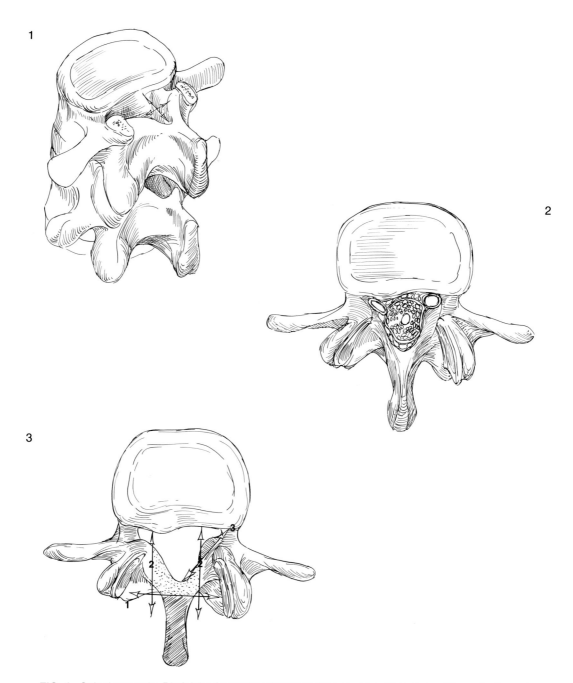

FIG. 1. Spinal stenosis. Diminished anteroposterior and transverse diameters of the spinal canal.

FIG. 2. Lateral recess stenosis.

FIG. 3. Numbers indicate three-stage laminectomy and joint excision. *1:* Coronal plane; resection of the spinous processes. *2:* Sagittal plane; resection of the laminae. *3:* Oblique plane; resection of the deep surface of the facet joints.

out of fifty he treated who developed frank instability, which was thought to be secondary in an unrelated traumatic event. Stabilization was not an issue, and fusion was unnecessary. However, the duration of follow-up was not specified. This favorable report has not been the experience of other authors, who describe clinically significant subluxation occurring in 20% of patients following wide decompression with sacrifice of the articular facets (see Chapter 90). Moreover, it has been the experience of many, particularly the Japanese, that the multiple-level decompression, combined with fusion in stenosis that involves two or more levels, has resulted in improved long-term results when compared to decompression alone. Rosomoff has since abandoned this technique.

However, the problems of providing a fusion following wide decompression are not insignificant, particularly because the limited area for bone grafting consists of only the lateral masses and transverse processes. The addition of internal fixation and, in particular, pedicle screw devices, has improved pseudarthrosis rates, which previously were reported to range from 5% to 40% (see Chapter 98). Moreover, the addition of a fusion with internal fixation may be time-consuming and is associated with considerable blood loss and an increased rate of infection.

As an alternative, some have utilized a posterior lumbar interbody fusion combined with posterior instrumentation following wide decompression for spinal stenosis (see Chapter 94). In our opinion, this may result in increased neurological risk in an already neurologically compromised patient suffering from spinal stenosis. Moreover, the addition of the interbody fusion considerably increases epidural scarring and increases the risk of arachnoiditis.

Because of these problems with wide decompression with or without fusion, laminoplasty is gaining increasing popularity as a means of preserving posterior stability as well as providing a greater bed for bone grafting.

Preservation of the posterior elements results in increased protection of the contents of the dura, and theoretically might be associated with less post-operative scarring.

TECHNIQUES

A variety of techniques have been described for laminoplasty of the thoracic and lumbar spine (Fig. 4). In the thoracic spine, the techniques as described for the cervical spine elsewhere in this text may apply. The open-book technique of Hirabayashi (2), which enlarges the canal by unilateral laminotomy and contralateral osteoplasty (Fig. 5), has been our preferred technique. The posterior arch is raised on one side en bloc and is hinged on the opposite side. The open side of the book is sutured to the muscles. This provides protection of the dural sheath and prevents secondary kyphosis. It has been our practice in the thoracic spine to use bone obtained either from the spinous processes or through the iliac crest as a graft on the side of the hinge. This technique has proven to be of value particularly in achondroplastic dwarfs,

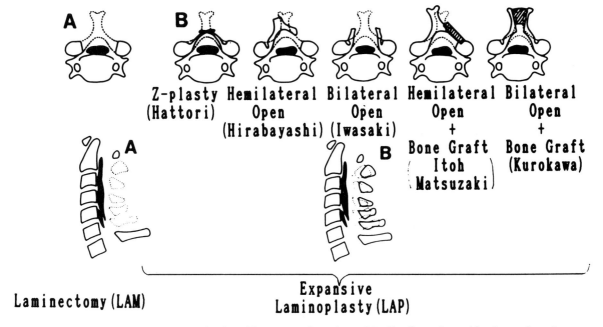

FIG. 4. Various cervical laminoplasties. These may be adapted to the thoracic and lumbar spine. **A:** Laminectomy. **B:** Expansive laminoplasty.

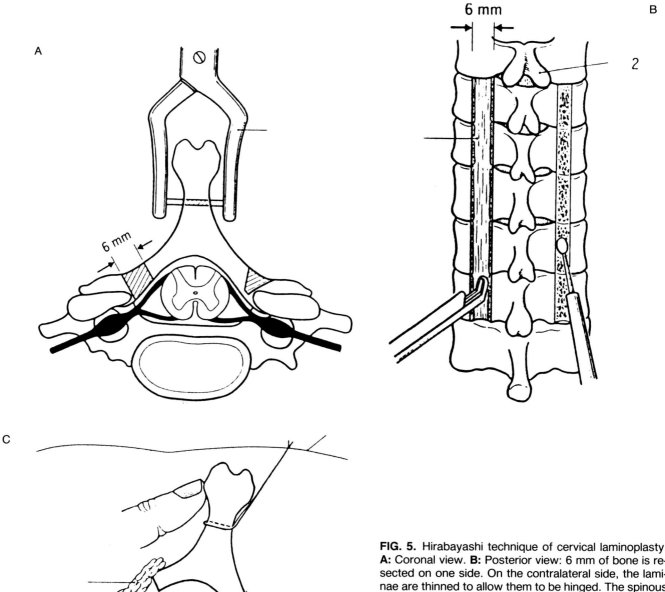

FIG. 5. Hirabayashi technique of cervical laminoplasty. **A:** Coronal view. **B:** Posterior view: 6 mm of bone is resected on one side. On the contralateral side, the laminae are thinned to allow them to be hinged. The spinous processes may be resected for bone graft and added to the side of the hinge. **C:** A free fat graft is placed over the open side. The laminae are sutured to the overlying soft tissue.

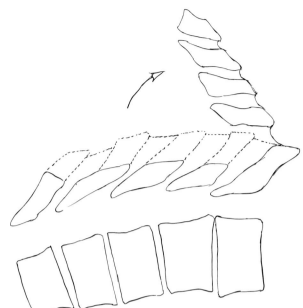

FIG. 6. The spinous process ligament complex is preserved before the laminectomy.

where it prevents development of an increasing kyphosis.

In the thoracic spine, an alternative is to remove the posterior lamina using the so-called lobster-shell technique described later. However, this technique is not without some risks because of the thoracic canal dimensions.

Tsuzuki et al. (12) have described a technique of laminopediculoplasty as a method of reconstructing the posterior elements of the thoracic spine. Access to the back of the thoracic vertebral bodies can be gained through a wide posterior approach. They described fifteen cases in which a periosteal iliac graft was used to re-establish stability and reconstruct the posterior elements. With their technique, a circumferential decompression of the thoracic cord may be achieved through a single posterior approach. They use this technique after excision of the posterior elements, including laminae, facet joints, and the medial two thirds of the pedicles (Fig. 6). The lateral third of the pedicle is preserved as a base for reconstruction. Preservation of the lateral wall with pedicle does not seem to restrict access to the cord except for its most anterior part. If the anterior central one third requires decompression, this is accomplished by first deepening the vertebral body with the use of an air drill. The base of the remaining bony mass is then removed, leaving untouched the part of the bone in contact with the anterior dura. Following this, the remaining portion of bone may be gently freed and resected. If the dural tube is ossified, the dural tube is opened and expanded with a fascial patch. In cases in which a simple posterior enlargement of the dural tube may not suffice, the dura is resected together with the areas of anterior ossification (Fig. 7). Reconstruction of the posterior elements is achieved by the use of a thin corticocancellous osteoperiosteal graft taken from the outer aspect of the iliac crest and bent into a semicircle approximately four centimeters in di-

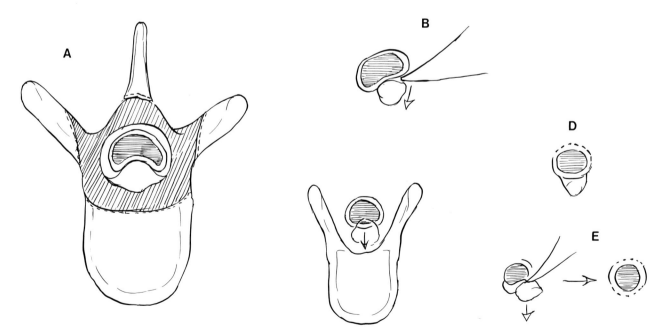

FIG. 7. Anterior decompression of the thoracic cord through the wide posterior approach. **A:** Area of bone resected. **B:** Bony remnant separated from the anterior dura. **C:** Where bony remnant cannot be separated from the dura, both are allowed to fall forward into prepared cavity. **D:** Expansion of involved dura with a patch. **E:** Resection of involved dura and posterior longitudinal ligament.

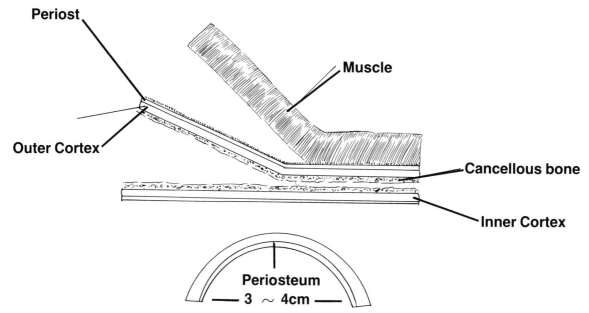

FIG. 8. Obtaining the osteoperiosteal graft. A thin corticocancellous graft with the periosteum intact is taken from the outer corticocancellous portion of the iliac wing.

ameter with the periosteum on the inside (Figs. 8 and 9A). If an anterior decompression has been undertaken, a posterior thoracic interbody fusion is then performed (Fig. 9B). The curved periosteal graft is fitted over the spinal cord between the two pedicles. If flexibility of the graft is a problem, the graft may be placed obliquely or transversely after reconstructing the pedicle with a peg. Further bone graft is then applied, and the posterior spinal ligamentous complex is reattached to the lamina above and below the decompression. More recently, Tsuzuki et al. (12) have advocated the use of posterior instrumentation to stabilize the spine from above and below the level of decompression, as this allows more rapid and early mobilization of the patient. All patients in their series fused, and no late bone formation was observed in the spinal canal. Neurological improvement occurred in 80% of their complex cases.

They have used this technique only in cases of thoracic myelopathy and report a marked improvement compared to Jefferson's (4) results. Those investigators advocated a unilateral wide posterior approach for removal of anterior structures causing spinal cord compromise. Tsuzuki's main complication was fracture of the graft intra-operatively while attempting to bend it. This was not a problem in the elderly patient, but in the younger patient it led them to use an oblique or transverse graft application after reconstructing the pedicles with a peg. In the younger person the graft may have to be fractured at a number of intervals in order to achieve the desired curve. To date, this technique has been applied to as many as three levels.

Eggshell Procedure

Heinig (1) has described the use of the eggshell procedure primarily for kyphotic deformities involving the thoracic, thoracolumbar, or lumbar spine if there is a need to decompress the spinal canal and its contents prior to correction of a kyphosis. His technique is limited to rigid kyphotic deformities involving one or two levels. The spine may be approached posteriorly or anteriorly; in some cases a combined approach may be necessary. Using the eggshell procedure (transpedicular vertebrectomy), the spinal column may be operated on from both back and front using a single posterior approach.

The term "eggshell" comes from the appearance of a vertebral body with the cancellous bone removed and the cortical shell intact. The technique utilizes the pedicle as a conduit to reach the anterior portion of the spine. The hollowed-out pedicle is used as a porthole to the vertebral body. Through this tube the cancellous bone is removed. Once sufficient decancellation has been achieved, the remaining cortical bone is either fractured or removed. This operative approach may be used to carry out a biopsy, decompression, osteotomy, or complete vertebrectomy. This technique has the advantage of using a posterior approach, which allows for the use of the widest variety of instrumentation systems. The single surgical wound and no need to reposition the patient are also advantages.

The patient is positioned on the OR table in the prone position. When correction of a deformity is to be carried out it is important to position the patient so that the apex

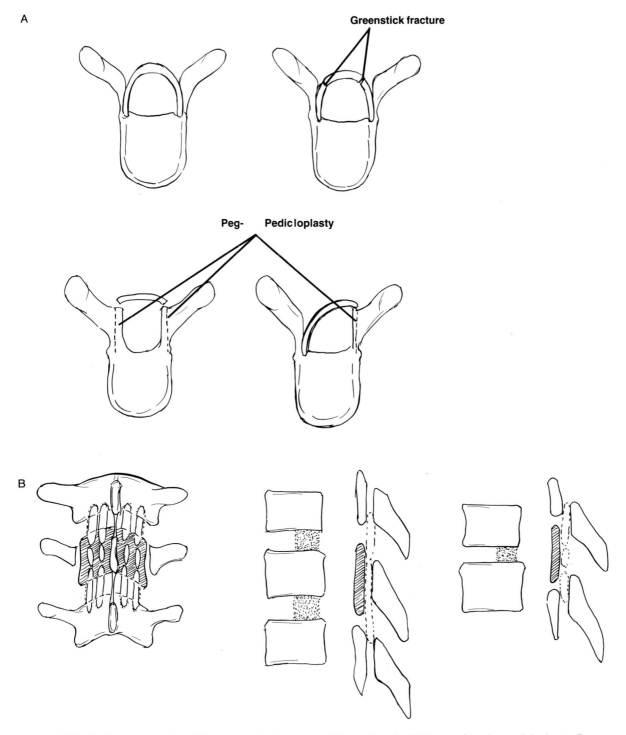

FIG. 9. Reconstruction of the posterior elements of the spine. **A:** Patterns of laminopedicloplasty. **B:** Sites for grafting. The spinous process ligament complex is replaced on a new lamina.

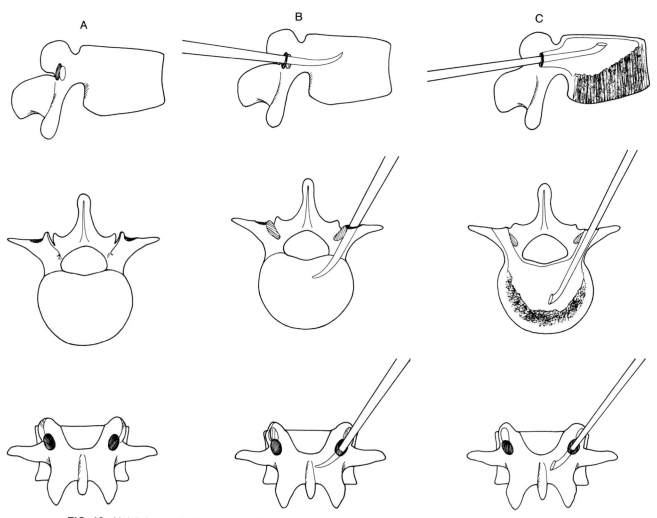

FIG. 10. Heinig's eggshell procedure. **This page, A:** Locate the pedicle. **B:** Remove cortical bone directly over the pedicle. Place a probe within the medullary canal of the pedicle. **C:** Use curettes and rongeurs to remove bone. (Opposite page, Figs. 10D–10E.)

of the curve is aligned with the mechanical break in the table. This allows for external corrective forces to be used in conjunction with internal instrumentation. Since this technique is used to address both sides of the neural tube, it may be prudent to use some form of neuromonitoring. This may be induced motor or sensory potentials. Neural function may be followed by observing the peripheral motor responses during the procedure. A wake up test may also be used to document the integrity of the neural system. Once the posterior spine has been exposed, the pedicle of the selected level is identified (Fig. 10A). The cortical bone directly over the pedicle is removed. The pedicle is a tubular bone with a cortical wall and cancellous center. A probe is placed in the intramedullary canal (Fig. 10B). Next, this canal is enlarged using progressively larger curettes. This hollow channel allows for access to the vertebral body (Fig. 10C). This may be all the surgery necessary if a biopsy or drainage is to be performed.

The following technique is used if decompression or osteotomy is to be carried out. The pedicle now provides a channel through which the cancellous bone may be removed with curettes and pituitary rongeurs (Fig. 10C). If a larger opening to the vertebral body is needed, the lateral wall of the pedicle may be fractured and allowed to retract laterally. This also allows the curette to be directed in a more lateral to medial direction. This is necessary to remove bone from directly anterior to the spinal canal. The pedicle on the opposite side is entered in the same fashion. The surgeon may use a curette to loosen the cancellous bone through one pedicle while an assistant uses suction and a rongeur to remove the loose fragments through the other pedicle. Once the desired amount of spongy bone has been removed, attention is directed to preparation of the posterior spine for the desired fixation device. At this point the spinal canal is still protected by the lamina, medial walls of the pedicles, and the posterior wall of the vertebral body. In the in-

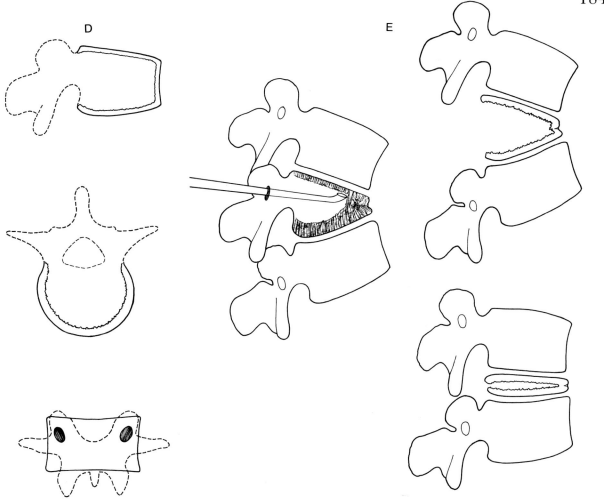

FIG. 10. *Continued.* **D:** Remove the posterior elements, pedicles, and posterior wall of the vertebral body. **E:** For correction of deformity: (1) Remove cancellous bone. (2) Remove posterior elements, pedicles, and posterior wall of the body. (3) Close the osteotomy.

stance of fracture with retropulsion of a bony fragment into the dura, the canal is decompressed by entering the canal through the medial pedicle wall. A long elevator is placed between the dura and the fragment. The retropulsed piece of bone is then forced anteriorly into the hollow vertebral body, away from the neural elements. Following internal fixation and transpedicular bone grafting, the wound is closed in the standard fashion.

If an osteotomy is to be performed, the same procedure as for a fracture is used to gain exposure. Instead of removing only the retropulsed fragment, the entire posterior arch, pedicle, and posterior wall of the vertebral segment may be removed (Fig. 10D). Further mobility of the spine may be obtained by disc removal. Even more correction is possible by fracturing the lateral vertebral body walls of the involved segment. This can be accomplished by using an osteotome to cut the side of the cortical shell. With this degree of mobility, fixed deformities of the spine can be satisfactorily corrected (Fig. 10E). Prior to closing the osteotomy or realigning the spine, it is necessary to ensure that there is no bony impingement to the neural elements. This may require removing the leading edge of the lamina above and below the osteotomy level.

Numerous techniques for laminoplasty have been described for the lumbar spine, including micro-laminoplasty, the lobster-shell technique, hemi-laminoplasty, and division of the pars interarticularis with temporary removal of the posterior neural arch and subsequent replacement. These techniques, with the exception of micro-laminoplasty, are usually combined with fusions.

Micro-Laminoplasty

Micro-laminoplasty or resculpturing of the lamina is a microsurgical technique designed for spinal canal stenosis and is fully described in Chapter 87. As noted by McCulloch in that chapter, only degenerative non-olisthetic spinal canal stenosis will respond to micro-

A

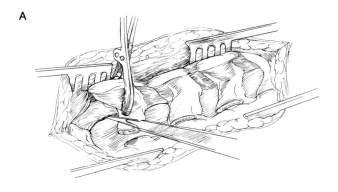

B

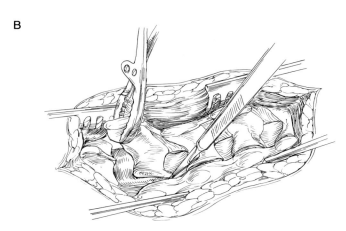

FIG. 11. Lobster shell technique. **A:** Division of the ligamentum flavum distally. **B:** Removal of posterior arches in one piece.

laminoplasty. The diagnosis is established based on a description of the patient's symptoms and investigative steps of a radiological nature.

Lobster-Shell Technique

Roy-Camille and Benazet (11) described this operation. They felt it to be faster and cause less bleeding as well as being less traumatic to the neural elements.

The first step consists of a resection of the posterior arch (Figs. 11A–11B). Roy-Camille and Benazet (11) have done this resection with an oscillating saw using a 15-millimeter blade or a high-speed micro burr. We feel that a burr is less traumatic because it does not introduce instrumentation between the lamina and the dura mater. Vertical cuts are made bilaterally. The yellow ligaments on the deeper aspect of the lamina prevent the saw or burr from going too deep. The cuts must not be done too far lateral as they will then enter the articular processes and the pedicles. We advocate making the verticle cut about three millimeters from the inferior articular process and about five millimeters from the facet joint space. Roy-Camille advocated its use only over two to four levels (Fig. 11A).

The second step consists of division of the ligamentum flavum, which is done using a scalpel (Fig. 11B). The third step consists of removal of the posterior arch, which is achieved by grasping the spinal process distally and pulling the laminae cranially. A small elevator is used to divide adhesions between the dura and the posterior arch and the ligamentum flavum laterally as the dissection is extended proximally. The proximal ligamentum flavum is again divided transversely. Following this maneuver, nerve roots may be freed through osseous resection of the inner part of the articular processes from inside outwards. Roy-Camille has not advocated replacement of posterior elements. We prefer to do this using interlaminar screw fixation and posterior decortication with a high-speed burr, with the addition of bone graft posteriorly and along the transverse processes (Figs. 12A and 12B). This allows for protection of the neural elements and enhances stabilization, which we feel is necessary when decompression is performed over two or more levels, and in particular if the articular processes are in any way damaged.

Pars Interarticularis Osteotomy

A similar technique may be carried out by doing an osteotomy through the pars interarticularis into the neural foramina. The ligamentum flavum is then divided distally. The facet capsules are then divided and the neural arch removed en bloc and preserved. The inside of the neural arch may be sculptured and soft tissue, primarily ligamentum flavum, removed. This may be carried out over as many levels as is desired. The arch is restored after removing the articular surfaces of the facets. The neural canal may be enlarged by applying a corticocancellous bone graft that is placed en bloc in the facets and fixed with a translaminar screw. This screw extends from the contralateral side of the spinous process through the lamina across the joint and graft into the base of the transverse process (Figs. 13A and 13B). We have used this technique for spinal stenosis, including multiple-level central and lateral recesses, as well as for cases of spondylolisthesis (Figs. 14A and 14B). Further bone graft may be added on the transverse processes. Magerl (7) and Jacobs (3) have shown that the addition of translaminar fixation enhances the rigidity and subsequent consolidation of the fusion (Fig. 15).

Hemi-Laminoplasty

When unilateral decompression is desired and limited to one or two levels, a hemi-laminoplasty may be performed. The ligamentum flavum is cut in the midline and a Gigli saw is passed underneath the neural arch in the midline. The pars interarticularis is cut, and the spi-

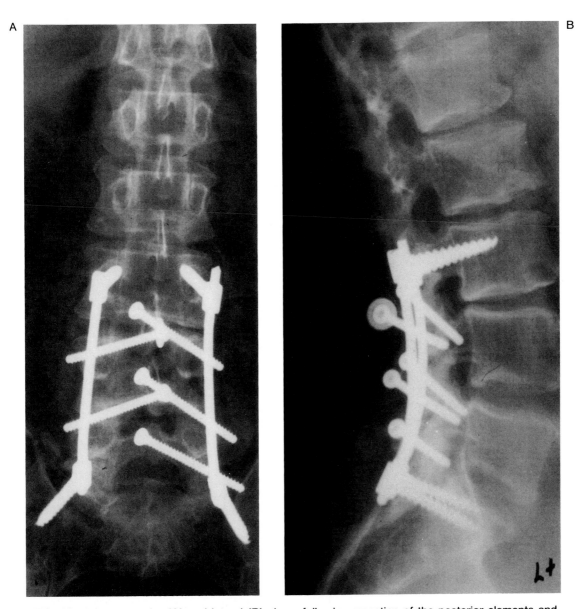

FIG. 12. Anteroposterior **(A)** and lateral **(B)** views following resection of the posterior elements and adequate neural decompression. The posterior elements are replaced and fixed with translaminar screws. Pedicle fixation was also added. The posterior elements and transverse processes are decorticated with a high speed burr and bone graft is added for fusion.

A

B

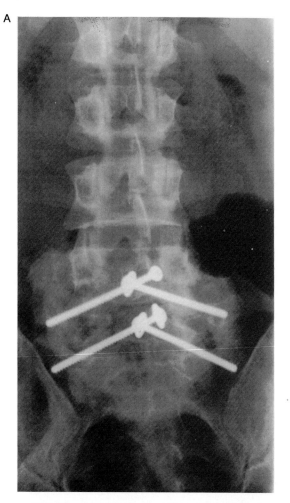
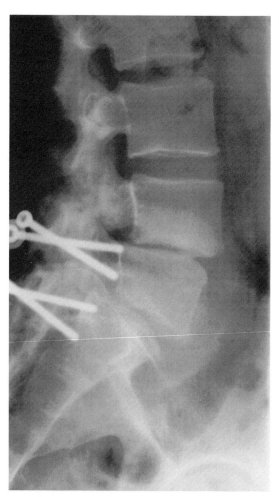

FIG. 13. Anteroposterior **(A)** and lateral **(B)** views of pars interarticular osteotomy. Patient suffered from spinal stenosis of L4-L5 with a mild L5-S1 spondylolisthesis. The posterior arches of L4 and L5 were removed en bloc by osteotomies through the pars interarticularis. Following decompression the posterior arches were replaced. They were built up by adding 0.5 cm graft in the facet joints and fixed with translaminar screws. Further transverse process graft was added.

nous process is then divided in the midline. The facet capsule is cut on the affected side and the hemi-lamina removed en bloc. The compression may then be carried out and the lamina restored after removing the articular surface. Stabilization is achieved again by translaminar screw.

We have used this technique or the technique previously described, replacing the lamina without doing a facet fusion, and fixing the pars with a screw. Articular motion may be preserved without doing a fusion by simply replacing the posterior elements. Union is achieved by a pars interarticularis reconstruction using either a screw across the pars or the hook screw reconstruction technique as described by Morscher (9) (Figs. 16A and 16B). However, we have usually done a facet and posterior posterolateral fusion in conjunction with these forms of laminoplasty, since in the majority of cases the articular cartilage of the facet joint is markedly degenerated.

Laminoplasty

Lozes, Fawaz, Herlan, and Jomin (5) have described a monoblock transversoarthropediculotomy.

This procedure may be unilateral or bilateral. It is described as a conservative removal of part or all of the posterior arch and is suitable when a posterolateral approach is indicated.

After exposure of the spine, the ligamentum flavum is excised superior and inferior to the desired level to be excised. The dural sac and nerve roots as they exit toward the foramen are protected. Three osteotomies are done using a fine oscillating saw or fine osteotomes (Fig. 17). The first osteotomy is made through pars interarticularis superior to the superior articular facet to be excised. The osteotomy is angled slightly down as it enters the intervertebral foramen.

A similar osteotomy is created through the distal pars interarticularis, and the direction is slightly up. This pro-

A

B

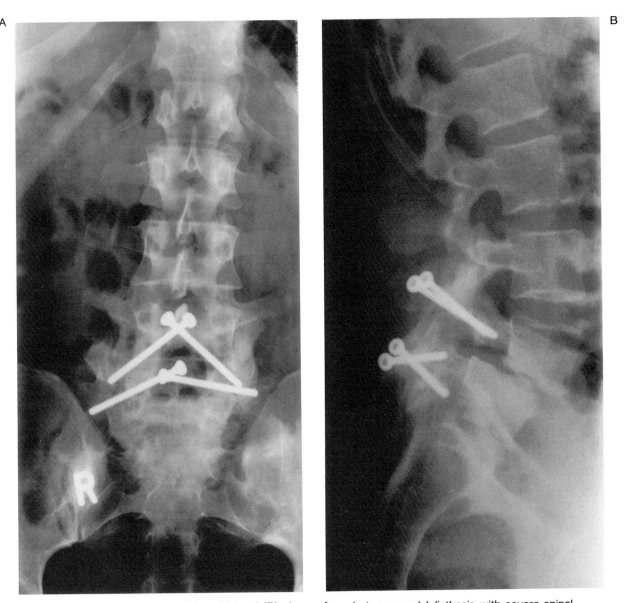

FIG. 14. Anteroposterior **(A)** and lateral **(B)** views of grade two spondylolisthesis with severe spinal stenosis fixed with translaminar screws after laminoplasty for decompression.

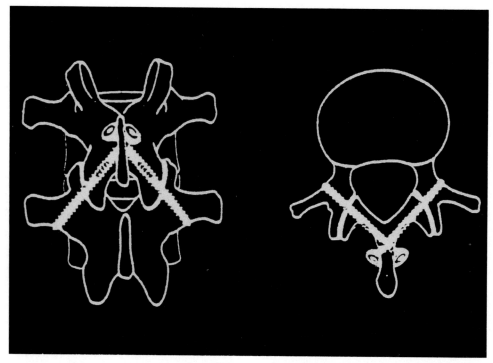

FIG. 15. AO (Magerl) translaminar screws (with permission from ref. 3).

duces a wedge effect for subsequent replacement of the bone fragment.

The third osteotomy is done in the frontal plane at the base of the pedicle.

If a unilateral resection is to be done, a further osteotomy in the sagittal plane is done through the spinous process removing one half of the posterior arch (Fig. 18). Following completion of the osteotomies, the hemi-arch or total arch may be removed in its entirety. Any adhesions of the ligamentum flavum are separated by sharp dissection. If the osteotomy through the pedicle is incomplete, gentle rotation in the axis of the pedicle will result in freeing up the monoblock.

The arch is then kept in physiological saline until the time comes to replace it. Because of the oblique cuts through the pars interarticularis, replacement of the fragment ensures some degree of stability. The joint is preserved. If internal fixation is desirable, the pars may be fixed with a screw directly or with the use of the spring hook device designed by Morscher (9) (Figs. 16A and 16B).

Morscher has described 35 cases. His indications were essentially those of a posterolateral approach to the lumbar spine or thoracic spine, including cases of trauma, thoracic disc herniation, thoracic meningioma, and foraminal neural compression. Non-unions were not reported, despite the absence of internal fixation. There were no complications noted, but the surgery was felt to be difficult to perform in obese people and in cases of re-operation or tumor.

RESULTS

Laminoplasty is a relatively new procedure and reports are few. In Tsuzuki's series, neurological improvement occurred in twelve of the fifteen cases (80%) (12). Mixed improvement and deterioration were noted in two cases; one patient was unchanged. A poor neurological outcome was associated with delayed surgery after the onset of symptoms. Indications included post-traumatic displacement, meningioma, ossification of the posterior longitudinal ligament, ossification of the ligamentum flavum, and osteochondroma. They also advocated possible use for chronic thoracic disc resulting in cord impingement.

Lozes performed his technique of transverse arthropediculotomy primarily in the lumbar spine but did perform it in the thoracic spine as well. Intervention was carried out in thirty-five patients between the ages of 16 and 58. Fifteen cases were for traumatic reasons, but he felt that it was particularly indicated in cases of trauma where the posterior arch was not injured. A major indication was for foraminal decompression. He also described its use for posterolateral disc herniation in the lumbar spine, while in the thoracic spine it was used for disc herniation. No non-unions were noted post-operatively. The procedure is not indicated in very obese patients or in cases of epidural scarring as a result of previous intervention. There were no post-operative neurological complications.

In twenty-two cases of pars interarticularis osteotomy

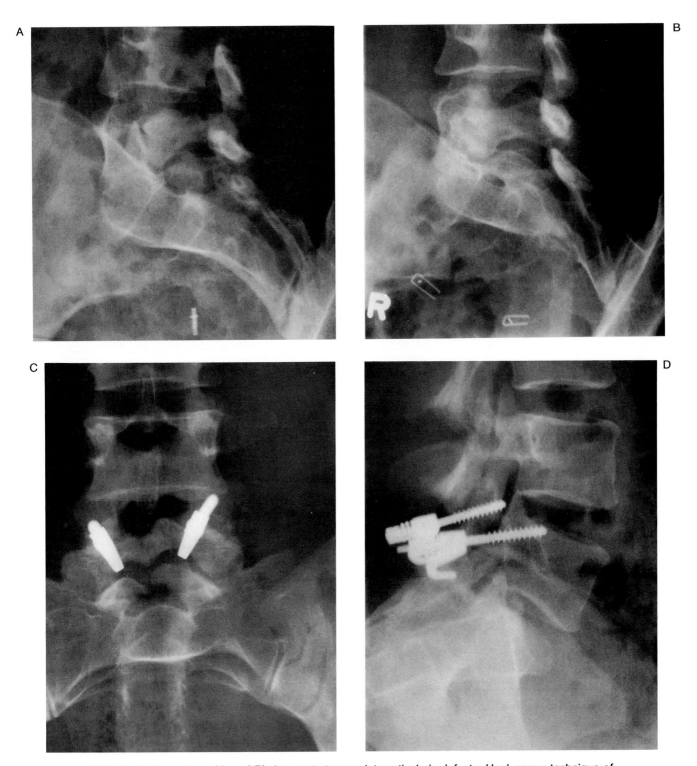

FIG. 16. Oblique views **(A and B)** demonstrate pars interarticularis defects. Hook screw technique of Morscher **(C and D)** for fixation of spondylolysis. The system is dynamized by the spring. The technique is preferable to screw fixation of a pars interarticularis defect or to the wire technique of Scott. The screw goes into the superior articular mass. The dynamized hook goes around the inferior aspect of the lamina.

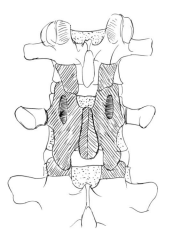

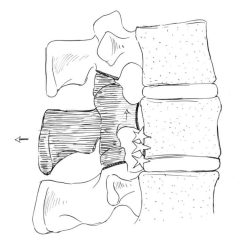

FIG. 17. Hemi-transversoarthropediculotomy osteotomies for foraminal disc herniation.

the posterior bony arch reunited in all patients when internal fixation was used. There were no associated neurological problems. The operative time for these procedures was no longer than routine laminectomy and posterolateral fusion with or without internal fixation.

Potential complications include neurological damage as a result of the various osteotomies performed, but this is the most inherent potential complication. Other potential complications include non-union of either of the pars or pseudarthrosis of the accompanying arthrodesis. Complications related to internal fixation are not as integral to this procedure as they are to the use of internal fixation for other reasons.

In summary, we feel that laminoplasty will have an increasing role to play in the thoracic and lumbar spine as it becomes better known, similar to the increasing role of laminoplasty in the cervical spine as described by Japanese authors.

The major advantage of laminoplasty is the possibility of preserving motion if fusion is not performed. Other advantages are the preservation of stability and protection of the neural elements from posterior injury. Replacement of posterior elements provides a greater area for fusion with increased stability. Another potential advantage is the prevention of extensive epidural scarring.

ACKNOWLEDGMENT

The author wishes to thank Drs. Samuel J. Chewning, Charles F. Heinig, and Todd M. Chapman for contributing the text and illustrations pertaining to the eggshell procedure.

REFERENCES

1. Heinig: Personal communication.
2. Hirabayashi K, Watanabe K, Wakano K, et al (1983): Expansive open-door laminoplasty for cervical spinal stenotic myelopathy. *Spine* 8:693–699.
3. Jacobs RR, Montesano PX, Jackson RP (1989): Enhancement of lumbar spine fusion by use of translaminar facet joint screws. *Spine* 14:12–15.
4. Jefferson A (1975): The treatment of thoracic intervertebral disc protrusions. *Clin Neurol Neurosurg* 78:1–9.
5. Lozes G, Fawaz A, Herlan M, Jomin M (1987): Abord des segments anterieurs et lateraux du rachis dorso-lombaire par transverso-arthro-pediculotomie conservatrice. *Neurochirurgie* 33:497–499.
6. Macnab I (1977): *Backache.* Baltimore: Williams & Wilkins.
7. Magerl FP (1983): Translaminar facet joint screw fixation. A.O. Spine Course, Davos, Switzerland.
8. Matsuzaki H (1986): Laminoplasty. Presentation, A.A.O.S. conference, Atlanta.
9. Morscher E (1985): Compression hook for the treatment of pars interarticularis defects. A.O. Spine Course, Davos, Switzerland.
10. Rosomoff H (1981): Neural arch resection for lumbar spinal stenosis. *Clin Orthop & Rel Res* (154):83–89.
11. Roy-Camille R, Benazet (1989): *Atlas of orthopaedic surgery.* Paris: Masson, pp. 439–441.
12. Tsuzuki N, Tanaka H, Seichi A (1989): Laminopediculoplasty: a new method of reconstructing the posterior elements of the thoracic spine. *International Orthopaedics* (SICOT) 13:39–45.

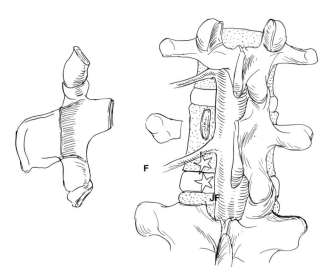

FIG. 18. Monobloc removed. Foraminal and juxtaforaminal neurogenic structures.

The Adult Spine: Principles and Practice,
J. W. Frymoyer, Editor-in-Chief.
Raven Press, Ltd., New York © 1991.

CHAPTER 89

The Management of Treatment Failures After Decompressive Surgery

Surgical Alternatives and Results

Kevin Gill and John W. Frymoyer

We in the industrialized societies have a significant burden. We must explain why the problem of chronic back disability in third world countries is virtually unknown. Have we the sophisticated, scientific physicians and surgeons created our own monster, the failed back syndrome?

Vert Mooney (35)

The spinal surgeon is faced with one of the most difficult problems in medicine when he confronts a patient whose symptoms are unchanged or have deteriorated following laminectomy or discectomy. The estimated rate of failure following decompressive surgery also varies widely and ranges from 5% to over 50% (41), with an average of 15% (60). These significant variations are the result of differing criteria used to measure success (23), the pathol-

K. Gill, M.D.: Clinical Associate Professor of Orthopaedic Surgery, University of Texas Southwestern Medical Center, 5920 Forest Park Road, Suite 400, Dallas, Texas, 75235.
J. W. Frymoyer, M.D.: Professor of Orthopaedics, Director, McClure Musculoskeletal Research Center, Department of Orthopaedics and Rehabilitation, University of Vermont, Burlington, Vermont, 05405.

ogy, the type of operation (i.e., simple disc excision versus extensive decompression), and the specific population being analyzed. For example, the extreme rate of failure (41) was reported in a cohort of workers' compensation patients.

Many words are used to describe this group of patients with failed spinal surgery, who represent the "Achilles heel" of spinal surgeons. Moreover, the surgeon who performed the initial operation is often in the worst position to make decisions about further surgery in one of his own patients. Although the goal is to correct a "failure," he must place himself in the more objective position of being a member of an evaluation team.

CAUSES OF FAILURE

There are three broad causes of failure following spinal decompression: improper pre-operative diagnosis, improper indications, or technical problems that complicate or limit the success of the procedure. From this broad perspective, failures are particularly likely to occur when inadequate pre-operative assessment is combined with the failure to understand the impact of psychosocial problems on the outcome. Even with today's sophisticated imaging techniques, the basic formula for success is well-correlated subjective pain complaints, objective physical findings, and confirmatory imaging studies. Even with this attention to pre-operative evaluation, failures may sometimes be out of the surgeon's control, such as the patient with a well-conceived and well-executed operation who then develops nerve root scarring either intrathecal or extradural.

A second broad perspective to the prevention of failure is the role of rehabilitation. From this perspective, surgery is viewed as part of a continuum of care rather than the sole event that will lead to functional restoration of the patient. Recognition of this issue is of even more crucial importance in planning an operative intervention in a patient who has already had one or more failures of decompression. In this setting, a thorough multidisciplinary evaluation is essential (29). It is also essential that repeat surgery, if indicated, is viewed as only one of many steps in the rehabilitation process, the ultimate goal of which is measured by pain relief, restoration of function, and patient satisfaction. Most, but not all, patients desire the ability to earn a wage and be drug free in today's society, particularly when faced with the full implications of lifelong low-back-related disability.

This chapter details the causes of failure in patients who have had decompressive operations of the lumbar spine and reviews solutions. Included in this analysis are what steps can be taken before the first operation to avoid operating on a patient who is a poor candidate for surgery (51). Second, what are the clinical presentations of patients with surgical failures? Third, what are the alternatives available to treat the patient when specific failures have occurred?

CLASSIFICATION OF FAILURES

Many schemes have been developed to classify failures of lumbar decompression (5,14,32). It is important to have a classification scheme that correlates the failures in a temporal context as shown in Table 1.

It is also convenient to divide this classification into conditions in which radiculopathy predominates and those in which low back pain is the major symptom (Table 2), although there is obviously considerable overlap in many patients. In general, the predictability of success is greater in those patients with persisting or recurrent radiculopathy.

In addition to these causes of failure, spinal decompression may be followed by serious complications, which in the viewpoint of the patient may create a problem as bad as or worse than the pain that led him to consider decompressive surgery. Many of these complications have been presented in other chapters, but a broad compilation will be given later in this chapter.

TABLE 1. *Classification of failures*

I. No improvement immediately following surgery with outright failure to improve mono- or polyradiculopathy.
   A. Wrong pre-operative diagnosis
      1. Tumor
      2. Infection
      3. Metabolic disease
      4. Psychosocial
      5. Discogenic pain
      6. Decompression done too late for disc sequestration (>6 months)
   B. Technical error
      1. Missed level or levels
      2. Failure to perform adequate decompression
         a. Missed fragment including foraminal disc
         b. Failure to recognize spinal stenosis as part of lumbar disc herniation
         c. Conjoined nerve root
II. Temporary relief but recurrence of pain
   A. Early recurrence of symptoms (within weeks)
      1. Infection
      2. Meningeal cyst
   B. Mid-term (within weeks to months)
      1. Recurrent disc prolapse
      2. Battered root
      3. Arachnoiditis
      4. Patient expectation
   C. Longer-term failures (within months to years)
      1. Recurrent stenosis or development of lateral stenosis from disc space collapse
      2. Instability

TABLE 2. *Causes of failure classified by the dominant symptom*

Radiculopathy predominant	Low back pain predominant
Neural tumors	Osseous tumors
Infections—Epidural abscess	Infections
Inadequate decompression	Discitis
Missed fragment	Osteomyelitis
Foraminal disc	Discogenic pain
Conjoined nerve root	Segmental instability
Recurrent disc prolapse	
Peridural fibrosis	
Meningeal cyst	
Arachnoiditis	

APPROACH TO THE PATIENT WITH A FAILURE OF SPINAL DECOMPRESSION

The clinical history is of major importance in assessing probable causation of the patient's continuing or recurrent symptoms, particularly when radiculopathy is the predominant complaint. Finnegan et al. (12) emphasized the importance of the timing of this assessment. They identified three typical pain syndromes:

1. The patient has no initial relief of symptoms or his symptoms are worse. It is likely that the wrong diagnosis was made or the wrong operation was performed.
2. The patient has initial relief, sometimes accompanied by increased numbness or even weakness, followed by gradual onset of recurrent radiculopathy over weeks to months. It is likely that nerve root injury has occurred with subsequent scarring.
3. The patient has complete relief of symptoms but later, over months to years, develops recurrent radiculopathy—often suddenly. It is likely that recurrent disc has occurred.

Frymoyer (16) also stressed the importance of longer-term failures, which are usually the manifestation of an ongoing degenerative process. All of these historical factors are less useful in assessing patients with the predominant complaint of continuing or recurrent low back pain. In patients who have undergone decompressions for radiculopathy, numerous studies attest to low back pain as a continued problem, regardless of whether or not fusion is performed. The patient's expectation of complete relief of all back symptoms was probably ill-founded. The great difficulty is establishing who has the usual expected back pain, and who has severe back pain for which an anatomic cause can be established.

Additional factors in the history are the presence of other systemic symptoms, a detailed psychosocial and work history, and the status of compensation or legal actions. Every effort must be made to obtain all prior operative and hospitalization records.

The physical examination may be less rewarding in establishing the precise cause of the patient's symptoms, particularly when low back pain is the predominant complaint. The interpretation of the neurologic findings may be difficult because of residual deficits from prior surgery. For example, 40% to 50% of patients with prior successful disc excision have residual alterations in reflex and sensation correspondent to the original level of root involvement (16,38). However, nerve root tension signs rarely persist after successful surgery and are a very useful sign when positive. In other instances, the nature of the pathology will tend to produce confusing findings. For example, patients with recurrent stenosis often have confusing or misleading physical findings, comparable to the clinical examination in patients who have not had prior surgery (54). The utilization of clinical tests such as those described by Waddell (56) provides a simple means to identify patients who have inappropriate pain response.

Modern imaging techniques have a high probability of clarifying the cause of symptoms. It is worth re-emphasizing that the probable cause should be apparent from the history or physical examination and, thus, the imaging study is a confirmation, rather than the dominant basis for diagnosis. In other chapters, detailed presentations have been made about the various imaging techniques and their limitations and interpretation. Although there is no unanimity of opinion, the enhanced MRI currently appears to be the most useful screening test. This technique is the most sensitive to possible inflammatory and neoplastic causations of symptoms. More important, it is the most sensitive test in differentiating scarring from recurrent pathology. As an adjunct to MRI, other modalities are important and should be used selectively. For example, in assessing the possibility of lateral or central stenosis as a cause of continued nerve root symptoms after lumbar decompression, the most powerful modality is myelographically enhanced multiplanar CT scan. In other cases, particularly when low back pain predominates, the discogram-CT scan may be useful, particularly because of the additional information derived from pain provocation.

Other techniques may also be employed, such as anesthetic blocks. Unfortunately, the facet block has been less useful than hoped in defining the role of those anatomic structures in the causation of pain (11), although in one series it did prove useful (10). In more difficult cases in which radiculopathy predominates, selective nerve root injections under radiographic control may also be useful (27,32).

Last, in approaching the patient with failed surgery, the importance of comprehensive evaluation must be emphasized again (29). Included in this evaluation may be other specialists such as internists, rheumatologists, and psychiatrists, as well as the use of psychologic tests such as the Beck Depression Inventory.

An analysis of each of the categories of failure as shown in Table 1 will help to further elucidate the causes of failure.

IMMEDIATE FAILURE

Wrong Diagnosis

It is well-recognized that sciatica or claudication has a variety of causes beyond lumbar disc herniation and spinal stenosis, although there is only limited information as to the incidence of these conditions. In a group of 5,362 patients Wiesel (61) found that 109 patients (2%) failed to improve. Of these 109 patients, only 14 ultimately were found to have an underlying disease, discovered by extensive multidisciplinary analyses. Schofferman (48) also emphasized occult infections as an important cause of symptoms in patients with low back pain and radiculopathies. Others have reported specific disease incidences such as spinal infection (including spinal epidural abscess—0.037/1,000), disc space infection (0.037/1,000), metastatic or vertebral neoplasms (0.12/1,000), and multiple myeloma (0.07/1,000) (7).

In the specific subset of patients with suspected lumbar disc herniations, neural tumors are reported to be present in 1% (30). Included in the differential diagnosis are epidural abscess, osteomyelitis (with or without accompanying disc space involvement), retroperitoneal tumors (including endometriosis), viral "plexorophies," and peripheral neuropathies of metabolic, viral, or traumatic etiologies. In addition, symptoms suggestive of spinal stenosis can arise from vascular disease, metastatic neoplasms, and arthritic conditions, particularly those affecting the hip. Most of these causes can be suspected from a complete history and thorough physical examination. For example, patients at risk for infection often are diabetics, are immunosuppressed from either prolonged high-dose steroids or cyclosporine, have acquired immunodeficiency syndrome, or have undergone recent urinary tract surgery (1,19,28).

Therapeutic Approaches

If the patient's condition requires surgery, it is tailored to the specific pathology identified. The principles and approaches have been covered in prior chapters (infection, bone, neurologic and metastatic tumors). Other patients will be best treated non-surgically, according to the principles detailed in those chapters (such as the patient who is discovered to have a metastatic neoplasm managed by radiation therapy).

Psychosocial Causes

The psychosocial determinants to failures in lumbar spinal surgery have been detailed in Chapter 12. This category, in fact, is a dominant cause in many surveys of failure of decompressive surgery (12,29,41,52). To recapitulate, the important factors in predicting failure are workers' compensation, job dissatisfaction, low education and income, heavy job requirements, cigarette smoking, psychologic disturbances, and litigation (9,21,51,60). In approaching the patient with a prior failure of decompression, these factors must be clearly understood through a detailed multidisciplinary evaluation (29). More important, a specific anatomic cause of pain must be identified if surgery is even remotely considered. The concept of "exploratory surgery" is outdated given today's imaging capability.

Therapeutic Approaches

Surgical intervention in these patients is inappropriate, unless they clearly have an additional, specific anatomic causation. It is now quite clear that prolonged rest (7) is inappropriate. The use of progressive exercise programs (31), aggressive rehabilitation programs (33), and pain clinics (36) (see Chapter 14) are alternatives that have proven to be successful in a significant number of these patients.

Discogenic Pain

The concept of discogenic pain has been carefully reviewed by Crock in Chapter 97 (4). Discography may duplicate the patient's symptoms and demonstrate morphologic disruption of the disc. In the opinion of Crock, the condition of internal disc derangement arises from significant compressive mechanical overload. In patients undergoing discography without prior surgery, a high degree of sensitivity and specificity for the procedure has been shown by Walsh and Weinstein et al. (57). Other authorities dispute the scientific evidence that supports the use of discography (37). This issue is even more difficult in the patient who has undergone a lumbar disc excision and had no relief or accentuation of his low back symptoms. In this instance the interpretation of the morphologic evidence of disc disruption is no longer valid, because the prior surgery disrupts the disc. Thus, the major information to be gained is from the reproduction of pain. However, if there is significant residual disc protrusion, the discography-CT may give important additional information. In primary cases, surgical successes of greater than 95% have been reported (6,41,45), while at least one study suggests that these primary results may be replicated in patients with prior failures (42).

Therapeutic Approaches

If the diagnosis of disc disruption is made and surgical intervention is deemed appropriate, there are four alternative approaches: anterior interbody fusion (5,6), posterior interbody fusion, posterolateral fusion (with or without instrumentation), or combined anterior and posterior fusion (either staged or performed simultaneously) (42) (see Chapter 95). The operative approaches are identical with those described in previous chapters, with the exception that when posterior interbody fusion is chosen, the operation may be significantly more difficult because of post-operative scarring. Thus, wider exposure and greater sacrifice of facet joints may be required to reduce risk of neurologic injury.

Internal Disc Disruption
After Decompression/Discectomy Surgery

Case Example

A 46-year-old female underwent three discectomies at L4–L5. On the third attempt no change in her pain occurred. Severe back and leg pain were still present. CT scan at L4–L5 (Fig. 1) showed no evidence of recurrent disc herniation. Sagittal MRI scan (Fig. 2) showed evidence of chronic vertebral end-plate changes consistent

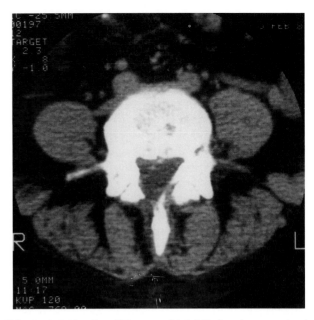

FIG. 1. Axial lumbar CT scan of L4–L5 showing post-laminectomy peridural and epidural fibrosis without evidence of recurrent disc herniation.

with internal disc disruption. Discogram confirmed the L4–L5 segment as the patient's pain source (Fig. 3).

Anterior lumbar interbody fusion at L4–L5 stabilized the motion segment, allowing the patient to return to

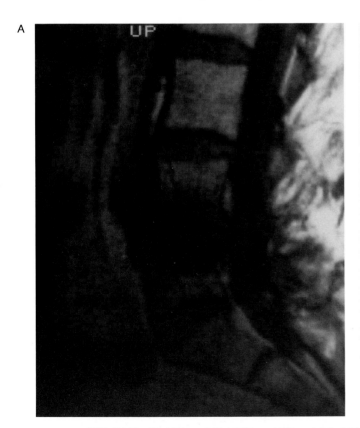

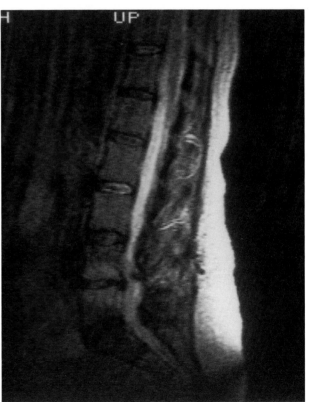

FIG. 2. Sagittal T1-weighted (**A**) and T2-weighted (**B**) MR images of L4–L5 showing endplate changes that demonstrate metabolic activity.

work in four months. She experienced marked reduction in low back pain.

Delayed Decompression

The patient who presents for surgery with a history of sciatica greater than 6 months with signs of limited SLR and perhaps mild motor weakness and sensory changes may not do as well following surgery, especially if the disc has been sequestered and there is considerable root scarring as a result. The delay is usually due to late referral or patient apprehension of surgery.

Another subset of patients includes those who underwent discotomy or decompression where the pre-operative symptoms included a long-standing history of low back pain with a more recent history of sciatica. If the back pain is predominant, discotomy or decompression is undertaken with the misconception on the part of both the surgeon and the patient that removal of a disc or decompression will also alleviate the back pain. Though the sciatica is relieved in whole or in part, back pain persists or may even be worse. If the condition is incapacitating and unrespondent to non-operative treatment modalities, and the instability is well-localized by such tests as dynamic radiographs, facet blocks, and discography, fusion may be considered.

Technical Error of Missed Level or Levels

In this instance, the actual level of involvement has been missed or the wrong side has been operated on. In patients with a primary disc prolapse or herniation, the following factors may be contributory:

1. Obesity or large patient size with inability to obtain adequate intra-operative radiographic confirmation (Fig. 4). This problem is of particular importance in microsurgical approaches.
2. Segmentation abnormalities that make the neurologic level of involvement different from the motion segment level (Fig. 5).
3. Inadequate pre-operative knowledge of the patient's side of involvement or mislabeled imaging studies.

Therapeutic Approaches

These patients require additional operative intervention, based on the premise that the original indications for surgery were well-founded. How soon the surgery should be performed is debatable, although unrelenting symptoms of more than two weeks post-operatively

should lead to re-evaluation for the possibility of a missed level or side. In a patient with a missed level or side, scarring is not a problem and, thus, the surgical approach should be identical with the surgeon's usual method for lumbar disc herniation. These approaches have been outlined in prior chapters.

Failure To Perform Adequate Decompression

The literature contains many references to "negative exploration" and its association with a high degree of failure (50). Many investigators, most notably Macnab (32), emphasized the importance of a diligent search for the sites of continued nerve root compression. The causes he found in his patient series are given in Table 3. In lumbar disc surgery, the typical pain pattern is that an L4–L5 disc herniation produces L5 pain, and the L5–S1 herniated disc produces S1 pain. However, there are significant variations in this classic pattern that may be overlooked, a point made historically by Dandy in the concept of the "hidden disc." The permutations of the more classic disc presentation may include a far lateral herniated nucleus pulposus; two-level disc herniations, which historically were thought to occur in as many as 10% of patients (43); a central disc herniation at L4–L5 producing S1 root symptoms; and a central disc herniation at L3–L4 producing a cauda equina syndrome (58) and the far out syndrome described by Wiltse. Adequate imaging studies prior to the first operation should identify these variations. Usually, failure occurs in these instances because the operative approach chosen for the operation did not permit a complete decompression. Specifically, the far lateral lesion is often at L5–S1, but can occur at levels above, e.g., the L4–L5 producing L4 root symptoms, and the L3–L4 producing L3 root symptoms. In each of these instances, the traditional intralaminar approach will be unsuccessful, particularly if there is an extruded, free fragment. The use of the extraforaminal approach popularized by McCullough in his chapter can be used successfully in either a primary or salvage case.

Far more common as a source of continuing radiculopathy is the failure to recognize foraminal stenosis as part of the causation of the patient's radiculopathy, with initial disc removal only, and inadequate decompression of the bony component. Burton (3) and Macnab (32) have suggested this is the single most common source of failure after lumbar disc surgery. This accounted for 58% of the cases treated by Burton. Although the usual causes are congenital (trefoil canal) or are due to facet hypertrophy, leading to superior articular facet impingement, Macnab (32) also pointed out the importance of the pedicle as an overlooked site of nerve root compression.

In the patient with multilevel spinal stenosis, the issue

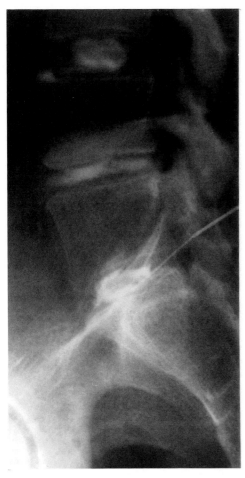

FIG. 3. Lateral L4–L5 lumbar discogram showing disc degeneration. This discogram reproduced the patient's pain.

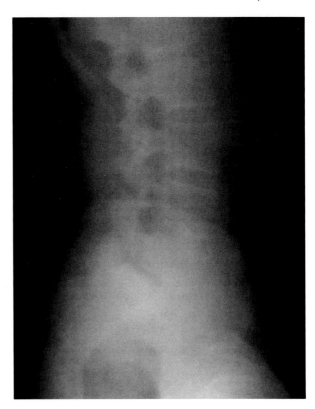

FIG. 4. Lateral lumbar radiograph in an obese (300 lb.) patient showing the difficulty in viewing the L5–S1 disc space.

of how many levels to decompress is even more difficult and, thus, it is easier to fail to adequately decompress the affected levels. The criteria that may be used in addition to the history, physical examination, and imaging studies include pre- and intra-operative somatosensory-evoked potentials (the sensitivity, specificity, and utility of this procedure remains debated) and the use of intra-operative criteria such as restoration of dural pulsations and possibly intra-operative ultrasound. Missed levels may also occur in degenerative spondylolisthesis or occasionally in patients decompressed for isthmic spondylolisthesis. In degenerative spondylolisthesis, decompression has been limited to the L5 roots, with failure to recognize common involvement of the L4 root in the lateral recess. In L5 isthmic spondylolisthesis, the usual cause of nerve root compression is at the L5 root from the bony excrescence rather than the presumed, but very uncommon, involvement of the S1 roots, as well as an unrecognized L4–L5 disc herniation proximal to an L5 spondylogenic spondylolisthesis, which may be a cause of continued sciatica and/or back pain.

Therapeutic Approaches

The overall objective is to adequately decompress the involved root(s), which may include the need to sacrifice the motion segment's stability. Because the prior surgery was at this level, some element of perineural scar should be anticipated. After a routine midline exposure, the margins of the old laminotomy (if previously performed) are carefully delineated using a curette (Fig. 6). Dorsal scar or fat graft can be debulked, but no attempt is made to expose the underlying dura. Using a Penfield or small curette, a dissection plane can usually be developed between the overhanging lamina laterally and inferiorly, and the Kerrison rongeur used to remove bone (Figs. 7 and 8). If there is substantial bony hypertrophy, a power

TABLE 3. Causes of continued radiculopathy in 68 cases

Causes	Number of cases
Facet impingement	19
Pedicular kinking	12
Foraminal migration	9
Spinal stenosis	8
Extraforaminal disc	2
No cause identified	18

Source: ref. 32.

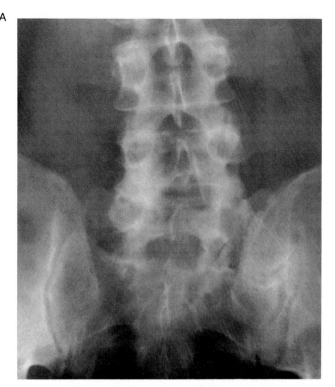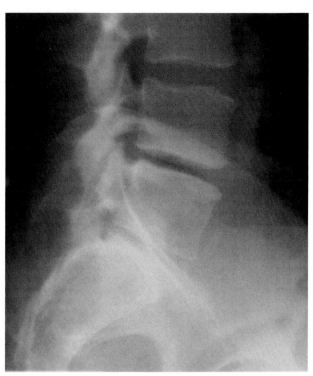

FIG. 5. AP (**A**) and lateral (**B**) lumbar radiographs showing the segmentation error that makes identification of the lumbosacral disc more difficult.

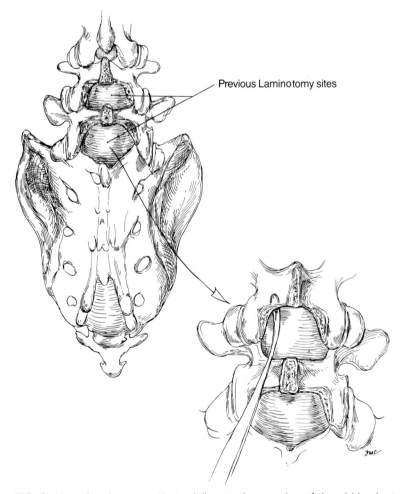

Previous Laminotomy sites

FIG. 6. Use of a sharp curette to delineate the margins of the old laminotomy.

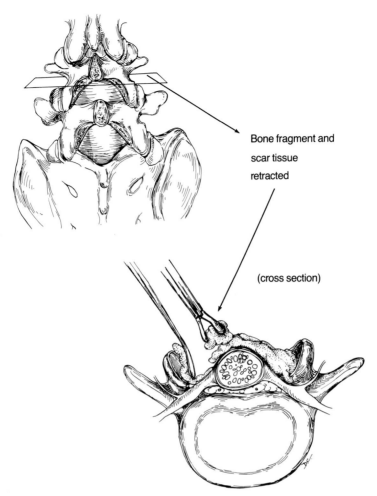

FIG. 7. Use of a Penfield and pituitary or Kerrison rongeur to define the lateral margin of the spinal canal.

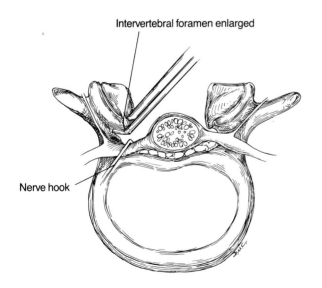

FIG. 8. Use of a 45° Kerrison rongeur to undercut the superior facet accomplishing a foraminotomy and nerve root decompression.

burr may be used to debulk the bone or to perform the dissection. Dependent on the magnitude of scar, two anatomic landmarks usually can be established, in either the pedicle laterally or the nerve root inferiorly. If the root is identified, dissection can then proceed proximally to the level of the pedicle. Conversely, if the lamina is the only identifiable landmark, dissection should proceed cautiously and distal until normal, unscarred nerve root is encountered. If possible, the facet should be undercut as shown in Figure 8, as advocated by Kirkaldy-Willis. The bony dissection should continue both laterally and proximally back to the root takeoff until it is clear the root has been unroofed. In assessing the adequacy of bony decompression, two criteria can be utilized—the root is free and easily retracted medially a minimum of 5 mm, or a probe can be passed into the foramina. We make no effort to expose or decompress the disc space, unless the pre-operative studies indicate the presence of residual disc material. The defect is then covered with a generous free fat graft and routine closure performed.

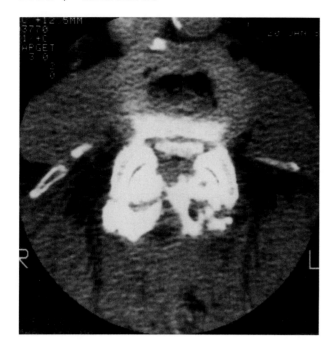

FIG. 9. Axial lumbar CT myelogram at the superior edge of L3–L4 foramina showing a narrowed canal.

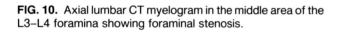

FIG. 10. Axial lumbar CT myelogram in the middle area of the L3–L4 foramina showing foraminal stenosis.

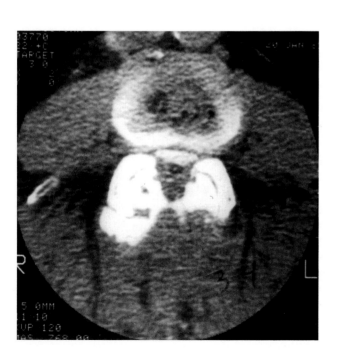

FIG. 11. Axial lumbar CT myelogram showing superior facet hypertrophy and foraminal stenosis.

Spinal Stenosis with Inadequate Nerve Root Decompression

Case Example

A 65-year-old man with a history of neurogenic claudication presented to a local physician, who performed a midline decompressive laminotomy without foraminotomy. Patient's symptoms did not change after surgery.

CT/myelogram (Figs. 9, 10, and 11) confirmed inadequate decompression of the foramina.

A second decompression with foraminotomy relieved his symptoms.

Conjoined Nerve Root

Anatomic studies indicate that from 2% to 14% of patients have a conjoined nerve root. Surgical decompression in patients with these congenital abnormalities has been associated with a higher than expected degree of failure. Failure to recognize the conjoined nerve root at the time of the initial surgery may have three consequences: The conjoined root may be avulsed, leading to an increased neurologic deficit; the conjoined nerve root may be "battered," leading to increased perineural scarring; or the portion of the nerve root that is compressed may be overlooked, leading to continued symptoms. Unfortunately, the first two conditions are more common than the third and are not amenable to further surgery. In the few cases we have encountered where continued symptoms occurred, the condition could have been suspected by the initial CT scan, MRI, or myelogram, but the images were interpreted as consistent with a disc herniation. The surgical approach in these instances is identical with that described for residual lateral stenosis.

TEMPORARY RELIEF FOLLOWED BY EARLY RECURRENCE OF PAIN (DAYS–WEEKS)

Infection

An infectious process after spinal decompression may include "discitis"; frank osteomyelitis most commonly involving the anterior and middle column, but occasionally involving the posterior column; and an epidural abscess. The reported rate of this complication is 0.5% to 2.7% (17,22,50).

Discitis

Discitis is characterized classically as producing intense back pain from 2 weeks to 3 months after an appar-

ently successful surgical intervention. The severity of back pain is noteworthy and is often described as similar to an intra-abdominal crisis. However, the physical findings, other than extreme discomfort and limited straight leg raising, are often unremarkable. Often spinal radiographs and white blood count and differential are normal, and the erythrocyte sedimentation rate is typically elevated. In the early phase, bone scan or MRI is most sensitive. Aspirations of the disc space frequently are sterile; the most common organism is *Staphylococcus*. For this reason, some investigators have suggested an autoimmune, rather than an infectious, etiology. However, animal models of this condition (13) show unequivocally the necessity of bacteria to produce the radiographic changes that accompany discitis. The later radiographic changes include striking disc space narrowing, end-plate erosions, and the development of marginal osteophytes. Later, spontaneous fusion of the disc space may occur in 50% of cases (Fig. 12).

Therapeutic Approaches

The management of discitis is somewhat controversial. Pilgaard (45) noted the absence of an organism in many cases, and many of his patients were successfully treated without antibiotics. However, a diligent search must be made, and treatment for 4 to 6 weeks with the appropriate intravenous antibiotic is advocated by many (see Chapter 38). Immobilization by spica cast appears to be the most effective means for pain relief and may be supplemented by a back brace as the patient becomes ambulatory. An uncomplicated discitis should not require surgery, as differentiated from frank osteomyelitis. The long-term results in Pilgaard's non-operatively treated series were excellent, most patients having gone on to spontaneous interbody fusion over a period of 6 months to 1 year.

Post-Operative Osteomyelitis

This complication may present initially much like discitis. However, the subsequent course is more likely to be characterized by increasing symptoms; systemic symptoms may also be more prominent (although this finding is absent in 50% of cases), and the sedimentation rate is elevated. This problem may be suspected by greater bony involvement seen in the initial imaging studies, but is often discovered only by serial radiographs demonstrating vertebral body collapse if the anterior and middle columns are involved. In these patients, an organism can usually be cultured. In the rarer instance of posterior column involvement, the wound may demonstrate the more typical signs of infection.

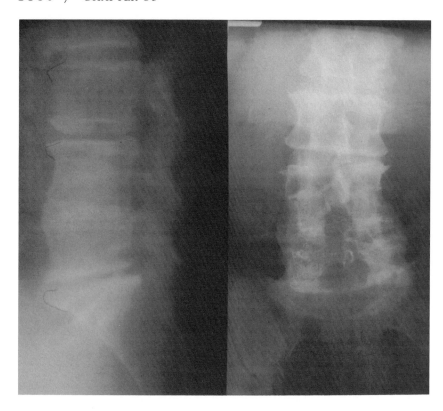

FIG. 12. A 30-year-old male had disc excision at L4–L5 followed in 3 weeks by intense low back pain. He was braced and the CSR slowly returned to normal. Twenty years later, he shows the solid interbody fusion.

Therapeutic Approaches

The approach is based on the organism, the response to antibiotics, evidence of continuing vertebral body collapse, or signs of new neurologic involvement. The principles of treatment are identical with the management of acute hematogenous vertebral body osteomyelitis (see Chapter 38). Antibiotic treatment alone, with appropriate immobilization, may be adequate. If there is progressive vertebral body collapse or changing neurologic signs, anterior debridement and bone graft are appropriate. If the infection is posterior, debridement alone with antibiotic management is usually preferred.

Epidural Abscess

An isolated epidural abscess following decompression is rare. This condition is suspect when a patient has increasing neurologic symptoms and signs in the early post-operative period, and may be difficult to separate from an expanding hematoma if systemic signs of infection are absent. The diagnostic test of choice is the MRI. Decompression and antibiotic management are mandatory. More often this condition arises in association with vertebral osteomyelitis and serves as one of the indications for early decompression.

Meningeal Cyst

Meningeal cysts are an uncommon cause of early, recurrent radiculopathy after disc excision and are re-

ported in less than 1% of patients who have had that operation. How this problem occurs after extensive decompressions for spinal stenosis is not known, but would be suspected to be more common than for disc excision. The possibility of their occurrence is definitely increased

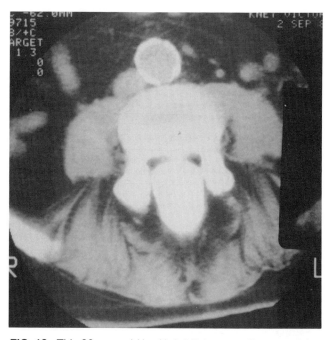

FIG. 13. This 60-year-old had L4–L5 degenerative spondylolisthesis. During decompression, durotomy occurred and was loosely closed. He presents with a palpable mass when standing, but minimal neurologic involvement. He refused surgical intervention.

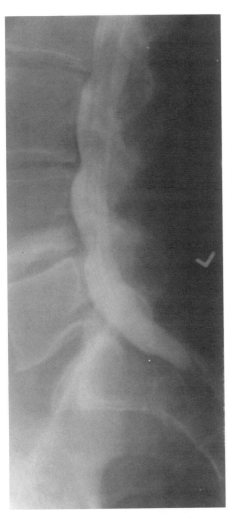

FIG. 14. Lateral view of lumbar myelogram showing a posterior displacement of the dye column at L4–L5 consistent with a herniated nucleus pulposus.

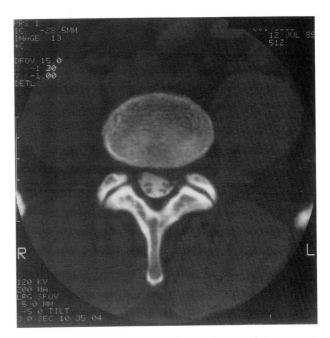

FIG. 15. Axial view at L4–L5 of a myelogram/CT scan confirming a herniated disc at that level.

when a decompression is performed in patients with prior surgery (34). Jones (26) has shown that an "incidental durotomy" accompanying a disc excision does not compromise the later results if the dural leak is recognized and closed. Unrecognized durotomy may lead to a "ball valve" phenomenon with a slowly expanding mass. In other instances, nerve root(s) may become part of the meningeal cyst, in which case nerve root pain is common.

The physical examination may reveal soft tissue bulging, particularly when the patient is standing. The important diagnostic test is myelographically performed with an adequate period of standing while the dye is in place (Fig. 13).

Therapeutic Approaches

Removal of the meningeal cyst involves careful dissection around the cyst and identification of the dural opening. The cyst should be opened before it is amputated because of the possibility it contains nerve roots. Closure can usually be accomplished by resuturing the dura or, in large defects, by using a fascial graft.

MID-TERM FAILURES (WEEKS–MONTHS)

Recurrent Disc Prolapse

A recurrent disc prolapse may occur on the same side and at the same level as the prior operation, on the opposite side at the same level, or at an entirely new level. In some series (16,22) this is reported as the most common failure. A compilation of 268 cases culled from the literature revealed that 43% of the failures were at the same level and 22% at a new level (14).

The literature contains many references to prevention of recurrences by performing a more vigorous evacuation of the disc at the time of surgery. However, anatomic studies simulating disc excision and follow-up studies of limited disc excision (51) indicate minimal evidence to support that assertion. Similarly, the notion that two-level bilateral decompressions were preventative has not been borne out and can be viewed as a historical perspective (43) rather than a current practice.

Typically, these patients have complete relief of their sciatica following the original decompression, are functioning well, and then have severe recurrent symptoms. The physical examination reveals typical signs of disc herniation with positive tension signs. As previously noted, the interpretation of the neurologic findings may be difficult because of residual deficits from the prior surgery.

Therapeutic Approaches

The alternative therapies are similar to those available for a patient with a primary disc protrusion or frank herniation. They include short-term bed rest, analgesics, non-steroidal anti-inflammatory drugs, epidural blocks, and graded exercise. There are no studies that have evaluated the non-operative outcomes of recurrent disc lesions. Theoretically, a recurrence at a new level or side opposite the original lesion should have the same rate of recovery as a primary lesion, where it is known that at least 70% to 80% function well without surgery (20,59). When the lesion is at the same level and side, some of us have a clinical impression that the probability of recovery with conservative management is less. Perhaps this is because the original annulotomy produces a situation in which a free fragment of disc is more often present.

The surgical alternatives and approaches for those patients who fail to respond to treatment are identical to those for primary disc lesions when the pathology is at a new side or level. In patients whose surgery is at the same side and level, percutaneous discectomy is inappropriate, and formal disc excision is required with or without microscopic enhancement. Our approach is identical with that described in patients with lateral recess stenosis, except that attempts are made to preserve the facets in their entirety and the nerve root may require greater

mobilization to identify the fragment. In some instances, the disc space may not be easily identified, and an intra-operative radiograph may be of great assistance.

The outcome of these procedures appears to be virtually identical to primary disc excision, as measured in long-term follow-up studies (16).

Recurrent Disc Herniation

Case Example

A 48-year-old man presented with a one-year history of severe left hip and radiating leg pain. Physical examination revealed weakness of left extensor hallicus longus. There was a positive root tension sign. Routine lumbar radiographs were unremarkable. Lateral lumbar myelogram (Fig. 14) showed a herniated L4–L5 disc. CT-myelogram (Fig. 15) confirmed the same findings with marked posterior displacement of the L5 nerve root.

The patient did very well after surgery. He experi-

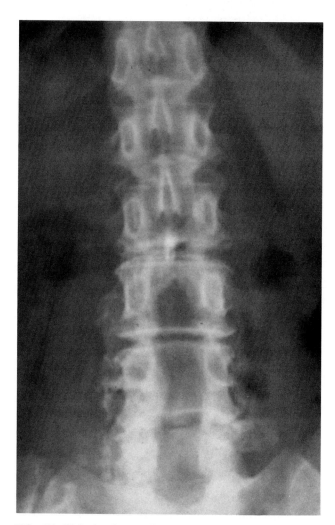

FIG. 17. Plain lumbar radiograph demonstrating wide decompressive laminectomy at L3–L5.

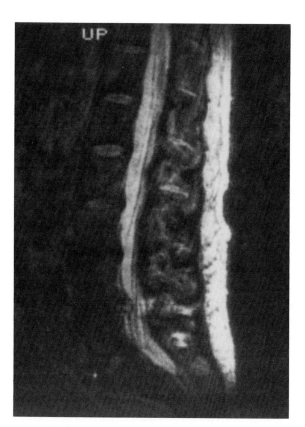

FIG. 16. Sagittal T2-weighted MR image of the lumbar spine confirmed a recurrent herniated disc at L4–L5.

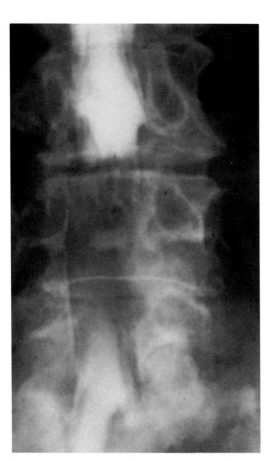

FIG. 18. Oblique lumbar myelogram demonstrating displacement of the dural column by epidural fibrosis.

enced complete relief of his leg pain and returned to work. Three months after surgery, while walking across a parking lot, sciatic pain returned. Lumbar MRI (Fig. 16) showed evidence of a recurrent disc herniation at L4–L5. Patient was treated non-surgically with resolution of his pain after six months.

Battered Root

Perineural scarring occurs to some degree in most spinal decompression and relates to the magnitude of the decompression. However, the magnitude of the problem as a causation of clinical failure in practice is small, and variously estimated to occur in 1% to 2% of patients undergoing disc excision (50). In one report (16), which culled 268 cases of failure from the literature, nerve root scarring accounted for 12% of all failures, while in Burton's study (2), 8% of failures were due to this cause. One of the presumed benefits of microscopic discectomy is reported to be reduction in the exposed neural surfaces, yet this assertion has never been proven in carefully controlled, prospective studies. Factors that predispose to such scarring are excessive bleeding, excessive retraction,

the presence of conjoined nerve roots, and possibly the use of cottonoid patties (24).

Watkins (58) has reviewed the factors important for prevention, which include proper training and experience, the recognition that there is no such thing as a "simple disc," proper lighting and magnification, the proper operative frame to promote decompression of the abdomen and secondarily of the epidural veins, proper instrumentation, proper assistance, and the careful analysis of one's own operative techniques and results to gain facility and effectiveness and minimize complications. To this list should be added the role for free fat grafts, which still remains controversial.

The clinical syndrome, as defined by Bertrand (1a) and Finnegan (12), is fairly classic. The immediate postoperative course may be benign, but more often is associated with incomplete resolution of sciatica, sometimes accompanied by an increased sensory or even motor deficit. At this point, the surgeon is hopeful the problem is nerve root swelling, rather than frank injury. Instead of undergoing complete recovery, the symptoms slowly increase over the next 3 to 6 months, with increasing sciatica and varying degrees of low back pain. The neurologic examination simply confirms the sensory and/or motor deficits, and the degree of elevation to produce sciatica is variable.

A variant of the battered root is the more dramatic and, from the patient's perspective, catastrophic frank nerve or caudal injury. Evidence of frank nerve root injury manifested in severe weakness is variously reported to occur in 0.4% to 4% of patients. The higher rates are derived from the historic literature. Caudal injury with sphincteric disturbance is rarely reported. Spangfort (50) identified 5 out of 2,504 cases who underwent disc excision. This condition has also been reported as a complication of free fat grafting, where the source of compression was from bleeding.

This same situation may occur at the root level or more diffusely, following decompression for spinal stenosis. When scarring is diffuse, the patient's stenotic symptoms recur, and imaging studies typically demonstrate a large dorsal mass of epidural scar.

Therapeutic Approaches

A variety of surgical therapies have been advocated, including removal of scar followed by use of a variety of interpositional membranes, radical decompression, longitudinal sectioning of scar over the nerve root, spinal fusion, and the implanting of a variety of electrical stimulators. These alternatives are presented by Wilkinson in Chapter 99. The most hotly debated treatment is extensive spinal fusion, which may include combined anterior-posterior techniques. To date, the absence of a well-documented series of patients treated by this technique leaves its benefits questionable.

The alternative treatments focus on functional restoration and pain management. The organization of these programs and their success in managing such complex patients have been detailed in Chapters 13 and 14.

Epidural Fibrosis

Case Example

A 62-year-old female with a history of discectomy/laminotomy L3–L4, L4–L5 in 1962 and 1968 (Fig. 17) had recurrent pain in 1980. The myelogram/CT demonstrated dense epidural fibrosis (Figs. 18 and 19). No new nerve root tension signs were seen on physical exam. Based on her history, physical examination, and CT/myelogram, a non-surgical course was elected. Patient's pain slowly improved over two years.

Arachnoiditis

This topic is presented in detail in Chapter 99 by Wilkinson. The important issues in prevention today are the avoidance of oil-based radiopaque contrast media, the avoidance of bleeding during myelography of any type, the avoidance of the use of intrathecal corticosteroids, and a non-traumatic surgical technique. With non-surgi-

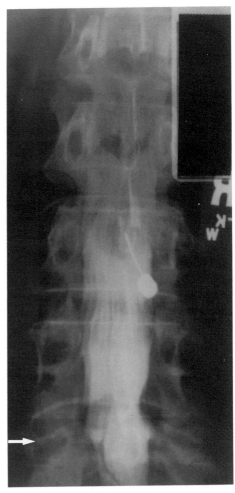

FIG. 20. Lumbar AP myelogram showing evidence of subarachnoid scarring consistent with arachnoiditis (arrow).

cal treatment, the long-term results of this condition may be more favorable than previously reported.

Guyer (18) reported 50 patients with follow-up ranging from 10 to 21 years. Ninety percent had prior pantopaque myelogram. All were found to have arachnoiditis at later follow-up, and the oil-based contrast media was strongly implicated in the etiology.

Over that follow-up period, no change in motor strength or incontinence was demonstrated. Fifty-seven percent of patients noted no change in pain, while 17% expressed slight improvement and 14% were slightly worse.

Pain was the sole reason for dysfunction, as 62% never worked again and 34% showed alcohol and/or drug abuse. There was only one suicide among the patients, but their life expectancy was shortened by 14 years, never due solely to the arachnoiditis.

Case Example

A 42-year-old female had a history of prior discectomy in 1962. Oil-soluble myelography was used at that time.

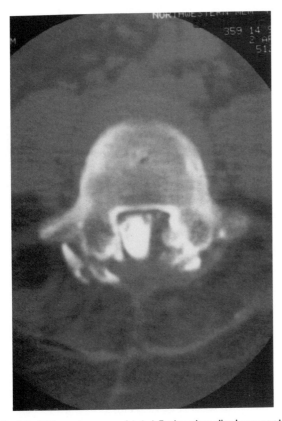

FIG. 19. CT myelogram of L4–L5 showing displacement of normal dural structures by epidural fibrosis.

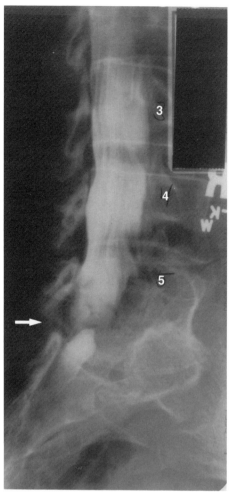

FIG. 21. Lumbar oblique myelogram showing arachnoiditis (arrow).

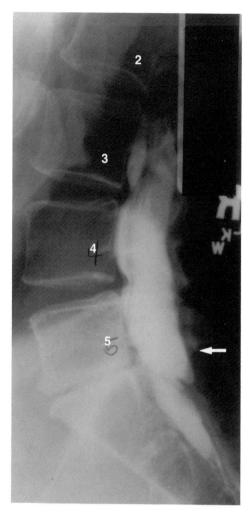

FIG. 22. Lumbar lateral myelogram showing arachnoiditis (arrow).

In 1982 she had recurrent sciatic symptoms, and a water-soluble myelogram/CT scan (Figs. 20, 21, 22, and 23) demonstrated examples of arachnoiditis.

A patient with whom the goals of surgery have not been adequately explained may experience good relief of pain from the placebo effect of intervention for a few weeks. With the passage of time, the patient realizes his goals have not been achieved. Treatment consists of careful consultation, explanation, and physical rehabilitation.

LONG-TERM FAILURES (MONTHS–YEARS)

Recurrence of symptoms months or years after surgery in many instances should not be considered a failure as much as the evolution of the degenerative process. However, the recognition that disease process may progress and be influenced by the surgical procedure chosen at the first operation is relevant, and in some instances, later failure can be prevented. Thus, the issue of accurate pre-operative assessment is important. When the patient

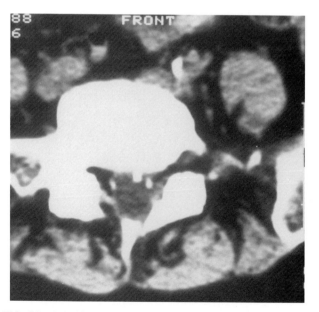

FIG. 23. Axial CT myelogram of L5 pedicle area showing an area of poor myelogram dye filling consistent with severe dense subarachnoid scarring.

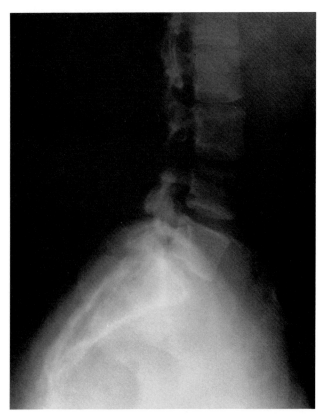

FIG. 24. Lateral lumbar radiograph showing normal L4–L5 disc space height at the time of initial discectomy.

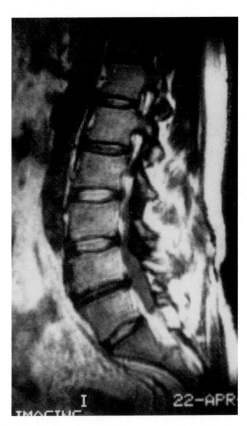

FIG. 25. Sagittal lumbar MR image showing disc degeneration and collapse at L4–L5.

has an isolated disc protrusion or extrusion, the addition of a spinal fusion cannot be considered preventative. The historic belief, particularly popular in the decade following World War II, was that the surgeon should routinely decompress both the L4–L5 and L5–S1 levels, bilaterally. In the era of inadequate imaging, this assertion may have had some validity, but with today's imaging sophistication, there should be minimal doubt about the cause of the patient's radiculopathy. Similarly, there has accumulated a body of clinical data that shows minimal, if any, benefit to routine spinal fusion in the improvement of clinical results (15) in patients with simple lumbar disc lesions. A particularly enlightening report showed in a series of workers' compensation cases a 100% failure rate for combined disc excision and fusion. This simply reminds us that fusion cannot overcome poor patient selection, no matter how meticulously the operation is done. However, the issues are considerably more complex when decompressions are being done for spinal stenosis.

Recurrent Stenosis or Development of Lateral Stenosis from Disc Space Collapse

As already noted previously, recognition of stenosis as a contributor to radiculopathy should be a high priority in pre-operative assessment. The group of patients who will be considered here are those who had initial adequate diagnosis and decompression and later developed recurrent symptoms, following either disc excision or prior decompression for stenosis.

Following lumbar disc excision, some reports indicate that virtually all patients will develop disc space narrowing (16,17,21,38), while other reports suggest a lower rate of 16% (40). This narrowing is commonly associated with the development of osteophytes and some degree of facet hypertrophy, but has little effect on the patient's outcome (16,21). Why some patients develop later stenotic symptoms and others do not is conjectural; the radiographic changes appear to be independent of sex, age, or occupation (16,39), but probably relate to the original canal dimensions (55) and other, as yet to be determined, congenital or structural predispositions (49). As a rarer problem, the patient may develop signs of central or mixed stenosis.

In the second group of patients, the presence of stenosis was recognized at the time of the original operation and corrected, but stenosis recurred at a new or the same site. Again, the identification of the patient at risk is unclear, unless the original surgical procedure produced instability (see below).

The clinical presentation of these patients typically is a long period of relief from sciatica, followed by the gradual recurrence of a mono- or polyradiculopathy. In the interval, there may have been slowly increasing chronic low back pain consistent with spinal osteoarthritis. The physical examination is consistent with patients, in general, with spinal stenosis who have not undergone operation, although the residual neurologic changes from prior surgery may confuse the clinical picture.

Therapeutic Approaches

The conservative approach to these patients is similar to that in cases of primary stenosis and includes short-term bed rest, non-steroidal anti-inflammatory medications, epidural blocks, and possibly flexion braces. Because walking may increase their symptoms, aerobic exercise is better performed using a bicycle or swimming programs. There are no prospective studies to date that have rigorously evaluated the outcome of patients with spinal stenosis treated by these conservative measures. If conservative management fails, the operative approach is identical with that previously described in this chapter.

Disc Space Collapse with Foraminal Stenosis After Discectomy

Case Example

A 42-year-old female underwent L4–L5 discectomy in 1982 for herniated disc. Lateral lumbar radiograph taken at that time indicates normal disc space height (Fig. 24).

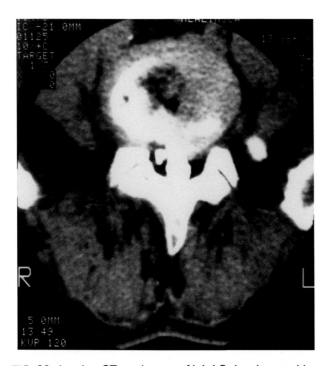

FIG. 26. Lumbar CT myelogram of L4–L5 showing combination of disc degeneration and bulging to compress the left L5 root and thecal sac.

In 1987, patient presented with recurrent sciatic pain involving the left leg. Sagittal MRI scan (Fig. 25) and axial CT/myelogram (Fig. 26) document disc space narrowing with disc bulging resulting in compression of the left L5 root. Posterior lumbar interbody fusion allowed relief of back and left leg pain.

Instability After Disc Excision

Segmental instability following spinal decompression has been reported to vary widely. The broad issues in segmental instability have been detailed in Chapter 90. Here, we will consider segmental instability following disc excision and after more extensive spinal decompression.

Instability is reported to be the third most common source of failure after lumbar disc excision and has been reported to account for 18% of the overall failures. Although there is no classic syndrome, most patients seem to have a gradual onset of low back pain following resolution of sciatica. As a possible cause of symptoms, segmental instability may be difficult to document. The problem is that some element of hypermobility is common in asymptomatic patients. In one series, evidence of instability (disc space narrowing, excessive translation, and traction spurs) was found in 20% of post-operative patients, most typically females, whose prior surgery was at L4–L5. Documentation that instability is in fact causing symptoms is, therefore, difficult (53) and seems minimally benefited by imaging studies, including motion radiography, unless the translations are of a large order of magnitude or by facet injections. The temporary use of fixators (10,44) has been promising as one part of the evaluation of these patients, but currently should be viewed as experimental.

Instability After Lumbar Decompression

More extensive decompressions have a higher probability of producing instability, and the criteria for prevention have become better established. Specifically, the elegant laboratory studies of Panjabi have shown that sacrifice of more than 50% of both facets, or the sacrifice of a single entire facet, significantly alters the motion segment kinematics. Occasionally a facet fracture may occur later and also produce instability (47). Factors that have been thought to influence later instability are patient age (the younger patient is at greater risk), female gender, disc space narrowing with osteophytes (the patient is at less risk), level of decompression (the L5–S1 level is less susceptible to later instability), pathology treated (a lesion with inherent instability is at greater risk, such as degenerative spondylolisthesis), and the extent of the decompression (the more radical the operation the higher the risk) (25).

Therapeutic Approaches

There are no studies that have looked at the outcome of conservative management in patients with suspected primary degenerative instability or in patients with prior decompression and failure thought to be due to instability. If instability is deemed to be present and can be confirmed by radiologic studies, the treatment of choice is spinal fusion. The technique used should be the one most comfortable for the surgeon, and may range from anterior interbody fusion in cases with extensive previous posterior operation to combined anterior posterior fusion with instrumentation. Although the evidence is not yet certain, the use of fixation devices, particularly pedicle fixation, appears most applicable to patients with extensive prior decompression. In one study the results of treatment with fusion were equivalent to the results of primary fusion (16) in carefully selected cases.

COMPLICATIONS

In addition to the specific problems that can produce failure after spinal decompression, local and general complications can compromise the short- and long-term results. Table 4 gives a compilation of these complications. Figure 27 presents a diagnostic algorithm for these cases.

SUMMARY

Failures in low back surgery can be avoided by multiple strategies. First, the original decision for surgical care should be based on valid criteria and a structured anatomic diagnosis, where the imaging studies are a confirmation of clinical acumen rather than the indication for the operation. At the completion of a successful operation, a clear focus should be kept on rehabilitation. Faced with a patient who has had a prior operation and continuing or recurrent symptoms, the surgeon has to

TABLE 4. *Complications of spinal decompression*

Complication	Reported rate
Superficial wound infection	0%–3.2%
Deep wound infection	0.5%–3.0%
Discitis	0.5%–2.7%
Meningitis	0.1%
Peripheral nerve compression (secondary to positioning)	0%–1.0%
Vascular complications (acute lacerations, false aneurysm, A-V fistulae, death)	0%–1.0%
Deep venous thrombosis	1.2%–3.0%
Pulmonary emboli	0.1%–1.2%
Visceral injury (bowel, kidney, ureter)	Sporadic case reports
Urinary tract infection	2.4%–10%
Urinary retention	0.5%–38%

return to the original operation and determine whether it was based on well-thought-out indications. If the answer is no and there are significant psychosocial issues, the probability that repeat surgery will solve the problem is low. If the answer is yes, then it is incumbent that the multiple possible causes be narrowed down through history, physical examination, and confirmatory imaging studies. If the second operation is well-founded, the probability of success is high and, in fact, approaches the success rate of primary, well-indicated surgical decompressions.

REFERENCES

1. Baker AS, Ojemann RG, Swartz MN, Richardson EP Jr (1975): Spinal epidural abscess. *N Engl J Med* 293:463–468.
1a. Bertrand G (1975): The "battered" root syndrome. *Orthop Clin North Am* 6(1):305–310.
2. Burton C (1981): The role of spine fusion: Question 4. *Spine* 6:291.
3. Burton CV, Kirkaldy-Willis WH, Yong-Hing K, Heithoff KB (1981): Causes of failure of surgery on the lumbar spine. *Clin Orthop* (157):191–199.
4. Crock HV (1970): A reappraisal of intervertebral disc lesions. *Med J Aust* 1:983–989.

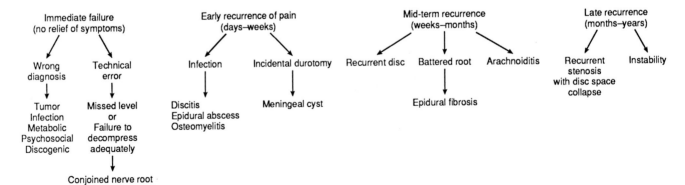

FIG. 27. Diagnostic algorithm for failures after decompressive surgery.

5. Crock HV (1976): Observations on the management of failed spinal operations. *J Bone Joint Surg* [Br] 58:193–199.

6. Crock HV (1986): Internal disc disruption: A challenge to disc prolapse fifty years on. *Spine* 11:650–653.

7. Deyo RA (1987): Reducing work absenteeism and diagnostic costs for backache. In: Hadler NM, ed. *Clinical concepts in regional musculoskeletal illness.* Orlando: Grune & Stratton, pp. 25–50.

8. Deyo RA, Diehl AK, Rosenthal M (1986): How many days of bedrest for acute low back pain? A randomized clinical trial. *N Engl J Med* 315:1064–1070.

9. Dvorak J, Valach L, Fuhrimann P, Heim E (1988): The outcome of surgery for lumbar disc herniation. II. A 4–17 years' follow-up with emphasis on psychosocial aspects. *Spine* 13:1423–1427.

10. Esses SI, Botsford DJ, Kostuik JP (1989): The role of external spinal skeletal fixation in the assessment of low-back disorders. *Spine* 14:594–601.

11. Fairbank JC, Park WM, McCall IW, et al. (1981): Apophyseal injection of local anesthetic as a diagnostic aid in primary low-back pain syndromes. *Spine* 6:598–605.

12. Finnegan WJ, Fenlin JM, Marvel JP, Nardini RJ, Rothman RH (1979): Results of surgical intervention in the symptomatic multioperated back patient. Analysis of 67 cases followed for three to seven years. *J Bone Joint Surg* [Am] 61:1077–1082.

13. Fraser RD, Osti OL, Vernon-Roberts B (1986): Discitis following chemonucleolysis: An experimental study. *Spine* 11:679–687.

14. Frymoyer JW (1981): The role of spine fusion. Question 3. *Spine* 6:284–290.

15. Frymoyer JW (1988): Back pain and sciatica. *N Engl J Med* 318:291–300.

16. Frymoyer JW, Hanley EN Jr, Howe J, Kuhlmann D, Matteri RE (1979): A comparison of radiographic findings in fusion and non-fusion patients, ten or more years following lumbar disc surgery. *Spine* 4(5):435–440.

17. Gurdjian ES, Webster JE, Ostrowski AZ, et al. (1961): Herniated lumbar intervertebral discs—An analysis of 1176 operated cases. *J Trauma* 1:158–176.

18. Guyer DW, Wiltse LL, Eskay ML, Guyer BH (1989): The long-range prognosis of arachnoiditis. *Spine* 14(12):1332–1341.

19. Hadler NM (1986): Regional back pain [editorial]. *N Engl J Med* 315:1090–1092.

20. Hakelius A (1970): Prognosis in sciatica. A clinical follow-up of surgical and non-surgical treatment. *Acta Orthop Scand* [Suppl] 129:1–76.

21. Hanley EN Jr, Shapiro DE (1989): The development of low-back pain after excision of a lumbar disc. *J Bone Joint Surg* [Am] 71:719–721.

22. Hirsch C, Nachemson A (1963): The reliability of lumbar disk surgery. *Clin Orthop* 29:189–194.

23. Howe J, Frymoyer JW (1985): The effects of questionnaire design on the determination of end results in lumbar spinal surgery. *Spine* 10:804–805.

24. Hoyland JA, Freemont AJ, Denton J, Thomas AM, McMillan JJ, Jayson MIV (1988): Retained surgical swab debris in post-laminectomy arachnoiditis and peridural fibrosis. *J Bone Joint Surg* [Br] 70:659–662.

25. Johnsson KE, Redlund-Johnell I, Uden A, Willner S (1989): Preoperative and postoperative instability in lumbar spinal stenosis. *Spine* 14:591–593.

26. Jones AA, Stambough JL, Balderston RA, Rothman RH, Booth RE Jr (1989): Long-term results of lumbar spine surgery complicated by unintended incidental durotomy. *Spine* 14:443–446.

27. Krempen JF, Smith BS (1974): Nerve root injection: A method for evaluating the etiology of sciatica. *J Bone Joint Surg* [Am] 56:1435–1444.

28. Liang M, Komaroff AL (1982): Roentgenograms in primary care patients with acute low back pain: A cost-effectiveness analysis. *Arch Intern Med* 142:1108–1112.

29. Long DM, Filtzer DL, BenDebba M, Hendler NH (1988): Clinical features of the failed-back syndrome. *J Neurosurg* 69:61–71.

30. Love JG, Rivers MH (1962): Spinal cord tumors simulating protruded intervertebral disks. *JAMA* 179:878–881.

31. McKenzie RA (1981): *The lumbar spine, mechanical diagnosis and therapy.* New Zealand: Spinal Publications.

32. Macnab I (1971): Negative disc exploration: An analysis of the causes of nerve-root involvement in 68 patients. *J Bone Joint Surg* [Am] 53:891–903.

33. Mayer TG, Gatchel RJ, Kishino N, Keeley J, Capra P, Mayer H, Barnett J, Mooney V (1985): Objective assessment of spine function following industrial injury: A prospective study with comparison group and one-year follow-up. *Spine* 10:482–493.

34. Miller PR, Elder FW Jr (1968): Meningeal pseudocysts (meningocele spurius) following laminectomy. *J Bone Joint Surg* [Am] 50:268–276.

35. Mooney V (1988): The failed back—an orthopaedic view. *Int Disabil Stud* 10:32–36.

36. Mooney V, Cairns D, Robertson J (1976): A system for evaluating and treating chronic back disability. *Western J Med* 124:370–376.

37. Nachemson A (1989): Lumbar discography—Where are we today? *Spine* 14:555–557.

38. Nashold BA Jr, Blaine S, Hrubec A (1971): *Lumbar disc disease: A twenty-year clinical follow up study.* St. Louis: C. V. Mosby.

39. Naylor A (1974): Late results of laminectomy for lumbar disc prolapse. A review after ten to twenty-five years. *J Bone Joint Surg* [Br] 56:17–29.

40. Naylor A, Shentall RD, Micklethwaite B (1977): An electron microscopic study of the segment long spacing collagen from the intervertebral disc. *Orth Clin North Am* 8:217–223.

41. Norton WL (1987): Chemonucleolysis versus surgical discectomy: Comparison of costs and results in workers' compensation claimants. *Spine* 11:440–443.

42. O'Brien JP, Dawson MH, Heard CW, et al. (1986): Simultaneous combined anterior and posterior fusion: A surgical solution for failed spinal surgery with a brief review of the first 150 patients. *Clin Orthop* (203):191–195.

43. O'Connell JEA (1951): Protrusions of the lumbar intervertebral discs. A clinical review based on five hundred cases treated by excision of the protrusion. *J Bone Joint Surg* [Br] 33:8–30.

44. Olerud S, Sjostrom L, Karlstrom G, Hamberg M (1986): Spontaneous effect of increased stability of the lower lumbar spine in cases of severe chronic back pain: The answer of an external transpeduncular fixation test. *Clin Orthop* (203):67–74.

45. Pilgaard S (1969): Discitis (closed space infection) following removal of lumbar intervertebral disc. *J Bone Joint Surg* [Am] 51:713–716.

46. Raugstad TS, Harbo K, Hogberg A, Skeie S (1982): Anterior interbody fusion of the lumbar spine. *Acta Orthop Scand* 53:561–565.

47. Sage FP (1975): Post-operative fracture in the lumbar facets following lumbar disc surgery. *J Bone Joint Surg* [Am] 57:1173.

48. Schofferman L, Schofferman J, Zucherman J, Gunthorpe H, Hsu K, Picetti G, Goldthwaite N, White A (1989): Occult infections causing persistent low-back pain. *Spine* 14:417–419.

49. Schonstrom N (1988): *The narrow lumbar spinal canal and the size of the cauda equina in man.* Department of Orthopaedics, Gothenburg University, Sahlgren Hospital, Goteborg, Sweden.

50. Spangfort EV (1972): The lumbar disc herniation: A computer-aided analysis of 2,504 operations. *Acta Orthop Scand* [Supp] 142:1–95.

51. Spengler DM (1982): Lumbar discectomy: Results with limited disc excision and selective foraminotomy. *Spine* 7:604–706.

52. Spengler DM, Freeman C, Westbrook R, Miller JW (1980): Low-back pain following multiple lumbar spine procedures. Failure of initial selection. *Spine* 5:356–360.

53. Stokes IA, Counts DF, Frymoyer JW (1989): Experimental instability in the rabbit lumbar spine. *Spine* 14:68–72.

54. van Akkerveeken PF (1989): Lateral stenosis of the lumbar spine. Libertas Drukwerkservice bv, Utrecht, The Netherlands.

55. Vanharanta H, Guyer RD, Ohnmeiss DD, Stith WJ, Sachs BL, Aprill C, Spivey M, Rashbaum RF, Hochschuler SH, Vedeman T, Selby DK, Terry A, Mooney V (1988): Disc deterioration in low-back syndromes. A prospective, multi-center CT/discography study. *Spine* 13:1349–1351.

56. Waddell G, McCulloch JA, Kummel E, Venner RM (1980): Non-organic physical signs in low-back pain. *Spine* 5:117–125.

57. Walsh TR, Weinstein JN, Spratt KF, Lehmann TR, Aprill CN, Sayre H, Found E (1989): Lumbar discography: A controlled, prospective study of normal volunteers to determine the false-positive

rate. Presented to the International Society for the Study of the Lumbar Spine.

58. Watkins RG (1987): Summary of etiologies of postlaminectomy syndrome. In: Watkins RG, Collis JS, eds. *Lumbar discectomy and laminectomy.* Rockville, Maryland: Aspen Publishers, Inc., pp. 267–269.

59. Weber H (1983): Lumbar disc herniation. A controlled, prospective study with ten years of observation. *Spine* 8:131–140.

60. Wiesel SW (1985): The multiply operated lumbar spine. *Instructional Course Lectures, XXXIV,* pp. 68–77.

61. Wiesel SW, Feffer HL, Borenstein DG (1988): Evaluation and outcome of low-back pain of unknown etiology. *Spine* 13:679–680.

Segmental Instability

The Adult Spine: Principles and Practice,
J. W. Frymoyer, Editor-in-Chief.
Raven Press, Ltd., New York © 1991.

CHAPTER 90

Segmental Instability

Overview and Classification

John W. Frymoyer

The normal functional spinal unit (FSU) is inherently a stable structure, whereas the spine as a whole is an unstable structure when divorced from its restraining muscles. This point is emphasized by the capacity of individual lumbar functional spinal units to withstand substantial compression, tension, torsional, and shear loads in laboratory experiments, as well as the capacity of the intact spine in living individuals to withstand both single and repetitive overloads. However, an intact spine stripped of its muscles can only withstand axial loads of 4 kg before buckling occurs (41). These later observations are important to the understanding of spinal deformities, particularly scoliosis and kyphosis associated with neuromuscular disorders, but have minimal relevance to the clinical diagnosis and treatment of most conditions affecting the adult lumbar spine. The most important issue has been to qualitatively and quantitatively describe what constitutes instability in individual spinal units and to apply this knowledge to clinical diagnosis and treatment.

This chapter will consider some of the available information regarding the definition, clinical classification, and treatment of segmental instabilities which affect the adult lumbar spine.

J. W. Frymoyer, M.D.: Professor of Orthopaedics; Director, McClure Musculoskeletal Research Center, Department of Orthopaedics and Rehabilitation, University of Vermont, Burlington, Vermont, 05405.

DEFINITION OF SPINAL INSTABILITY

A myriad of biomechanical and clinical definitions have been developed to describe spinal instability. At the most simplistic level instability is a lack of stability, which in mechanical terms means decreased stiffness of the FSU, increased mobility, or abnormal motions. These descriptors are implicit in the definition given by the American Academy of Orthopaedic Surgeons which states: "Segmental instability is an abnormal response to applied loads, characterized by motion in motion segments beyond normal constraints" (3). Pope and Panjabi (65) graphically described these attributes as shown in Figure 1. To this definition has often been added the concept that alterations in spinal mechanics place neurologic structures at risk. This later conceptualization is implicit in Hippocrates's early observation: "When a gibbosity seizes a person, it occasions a crisis of the then existing disease" (Hippocrates, *On Articulations*).

The mechanical attributes of decreased stiffness and the risk to neurologic structures have been combined in the clinical checklist for spinal stability developed by Posner et al. (66). These investigators sectioned posterior structures of the FSU and determined the resultant instability in carefully controlled biomechanical experiments. Their clinical scoring method which has particular applicability to lumbar spine trauma is shown in Table 1. Others have used somewhat similar biomechanical experiments to study spinal destabilization and re-

TABLE 1. *Clinical checklist for lumbar spine trauma*

Element	Point value[a]
Cauda equina damage	3
Relative flexion sagittal plane translation > 8% or extension sagittal plane translation > 9%	2
Relative flexion sagittal plane rotation < −9%	2
Anterior elements destroyed	2
Posterior elements destroyed	2
Dangerous loading anticipated	1

With permission from ref. 66.
[a] Total of 5 or more = clinically unstable.

stabilization. For example, McAfee and associates (42) have developed animal models of instability, which are based on removal of the vertebral body to simulate anterior column disruption, resection of the anterior column and removal of posterior spinal ligaments to simulate combined anterior and posterior column destabilization. Based on the analysis of CT scans McAfee et al. (42) have also argued for the importance of the anterior, posterior, and middle columns to stability. However, these experiments have proven less satisfactory in the definition of instabilities associated with spondylolisthesis and spinal degeneration. In these later conditions, acute disruption of spinal structures has not occurred; instead there is a slow evolution of an unstable condition, most

TABLE 2. *Lumbar segmental instabilities*

I. Fractures and fracture-dislocations

II. Infections involving anterior columns
  A. With progressive loss of vertebral body height and deformity despite treatment with antibiotics
  B. With progressing neurologic symptoms despite treatment with antibiotics (if accompanied by progressive loss of vertebral body height and deformity)

III. Primary and metastatic neoplasms
  A. With progressive loss of vertebral body height and deformity
  B. With progressing neurologic symptoms not resulting from direct tumor involvement of the spinal cord, cauda equina, or nerve roots (e.g., caused by progressive loss of vertebral body height and deformity)
  C. Post-surgical (after resection of neoplasm)

IV. Spondylolisthesis
  A. Isthmic spondylolisthesis
    1. L5–S1 progressive deformity in a child, particularly when accompanied by radiographic risk signs (this lesion is rarely unstable in adults)
    2. L4–L5 deformity (probably unstable in adults)

V. Degenerative instabilities

VI. Scoliosis (any progressive deformity in a child—subclassified by the criteria of the Scoliosis Research Society)

Modified with permission from ref. 26.

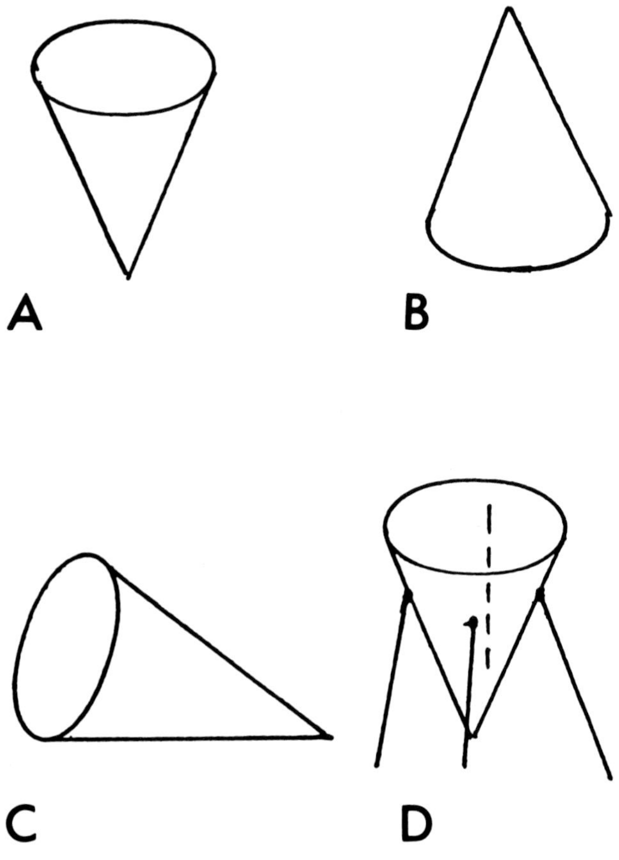

FIG. 1. The concept of instability as illustrated by a series of cones. **A:** If the cones are slightly displaced, cone A will move into a new position of equilibrium (unstable equilibrium). **B:** Cone B will return to the same position (stable equilibrium). **C:** Cone C will stay in the displaced position (neutral equilibrium). **D:** The unstable cone is made stable by the addition of guy wires to hold it in position (with permission from ref. 65).

likely the result of subacute, chronic, repetitive mechanical overloads. Because of the subtle nature of the mechanical forces, these conditions have proven to be far more elusive to define in biomechanical and clinical terms. My definition (21) combines many previously described attributes:

> Segmental instability is a loss of spinal motion segment stiffness, such that force application to that motion segment produces greater displacement(s) than would be seen in a normal structure, resulting in a painful condition, the potential for progressive deformity, and neurologic structures at risk.

CLINICAL CLASSIFICATION OF SPINAL INSTABILITY

An overall classification of segmental instability is given in Table 2 (26). The clinical and radiologic descriptions of instabilities associated with trauma, tumors, infections, and spondylolisthesis will be found in other chapters, as well as the pattern of involvement of the anterior, middle, and posterior columns which produce these conditions. In general, tumors, infections, and trauma produce mechanical weakening of the anterior and middle columns (Fig. 2). As previously noted, the instability associated with trauma can be well-defined in biomechanical and clinical terms, because the condition

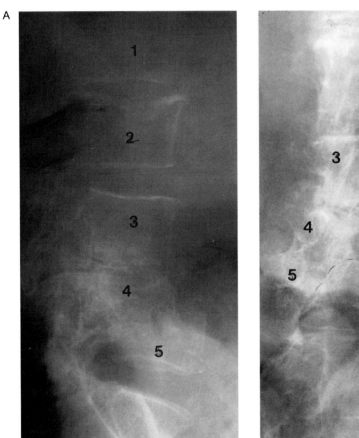
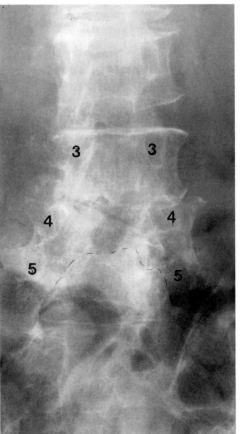

FIG. 2. This patient illustrates dramatically an unequivocal instability. She had undergone decompression three months earlier followed by progressive back pain. She was transferred to our hospital with impending cauda equina syndrome, and the AP **(A)** and lateral **(B)** radiographs are shown here. The body of L4 is totally destroyed and its remnants displaced posteriorly on L5. She was treated by anterior debridement and bone grafting, followed two weeks later by posterior fusion with pedicle fixation.

is easily simulated under experimental conditions. Moreover, the principles derived from traumatic conditions are generally transferable to infection and tumors. The remaining subgroups of instability, particularly those associated with spinal degeneration, are more difficult to define rigorously in mechanical and clinical terms.

DEGENERATIVE INSTABILITIES

Knutsson first observed in 1944 that degeneration of the lumbar intervertebral disc was associated with increased translations of the affected spinal motion segment, as measured by flexion/extension radiographs (2,34). Later, other investigators replicated his experiments and added other directions for the applied stress such as lateral bending (39). By 1957, Morgan and King (49) concluded that 25% of all back pain was the result of segmental instability. It was also generally accepted, after Mixter and Barr's (48) description of the clinical syndrome of lumbar disc herniation, that surgical removal of a disc weakened ("destabilized") a motion segment; this general conceptualization formed the rationale for spinal fusion in those patients. The seminal work of Kirkaldy-Willis (33) added greater credence to concepts of instability. Based on detailed anatomic and pathologic experiments, he concluded the degenerative process occurred in three sequential phases: dysfunction, instability, and restabilization. The dysfunctional phase was least well-defined, and includes annular tears and earlier nuclear degeneration, sometimes in combination with early osteoarthritic changes in the cartilage of the articular facets. The unstable phase includes reduction of the disc height, gross morphologic changes consistent with disc degeneration, laxity of the spinal ligaments and facet joints, and results in "increased and abnormal range of movement." The later physiologic changes in the disc, such as increased collagen and decreased mucopolysaccharides, decreased water content, and spinal osteophytes tend to reverse this process and result in increased spinal stiffness, i.e., restabilization. In this last stage, spinal stenosis is a possible clinical sequela.

Biomechanical studies in vivo and in vitro have provided some confirmation of Kirkaldy-Willis' overall description. The basic laboratory studies, in general, have involved an analysis of repetitively loaded functional spinal units, or the analysis of the mechanical behavior of degenerative specimens. Loss of stiffness, accompanied by annular tears, or even nuclear disruption, have been produced in the laboratory by repetitive loading cycles which simulate normal human exposures (1,8,40). In other experiments, load applications to degenerative segments have revealed loss of stiffness which in some specimens is quite dramatic (81). Similar observations have

been made by other investigators (13,32,50,60). Mathematical models have also been devised to study how the experimental observations might be modified by the presence of active muscle vectors (61). Holmes and associates (28) have attempted to quantify these alterations in mechanical behavior in vitro and in patients undergoing spinal surgery. They have reported alterations in the stiffness as a function of disc degeneration (Fig. 3).

The difficulty has been to translate these elegant observations into clinical, radiographic, or biomechanical descriptions that could serve as a basis for rational treatment. This problem is detailed by Dupuis et al. (11), who reported, "Little is known about the true clinical presentation of motion segment laxity." In an attempt to overcome this problem, Kirkaldy-Willis and Farfan (33) suggest we have unduly complicated the clinical definition, and define its existence as a condition when "minor perturbations produce acute pain." To describe this situation they used a "catastrophe fold" (Fig. 4). We have not found this description to be particularly useful in clinical practice, particularly as a guide to treatment. The nonspecific symptoms include low back pain, sclerotomatous pain radiating into the upper thighs, dynamic root entrapments, i.e., recurrent sciatica which is positional, catching sensations in the spine, and intermittent postural scoliosis. These symptoms, as will be seen in other chapters, are also associated with discogenic low back pain, the facet syndrome and central lumbar disc herniations, as well as non-specific lumbosacral strains and sprains.

Clinical signs have included deformity such as inter-

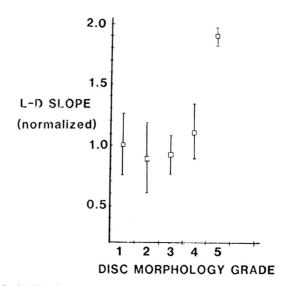

FIG. 3. The force necessary to distract vertebral specimens (L-D, load deflection) compared with disc morphology. Note loss of stiffness in Grades 2 and 3, while in Grade 4 stiffness is restored (with permission from ref. 28).

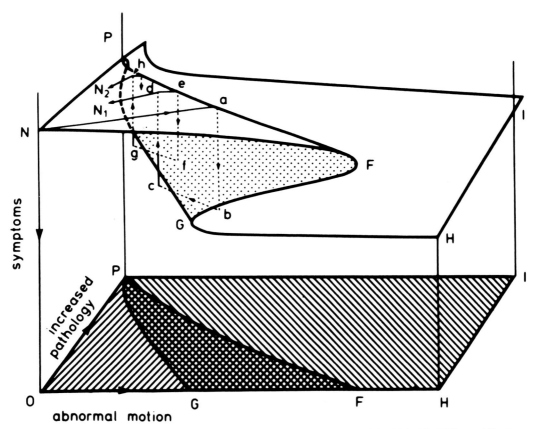

FIG. 4. The catastrophe fold theory of segmental instability proposed by Kirkaldy-Willis and Farfan graphically demonstrates that minimal changes in an unstable system can be accompanied by major changes in function (with permission from ref. 33).

mittent rotoscoliosis, disruptions in the normal smooth arc of lumbar flexion and extension (the "instability" catch) (51), and the intermittent presence of objective neurologic signs such as depressed reflexes. Some observers have noted the presence of a step deformity or the palpation of abnormal motions during flexion and extension, and hypertrophied bands of muscle at the affected level(s) (64). Attempts to establish intra- and interobserver reliability for such observations have not proven successful in some clinical studies (54).

Radiologic observations and measurements have been the most consistently reported methods to establish instability, but again there is considerable controversy. These findings include disc space narrowing, which is without doubt a sign of significant morphologic degeneration. Asymmetric disc space narrowing is an additional observation of questionable significance. However, neither of these findings have proven particularly reliable, because of the common age-related finding of disc space narrowing in asymptomatic individuals (18).

A second radiographic observation has been the presence of traction spurs, as described by Macnab (Fig. 5) (45). Based on the analysis of spinal anatomy, he sug-

gested the traction spur resulted from tensile stresses being applied by the outer annular fibers which attach to the vertebral body. The claw spur was hypothesized to be the result of compressive overloads and a benign finding. This conceptualization is consistent with epidemiologic studies (29) as well as analysis of anatomic specimens (52), which indicate the claw spur is an adaptive and mechanically advantageous response to spinal overloads. However, more detailed clinical studies have shown traction spurs to be a variable finding (74).

The third and probably most significant observation has been the presence of spinal malalignments, particularly when these were observed to progress in spinal sequential radiographs of patients with increasing symptoms. The two best examples of this condition are degenerative spondylolisthesis and degenerative scoliosis. In the first instance, Junghann's (31) original anatomic descriptions and Macnab's (44) subsequent clinical and radiographic analysis strongly implied that degenerative spondylolisthesis was a progressive deformity. Newman and Stone (53) measured these changes which averaged 2 mm every four years. Similar observations have been made about the progression of adult de-

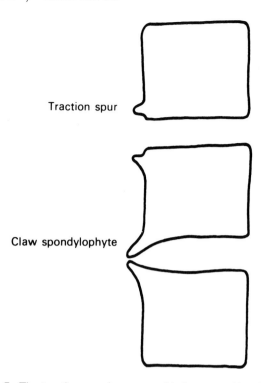

Traction spur

Claw spondylophyte

FIG. 5. The traction spur is proposed to be caused by abnormal tension on the outer annular fibers resulting from shear stresses. This appearance is different from that of the claw spur, which is thought to be a physiologic response to compression stresses (with permission from ref. 45).

generative scoliosis (25), and to a lesser degree with retrolisthetic deformities. However, the more common assessment of instability has been based on the early radiographic observations of Knutsson (34). He defined instability as 3 mm or more of anterior translation measured between flexion and extension radiographs. A variety of methods have been developed to more precisely quantify these displacements including those of Frymoyer and associates (17), Arkin (5), Lindahl (39), and Dupuis (11) (Fig. 6). Most recently Woody et al. (82) determined the intra- and inter-observer errors for such measurements and concluded that a minimum of 4 mm forward displacement was necessary at the L3–L4 and L4–L5 levels to define instability, while at the L5–S1 level, displacements of greater than 5 mm were necessary for accurate measurement. Others have noted that greater accuracies may be possible and that only 7% of normal subjects had displacements of 3 mm (6).

It has been suggested that the large magnitudes of displacements necessary to measure instability by simple flexion/extension radiographs are too specific. In this perspective, instability may be too subtle a displacement to be identified and measured. Thus, attempts have been made to identify these proposed subtle patterns of three-dimensional spine motion. The earlier attempts to quantify spinal motion more precisely were based on biplanar radiographs which allow accurate measurement of 1 mm

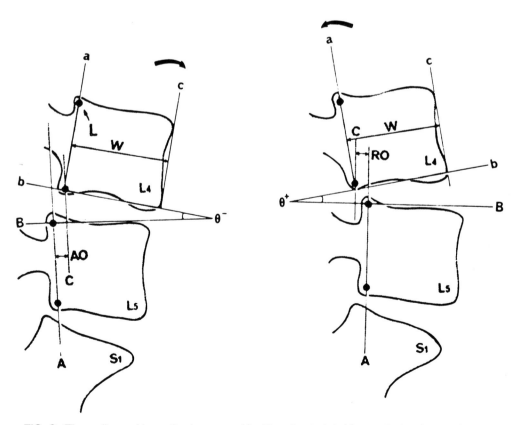

FIG. 6. The radiographic method proposed by Dupuis et al. (with permission from ref. 11).

translations and 2 degree rotations (57,59,70,80). Despite intensive research in this area, in general this technique has produced disappointing and non-useful clinical tools (74). An even greater level of accuracy is made possible by the implantation of small, target metallic markers (57–59). When this technique is combined with biplanar radiography, resolution at a level of 0.1 to 0.2 mm is possible. To date, such techniques have not been applied to a series of patients with suspected segmental instabilities.

It has also been suggested that many instabilities do not occur at the extremes of flexion and extension, which is the usual technique utilized in routine clinical examination and biplanar radiographic studies. This notion is strengthened by the clinical observation that the "instability catch" occurs during the mid-range of flexion or extension. It is also postulated that muscle splinting to maintain the flexed or extended posture might also reduce the unstable segments. Attempts to overcome this barrier have included other forms of static loading, dynamic sequential radiographs, and cinefluo-

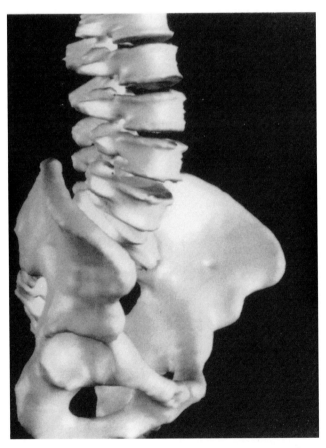

FIG. 7. Computer-generated model of the spine taken from spinal motion radiographs. Using these models, the goal is to measure precisely three-dimensional spinal motion (with special permission from Herbert M. Reynolds, Ph.D., and Richard Hallgren, Ph.D., Department of Biomechanics, College of Osteopathic Medicine, Michigan State University).

rography. Friberg (16) studied patients with degenerative spondylolisthesis and retrospondylolisthesis by first applying traction, and then a standard axial compressive load. He observed all 7 patients with degenerative spondylolisthesis and 37 out of 65 patients with retrospondylolisthesis had increased displacements when the traction (reducing force) was compared with the axial compressive (displacing force) loading condition. He also observed that patients who underwent displacement had a greater severity of symptoms. These observations have been subjected to a rigorous analysis, which concluded that the observed displacements were within the measurement error of the technique and, thus, invalid.

The second method of dynamic sequential radiographs at 5 to 10 degree increments through a complete arc of motion has been promoted in particular by Gertzbein (22). He devised an elegant system of measurement based upon the centrode of motion. In early laboratory and clinical experiments this method appeared to be extremely promising. Later analyses of his clinical technique has led him to abandon this approach and undertake other measurements of centrode displacement, the value of which remains uncertain (23).

As an extension of biplanar radiography, biplanar cinefluorography has been combined with sophisticated image reconstruction to provide three-dimensional representations of spinal motion segments moving in space (Fig. 7). To date, the possible clinical value is uncertain.

In addition to these general technical problems, the other major difficulty in assessing degenerative instabilities has been the presence of the radiographic signs of instability in asymptomatic individuals. For example, Valkenburg and Haanen (76) have demonstrated that as many as 10% of female patients over the age of 60 have grade 2 or greater degenerative spondylolisthesis, yet the majority have not experienced symptoms. This general problem is not unique to segmental instability, as noted in other chapters in this book.

Lastly, it has been proposed that a trial of bracing should produce relief in a patient with instability. In general, the results have been non-diagnostic, possibly because customary spinal braces produce little or no spinal immobilization (15). A more definitive immobilization has been accomplished by the use of external fixators as proposed by Olerud (57). He reported significant pain reduction by this technique was followed by improved clinical results in patients who subsequently underwent spinal fusion. This result has been replicated by others, but seems applicable to only a small subgroup of patients with unrelenting and severely disabling symptoms, most of whom have undergone previous spinal surgery (56).

Despite these major problems in clinical and radiographic definition, the diagnosis of instability can be considered in patients with continuing mechanical low back pain, particularly when the symptoms, signs, and radiographic findings are well correlated. In other publica-

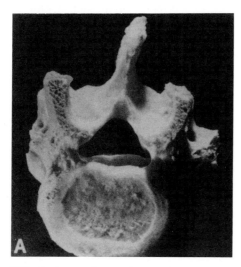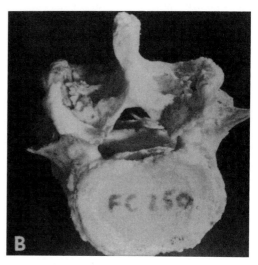

FIG. 8. Anatomic specimen of degenerative spondylolisthesis demonstrating the rotational deformity best appreciated on these **(A and B)** axial views (with permission from ref. 12).

tions, I have proposed a classification and criteria for degenerative segmental instabilities, which represents an expansion of an earlier classification system (Table 3) (19).

1. The patient has a deformity apparent on static radiographs which increases during spinal motion or compressive/tension loads beyond normal measurement errors, or can be documented to increase on serial radiographs, in association with progressive symptoms. Conversely, non-specific findings include disc space narrowing seen in plain radiographs, diffuse disc bulge observed in CT and MRI, or altered T2 signal intensity on MRI.

2. The patient's clinical symptoms and signs are con-

TABLE 3. Degenerative segmental instabilities

Primary instabilities
1. Axial rotational instability
2. Translational instability
3. Retrolisthetic instability
4. Progressing degenerative scoliosis
5. Disc disruption syndrome

Secondary instabilities
1. Post-disc excision—Subclassified according to the pattern of instability as described under primary instabilities
2. Post-decompressive laminectomy
    A. Accentuation of pre-existent deformity
    B. New deformity, i.e., no deformity existed at the time of original decompression. Further subclassified as for primary instabilities
3. Post-spinal fusion
    A. Above or below a spinal fusion, subclassified as for primary instabilities
    B. Pseudarthrosis
4. Post-chemonucleolysis

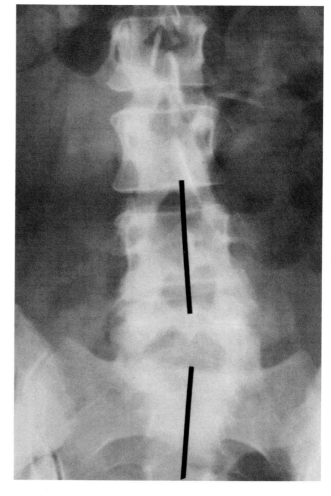

FIG. 9. An AP radiograph of a patient with suspected instability at L4-L5 demonstrating the misalignment of the spinous processes of L3-L4 with those of L5-S1-S2.

sistent with the lumbar segment which appears unstable. Strongly suggestive findings would be recurrent sciatica with accompanying neurologic findings consistent with that level. Less certain, but suggestive findings incorporate Kirkaldy-Willis and Farfan's (33) observation that the history should be characterized by recurrent, usually acute episodes of low back pain produced by mechanical stresses of diminishing magnitude. The importance of rotoscoliosis and instability catches are uncertain symptoms and signs.

3. The complaints of low back pain or pain on spinal motion are non-specific symptoms.

SPECIFIC PATTERNS OF INSTABILITY ASSOCIATED WITH SPINAL DEGENERATION

Despite the hope that sophisticated radiographic analyses might further refine the diagnosis of segmental instability (19), clinical syndromes have yet to be correlated with a specific radiologic pattern of instability (11,74). The classification given, therefore, is based on a combina-

tion of the radiographic finding and other determining factors such as prior decompressive surgery.

Primary Instabilities

A primary instability is one where there has been no prior intervention or treatment which might account for the observed deformity.

Type I: Axial Rotational Instability

Farfan's research has demonstrated that torsional stresses are associated with increased laxity of the facet joints or crumpling of the neural arch (12). His anatomic studies have also demonstrated that rotational deformities accompany degenerative spondylolisthesis (Fig. 8). Therefore, it is quite possible that type I and type II are identical lesions (12). It has been hoped that abnormal torsional motions might be identified by biplanar radiography before a more obvious deformity is present. This

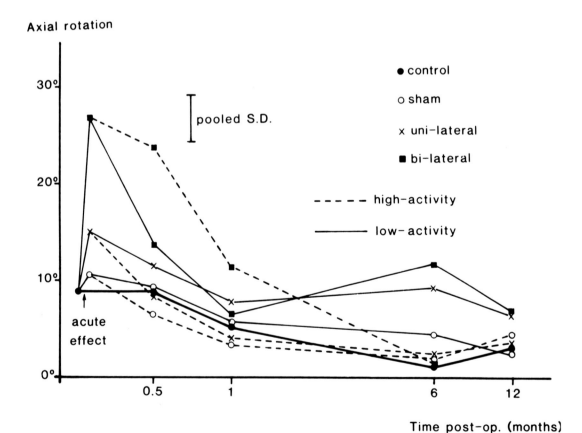

FIG. 10. Rabbits have undergone unilateral facetectomies at the opposite side above and below the disc space level in question, while others have undergone bilateral facetectomies at the same level. The recovery is plotted for the experimental groups, a sham operated group, and a non-operated control group, subjected to high and low activity. Note that initial instability is produced, followed by evidence of restabilization, which is greatest in those animals who undergo higher levels of exercise (with permission from ref. 74).

hope was not realized in one clinical study (79). However, Mimura et al. (47) demonstrated the average rotation was 35% of the total lumbar motion in patients with degenerative spondylolisthesis, whereas the comparable percentage was 15% in normal subjects. Kirkaldy-Willis and Farfan (33) have also reported dynamic CT scans taken with imposed axial rotatory stresses may define instability. A suggestive plain radiographic finding for a rotational deformity is a malalignment of the spinous processes as seen on anteroposterior radiographs (Fig. 9). Myelograms have shown a pedicle to pedicle defect. Based on his analysis of the pathoanatomy of this lesion, Farfan believes a derotation fusion technique is necessary. He distracts the facet and inserts a bone block on the side towards which axial rotation is directed.

Attempts to produce this deformity in animal models have also produced varied results. Sullivan and Farfan (75) demonstrated radiographic evidence of instability after excision of contralateral facets, above and below the disc level of interest in rabbits. Cauchoix and associates (9) showed histologic evidence of disc degenera-

tion using the same model. However, Stokes and Frymoyer (74) could not demonstrate biochemical evidence of degeneration in the disc with this animal model, despite the presence of instability. Restabilization was identified when the animals were analyzed six months after the surgical intervention (Fig. 10).

Type II: Translational Instability

Translational instability represents degenerative spondylolisthesis, and a positive Knutsson's sign is thought to be the earliest radiographic sign. In addition, disc space narrowing and traction spurs have been observed preceding or accompanying the actual deformity (45). Additional signs may include segmentation abnormality or elongation of the L5 transverse process, which effectively

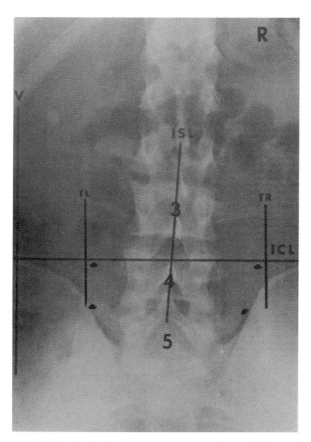

FIG. 11. A variety of measurements may be made from AP radiographs which have been thought to have significance to spinal stability, particularly at the L4-L5 interspace. The most important is the interaction of the intercristal line (**ICL**) with the lumbar vertebral bodies. When the line interacts with the body of L4, the spine is relatively deep seated and the L4-L5 interspace well protected (with permission from ref. 18).

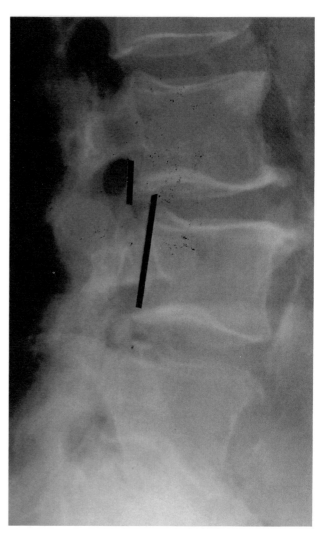

FIG. 12. An extension lateral lumbar radiograph of a man with increasing low back pain, accompanied by pain most consistent with L4 nerve root irritation. Note the posterior displacement occurring at the L3-L4 level, accompanied by spurs, which at this point appear to be claw in characteristic.

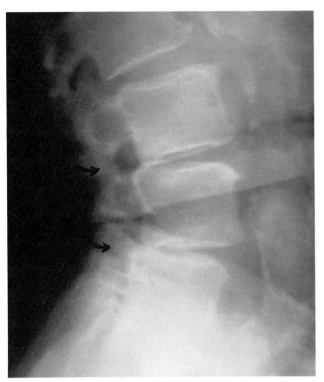

FIG. 13. This 70-year-old female had undergone disc excision at L4-L5 13 years earlier. Here she presents with low back pain and predominantly neurologic evidence of L3-L4 disc disease. Note the anterior translational deformities occurring both at L3-L4 and at L4-L5, paradoxically with extension. After investigation, it was concluded that L3-L4 was the dominant source of symptoms.

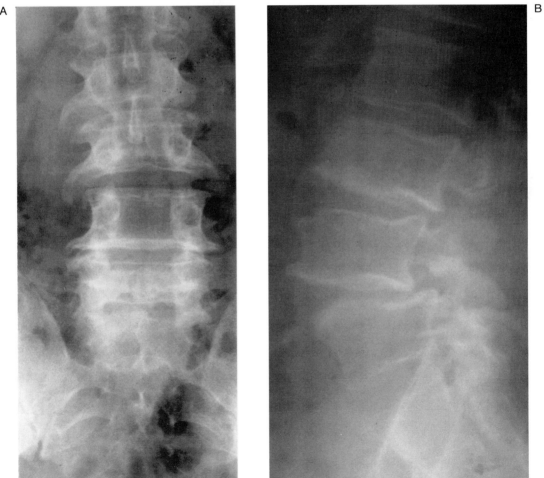

A

B

FIG. 14. Anteroposterior **(A)** and lateral **(B)** radiographs of a 60-year-old male who underwent extensive laminectomies. He presents with increasing pain. The AP film demonstrates the extent of decompression, while on the lateral an accentuation of a pre-existent spondylolisthesis is seen at L4-L5, accompanied by a new retrolisthetic deformity at L3-L4.

stabilizes the L5–S1 level and exposes the L4–L5 level to greater stresses (Fig. 11) (43,69). These same findings are also reported in association with type I.

Females are at additional risk because they are four times more likely to require surgical intervention (69), even though the deformity is only two times more common in the general population (76). Diabetics are also reported to be at greater risk (69). This is of particular interest because diabetic animals demonstrate greater disc degeneration than their non-diabetic controls (27). However, animal models used to simulate this deformity have not produced a progressive instability (74). Other explanations for the deformity have included abnormal and increased facet angles, interpreted to be a congenital dysplasia of those joints (4).

Type III: Retrolisthetic Instability

Retrolisthetic instability is most common at the L5–S1 levels. Lehmann and Brand (37) observed 30% of their male subjects with low back pain had increased retrolisthesis on spinal extension (Fig. 12). In later stages,

degeneration of the facet joints may lead to symptoms of lateral spinal stenosis. This deformity is thought by some to be best treated by a distraction device such as Knodt rods (20) (see Chapter 95).

Type IV: Degenerative Scoliosis

Development de novo of a scoliotic deformity in late adulthood has become more appreciated in the past 5 years (25). Lateral deviation of the spine is associated with significant rotational deformities and symptoms of central or lateral recess spinal stenosis or back pain are common indications for spinal surgery (see Chapter 65). Recent reviews indicate decompression alone is insufficient treatment in many patients (25,71). Spinal fusion with pedicle fixation is recommended by some authors.

Type V: Internal Disc Disruption

Internal disc disruption will be considered in depth in Chapter 97. It is questionable if this condition is unstable.

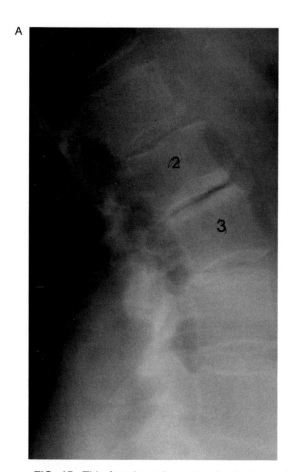 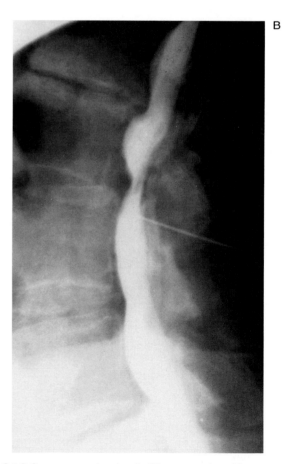

FIG. 15. This female underwent a laminotomy at L2-L3 2 years previously. **A:** She presents with an increasing scoliosis, pain, recurrent radiculopathy, and a retrolisthetic slip at L2-L3, with minor forward slip at L3-L4. **B:** A myelogram shows wasting at both L2-L3 and L3-L4.

Secondary Instabilities

Type I: Post-Disc Excision

A positive Knutsson's sign has been observed in 20% of patients who have undergone post-disc excision, but the majority are asymptomatic (17). The finding is most common at the L4–L5 level and in females, thus sharing a similarity with type II, primary lesions (Fig. 13). Symptoms sufficient to require later stabilization occurred in only 3% of the patients. Retrolisthetic deformities may also occur after simple disc excision. Although there is no definite data, the clinical impression is that L5–S1 levels are more commonly affected. These lesions seem relatively uncommon.

Type II: Post-Decompressive Laminectomy

A. Accentuation of Pre-Existent Deformity

After extensive spinal decompression, accentuation of the pre-existent deformity is sometimes observed, but it is uncertain how often this event occurs (Fig. 14). Fur-thermore, accentuation of the deformity is often asymptomatic. Reynolds and Wiltse (67) and Johnsson (30) noted radical facetectomy for degenerative spondylolisthesis always was followed by increased deformity, but frequently was unassociated with symptoms. A similar observation was made by Feffer et al. (14), although they thought the clinical results were somewhat improved if fusion was performed. Predispositions to increased deformity include a greater disc space height at the time of decompression, the absence of claw osteophytes, the removal of the disc at the time of decompression, and a younger age group (67). The presence of these predictive factors has been used as an indication for fusion at the time of decompression.

B. Development of a New Deformity After Laminectomy

The development of a new deformity after laminectomy is reported to be most common in young patients who have undergone extensive decompression for congenital or mixed spinal stenosis (Fig. 15) (30). In one clinical report, the likelihood of this occurrence was much greater than the 3.7% reported by Lee (36). There

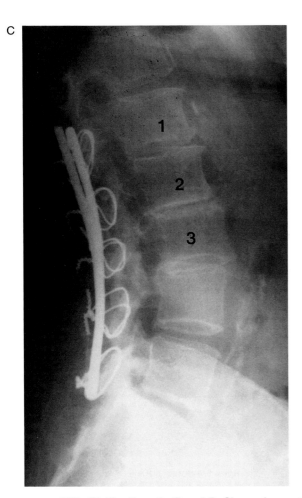
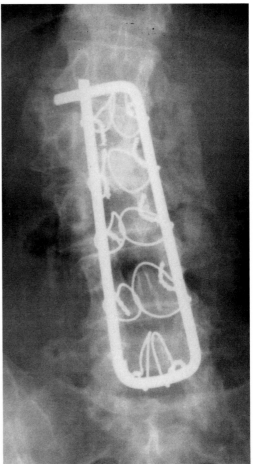

FIG. 15 *(Continued).* **C and D:** She underwent decompression and fusion with Luque rods.

is now sufficient biomechanical data to predict which patients are at risk. Panjabi et al. (62) have demonstrated 50% of both facets or 100% of one facet can be excised without significantly altering the stiffness of human intervertebral segments. This is significantly greater than the traditional teaching that only one-third of each facet could be removed without altering stability. Furthermore, Panjabi's studies of facetectomy in a canine model mimic the results seen in the previously illustrated rabbit model (63). Thus, these studies indicate there may be a significant stabilization possible even in significantly destabilized segments probably from scar formation.

Type III: Post-Spinal Fusion

A. Above or Below a Fusion

Spinal fusion increases the shear stress in the next mobile vertebral segment based upon biomechanical and clinical studies. However, there is a poor correlation between the radiologic appearance and the clinical symptoms reported by the patient. Despite the fact that 20% of patients who had undergone L4 to sacrum fusions had a positive Knutsson's sign, only 4% of our patients had required an extension of their fusion at a mean follow-up of 13.7 years (Fig. 16) (17). In contrast, 20% of a small patient subset who had undergone L5 to sacrum fusion had required extension of their fusion. A similar obser-

vation was also made by Lehmann et al. (38) in their lengthy follow-up analysis. They noted 45% of the patients had instability but most were asymptomatic. It is debatable what is the greater cause of symptoms, stenosis or instability. Brodsky (7) reported stenosis was the major problem, whereas Lehmann et al. (38) reported stenosis was usually associated with instability.

Biomechanical data gives a scientific basis for the development of instability. Studies that utilized biplanar radiography have demonstrated increased shear forces at the first mobile segment above a fusion (70), a point confirmed by in vitro biomechanical analyses (67), and biomechanical modeling (55). In the studies by Nolte et al. (55) these stresses were reduced by placing the fusion mass closer to the anatomic center of vertebral rotation such as transverse process fusion. Based on uncontrolled clinical experiments (35), it is also suggested that the rigidity of the fixation, such as the use of pedicle screws, increases the risk of accelerated degeneration.

B. Pseudarthrosis

It can be debated if pseudarthrosis represents an unstable spinal condition, except in those instances where facet excision in combination with fusion has failed. In patients fused for lumbar disc protrusion, failures of the fusion are identified in as many as 30%, but less than half are symptomatic (10,17,38). If low back symptoms are

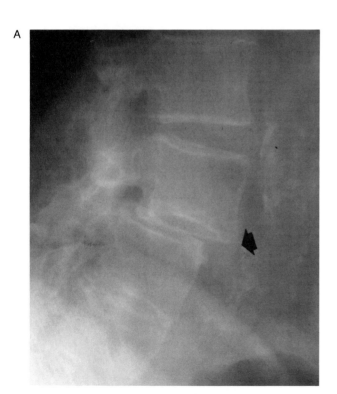

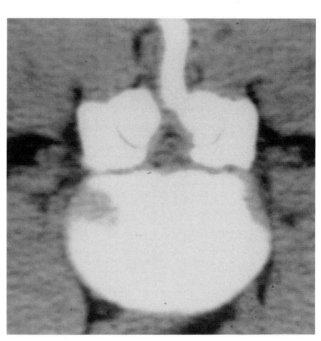

FIG. 16. Female patient who underwent fusion L4 to sacrum many years previously. She now presents with symptoms of L3-L4 stenosis and back pain. The lateral radiograph **(A)** shows the slip L3 on L4 that has occurred. The CT scan **(B)** demonstrates stenosis at the affected L3-L4 level.

significant, the role of pseudarthrosis in pain production can be tested by local anesthetic injections or discography (46). The sensitivity and specificity of those diagnostic tests, however, have not been subjected to rigorous evaluation. This observation may be of significance because successful repair of the fusion leads to symptom relief in only 50% of the patients we studied (17).

C. Acquired Spondylolysis

Acquired spondylolysis is almost exclusively a problem with posterior midline fusion, where it occurs in 1% of patients. Rolander's (68) biomechanical studies would suggest it is the result of abnormal mechanical stresses,

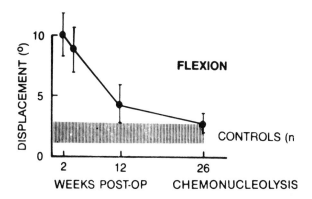

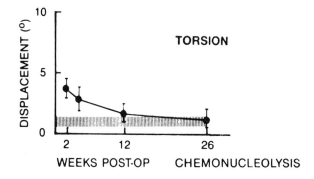

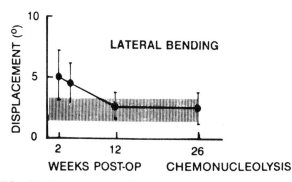

FIG. 17. Displacement after chemonucleolysis for flexion, torsion, and lateral bending. Note that the initial displacements (instability) recover over time (with permission from ref. 73).

but clinical analyses suggest it may be the result of decortication at the pars interarticularis (17).

Type IV: Instability Following Chemonucleolysis

Significant low back pain is recorded in 20% to 67% of patients who undergo chymopapain injections (72). Although the usual duration is 6 weeks, Spencer found 41% of patients have continued complaints 6 months after the injection. To test the hypothesis that chymopapain induces "instability," experiments were conducted in dogs. Figure 17 demonstrates the altered mechanics of the functional spinal units of injected animals, indicating the initial instability is followed by restabilization (73). In their long-term follow-up analysis of chymopapain versus disc excision, Weinstein and associates (77) found little difference in symptoms between the two treatment protocols, but spinal radiographs were not included as part of their analysis. Their clinical results do suggest chymopapain-induced instability is probably no greater in surgical and chymopapain treated patients than in lumbar disc hernias.

Spondylolisthesis

The issue of instability in the various forms of spondylolisthesis is discussed in Chapter 78. In the adult with L5–S1 isthmic spondylolisthesis the lesion would appear to be relatively stable, but when the L4–L5 level is involved, there is a significantly greater likelihood of progression over time, or abnormal and increased motions at the affected level (Fig. 18) (24). It is uncertain if other congenital deformities may present in adulthood with instability (Fig. 19).

SUMMARY

At the current time, there are well-established experimental models of spinal instability associated with fracture, which are generalizable to infections and tumors. This has resulted in mechanical criteria easily utilized in clinical settings. However, the definition of degenerative instability has been more elusive. Experimental animal models which initially demonstrate instability are usually followed by physiologic restabilization. Biomechanical experiments have given considerable insight into the mechanical behavior of degenerative motions and have also demonstrated how chronic, repetitive force applications can produce tissue injury. However, this modest amount of new information has been applicable only to clinical diagnosis. Particularly troubling is the presence of radiographic instability in patients who have no clinical syndromes. Despite these limitations, instability can be identified by radiographic criteria and

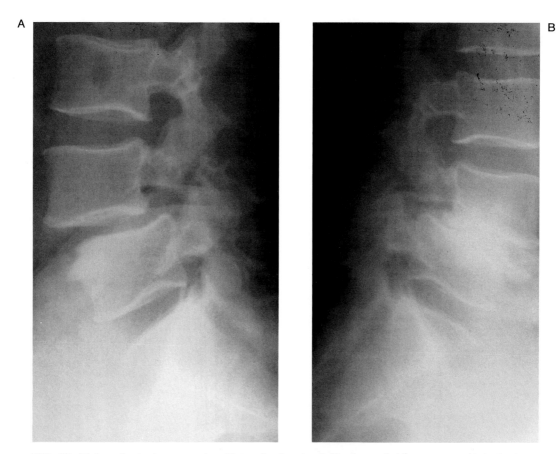

FIG. 18. Male patient who presents with low back pain. **A:** Radiograph 10 years ago. Note the large traction spur and the presence of an isthmic defect at L4-L5. **B:** He now presents with increasing pain and signs of spinal stenosis. Note the modest increase in the slip and the profound disc space narrowing.

A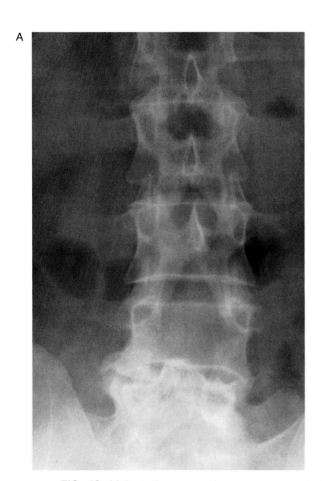

B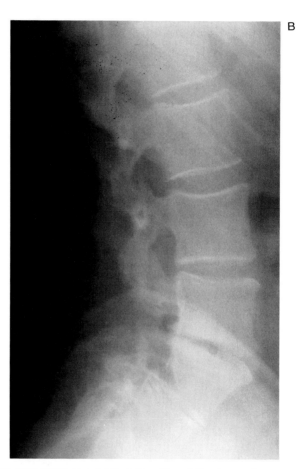

FIG. 19. Male patient treated at another hospital for increasing low back pain with subtle signs of radiculopathy. At operation a duplicated nerve root was found as well as congenital absence of the facet at L4-L5 on the right, and anomalous facet at L4-L5 on the left. His symptoms have worsened. The AP **(A)** shows the laminotomy. The absent facet is not surgically produced. The lateral **(B)** shows the large posterior osteophyte, vacuum sign, and anomalous L5 vertebra. Motion radiography shows decreased movements. The question is whether this represents an instability.

can occur as part of the evolution of the degenerative process, as well as after the surgical and chemical treatment of degenerative disorders. Although these radiographic patterns of instability are not strictly correlated with unique clinical syndromes, recognition of these patterns is important to surgical treatment in the small subset of patients who fail to respond to conservative management.

REFERENCES

1. Adams MA, Hutton WC (1982): Prolapsed intervertebral disc: A hyperflexion injury. *Spine* 7:184–191.
2. Allbrook D (1957): Movements of the lumbar spinal column. *J Bone Joint Surg* [Br] 39:339–345.
3. American Academy of Orthopaedic Surgeons: A glossary on spinal terminology. Chicago: American Academy of Orthopaedic Surgeons, p. 34.
4. Arima T, Mochida J, Nakesko J, Chiba M (1989): A study of the intervertebral joint suggestive of development of degenerative spondylolisthesis. Presented at the meeting of the International Society for the Study of the Lumbar Spine, Kyoto, Japan.
5. Arkin AM (1950): The mechanism of rotation in combination with lateral deviation in the normal spine. *J Bone Joint Surg* [Am] 32:180–188.
6. Boden SD, Wiesel WS (1989): Lumbosacral segmental motion in normal individuals. Presented at the meeting of the International Society for the Study of the Lumbar Spine, Kyoto, Japan.
7. Brodsky AE (1976): Post-laminectomy and post-fusion stenosis of the lumbar spine. *Clin Orthop* 115:130–139.
8. Brown T, Hansen RJ, Yorra AJ (1957): Some mechanical tests on the lumbosacral spine with particular reference to the intervertebral discs: A preliminary report. *J Bone Joint Surg* [Am] 39:1135–1164.
9. Cauchoix J, Yaacubi E, Romero CG, et al (1984): An experimental model of lumbar degenerated discs in rabbits. Presented at the tenth meeting of the International Society for the Study of the Lumbar Spine, Montreal, Canada.
10. DePalma AF, Rothman RH (1968): The nature of pseudarthrosis. *Clin Orthop* 59:113–118.
11. Dupuis PR, Young-Hing K, Cassidy JD, Kirkaldy-Willis WH (1985): Radiologic diagnosis of degenerative lumbar spinal instability. *Spine* 10:262–276.
12. Farfan HF (1980): The pathological anatomy of degenerative spondylolisthesis: A cadaver study. *Spine* 5:412–418.
13. Farfan HF, Gracovetsky S (1984): The nature of instability. *Spine* 9:714–719.
14. Feffer HL, Wiesel SW, Cuckler JM, Rothman RH (1985): Degenerative spondylolisthesis. To fuse or not to fuse. *Spine* 10:287–289.
15. Fidler MW, Plasmans CM (1983): The effect of four types of support on the segmental mobility of the lumbosacral spine. *J Bone Joint Surg* [Am] 65:943–947.
16. Friberg O (1987): Lumbar instability: A dynamic approach by traction—Compression radiography. *Spine* 12:119–129.
17. Frymoyer JW, Hanley EN Jr, Howe J, Kuhlmann D, Matteri RE (1979): A comparison of radiographic findings in fusion and non-fusion patients, ten or more years following lumbar disc surgery. *Spine* 4:435–440.
18. Frymoyer JW, Newberg A, Pope MH, Wilder DG, Clements J, MacPherson B (1984): Spine radiographs in patients with low-back pain. *J Bone Joint Surg* [Am] 66:1048–1055.
19. Frymoyer JW, Selby DK (1985): Segmental instability: Rationale for treatment. *Spine* 10:280–286.
20. Frymoyer JW, Krag MH (1986): Spinal stability and instability: Definitions, classification, and general principles of management. In: Dunsker SB, Schmidek HH, Frymoyer J, Kahn A, eds. *The unstable spine*. New York: Grune & Stratton.
21. Frymoyer JW (1990): Segmental instability. In: Weinstein JN, Wiesel SW, eds. *The lumbar spine.* International Society for the Study of the Lumbar Spine. Philadelphia: WB Saunders.
22. Gertzbein SD, Seligman J, Holtby R, Chan KH, Kapasouri A, Tile M, Cruickshank B (1985): Centrode patterns and segmental instability in degenerative disc disease. *Spine* 10:257–261.
23. Gertzbein SD, Wolfson N, King G (1988): The diagnosis of segmental instability in vivo by centrode length. Presented at the meeting of the International Society for the Study of the Lumbar Spine, Miami, Florida.
24. Grobler L, Haugh L, Wiltse L, Frymoyer J (1989): L4-5 Isthmic spondylolisthesis: Clinical and radiological review of 52 cases. Presented at the meeting of the International Society for the Study of the Lumbar Spine, Kyoto, Japan.
25. Grubb SA, Lipscomb HJ, Coonrad RW (1988): Degenerative adult onset scoliosis. *Spine* 13:241–245.
26. Hazlett JW, Kinnard P (1982): Lumbar apophyseal process excisions and spinal instability. *Spine* 7:171–176.
27. Holm S (1989): Does diabetes induce degenerative processes in the lumbar intervertebral disc? Presented at the meeting of the International Society for the Study of the Lumbar Spine, Kyoto, Japan.
28. Holmes DC, Brown MD, Eckstein EC, et al (1988): Instability assessment of the lumbar functional spinal unit. Presented at the meeting of the International Society for the Study of the Lumbar Spine, Miami, Florida.
29. Hult L (1954): Cervical, dorsal, and lumbar spinal syndromes. *Acta Orthop Scand* 24:174–175.
30. Johnsson KE, Willner S, Johnsson K (1986): Postoperative instability after decompression for lumbar spinal stenosis. *Spine* 11:107–110.
31. Junghanns H (1930): Spondylolisthesen ohne Spalt in Zwischengelenkstueck. *Archiv fuer Orthopadische Unfallchirurgie* 29:118–127.
32. Kazarian LE (1975): Creep characteristics of the human spinal column. *Orthop Clin North Am* 6:3–18.
33. Kirkaldy-Willis WH, Farfan HF (1982): Instability of the lumbar spine. *Clin Orthop* 165:110–123.
34. Knutsson F (1944): The instability associated with disc degeneration in the lumbar spine. *Acta Radiol* 25:593–609.
35. Krag MH, Weinstein JN, Brown MD, Zindrick M, Callahan T (1989): Clinical and scientific rationale for pedicle fixation of the spine. Presented at the American Academy of Orthopaedic Surgeons meeting, Las Vegas, Nevada.
36. Lee C (1983): Lumbar spinal instability (olisthesis) after extensive posterior spinal decompression. *Spine* 8:429–433.
37. Lehmann T, Brand R (1983): Instability of the lower lumbar spine. *Orthop Trans* 7:97.
38. Lehmann TR, Spratt KF, Tozzi JE, Weinstein JN, Reinarz SJ, El-Khoury GY, Colby H (1987): Long-term follow-up of lower lumbar fusion patients. *Spine* 12:97–104.
39. Lindahl O (1966): Determination of the sagittal mobility of the lumbar spine. *Acta Orthop Scand* 37:241–254.
40. Liu YK, Goel VK, DeJong A, Njus GO, Wu HC (1983): Torsional fatigue of the lumbar intervertebral joints. In: *Proceedings of the International Society for the Study of the Lumbar Spine.* Cambridge, England.
41. Lucas D, Bresler B (1961): Stability of ligamentous spine. In: *Biomechanics Laboratory Report 40.* San Francisco: University of California.
42. McAfee PC, Yuan HA, Fredrickson BE, Lubicky JP (1983): The value of computed tomography in thoracolumbar fractures. *J Bone Joint Surg* [Am] 64:461–473.
43. MacGibbon B, Farfan HF (1979): A radiologic survey of various configurations of the lumbar spine. *Spine* 4:258–266.
44. Macnab I (1950): Spondylolisthesis with an intact neural arch—The so-called pseudo-spondylolisthesis. *J Bone Joint Surg* [Br] 32:325–333.
45. Macnab I (1971): The traction spur: An indicator of segmental instability. *J Bone Joint Surg* [Am] 53:663–670.
46. Macnab I, Johnson RG (1985): Localization of symptomatic lumbar pseudarthroses by use of discography. *Clin Orthop* 197:164–170.
47. Mimura M, Moriya K, Takahashi M, et al (1989): Rotational instability in degenerative spondylolisthesis—A possible mechanical etiology of the disease. Presented at the meeting of the International Society for the Study of the Lumbar Spine, Kyoto, Japan.
48. Mixter WJ, Barr JS (1934): Rupture of the intervertebral disc with involvement of the spinal canal. *N Engl J Med* 211:210–215.

49. Morgan FP, King T (1957): Primary instability of lumbar vertebrae as a common cause of low-back pain. *J Bone Joint Surg* [Br] 39:6–22.
50. Nachemson AL, Schultz AB, Berkson MH (1979): Mechanical properties of human lumbar spine motion segments: Influence of age, sex, disc level, and degeneration. *Spine* 4:1–8.
51. Nachemson A (1985): Lumbar spine instability. A critical update and symposium summary. *Spine* 10:290–291.
52. Nathan H (1962): Osteophytes of the vertebral column. An anatomical study of their development according to age, race, and sex with considerations as to their etiology and significance. *J Bone Joint Surg* [Am] 44:243–268.
53. Newman PH, Stone KH (1963): The etiology of spondylolisthesis. *J Bone Joint Surg* [Br] 45:39–59.
54. Nelson RM (1989): *Low back atlas of standardized tests/measures.* NTIS Publication PB 89-165-096.
55. Nolte LP, Hedtmann A, Kramer J, Pingel T (1989): Biomechanical analysis of juxta-fused lumbosacral segments. Presented at the meeting of the International Society for the Study of the Lumbar Spine, Kyoto, Japan.
56. North A, Wilde P, Mulholland A, Webb R (1989): External fixation of the lumbar spine as a predictor of the outcome of spinal fusion. Presented at the meeting of the International Society for the Study of the Lumbar Spine, Kyoto, Japan.
57. Olerud S, Sjostrom L, Karlstrom G, Hamberg M (1986): Spontaneous effect of increased stability of the lower spine in cases of severe chronic back pain—The answer of an external transpeduncular fixation test. *Clin Orthop* 203:67–74.
58. Olsson TH, Selvik G, Willner S (1976): Kinematic analysis of posterolateral fusion in the lumbosacral spine. *Acta Radiologica (Diagnostica)* 17:519–530.
59. Olsson TH, Selvik G, Willner S (1977): Mobility in the lumbosacral spine after fusion studied with the aid of roentgen stereophotogrammetry. *Clin Orthop* 129:181–190.
60. Panjabi MM, Goel V, Summers D (1982): Relationship between chronic instability and disc degeneration. Presented at the meeting of the International Society for the Study of the Lumbar Spine, Toronto, Canada.
61. Panjabi MM, Abumi K, Duranceau J (1988): Spinal stability and intersegmental muscle forces. Presented at the meeting of the International Society for the Study of the Lumbar Spine, Miami, Florida.
62. Panjabi MM, Duranceau JS, Kramer K (1988): Lumbar facetectomies leading to spinal instability. Presented at the meeting of the International Society for the Study of the Lumbar Spine, Miami, Florida.
63. Panjabi MM, Pelker R, Crisco JJ, Thibodeau L, Yamamoto I (1988): Biomechanics of healing of posterior cervical spinal injuries in a canine model. *Spine* 13:803–807.
64. Paris SV (1985): Physical signs of instability. *Spine* 10:277–279.
65. Pope MH, Panjabi M (1985): Biomechanical definitions of spinal instability. *Spine* 10:255–256.
66. Posner I, White AA, Edwards WT, et al (1982): A biomechanical analysis of the clinical stability of the lumbar and lumbosacral spine. *Spine* 7:374–389.
67. Reynolds JB, Wiltse LL (1979): Surgical treatment of degenerative spondylolisthesis. *Spine* 4:148–149.
68. Rolander SD (1966): Motion of the lumbar spine with special reference to the stabilizing effect of posterior fusion. *Acta Orthop Scand Suppl* 90:1–144.
69. Rosenberg NJ (1975): Degenerative spondylolisthesis: Predisposing factors. *J Bone Joint Surg* [Am] 57:467–474.
70. Selby D (1986): Internal fixation with Knodt's rods. *Clin Orthop* 203:179–184.
71. Simmons EH, Capicotto WN (1988): Posterior transpedicular Zielke instrumentation of the lumbar spine. *Clin Orthop* 236:180–191.
72. Spencer DL, Watt DL, Miller JAA (1984): Chymopapain chemonucleolysis: A clinical study of results and correlation with size of disc protrusion and post-injection disc space narrowing. Presented at the 51st annual meeting of the American Academy of Orthopaedic Surgeons, Atlanta, Georgia.
73. Spencer DL, Miller JA, Schultz AB (1985): The effects of chemonucleolysis on the mechanical properties of the canine lumbar disc. *Spine* 10:555–561.
74. Stokes IA, Counts DF, Frymoyer JW (1989): Experimental instability in the rabbit lumbar spine. *Spine* 14:68–72.
75. Sullivan JD, Farfan HF, Kahn DS (1971): Pathologic changes with intervertebral joint rotational instability in the rabbit. *Can J Surg* 14:71–79.
76. Valkenburg HA, Haanen HCM (1982): The epidemiology of low back pain. In: White AA III, Gordon SL, eds. *American Academy of Orthopaedic Surgeons symposium on idiopathic low back pain.* St. Louis: C. V. Mosby, pp. 9–22.
77. Weinstein J, Spratt KF, Lehmann T, McNeill T, Hejna W (1986): Lumbar disc herniation: A comparison of the results of chemonucleolysis and open discectomy after ten years. *J Bone Joint Surg* [Am] 68:43–54.
78. Weinstein JN, Wiesel SW, eds. (1990): *The lumbar spine.* International Society for the Study of the Lumbar Spine. Philadelphia: WB Saunders.
79. White AA III, Panjabi MM, eds. (1978): *Clinical biomechanics of the spine.* Philadelphia: J. B. Lippincott.
80. Wilder DG (1986): On loading of the human lumbar intervertebral motion segment. Dissertation for degree of Doctor of Philosophy, Mechanical Engineering, Civil and Mechanical Engineering Department, University of Vermont, October 1985. *Dissertation Abstracts International* 46(12):4328-B. Ann Arbor: University Microfilms International, manuscript DA8529728.
81. Wilder DG, Pope MH, Frymoyer JW (1988): The biomechanics of lumbar disc herniation and the effect of overload and instability. *J Spinal Disorders* 1:16–33.
82. Woody J, Lehmann T, Weinstein J, et al (1988): Excessive translation on flexion-extension radiographs in asymptomatic populations. Presented at the meeting of the International Society for the Study of the Lumbar Spine, Miami, Florida.

The Adult Spine: Principles and Practice,
J. W. Frymoyer, Editor-in-Chief.
Raven Press, Ltd., New York © 1991.

CHAPTER 91

Who Should Be Fused?

Edward N. Hanley, Jr., Eric D. Phillips, and John P. Kostuik

BACKGROUND AND HISTORY OF LUMBAR SPINAL FUSION

The historic role of fusion has been to treat painful joints and to augment the correction of deformity and prevent its recurrence. Pain of musculoskeletal origin arises from complex neural networks, beginning with the peripheral stimulation of nociceptors. The inciting stimulus may be from endogenously released chemicals, heat, or mechanical deformations (112). Although the precise mecha-

nisms involved in spinal pain have yet to be clearly elucidated, motion, particularly when it is abnormal in character or degree, often is a potent stimulus to peripheral nociception. Deformity and loss of structural integrity may also contribute to abnormal motion and mechanical stresses, further activating nociceptors with resultant pain.

When pathologic motion is eliminated by immobilization or arthrodesis, pain relief may follow. When deformity is corrected, fusion maintains skeletal alignment and prevents recurrence. Based on these general premises, spinal arthrodesis has been employed to control pain attributed to unstable motion or mechanical insufficiency produced by traumatic, degenerative, inflammatory, neoplastic, and infectious processes. Likewise, spinal fusion has been used to maintain the correction of spinal deformities associated with these same pathologic processes as well as progressive deformity secondary to congenital and developmental conditions.

E. N. Hanley, Jr., M.D.: Chairman, Department of Orthopaedic Surgery, Carolinas Medical Center, Charlotte, North Carolina, 28232.

E. D. Phillips, M.D.: Medical Director, Kansas City Spine Center, Baptist Medical Center, Kansas City, Missouri, 64131.

J. P. Kostuik, M.D., F.R.C.S.(C): Professor of Orthopaedics, University of Toronto, Toronto, Ontario; Director, Spinal Surgery; Director, Biomechanics Laboratory, The Toronto Hospital, Toronto, Ontario, M5G 2C4.

A

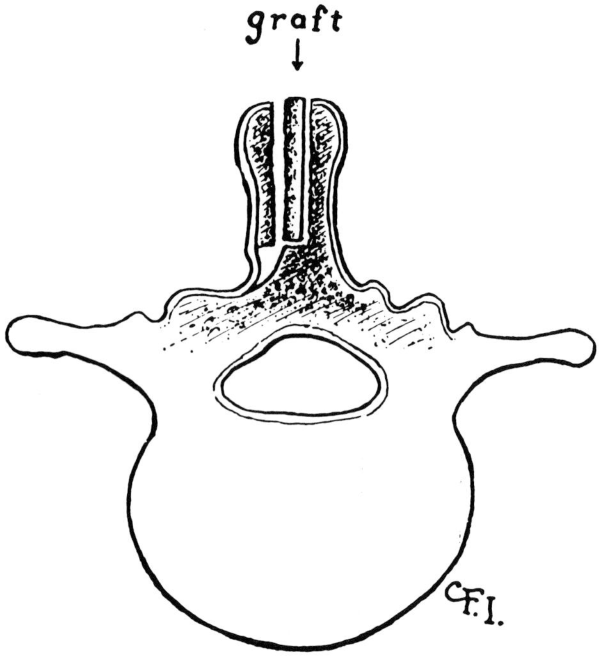

graft

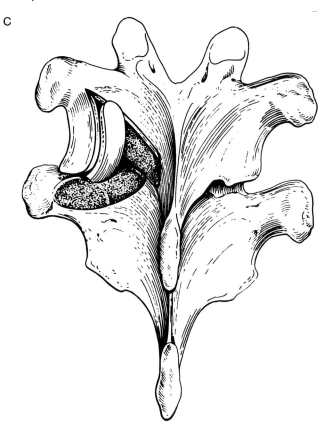

FIG. 1A: Albee fusion technique. **B–D:** Hibbs fusion technique.

B

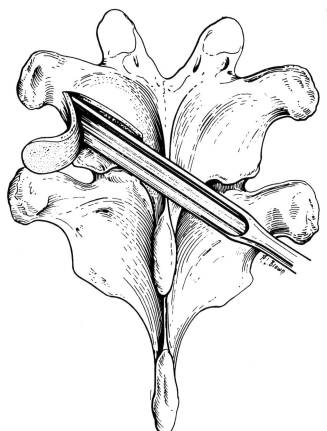

FIG. 1B: Decortication.

C

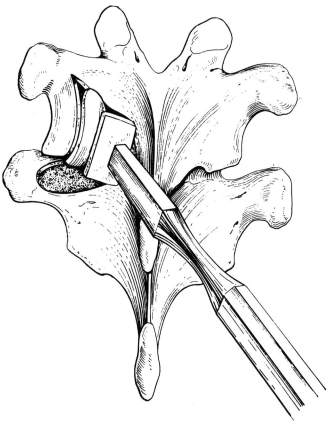

FIG. 1C: Decortication of superior and inferior laminae. Petalled fragments overlap.

D

FIG. 1D: Bone graft is added and impacted, which may include the addition of facet joint decortication.

The first clinical reports of spinal fusion were in 1911 by Hibbs and Albee (1) who used this technique for the treatment of Pott's disease (Fig. 1). Hibbs observed the natural ankylosis of the infected spine and reasoned that the surgical acceleration of this process might result in more rapid and certain healing. Albee (1) implanted a tibial graft in the spinous processes, which he thought might provide an internal splint and hasten stabilization of the spine. In 1917, DeQuervain and Hoessly (19) and others (56) made use of the scapular spine as an internal splint and source of bone graft. In the same year Hibbs (52) reported on spinal fusion to prevent the increasing deformity of scoliosis. No internal fixation was used even though Hadra in 1891 (37) had reported a technique for wiring the spine, and Lange in 1902 (67) had developed a system of steel rods combined with a celluloid cylinder.

Modification and broadening application of the more popular Hibbs technique ensued in the next 30 years (7). In addition to infection and scoliosis, fractures and developmental deformities were managed by this technique. In 1929, Hibbs and Swift (53) reported their follow-up of lumbosacral fusions performed for degenerative conditions. Later in 1943, Howorth (58) broadened the indications for fusion as an adjunctive method for the treatment of a ruptured nucleus pulposus. He concluded that fusion "may be the quickest and most economical method of relief, in this way offering a financial advantage to patient, hospital, and community."

In recent decades, the broad indications for spinal fusion have changed little, with the exception of a dwindling enthusiasm for its use in conjunction with excision of lumbar disc hernias. However, the techniques have evolved to include a wide variety of internal fixation devices in an attempt to provide greater correction of deformities when they exist, to enhance stabilization, and, it is hoped, to increase the rate of bony consolidation. Anterior spinal fusion has permitted more direct access to anterior column pathology. Fusions performed by this route may also be used to supplement posterior arthrodesis when there is circumferential disease or when the spinal condition is very unstable. The search for improved bone grafting material has continued parallel with the development of stabilization devices. Advances are constantly being made in pre- and intra-operative imaging techniques, operating room facilities, and surgical instruments and techniques. Despite these technical developments, it is evident that the single most important determinant of success in surgical arthrodesis is appropriate patient selection.

In this chapter we will review indications for lumbar spinal fusion from the perspective of spinal pathology, as well as consider those anatomic and psychosocial factors which determine success or failure. We will also review the common surgical constructs which are used in spinal fusion as a backdrop to later chapters which detail some

of the more sophisticated approaches that may be used to manage specific pathologic conditions including failures of previous spinal fusion (see Chapters 92–98).

ANATOMIC INDICATIONS FOR SPINAL FUSION

The basic indications for spinal fusion are related to instability or deformity. The broad biomechanical, clini-

TABLE 1. *Possible indications for lumbar spinal fusion*

Indications	Discussion
Congenital and Acquired Deformities	
Scoliosis	see Chapter 65
Kyphosis	see Chapter 64
Kyphoscoliosis	see Chapters 64, 65
Spondylolisthesis	see Chapters 78, 91
Traumatic	
Unstable fractures	see Chapter 33
Fracture dislocations	see Chapter 33
Spondylolisthesis	see Chapter 78
Inflammatory—Infectious	
Unstable and progressing disc space infection	see Chapter 38
Unstable and progressing vertebrae osteomyelitis	see Chapter 38
Tuberculosis	see Chapter 38
Some fungal infections	see Chapter 38
Inflammatory—Non-Infectious	
Spondyloarthropathies	see Chapter 36
Metabolic	
Osteoporosis (rare as primary indication)	see Chapter 64
Neoplasms	
Primary neoplasms	see Chapter 41
Secondary neoplasms	see Chapter 42
Degenerative	
Degenerative spondylolisthesis	see Chapter 78
Degenerative segmental instability	see Chapter 31
Spinal stenosis	
Degenerative scoliosis	see Chapter 65
Disc disruption after primary lumbar disc excision (rare)	see Chapter 97
Iatrogenic and Fusion Failures	
Primary: following sacrifice of greater than 50% of both facets	see Chapter 90
After failed disc excision	see Chapter 89
After failed chymopapain	see Chapter 90
Above prior fusion	
Pseudarthrosis repair	
Acquired spondylolysis above fusion	see Chapter 78
Failed low back surgery (syndrome)	see Chapter 95

cal, and radiologic issues relating to the definition of instability are discussed in Chapter 90. Here we will detail some of the more common indications as they relate to spinal pain. Topics such as scoliosis, trauma, infections, and tumors have been presented in other chapters and will not be reviewed. However, it is worth remembering that these conditions constitute a minority of indications for spinal arthrodesis (Table 1), and the majority are done for one or another form of segmental instability.

SPONDYLOLISTHESIS

Chapter 78 discusses spondylolisthesis in detail. In this section we have focused on the issue of children and young adults to emphasize that the surgical management of this condition is a continuum. Furthermore, it raises the question: Can low back pain in the adult be prevented by early fusion?

Isthmic and congenital spondylolisthesis is found in 5% of the American population (9,24,117). Although this condition may be seen at any level of the lumbar spine, the level predominantly affected is L5-S1. The natural history indicates that patient age and the degree of slippage observed at the time of diagnosis are the most important prognosticators for future low back pain (96) (Fig. 2). The majority of high-grade isthmic slips develop from age 10 to 14 and significant increases are unusual in adulthood, with the exception of lesions involving the L4-L5 level (34). When the slip is less than 10%, the likelihood of future back problems is similar to that for the general population. When the slippage progresses beyond 25%, there appears to be an increased risk for future back pain (100). Beyond these characteristics, it has been difficult to quantify precisely what are the risk factors for slip progression, back pain, or the later development of associated degenerative changes (48).

Symptoms at presentation may include back or lower extremity pain, often accompanied by hamstring tightness in the child which may alter the gait pattern. Three general types of pain presentation and neurologic abnormalities may occur. The patient may have back pain only, back and extremity pain without neurologic findings, or back and extremity pain with neurologic dys-

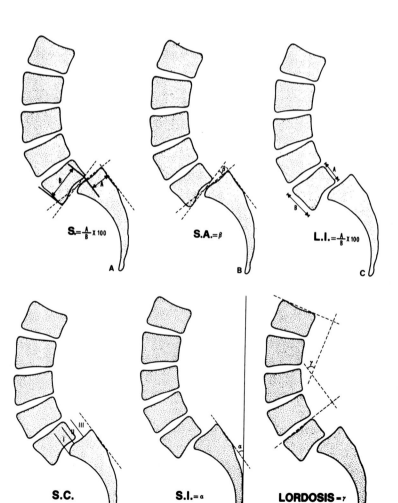

FIG. 2. Common measurements made in spondylolisthesis. **A:** *S*, percentage slip. **B:** *S.A.*, slip angle. **C:** *L.I.*, lumbar index. **D:** *S.C.*, slip classification. **E:** *S.E.*, sacral inclination. **F:** *Lordosis*, L1-L5 and L1-S1. For a more detailed explanation see Chapter 78.

function. The etiology of back pain with spondylolisthesis is believed to be due to mechanical and/or chemical activation of primary sensory neurons located in the outer fibers of the annulus fibrosus or posterior longitudinal ligament, both of which are placed under stress by the slip (112). The posterior elements, usually the pars interarticularis, may also be involved in the production of pain, particularly when there are nerve root symptoms. Radiculopathy, most often involving the fifth lumbar nerve root, has been attributed to nerve root irritation or displacement by hypertrophic fibrocartilaginous tissue present at the pars defect, or less likely, from entrapment of the L5 root between the L5 pedicle and the sacrum when the L5-S1 disc degenerates. A mobile olisthetic segment may also apply abnormal stresses on the spinal nerve root.

SURGICAL INDICATIONS

Radiographic criteria on which to base treatment include the degree of slippage and the slip angle (79). Saraste (100) demonstrated the radiographic findings of lumbosacral instability and early disc degeneration which correlated strongly with symptoms and abnormal clinical signs in adults with spondylolisthesis. Hensinger (48) concluded that most symptomatic children and teenagers with grade II or more slippage will eventually require surgical intervention to control symptoms. He noted non-operative measures were unsuccessful in greater than 50% of patients when a grade III or IV slippage had been reached. He recommended that patients with this degree of slip and pain which interferes with lifestyle and is unresponsive to non-operative treatment could be successfully managed by *in situ* fusion (17,44,63,115) (Fig. 3).

Many other authors have used the potential risk of future slippage as a surgical indication, but the documentation to support this belief has been incomplete (8,17,43,68,73,107). These issues are even more complex in adults where progressive slippage of the typical L5-S1 lesion rarely occurs, even when a high-grade olisthesis is present.

Even more complex is what to do in a child with a slip greater than 50% when symptoms are not present. One indication which has been used is the presence of a gait disturbance in a child whose spondylolisthesis is progressing, but who has no other symptoms (8,9,17,43,47). In fact, Hensinger recommends that children with slips greater than 50% be fused, whether or not symptoms are present, in order to prevent progression. He also includes as an indication for surgery a growing child with a pathologic spondylolisthesis and kyphosis. His views are also consistent with those of Laurent and Osterman (68) who were even less stringent and recommended early fusion for growing children with evidence of slip progression

greater than one third, even when they were symptom-free. Many of these studies have shown good or excellent results with complete resolution of pre-operative symptoms after successful *in situ* fusion. Furthermore, a much better long-term prognosis is noted if arthrodesis is performed in childhood rather than after skeletal maturity has been obtained (40,48). This lends additional credence to an aggressive surgical approach in children, but not necessarily in adults. However, not all authorities agree with this philosophy.

Long-term follow-up studies by Apel et al. (2) and Fredrickson et al. (24) defend the position of non-operative treatment for the vast majority of children, teenagers, and adults with non-disabling low back pain and lower grades of slippage. Even individuals with higher grades of spondylolisthesis can be treated conservatively with success. In Harris and Weinstein's study (44), patients treated non-operatively were found to remain active and require only minor adjustments in their lifestyles to cope with mild symptoms. They concluded that aggressive, conservative treatment usually was effective in both adults and children, and reserved surgical treatment for those whose symptoms were incapacitating, thus placing minimal importance on radiographic criteria.

RESULTS OF SURGICAL INTERVENTION

There is a great variation in the results of surgical treatment of spondylolisthesis, even when the procedure is relatively standardized. In a review of patients of all ages who underwent lumbosacral arthrodesis for isthmic spondylolisthesis, Hanley and Levy (40) reported excellent (100%) success in patients under age 20. Older patients fared less well and the success rate ranged from 27% to 73%. The worse results were obtained in adults who had compensable, work-related symptoms. In this cohort, success was achieved in only 39% of patients as compared to the 83% success achieved when compensation was not present. The results were independent of the degree of slip.

AUTHORS' INDICATIONS FOR SPINAL FUSION FOR SPONDYLOLISTHESIS

At the present time our indications for surgical stabilization for this condition and fusions include:

1. Persistence of painful mechanical or neurologic symptoms in a child despite an appropriate course of non-operative treatment.
2. Documentation of progressive and symptomatic slippage in a child beyond 33% of vertebral body width.
3. Initial presentation in a child with a symptomatic slip of greater than 50%.

4. A lumbar disc herniation in an adult at L4-L5 or more rarely at L5-S1, in association with spondylolisthesis (see Fig. 3).

5. Progressive slip and pain in an adult with an L4-L5 isthmic spondylolisthesis (34).

A relative, but not absolute, contraindication is an adult with predominantly low back pain, a slip of less than 50%, and a compensation claim. These patients require careful and comprehensive analysis before surgery is to be recommended.

The issue of who should not be fused when neurological symptoms predominate is more controversial. A generally accepted school of thought has argued for fusion in all patients (47,102). The basis for that opinion was the increased propensity for slips to increase even in adults after decompression alone. In these patients, a secondary fusion was frequently advised because of this progression or for incapacitating back symptoms (88). We agree with

this general philosophy, with the possible exception of patients over the age of 65 who have neurologic symptoms exclusively. Even some patients in this age group will exhibit further slippage and require later fusion (32).

DEGENERATIVE CONDITIONS

Here we will consider the various degenerative conditions for which fusion might be recommended and at the end of this section will give our current indications.

Degenerative Spondylolisthesis

Degenerative spondylolisthesis is an acquired condition thought to be secondary to disc degeneration and long-standing intersegmental instability (23). Facet tropism and rotatory instability are essential features of the

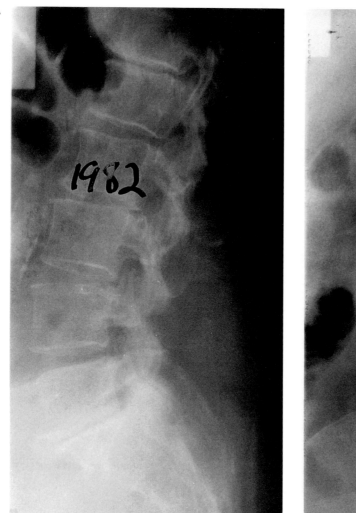

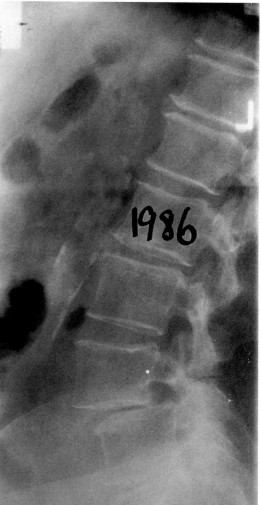

FIG. 3. A: Pre-operative lateral view in 1982 demonstrates a mild L4-L5 slip. **B:** Following decompression, the slip L4-L5 increased remarkably with severe neurological symptoms and back pain. (Fig. 3C follows.)

pathologic process (21,96). Slippage most often occurs at L4-L5, and seldom progresses to more than 33% of vertebral body width. As the olisthesis progresses, patients may present with sciatica or claudication. Back pain is frequently present but seldom predominates. The lesion is very common in the elderly population and many patients can be treated non-operatively. Surgical treatment is indicated when the disease becomes functionally incapacitating or when neurologic dysfunction is progressive.

Surgical treatments have consisted of decompression or arthrodesis or a combination of the two operations. Studies where comparable treatment groups have been analyzed have not shown statistical differences to support the benefit of the different operative techniques (22,93). Lombardi et al. (71) concluded that the decompression-with-fusion group "continued to feel better and stronger with time." Feffer et al. (22) noted that those who had decompression accompanied by fusion had qualitatively more favorable outcomes than those treated with decompression alone. Rosenberg (97) noted

C

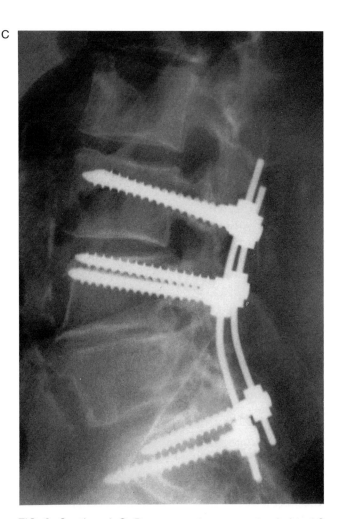

FIG. 3. *Continued.* **C:** Decompression was extended to L3, which was also severely stenotic. Fusion with Zielke instrumentation was done from L3-S1 with a good result.

that back symptoms presumed to be due to instability after decompression diminished with time. His patients generally were able to accommodate functionally to their back symptoms and later fusion was rarely necessary. Similarly, Herron and Trippi (49) concluded that fusion was not routinely necessary if pre-operative radiographs did not show instability and if structural integrity remained after the decompressive procedure.

Reynolds and Wiltse (93) attempted to further refine the analysis by considering the results in those under and over age 65. They concluded that fusion was beneficial in those patients under 65 and in good health. Many surgeons have tended to selectively fuse only younger patients or those who required extensive laminectomy including facetectomy (23,115,116). Waiting to see whether progressive spondylolisthesis and symptoms develop before proceeding with arthrodesis has also been recommended (13,97). However, a successful arthrodesis will predictably provide long-term stability to resist further torsion or translation in those patients who are decompressed extensively or in younger patients with back pain and instability as their predominant symptoms (38,64,101).

Segmental Instability

The indications for spinal fusion in the treatment of "disc disease" are controversial. The basic problem lies in the definition of degenerative instability, a topic considered at length in Chapter 90. There now exist many theories that attempt to correlate both radiographic and biomechanical criteria with this condition. Further confounding the issue is the realization that the typical symptoms of motion segment instability have yet to be defined. A key premise is that selective fusion of an "unstable motion segment" has a high probability of relieving symptoms if a diagnosis can be made with certainty (26). To make this definition, many classifications have been proposed, including biomechanical, clinical, and radiographic criteria (30,82,90,114). Frymoyer and Selby (30) attempted to divide segmental instabilities into subtypes based on the deformity which would produce symptoms if progression occurred. They also proposed tailoring a specific fusion technique to the type of instability as a means of reducing the failure rate. In a later publication, Stokes and Frymoyer (106) concluded that this classification could not be used with clinical success even when sophisticated biplanar radiographs were used in the evaluation.

Despite these concerns, there is a generally held belief that patients do exist with degenerative instabilities, and a classification is presented in Chapter 90. Radiographic signs such as the traction spur (74) and abnormal translational and angulatory motions (89) continue to be used as clinical criteria for the diagnosis. Additional attempts based on cadaveric studies have been made to more precisely quantify the type of magnitude of motion which occurs (90) or to define the source of pain through facet blocks (81) or discometry (36). More recently a trial of short-term external fixation (20) has shown promise in determining those patients who will benefit from fusion.

Spinal Stenosis and Degenerative Scoliosis

Degenerative scoliosis may develop de novo without any pre-existing deformity. Grubb et al. (35) analyzed a group of adults who developed scoliosis and an associated round back deformity with loss of lumbar lordosis. These patients were different from the usual adults with pre-existent idiopathic scoliosis, who typically are female, 20 to 50 years of age, and have predominantly low back complaints. In degenerative scoliosis the patients are older, the female to male ratio is equal, and there is an absence of the bony structural changes characteristic of idiopathic scoliosis. Moreover, the clinical and radiographic presentation often includes significant osteoporosis (see Chapter 65).

The symptom complex of acquired degenerative scoliosis is a combination of back pain and spinal stenosis, although patients often do not get relief of their stenotic symptoms by sitting. Spinal collapse is the result of hypertrophic changes of the apophyseal joints, translational and rotational deformities, and sometimes osteoporosis. These bony changes in combination with pathologic motion may diminish canal dimensions and limit the space available for exiting nerve roots, as well as the cauda equina. Contrary to common belief, traction may be placed on the nerve roots exiting on the convex side of the curve and, as a result, the initial neural symptoms most often are reported on the ipsilateral lower extremity (39).

Non-operative treatment of this condition is limited in its effectiveness, but a trial of non-steroidal, anti-inflammatory medication, rest, and epidural blocks may be tried. Corsets usually do not provide adequate immobilization and more rigid braces are poorly tolerated in the elderly. Therefore, surgical decompression combined with internal stabilization may be warranted.

However, Nachemson in 1979 (82) suggested that not all patients required stabilization and that decompression alone would suffice in many. Despite the deformity, his recommendation would parallel the experience of others in the surgical management of multilevel spinal stenosis without deformity. Similarly, San Martino et al. (99) studied 20 patients with radicular compression caused by degenerative scoliosis. Pain relief and restored function were noted in all after surgical decompression was performed along the curve concavity. Fusion was not performed and no patient suffered a recurrence of major symptoms.

On the other hand, Lonstein (72) and Benner and Ehri (5) pointed out that not all patients do well without fusion and emphasized the need to assess curve stability pre-operatively (Fig. 4). An even more aggressive approach has been recommended by Jackson et al. (60) who advocated routine stabilization using devices such as the Zielke apparatus. This same approach is advocated by Kostuik (65,66) and is presented in Chapters 33, 64, and 65.

Iatrogenic Instability

An easier problem than the primary diagnosis of segmental instability is the intra-operative definition that decompression has produced an unstable motion segment. Recent sophisticated biomechanical analyses have shown that sacrifice of more than 50% of both facets or the sacrifice of one entire facet will produce significant loss of mechanical integrity (114). This research has tended to confirm the clinical experience of others such as Booth (6). However, Hazlett and Kinnard (46) reported on 33 patients in whom at least one entire facet was removed in the process of lumbar decompression. Only 4 of these 33 patients showed radiographic signs of instability, though all had multiple level excisions of the facet joints. Despite radiographic signs of post-operative instability, 2 of the 4 had acceptable clinical results. Similarly, Lee (69) reviewed 27 patients after extensive posterior decompression and found progressive slippage occurred in only 3.7%.

This clinical experience would indicate that other factors may influence the long-term result. The presence of advanced age, marked disc space narrowing, and osteophytes are generally thought to reduce the need for fusion because of the additional stiffness they produce in the motion segment. On the other hand, operations in a younger patient, particularly when radical facet resections are performed, can lead to a spine which is dramatically unstable (119). If disc excision is performed in conjunction with the decompression, this may further increase the instability (109) (Fig. 5).

Discogenic Low Back Pain

Perhaps the greatest debate with regard to spine fusion has been generated by the use of discography as a diagnostic criterion. In a 1988 poll (92) of 297 members of the North American Spine Society (NASS), 227 responded in the affirmative to the question "Do you perform fusion for back pain?" Of equal interest was that 157 of the respondents used discography as a significant determinant of the fusion levels. A position statement by that organization (86) supported the diagnostic value of discography, but in a rebuttal Nachemson (83) suggested that the technique be limited to prospective studies con-

A
B

C

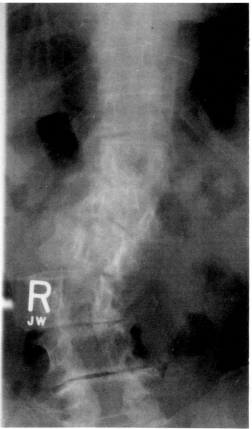
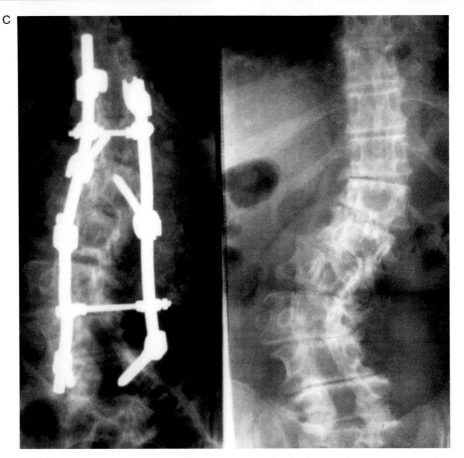

FIG. 4. A: A 62-year-old female had marked symptoms of spinal stenosis, secondary to degenerative spondylolisthesis and scoliosis. She was unaware of her deformity but had lost height. Back pain was mild. **B:** Following decompression, the curve progressed from 22 degrees to 33 degrees and back pain was severe. **C:** The deformity increased to 50 degrees with increasing back pain and sciatica. Stabilization and fusion with restoration of lordosis resulted in marked relief of all symptoms.

A

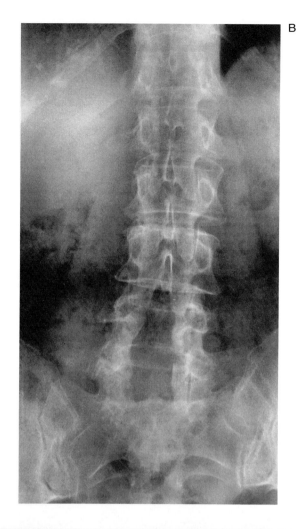

B

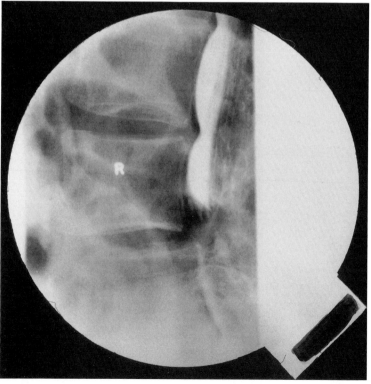

C

FIG. 5. A: A 61-year-old female with spinal stenosis at L4-S1 and L5-S1. **B:** Decompression was performed at L4-S1.5. **C:** One year later, slip developed at L3-L4 with a myelographic block and severe spinal stenosis. (Fig. 5D follows.)

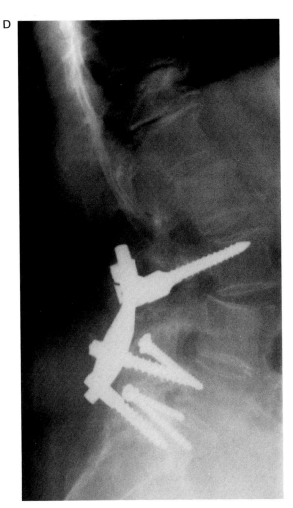

D

FIG. 5. *Continued.* **D:** Post-operative lateral view following decompression and fusion from L3 to S1 using pedicle fixation and facet screws.

ducted in large spinal centers. At the heart of this debate are two questions. First, is discography a specific test on which therapeutic decisions can be made? Second, is there a specific pathologic condition which is often termed "disk disruption"? The NASS position cited numerous studies which would support an affirmative answer to these two questions, although Nachemson (83) could persuasively argue to the contrary. Recent evidence presented by Weinstein and Rydevik (112) suggests that in fact, discography is a reliable means to assess pain originating from the intervertebral disc. Whether fusion will alleviate such pain continues to be controversial, but many believe it does.

FUSION AFTER EXCISION FOR LUMBAR DISC HERNIATION

Strangely, the least debated issue for the use of spinal fusion in degenerative conditions now appears to be its routine use in lumbar disc excision where the major sur-

gical indication is radiculopathy. This is interesting because this topic was hotly debated for many decades. A variety of retrospective studies (3,27,84) showed little benefit from fusion as a routine adjunct to disc excision. In fact, the current trends have been toward less invasive procedures such as chymopapain, microdiscectomy, and suction discectomy. Nevertheless, a recent study by Vaughan (108) supports the selective use of the fusion procedure when the L4-L5 disc level is involved. He reported 85% satisfactory results when fusion was combined with disc excision, but only 39% of patients who were not fused had a successful outcome. Of the 33 fusion patients, the operation was restricted to L4-L5 alone, while in 19, L5-S1 was included. A number of features of this clinical study deserve attention. First, discography and radiography were used to evaluate the adjacent levels pre-operatively. They performed total disc excisions which may be associated with a high rate of later back pain. His results also contradict those of Spangfort (103), Frymoyer et al. (28), and others who have shown little difference in the surgical results obtained at L4-L5 and L5-S1 when disc herniation with radiculopathy is the sole indication for operative intervention.

FAILED PRIOR FUSION

A wide set of indications and operative approaches are used for the patient who has had failure of a prior fusion performed for a multiplicity of causes. These issues are detailed in Chapter 98.

AUTHORS' INDICATIONS FOR FUSION IN DEGENERATIVE DISEASES

Although there is controversy, we have adopted the following general indications for fusion in degenerative spinal conditions.

Degenerative Spondylolisthesis

We advocate fusion in combination with stabilization for the majority of patients who require decompression. A poor medical status, the very elderly, or patients with extensive osteophytes accompanied by disc narrowing, particularly where minimal facets are sacrificed during surgery, may be exempt from this recommendation.

Multilevel Spinal Stenosis

Because the results obtained with multilevel decompression in spinal stenosis show only marginal improvement with fusion, we reserve the operation for those whose surgery requires sacrifice of either one entire facet or more than 50% of both facets at more than one level.

Degenerative Scoliosis

We advocate fusion in combination with decompression, except in those patients where single root involvement with radiculopathy is present or where the patient's overall medical status precludes surgery of this magnitude and a procedure is performed in which stability can be maintained.

Primary Segmental Instability

Because the diagnostic criteria for this condition are uncertain before a deformity is present, we are conservative in advocating fusion for these patients. However, excessive translation (greater than 4 mm), relief of pain by facet blocks, or faithful reproduction of pain by discography may on occasion serve as relative indications in patients with a stable psychosocial profile.

Iatrogenic Segmental Instability

We are aggressive in advocating prophylactic fusion when there is sacrifice of more than 50% of both facets or complete removal of one facet, particularly when more than one level is involved. The exceptions to this statement in multilevel decompression for spinal stenosis and degenerative scoliosis have been noted previously in this chapter.

Discogenic Low Back Pain

Although the indication is controversial, we may fuse patients who fulfill Crock's (16) clinical criteria, where the discogram faithfully reproduces the patient's symptoms and morphologic evidence of advanced degeneration is present on a subsequent enhanced CT scan. The pattern of dye extravasation is particularly useful when it is to the side of the patient's reported leg symptoms.

ROUTINE DISC EXCISION

We find little compelling evidence to perform a primary spinal fusion in patients with the typical symptoms of monoradiculopathy and a confirmatory image for lumbar disc herniation. In doing so, we accept a 10% to 15% incidence of significant post-operative low back pain (41) and the possibility that fusion may be required for later disc degeneration (27).

FAILURE TO ACHIEVE THE GOAL OF STABILIZATION

Determinants of Success and Failure

Although spinal fusion is an important technique in lumbar surgery, the outcome is by no means successful in all patients. The broad issues surrounding failures and complications of lumbar spinal fusion will be presented in Chapter 98. If the indications for fusion are to stabilize unstable segments and to relieve pain, success should be measured by satisfactory fulfillment of these criteria.

The first goal of spine fusion procedures is successfully to produce arthrodesis of those spinal segments involved in the disease process. Lack of success is pseudarthrosis, which occurs in 5% to 60% of fusions performed in the lumbar spine. Numerous factors exist to increase or decrease the probability of this failure, although it must be emphasized that not all pseudarthroses will produce pain. A discussion of the determining factors follows.

Number of Levels Fused

This is the single best predictor for failure of arthrodesis and is common to all techniques used.

Type of Operation

Advocates of various operative approaches have suggested that their techniques produced the highest rate of arthrodesis. However, true comparisons are almost impossible to make because so many other variables may have influenced the results, ranging from patient selection to operative technique. Naturally, each author believes his results are due to meticulous technique, which perhaps is true.

A few general conclusions do seem substantiated based on a general overview of the literature.

1. Posterior midline fusions have the lowest fusion rate, particularly when they are extended over more than one level. There are important reasons for this failure. The position of the graft is mechanically poor because the fusion is posterior to the center of rotation, and subject to greater tensile forces (94). The vascular bed for the fusion is tenuous because of the absence of a large mass of surrounding musculature, and limited blood supply (75). For these reasons, intertransverse process fusion has virtually supplanted the posterior midline technique.

2. Interbody fusion techniques seem most dependent on operative technique, although a caveat to this statement is that the criteria for solid fusion are debated and often different when surgical results are reported. This general conclusion is based on the observation that the greatest range of pseudarthrosis is reported with inter-

body techniques, seemingly independent of other factors which might have influenced the result. The reports of successful fusion range from 20% to 96% (15,25,33, 42,54,105). For example, Stauffer and Coventry (105) reported a low rate of fusion with anterior interbody techniques because of graft crumbling, whereas others, such as Crock (15), report this to be rarely a problem. To overcome this perceived high rate of graft failure, some are now advocating the circumferential fusion (see Chapter 95). Contributing to this problem may be that many surgeons use this technique infrequently. Other interbody techniques such as posterior interbody fusion are technically demanding.

3. The addition of stable fixation may increase the rate of fusion. This statement is based on recently reported animal experiments (77) rather than on controlled clinical studies, and should not be construed to mean internal fixation is necessary or even desirable in all patients. In fact, there is no available, controlled study to prove the benefits of internal fixation in many spinal pathologies. A comparative study of internal fixation with Magerl screw and no internal fixation suggested but did not prove either an increased rate or eventual consolidation of fusion with one or the other technique (61). Most would agree that internal fixation is desirable when fusion is performed for fractures and other obvious instabilities, or when correction of deformity is an objective.

Source of Graft Material

The controversy regarding the choice of graft material is mounting. A general belief is that autologous graft is optimum, but comparable rates of fusion are reported in some series with allograft (85). The biologic issues are discussed in detail in Chapter 28.

Pathology

The rate of fusion does relate to pathology in the general sense that more unstable conditions (e.g., fractures and fracture dislocations) are more difficult to stabilize than stable lesions (e.g., an adult with grade I, L5-S1 isthmic spondylolisthesis). The pathology is also the most important factor in determining which of the wide menu of fusion techniques is most appropriate. These issues are discussed in detail in later chapters. A rare, particularly potent, and overlooked cause of pseudarthrosis is the Charcot spine (10).

Constitutional Factors

It is generally believed but often unclear what role is played by age, sex, and osteoporosis. Goldner (33) in particular reports that the post-menopausal female has the poorest rate of fusion, which led him to advocate anterior interbody and even combined anterior and posterior operations. More certain is the role of cigarette smoking. Brown et al. (11) have shown the fusion rate using an intertransverse process technique from L4-sacrum was 90% in non-smokers and 63% in smokers. Similar results have been reported by Hanley and Levy (40) for fusion for spondylolisthesis.

External Support

The stabilization afforded by braces and corsets has been presented in detail in Chapter 74. Although many surgeons insist on external stabilization, it is conjectural whether these influence the rate of fusion. Certainly, the biomechanical information presented in Chapter 74 indicates minimal mechanical support by most commonly employed devices.

Assessment of Fusion

Cleveland et al. (14) deserve much of the credit for stressing that plane radiographs will not reveal pseudarthrosis. They advocated flexion-extension (dynamic) radiography to make the determination. In their report, plane films revealed a pseudarthrosis in 11.8%, but when motion films were included, 21% were then found to have failed. We strongly advocate this approach, but point out motion of 2 to 3 degrees is common due to "springiness" of the graft (27). A more difficult problem in assessing fusion is seen with interbody techniques and when there is rigid internal fixation.

It is evident from this presentation that the surgeon and patient can control the fusion success to a significant degree. This leads to a general statement that the number of vertebrae fused should be limited to only those in which the disease process exists. Conversely, the fusion should encompass those segments which are pain productive. The decision, therefore, should include some objective measurements. This may be easy when the pathologic process is acute and obvious (e.g., infection, tumor, or gross instability), or may be difficult when the pathologic process is more diffuse (e.g., degenerative scoliosis). Historically these decisions have been based on plain radiographic studies, which are a poor predictor of painful spinal segments. More recently, magnetic resonance imaging is being used as a sensitive sign of advanced spinal degeneration. However, many surgeons now think discography is the method of choice as this technique not only gives important morphologic information, but also is pain provocative in symptomatic degenerative discs. However, this is a controversial issue (83).

PAIN RELIEF

Spinal pain is a complex neurophysiologic, mechanical, and psychologic phenomenon, as emphasized in previous chapters. Not only is pain impossible to quantify, but a major problem in spinal surgery is the divergence between the patient's and the surgeon's expectations. The patient may expect to be pain-free and return to a high functional level, which in today's world frequently includes sports participation. On the other hand, the surgeon simply hopes to alleviate some of the pain and improve modestly the patient's function. Each perspective is valid.

The problem of chronic back pain has confounded clinicians for some time. Following the classic description of Mixter and Barr in 1934 (80), great enthusiasm was generated for the relief of back pain and sciatica by lumbar operations. Subsequent studies have revealed that removal of an offending disc herniation frequently did not produce relief of pre-existing symptoms, particularly low back pain. As early as 1951, Barr discussed a group of patients who had persistent low back pain or sciatica despite the fact that a technically satisfactory operation had been performed, and pathology had been discovered adequate to explain the symptoms. Long-term studies by Weber (111) have shown that the short-term results of disc excision produce more rapid functional recovery than conservative management, but that over time the two approaches produce virtually identical results.

Despite the hope that spine fusion, in conjunction with disc excision, would reduce the rate of back pain, this assertion has not been borne out in long-term studies (18,28,84). Similarly, successful arthrodeses for a variety of other spinal pathologies have not uniformly been associated with symptomatic relief. These failures emphasize the need for understanding spinal pain not only as an anatomic problem, but as a complex psychologic and environmentally modified experience.

Wing et al. (118), Spengler et al. (104), Waddell et al. (109), Frymoyer et al. (29), Hurme and Alaranta (59), and Herron et al. (50), among others, have demonstrated the importance of psychologic factors in predicting the outcome of decompression and fusion procedures. Emphasis has been placed on the importance of understanding not only the anatomic sources of pain, but the psychologic factors which will influence the results. It has been shown that the success of a lumbar operation in general and fusions correlates with certain personality traits, including low ego strength, hypochondriasis, depression, and hysteria, all of which predict poor outcomes. The importance of these factors is also suggested by the disproportionate number of patients with failed fusions who enter rehabilitation programs after numerous attempts at surgical intervention (4,45,76). Of course, the question of which came first is always raised: the failure then the psychologic problems, or were the psychologic problems present at the time of operation, which would have predicted the failure? The problem becomes even more of an issue when the patient has chronic disabling low back pain prior to the first operation.

Because of these problems, it has become increasingly recognized that the evaluation of a patient for lumbar surgery should include a careful assessment of not only anatomic causations, but psychosocial issues as well. Some of the important factors to be considered are the history of disability, the presence of compensation, and drug and alcohol abuse. The use of psychologic tests rises dramatically in a patient who has chronic disability with an uncertain pathoanatomic cause for pain. The importance of this principle is underscored by the observation that only 20% of patients with disabling back pain and uncertain anatomic causation for their pain will be relieved by spinal fusion.

If a patient is shown to have significant psychologic dysfunction, it can be argued that surgery should be performed only when the pathology is grossly apparent from the history, physical examination, and imaging studies, and that all other patients should be entered into a comprehensive rehabilitation program. The dilemma is that some patients who have completed these programs and shown improvement may, nevertheless, have continuing pain complaints and later be shown to return to function after surgery.

Not only is the psychologic condition important, but the presence of compensation is an additional variable determining success. Earlier in this chapter it was shown that the results of fusion for spondylolisthesis are more influenced by compensation than by the magnitude of deformity (40). A similar conclusion was reached by Norton (87), who demonstrated the socioeconomic consequences of failed laminectomy and chemonucleolysis in patients with lumbar disc herniations.

Waddell, both in Chapter 10 (this text) and in other publications (109), has considered these issues and pointed out that the surgeon is most influenced in his assessment of results by post-operative pain, disability, and physical impairment, rather than by the original diagnosis. The patient is influenced by his perception of residual physical impairment, disability status, and the type of surgery that he perceives has been performed. The other outcome measure Waddell emphasized was return to work, which was moderately influenced by post-operative disability but even more so by social and work-related factors. Again, these differences indicate that anatomic factors are but a small part of the eventual outcome which is achieved, and that psychosocial factors are a major determinant. These issues are equivalently important when the published surgical results for lumbar fusion are analyzed. As one reviews the results presented by other authors in this section, a few general queries serve as important guidelines to the evaluation of the presented data.

1. Was the post-operative assessment performed by an independent observer or did the surgeon determine the results? In general, independent observers find poorer results than does the operating surgeon.
2. How was the patient's pain measured? Was this simply a question about pain improvement, or were objective criteria employed (e.g., medication needs, further treatment, etc.)?
3. What was the patient's functional status? It is argued in a number of chapters that return to work may not be a valid outcome criterion after spinal fusion, and pain relief is all that could be expected. Some of us believe that return to work in an individual who is in the working age category is an important criterion, except in severe life or neurologically threatening conditions.

Waddell noted no absolute relationships among the three measures of outcome and emphasized that return to work was most influenced by the post-operative rather than the pre-operative state. In other words, the severity of pre-operative symptoms was not the major determinant. Other demographic factors such as age and sex had minimal influence, while the nature of the patient's occupation was a major determinant. In fact, he attempted to quantify these outcome determinants using a numerical rating scale, employing both the observer and patient's perceptions.

For the patients, three points indicated the result:

0 denoted a patient who assessed the outcome as not worthwhile.
1 denoted a patient who assessed the outcome as doubtful.
2 denoted a successful or good result.

The observers were similarly rated:

0 denoted a poor result.
1 denoted a fair result.
2 denoted a good result.

The patient and observer scores were then added. Three or more was taken as success; two or less was a failure. Using this approach, Waddell found that the post-operative pain score and physical impairments were the most potent determinants of success. A somewhat convoluted analysis then led to a numerical value where post-operative outcome equaled one quarter times the pain percentage minus eight. A positive result was indicated as a failure, a negative result was graded as a success. He reports that this numerical rating correlated with the total clinical assessment in nearly all of the cases that he analyzed.

Others such as Prolo et al. (91) and Howe and Frymoyer (57) have attempted to combine anatomic and other post-operative indicators to assess the contribution of pre-operative pathology and psychosocial and work factors to the end results. For example, Prolo et al. (91) attempted to semi-qualitatively delineate the pre- and post-operative condition of patients. The economic grade of the patient expressed the patient's capacity for meaningful employment, or alternative comparable pursuits such as household work or retirement activities. The functional grade of the patient's pain response expressed the effect of pain on the activities of living. Each grade consisted of five reproducible criteria that could be assessed pre- and post-operatively. The assembly of responses from these two scales ranged from a perfect 10 to complete incapacity, which was rated as 2. Excellent results were scored as 10 and 9, good as 8 and 7, fair as 6 and 5, and poor was 2. Anatomic criteria included the quality and presence of a fusion. Other criteria included the presence of a problem proximal to the fusion. He noted little correlation between the economic and functional results and the fusion.

These studies simply underscore important principles in all lumbar surgery, including fusion. The following conclusions can be reached:

1. The success or failure of a fusion is dependent on a careful assessment of the anatomic causation of pain. The more certain the diagnosis, the more likely the positive outcome.
2. The success or failure is equivalently dependent on complex psychosocial and workplace factors, particularly when functional criteria are included as an important determinant of success or failure.
3. A meticulously performed and technically successful fusion which subsequently becomes solid is not necessarily synonymous with clinical success; nor is pseudarthrosis synonymous with failure.
4. For the majority, but not all, of patients for whom spinal fusion might be considered, the operation should be viewed as elective and, therefore, both the anatomic and psychosocial/work factors must be weighed before an operative decision is made. The exception is the patient whose pathology or deformity is a major threat to neurologic function, or where the known natural history of the disorder will inevitably cause functional deterioration over time.
5. When in doubt, a multi-disciplinary evaluation is warranted. This should analyze completely both the anatomic and psychosocial dimensions of the patient's pain problem. One approach to this issue is described in Chapter 95, which deals with the complex group of patients being considered for circumferential fusion. Similarly, in Chapter 13 an alternative approach to managing these patients by non-operative methods is outlined.

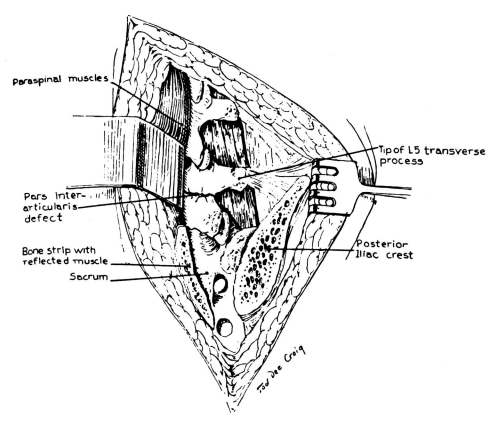

FIG. 6. Fusion bed for intertransverse fusion. The facet joints, pars interarticularis, lateral aspects of the pedicles, and transverse processes are included. This provides more stability to resist translational and rotary forces than does a posterior arthrodesis (adapted with permission from ref. 110).

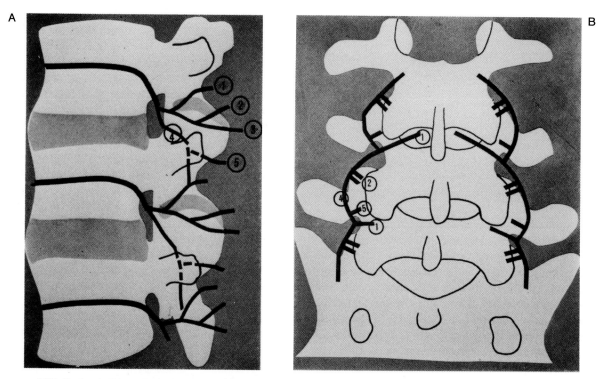

FIG. 7. A: *1:* Interarticular artery. *2–3:* Superior articular arteries. *4:* Communicating branch. *5:* Inferior articular artery. **B:** *1:* Interarticular artery lateral to pars. *2–3:* Superior articular arteries. *4:* Communicating artery. *5:* Inferior articular artery (with permission from ref. 75).

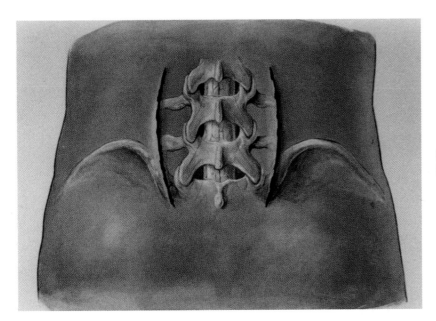

FIG. 8. Bilateral paraspinal lumbosacral approach.

SELECTION OF APPROPRIATE FUSION TECHNIQUE

The selection of an appropriate fusion technique follows the complete evaluation of the patient. Ideally, an operation should be chosen which is tailored to the pathology being treated, once the decision has been made that fusion is indicated. Here, we will detail the most common fusion techniques employed, as well as the technical details of these procedures. We will not, however, review the issues of failed arthrodesis (see Chapter 98) or the issues of internal fixation devices, which will be covered in Chapter 92.

COMMON FUSION TECHNIQUES

Spinal fusion techniques have been modified over the years since the first reported case by Hibbs in 1911 (51) (see Figs. 1B–1D). His technique of posterior fusion was performed through a longitudinal incision allowing the removal of the spinous processes to be applied to the lamina as a local autogenous graft. This technique is now rarely used alone, as a high pseudarthrosis rate was encountered. Cleveland et al. in 1948 (14) described the use of a more laterally placed bone graft as a method of treatment of pseudarthrosis of a posterior spinal fusion. This technique was popularized in 1953 by Watkins (110) who used a posterolateral approach to the spine, thus gaining direct access to the posterior articulations, pars interarticularis, and transverse processes (Fig. 6). Macnab and Dall (75) described an anatomic study of the blood supply to the region of the intertransverse lumbar fusion. These important observations provided a basis for eliminating the disadvantages of profuse bleeding found by many with the intertransverse fusion technique (Fig. 7).

Intertransverse arthrodesis of the lumbar spine is performed either through a midline or paraspinal approach (Fig. 8). The posterior facet joints, pars interarticularis, and transverse processes encompass the fusion bed which is prepared by excising soft tissue and turning up chips of bone from their surfaces. Corticocancellous and cancellous bone grafts obtained from the iliac crest or other sites are firmly placed into the area bridging the decorticated surfaces between levels (Fig. 9). Upon wound enclosure, the graft (covered by muscle) sits snugly over the lateral aspects of the spinal column.

The posterior intertransverse process fusion is indicated for most primary fusion procedures in the lumbosacral spine. Its occasional use in difficult salvaged spine surgery is also advocated. An excellent rate of solid arthrodesis with few operative complications supports the use of this technique in primary procedures for disorders of the lumbosacral spine, particularly spondylolisthesis (95).

Many variations of the posterior and posterolateral fusion techniques exist. The importance of the facet joint was stressed by McBride in 1949 (78) when he described his results with a mortised transfacet bone block for lumbosacral fusion. This simple technique attempted to eliminate intervertebral motion at the facet articulation. The technique is performed by excavating a rectangular mortise and impacting a dovetailed graft into this, using interspinous distraction to assist with graft placement (Fig. 10). Additional bone graft may be placed at the intertransverse fusion site. The bone block grafts are taken from the spinous processes, with each process furnishing material for two blocks. The prominence at the

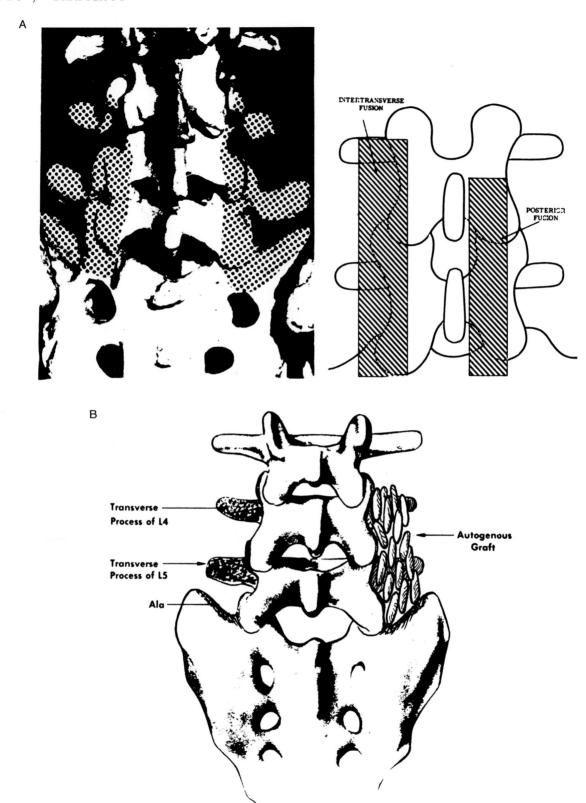

FIG. 9. Technique of intertransverse lumbar fusion. **A:** The area of the transverse process fusion compared to a midline fusion. **B:** Cancellous and corticocancellous bone strips should bridge the fusion area (redrawn with permission from ref. 75).

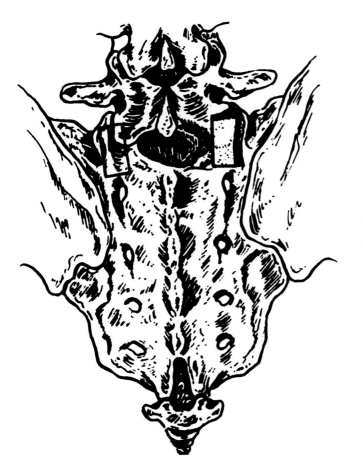

FIG. 10. The technique of facet fusion as described by McBride. Distraction is applied prior to placement of the block grafts to permit their impaction (with permission from ref. 78).

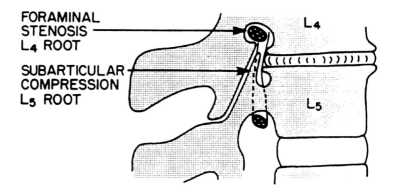

FORAMINAL STENOSIS L₄ ROOT

SUBARTICULAR COMPRESSION L₅ ROOT

L₄

L₅

FIG. 11. Posterior lumbar interbody fusion. This technique is demanding. Theoretically, it can restore intervertebral disc space height, thus opening the neural foramen (with permission from ref. 70).

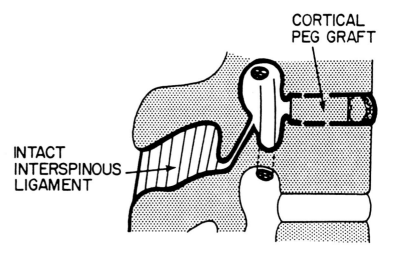

CORTICAL PEG GRAFT

INTACT INTERSPINOUS LIGAMENT

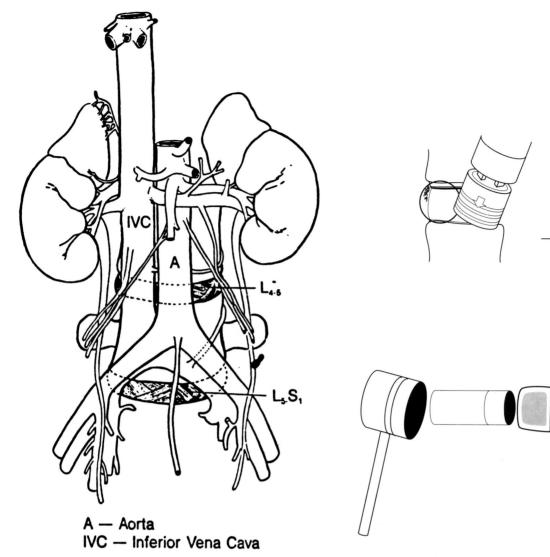

A — Aorta
IVC — Inferior Vena Cava

FIG. 12. Anatomical considerations in anterior lumbar fusion. A left-sided approach is generally preferred.

FIG. 13. A and B: Crock's technique for anterior interbody fusion using a dowel.

posterior spine of the ilium may be used if thicker, heavier bone is desired.

Interbody grafting techniques are advocated because they place the fusion closer to the center of vertebral motion, thus achieving greater stiffness when arthrodesis has occurred. Both anterior and posterior interbody fusion techniques have been popularized.

Posterior lumbar interbody fusion was first described by Jaslow in 1946 (62). The technique for this procedure stresses the need for bony exposure with removal of adequate amounts of the posterior elements to allow epidural hemostasis and complete disc removal. Facetectomy and foramenotomy are routine. Decortication of the end plates is essential. Many surgeons undercut the vertebral end plates to minimize the possibility of posterior graft migration. Both autogenic and allogenic bone grafts have been used and are typically inserted after distrac-

tion of the disc space with a laminar spreader or other device. Specialized instrumentation exists to perform this type of fusion with greater technical ease (Fig. 11). The technical details of this procedure are presented extensively in Chapter 94.

Burns (12) was the first to describe the anterior lumbar interbody fusion. He utilized this for the treatment of spondylolisthesis. Crock (15) described an anterior interbody fusion technique which has been among the most popular. Through an extraperitoneal exposure to the spine, the appropriate disc space is isolated, protecting the major vessels and the sympathetic trunk (Fig. 12). The disc is removed by use of elevators, rongeurs, and curettes, and its dimensions are determined. In the Crock technique (see Chapter 97), dowel cutters are used to ream a circular cut across the intervertebral space. Later a dowel cutter is used to remove a tricortical graft

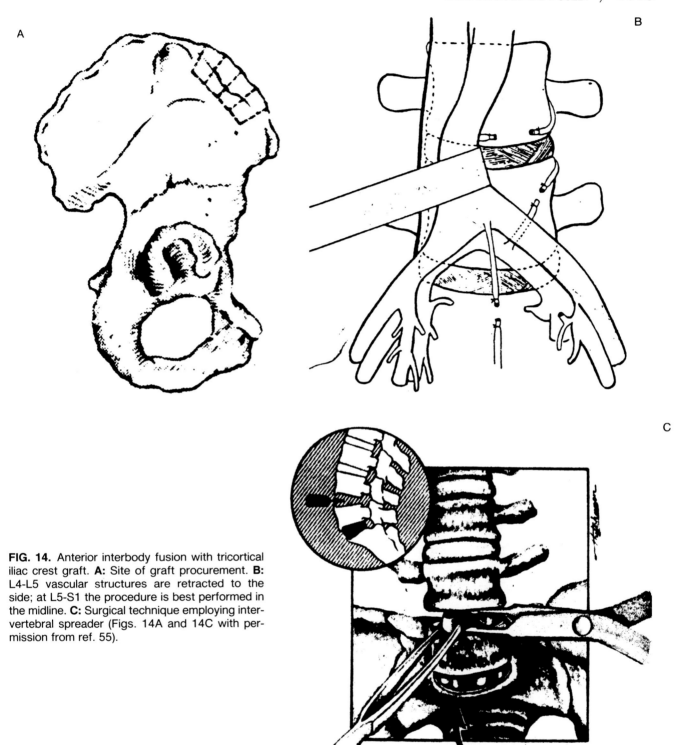

FIG. 14. Anterior interbody fusion with tricortical iliac crest graft. **A:** Site of graft procurement. **B:** L4-L5 vascular structures are retracted to the side; at L5-S1 the procedure is best performed in the midline. **C:** Surgical technique employing intervertebral spreader (Figs. 14A and 14C with permission from ref. 55).

A

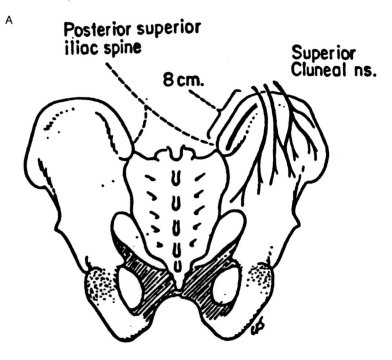

Posterior superior iliac spine

8 cm.

Superior Cluneal ns.

B

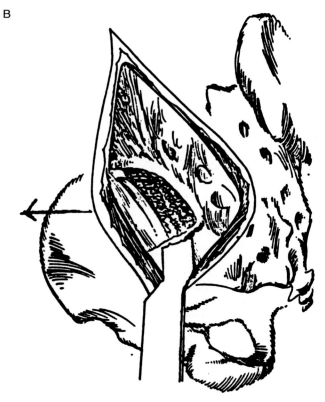

FIG. 15. A: Site of posterior iliac bone graft incision. Avoid the cluneal nerves (with permission from ref. 31). **B:** Method of obtaining bone graft. Procedure is most easily performed on the left side of the patient. The use of gouges in a horizontal medial to lateral orientation facilitates the procurement of graft "strips" and avoids the sciatic notch (with permission from ref. 98).

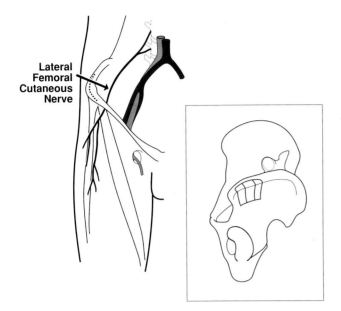

Lateral
Femoral
Cutaneous
Nerve

FIG. 16. Left: Site of incision for anterior iliac bone graft. Note lateral femoral cutaneous nerve (with permission from ref. 31). **Inset:** Method of obtaining graft from outer table of ilium. Tricortical grafts may also be obtained by this method, but this may result in a painful or cosmetically unappealing defect. An alternate technique is to remove a window of bone approximately 8 to 10 mm thick, leaving the top of the iliac crest intact. This provides a bicortical graft.

from the adjacent iliac crest. Graft is impacted into place and recessed slightly (Figs. 13A and 13B). An alternative technique includes the use of tricortical blocks of bone graft in the recipient's site with the anterior surface of the grafts flush with the cortices of the vertebral body (Figs. 14A and 14B).

Autogenous bone graft of sufficient quality and quantity is most easily obtained from either the posterior or anterior iliac crest. When approaching the posterior ilium, the superior cluneal nerves and the sciatic notch should be avoided. Typically, the outer table provides a large amount of corticocancellous and cancellous bone graft for posterior spinal procedures. Full thickness grafts, if obtained posteriorly, should avoid the region of the sacroiliac joint and the ligamentous complex, which provide a majority of its stability (Figs. 15A and 15B). Anterior bone grafts are best taken through an incision which should be placed lateral on the anterior superior iliac spine to avoid the lateral femoral cutaneous nerve. The outer table of bone is typically used for cannulous bone graft, leaving the inner cortex to protect the vascular and visceral structures. Full thickness grafts (bicortical or tricortical), however, may be taken after subperiosteal dissection of the inner table (Fig. 16).

REFERENCES

1. Albee FH (1911): Transplantation of a portion of the tibia into the spine for Pott's disease. *JAMA* 57:885–886.
2. Apel DM, Lorenz MA, Zindrick MR (1989): Symptomatic spondylolisthesis in adults: Four decades later. *Spine* 14:345–348.
3. Barr JS, Kubik GS, Molloy MK, et al (1967): Evaluation of end results in treatment of ruptured lumbar intervertebral discs with protrusion of nucleus pulposus. *Surg Gynecol Obstet* 125:250–256.
4. Beals RK, Hickman NW (1972): Industrial injuries of the back and extremities. Comprehensive evaluation—An aid in prognosis and management: A study of one hundred and eighty patients. *J Bone Joint Surg* [Am] 54:1593–1611.
5. Benner B, Ehri G (1979): Degenerative lumbar scoliosis. *Spine* 4:548–552.
6. Booth RE Jr (1986): Spinal stenosis. In: *Instructional course lectures XXXV.* American Academy of Orthopaedic Surgeons. St. Louis: C.V. Mosby.
7. Bosworth DM (1948): Technique of spinal fusion: Pseudoarthrosis and method of repair. In: American Academy of Orthopaedic Surgeons. *Instructional Course Lectures V.* St. Louis: C.V. Mosby, pp. 295–313.
8. Boxall D, Bradford DS, Winter RB, Moe JH (1979): Management of severe spondylolisthesis in children and adolescents. *J Bone Joint Surg* [Am] 61:479–495.
9. Bradford DS (1985): Spondylolysis and spondylolisthesis in children and adolescents. In: Bradford DS, Hensinger RN, eds. *Pediatric spine.* New York: Thieme and Stratton, Chapter 28.
10. Briggs JR, Freehafer AA (1967): Fusion of the Charcot spine. Report of three cases. *Clin Orthop* (53):83–93.
11. Brown CW, Orme TJ, Richardson JD (1986): The rate of pseudoarthrosis (surgical nonunion) in patients who are smokers and patients who are nonsmokers: A comparison study. *Spine* 11:942–943.
12. Burns BH (1933): An operation for spondylolisthesis. *Lancet* 1:1233.
13. Cauchoix J, Benoist M, Chassaing V (1976): Degenerative spondylolisthesis. *Clin Orthop* (115):122–129.
14. Cleveland M, Bosworth DM, Thompson F (1948): Pseudoarthrosis in the lumbosacral spine. *J Bone Joint Surg* [Am] 30:302–311.
15. Crock HV (1982): Anterior lumbar interbody fusion: Indications for its use and notes on surgical technique. *Clin Orthop* (165):157–163.
16. Crock HV (1986): Internal disc disruption: A challenge to disc prolapse fifty years on. *Spine* 11:650–653.
17. Dandy DJ, Shannon MJ (1971): Lumbo-sacral subluxation. *J Bone Joint Surg* [Br] 53:578–595.
18. DePalma AF, Rothman RH (1968): The nature of pseudoarthrosis. *Clin Orthop* (59):113–118.
19. DeQuervain F, Hoessly H (1917): Operative immobilization of the spine. *Surg Gynecol Obstet* 24:428–436.
20. Esses SI, Botsford DJ, Kostuik JP (1989): The role of external

spinal skeletal fixation in the assessment of low back disorders. *Spine* 14:594–601.

21. Farfan HF (1980): The pathological anatomy of degenerative spondylolisthesis: A cadaver study. *Spine* 5:412–418.

22. Feffer HL, Wiesel SW, Cuckler JM, Rothman RH (1985): Degenerative spondylolisthesis: To fuse or not to fuse. *Spine* 10:287–289.

23. Fitzgerald JA, Newman PH (1976): Degenerative spondylolisthesis. *J Bone Joint Surg* [Br] 58:184–192.

24. Fredrickson BE, Baker D, McHolick WJ, Yuan H, Lubicky JP (1984): The natural history of spondylolysis and spondylolisthesis. *J Bone Joint Surg* [Am] 66:699–707.

25. Freebody D, Bendall R, Taylor RD (1971): Anterior transperitoneal lumbar fusion. *J Bone Joint Surg* [Br] 53:617–627.

26. Frymoyer JW (1981): The role of spine fusion, question 3. *Spine* 6(3):284–290.

27. Frymoyer JW, Hanley E, Howe J, Kuhlman D, Matteri R (1978): Disc excision and spine fusion in the management of lumbar disc disease: A minimum ten-year follow-up. *Spine* 3:1–6.

28. Frymoyer JW, Matteri RE, Hanley EN, Kuhlman D, Howe J (1978): Failed lumbar disc surgery requiring second operation: A long-term follow-up study. *Spine* 3(1):7–11.

29. Frymoyer JW, Rosen JC, Clements J, Pope MH (1985): Psychologic factors in low-back pain disability. *Clin Orthop* (195):178–184.

30. Frymoyer JW, Selby DK (1985): Segmental instability: Rationale for treatment. *Spine* 10:280–286.

31. Garfin SR (1989): *Complications of spine surgery.* Baltimore: Williams & Wilkins.

32. Gill GG, Manning JG, White HL (1955): Surgical treatment of spondylolisthesis without spine fusion. *J Bone Joint Surg* [Am] 37:493–520.

33. Goldner JL (1981): The role of spine fusion: Question 6. *Spine* 6:293–303.

34. Grobler LJ, Haugh L, Wiltse LL, Frymoyer JW (1989): L4-5 isthmic spondylolisthesis: Clinical and radiological review of 52 cases. Presented at the Meeting of the International Society for the Study of the Lumbar Spine, Kyoto, Japan.

35. Grubb SA, Lipscomb HJ, Conrad RW (1988): Degenerative adult onset scoliosis. *Spine* 13:241–245.

36. Grubb SA, Lipscomb HJ, Guilford WB (1987): The relative value of lumbar roentgenograms, metrazamide myelography, and discography in the assessment of patients with chronic low-back syndrome. *Spine* 12:282–286.

37. Hadra B (1891): Wiring of the vertebrae as a means of immobilization in fracture and Pott's Disease. *Am Orthop Assn Trans* 4:206.

38. Hanley EN Jr (1986): Decompression and distraction-derotation arthrodesis for degenerative spondylolisthesis. *Spine* 11:269–276.

39. Hanley EN Jr, Eskay ML (1985): Degenerative lumbar spinal stenosis. *Adv Orthop Surg* 8(6):396–403.

40. Hanley EN Jr, Levy JA (1989): Surgical treatment of isthmic lumbosacral spondylolisthesis: Analysis of variables influencing results. *Spine* 14:48–50.

41. Hanley EN Jr, Shapiro DE (1989): The development of low-back pain after excision of a lumbar disc. *J Bone Joint Surg* [Am] 71:719–721.

42. Harmon PD (1960): Anterior extraperitoneal lumbar disc excision and vertebral body fusion. *Clin Orthop* (18):169–184.

43. Harrington PR, Tullos HS (1971): Spondylolisthesis in children: Observations and surgical management. *Clin Orthop* (79):75–84.

44. Harris IE, Weinstein SL (1987): Long-term follow-up of patients with grade III and IV spondylolisthesis. Treatment with and without posterior fusion. *J Bone Joint Surg* [Am] 69:960–969.

45. Hazard RG, Fenwick JW, Kalisch SM, et al (1989): Functional restoration with behavioral support: A one-year prospective study of patients with chronic low back pain. *Spine* 14:157–161.

46. Hazlett JW, Kinnard P (1982): Lumbar apophyseal process excision and spinal instability. *Spine* 7:171–176.

47. Hensinger RN (1983): Spondylolysis and spondylolisthesis in children. In: American Academy of Orthopaedic Surgeons. *Instructional course lectures.* St. Louis: C.V. Mosby 32:132–151.

48. Hensinger RN (1989): Current concepts review: Spondylolysis and spondylolisthesis in children and adolescents. *J Bone Joint Surg* [Am] 71:1098–1107.

49. Herron LD, Trippi AC (1989): L4-5 degenerative spondylolisthesis: The results of treatment by decompressive laminectomy without fusion. *Spine* 14:534–538.

50. Herron LD, Turner J, Clancy S, Weiner P (1986): The differential utility of the Minnesota Multiphasic Personality Inventory. A predictor of outcome in lumbar laminectomy for disc herniation versus spinal stenosis. *Spine* 11:847–850.

51. Hibbs RA (1911): An operation for progressive spinal deformities. *NY Med J* 93:1013–1016.

52. Hibbs RA (1917): Treatment of deformities of the spine caused by poliomyelitis. *JAMA* 69:787–796.

53. Hibbs RA, Swift WE (1929): Developmental abnormalities at the lumbosacral juncture causing pain and disability. *Surg Gynecol Obstet* 48:604–612.

54. Hodgson AR, Wong SK (1968): A description of a technique and evaluation of anterior spinal fusion for deranged intervertebral discs and spondylolisthesis. *Clin Orthop* (56):133–162.

55. Hoover NW (1968): Methods of lumbar fusion. *J Bone Joint Surg* [Am] 50:200–210.

56. Howarth F, Hoessly H (1917): Operative immobilization of the spine. *Surg Gynecol Obstet* 24:428.

57. Howe J, Frymoyer JW (1985): The effects of questionnaire design on the determination of end results in lumbar spinal surgery. *Spine* 10:804–805.

58. Howorth MB (1943): Evolution of spinal fusion. *Ann Surg* 117:278–289.

59. Hurme M, Alaranta H (1987): Factors predicting the result of surgery of lumbar intervertebral disc herniation. *Spine* 12:933–938.

60. Jackson RP, Simmons EH, Stripinis D (1983): Incidence and severity of back pain in adult idiopathic scoliosis. *Spine* 8:749–756.

61. Jacobs RR, Montesano PX, Jackson RP (1989): Enhancement of lumbar spine fusion by use of translaminar facet joint screw. *Spine* 14:12–15.

62. Jaslow IA (1946): Intercorporal bone graft in spinal fusion after disc removal. *Surg Gynecol Obstet* 82:215–218.

63. Johnson JR, Kirwan EO (1983): The long-term results of fusion in situ for severe spondylolisthesis. *J Bone Joint Surg* [Br] 65:43–46.

64. Knox BD, Harvell JL, Nelson PB, Hanley EN (1989): Decompression and Luque rectangle fusion for degenerative spondylolisthesis. *J Spinal Disord* 2:223–228.

65. Kostuik JP (1979): Decision making in adult scoliosis. *Spine* 4:521–525.

66. Kostuik JP (1980): Recent advances in the treatment of painful adult scoliosis. *Clin Orthop* (147):238–252.

67. Lange F (1910): Support for the spondylitic spine by means of buried steel bars attached to the vertebrae. *Am J Orthop Surg* 8:344.

68. Laurent LE, Osterman K (1976): Operative treatment of spondylolisthesis in young patients. *Clin Orthop* (117):85–91.

69. Lee CK (1983): Lumbar spinal instability (olisthesis) after extensive posterior spinal decompression. *Spine* 8:429–433.

70. Lin PM, Gill K (1989): *Principles and techniques in spine surgery.* Rockville, Maryland: Aspen, p. 40.

71. Lombardi JS, Wiltse LL, Reynolds J, Widell EH, Spencer C 3rd (1985): Treatment of degenerative spondylolisthesis. *Spine* 10:821–827.

72. Lonstein J (1987): Adult scoliosis. In: Bradford D, Lonstein J, Ogilvie T, Winter R, eds. *Moe's textbook of scoliosis and other spinal disorders, 2nd ed.* Philadelphia: W.B. Saunders.

73. Luskin R (1965): Pain patterns in spondylolisthesis: A correlation of symptoms, local pathology, and therapy. *Clin Orthop* (40):123–136.

74. Macnab I (1971): The traction spur. An indicator of segmental instability *J Bone Joint Surg* [Am] 53:663–670.

75. Macnab I, Dall D (1971): The blood supply of the lumbar spine and its application to the technique of intertransverse lumbar fusion. *J Bone Joint Surg* [Br] 53:629–638.

76. Mayer TG, Gatchel RJ, Kishino N, et al (1985): Objective assessment of spine function following industrial injury: A prospective study with comparison group and one-year follow-up. *Spine* 10:482–493.

77. McAfee PC, Farey ID, Sutterlin CE, Gurr KR, Warden KE, Cun-

ningham BW (1989): 1989 Volvo award in basic science. Device-related osteoporosis with spinal instrumentation. *Spine* 14:919–926.

78. McBride ED (1949): A mortised transfacet bone block for lumbosacral fusion. *J Bone Joint Surg* [Am] 31:385–393.

79. Meyerding HW (1932): Spondylolisthesis: Surgical treatment and results. *Surg Gynecol Obstet* 54:371–377.

80. Mixter WJ, Barr JS (1934): Rupture of the intervertebral disc with involvement of the spinal canal. *N Engl J Med* 211:210–215.

81. Mooney V (1981): The role of spine fusion. Question 7. *Spine* 6:304–305.

82. Nachemson A (1979): Adult scoliosis and back pain. *Spine* 4:513–517.

83. Nachemson A (1989): Editorial comment: Lumbar discography —Where are we today? *Spine* 14:555–557.

84. Nachlas IW (1952): End-result study of treatment of herniated nucleus pulposus by excision with fusion and without fusion. *J Bone Joint Surg* [Am] 34:981–988.

85. Nasca RJ, Whelchel JD (1987): Use of cryopreserved bone in spinal surgery. *Spine* 12:222–227.

86. North American Spine Society (1988): Position statement on discography. *Spine* 13:1343.

87. Norton WL (1986): Chemonucleolysis versus surgical discectomy: Comparison of costs and results in workers' compensation claimants. *Spine* 11:440–443.

88. Osterman K, Lindholm TS, Laurent LE (1976): Late results of removal of the loose posterior element (Gill's operation) in the treatment of lytic lumbar spondylolisthesis. *Clin Orthop* (117):121–128.

89. Penning L, Blickman JR (1980): Instability in lumbar spondylolisthesis: A radiologic study of several concepts. *AJR* 134:293–301.

90. Posner I, White AA III, Edwards WT, Hayes WC (1982): A biomechanical analysis of the clinical stability of the lumbar and lumbosacral spine. *Spine* 7:374–389.

91. Prolo DJ, Oklund SA, Butcher M (1986): Toward uniformity in evaluating results of lumbar spine operations. *Spine* 11:601–606.

92. Ray CD (1989): The tabulator: Results from questionnaire #1, October 1988. *NASS News* 3(1):7.

93. Reynolds JB, Wiltse LL (1977): Surgical treatment of degenerative spondylolisthesis. *Spine* 4:148–149.

94. Rolander SD (1966): Motion of the lumbar spine with special reference to the stabilizing effect of posterior fusion. An experimental study on autopsy specimens. *Acta Orthop Scand (Suppl)* 90:1–44.

95. Rombold C (1966): Treatment of spondylolisthesis by posterolateral fusion, resection of the pars interarticularis and prompt mobilization of the patient. *J Bone Joint Surg* [Am] 48:1282–1300.

96. Rosenberg NJ (1975): Degenerative spondylolisthesis: Predisposing factors. *J Bone Joint Surg* [Am] 57:467–474.

97. Rosenberg NJ (1976): Degenerative spondylolisthesis: Surgical treatment. *Clin Orthop* (117):112–120.

98. Rothman R, Simeone F (1975): *The spine.* Philadelphia: W.B. Saunders, p. 495.

99. San Martino A, D'Andria FM, San Martino C (1983): The surgical treatment of nerve root compression caused by scoliosis of the lumbar spine. *Spine* 8:261–265.

100. Saraste H (1987): Long term clinical and radiological follow-up of spondylolysis and spondylolisthesis. *J Pediatr Orthop* 7:631–638.

101. Selby DK (1983): When to operate and what to operate upon. *Orthop Clin North Am* 14:577–588.

102. Sherman FC, Rosenthal RK, Hall JE (1979): Spine fusion for spondylolysis and spondylolisthesis in children. *Spine* 4:59–66.

103. Spangfort EV (1972): The lumbar disk herniation. A computer aided analysis of 2,504 operations. *Acta Orthop Scand (Suppl)* 142:1–95.

104. Spengler DM, Freeman C, Westbrook R, Miller JW (1980): Low back pain following multiple lumbar spine procedures: Failure of initial selection. *Spine* 5:356–360.

105. Stauffer RN, Coventry MB (1972): Posterolateral lumbar-spine fusion. Analysis of Mayo Clinic series. *J Bone Joint Surg* [Am] 54:1195–1204.

106. Stokes IA, Frymoyer JW (1987): Segmental motion and instability. *Spine* 12:688–691.

107. Turner RH, Bianco AJ Jr (1971): Spondylolysis and spondylolisthesis in children and teenagers. *J Bone Joint Surg* [Am] 53:1298–1306.

108. Vaughan PA, Malcolm BW, Maistrelli GL (1988): Results of L4-L5 disc excision alone versus disc excision and fusion. *Spine* 13:690–695.

109. Waddell G, Kummel EG, Lotto WN, Graham JD, Hall H, McCulloch JA (1979): Failed lumbar disc surgery and repeat surgery following industrial injuries. *J Bone Joint Surg* [Am] 61:201–207.

110. Watkins MB (1959): Posterolateral bone-grafting for fusion of the lumbar and lumbosacral spine. *J Bone Joint Surg* [Am] 41:388–396.

111. Weber H (1983): Lumbar disc herniation. A controlled prospective study with ten years of observation. *Spine* 8:131–140.

112. Weinstein J, Rydevik B (1989): The pain of spondylolisthesis. *Semin Spine Surg* 1(2):100–105.

113. White AA 3rd, Panjabi MM (1978): *Clinical biomechanics of the spine.* Philadelphia: J.B. Lippincott, pp. 159–261.

114. White AA 3rd, Panjabi MM, Posner I, Edwards WT, Hayes WC (1981): Spinal stability: Evaluation and treatment. In: American Academy of Orthopedic Surgeons. *Instructional course lectures, 30.* St. Louis: C.V. Mosby, pp. 457–483.

115. Wiltse LL, Hutchinson RH (1967): Surgical treatment of spondylolisthesis. *Clin Orthop* (35):116–135.

116. Wiltse LL, Kirkaldy-Willis WH, McIvor GW (1976): The treatment of spinal stenosis. *Clin Orthop* (115):83–91.

117. Wiltse LL, Newman PH, Macnab I (1976): Classification of spondylolysis and spondylolisthesis. *Clin Orthop* (117):23–29.

118. Wing PC, Wilfling FJ, Kokan PJ (1973): Psychological demographic and orthopaedic factors associated with prediction of outcome of spinal fusion. *Clin Orthop* (90):153–160.

119. Wisneski RJ (1989): Surgical treatment: The role of fusion in lumbar disc disease. *Semin Spine Surg* 1(1):60–67.

The Adult Spine: Principles and Practice,
J. W. Frymoyer, Editor-in-Chief.
Raven Press, Ltd., New York © 1991.

CHAPTER 92

Spinal Fusion

Overview of Options
and Posterior Internal Fixation Devices

Martin H. Krag

A major component of orthopedic surgery is to eliminate pain originating from joints. Two major approaches to achieving this goal are obliteration of motion by arthrodesis or joint replacement by arthroplasty. For the spine, efforts at developing clinically useful arthroplasty have either been unsuccessful (108,109) or are still experimental (see Chapter 96). Thus, fusion remains the method of choice for surgically relieving spinal pain.

Bone grafting alone has a number of drawbacks. First, most grafting techniques have limited or no capacity to correct spinal deformity (but may arrest progression). Second, most posterior grafting techniques do not provide early control of motion, which does not occur until after graft consolidation. Third, pseudarthrosis occurs with an unacceptable frequency, particularly when multiple levels are incorporated in the fusion. For these reasons, orthopedists have searched for adjuncts to bone grafting such as electrical stimulation (26,92,160,161,

244,312) or internal fixation devices, which would reduce the magnitude of or eliminate these three problems. In the past decade, posterior fixation devices have achieved increasing popularity because of their capacity to correct spinal deformity and provide early stabilization. There is substantial evidence, if not yet extensive proof, that they also increase the rate of solid arthrodesis, particularly when multiple motion segments are included in the fusion area.

EVOLUTION AND TYPES OF IMPLANTS

The earliest reports of attempted internal fixation for the spine were by Hadra in 1889 (134,135) and Lange in 1910 (195,196) (see also 31), and preceded by two decades the first reports of successful spinal fusion by Albee (6) and Hibbs (148,149). Over the next five decades the greatest attention was paid to developing improved methods of graft placement. Initially the spinous processes were used (6,36–38,125), but to improve fusion rates and to avoid spondylolysis development above the graft mass (9,29,33,49,54,77,116,141,283,309,321,

M. H. Krag, M.D.: Associate Professor, McClure Center for Musculoskeletal Research, Vermont Rehabilitation Engineering Center, Department of Orthopaedics and Rehabilitation, University of Vermont, Burlington, Vermont, 05405.

324,334,340), transverse processes were included as well (55,60,227,231,332,339,348–350). Also during this time various incisions were tried, partly to decrease soft tissue trauma (190,362–365). More recently, a variety of bone grafting methods or substitutes have been tried such as vascularized grafts (42,86,142,154,163,229,285,308), allograft (22,84,147,176,208,224,232,243,298), decalcified bone matrix (250,270,341), periosteal strips (258), or ceramics (129,346). Despite this extensive clinical research, posterior lumbar spinal fusion attempts continued to result in significant clinical and biological failure. Certain aspects of this topic, which are reviewed in detail in Chapter 98, were central to the development of posterior fixation devices.

Cause of Low Back Symptoms Often Unknown

Although very convincing evidence exists that mechanical factors are the major causation of back symptoms (13,67,68,91,105,106,114,118,119,150,171,217, 268), there has been a great deal of difficulty devising diagnostic criteria for conditions such as "instability." This is largely because of our lack of understanding of how these mechanical abnormalities actually develop. It is also because explicit quantifiable definitions of "instability" have not been agreed on. Furthermore, the roles of neurophysiologic, autoimmune, biochemical, and hormonal influences are only now becoming understood.

Pseudarthrosis

This topic is extensively considered in Chapters 91 and 98. The summary of the data presented there is that the incidence of pseudarthrosis is affected by the surgical construct, graft source, number of levels fused, and pathology being treated, and is increased by cigarette smoking. One of the perplexing issues is that pseudarthrosis is not predictably painful, particularly when the pre-existent condition was stable (37,116,287,350,372). Pseudarthrosis can be quite difficult to detect, as evidenced by the number of different methods that have been studied (59,74,78,113,115,191,194,240,255–257,274,314, 323).The relationship between bracing and pseudarthrosis development has received surprisingly little study (315,325).

Persistent Pain Despite Solid Fusions

There are numerous reasons why a solid fusion may not be followed by pain relief. These have been elucidated partly as a result of studies comparing grafting to non-grafting after partial discectomy either retrospectively (25,116,280,338,343) or prospectively (354).

Other extensive retrospective studies (155,172,203, 269,309,315,344) have also been reported. The reasons for failure include incorrect diagnosis or an inadequate length of fusion to bridge all the pain sources (106,127,238,241,368). A more subtle cause is the presence of excessive springiness or deflection despite the presence of a continuous arthrodesis (202,282,351,370). This tends to occur to a greater extent when the bone graft is placed more posteriorly. Conversely, intertransverse process or interbody grafts are less subject to this problem since the lever arm between graft and loading axis is less (282).

Others have suggested that non-osseous spinal structures are the source of the residual pain. Proposed structures include the supraspinous and interspinous ligaments (67,68,365); posterior primary rami which supply muscles, facet joints, and the neural arch (166,218,365); facet joint capsules (105,166,218) or muscles damaged intra-operatively mechanically or by retractor-induced ischemia (67,365); graft impingement on adjacent facets (68,188,328) or nerve roots (365); laminar hypertrophy (40,353); or continued presence of the degenerated disc itself (246,247).

Late onset pain may result from accelerated degeneration adjacent to the arthrodesis (40,45,115,143,200, 206,210,233,371). Such degeneration does not necessarily occur, which has allowed "floating fusions" to be used (45,46). The biomechanical events which promote this accelerated breakdown have been studied both in vitro (202,273,370) and in vivo (262,318). The biochemical aspects of this problem have been studied in animals (61,237,313,322,359).

The development of internal fixation devices was directly stimulated by the problem of pseudarthrosis, particularly in patients with mechanical insufficiencies, deformities, or multilevel problems. Recently, external fixation devices (102,164,251,253) have been used as a diagnostic tool to establish pre-operatively if temporary spinal stabilization eliminates or reduces pain. The following information details the historical types of spinal fixation. Because there have been many different stabilization devices used in clinical practice, these will be presented in groups organized by the site of vertebral attachment: facet joint, spinous process, lamina, and pedicle. The major focus of the remainder of this chapter will be on the pedicle screw since this is the dominant theme in today's fixation devices.

SPINAL FIXATION DEVICES

Extensive development of internal fixation devices for the lumbar and lumbosacral spine has occurred in the past 15 years. The most common rationale for using such devices is to reduce the incidence of pseudarthrosis after bone grafting. Another rationale (typically for trauma management) is to maintain intervertebral align-

1982 -5

ment until spontaneous healing occurs. Most recently, fixation devices (albeit external ones) have been used diagnostically to help determine whether fusion will provide pain relief. The development of these devices, their current uses, and various relevant issues are discussed below.

Facet Joint Fixation Screws

One of the early fixation methods was placement of screws obliquely across each facet joint involved in the grafting. This was described by Toumey (335) and then one year later by King (169). From these authors as well as others using this method (23,168,333) the pseudarthrosis rate for L5-S1 grafts was 9% to 12%, but for L4-S1 grafts the rate was still high at 55%.

1959 Boucher (39) attempted to reduce this unacceptable pseudarthrosis rate by using longer screws directed more medially, through the inferior articular process, across the facet joint, then across the superior articular process and part way into the pedicle of the subjacent vertebra. It should be noted that this technique is quite different from that used for a transpedicular screw, which is directed into the vertebral body but does not cross the facet joint, and thus functions as a handle or rigid extension of a single vertebra. Boucher's modification reduced his pseudarthrosis rate to 1% overall, and in Pennal's series (264) the rate was 2% for L5-S1 grafts and 16% for L4-S1 grafts. Recently, Andrew et al. (10) have reported similar results with Boucher's technique.

Much later Magerl (219–222) used yet another screw placement. The screw enters through the contralateral cortex of the base of the spinous process; proceeds caudally, laterally, and anteriorly across the facet joint; then exits along the caudal edge of the base of the ipsilateral transverse process. Kornblatt et al. (179) report a 13% pseudarthrosis rate with this technique combined with bilateral posterolateral grafting. Various authors (157, 319) have used this method to supplement their posterior interbody grafts and have reported a favorable preliminary experience.

Spinous Process Plates

While screw techniques were being developed in the 1940s, plates attached to the spinous processes were also being tried for lumbar and lumbosacral fusions. The first experience with these was reported by Straub (320) and '52 Wilson and Straub (361), who bolted plates which were curved in the sagittal plane onto both sides of the spinous processes of L4, L5, S1, and S2 (Fig. 1). Their pseudarthrosis rate was 15% in 101 graftings. This device differed from the plates described by Williams (360) or Reimers (278) which were straight and meant for thoracolumbar fracture-dislocations, rather than curved to fit the lumbosacral lordosis. Later, Cabot et al. (52,53) described a "crab plate" which crimps onto the lumbosacral spinous processes. In a series of 110 patients (52), they had a 6% pseudarthrosis rate. Other plates have also been tried (267).

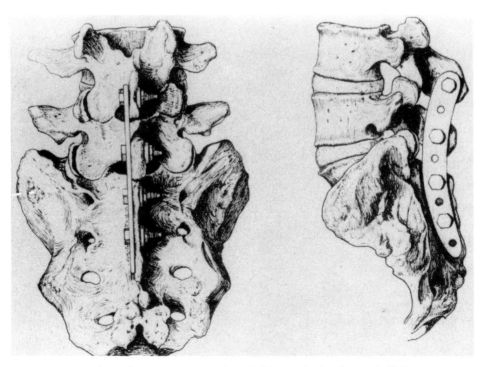

FIG. 1. Spinous process plates (with permission from ref. 361).

Laminar Hooks and Rods

The earliest description of this method appears to be by Knodt and Larrick (177) in 1964. This device consists of a hook on each end of a threaded rod (right hand thread on one end, left hand thread on the other), which when turned causes the hooks to spread apart (Fig. 2). Knodt and Larrick (177) provided no data on their 89 patients, but Beattie (27) reported an overall 14% pseudarthrosis rate at the L4-L5 and 11% at the L5-S1 levels. Others (43,73,306,326,355) have described pseudarthrosis rates ranging from 7% to 18%. Dubuc (90) reported a high rate of complications, which required rod removal. Lee and deBari (201) carefully studied the extent to which foraminal enlargement occurred, since this was hypothesized to be an important effect of Knodt rods (27,177). Enlargement was in fact produced, but did not correlate at all with clinical outcome.

The most widely used and well-known internal fixation device, Harrington distraction rods (Fig. 3A), was originally devised for scoliosis treatment (136,138) for which implantation down to the sacrum had been performed (41,180). Their use has been extended to treatment of other conditions such as spondylolisthesis (43, 48, 51, 137, 139, 140, 162, 179, 225, 299, 356, 374) and trauma (5,12,48,64,111,137), and various modifications of the implant have evolved (32,35,50,63,76,96,97,98, 112,121,156,159,242,266,286,304,327,336,337,369). However, there have been few reports of their use for lumbar degenerative problems (179,356) as shown in Figure 3B. Special problems associated with Harrington rod use in the lumbosacral area include attachment of the lower end (48,139,140,225,299,374) and the loss of lumbar lordosis ("flatback") that tends to occur with a poste-

rior distraction device (57,193,236,366). Various other complications have been noted (e.g., 124,286).

The Harrington compression rods (Fig. 4) apply force opposite to the distraction devices. Their application has been widespread for treatment of spinal deformities, but less so for lumbar degeneration because of their tendency to produce lumbar extension—just the opposite of the flatback produced by the distraction rods. The concern with extension is not the postural change itself, but rather the decrease in foraminal height and possible nerve root encroachment. Despite this tendency, Attenborough and Reynolds (21) reported good results with a similar compressing device, and Lee and deBari (201), as noted above, did not find that distraction with Knodt rods predictably provided any benefit.

"Segmental" Wires and Smooth Rods

Instead of being used to produce either distraction or compression forces, these implants are used to resist flexion, extension, or lateral bending. These were initially reported by Resina and Alves (279), as shown in Figure 5, and later by Luque et al. (211–214) who used wires around the entire lamina. These have had their greatest application in scoliosis, particularly in paralytic curves (7,8,180,230), and also have been used for conditions such as trauma (44), tumors (276), and degenerative spondylolisthesis and disc disruption (213,248) (see also Chapters 91 and 97). Various methods for attaching the rods to the sacrum are described by Luque (213). The wire which attaches the rod to the lamina controls lateral bending or flexion-extension of a multivertebrae segment, but cannot resist axial compression/distraction, axial rotation, or local flexion of a single vertebra about the point of contact between rod and lamina. A variation of this method that is significantly stiffer is to replace the two rods with a single rectangle, shaped to be planar (110,248) or peaked at the midline to provide clearance of midline structures and improved attachment to bone (88).

One of the significant risks of circumlaminar wires is dural or cord injury during either wire placement (66,88,126), or removal (254). Careful technique is essential, and use of soft, flexible Mersilene tapes instead of wire (120,128) has proven to be a quite useful alternative. Another approach to increase safety is to wire the rods to the base of the spinous process, rather than to the lamina (89,165).

Transpedicular Screw-Based Devices

The major recent advance in spinal implants has been the use of transpedicular screws as a method for attachment to the vertebrae. This method has provided for the first time a "grip" on the vertebra which resists loads of any type, not just a few special types. Although the pedi-

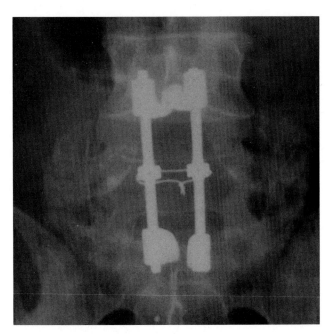

FIG. 2. Knodt rods.

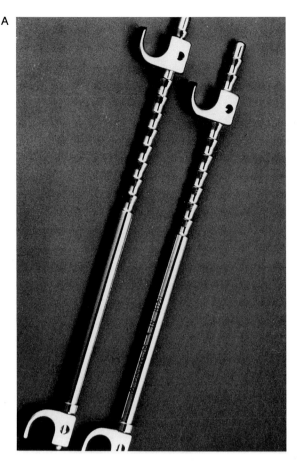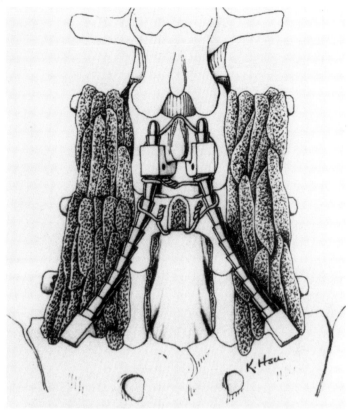

FIG. 3. Harrington distraction rods. **A:** Undeformed implant. **B:** Implementation from L3 to sacrum (with permission from ref. 353).

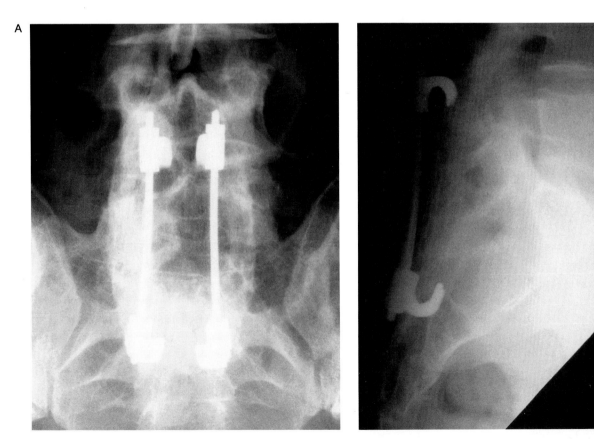

FIG. 4. Bilateral Harrington compression rods (⅛″ diameter) for treatment with supplemental bone graft of an L5-S1 pseudarthrosis. Lower hooks are placed into a window cut into the dorsal cortex of the original graft mass. **A:** AP view. **B:** Lateral view.

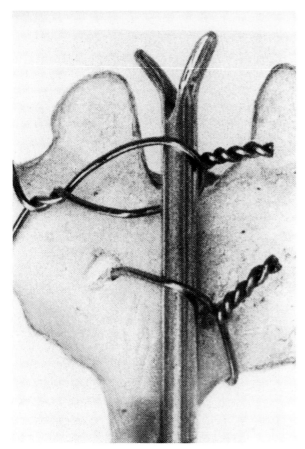

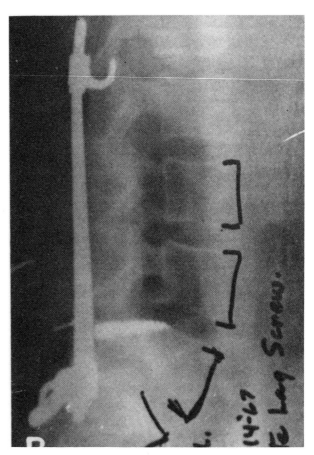

FIG. 5. Close-up of segmental wires as described by Resina and Alves (1977) (ref. 279), similar to circumlaminar wires described later by Luque (1982) (ref. 211) (with permission from ref. 279).

FIG. 6. Initially published case of transpedicular screw implantation by Harrington and Tullos (1969) (ref. 140). Wires from the L5 screws were used to produce further reduction of the spondylolisthesis beyond that already produced by the distracting rods (with permission from ref. 140).

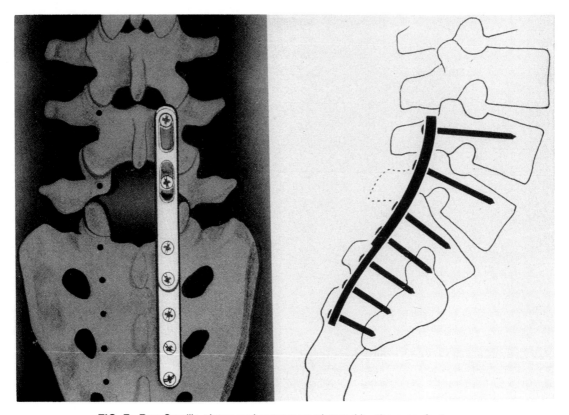

FIG. 7. Roy-Camille plates and screws as pictured by the manufacturer.

cle had been used earlier as a route for vertebral body biopsy (65,234) and also had been used for placement or removal of bone from the vertebral body (69,70–72,144), its first use as a route for placement of a truly transpedicular screw was not reported until 1969 by Harrington and Tullos (140) who used it for attempting reduction of L5 spondylolisthesis (Fig. 6).

Subsequently it was Roy-Camille who developed the first practical method of pedicle screw fixation. He acquired extensive experience with his plate and screw system (288–296) as have others (167,170) (Fig. 7). Substantial positional control can be achieved with these plates, but if any bone resorption or compression occurs under the plate, the "toggle" of the screws within the plate holes still allows some motion to take place (34,170). In addition, the loading on the screw will change from tensile to cantilever bending if any slippage occurs between the smooth plate and underlying vertebra (62,146,181,226,261,265,373), probably contributing to the fairly high screw breakage rate with this system (289,296). Similar problems have been seen with other types of plates with "free" screws (209,330).

To try to solve the problem of screw toggle, Steffee et al. (316,317) provided a means to attach the screw rigidly in a perpendicular position to the plate (Fig. 8). However, with this linkage, if the screw is not initially perpendicular to the segment of plate through which it passes, either the screw shaft tends to be bent as the nut is tight-ened [which increases the chance of breakage (152,239,317,357,379)], or the screw is not seated securely against the plate (152,277,316).

There are under investigation other systems which also require bending in order to achieve three-dimensional adjustability between the screws and longitudinal linking members. Experience with a device designed by Wiltse (Fig. 9) has been reported by various authors (132,151,263,331). Zielke screws, linked by a solid rod rather than a cable, also have been used posteriorly (272,311,374). The Cotrel-Dubousset system (Fig. 10) (63) has been reported to be useful for lumbosacral fusion revisions (104) and various other conditions (130). Edwards et al. (93,94,95,99) have developed a system (Fig. 11) combining pedicle screws and ratcheted rods. Schreiber et al. (305) reported on the Balgrist system and Puno et al. (271) described mechanical testing of their system.

Quite different from the above has been the development of implants that have both truly three-dimensional adjustability and three-dimensional positional control between each screw and its longitudinally linking rod.

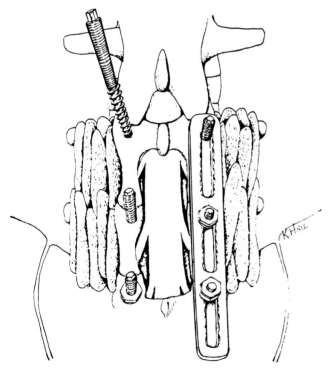

FIG. 8. Steffee plates and screws, L4-S1 implantation. Steps involved are shown sequentially (tap, screw insertion, ventral nut, plate, dorsal nut, locking nut) (with permission from ref. 353).

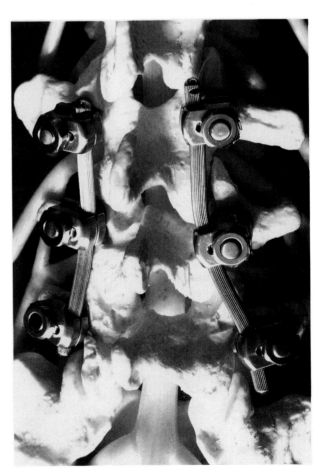

FIG. 9. Wiltse system (courtesy of Leon L. Wiltse, M.D.).

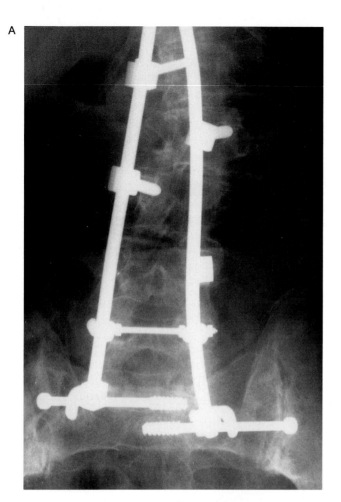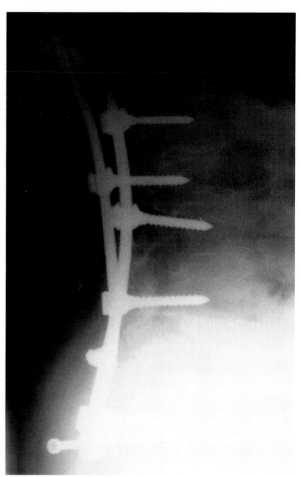

FIG. 10. Cotrel-Dubousset system, AP **(A)** and lateral **(B)** views.

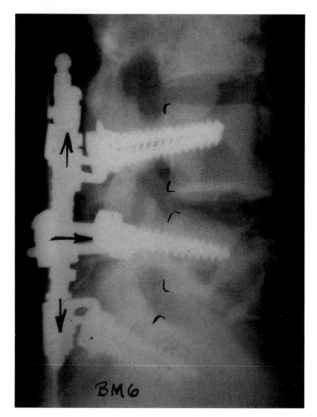

FIG. 11. Edwards system.

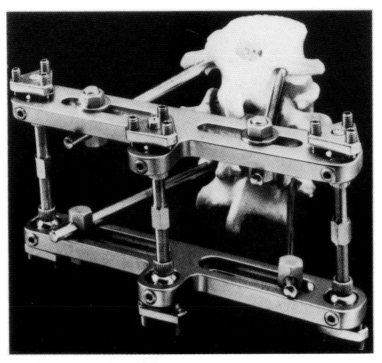

FIG. 12. Magerl external spinal fixator (with permission from ref. 221).

The usefulness of this approach is exemplified by modern-day external fixators for limb and pelvis applications, which also have these features of three-dimensional adjustability and control. It was only logical to extend the use of external fixators from the limbs to the spine. This was pioneered starting in 1977 by Magerl (Fig. 12) (219–222), who used external fixators for various purposes, including lumbosacral spine operations. Others (70,102,175) have also reported their experience with the Magerl fixator. Arnold (14,15) also has designed and used a similar device. Ölerud et al. (164,251,253) developed the direct but novel approach of using a somewhat different external fixator as a "dry run" for surgery: by placing the fixator across various motion segments one at a time, the abnormal level(s) could be identified by the pain relief produced. Additional experience with this approach was reported by Esses et al. (102).

The next logical development was to "internalize" the external fixator, and this began almost simultaneously along two separate lines which have proceeded independently. Magerl, according to Dick (79,80), suggested such an internal fixator which was subsequently designed in 1982 by Dick and co-workers, first implanted in 1983, and reported in 1984 (80,81). This is shown in Figure 13. The various components comprising the articulating linkage at each screw may be seen in Figure 13A. The overall size of the device may be seen in Figure 13B. Clinical experience has accumulated since then (2,3,70,79,82,102,223,329). Kluger and Gerner de-

scribed a modification of this device (175), which has been also used by others (34). A more complex modification (Fig. 14), apparently in use since 1985, has been described by Ölerud et al. (252).

The other line of internal fixator development occurred at the University of Vermont and was stimulated in 1981 by Magerl's research concerning his external fixator and by experience with the Roy-Camille plate and screw system. At that time even the basic morphometric issues needed further research, so a program was begun of anatomic studies (185,189), screw design (185), and mechanical testing (181,183–186,188), leading to initial clinical implantation in 1986 (182). The major design objectives for the Vermont Spinal Fixator or VSF (Fig. 15) were very few component parts for simple, easy assembly (low "fiddle factor") and overall small size to reduce adjacent tissue irritation, especially to the adjacent upper facet joint (Fig. 15B). The recess on each side of the screw head provides a means for intra-operative attachment of a reduction frame to allow multidirectional realignment, after which the locking bolts are tightened and the reduction frame is removed. This approach helps maintain the small size and simplicity of the implanted components.

Figures 16A and 16B show the VSF used for degenerative scoliosis from L3 to S1. Note the rods do not need to be contoured since only two screws are used on each side (interposed vertebrae need not be instrumented). Also note the rods do not contact the lamina, thus bone graft placement is not restricted. Figures 16C and 16D show a

A

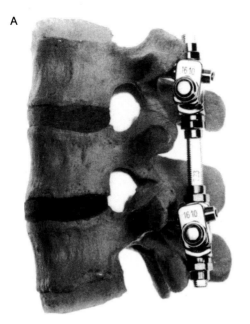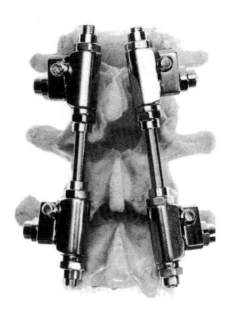

FIG. 13. Dick internal spinal fixator. **A:** Lateral and posterior photographic views. **B:** Lateral x-ray view (with permission from ref. 80).

B

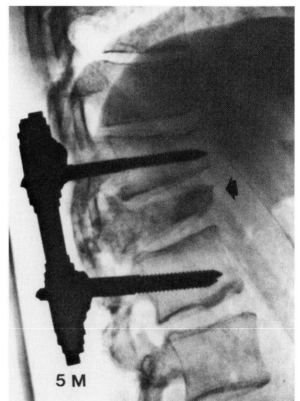

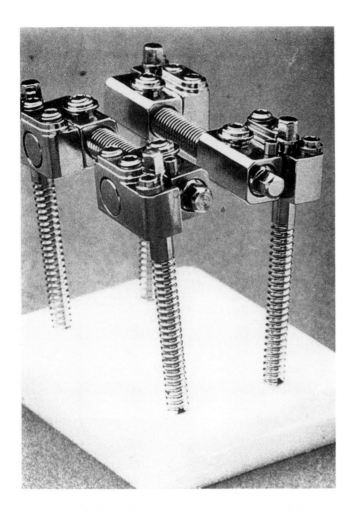

FIG. 14. Ölerud internal fixator shown attached to a plastic block. The various adjusting and locking screws for each transpedicular screw may be seen (with permission from ref. 164a).

A

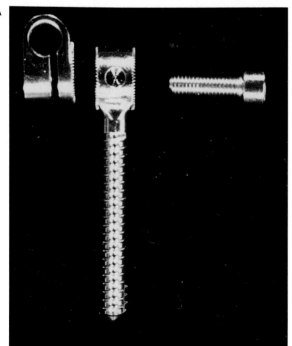

B

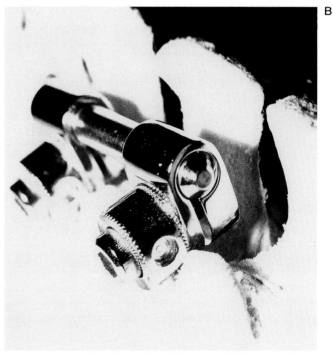

FIG. 15. Vermont spinal fixator device. **A:** Components: screw, clamp, locking bolt (rod, not shown, slides into clamp). **B:** Assembled implant spanning a single motion segment, on the right side of plastic spine model, seen from the right, cephalo-dorsal view. Note that the right cephalad facet joint (lower right hand corner) is unconstrained by the implant (with permission from ref. 182).

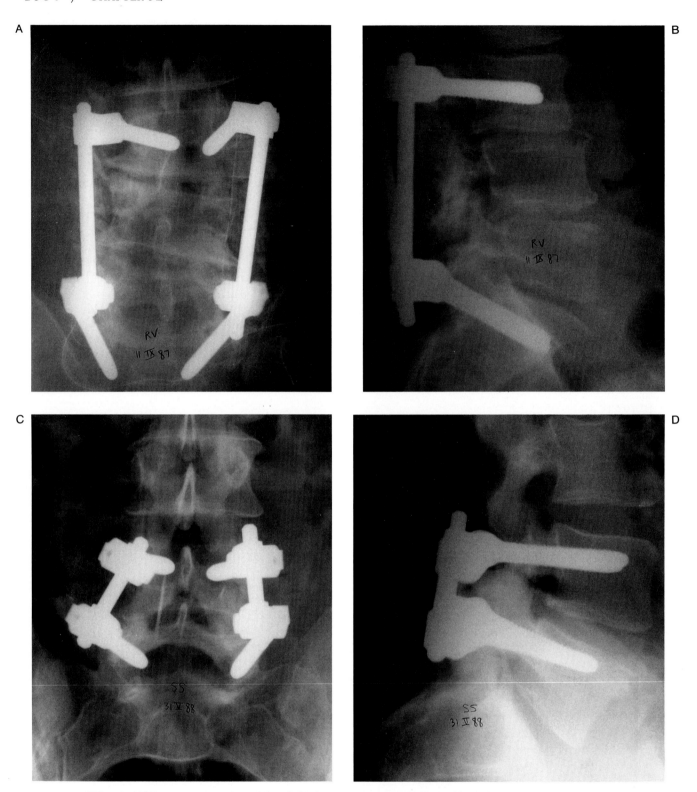

FIG. 16. VSF implantation. **A and B:** L3-S1 for degenerative scoliosis. Note that the rod need not be contoured and L4 and L5 are not instrumented. **C and D:** L4-L5 for single-level disc degeneration. This may be readily accomplished because of the compact size of the articulating clamp.

case of a single segment L4-L5 "floating fusion," which is easily accomplished due to the small size of the articulating linkage. No cross-linking is used because of the resistance to lateral "pushover" that results from oblique screw placement, discussed further below.

Comparative Mechanical Testing of Devices

All of these studies have been performed in vitro using either human or non-human cadaveric specimens. A wide variety of vertebral levels, loading methods, performance parameters, and device comparisons have been used. These studies have been reviewed elsewhere (181), therefore only the more recent studies will be briefly presented here, with the emphasis on devices which involve transpedicular screws. Articles which discuss the general approach to this testing are also available, such as Panjabi et al. (259) and Ashman et al. (19).

Studies of posterior non-transpedicular implants have been performed using experimental models of trauma (158,192,260,271), spondylolysis (19,145) and scoliosis (19,271,369). Lumbosacral devices have been the particular focus of a number of other studies (19,58,133,249). Comparisons have also included anterior implants (1,19,103,192).

The major findings from the studies involving transpedicular screw-based devices that were applied above the sacrum are as follows. Abumi et al. (1) found that an Ölerud external fixator, compared to three other non-pedicular devices (Harrington compression rods, Luque rectangle, and Kaneda anterior screws and rods), was the "only device that provided sufficient stability . . . for all load types." Akbarnia et al. (5) rank ordered the stiffness of various implants (Harrington rods without and with Edwards sleeves or wires, Luque rectangle, anterior Kaneda device without or with crosslink, and Steffee plates) applied to calf spines. The overall greatest stiffness was from the Steffee plates. Ashman et al. (20) compared five different implants and found that all were approximately equally stiff, but that higher strains were produced on those screws that were securely attached to their longitudinal linking element, compared to those where some motion could occur at this junction. Falahee et al. (103) reported that supplementation with transfacet screws was needed to bring the stiffness of the Syracuse "I" anterior plate construct up to that produced by the Dick internal fixator. Ferguson et al. (107) found that a "one above–one below" VSF provided as much stiffness as "two above–two below" Jacobs rods or Harrington rods with circumlaminar wiring. In addition, they showed that the Roy-Camille plates were stiffer than the VSF rods, and that both of these devices, unlike the rod and hook systems tested, were able to maintain lateral stability after cyclic loading. Gurr et al. (131) showed that a "one above–one below" Cotrel-Dubousset transpedicular implant with a rigid screw-rod connection applied to a highly unstable "posterior instability" model returned

the overall construct stiffness back to normal. They also found that a "two above–two below" implant was even stronger than the intact state. Wörsdörfer et al. (367) found that the Magerl external fixator provided greater overall positional control than any of the other non-pedicle implants studied.

Only two studies have been done specifically on lumbosacral implantation of transpedicular screw-based devices. Asazuma et al. (16) used intact porcine L5, L6, L7, S1 specimens, and compared Harrington distraction rods, Luque rods (Galveston technique), Steffee plates, VSF, and Zielke screw and rods without and with a Luque rectangle. They state that the VSF was "the most rigid construct overall . . .", even though the screws were only placed into L5 and S1 (and not into the interposed L6 and L7 vertebrae). Puno et al. (271) compared Luque rods (Galveston technique), Luque rectangle, Steffee plates (without and with S2 screws), and three experimental screw and rod devices. Major findings included a troublesome bulkiness to the experimental articulated fixator, and a substantial increase in stiffness of the Steffee plate construct from addition of a screw into the S2 lateral mass.

Unresolved Issues for Transpedicular Screw Use

What Is the Optimal Thread Design?

Although a number of biomechanical comparisons of bone screws have been made for limb bones (11,28,75,83,178,216,300), few have been done for transpedicular screws (122,185,207) and only one of these (185) systematically varied pitch, minor diameter, and tooth profile, which allowed separation of the effects of each variable. This study showed no benefit of buttress over "V" threads in pullout, and showed that shallower threads (larger minor diameter) produced little loss in pullout strength and a large gain in bending strength. However, in that study the number of specimens and the ranges of the controlled variables were not large. Sell et al. (307) showed no difference between pullout strength of three different screw types inserted to a depth of 30 mm, but here too specimen number was small.

What Is the Optimal Position for Screw Placement?

The alternatives for entry site and orientation (Fig. 17) are to go "straight ahead" (291,292,295,296), "inward" (2,3,79–81,185,186,188,219–222,352), or "up and in" (181). The orientations of the pedicle axes are shown in Figure 18, and the lengths of screws that may be placed without anterior cortex penetration are shown in Figure 19. The benefits of the more oblique orientation are: a) less interference with the superjacent facet joint

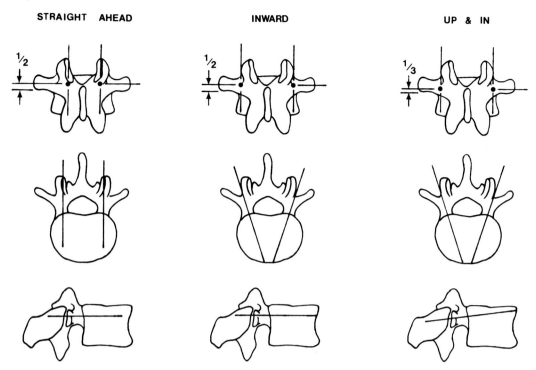

STRAIGHT AHEAD   INWARD   UP & IN

FIG. 17. Transpedicular screw entry site and orientation alternatives.

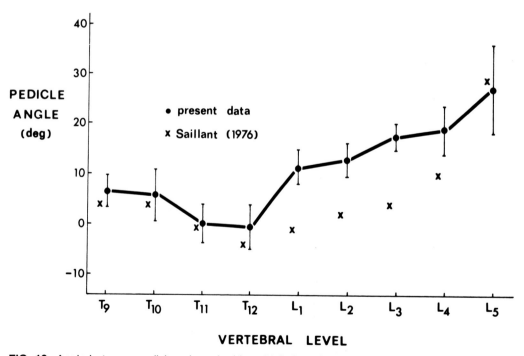

PEDICLE
ANGLE
(deg)

• present data
x Saillant (1976)

VERTEBRAL LEVEL

FIG. 18. Angle between pedicle axis and mid-sagittal plane (measured in the transverse plane) for T9-L5. Means and standard deviations are shown, as well as comparison to data of Saillant (1976) (ref. 297) (with permission from ref. 185).

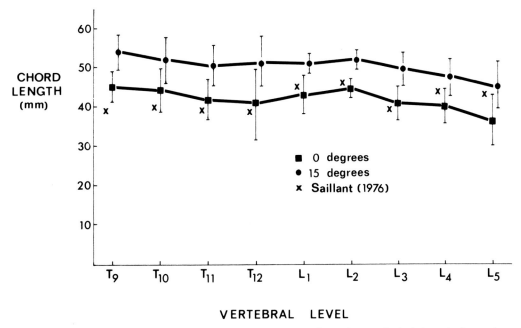

FIG. 19. Path length (*chord length*) from posterior cortex of pars interarticularis to anterior cortex of vertebral body. Measurements at both 0° and 15° relative to the sagittal plane are provided to indicate the dependence upon orientation. Means and standard deviations, as well as the means from Saillant (1976) (ref. 297) are shown. This defines the upper level of screw length for T9-L5 (with permission from ref. 185).

(181,182,205), b) a longer screw may be used (185,189) thereby providing a stronger grip on the vertebra (183), and c) a three-dimensional locking effect ("toe nailing") is produced by the oblique orientation of right and left implants, which produces resistance to lateral shifting (Fig. 20) (181) even without transverse connectors (17,56,174).

Two commonly used orientations for screw placement into the sacrum are anteromedially (toward the sacral promontory) or anterolaterally (toward the sacral ala) as shown in Figure 21. There are proponents of each method, but facts on this subject are few. Anatomic data are reported by Asher and Strippgen (18) and Dohring et al. (85). Bone-screw interface strengths are reported by

Zindrick (377,378) who reported the strength of alar screws to be somewhat stronger than that of promontory screws. However, the load type was pullout along the screw axis, no right-left comparisons were made, and the interspecimen variability was high. Testing from our laboratory (85) involved flexion loading, which we believe is the more important load type in vivo, and right-left comparisons were made between the promontory and alar screw positions. Each screw was inserted to the anterior cortex or to a depth of 55 mm, whichever occurred first. Displacement was measured directly between the ventral tip of the screw and the superior end plate of S1. Two measures of screw-bone interface failure were used, namely the loads required to rotate the screw through 0.1

STRAIGHT AHEAD   **UP & IN**

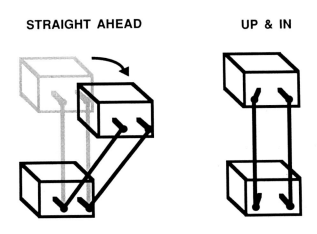

FIG. 20. The 3D locking effect ("toe nailing") produced by obliquely oriented right and left implants, which produce resistance to lateral "pushover," even without cross-linking. Pushover can easily occur when the screws are oriented straight ahead, since all 4 screws are parallel (with permission from ref. 181).

degree and through 1.0 degree. This testing showed that the torque required to produce 0.1 degree rotation of the promontory screws is not significantly different than for alar screws. However, for 1.0 degrees the torque is significantly greater for the promontory screws (15 Nm vs. 6 Nm, $p < .01$).

What Is the Optimal Method for Monitoring Screw Placement?

Locating the pedicle can be done by direct visualization after partial resection of posterior elements (although this weakens the screw site), by palpation of the inferolateral portion of the pedicular cortex, by use of surface landmarks [although substantial anatomical variability does exist (24,30,185,186,189,235,239,297, 376)], or by intra-operative visualization radiographically, done most conveniently with a "C"-arm image intensifier. Although the traditional anteroposterior and lateral views have been shown to be not very safe as defined by pedicle "miss" rate (199,281,288,352,388), an oblique view along the axis of the pedicle [the "bulls-eye" or "pedicle coaxial" x-ray (181–183)] shown in Figure 22 provides direct confirmation of correct drill bit or screw orientation and location even before any bone entry.

What Is the Optimal Depth of Screw Insertion?

A variety of clinically based opinions have been expressed concerning penetration depth, ranging from screw placement just deep enough to reach into the body (291–293,295,296) all the way to screw placement contacting the anterior cortex (79–81,188,219–222). Relevant anatomic data are shown in Figure 19. A significant relation between strength and depth of insertion has been reported (183,198,378) as shown in Figure 23, but the clinical importance of this has not yet been established.

To decrease the likelihood of unintentional penetration of the anterior cortex, use of a "near approach" or obliqued lateral x-ray view has been recommended (181,188,358). This view is tangential to the anterior cortex of the vertebra at that location at which cortical penetration would occur if the drill were inserted too far. On this view, the tip of the drill appears on x-rays to most nearly approach the anterior cortex. This same approach has earlier been applied to the knee (100) and hip (47,204,284,310,345,347).

How Should the Screw Hole Be Prepared?

There are proponents for the use of a drill bit (152,181,182,188,219–222,291–293,295,296), curet

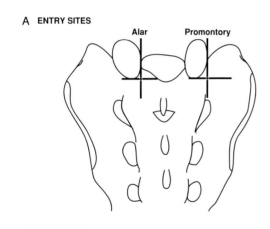

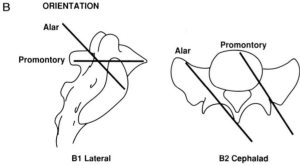

FIG. 21. Two commonly used sacral screw placements: anterolaterally into the ala or anteromedially into the promontory. **A:** Posterior view. **B:** Lateral and cephalad views.

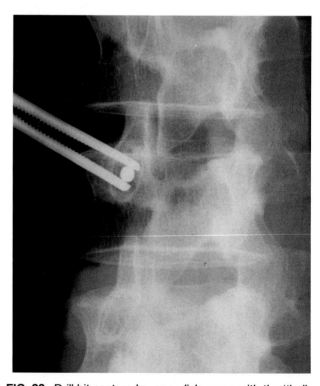

FIG. 22. Drill bit centered over pedicle, seen with the "bulls-eye" or "pedicle coaxial" x-ray view. The image intensifier axis is rotated to align with the pedicle axis, and the drill bit is held end-on, centered over the pedicle with a long handled surgical clamp. Correct placement is seen even before drill insertion is performed (with permission from ref. 181).

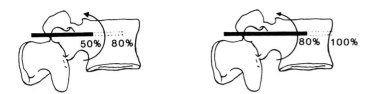

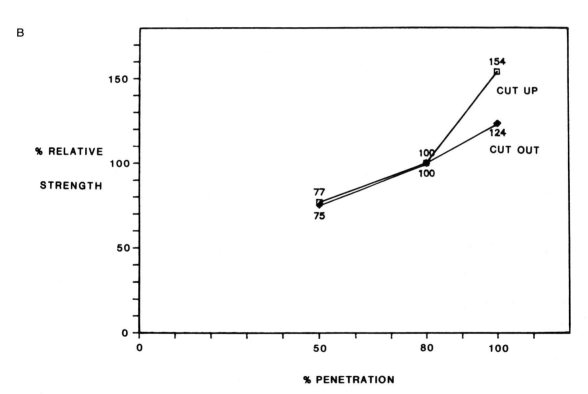

FIG. 23. Increased strength of transpedicular screw with increased depth of insertion. **A:** Experimental method: comparison of 80% versus 50% and 80% versus 100% depth of penetration, for both flexion and torsion load types (with permission from ref. 183).

FIG. 23. *Continued.* **B:** Strength (relative to that of the 80% depth screw) versus depth of penetration. This relationship is approximately linear.

(95,197), curved flat probe (132,316), and straight probe (252). Two reports have compared these methods biomechanically. George et al. (123) showed no difference in screw pullout strength from holes prepared by drill bit versus straight conical-tipped probe. Although Moran et al. (239) reported significantly less strength (84%, $p <$ .04) for the drilled hole compared to the probed hole based upon a one-tailed t statistic, the more appropriate two-tailed statistic shows no significant difference in strength (123).

Although tapping is advised by some authors, the evidence, although not weighty, seems to be against it. Zindrick et al. (377) from cadaver testing of tapped versus non-tapped screws found little difference overall, and weakening in some specimens with the use of a tap. This is similar to data from bovine cancellous bone (245) and femoral diaphyseal bone (178,342).

How Long a Spine Segment Should Be Instrumented?

The uniqueness of transpedicular screws for vertebral attachment is that they can provide a three dimensionally controlling "grip" on the vertebra, unlike hooks (e.g., a distraction hook can only resist compression and anterior translation) or wires (e.g., circumlaminar wires cannot prevent compression or rotation). It is this feature that prevents the need for any "extra" vertebrae to be instrumented, and allows a "one above–one below" approach to work (assuming the screw can be attached in a three-dimensionally secure manner to the rod or plate).

However, this requires that the screw bone interface be strong enough to deal with the full range of in vivo loads. As described earlier, strength is affected by depth of screw insertion (182,188) and by bone quality (e.g., osteopenia). Reliable provision of adequate strength, especially in osteopenic bone, remains a challenge for transpedicular screws, especially in situations where load-sharing anteriorly through the vertebral bodies is limited.

Polymethylmethacrylate can be used to strengthen the screw site (173,375), but extrusion against cord or roots, infection, and difficulty of removal should be kept in mind. Screw strength has been increased by improvements in design (184,185) and material (207), but some screw breakage still occurs. One of the major challenges to optimizing screw design is that the loads acting upon the implant are not well known (183,187). A few in vivo measurements have been obtained by means of a strain-gauged Magerl external fixator (301–303), but full separation of the individual load components (e.g., compressive force from flexion moment) remains to be accomplished.

If the linkage between longitudinal element and screw is not three dimensionally secure (e.g., a screw which can toggle within a plate), then either an immediate load-bearing interbody graft can be used (which prevents ante-

rior compressive forces from producing bending moments on the screw) or an additional vertebra above and below ("two above–two below") can be instrumented. The screw in the "second-above" vertebra in effect protects the screw in the "first-above" vertebra from the bending moment, although the problem has now been shifted to the second screw. This explains in part why almost all of the screw breakages in such plate and screw systems are at the uppermost or lowermost screws (296). The drawback to this "two above–two below" solution is the longer fusion length, the particular avoidance of which has been one of the major incentives to pedicle screw device development.

How Important Is "Crosslinking"?

The rationale for crosslinking the right and left implant components is to improve the mechanical performance of the overall construct. Initially spinal implant crosslinking was performed to improve curve correction for scoliosis, and this has been shown to be quite effective. More recently the focus for crosslinking has been to increase overall stiffness or positional control, but for this the effectiveness is not yet well established.

Gurr and McAfee (130) crosslinked Cotrel-Dubousset rods attached to transpedicular screws inserted into calf spine specimens. They found no significant increase in stiffness. Kling et al. (174) studied screw pullout from calf vertebrae. They found that crosslinked right and left screws were more than twice as strong as a single screw. This increase was 30% for 4 mm diameter screws and 16% for 5 mm screws. Intraspecimen controls and statistical analysis of significance were not reported. Wörsdörfer (367) performed a similar experiment using 5 mm Schanz screws in human vertebrae and did not find such a strengthening effect. Unfortunately, there was high interspecimen variation and no right-left comparison or statistical analysis.

Carson et al. (56) measured the strains on the screws of Steffee implants in human cadaveric specimens. They found little or no reduction in screw strain from crosslinking the plates when the screws were oriented 15 degrees or more away from the sagittal plane. Only when the screws were less oblique than this did major strain reductions occur from crosslinking. In the lower lumbar spine, the pedicle axis is typically oriented at least 15 degrees away from the sagittal plane. Thus, as long as the implant design does not prevent oblique screw placement along the pedicle axis, the implant-vertebra construct can resist substantial lateral loads (181) without the additional complexity and bulk of a crosslinking component (Fig. 18). Clinical reports so far have not described problems in the lumbar or lumbosacral region due to the absence of crosslinking, although further experience will be useful.

What Are the Optimal Mechanical Characteristics of Transpedicular Implants?

Given the variety of implants presently evolving, it may be useful to consider certain general mechanical characteristics in comparing implants. Positional adjustability affects the ease and extent to which the implant allows screw placement to match anatomical constraints, and the ease with which intervertebral realignment can be accomplished. Positional control affects maintenance of reduction and achievement of solid fusion. We do not yet know which is best: a fair amount of "toggle" between screw and plate (215,296), a small "jog" of motion between screw and rod (271) or no slippage at all (79,185).

The biological effects of implant stiffness, which vary widely across available devices, are not fully understood. McAfee et al. (228) have shown stress-shielding–induced osteopenia with the stiffer implants, but also a higher rate of union. Hsu et al. (153) have conjectured that the more rapid onset of degeneration in discs adjacent to fusions with Steffee plates (relative to those with no hardware) is due to the stiffness of the plates. However, a more plausible explanation is the impingement of the upper screw and plate end on the upper non-grafted facet joint.

Implant bulk and ease of assembly and implantation ("fiddle factor") are not readily quantified, but there certainly is a spectrum among current devices. The optimal balance between these various features and the performance of each device will become more clear with time.

Clinical Experience with Transpedicular Fixation

The major hoped-for benefits from use of these devices are improved fusion rates, improved ability to obtain reduction, and improved maintenance of reduction, all of which ideally would be obtained without any significant increased biological cost.

Solidity of fusion is much more difficult to establish with hardware in place than without. Most of the clinical studies reported to date have not involved routine hardware removal, and thus have inferred fusion solidity from one or more of the following: relief of pre-operative pain, absence of screw breakage, absence of lucency about the screws, and absence of motion on flexion/extension x-rays. How reliable those indicators are is not yet well established, thus these reported pseudarthrosis rates must be interpreted carefully.

Despite this caveat, the results look quite promising. For series of patients for which the diagnoses are mostly or only degenerative, there are a number of reports of fusion rates from 90% to 100% (79,101,151,277,357). For patients with pseudarthroses, the results are also encouraging. Thalgott et al. (330) report a 76% union rate

for interbody and 80% for posterior graft pseudarthroses. Edwards and Weigel (99) report 100% for 1-level and 81% for 2- and 3-level pseudarthroses.

Deformity reduction is certainly achievable using transpedicular screws: they provide a three dimensionally rigid "grip" on the vertebra by means of which realignment can be potentially effected. The reduction can be accomplished either to a limited extent by pre-bending the plate or rod, or more thoroughly by means of an adjustable linkage between upper and lower screws and a mechanism for producing the realignment (79,175, 183,187,252). For spondylolisthesis, Dick and Schnebel (82) reduced the mean slip from 72% to 36%, which only increased to 39% at follow-up. For fractures, realignment to within a few degrees of neutral has been reported by various authors (3,79,101). The increase in kyphosis between immediate post-operation and follow-up was small: for the fixators 2.8 degrees mean (3) and 4.0 degrees mean (79), and for unconstrained screw and plates a slightly longer 6.5 degrees mean (296).

Is the biological cost acceptable? A simple answer does not exist, although for complex deformities, highly "unstable" conditions, or pseudarthroses the answer seems to be "yes." For single-level problems without previous bone grafting efforts, this is far less clear. The major biological complications are infection or increased neurologic deficit. The former in a number of series has been disturbingly high [5.3% to 6.0% for Roy-Camille (296); Steffee et al. (316); Thalgott et al. (330); and Zucherman et al. (379)], although these patients were largely high risk because of multiple previous operations. Later experience has been more favorable. In series of patients that have not had previous operations, the rates are substantially lower [0% to 1.1% for Aebi et al. (3), Dick (79), and Louis (209)].

Major increased neurologic deficit has been very low in the lumbar spine: the absence of spinal cord and presence of large pedicles are helpful factors in this regard. However, nerve root irritation or transient weakness has been fairly high in some series [5.0% to 12% for Roy-Camille (296), Reed and Wagner (277), Thalgott et al. (330), Zucherman et al. (379), and Whitecloud et al. (358)]. Related to this is the incidence of pedicle cortical disruptions which in some reports is disturbingly high (199,281,288,352,358). Although pedicle disruption does not necessarily cause neural deficit, keeping the screw contained within the pedicle is one sure way to prevent it. With careful attention to screw placement, nerve root irritation can be kept to a minimum [0% for Dick (79) and for Horowitch et al. (151)].

The major reduction in biological cost brought by transpedicular screw fixation is the greater security of attachment (fewer hardware failures) and the shorter length of fusion needed to accomplish positional control. Hook dislocations of 5% to 10% and fusion lengths of five, six, or even seven vertebrae such as with Harrington distraction rods have been substantially improved on by transpedicular screw-based fixation devices.

REFERENCES

1. Abumi K, Panjabi MM, Duranceau J (1989): Biomechanical evaluation of spinal fixation devices: Part III. Stability provided by six spinal fixation devices and interbody bone graft. *Spine* 14:1249–1255.
2. Aebi M, Etter C, Kehl T, Thalgott J (1988): The internal skeletal fixation system: A new treatment of thoracolumbar fractures and other spinal disorders. *Clin Orthop* 227:30–43.
3. Aebi M, Etter C, Kehl T, Thalgott J (1987): Stabilization of the lower thoracic and lumbar spine with the internal spinal skeletal fixation system: Indications, techniques, and first results of treatment. *Spine* 12:544–551.
4. Akbarnia BA, Fogarty JP, Tayob AA (1984): Contoured Harrington instrumentation in the treatment of unstable spinal fractures: The effect of supplementary sublaminar wires. *Clin Orthop* 189:186–194.
5. Akbarnia BA, Merenda JT, Keppler L, Gaines RW Jr, Lorenz M (1987): Surgical treatment of fractures and fracture dislocations of thoracolumbar and lumbar spine using pedicular screw and plate fixation. Proceedings of the American Academy of Orthopedic Surgeons, 54th Annual Meeting, San Francisco, California.
6. Albee FH (1911): Transplantation of a portion of the tibia into the spine for Pott's disease. *JAMA* 57:885–886.
7. Allen BL Jr, Ferguson RL (1982): Galveston technique for L rod instrumentation of the scoliotic spine. *Spine* 7:276–284.
8. Allen BL, Ferguson RL (1988): The Galveston experience with L-rod instrumentation for adolescent idiopathic scoliosis. *Clin Orthop* 229:59–69.
9. Anderson CE (1956): Spondyloschisis following spine fusion. *J Bone Joint Surg* [Am] 38:1142–1146.
10. Andrew TA, Brooks S, Piggott H (1986): Long-term follow-up evaluation of screw-and-graft fixation in the lumbosacral spine. *Clin Orthop* 203:113–119.
11. Ansell RH, Scales JT (1968): A study of some factors which affect the strength of screws and their holding power in bone. *J Biomech* 1:279–302.
12. Armstrong GWD (1976): Harrington instrumentation for spinal fractures. Proceedings of the Scoliosis Research Society Annual Meeting.
13. Armstrong JR (1965): Lumbar disc lesions: Pathogenesis and treatment of low back pain and sciatica. Baltimore: Williams and Wilkins.
14. Arnold W (1985): Early surgical treatment using an external fixation device in traumatic paraplegia. *Beitr Orthop Traumatol* 32:6–14.
15. Arnold W (1985): Early surgical treatment of traumatic paraplegia with an external fixation device and diagonal vertebroplasty. *Der Unfallchirurg* 88:293–298.
16. Asazuma T, Stokes IAF, Moreland MS, Suzuki N (1989): An intersegmental spinal flexibility with lumbosacral instrumentation: In vitro biomechanical investigation. Proceedings of the International Society for Study of the Lumbar Spine, Kyoto, Japan.
17. Asher M, Carson W, Heinig C (1988): A modular spinal rod linkage system to provide rotational stability. *Spine* 13:272–277.
18. Asher MA, Strippgen WE (1986): Anthropometric studies of the human sacrum relating to dorsal transsacral implant designs. *Clin Orthop* 203:58–62.
19. Ashman RB, Birch JG, Bone LB, Corin JD, Herring JA, Johnston CE, Ritterbush JF, Roach JW (1988): Mechanical testing of spinal instrumentation. *Clin Orthop* 227:113–125.
20. Ashman RB, Galpin RD, Corin JD, Johnston CE II (1989): Biomechanical analysis of pedicle screw instrumentation systems in a corpectomy model. *Spine* 14:1398–1405.
21. Attenborough CG, Reynolds MT (1975): Lumbosacral fusion with spring fixation. *J Bone Joint Surg* [Br] 57:283–288.
22. Aurori BF, Weierman RJ, Lowell HA, Nadel CI, Parsons JR (1985): Pseudarthrosis after spinal fusion for scoliosis: A comparison of autogenous and allogenic bone grafts. *Clin Orthop* 199:153–158.
23. Baker LD, Hoyt WA (1948): The use of interfacet vitalium screws in the Hibbs fusion. *South Med J* 41:419–426.
24. Banta CJ, King AG, Dobezies EJ, Liljeberg BS (1989): Measurement of effective pedicle diameter in the human spine. *Orthopaedics* 12:939–942.
25. Barr JS, Kubik CS, Molloy MK, McNeil JM, Riseborough EJ, White JC (1967): Evaluation of end-results in the treatment of ruptured lumbar intervertebral discs. *Surg Gynecol Obstet* 125:250–256.
26. Bassett CA (1984): The development and application of pulsed electromagnetic fields (PEMFS) for ununited fractures and arthrodeses. *Orthop Clin North Am* 15:61–87.
27. Beattie FC (1969): Distraction rod fusion. *Clin Orthop* 62:218–222.
28. Bechtol CO (1959): Internal fixation with plates and screws. In: Bechtol CO, Ferguson AB Jr, Laing PB, eds. *Metals and engineering in bone and joint surgery.* Baltimore: Williams and Wilkins, pp. 152–171.
29. Beller HE, Kirsh D (1964): Spondylolysis and spondylolisthesis following low back fusions. *South Med J* 57:783–786.
30. Berry JL, Moran JM, Berg WS, Steffee AD (1987): A morphometric study of human lumbar and selected thoracic vertebrae. *Spine* 12:362–367.
31. Bick EM (1964): An essay on the history of spine fusion operations. *Clin Orthop* 35:9–15.
32. Birch JG, Herring JA, Roach JW, Johnston CE (1988): Cotrel-Dubousset instrumentation in idiopathic scoliosis. *Clin Orthop* 227:24–29.
33. Blasier RD, Monson RC (1987): Acquired spondylolysis after posterolateral spinal fusion. *J Pediatr Orthop* 7:215–217.
34. Blauth M, Tscherne H, Haas N (1987): Therapeutic concept and results of operative treatment in acute trauma of the thoracic and lumbar spine: The Hannover experience. *J Orthop Trauma* 1:240–252.
35. Bobechko WP (1981): The instant Harrington. Proceedings of the Scoliosis Research Society Annual Meeting.
36. Bosworth DM (1945): Clothespin graft of the spine for spondylolisthesis and laminal defects. *Am J Surg* 67:61–67.
37. Bosworth DM (1948): Techniques of spinal fusion. Pseudarthrosis and method of repair. American Academy of Orthopaedic Surgeons *Instructional Course Lectures* 5:295–313.
38. Bosworth DM, Levine J (1949): Tuberculosis of the spine. An analysis of cases treated surgically. *J Bone Joint Surg* [Am] 31:267–274.
39. Boucher HH (1959): A method of spinal fusion. *J Bone Joint Surg* [Br] 41:248–259.
40. Boumphrey FRS (1982): Fusions in the lumbar spine. In: Hardy RW Jr, ed. *Lumbar disc surgery.* New York: Raven Press, p. 186.
41. Bradford DS (1988): Adult scoliosis: Current concepts of treatment. *Clin Orthop* 229:70–87.
42. Bradford DS (1980): Anterior vascular pedicle bone grafting for the treatment of kyphosis. *Spine* 5:318–323.
43. Bradford DS, Gotfried Y (1987): Staged salvage reconstruction of grade IV and V spondylolisthesis. *J Bone Joint Surg* [Am] 69:191–202.
44. Bridwell KH (1984): The treatment of flexion/distraction spinal fractures with SSI and Luque Rectangles. Proceedings of the Scoliosis Research Society 19th Annual Meeting.
45. Brodsky AE (1976): Post-laminectomy and post-fusion stenosis of the lumbar spine. *Clin Orthop* 115:130–139.
46. Brodsky AE, Hendricks RL, Khalil MA, Darden BV, Brotzman TT (1989): Segmental ("floating") lumbar spine fusions. *Spine* 14:447–450.
47. Brodsky JW, Barnes DA, Tullos HS (1984): Unrecognized pin penetration of the hip joint. *Contemp Orthop* 9:13–20.
48. Brown CW, Donaldson DH, Odom JA (1984): A new approach to low lumbar fractures. Proceedings of the Scoliosis Research Society 19th Annual Meeting, p. 126.
49. Brunet JA, Wiley JJ (1984): Acquired spondylolysis after spinal fusion. *J Bone Joint Surg* [Br] 66:720–724.
50. Bryant CE, Sullivan JA (1983): Management of thoracic and lumbar spine fractures with Harrington distraction rods supplemented with segmental wiring. *Spine* 8:532–537.
51. Bunch WH, Vanderby R, Stonecipher TK (1981): Segmental instrumentation in the reduction of spondylolisthesis—A biome-

chanical analysis and case report. Proceedings of the 16th Annual Meeting of the Scoliosis Research Society (in *Orthop Trans* 6:2–3, 1982).

52. Cabot JR, Fairén M, Roca J, Tur J, Blaimont P, Van Elegem P, Libotte M (1981): La panarthrodèse lumbo-sacrée avec la plaque crabe. *Acta Orthop Belg* 47(4–5):657–666.

53. Cabot J, Roca J, Fernandez-Fairén M, Alvarez SA (1976): Etude mécanique de la plaque de Cabot pour arthrodèse lombo-sacrée. *Acta Orthop Belg (Suppl 1)* 42:22–28.

54. Calabrese AS, Freiberger RH (1963): Acquired spondylolysis after spinal fusion. *Radiology* 81:492–494.

55. Campbell WC (1927): An operation for extra-articular fusion of sacro-iliac joint. *Surg Gynecol Obstet* 45:218–219.

56. Carson WL, Duffield RC, Arendt M, Ridgely BJ, Gaines RW Jr (1989): Internal forces and moments on transpedicular spine instrumentation—The effect of pedicle screw angle and transfixation: The 4R-4 bar linkage concept. Proceedings of the Scoliosis Research Society 24th Annual Meeting, pp. 465–466.

57. Casey MP, Asher MA, Jacobs RR, Orrick JM (1987): The effect of Harrington rod contouring on lumbar lordosis. *Spine* 12:750–753.

58. Casey MP, Jacobs RR (1984): Internal fixation of the lumbosacral spine: A biomechanical evaluation. Proceedings of the Annual Meeting of the International Society for the Study of the Lumbar Spine, Montreal.

59. Chafetz N, Cann CE, Morris JM, Steinbach LS, Goldberg HI (1987): Pseudarthrosis following lumbar fusion: Detection by direct coronal CT scanning. *Radiology* 162:803–805.

60. Cleveland M, Bosworth DM, Thompson FR (1948): Pseudarthrosis in the lumbosacral spine. *J Bone Joint Surg [Am]* 30:302–312.

61. Cole TC, Ghosh P, Hannan NJ, Taylor TKF, Bellenger CR (1987): The response of the canine intervertebral disc to immobilization produced by spinal arthrodesis is dependent on constitutional factors. *J Orthop Res* 5:337–347.

62. Cordey J, Perren SM (1985): Limits of plate on bone friction in internal fixation of fractures. Proceedings of the Orthopaedic Research Society Annual Meeting, Las Vegas, Nevada, p. 186.

63. Cotrel Y, Dubousset J, Guillaumat M (1988): New universal instrumentation in spinal surgery. *Clin Orthop* 227:10–23.

64. Court-Brown CM, Gertzbein SD (1987): The management of burst fractures of the fifth lumbar vertebra. *Spine* 12:308–312.

65. Craig FS (1956): Vertebral body biopsy. *J Bone Joint Surg [Am]* 38:93–102.

66. Crawford RJ, Sell PJ, Ali MS, Dove J (1989): Segmental spinal instrumentation: A study of the mechanical properties of materials used for sublaminar fixation. *Spine* 14:632–635.

67. Crock HV (1983): *Practice of spinal surgery.* New York: Springer-Verlag.

68. Crock HV (1976): Observations on the management of failed spinal operations. *J Bone Joint Surg [Br]* 58:193–199.

69. Curran JP, McGaw WH (1968): Posterolateral spinal fusion with pedicle grafts. *Clin Orthop* 59:125–129.

70. Daniaux H (1986): Transpedikuläre Reposition und Spongioplastik bei Wirbel-körperbruchen den unteren Brust- und Lendenwirbelsäule. *Unfallchirurgie* 89:197–213.

71. Daniaux H (1983): Technik und Ergebnisse der transpedikulären Spongiosaplastik bei Brüchen im thorakolumbalen Übergangs- und Lendenwirbelsäulenbereich. *Hefte Unfallheilkunde* 165:182.

72. Daniaux H (1982): Technik und Erste Ergebnisse der transpedikulären Spongiosaplastik bei Kompressionsbrüchen im Lendenwirbelsäulebereich. *Acta Chirurgica Aust (Suppl)* 43:79.

73. Davis GW (1980): Posterior lumbar interbody fusion enhancement by Knodt rods. *J Neuro Orthop Surg* 1:279–283.

74. Dawson EG, Clader TJ, Bssett LW (1985): A comparison of different methods used to diagnose pseudarthrosis following posterior spinal fusion for scoliosis. *J Bone Joint Surg [Am]* 67:1153–1159.

75. DeCoster T, Heetderks DB, Downey DJ, Ferries JS, Jones W (1990): Optimizing bone screw pullout force. *J Orthop Trauma* 4:169–174.

76. Denis F, Ruiz H, Searls K (1984): Comparison between square-ended distraction rods and standard round-ended distraction rods in the treatment of thoracolumbar spinal injuries: A statistical analysis. *Clin Orthop* 189:162–167.

77. DePalma AF, Marone PJ (1959): Spondylolysis following spinal fusion. *Clin Orthop* 15:208–211.

78. DePalma A, Rothman R (1968): The nature of pseudarthrosis. *Clin Orthop* 59:113–118.

79. Dick W (1987): The "fixateur interne" as a versatile implant for spine surgery. *Spine* 12:882–900.

80. Dick W (1984): Innere Fixation von Brust—und Lendenwirbelfrakturen. Bern, Switzerland: Hans Huber Verlag.

81. Dick W, Kluger P, Magerl F, Wörsdörfer O, Zäch G (1985): A new device for internal fixation of thoracolumbar and lumbar spine fractures: The "fixateur interne". *Paraplegia* 23:225–232.

82. Dick WT, Schnebel B (1988): Severe spondylolisthesis: Reduction and internal fixation. *Clin Orthop* 232:70–79.

83. Diehl K, Hanser U, Hort W, Mittelmeier H (1974): Biomechanische Untersuchungen uber die maximalen Vorspannkräfte der Knochenschrauben in verschiedenen Knochenabschnitten. *Acta Orthop Unfallchirurgie* 80:89.

84. Dodd CA, Fergusson CM, Freedman L, Houghton CR, Thomas D (1988): Allograft versus autograft bone in scoliosis surgery. *J Bone Joint Surg [Br]* 70:431–434.

85. Dohring EJ, Krag MH, Johnson CC (1990): Sacral screw fixation: A morphologic, anatomic and mechanical study. Proceedings of the North American Spine Society Annual Meeting, Monterey, California.

86. Doi K, Kawai S, Sumiura S, Sakai K (1988): Anterior cervical fusion using the free vascularized fibular graft. *Spine* 13:1239–1244.

87. Dove J (1989): Segmental wiring for spinal deformity: A morbidity report. *Spine* 14:229–231.

88. Dove J (1986): Internal fixation of the lumbar spine: The Hartshill Rectangle. *Clin Orthop* 203:135–140.

89. Drummond DW, Guadagni J, Keene JS, Breed A, Narechania R (1984): Interspinous process segmental spinal instrumentation. *J Pediatr Orthop* 4:397–404.

90. Dubuc F (1975): Knodt rod grafting. *Orthop Clin North Am* 6:283–287.

91. Dunsker SB, Schmidek HH, Frymoyer J, Kahn A III (1986): *The unstable spine.* New York: Grune & Stratton.

92. Dwyer AF (1974): Direct current stimulation in spinal fusion. *Med J Austr* 1:73–75.

93. Edwards CC (1986): New method for direct sacral fixation: Rationale and clinical results. International Society for the Study of the Lumbar Spine, Dallas, Texas.

94. Edwards CC (1984): Sacral fixation device: Design and preliminary results. Proceedings of the 19th Annual Meeting of the Scoliosis Research Society.

95. Edwards CC (1986): Spinal screw fixation of the lumbar and sacral spine: Early results treating the first 50 cases. Proceedings of the 21st Annual Meeting of the Scoliosis Research Society, p. 99.

96. Edwards CC, Griffith P, Levine AM, DeSilva JB (1982): Early clinical results using the spinal rod sleeve method for treating thoracic and lumbar injuries. Proceedings of the American Academy of Orthopaedic Surgeons Annual Meeting.

97. Edwards CC, Levine AM (1986): Early rod-sleeve stabilization of the injured thoracic and lumbar spine. *Orthop Clin North Am* 17:121–145.

98. Edwards CC, Levine AM, York JJ, Holt ES (1984): A new spinal hook: Rationale and clinical trials. Proceedings of the Scoliosis Research Society 19th Annual Meeting.

99. Edwards CC, Weigel MC (1988): A prospective study of 51 low lumbar nonunions. Proceedings of the International Society for the Study of the Lumbar Spine, Miami, Florida.

100. El-Khoury GY, McWilliams FE (1978): A simple radiological aid in the diagnosis of small avulsion fractures of the knee. *J Trauma* 18:275–277.

101. Esses SI (1989): The AO spinal internal fixator. *Spine* 14:373–378.

102. Esses SI, Botsford DJ, Kostuik JP (1989): The role of external spinal skeletal fixation in the assessment of low-back disorders. *Spine* 14:594–601.

103. Falahee M, Mann K, Yuan H, Fredricksen B, Lubicky J, Albanese S, McGowan D (1988): Biomechanical evaluation of augmented anterior and posterior short segment internal fixation for thoracolumbar burst fractures. Proceedings of the International Society for the Study of the Lumbar Spine, Miami, Florida.

104. Farcy JP, Roye DP, Weidenbaum M (1987): Cotrel-Dubousset instrumentation technique for revision of failed lumbosacral fusion. *Bull Hosp J Dis Orthop Inst* 47:1–12.

105. Farfan HF (1973): *Mechanical disorders of the low back.* Philadelphia: Lea & Febiger.

106. Farfan HF, Kirkaldy-Willis WH (1981): The present status of spinal fusion in the treatment of lumbar intervertebral joint disorders. *Clin Orthop* 158:198–214.

107. Ferguson RL, Tencer AF, Woodard P, Allen BL Jr (1988): Biomechanical comparisons of spinal fracture models and the stabilizing effects of posterior instrumentations. *Spine* 13:453–460.

108. Fernström U (1972): Der Bandscheibenersatz mit Erhaltung der Beweglichkeit. *Die Wirbelsäule in Forschung und Praxis* 55:125–130.

109. Fernström U (1966): Arthroplasty with intercorporal endoprosthesis in herniated disc and in painful disc. *Acta Chir Scand Suppl* 357:154–159.

110. Flatley TJ, Derderian H (1985): Closed loop instrumentation of the lumbar spine. *Clin Orthop* 196:273–278.

111. Fredricksen BE, Yuan HA, Miller H (1982): Burst fractures of the fifth lumbar vertebra: A report of four cases. *J Bone Joint Surg* [Am] 64:1088–1094.

112. Freedman LS, Houghton GR, Evans M (1986): Cadaveric study comparing the stability of upper distraction hooks used in Harrington instrumentation. *Spine* 11:579–582.

113. Froning EC, Frohman B (1968): Motion of the lumbosacral spine after laminectomy and spine fusion: Correlation of motion with the result. *J Bone Joint Surg* [Am] 50:897–918.

114. Frymoyer JW, Gordon SL (1989): Research perspectives in low-back pain: Report of a 1988 workshop. *Spine* 14:1384–1390.

115. Frymoyer JW, Hanley EN, Howe J, Kuhlmann D, Matteri RE (1979): A comparison of radiographic findings in fusion and non-fusion patients ten or more years following lumbar disc surgery. *Spine* 4:435–440.

116. Frymoyer JW, Hanley E, Howe J, Kuhlmann D, Matteri R (1978): Disc excision and spine fusion in the management of lumbar disc disease: A minimum ten-year follow-up. *Spine* 3:1–6.

117. Frymoyer JW, Howe J, Kuhlmann D (1978): Long term effects of spinal fusion in the sacroiliac joints and ilium. *Clin Orthop* 134:196–201.

118. Frymoyer JW, Krag MH (1986): Spinal stability and instability: Definitions, classification, and general principles of management. Chapter 1. In: Dunsker SB, Schmidek HH, Frymoyer JW, Kahn A III, eds. *The unstable thoracic and lumbosacral spine.* New York: Grune & Stratton.

119. Frymoyer JW, Selby DK (1985): Segmental instability. Rationale for treatment. *Spine* 10:280–286.

120. Gaines RW Jr, Abernathie DL (1986): Mersilene tapes as a substitute for wire in segmental spinal instrumentation for children. *Spine* 9:907–913.

121. Gaines RW, Breedlove RF, Munson G (1984): Stabilization of thoracic and thoracolumbar fracture—Dislocations with Harrington rods and sublaminar wires. *Clin Orthop* 189:195–203.

122. Geiger JM, Udovic NA, Berry JL (1989): Bending and fatigue of spine plates and rods, and fatigue of pedicle screws. Proceedings of the American Academy of Orthopaedic Surgeons Annual Meeting.

123. George DC, Krag MH, Johnson CC, Van Hal ME, Haugh LJ, Grobler LJ (in press): Hole preparation techniques (drill versus probe) for transpedicular screws: Effect upon pullout strength from human cadaveric vertebrae.

124. Gertzbein SD, MacMichael D, Tile M (1982): Harrington instrumentation as a method of fixation in fractures of the spine: A critical analysis of deficiencies. *J Bone Joint Surg* [Br] 64:526–529.

125. Ghormley RK (1933): Low back pain with special reference to the articular facets with presentation of an operative procedure. *JAMA* 101:1773–1777.

126. Goll SR, Balderston RA, Stambough JL, Booth RE Jr, Cohn JC, Pickens GT (1988): Depth of intraspinal wire penetration during passage of sublaminar wires. *Spine* 13:503–509.

127. Goldner JL: Symposium: Role of spine fusion: Question #6. *Spine* 6:293–303.

128. Grobler LJ, Kempff PG, Gaines RW Jr (1987): Comparing Mer-silene tape (M.T.) and stainless steel wire (S.S.W.) during segmental spinal instrumentation—Evaluation of the macroscopical and microscopical tissue response in the baboon (*Papio urinus*). Proceedings of the Scoliosis Research Society Annual Meeting, Vancouver, British Columbia.

129. Grobler LJ, Neale G, Wilder DG, Pope MH, Waisbrod H (1990): Anterior interbody stabilization with metal molds and cadaveric (allograft) bone: An experimental comparative investigation (6 month followup). Proceedings of the American Academy of Orthopedic Surgeons Annual Meeting, New Orleans, Louisiana.

130. Gurr KR, McAfee PC (1988): Cotrel-Dubousset instrumentation in adults: A preliminary report. *Spine* 13:510–520.

131. Gurr KR, McAfee PC, Shih CM (1988): Biomechanical analysis of posterior instrumentation systems following decompressive laminectomy: An unstable calf model. *J Bone Joint Surg* [Am] 70:680–691.

132. Guyer DW, Wiltse LL, Peek RD (1988): The Wiltse pedicle screw fixation system. *Orthopaedics* 11:1455–1460.

133. Guyer DW, Yuan HA, Werner FW, Frederickson BE, Murphy D (1987): Biomechanical comparison of seven internal fixation devices for lumbosacral junction. *Spine* 12:569–573.

134. Hadra BE (1981): Wiring of the spinous process in injury and Pott's disease. *Trans Am Orthop Assoc* 4:206.

135. Hadra BE (1975): The classic: Wiring of the vertebrae as a means of immobilization in fractures and Pott's disease. *Clin Orthop* 112:4–8.

136. Harrington PR (1973): The history and development of Harrington instrumentation. *Clin Orthop* 93:110–112.

137. Harrington PR (1967): Instrumentation in spine instability other than scoliosis. *S Afr J Surg* 5:7–12.

138. Harrington PR (1962): Treatment of scoliosis. Correction and internal fixation by spine instrumentation. *J Bone Joint Surg* [Am] 44:591–610.

139. Harrington PR, Dickson JH (1976): Spinal instrumentation in the treatment of severe progressive spondylolisthesis. *Clin Orthop* 117:157–163.

140. Harrington PR, Tullos HS (1969): Reduction of severe spondylolisthesis in children. *South Med J* 62:1–7.

141. Harris RI, Wiley JJ (1963): Acquired spondylolysis as a sequel to spine fusion. *J Bone Joint Surg* [Am] 45:1159–1170.

142. Hartman JT, McCarron RF, Robertson WW (1983): A pedicle bone grafting procedure for failed lumbosacral spinal fusion. *Clin Orthop* 178:223–227.

143. Hayes MA, Tompkins SF, Herndon WA, Gruel CR, Kopta JA, Howard TC (1988): Clinical and radiological evaluation of lumbosacral motion below fusion levels in idiopathic scoliosis. *Spine* 10:1161–1167.

144. Heinig CF, Boyd BM Jr (1984): One stage vertebrectomy or eggshell procedure. Proceedings of the Scoliosis Research Society Annual Meeting, p. 116.

145. Herring JA, Ashman RB (1986): Biomechanical testing of instruments for the fixation of spondylolisthesis. Proceedings of the Scoliosis Research Society 21st Annual Meeting.

146. Herrmann HD (1979): Transarticular (transpedicular) metal plate fixation for stabilization of the lumbar and thoracic spine. *Acta Neurochir (Wien)* 48(1–2):101–110.

147. Herron LD, Newman MH (1989): The failure of ethylene oxide gas-sterilized freeze-dried bone graft for thoracic and lumbar spinal fusion. *Spine* 14:496–500.

148. Hibbs RA (1924): A report of fifty-nine cases of scoliosis treated by fusion operation. *J Bone Joint Surg* 6:3–37.

149. Hibbs RA (1911): An operation for progressive spinal deformities. *NY Med J* 93:1013–1016.

150. Hopp E, Tsou PM (1988): Postdecompression lumbar instability. *Clin Orthop* 227:143–151.

151. Horowitch A, Peek RD, Thomas JC, Widell EH Jr, DiMartino PP, Spencer CW III, Weinstein J, Wiltse LL (1989): The Wiltse pedicle screw fixation system: Early clinical results. *Spine* 14:461–467.

152. Hsu K, Zucherman JF, White AH, Wynne G (1987): Internal fixation with pedicle screws. In: White AH, Rothman RH, Ray CD, eds. *Lumbar spine surgery: Techniques and complications.* St. Louis: C.V. Mosby.

153. Hsu KY, Zucherman J, White A, Wynne G, Reynolds J, Goldthwaite N, Schofferman J (1988): Deterioration of motion seg-

ments adjacent to lumbar spine fusions. Proceedings of the North American Spine Society Annual Meeting, Colorado Springs, Colorado.

154. Hubbard LF, Herndon JH, Buonanno AR (1985): Free vascularized fibula transfer for stabilization of the thoracolumbar spine. A case report. *Spine* 10:891–893.

155. Jackson RK, Boston DA, Edge AJ (1985): Lateral mass fusion. A prospective study of a consecutive series with long-term follow-up. *Spine* 9:828–832.

156. Jacobs RR, Dahners LE, Gertzbein SD, Nordwall A, Mathys R Jr (1983): A locking hook-spinal rod: Current status of development. *Paraplegia* 21:197–200.

157. Jacobs RR, Montesano PX, Jackson RP (1989): Enhancement of lumbar spine fusion by use of translaminar facet joint screws. *Spine* 14:12–15.

158. Jacobs RR, Nordwall A, Nachemson A (1982): Stability and strength provided by internal fixation systems for dorso-lumbar spinal injuries. *Clin Orthop* 171:300–308.

159. Jacobs RR, Schlaepfer F, Mathys, R Jr, Nachemson A, Perren SM (1984): A locking hook spinal rod system for stabilization of fracture-dislocations and correction of deformities of the dorso-lumbar spine: A biomechanic evaluation. *Clin Orthop* 189:168–177.

160. Kahanovitz N, Arnoczky SP, Hulse D, Shires PK (1984): The effect of postoperative electromagnetic pulsing on canine posterior spinal fusions. *Spine* 3:273–279.

161. Kane WJ (1988): Direct current electrical bone growth stimulation for spinal fusion. *Spine* 3:363–365.

162. Kaneda K, Kazama H, Satoh S, Fujiya M (1986): Follow-up study of medial facetectomies and posterolateral fusion with instrumentation in unstable degenerative spondylolisthesis. *Clin Orthop* 203:159–167.

163. Kaneda K, Kurakami C, Minami A (1988): Free vascularized fibular strut graft in the treatment of kyphosis. *Spine* 13:1273–1277.

164. Karlström G, Ölerud S, Sjöström L (1988): Transpedicular segmental fixation: Description of a new procedure. *Orthopaedics* 11:689–700.

164a. Karlström G, Ölerud S, Sjöström L (1990): Transpedicular fixation of thoracolumbar fractures. *Contemp Orthop* 20:285–300.

165. Keene JS, Drummond DS, Narechania RG (1980): Mechanical performance of the Wisconsin compression system. Proceedings of the Orthopaedic Research Society 26th Annual Meeting, Atlanta, Georgia.

166. Keene JS, Kling TE Jr (1989): Surgical treatment of grades I-III spondylolisthesis in athletes. *Surg Rounds Orthop* Aug., pp. 27–35.

167. Kempf I, Jaeger JH, Ben Abid M, LeMaquet A, Renault D (1979): Osteosynthesis of dorso-lumbar spinal fractures. Biomechanical approach and comparative study: Reversed Harrington pins and hooks. Roy-Camille bone plates. *Rev Chir Orthop* 65(11):43–46.

168. King D (1948): Internal fixation for lumbosacral spine fusions. *J Bone Joint Surg* [Am] 30:560–565.

169. King D (1944): Internal fixation for lumbosacral fusion. *Am J Surg* 66:357–361.

170. Kinnard P, Ghibely A, Gordon D, Trias A, Basora J (1986): Roy-Camille plates in unstable spinal conditions: A preliminary report. *Spine* 11:131–135.

171. Kirkaldy-Willis WH (1988): *Managing low back pain.* New York: Churchill Livingstone.

172. Kiviluoto O, Santavirta S, Salenius P, Morri P, Pyllkänen P (1985): Posterolateral spine fusion. A 1–4 year follow-up of 80 consecutive patients. *Acta Orthop Scand* 56:152–154.

173. Kleeman BC, Gerhart TN, Hayes WC (1987): Augmenting screw fixation in osteopenic trabecular bone. Proceedings of the Society of Biomaterials Annual Meeting.

174. Kling TF Jr, Vanderby R Jr, Belloli DM, Thomsen EL (1986): Cross-linked pedicle screw fixation in the same vertebral body: A biomechanical study. Proceedings of the 21st Annual Meeting of the Scoliosis Research Society.

175. Kluger P, Gerner HJ (1986): Das mechanische Prinzip des Fixateur Externe zur dorsalen Stabilisierung der Brust- und Lendenwirbelsäule. *Unfallchirurgie* 12:68–79.

176. Knapp DR Jr, Jones ET (1988): Use of cortical cancellous allograft for posterior spinal fusion. *Clin Orthop* 229:99–106.

177. Knodt H, Larrick RB (1964): Distraction fusion of the spine. *Ohio State Med J* 60:1140–1142.

178. Koranyi E, Bowman CE, Knecht CD, Janssen M (1970): Holding power of orthopaedic screws in bone. *Clin Orthop* 72:283–286.

179. Kornblatt MD, Casey MP, Jacobs RR (1986): Internal fixation in lumbosacral spine fusion: A biomechanical and clinical study. *Clin Orthop* 203:141–150.

180. Kostuik JP, Hall BB (1983): Spinal fusion to the sacrum in adults with scoliosis. *Spine* 8:489–500.

181. Krag MH (1990): Biomechanics of transpedicle spinal fixation. In: Weinstein JN, Wiesel S, eds. *The lumbar spine.* Philadelphia: W.B. Saunders. pp. 916–940.

182. Krag MH (1988): Lumbosacral fixation with the Vermont Spinal Fixator. In: Lin PM, Gill K, eds. *Lumbar interbody fusion: Principles and techniques of spine surgery.* Rockville, Maryland: Aspen Publishers.

183. Krag MH, Beynnon BD, DeCoster TA, Pope MH (1988): Depth of insertion of transpedicular vertebral screws into human vertebrae: Effect upon screw-vertebra interface strength. *J Spinal Disord* 1:287–294.

184. Krag MH, Beynnon BD, Frymoyer JW, Haugh LD (1987): Fatigue testing of an internal fixator for posterior spinal stabilization. Proceedings of the American Academy of Orthopaedic Surgeons 54th Annual Meeting, San Francisco, California.

185. Krag MH, Beynnon BD, Pope MH, Frymoyer JW, Haugh LD, Weaver DL (1986): An internal fixator for posterior application to short segments of the thoracic, lumbar, or lumbosacral spine: Design and testing. *Clin Orthop* 203:75–98.

186. Krag MH, Frymoyer JW, Beynnon BD, Pope MH (1987): An internal fixator for posterior application to short segments of the thoracic, lumbar, or lumbosacral spine: Design and testing. In: White AH, Rothman RH, Ray CD, eds. *Lumbar spine surgery: Techniques and complications.* St. Louis: C.V. Mosby, pp. 339–367.

187. Krag MH, Pope MH, Wilder DG (1986): Mechanisms of spine trauma and features of spinal fixation methods. Part I: Mechanisms of injury. In: Ghista D, ed. *Spinal cord medical engineering.* Springfield: Charles C Thomas, pp. 133–157.

188. Krag MH, Van Hal ME, Beynnon BD (1989): Placement of transpedicular vertebral screws close to anterior vertebral cortex: Description of methods. *Spine* 14:879–883.

189. Krag MH, Weaver DL, Beynnon BD, Haugh LD (1988): Morphometry of the thoracic and lumbar spine related to transpedicular screw placement for surgical spinal fixation. *Spine* 13:27–32.

190. Kurz LT, Garfin SR, Booth RE Jr (1989): Harvesting autogenous iliac bone grafts: A review of complications and techniques. *Spine* 14:1324–1331.

191. Laasonen EM, Soini J (1989): Low-back pain after lumbar fusion: Surgical and computed tomographic analysis. *Spine* 14:210–213.

192. Laborde JM, Bahniuk E, Bohlman HH, Samson B (1980): Comparison of fixation of spinal fractures. *Clin Orthop* 152:303–310.

193. La Grone MO (1988): Loss of lumbar lordosis. A complication of spinal fusion for scoliosis. *Orthop Clin North Am* 19:383–393.

194. Lang P, Genant HK, Chafetz N, Steiger P, Morris JM (1988): Three-dimensional computed tomography and multiplanar reformations in the assessment of pseudarthrosis in posterior lumbar fusion patients. *Spine* 13:69–75.

195. Lange F (1910): Support for the spondylytic spine by means of buried steel bars attached to the vertebrae. *Am J Orthop Surg* 8:344–361.

196. Lange F (1986): Support for the spondylytic spine by means of buried steel bars attached to the vertebrae (*reprinted from the original*). *Clin Orthop* 203:3–6.

197. Lavaste F (1980): Biomechanique du rachis dorso-lombaire. *Deuxieme Journées d'Orthopedie de la Pitie* 19–23.

198. Lavaste F (1977): *Étude des implants rachidiens. Mémoire de biomechanique.* Thesis "Ingeneur" Ecole Natl Supér des Arts et Metiers à Paris, 1977.

199. Laville C (1989): Technique of spine plate fixation of the lumbosacral spine. Transpedicular fixation of the spine: International Symposium. Medical College of Ohio, Continuing Medical Education, Toledo, Ohio.

200. Lee CK (1988): Accelerated degeneration of the segment adjacent to a lumbar fusion. *Spine* 13:375–377.
201. Lee CK, deBari A (1986): Lumbosacral spinal fusion with Knodt distraction rods. *Spine* 11:373–375.
202. Lee CK, Langrana NA (1984): Lumbosacral spinal fusion: A biomechanical study. *Spine* 9:574–581.
203. Lehmann TR, Spratt KF, Tozzi JE (1987): Long-term follow-up of lower lumbar fusion patients. *Spine* 12:97–104.
204. Lehman WB, Grant A, Rose D, Pugh J, Norman A (1984): A method of evaluating possible pin penetration in slipped capital femoral epiphysis using a cannulated internal fixation device. *Clin Orthop* 186:65–70.
205. Levine AM, Edwards CC (1988): Low lumbar burst fractures. *Orthopaedics.* 11:1427–1432.
206. Lipscomb HJ, Grubb SA, Talmage RV (1989): Spinal bone density following spinal fusion. *Spine* 14:477–479.
207. Liu YK, Njus GO, Bahr PA, Geng P (1990): Fatigue life improvement of nitrogen-ion implanted pedicle screws. *Spine* 15:311–317.
208. Lonstein JE (1984): Use of bank bone for spinal fusions. Proceedings of the Scoliosis Research Society Annual Meeting.
209. Louis R (1986): Fusion of the lumbar and sacral spine by internal fixation with screw plates. *Clin Orthop* 203:18–33.
210. Luk KD, Lee FB, Leong JCY, Hsu LCS (1987): The effect on the lumbosacral spine of long spinal fusion for idiopathic scoliosis: A minimum 10-year follow-up. *Spine* 12:996–1000.
211. Luque ER (1982): Anatomic basis and development of segmental spinal instrumentation. *Spine* 7:256–259.
212. Luque ER (1986): Interpeduncular segmental fixation. *Clin Orthop* 203:54–57.
213. Luque ER (1986): Segmental spinal instrumentation of the lumbar spine. *Clin Orthop* 203:126–135.
214. Luque ER, Cassis N, Ramirez-Wiella G (1982): Segmental spinal instrumentation in the treatment of fractures of the thoracolumbar spine. *Spine* 7:312–317.
215. Luque ER, Rapp GF (1988): A new semirigid method for interpedicular fixation of the spine. *Orthopaedics* 11:1445–1450.
216. Lyon WF, Cochran JR, Smith L (1941): Actual holding power of various screws in bone. *Ann Surg* 114:376–384.
217. Macnab I (1977): *Backache.* Baltimore: Williams and Wilkins.
218. Macnab I, Dall D (1971): The blood supply of the lumbar spine and its application to the technique of intertransverse lumbar fusion. *J Bone Joint Surg [Br]* 53:628–638.
219. Magerl F (1983): Clinical application on the thoracolumbar junction and the lumbar spine. In: Mears DC, ed. *External skeletal fixation.* Baltimore: Williams and Wilkins.
220. Magerl F (1982): External skeletal fixation of the lower thoracic and the lumbar spine. In: Uhthoff HK, Stahl E, eds. *Current concepts of external fixation of fractures.* New York: Springer-Verlag, pp. 353–366.
221. Magerl F (1985): External spinal skeletal fixation. In: Weber BG and Magerl F, eds. *The external fixator.* New York: Springer-Verlag, pp. 290–365.
222. Magerl FP (1984): Stabilization of the lower thoracic and lumbar spine with external skeletal fixation. *Clin Orthop* 189:125–141.
223. Magerl F, Coscia MF (1988): Total posterior vertebrectomy of the thoracic or lumbar spine. *Clin Orthop* 232:62–69.
224. Malinin TI, Brown MD (1981): Bone allografts in spinal surgery. *Clin Orthop* 154:68–73.
225. Manaresi C (1979): A new type of distractor for the surgical correction of scoliosis and spondylolisthesis. *Ital J Orthop Traumatol* 5(3):267–272.
226. Martin D, Cordey J, Rahn BA, Perren SM (1979): Bone screw displacement under lateral loading. Proceedings of the 2nd Meeting of the European Society of Biomechanics, Strasbourg.
227. Mathieu P, Demirleau J (1936): Traitment chirurgical du spondylolisthésis douloureux. *Rev Chir Orthop* 23:352–363.
228. McAfee PC, Farey ID, Sutterlin CE, Gurr ICR, Warden KE, Cunningham BW (1989): Device-related osteoporosis with spinal instrumentation. *Spine* 14:919–926.
229. McBride GG, Bradford DS (1983): Vertebral body replacement with femoral neck allograft and a vascularized rib strut graft. *Spine* 8:406–415.
230. McCarthy RE, Dunn H, McCullough FL (1989): Luque fixation to the sacral ala using the Dunn-McCarthy modification. *Spine* 14:281–283.
231. McElroy KD (1964): Technique for bilateral lateral lumbosacral fusion. *J Bone Joint Surg [Am]* 46:461.
232. McMurray GN (1962): The evaluation of Kiel bone in spinal fusions. *J Bone Joint Surg [Br]* 64:101–104.
233. Michel CR, Lalain JJ (1985): Late result of Harrington's operation. Long term evolution of the lumbar spine below the fused segments. *Spine* 10:414–420.
234. Michele AA, Kruger FJ (1949): Surgical approach to the vertebral body. *J Bone Joint Surg [Am]* 31:873–878.
235. Misenhimer GR, Peek RD, Wiltse LL, Rothman SL, Widell EH Jr (1989): Anatomic analysis of pedicle cortical and cancellous diameter as related to screwsize. *Spine* 14:367–372.
236. Moe JH, Denis F (1977): The iatrogenic loss of lumbar lordosis. Proceedings of the Scoliosis Research Society 11th Annual Meeting, 1976 (in *Orthop Trans* 1:131).
237. Moon MS, Ok IY, Ha KY (1986): The effect of posterior spinal fixation with acrylic cement on the vertebral growth plate and intervertebral disc in dogs. *Int Orthop* 10:69–73.
238. Mooney V (1981): Symposium: Role of spine fusion: Question #7. *Spine* 6:304–305.
239. Moran JM, Berg WS, Berry JL, Geiger JM, Steffee AD (1989): Transpedicular screw fixation. *J Orthop Res* 7:107–114.
240. Morris J, Chafetz N, Baumrind S, Genant HK, Korn E (1985): Stereophotogrammetry of the lumbar spine: A technique for the detection of pseudarthrosis. *Spine* 10:368–375.
241. Nachemson AL (1985): Fusion for low back pain and sciatica (editorial). *Acta Orthop Scand* 56:285–286.
242. Nasca RJ, Johnson LP (1988): Harrington-Bobechko instrumentation in the treatment of scoliosis: A preliminary report. *Spine* 13:246–249.
243. Nasca RJ, Whelchel JD (1987): Use of cryopreserved bone in spinal surgery. *Spine* 12:222–227.
244. Nerubay J, Marganit B, Bubis JJ, Tadmor A, Katznelson A (1986): Stimulation of bone formation by electrical current on spinal fusion. *Spine* 11:167–169.
245. Nunamaker DM, Perren SM (1976): Force measurements in screw fixation. *J Biomech* 9:669–675.
246. O'Brien JP (1983): The role of fusion for chronic low back pain. *Orthop Clin North Am* 14:639–647.
247. O'Brien JP (1979): Anterior spinal tenderness in low back pain syndromes. *Spine* 4:85–88.
248. Ogilvie JW, Bradford DS (1984): Lumbar and lumbosacral fusion with segmental fixation. Proceedings of the Scoliosis Research Society 19th Annual Meeting, p. 166.
249. Ogilvie JW, Schendel M (1986): Comparison of lumbosacral fixation devices. *Clin Orthop* 203:120–125.
250. Oikarinen J (1982): Experimental spinal fusion with decalcified bone matrix and deep-frozen allogenic bone in rabbits. *Clin Orthop* 162:210–218.
251. Ölerud S, Hamberg M (1986): External fixation as a test for instability after spinal fusion L4-S1: A case report. *Orthopaedics* 9:547–549.
252. Ölerud S, Karlström G, Sjöström L (1988): Transpedicular fixation of thoracolumbar vertebral fractures. *Clin Orthop* 227:44–51.
253. Ölerud S, Sjöström L, Karlström G, Hamberg M (1986): Spontaneous effect of increased stability of the lower lumbar spine in cases of severe chronic back pain: The answer of an external transpeduncular fixation test. *Clin Orthop* 203:67–74.
254. Olson SA, Gaines RW (1987): Removal of sublaminar wires after spinal fusion. *J Bone Joint Surg [Am]* 69:1419–1422.
255. Olsson TH, Selvik G, Willner S (1977): Mobility in the lumbosacral spine after fusion studied with the aid of roentgen stereophotogrammetry. *Clin Orthop* 129:181–190.
256. Olsson TH, Selvik G, Willner S (1976): Kinematic analysis of posterolateral fusion in the lumbosacral spine. *Acta Radiol (Diagn)* 17:519–530.
257. Olsson TH, Selvik G, Willner S (1976): Kinematic analysis of spinal fusions. *Invest Radiol* 11:202–209.
258. Osterman K, Snellman O, Poussa M, Ritsilä V (1981): Treatment of lumbar lytic spondylolisthesis using osteoperiosteal transplants in young patients. *J Pediatr Orthop* 1:289–294.
259. Panjabi MM (1988): Biomechanical evaluation of spinal fixation devices. I. A conceptual framework. *Spine* 13:1129–1134.
260. Panjabi MM, Abumi K, Duranceau J, Crisco JJ (1988): Biome-

chanical evaluation of spinal fixation devices. II. Stability provided by eight internal fixation devices. *Spine* 13:1135–1140.

261. Pawluk RJ, Musso E, Tzitzikalakis GI, Dick HM (1985): Effects of internal fixation techniques on altering plate screw strain distribution. Proceedings of the Orthopaedic Research Society Annual Meeting, Las Vegas, Nevada, p. 185.

262. Pearcy M, Burrough S (1982): Assessment of bony union after interbody fusion of the lumbar spine using a biplanar radiographic technique. *J Bone Joint Surg* [Br] 64:228–232.

263. Peek RD, Thomas JC Jr, Weinstein J, Wiltse LL, Widell EH Jr, DiMartino PP, Spencer CW III (1988): Lumbar spine fusion with pedicle screw and rods. Proceedings of the International Society for the Study of the Lumbar Spine, Dallas Texas, p. 74.

264. Pennal GF, McDonald GA, Dale GG (1964): Method of spinal fusion using internal fixation. *Clin Orthop* 35:86–94.

265. Perren SM, Cordey J, Enzler M, Matter P, Rahn BA, Schläpfer F (1978): Mechanics of bone screw with internal fixation plates. *Unfallheilkunde* 81:211–218.

266. Phillips WA, Hensinger RN (1988): Wisconsin and other instrumentation for posterior spinal fusion. *Clin Orthop* 229:44–51.

267. Pietruszka I (1980): Early rehabilitation after fracture fixation using Daab's serrate plate and cancellous autotransplants. *Chir Narzadow Ruchu Ortop Pol* 45:507–510.

268. Pope MH, Frymoyer JW, Andersson G (1984): *Occupational low back pain.* New York: Praeger.

269. Pouget G, Chaboche P, Servant J, Schifrine P, Cauchoix J (1979): Postero-lateral bone grafting in the lumbar and lumbo-sacral spine. *Rev Chir Orthop* 65:365–372.

270. Prolo DJ, Rodrigo JJ (1985): Contemporary bone graft physiology and surgery. *Clin Orthop* 200:322–342.

271. Puno RM, Bechtold JE, Byrd JE, Winter RB, Ogilvie JW, Bradford DS (1987): Biomechanical analysis of five techniques of fixation for the lumbosacral junction. Trans Orthopaedic Research Society 33rd Annual Meeting, San Francisco, California, p. 366.

272. Puschel J, Zielke K (1984): Transpedicular vertebral instrumentation using VDS instruments in ankylosing spondylitis. Proceedings of the Scoliosis Research Society 19th Annual Meeting.

273. Quinnell RC, Stockdale HR (1981): Some experimental observations of the influence of a single lumbar floating fusion on the remaining lumbar spine. *Spine* 6:263–267.

274. Ralston EL, Thompson WAL (1949): The diagnosis and repair of pseudarthrosis of the spine. *Surg Gynecol Obstet* 89:37–42.

275. Ray CD (1987): The paralateral approach to decompression for lateral stenosis and far lateral lesions of the lumbar spine. In: Collis EW, ed. *Lumbar discectomy and laminectomy.* Rockville, Maryland: Aspen Publishers, pp. 217–227.

276. Ray RC, Wiese GM, Wohns RNE (1984): Stabilization of metastatic tumors of the spine. Proceedings of the 19th Annual Meeting of the Scoliosis Research Society, p. 172.

277. Reed S, Wagner T (1986): Preliminary report on lumbo-sacral fusion with pedicle screws and Steffee plates. Proceedings of the Scoliosis Research Society 21st Annual Meeting.

278. Reimers C (1956): Die dorsale Spannverstrebung von Wirbelsäulenabschnitten mittels innerer Schienung. *Chirurgie* 17:10–16.

279. Resina J, Alves AF (1977): Technique of correction and internal fixation for scoliosis. *J Bone Joint Surg* [Br] 59:159–165.

280. Rish BL (1985): Comparative evaluation of posterior lumbar interbody fusion for disc disease. *Spine* 10:855–857.

281. Robbins S, Gertzbein S (1987): Accuracy of pedicle screw placement in vivo. Proceedings of the Orthopaedic Trauma Association Annual Meeting, Dallas, Texas, pp. 27–28.

282. Rolander SD (1966): Motion of the lumbar spine with special reference to the stability effect of posterior fusion. *Acta Orthop Scan Suppl* 90:1–143.

283. Rombold C (1965): Spondylolysis: A complication of spine fusion. *J Bone Joint Surg* 47:1237–1242.

284. Rooks MD, Schmitt EW, Drvaric DM (1988): Unrecognized pin penetration in slipped capital femoral epiphysis. *Clin Orthop* 34:82–89.

285. Rose GK, Owen R, Sanderson JM (1975): Transposition of rib with blood supply for the stabilization of spinal kyphosis. *J Bone Joint Surg* [Br] 57:112.

286. Rossier AB, Cochran TP (1984): The treatment of spinal fractures with Harrington compression rods and segmental sublaminar wiring: A dangerous combination. *Spine* 9:796–799.

287. Rothman RH, Booth R (1975): Failures of spinal fusion. *Orthop Clin North Am* 6:299–304.

288. Roy-Camille R (1987): Experience with Roy-Camille fixation for the thoracolumbar and lumbar spine. Acute spinal injuries: Current management techniques. University of Massachusetts Continuing Medical Education Course, Sturbridge, Massachusetts.

289. Roy-Camille R, Demeulenaere C (1970): Ostéosynthèse du rachis dorsal, lombaire et lombo-sacré par plaque métalliques vissées dans les pédicules vertébraux et es apophyses articulaires. *Presse Méd* 78:1447–1448.

290. Roy-Camille R, Roy-Camille M, Demeulenaere C (1972): Fixation par plaques des métastases vertébrales dorso-lombaires. *Nouv Presse Med* 1:2463–2466.

291. Roy-Camille R, Saillant G, Berteaux D, Marie-Anne S (1979): Early management of spinal injuries. In: McKibbin B, ed. *Recent advances in orthopaedics.* New York: Churchill Livingstone.

292. Roy-Camille R, Saillant G, Berteaux D, Marie-Anne S, Mamoudy P (1979): Vertebral osteosynthesis using metal plates. Its different uses. *Chirurgie* 105(7):597–603.

293. Roy-Camille R, Saillant G, Berteaux D, Salgado V (1976): Osteosynthesis of thoraco-lumbar spine fractures with metal plates screwed through the vertebral pedicles. *Reconstr Surg Traumatol* 15:2–16.

294. Roy-Camille R, Saillant G, Bisserie M (1984): Surgical treatment of spinal metastatic tumors by posterior plating and laminectomy. Proceedings of the American Academy of Orthopaedic Surgeons Annual Meeting.

295. Roy-Camille R, Saillant G, Marie-Anne S, Mamoudy P (1980): Behandlung von Wirbelfrakturen und -luxation am thorakolumbalen Übergang. *Orthopaedie* 9:63–68.

296. Roy-Camille R, Saillant G, Mazel C (1986): Internal fixation of the lumbar spine with pedicle screw plating. *Clin Orthop* 203:7–17.

297. Saillant G (1976): Étude anatomique des pédicules vertébraux: Application chirurgicale. *Rev Chir Orthop* 62(2):151–160.

298. Salama R (1983): Xenogeneic bone grafting in humans. *Clin Orthop* 174:113–121.

299. Scaglietti O, Frontino G, Bartolozzi P (1976): Technique of anatomical reduction of lumbar spondylolisthesis and its surgical stabilization. *Clin Orthop* 117:164–175.

300. Schatzker J, Sanderson R, Murnaghan PJ (1975): The holding power of orthopaedic screws in vivo. *Clin Orthop* 108:115–126.

301. Schläpfer F, Magerl F, Jacobs R, Perren SM, Weber BG (1980): *In vivo* measurements of loads on an external fixation device for human lumbar spine fractures. Institute of Mechanical Engineers. C131/80:59–64.

302. Schläpfer F, Wörsdörfer O, Magerl F, Perren SM (1980): Measurements of in vivo load supported by the skeletal external fixation device for spinal fractures. Proceedings of the Annual Meeting of the International Society of the Study of the Lumbar Spine, New Orleans, Louisiana.

303. Schläpfer F, Wörsdörfer O, Magerl F, Perren SM (1982): Stabilization of the lower thoracic and lumbar spine: Comparative in vitro investigation of an external skeletal and various internal fixation devices. In: Uhthoff HK, Stahl E, eds. *Current concepts of external fixation of fractures.* New York: Springer-Verlag.

304. Schlicke L, Schulak J (1980): The simultaneous use of Harrington compression and distraction rods in a thoracolumbar fracture-dislocation. *J Trauma* 20:177–179.

305. Schreiber A, Suezawa Y, Jacob HAC (1986): Preliminary report of 40 patients. Dorsal spinal fusion with a transpedicular distraction and compression system. *Orthop Rev* 15:93–96.

306. Selby D (1986): Internal fixation with Knodt's rods. *Clin Orthop* 203:179–184.

307. Sell P, Collins M, Dove J (1988): Briefly noted. Pedicle screws: Axial pullout strength in the lumbar spine. *Spine* 13:1075–1076.

308. Shaffer JW, Davy DT, Field GA, Bensusan JS (1989): Temporal analysis of vascularized and nonvascularized rib grafts in canine spine surgery. *Spine* 14:727–732.

309. Shaw EG, Taylor JG (1956): The results of lumbo-sacral fusion for low back pain. *J Bone Joint Surg* [Br] 38:485–497.

310. Shaw JA (1984): Preventing unrecognized pin penetration into hip joint. *Orthop Rev* 13:142–152.

311. Simmons EH, Capicotta WN (1988): Posterior transpedicular

Zielke instrumentation of the lumbar spine. *Clin Orthop* 236:180–191.

312. Simmons JW (1985): Treatment of failed posterior lumbar interbody fusion (PLIF) of the spine with pulsing electromagnetic fields. *Clin Orthop* 193:127–132.

313. Slater R, Nagel D, Smith RL (1988): Biochemistry of fusion mass consolidation in the sheep spine. *J Orthop Res* 6:138–144.

314. Slizofski WJ, Collier BD, Flatley TJ, Carrera GF, Hellman RS, Isitman AT (1987): Painful pseudarthrosis following lumbar spinal fusion: Detection by combined SPECT and planar bone scintigraphy. *Skeletal Radiol* 16:136–141.

315. Stauffer RN, Coventry MB (1972): Posterolateral lumbar spine fusion: Analysis of Mayo Clinic series. *J Bone Joint Surg* [Am] 54:1195–1204.

316. Steffee AD, Biscup RS, Sitkowski DJ (1986): Segmental spine plates with pedicle screw fixation: A new internal fixation device for disorders of lumbar and thoracolumbar spine. *Clin Orthop* 203:45–53.

317. Steffee AD, Sitkowski DJ (1988): Posterior lumbar interbody fusion and plates. *Clin Orthop* 227:99–102.

318. Stokes IAF, Wilder DG, Frymoyer JW, Pope MH (1981): Assessment of patients with low back pain by biplanar radiographic measurement of intervertebral motion. *Spine* 6:233–239.

319. Stonecipher T, Wright S (1989): Posterior lumbar interbody fusion with facet-screw fixation. *Spine* 14:468–471.

320. Straub LR (1949): Lumbosacral fusion by metallic fixation and grafts. *J Bone Joint Surg* [Br] 31:478.

321. Sullivan CR, Bickell WH (1960): The problems of traumatic spondylolysis: A report of three cases. *Am J Surg* 100:698–708.

322. Sullivan CR, McCaslin FE (1960): Further studies on experimental spondylitis and intercorporeal fusion of the spine. *J Bone Joint Surg* [Am] 42:1339–1347.

323. Suzuki T, Pearcy MJ, Tibrewal SB, Wilson D, Duthie RB (1985): Posterior intertransverse fusion assessed clinically and with biplanar radiography. *Int Orthop* 9:11–17.

324. Taillard W (1957): *Les spondylolisthesies.* Paris: Masson et Cie.

325. Taylor GJ, Laing PL (1986): The role of the plaster bed after spinal fusion. *Spine* 11:161–164.

326. Taylor LJ, Gardner ADH (1984): Knodt rod fusion of the lumbar spine. *Acta Orthop Scand* 55:542–544.

327. Tello CA (1984): Early results with a variation of spinal instrumentation. Proceedings of the Scoliosis Research Society Annual Meeting.

328. Terry A, McCall IW, O'Brien JP, Park WM (1981): Graft impingement following postero-lateral fusion. Proceedings of the International Society for Study of the Lumbar Spine.

329. Thalgott JS, Aebi M, LaRocca H (1988): Internal spinal skeletal fixation system. *Orthopaedics* 11:1465–1468.

330. Thalgott JS, LaRocca H, Aebi M, Dwyer AP, Razza BE (1989): Reconstruction of the lumbar spine using AO DCP plate internal fixation. *Spine* 14:91–95.

331. Thomas JC Jr, Haye W, Wiltse LL, Widell EC Jr, Spencer CW III, DiMartino PP, Peek RD (1988): Review of deep wound infection complicating pedicle screw fixation of the lumbar spine. Proceedings of the International Society for the Study of the Lumbar Spine, Miami, Florida.

332. Thompson WA (1974): Lumbosacral spine fusion: Method of bilateral posterolateral fusion combined with a Hibbs fusion. *J Bone Joint Surg* [Am] 56:1643–1647.

333. Thompson WAL, Ralston EL (1949): Pseudarthrosis following spine fusion. *J Bone Joint Surg* [Am] 31:400–405.

334. Tietjen R, Morgenstern JM (1976): Spondylolisthesis following surgical fusion for scoliosis: A case report. *Clin Orthop* 117:176–178.

335. Toumey JW (1943): Internal fixation in fusion of the lumbo-sacral joints. *Lahey Clin Bull* 3:188–191.

336. Trias A, Bourassa P, Massoud M (1979): Dynamic loads experienced in correction of idiopathic scoliosis using two types of Harrington rods. *Spine* 4:228–235.

337. Trias A, Massoud M, Ghibely A (1982): Modified Harrington rod. Proceedings of the 17th Annual Meeting of the Scoliosis Research Society, Denver, Colorado.

338. Tria AJ Jr, Williams JM, Harwood D, Zawadsky JP (1987): Laminectomy with and without spinal fusion. *Clin Orthop* 224:134–137.

339. Truchly G, Thompson WAL (1962): Posterolateral fusion of the lumbosacral spine. *J Bone Joint Surg* [Am] 44:505–512.

340. Unander-Scharin L (1950): Case of spondylolisthesis lumbalis acquisita. *Acta Orthop Scand* 19:536–544.

341. Urist MR, Dawson E (1981): Intertransverse process fusion with the aid of chemosterilized autolyzed antigen-extracted allogeneic (AAA) bone. *Clin Orthop* 154:97–113.

342. Vangsness CT, Carter DR, Frankel VH (1981): In vitro evaluation of the loosening characteristics of self-tapped and non–self-tapped cortical bone screws. *Clin Orthop* 157:279–286.

343. Vaughan PA, Malcolm BW, Maistrelli GL (1988): Results of L4-L5 disc excision alone versus disc excision and fusion. *Spine* 13:690–695.

344. Vincent A, Tshiakatumba ML, DeNayer P, Lokietek W, Maldague B, Malghem J, Rombouts JJ (1981): Postero-lateral arthrodesis of the lumbar spine. Long-term results. *Acta Orthop Belg* 47:619–635.

345. Volz RG, Martin MD (1977): Illusory biplane radiographic images. *Radiology.* 122:695–697.

346. Waisbrod H, Gershagen HU (1986): A pilot study of the value of ceramics for bone replacement. *Arch Orthop Trauma Surg* 105:298–301.

347. Walters R, Simon SR (1980): Joint destruction: A sequel of unrecognized pin penetration in patients with slipped capital femoral epiphysis. *Proceedings of the Eighth Open Scientific Meeting of the Hip Society.* St. Louis: C.V. Mosby.

348. Watkins MB (1953): Posterior lateral fusion of the lumbar and lumbosacral spine. *J Bone Joint Surg* [Am] 35:1014–1018.

349. Watkins MB (1959): Posterolateral bone-grafting for fusion of the lumbar spine. *J Bone Joint Surg* [Am] 41:388–396.

350. Watkins MB, Bragg EC (1956): Lumbosacral fusion results with early ambulation. *Surg Gynecol Obstet* 102:604–606.

351. Weatherley CR, Prickett CF, O'Brien JP (1986): Discogenic pain persisting despite solid posterior fusion. *J Bone Joint Surg* [Br] 68:142–143.

352. Weinstein JN, Spratt KF, Spengler D, Brick C (1988): Spinal pedicle fixation: Reliability and validity of roentgenogram-based assessment and surgical factors on successful screw placement. *Spine* 13:1012–1018.

353. White AH, Rothman RH, Ray CD (1987): *Lumbar spine surgery.* St. Louis: C.V. Mosby, p. 277.

354. White AH, Von Rogov P, Zucherman J, Heiden D (1987): Lumbar laminectomy for herniated disc: A prospective controlled comparison with internal fixation fusion. *Spine* 12:305–307.

355. White AH, Wynne G, Taylor LW (1983): Knodt rod distraction lumbar fusion. *Spine* 8:434–437.

356. White AH, Zucherman JF, Hsu K (1986): Lumbosacral fusions with Harrington rods and intersegmental wiring. *Clin Orthop* 203:185–190.

357. Whitecloud TS III, Butler JC, Cohen JL, Candelora PD (1989): Complications with the variable spinal plating system. *Spine* 4:472–476.

358. Whitecloud TS III, Skalley TC, Cook SD, Morgan EL (1989): Roentgenographic measurement of pedicle screw penetration. *Clin Orthop* 245:57–68.

359. Whitehill R, Barry JC (1985): The evolution of stability in cervical spinal constructs using either autogenous bone graft or methylmethacrylate cement. A follow-up report on a canine in vivo model. *Spine* 10:32–41.

360. Williams EWM (1963): Traumatic paraplegia. In: Matthews DN, ed. *Recent advances in surgery of trauma.* New York: Churchill Livingstone, pp. 171–186.

361. Wilson PD, Straub LR (1952): Lumbosacral fusion with metallic-plate fixation. *American Academy of Orthopaedic Surgeons Instructional Course Lectures.* 9:53–57.

362. Wiltse LL, Bateman JG, Duey R (1962): Experiences with transverse process fusions in the lumbar spine. *J Bone Joint Surg* [Am] 44:1013–1014.

363. Wiltse LL, Bateman G, Hutchinson RH, Nelson WE (1968): The paraspinal sacrospinalis-splitting approach to the lumbar spine. *J Bone Joint Surg* [Am] 50:919–926.

364. Wiltse LL, Hutchinson RH (1964): Surgical treatment of spondylolisthesis. *Clin Orthop* 35:116–135.

365. Wiltse LL, Spencer CW III (1988): New uses and refinements of the paraspinal approach to the lumbar spine. *Spine* 13:696–706.

366. Winter RB (1986): Harrington instrumentation into the lumbar spine. Technique for preservation of normal lumbar lordosis. *Spine* 11:633–635.

367. Wörsdörfer O (1981): Operative Stabilisierung der thorakolumbalen und lumbalen Wirbelsäule: Vergleichende biomechanische Untersuchungen zur Stabilität und Steifigkeit verschiedener dorsaler Fixations-Systems. Thesis, Medizinisch-Naturwissenschaftliche Hochschule der Universität Ulm.

368. Wright AM (1981): Symposium: Role of spine fusion: Question #5. *Spine* 6:292.

369. Yamagata M (1984): Biomechanical study of posterior spinal instrumentation for scoliosis. *J Jap Orthop Ass* 58:523–534.

370. Yang SW, Langrana NA, Lee CK (1986): Biomechanics of lumbosacral spinal fusion in combined compression-torsion loads. *Spine* 11:937–941.

371. Yglesias L (1933): Lumbosacral facetectomy for post-fusion persistent sciatica. *J Bone Joint Surg* 15:579–590.

372. Young HH, Love JG (1959): End-results of protruded lumbar

370. Yang SW, Langrana NA, Lee CK (1986): Biomechanics of lumbosacral spinal fusion in combined compression-torsion loads. *Spine* 11:937–941.

371. Yglesias L (1933): Lumbosacral facetectomy for post-fusion persistent sciatica. *J Bone Joint Surg* 15:579–590.

372. Young HH, Love JG (1959): End-results of protruded lumbar

intervertebral discs with and without fusion. American Academy of Orthopaedic Surgeons Instructional Course Lecture 16:13–16.

373. Zand MS, Goldstein SA, Matthews LS (1983): Fatigue failure of cortical bone screws. *J Biomech* 16:305–312.

374. Zielke K, Strempel AV (1986): Posterior lateral distraction spondylodesis using the twofold sacral bar. *Clin Orthop* 203:151–158.

375. Zindrick MR, Patwardhan A, Lorenz M (1986): Effect of methylmethacrylate augmentation upon pedicle screw fixation in the spine. Proceedings of the International Society for the Study of the Lumbar Spine, Dallas, Texas.

376. Zindrick MR, Wiltse LL, Doornik A, Widell EH, Knight GW, Patwardhan AG, Thomas JC, Rothman SL, Fields BT (1987): Analysis of the morphometric characteristics of the thoracic and lumbar pedicles. *Spine* 12:160–166.

377. Zindrick MR, Wiltse LL, Holland WR, Widell EH, Thomas JC, Spencer CW (1985): Biomechanical study of intrapedicular screw fixation in the lumbosacral spine. Proceedings of the International Society for the Study of the Lumbar Spine Annual Meeting, Sydney, Australia.

378. Zindrick MR, Wiltse LL, Widell EH, Thomas JC, Holland WR, Field BT, Spencer CW (1986): Biomechanical study of interpedicular screw fixation in the lumbosacral spine. *Clin Orthop* 203:99–111.

379. Zucherman J, Hsu K, White A, Wynne G (1988): Early results of spinal fusion using variable spine plating system. *Spine* 13:570–579.

The Adult Spine: Principles and Practice,
J. W. Frymoyer, Editor-in-Chief.
Raven Press, Ltd., New York © 1991.

CHAPTER 93

Anterior Interbody Fixation Devices

John Schlegel, Hansen A. Yuan, and Bruce Fredricksen

A variety of difficult pathologic conditions affect the lumbar spine and are best approached by anterior debridement, fusion, and supplemental anterior instrumentation. This chapter presents the various devices currently available, their indications for use, the technique and approach for their insertion, the results obtained, and the potential complications.

HISTORY

The clinical use of spinal fusion is traced to Hibbs (23) and Albee (1) who separately described their techniques in 1911. Prior to those reports, posterior fixation devices had been described by Hadra in 1891 and Lange in 1909 (2). Less well known is the fact that Muller of Germany described the anterior approach and fusion of the spine in 1906, but the work of Hibbs and Albee largely overshadowed his contribution. Posterior surgery was the procedure of choice until 30 years later. During the 1930s, anterior surgery became an accepted procedure, largely to address the problems of spondylolisthesis and Pott's disease.

J. Schlegel, M.D.: Assistant Professor, Department of Orthopaedics, University of Texas Southwestern Medical Center, Dallas, Texas, 74235.
H. A. Yuan, M.D., Professor and Chairman; B. Fredricksen, M.D., Associate Professor: Department of Orthopaedic Surgery, State University of New York, Health Sciences Center at Syracuse, Syracuse, New York, 13202.

Capener first described anterior interbody fusion for spondylolisthesis in 1932 (8). Subsequent reports followed from Mercer (47), Jenkins (29), Burns (6), and Speed (56). In 1934, Ito and colleagues described the technique for anterior spinal cord decompression (27). He was also one of the first investigators to describe a pararectus extra-peritoneal approach. Following World War II, Lane and Moore (40) reported on results of anterior fusion for degenerative lumbar disc lesions and gave their classic description of the transperitoneal anterior approach. Subsequently, larger series were presented by Hodgson and Stock (25), Harmon (22), Sacks (53), Hodgson (24), Taylor (58), and Freebody (20). The indications for anterior fusion varied from the treatment of spinal tuberculosis (25) to the management of degenerative spine disease (22).

Although the use of supplemental internal fixation for posterior fusion was common from 1940 to the present, anterior internal fixation was and still is not as widely accepted. Humphries and Hawk (26) developed a slotted plate that was contoured and placed directly over the anterior lower lumbar spine. They reported the aorta and vena cava needed no protection and had no vascular complications. Though their laboratory studies showed adequate stabilization, their clinical results in 27 patients were less acceptable. Thirty percent of their patients were unimproved, which they interpreted as a failure of proper patient selection. Werlinich (61) reported good results in 127 patients treated with anterior fusion and fixation with a serrated staple. More recent devices have been developed by Dwyer (15), Zielke, Dunn (12–14), Yuan et al. (63), Ryan et al. (52), Black et al. (3), Kostuik (32–38), and Kaneda (30). The design characteristics will be discussed later in the chapter. With the exception of the Dunn device, all are presently in use for anterior spinal surgery.

Historically, the indications for and role of anterior spinal surgery of the lumbar spine are at best controversial, particularly for degenerative conditions. Comparisons between large studies are difficult secondary to variation in techniques and surgical indications. Nevertheless, positive results have been reported by Harmon (95% fusion, 90% good or excellent clinical results) (22), Hodgson (77% fusion, 93% excellent results) (24), Crock (10), and Selby. When supplemental fixation is added, positive results have been shown by Kostuik (32–38) and Kaneda (30,31). Conversely, negative reports from Calandruccio and Benton (19% fusion, 56% good results) (7), Taylor (44% fusion) (58), Stauffer and Conventry (56% fusion, 14% excellent results) (57), and Flynn (56% fusion, 52% excellent results) (19) exist. Obviously, with history as a guide, one should proceed cautiously with both technique and patient selection.

ROLE OF ANTERIOR FUSION WITH INTERNAL FIXATION

At present, techniques and indications for anterior lumbar surgery are well known and, as shown in other chapters, include selected neoplastic, infectious, and degenerative conditions. The use of supplemental anterior internal fixation devices is presently not well established and accepted in all centers. The overall potential goals and benefits for the use of internal fixation in spinal fusion are: (a) correct deformity if present and reduce risk of late neurologic sequelae, (b) maintain rigidity and anatomic alignment, (c) decrease pseudarthrosis rate, and (d) enhance post-operative management. In conjunction with these general principles, the authors feel that certain specific and relative indications exist for anterior internal fixation and fusion.

These specific indications include: (a) symptomatic post-traumatic kyphosis with or without neurologic sequelae, (b) iatrogenic lumbar kyphosis (flatback syndrome), and (c) painful lumbar degenerative scoliosis with disc disease. In addition, painful iatrogenic kyphosis and degenerative lumbar scoliosis requiring fusion to the sacrum requires the combination of anterior and posterior stabilization with fusion.

Relative indications for anterior internal fixation and fusion include: (a) repair of failed posterior fusion, (b) instability secondary to wide laminectomy and posterior decompression, (c) high grade spondylolisthesis or spondyloptosis, and (d) spinal osteotomy.

The importance of careful patient evaluation and assessment must be stressed when the above difficult decision making is considered. This will be discussed in more detail later in the chapter.

PLACEMENT OF THE DEVICE

Device placement is initiated by exposing the lateral aspect of the spine by one of the methods described in the previous section. After the approach is completed, palpation will allow identification of the discs (hills) and the vertebral bodies (valleys). The aorta should be palpable anteriorly and must not be retracted too vigorously until the segmental vessels are ligated. X-rays should be used to identify appropriate levels since the anatomy may be distorted, though counting up from the sacrum promontory is usually reliable. After landmarks are identified, the overlying fascia is picked up with forceps and split sharply in a longitudinal plane in the mid-lateral portion of the spine. The segmental vessels are then identified. These are located in the midportion of the vertebral bodies (valleys) (Fig. 1). They are dissected with a right angle clamp and ligated at the midportion of the vertebral body. It is advisable not to ligate these segmental vessels too close to the aorta and not to place excessive retraction on them because avulsion may occur. Segmental vessels spanning the entire length of the instrumentation will need to be ligated (usually at least three vessels) (Fig. 2). Ligation at one of two levels (proximal or distal) will allow the vascular structures to fall away from the spine and help prevent possible vascular impingement on the fixation devices.

A Cobb elevator is used to reflect and expose the lateral spine subperiosteally (Fig. 3). If vertebrectomy is required, the procedure is as follows: The disc spaces above and below the vertebral body are identified and a large window is made in each. The contents of both discs are carefully removed with a rongeur at least as far back as the posterior longitudinal ligaments. An elevator is used to dissect the cartilaginous end plates. The bulk of the anterior and middle portions of the vertebral body is carefully removed with either a sharp rongeur or a burr. Posteriorly, the pedicle is palpated. If possible, the exiting nerve root should be visualized and followed to the thecal sac. A portion of the pedicle and posterior body is removed as is the posterior longitudinal ligament with a 45 degree Kerrison rongeur and curets. The thecal sac should be visualized at all times, and a small freer elevator should frequently be used to clear bone and ligament from underlying dura. Once decompression is complete, the vertebral end plates are debrided with curets and slots are made for the acceptance of the graft. The authors prefer the tricortical iliac crest with the tricortical portion placed posteriorly. Usually two pieces of graft can be introduced.

Accurate placement of the fixation device of choice is critical to success. As shown in Figure 4, only a small margin of safety is available. The device should be centered directly laterally. If it is placed too far anteriorly, it can abut the great vessels or the screws can penetrate the opposing foramen. Placement too far posteriorly can have obvious ill consequences including neural impingement.

TYPES OF DEVICES

Plate Systems

With adequate technique and exposure, plates can be easily and safely applied to the lumbar spine. Conventional DCP plates can be used as advocated by proponents of the AO system. In 1986, Ryan et al. (52) reported their technique and results utilizing a bolt plate fixation device for anterior fusion. This device consists of two transvertebral bolts placed in the coronal plane and connected by one lateral slotted plate. The system is made of pure titanium. It can be used for stabilization after discectomy or one level vertebrectomy. A post-operative orthosis is required, and only one device failure has been reported.

In 1988, Black et al. (3) described a low profile longitudinal rectangular plate which could span two or three adjacent vertebrae (Fig. 5). The plate is made of 316 LVM and contours easily to the vertebral bodies. Early results with its use in seven patients were encouraging.

The early experience with the Syracuse I plate has equally been positive (63). The device is a 3.5 mm stainless steel plate in the shape of an "I" that is attached to the vertebral body with four 6.5 mm cancellous screws. Clinical experience with its use has been reported in 16 cases with no major complications. An illustrative case is presented in Figure 6.

Plate systems have an important use in anterior spinal fixation when they span two or three vertebral segments. However, reduction of deformity must be carried out manually. They have application in post-traumatic kyphosis, iatrogenic flatback deformity, and failed posterior surgery or pseudarthrosis. They have no place in scoliotic or rotational deformities.

The major difficulty with plates is screw backout even after solid arthrodesis has been achieved. With the I plate the proximal part of the screw (distal to the head) completely fills the plate screw hole producing a "press-cold weld" fit and decreases the incidence of screw backout noted with other 6.5 mm cancellous screws.

Cable Systems

In 1964, Dwyer first used a cable system for anterior spinal instrumentation (Fig. 7) (21). Developed largely for scoliosis, the system gained widespread popularity. A special screw-staple assembly was drilled into each vertebral body on the convex side of the curvature. A braided titanium cable was passed through the screw heads and tension was applied. This device was a major conceptual breakthrough in anterior spine surgery and has been used extensively. Excellent results have been reported with its use (15,16). Dwyer reported only two cases of pseudarthrosis in 51 patients. Simmons et al. reported on over 80 patients with Dwyer instrumentation (54). Unfortunately, problems and complications have been presented. Dwyer reported a 43% complication rate in 77 patients (17) including progressive kyphosis (18 patients), loss of correction (22 patients), nonunion (15 patients), implant failure (5 patients), and deep paravertebral infection (3 patients). The pull-out strength of the screw system, especially in osteoporotic bone, has also been questioned. Finally, serious vascular and urologic complications have been documented (46).

The authors currently believe that lumbar degenerative curves that are symptomatic are still well treated by the Dwyer technique. Pre-operative evaluation with discography and facet blocks is mandatory to determine exact fusion levels. Since the device is a "tension" system, it can produce relative kyphosis; therefore any kyphosis in itself is a contraindication to the procedure. More specifically, it has no use in post-traumatic kyphosis, iatrogenic flatback deformity, deficient posterior elements with associated kyphosis, or where solid Dwyer body grafts are used.

Rod Systems

Zielke Device

In 1975 Zielke modified the Dwyer system (9). This system was made of stainless steel rather than titanium and appeared to have better pull-out characteristics (Fig. 8). The screws have slotted heads and are either top-opening (in between vertebra) or side-opening (top and bottom vertebra). A threaded 3.2 mm diameter flexible rod is attached to the screws. An outrigger device can be applied to produce lordosis (or reduce iatrogenic kyphosis) during curve correction, which is a distinctive benefit not available with plate systems.

During curve correction, compression is initiated at the apex of the curve. The nuts on the compression side of the device are then tightened and the surgeon works sequentially away from the apex of the curve. The screws must be inserted slightly posteriorly in the body because anterior placement will accentuate kyphosis. A 10% to 15% correction per disc level of scoliosis can be obtained in most cases.

We believe this implant is probably the implant of choice for correction of lumbar degenerative scoliosis (5). Moe et al. (48a) reported its use in 66 patients. Kaneda reported its use with 31 patients (only 8 adults) (31). A 59% correction of curve was obtained in the adult

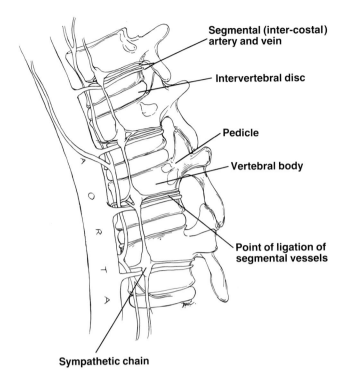

FIG. 1. Location of the segmental vessels at the mid portion of the vertebral bodies.

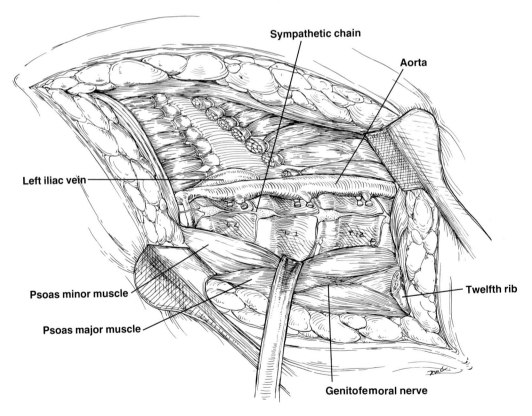

FIG. 2. Segmental vessels are ligated at the mid portion of the lateral aspect of the vertebral bodies.

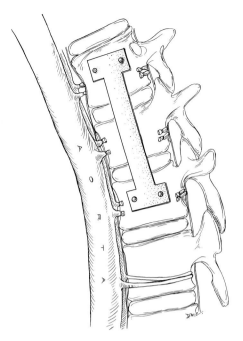

FIG. 3. Subperiosteal dissection exposes the anterior and lateral aspect of the spine.

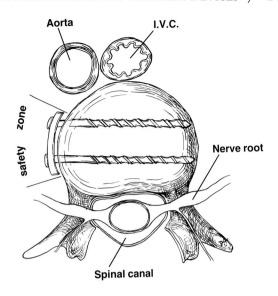

FIG. 4. Exact lateral placement of the device is a necessity. Only a small margin of safety is present as shown.

population. Kyphosis was also corrected (21 degrees to 8 degrees). Two of the adult patients later developed pseudarthrosis with its use. No major complications were encountered.

Kostuik feels the Zielke instrumentation is useful for symptomatic pseudarthrosis after attempted posterolateral fusion (36). He recommends the placement of two parallel Zeilke rods under compression.

The Zielke system is best used where the system is under tension and the bone is under compression as in scoliosis surgery. Used as a stabilizing device only, Kostuik noted an 18% incidence of pseudarthrosis with single rods, and a 9% incidence with double rods where interbody grafts were used in cases of salvage low back surgery.

Kostuik-Harrington Device

Kostuik has developed and extensively used an anterior modification of the classic posterior Harrington instrumentation (32–38). In this procedure, Kostuik spinal screws are inserted into the appropriate vertebral bodies, and a Harrington distraction rod placed through the screw holes and distracted in the usual fashion (Fig. 9). When optimal distraction is maintained, C-washers lock the rod into place. A second, heavier Harrington compression rod is then placed posteriorly to the first rod. This was his classical description in the treatment of burst fractures. The system is adaptable and can be used for distraction, compression, or stabilization alone.

Its use has been reported extensively and is an excel-

lent method for treating kyphotic and flatback deformities. Kostuik has reported 279 cases using this technique (35). Complications have included 35 screw breakages (12.5%) (24 of these were with the older, thin shanked screw), two distraction rods fractured (0.7%), two compression rods fractured (0.7%), and vertebral body fracture occurred in 8 cases (2.8%) without untoward effects. No vascular or neurologic injuries were reported. This device is a very acceptable system for the treatment of post-traumatic kyphosis, pseudarthrosis, iatrogenic flatback, and burst fractures.

Kaneda Device

In 1984, Kaneda et al. reported a series of unstable lumbar fractures treated with a new device (30). This device consists of two vertebral plates of a trapezoidal configuration each having four spikes (Fig. 10). Two screws pass through each plate, securing it to the appropriate vertebra (one above and one below). A vertebral body spreader can be placed between the screw heads to assist with reduction. Two rigid threaded rods with eight nuts (four nuts to each rod) are then used to connect the rods to the screws. The nuts can also be adjusted to allow for curve correction or compression. This device holds up well under biomechanical testing and would appear to be a good option for degenerative one or two level deformity (kyphosis, pseudarthrosis, and burst fracture).

Slot-Zielke Device

Slot of Holland described the use of a heavy single rod device, fixed to Zielke screws for the anterior correction

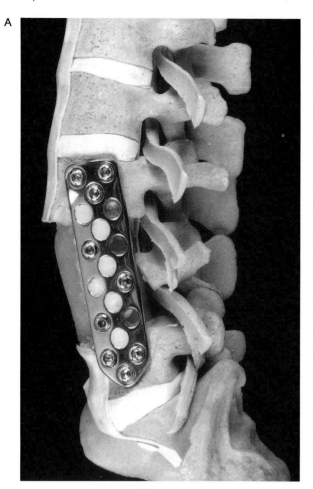
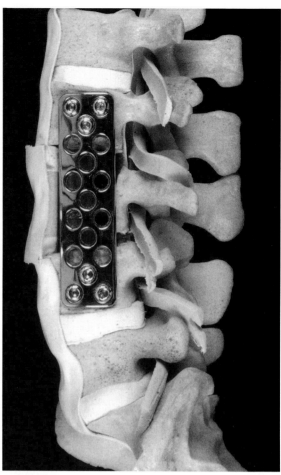

FIG. 5 (A and B). The Contoured Anterior Spinal Fixation System.

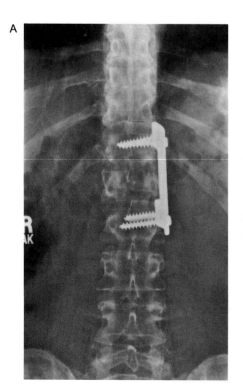
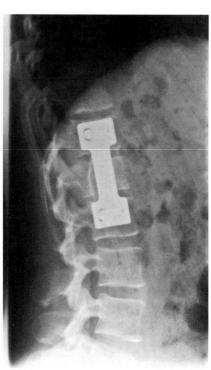

FIG. 6 (A and B). A 29-year-old male with a traumatic kyphotic deformity at L1. Note the exact lateral placement of the device.

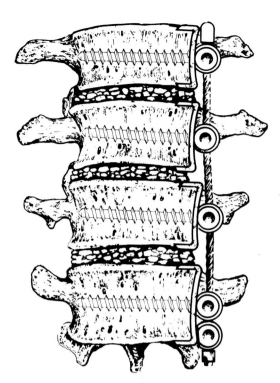

FIG. 7. The Dwyer Cable System.

of kyphotic deformities. Its design suffers from the use of only one rod that does not control rotational forces well. Gardener of England has used a similar device as has Pinto of Argentina. Currently considerable interest is being evoked in the development of anterior fixation devices.

BIOMECHANICS OF THE DEVICE

The underlying biomechanical concept of anterior fusion surgery is that compression is placed directly on the graft material. Posterior fusion, especially in kyphotic

situations, is under tension and this is subject to plastic deformation, fracture, or pseudarthrosis. Although the benefit of anterior bone grafting and fusion is through compressive forces, the loads in the lumbar spine can sometimes approach three times the body's weight. In certain pathologic conditions, we feel this is an excessive load to be placed on the graft material and that internal fixation is necessary to enhance stability. However, limited comparative biomechanical data exists to prove our assertion. Mann et al. (43) performed a laboratory evaluation of anterior fixation devices. Anterior vertebrectomy (with preservation of the anterior longitudinal ligament) was performed in nine fresh cadaver specimens. The grafted specimen alone, along with specimens internally fixed with the Kostuik device, Kaneda device, and I plate systems were compared with the intact spine in flexion, extension, and right and left lateral bending. The relative stability of each device is shown in Table 1. We believe these results indicate the use of bone graft without additional instrumentation does not provide adequate support to the spine with the gross instability produced by vertebrectomy. All of the devices tested returned stability to at least that of the intact spine. The Kaneda device and I plate provided the greatest increase in stiffness. Supplemental work by McGowan et al. (45) shows that if significant posterior element disruption is present, then anterior instrumentation alone does not provide appropriate support, and additional posterior fixation will be required. This is also supported by the clinical work of Kostuik.

Kostuik has also shown that the holding power of screws in vertebral bodies is doubled if the contralateral cortex of the vertebral body is perforated. A 6.5 mm cancellous thread is preferable. In osteoporotic bone, the addition of bone cement will greatly enhance the fixation of the screws.

INDICATIONS

Post-Traumatic Kyphosis

Late post-traumatic problems following fracture or injury to the thoracolumbar spine are not uncommon (Table 2). McAfee et al. (44) reported excellent results with

TABLE 1. *Bending moments of the average percent increase in stiffness of each device over the normal spine in each of the tested modes. Results for the grafted spine alone without instrumentation are included*

	Flexion (14 N-m)	Extension (12 N-m)	RL bend (10 N-m)	LL bend (10 N-m)
Graft	−6.8% (NS)	−10.0% (NS)	−48.6% (p < .0025)	−12.2% (p < 0.1)
Kostuik	−24.2% (p < 0.1)	5.3% (NS)	7.5% (NS)	20.1% (p < .05)
Kaneda	9.6% (NS)	3.3% (NS)	16.1% (p < .02)	37.2% (p < .01)
I Plate	12.4% (p < 0.15)	8.6% (NS)	6.8% (NS)	25.5% (p < .01)
Revised I-Plate	16.3% (p < 0.1)	8.7% (NS)	16.9% (p < .01)	29.0% (p < .01)

A negative number would indicate a percent decrease in stiffness when compared to the intact spine. Statistical significance levels when compared to the normal spine are listed in parentheses.
RL, right lateral; LL, left lateral; NS, not significant.

TABLE 2. *Degenerative conditions and corresponding fixation devices*

Degenerative condition	Implant of choice (in order of preference)
Post-traumatic kyphosis	Distraction rod systems Plate systems
Degenerative lumbar scoliosis	Rod systems (rotational correction) Cable systems
Iatrogenic lumbar kyphosis (flat back syndrome)	Distraction rod systems Plate systems
Failed posterior surgery/ pseudarthrosis	Plate systems Rod systems

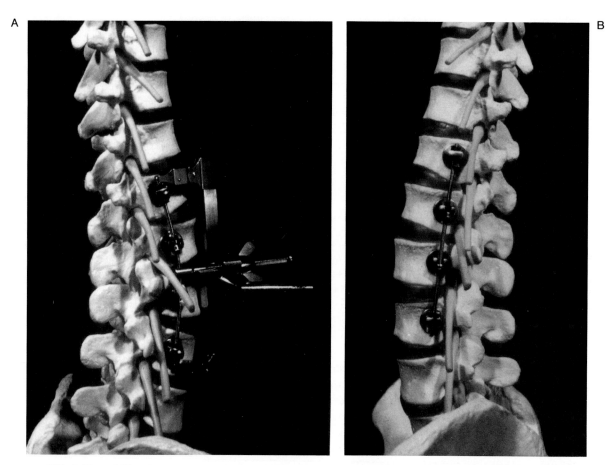

FIG. 8 (A and B). Zielke instrumentation with application of the derotating bar and outrigger. Note the top opening screws in the more central vertebra and the side opening screws in the most proximal and distal vertebra. Also note the slight posterior screw placement, especially in the more apical vertebra.

anterior decompression in patients with incomplete neurologic lesions, both acute and chronic. Although some authorities still advocate conservative acute management of spinal fractures (39), other reports document problems with late post-traumatic pain and neurologic compromise (35,38,42,49,51,62).

Malcolm and Bradford (42) reported their results of 48 patients surgically treated for post-traumatic kyphosis. Their indications for surgery were a painful deformity (greater than 50 degrees kyphosis), instability, and/or neurologic compromise. Twenty-four of the patients had a previous laminectomy (50%). Anterior fusion alone was performed on 12 patients with 6 failures out of 12 occurring (50%). No internal fixation was employed, and the patients were ambulated early (one week). Roberson and Whitesides (51) reviewed 34 patients with late post-traumatic kyphosis. Both anterior and posterior approaches were utilized. They felt that posterior fusion alone was usually not sufficient treatment and that it did not fully address the problem. Eighteen of these patients had anterior fusion alone with 17 of the patients obtaining solid fusion with no evidence of a further progression of the kyphosis. Roberson and Whitesides recommended 2 to 3 months of post-operative recumbency, but emphasized that internal fixation could significantly improve the post-operative rehabilitation. Kostuik has done extensive work with post-traumatic kyphosis. He has reported on 45 patients with post-traumatic kyphosis treated with anterior surgery and instrumentation with Kostuik-Harrington system. Pain relief was good or excellent in 37 out of 45 patients (82%). Screw breakage occurred in 3 out of 45 patients (6.6%). Four out of 10 residual paraparetics improved greater than one Frankel grade after surgery.

The present indications for surgery in cases of post-traumatic kyphosis are significant back pain, deformity, instability, progression of deformity, or current or progressing neurologic compromise. Supplemental posterior surgery does not need to be considered unless significant posterior instability is present. Rod systems (Kostuik, Kaneda, Zielke) are the preferable devices because they provide distraction forces for reduction of the kyphosis. Plates are also very applicable though the reduction must be done manually and no more than 2 or 3 segments can be bridged.

Iatrogenic Lumbar Kyphosis (Flatback Deformity)

Iatrogenic loss of lumbar lordosis following posterior distraction instrumentation and fusion for scoliosis has been well documented (35,37) and presents a major functional problem in those patients with posterior fusion that extends to the lower lumbar spine or sacrum. Extension osteotomy is the accepted procedure of choice when these patients become symptomatic. Classically,

these patients complain of back pain with an inability to stand erect without flexing the knees and hips. With fusion to the sacrum, Kostuik (37) reported a 49% loss of lordosis following Harrington instrumentation. He also noted that treatment by posterior osteotomy alone showed excellent early correction but that 50% of patients later showed loss of correction.

Because of these problems, the symptomatic patient with flatback deformity is better treated by single stage anterior opening wedge osteotomy with internal fixation followed by posterior closing wedge osteotomy. Kostuik reported significant pain relief in 90% of patients treated by this approach. The acceptable devices are the distraction rod systems (Kostuik, Kaneda, Zielke). Plating systems can also be used, but as mentioned previously have the disadvantages that the reduction and positioning must be done manually.

Lumbar Scoliosis

Degenerative scoliosis of the adult lumbar spine can be a disabling and painful condition (see Chapter 65). Posterior surgery alone is often insufficient to correct the curve and has a high rate of pseudarthrosis. Posterior distraction instrumentation and fusion to L4 or below are contraindicated especially in those patients with thoracic hypokyphosis. Because pain is the major disabling complaint of these patients, careful pre-operative evaluation is very important. Facet blocks and discography are used to identify the possible sources of pain and to accurately plan the levels of fusion. Bradford (5), Kostuik (35,36), and Kaneda (31) have all reported and recommended anterior instrumentation and fusion for painful lumbar scoliosis.

Painful adult scoliosis greater than 40 to 50 degrees or painful progressive scoliosis of the lumbar spine should be managed with anterior instrumentation and fusion after careful pre-operative evaluation and counseling. For curves greater than 80 degrees, a combination of anterior and posterior procedures may be needed. The preferred implant system anteriorly is the Zielke implant. Ten to fifteen degrees of curve correction per disc level can usually be obtained, although this varies as a function of age, spinal stiffness, and neurologic symptoms.

Failed Posterior Surgery

Much attention is focused on those unfortunate patients with failed posterior surgery (Chapter 98). Failed posterior surgery is a major cause of disability in this country. With the popularity of pedicle screw fixation and the 360 degree technique of fusion (50), anterior internal fixation is now rarely required. Nevertheless, in cases of significant posterior adhesion formation, extensive laminectomy, and loss of bone stock or posterior pseudarthrosis (11) anterior internal fixation and fusion remains a viable option (35,36). Anterior fusion and instrumentation have particular utility in those cases with associated kyphosis or deformity that needs correction. Both rod systems or plate systems can be utilized dependent on the extent and type of deformity. Long-term clinical trials in this population, however, are presently lacking.

Other Indications

Spondylolisthesis and degenerative disc lesions can be approached anteriorly with some success (10,20,22,24). No large series using internal fixation are currently available, nor do we believe there are obvious indications at the present time to support the use of internal fixation devices and anterior lumbar surgery in this setting.

COMPLICATIONS

Throughout this chapter, we have stressed the potential complications associated with the various fixation devices (Table 3) and paid particular attention to operative technique and device placement. The most devastating complications are vascular and neurologic. Kostuik reported 2 iliac vein lacerations in 79 patients treated with anterior decompression (2.5%) (32). In a larger series of patients (279) treated for a variety of kyphotic deformities, he reported 3 cases of vascular insult (1.1%) and 2 cases of neurologic deterioration (0.7%) (35). The vascular injuries occurred during surgery and were not

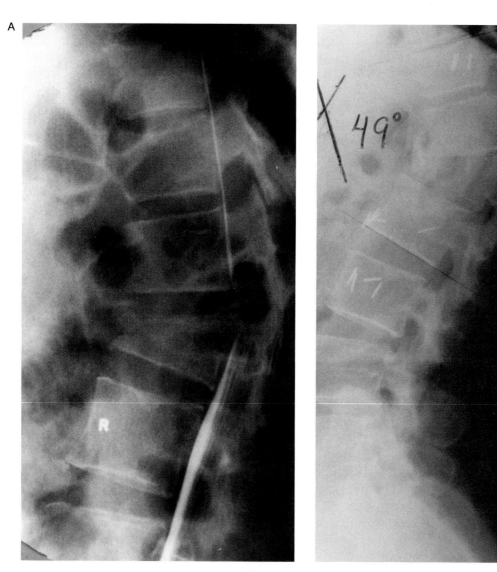

FIG. 9. A 32-year-old female suffered an acute traumatic injury to her thoracolumbar junction. **A:** Initial myelogram. The patient underwent anterior decompression and interbody grafting with neurologic recovery (Frankel D → Frankel E). **B:** Unfortunately, the graft collapsed and the patient deteriorated neurologically (Frankel D). (Figs. 9C–9D follow.)

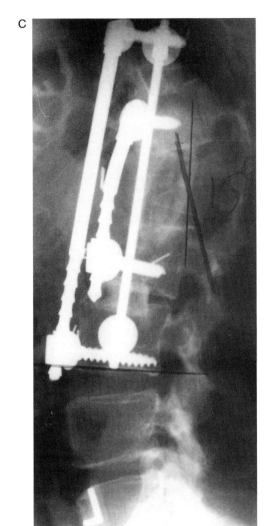

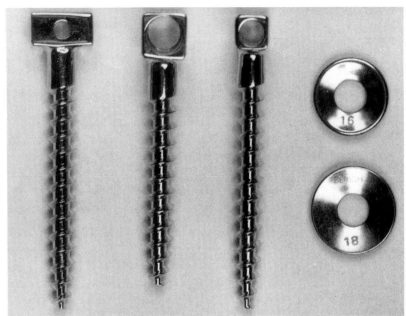

FIG. 9. *Continued.* **C:** Pre-operative discography revealed painful motion segments at the 2 adjacent disc levels. She underwent decompression and instrumentation with the Kostuik-Harrington System. She presently is neurologically intact and working in a factory. **D:** Kostuik screws (both ratchet and collar ended).

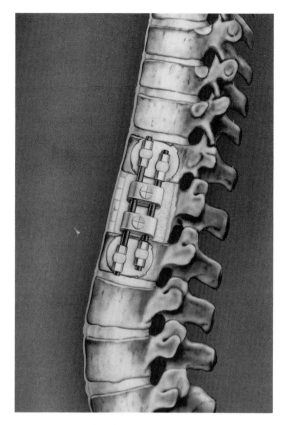

FIG. 10. Kaneda Device.

due to the fixation devices. However, significant vascular injuries led to the removal of the Dunn device from widespread commercial use (25). Whether technical or implant design features (or both) were responsible for these are not known. Urologic complications have been documented after Dwyer instrumentation (46), though the one case presented involved obstruction of the left ureter by scar tissue, and not by the device itself.

Prevention of complications is essential. Meticulous placement of the device with mobilization of the great vessels and adequate neurologic decompression are mandatory. Spinal cord monitoring or the wake up test should be routinely used. Careful pre-operative planning and patient selection cannot be overemphasized.

TABLE 3. *Potential complications associated with various fixation devices*

Retroperitoneal fibrosis
Urologic dysfunction
Major vascular injury/aneurysm
Neurologic impairment
Implant failure
Sympathetic nerve injury
Infection
Graft migration
Pseudarthrosis
Deep venous thrombosis/embolism

SUMMARY

Internal fixation in general is widely accepted by orthopedic surgeons to provide rigidity, improve fusion rates, reduce post-operative morbidity, and to correct deformity. Anterior lumbar surgery for a variety of indications has gained popularity in most centers throughout the world. The indications presently for anterior lumbar surgery augmented with internal fixation are small, but when indicated, are invaluable in dealing with very difficult surgical problems. Detailed knowledge of the approach, indications, and implant characteristics are most important. Even more important is careful patient evaluation, selection, and documentation. Further scientific investigation with implant and technical modification will help make anterior internal fixation a more acceptable, safer procedure in the future.

REFERENCES

1. Albee FH (1911): Transplantation of a portion of the tibia into the spine for Pott's disease. *JAMA* 57:885–886.
2. Bick EM (1964): An essay on the history of spine fusion operations. *Clin Orthop* 35:9–15.
3. Black RC, Gardner VO, Armstrong GWD, Oneil J, St. George M (1988): A contoured anterior spinal fixation plate. *Clin Orthop* 227:135–142.
4. Bohlman HH (1985): Treatment of fractures and dislocations of the thoracic and lumbar spine. *J Bone Joint Surg* [Am] 67:165–169.
5. Bradford DS (1986): Instrumentation of the lumbar spine. *Clin Orthop* 203:209–218.
6. Burns BH (1933): Operation for spondylolisthesis. *Lancet* 1:1233.
7. Calandruccio RA, Benton BF (1964): Anterior lumbar fusion. *Clin Orthop* 35:63–68.
8. Capener N (1932): Spondylolisthesis. *Br J Surg* 19:374–386.
9. Chan DP (1983): Zielke instrumentation. *AAOS Instructional Course Lectures* 32:208–209.
10. Crock HV (1977): Current views on the role of lumbar interbody fusion operations in the management of back and leg pain. *J Bone Joint Surg* [Br] 59:122–123.
11. DePalma AF, Rothman RH (1968): The nature of pseudarthrosis. *Clin Orthop* 59:113–118.
12. Dunn HK (1983): Spinal instrumentation. I. Principles of anterior and posterior instrumentation. *AAOS Instructional Course Lectures* 32:192–202.
13. Dunn HK (1984): Anterior stabilization of thoracolumbar injuries. *Clin Orthop* 189:116–124.
14. Dunn HK (1986): Anterior spine stabilization and decompression for thoracolumbar injuries. *Orthop Clin North Am* 17:113–119.
15. Dwyer AF, Newton NC, Sherwood AA (1969): An anterior approach to scoliosis. *Clin Orthop* 62:192–202.
16. Dwyer AF (1970): Anterior instrumentation in scoliosis. *J Bone Joint Surg* [Br] 52:782–783.
17. Dwyer AP, O'Brien JP, Seal PP, et al. (1977): The late complications after the Dwyer anterior spinal instrumentation for scoliosis. *J Bone Joint Surg* [Br] 59:117.
18. Fang HS, Ong GB, Hodgson AR (1964): Anterior spinal fusion. The operative approaches. *Clin Orthop* 35:16–33.
19. Flynn JC, Hoque MA (1979): Anterior fusion of the lumbar spine. *J Bone Joint Surg* [Am] 61:1143–1150.
20. Freebody D, Bendall R, Taylor RD (1971): Anterior transperitoneal lumbar fusion. *J Bone Joint Surg* [Br] 53:617–627.
21. Hall JE (1981): Dwyer instrumentation in anterior fusion of the spine. *J Bone Joint Surg* [Am] 63:1188–1190.

22. Harmon PH (1963): Anterior excision and vertebral body fusion operation for intervertebral disk syndromes of the lower lumbar spine. *Clin Orthop* 26:107–127.

23. Hibbs RA (1964): An operation for progressive spinal deformities. *Clin Orthop* 35:4–8.

24. Hodgson AR (1966): Results of anterior fusion. *J Bone Joint Surg* [Br] 48:595.

25. Hodgson AR, Stock FE (1956): Anterior spinal fusion. A preliminary communication on radical treatment of Pott's disease and Pott's paraplegia. *Br J Surg* 44:266–275.

26. Humphries AW, Hawk WA, Berndt AL (1961): Anterior interbody fusion of lumbar vertebrae: a surgical technique. *Surg Clin North Am* 41:1685–1700.

27. Ito H, Tsuchiya J, Asami G (1934): A new radical operation for Pott's disease. *J Bone Joint Surg* 16:499–515.

28. Jendrisak MD (1986): Spontaneous abdominal aortic rupture from erosion by a lumbar spine fixation device: A case report. *Surg* 99:631–633.

29. Jenkins JA (1936): Spondylolisthesis. *Br J Surg* 24:80–85.

30. Kaneda K, Abumi K, Fujiya M (1984): Burst fractures with neurologic deficits of the thoracolumbar-lumbar spine. *Spine* 9:788–795.

31. Kaneda K, Fujiya N, Satoh S (1986): Results with Zielke instrumentation for idiopathic thoracolumbar and lumbar scoliosis. *Clin Orthop* 205:195–203.

32. Kostuik JP (1983): Anterior spinal cord decompression for lesions of the thoracic and lumbar spine, techniques, new methods of internal fixation results. *Spine* 8:512–531.

33. Kostuik JP (1984): Anterior fixation for fractures of the thoracic and lumbar spine with or without neurologic involvement. *Clin Orthop* 189:103–115.

34. Kostuik JP (1988): Anterior fixation for burst fractures of the thoracic and lumbar spine with or without neurological involvement. *Spine* 13:286–293.

35. Kostuik JP (1989): Anterior Kostuik-Harrington distraction systems for the treatment of kyphotic deformities. *Iowa Orthop J* 8:68–77.

36. Kostuik JP, Errico TJ, Gleason TF (1986): Techniques of internal fixation for degenerative conditions of the lumbar spine. *Clin Orthop* 203:219–231.

37. Kostuik JP, Maurais GR, Richardson WJ, Okajima Y (1988): Combined single stage anterior and posterior osteotomy for correction of iatrogenic lumbar kyphosis. *Spine* 13:257–266.

38. Kostuik JP, Matsusaki H (1989): Anterior stabilization, instrumentation, and decompression for posttraumatic kyphosis. *Spine* 14:379–386.

39. Krompinger WJ, Fredrickson BE, Mino DE, Yuan HE (1986): Conservative treatment of fractures of the thoracic and lumbar spine. *Orthop Clin North Am* 17(1):161–170.

40. Lane JD Jr, Moore ES Jr (1948): Transperitoneal approach to the intervertebral disc in the lumbar area. *Annals Surg* 127:537–551.

41. Macnab I, Dall D (1971): The blood supply of the lumbar spine and its application to the technique of intertransverse lumbar fusion. *J Bone Joint Surg* [Br] 53:628–638.

42. Malcolm BW, Bradford DS, Winter RB, Chou SN (1981): Posttraumatic kyphosis. *J Bone Joint Surg* [Am] 63:891–899.

43. Mann KA, Found EM, Yuan HA, Fredrickson BE, Lubicky J (1987): Biomechanical evaluation of the effectiveness of anterior spinal fixation systems. Presented at the Orthopaedic Research Society 33rd annual meeting, San Francisco.

44. McAfee PC, Bohlman HH, Yuan HA (1985): Anterior decompression of traumatic thoracolumbar fractures with incomplete neurological deficit using a retroperitoneal approach. *J Bone Joint Surg* [Am] 67:89–104.

45. McGowan DP, Mann KA, Yuan HA, Fredrickson BE, Albanese SA (1987): A biomechanical study of anterior spinal fixation for thoracolumbar burst fractures with varying degrees of posterior disruption. Presented at International Society for the Study of the Lumbar Spine, 1987.

46. McMaster WC, Silber I (1975): An urological complication of Dwyer instrumentation. *J Bone Joint Surg* [Am] 57:710–711.

47. Mercer W (1936): Spondylolisthesis. *Edinburgh Medical Journal* 43:545–572.

48. Mirbaha MM (1973): Anterior approach to the thoraco-lumbar junction of the spine by a retroperitoneal–extrapleural technic. *Clin Orthop* 91:41–47.

48a. Moe JH, Purcell GA, Bradford DS (1973): Zielke instrumentation (VDS) for the correction of spinal curvature: Analysis of results in 66 patients. *Clin Orthop* 93:207.

49. Myllynen P, Bostman O, Riska E (1988): Recurrence of deformity after removal of Harrington's fixation of spine fracture. *Acta Orthop Scand* 59:497–502.

50. O'Brien JP, Dawson MHO, Heard CW, Momberger G, Speck G, Weatherley CR (1986): Simultaneous combined anterior and posterior fusion. *Clin Orthop* 203:191–195.

51. Roberson JR, Whitesides TE (1985): Surgical reconstruction of late posttraumatic thoracolumbar kyphosis. *Spine* 10:307–312.

52. Ryan MD, Taylor TKF, Sherwood AA (1986): Bolt-plate fixation for anterior spinal fusion. *Clin Orthop* 203:196–202.

53. Sachs S (1965): Anterior interbody fusion of the lumbar spine. *J Bone Joint Surg* [Br] 47:211–223.

54. Simmons EH, Sue-A-Quan EA, O'Leary PF, Garside HJ (1977): An analysis of Dwyer instrumentation of the spine with assessment of its place in spinal surgery. *J Bone Joint Surg* [Br] 59:117.

55. Southwick WO, Robinson RA (1957): Surgical approaches to the vertebral bodies in the cervical and lumbar regions. *J Bone Joint Surg* [Am] 39:631–644.

56. Speed K (1938): Spondylolisthesis. *Arch Surg* 37:175–189.

57. Stauffer RN, Coventry MB (1972): Anterior interbody lumbar spine fusion. *J Bone Joint Surg* [Am] 54:756–768.

58. Taylor TK (1970): Anterior interbody fusion in the management of disorders of the lumbar spine. *J Bone Joint Surg* [Br] 52:784.

59. Thomasen E (1985): Intercorporal lumbar spondylodesis. *Acta Orthop Scand* 56:287–293.

60. Watkins RG (1983): *Surgical approaches to the spine.* New York: Springer-Verlag.

61. Werlinich M (1974): Anterior interbody fusion and stabilization with metal fixation. *International Surg* 59:269–273.

62. Whitesides TE Jr (1977): Traumatic kyphosis of the thoracolumbar spine. *Clin Orthop* (128):78–92.

63. Yuan HA, Mann KA, Found EM, Helbig TE, Fredrickson BE, Lubicky JP, Albanese SA, Winfield JA, Hodge CJ (1988): Early clinical experience with the Syracuse I-plate: An anterior spinal fixation device. *Spine* 13:278–285.

The Adult Spine: Principles and Practice,
J. W. Frymoyer, Editor-in-Chief.
Raven Press, Ltd., New York © 1991.

CHAPTER 94

Posterior Lumbar Interbody Fusion

(PLIF)

James W. Simmons

> Throughout the centuries there were men who took first steps down new roads armed with nothing but their own visions.
>
> —Ayn Rand

Posterior lumbar interbody fusion (PLIF) has been considered by surgeons and researchers dealing with the spine since the advent of adequate anesthesia and the ability to replace the significant quantities of blood sometimes lost during the procedure. Considerations of the history of a given procedure must be taken into account before one embarks upon a new idea or modification of an old idea.

The stabilization of the spine was first introduced by Hibbs and Albee in 1911 (23). The advent of the intervertebral disc as producing a definite pathological entity was described by Mixter and Barr in 1934 (41). Putti in 1927, however, realized another common cause of sciatica, that being stenosis secondary to abnormalities of the facet joints and the need for bony decompression to alleviate the associated "sciatic pain" (46). The decompressive procedures done by removing these offending bony elements (facets) and soft tissue elements (intervertebral discs) inadvertently led to problems associated with an unstable segment.

The interlaminar fusion of the lumbar spine, originally described by Hibbs and Albee in 1911, became the standard fusion technique. Although originally performed for tuberculosis, it was subsequently extended to

include many other pathological conditions in the cervical, thoracic, and lumbar spines. In 1936, Mercer suggested that "the ideal operation for fusing the spine would be an interbody fusion, but the surgical difficulties encountered in performing such a feat would make the operation technically impossible (40). The procedure, posterior interbody fusion, following lumbar disc removal was reported by Jaslow in 1946 (27). The use of the interbody fusion was further extended by the application, anteriorly, by Hodgson and Stock (24). Based on individual need, as well as innovative genius, many variations of the PLIF have been used. Briggs (5) reported packing of bone chips between the vertebral bodies to obtain an intercorpus fusion. The use of autogenous corticocancellous chips from the posterior elements for a body-to-body fusion was reintroduced by Simmons in 1985 (48). Ovens and Williams (42) placed a portion of the spinous process elements in the intervertebral disc space, reported in 1945. Jaslow (27) used a peg of bone in the intervertebral disc space and bone chips placed posteriorly from the posterior elements for a segmental fusion, reported in 1946.

Ralph Cloward, however, has been the prime proponent and propagator of the PLIF. In 1945, he devised "the treatment of ruptured lumbar disc by intervertebral fusion—report of 100 cases," and reported his series at the Harvey Cushing Society meeting in Hot Springs, Virginia, in November of 1947 (9). Crock (13) indicated that the ideal operation for isolated lumbar disc resorption is the PLIF, allowing bilateral nerve root canal decompression. James and Nisbet (26) used the procedure

J. W. Simmons, M.D.: South Texas Surgical and Medical Center, San Antonio, Texas, 78229.

primarily for spondylolisthesis, but also for patients with prolapsed discs. LeVay (34) stated that the PLIF is favored by neurosurgeons in England. Junghanns and Schmorl (28) are advocates of Cloward's concept of the PLIF. Junghanns (29) suggested a phenomenon of an operative unfolding (distraction) of the disc space: "In the lumbar spine this only could be achieved posteriorly by removing disc tissue, eliminating the cartilaginous end plate, unfolding (distraction) of the disc space and positioning of the osseous packs." Wiltberger (53,54) uses a dowel graft through the facets. Christoferson (8) places a portion of the lamina removed during exposure of the intervertebral disc, in the intervertebral disc space following discectomy. Lin (35) modified Cloward's technique advocating the need for complete filling of the intervertebral disc space with bone.

INDICATIONS

The phenomenon of spinal stenosis following discectomy has been described by Kirkaldy-Willis (32), Farfan (16), Crock (13), Finneson (19), and Cauthen (6). Symptomatic spinal stenosis and/or instability, with or without sciatica, are the basic indications for PLIF. Various aspects of intervertebral disc disease as definitive indication for PLIF have been proposed by several authors. Collis's indications (12) are lumbar pain with or without sciatica, a degenerative disc with or without a protrusion, a midline disc protrusion, post-lumbar laminectomy/discectomy syndrome, a recurrent soft tissue protrusion, spondylolisthesis, grade I or grade II, a reverse spondylolisthesis, or any combination of the preceding seven conditions. Keim (30) has listed ten indications, such as unstable joint complex associated with long history of low back pain, spondylolisthesis with or without spondylolysis, congenital anomalies such as a transitional transverse process or spondylolysis without spondylolisthesis, localized lateral spinal stenosis or spondylosis at one level. Some of his other indications are facet resection from previous surgery, heavy labor or sports activity associated with simple disc herniation with or without degenerative change, bilateral disc herniation or massive midline herniation, previous disc surgery at the sympptomatic level, reconstructive procedures for failed back surgery syndrome (FBSS), including pseudarthrosis from lateral fusion; and his last indication is in obese patients with bilaterally extruded discs, preventing rapid post-operative settling of the disc space. Lin's indications (36) are quite similar to those listed by Keim. Crock (13) has also listed similar indications. Clowards's indications (9) have not changed after 45 years of experience: that is, "the treatment of low back pain with or without sciatica due to lumbar disc disease."

This author's indications are based on a combination of pathophysiology, musculoskeletal dsyfunction, and significantly impaired lifestyle. Specific indications are spinal stenosis not responding to non-operative measures, spinal instability not responding to job or activity modifications, and discogenic disease that likewise has not responded to non-operative measures. Discogenic disease, admittedly, is a medical colloquialism commonly used to describe the morphologic, histologic, and chemical abnormalities of the intervertebral disc with traumatic or aging characteristics not of infectious, tumor, metabolic, or inflammatory etiology.

Discogenic disease is used generically when covering the broad spectrum extending from the initial stage of dysfunction to the final stage of stabilization as described by Kirkaldy-Willis and Farfan (31). Otherwise more definitive diagnosis should be made relating to the anatomical structure involved, the lesion, the morphologic changes, instability, and extent of neurological involvement.

Defining and then identifying lumbar spinal instability is a crucial though difficult task when considering a patient for posterior lumbar interbody fusion. In a broad conceptual sense, instability has been defined as

> the loss of the ability of the spine under physiological load to maintain relationship between vertebrae in such a way that there is neither initial damage nor subsequent irritation to the spinal cord or nerve root and, in addition, there is no development of incapacitating deformity or pain to the structural changes (52).

In a narrow patient specific sense instability is more elusive. Both clinical and radiographic criteria are hazy if not contradictory.

Adding to the dilemma is the need to distinguish between instability and physiologic hypermobility. Normative values of intervertebral mobility in asymptomatic patients may present ranges of translation which exceed criteria for pathologic instability (22,33,45). This emphasizes the need to correlate both clinical and radiographic findings. More sophisticated techniques, i.e., centrode measurement (21) and biplane measurement (50,51), may not be useful in daily clinical practice.

Clinically, instability has been defined as "the patient with back problems who with the least provocation steps from the mildly symptomatic to the severe episode" (31). The patient may complain of "giving way" or "slipping out" (43). There may be a series of recurrent torsional type injury mechanisms (17,18). On exam a positive "torsion test" (18) may be found. Others have identified hypertrophied muscle, palpable catches on flexion, and uncoordinated muscle contractions as physical signs (43). All of these may be elusive and non-specific to the average clinician. Abnormal lumbar motion may be either translational or rotational (18,33,43). In addition, instability may be apparent in quality or coupling of movements rather than quantity (14,52).

Abnormal translation has been used to identify lumbar instability most frequently. Knutsson found more than 3 mm of translation in the sagittal plane to be abnormal (33). Posner found absolute values somewhat less and also defined percentage translational values: flexion, L1 to L5, 8%; flexion, L5 to S1, 6%; extension, all levels, 9% (45).

Rotational abnormalities may appear as a double density of the uncinate processes on the lateral projection (14). This finding at an isolated lumbar segment may indicate rotational instability. Side-bending x-rays may also demonstrate abnormal rotation with the spinous process at the abnormal segment rotating towards the convexity (14). An abnormal translational lateral shear may also be seen. The coupling of translation and rotation may obscure segmental instability and may make attempts to quantify it impossible. Abnormal coupling of movements therefore may be indicative of lumbar instability in quality only (14,52).

Because of these problems with primary radiographic signs, secondary findings should be considered (3). In my view, the vacuum gas sign, Macnab traction spur (39), spondylolisthesis (44), retrolisthesis (20), or previous total laminectomy (2) are all evidence of segmental instability.

BIOMECHANICAL ADVANTAGES

Junghanns and Schmorl (28) first described the lumbar intervertebral disc as a part of the motion segment. It has been well established that PLIF is the most biomechanically sound stabilizing procedure. Evans (15) has proposed a flagpole concept to explain the biomechanical rationale for performing posterior interbody fusions rather than a technically less demanding procedure. In his model, ultimate stability is obtained through the balance of compressive and torsional forces. The flagpole, or central compression force, represents the intervertebral graft placement, while the surrounding guidewires represent posterior facet joints, supraspinous and intraspinous ligaments, and anterior annulus. The advantages of a posterior interbody fusion are that the intervertebral positioning of the grafts optimizes the load bearing capacity of the vertebral segment and that lateral placement of the grafts produces stability. Evans further states that the uniform distribution of compressive interbody forces over the end plate helps prevent graft host collapse.

Evans's model relies on the preservation or reconstruction of posterior ligamentous structures since disc space distraction places tension on the remaining annulus fibrosus and posterior ligamentous structures. He further recommends that if structures are deficient, internal fixation may be necessary to balance the construct and prevent graft dislodgment. In addition, disc space distraction helps decompress foraminal encroachment of the nerve root.

The advantages of the PLIF have been posed by James and Nisbet (26), Keim (30), Evans (15), Lin (36), and Cautilli (7). The PLIF is demanding surgically, requiring meticulous surgical technique and a thorough knowledge of anatomy and pathophysiology. The PLIF accomplishes all of the needs of a compromised lumbar spinal segment allowing for extensive decompression and stabilization at the same operation with minimal dissection.

PLIF TECHNIQUE

After the usual preparation and preliminary soft tissue dissection exposing the posterior elements, an osteotome is used to remove the inferior border of the superior lamina of the segment involved. The medial portion of the medial facets is removed along with the exostosis present in the case of tropism causing spinal stenosis (Fig. 1). The medial border of the lateral facet is then quite well exposed (Fig. 2). Removing the medial border of the lateral facets out to the pedicle gives excellent visualization of the segmental nerve root (Fig. 3). By using lamina spreaders, the superior portion of the lateral facet is quite well exposed for removal if causing narrowing of the foramina and/or nerve root impingement (Fig. 4).

An osteotome is then used to take down the posterior annulus and the end plates (Fig. 5). Curettes are used quite extensively in cleaning out the intervertebral disc space (Fig. 6). The disc is removed to the lateral and anterior edges of the annulus, including the cartilaginous end plate (Fig. 7). Using a lamina spreader, excellent visualization can be obtained (Fig. 8). With some end plate remaining for support, a punch is used to puncture the end plate to obtain a bleeding surface for the bone plugs (Fig. 9). Spanners are used to measure the width and depth of the intervertebral disc space with moderate distraction being placed with the lamina spreaders (Fig. 10). A spacer of the appropriate size is then placed on one side of the intervertebral disc space to maintain the distraction (Fig. 11). An appropriate size allograft bone plug is then fashioned to fit the side opposite the spacer. This is placed in the intervertebral disc space with very little resistance to impaction (Fig. 12).

Text continues on page 1968.

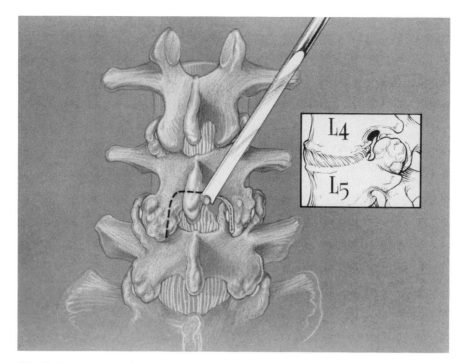

FIG. 1. An osteotome is used to remove the inferior border of the superior lamina and offending part of the inferior medial facet.

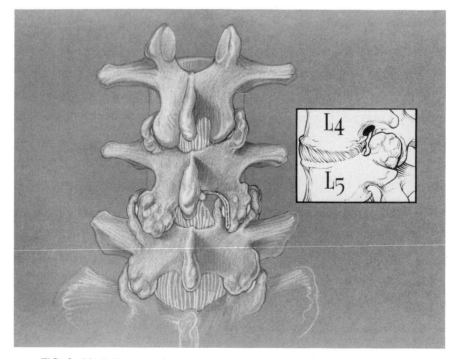

FIG. 2. Medial border of the superior lateral articular process is exposed.

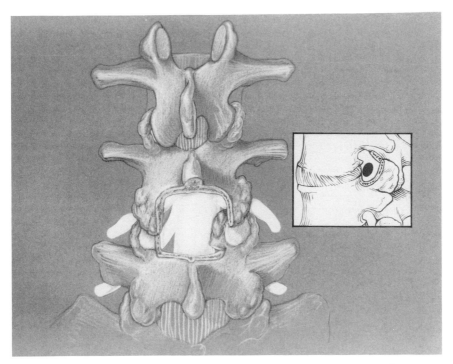

FIG. 3. Comparison between compressed and decompressed nerve root after resection of medial border of the superior lateral articular process.

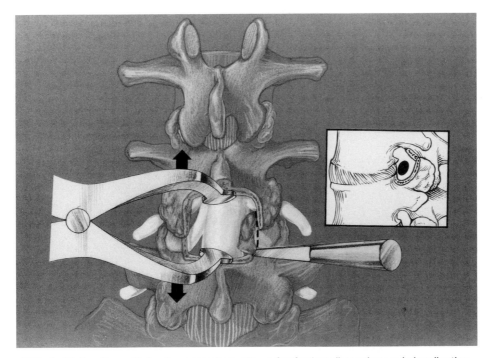

FIG. 4. Distraction with lamina spreaders allows for further dissection and visualization.

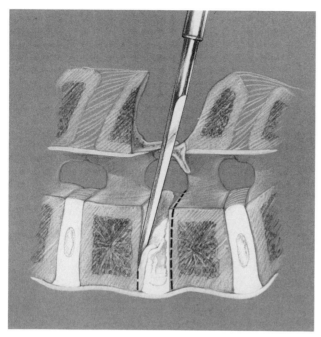

FIG. 5. An osteotome is used to remove the annulus and cartilaginous end plates.

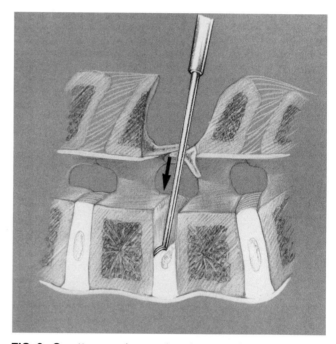

FIG. 6. Curettes are also used to clean out the intervertebral disc space.

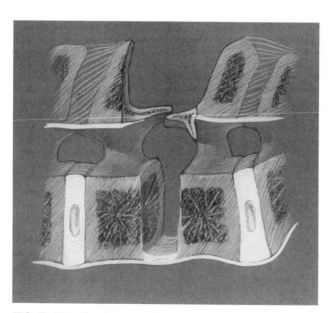

FIG. 7. The disc is removed and the site is ready for bone block.

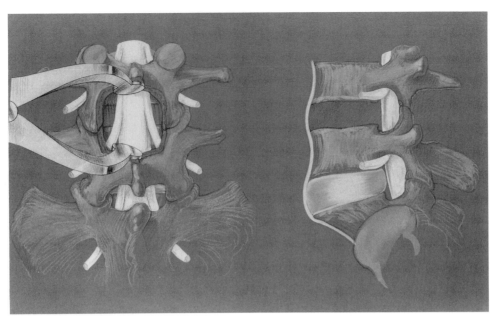

FIG. 8. Lamina spreaders allow excellent visualization.

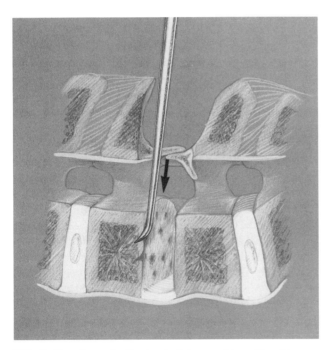

FIG. 9. Punctures to the end plate provide a bleeding surface.

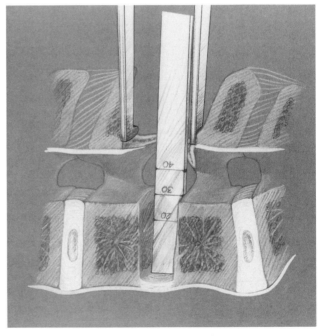

FIG. 10. Spanners are used to determine depth of disc space.

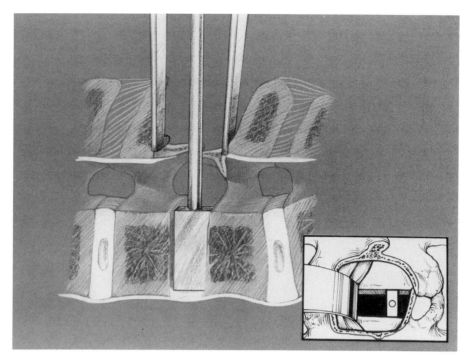

FIG. 11. A spacer is placed to maintain the distraction.

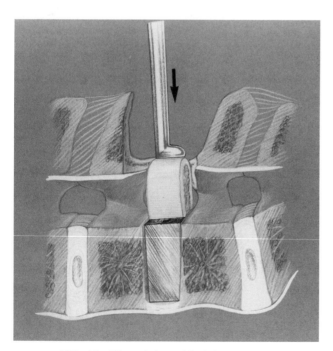

FIG. 12. Allograft bone block is inserted.

A second bone block may be inserted by moving the first bone block medially with the Puka chisels (Figs. 13, 14, 15, and 16). The spacer is then removed (Fig. 17). With the previous bone block acting as a spacer, block(s) are fashioned for the side from which the spacer was removed (Fig. 18). Puka chisels are used to "walk" the bone blocks to the midline using the pedicle as leverage (Figs. 19 and 20). Three to four tricortical or bicortical allograft blocks from cadaveric iliac crest are usually accepted by the intervertebral disc space. These should lie comfortably in the intervertebral disc space, 2–4 mm below the posterior border of the vertebral body (Fig. 21). The graft produces good stability and the neural elements are not compromised following placement of the allograft bone blocks (Fig. 22). A fat graft is placed anteriorly between the dura and the allograft blocks and posterior over the dura (Figs. 23 and 24).

Text continues on page 1973.

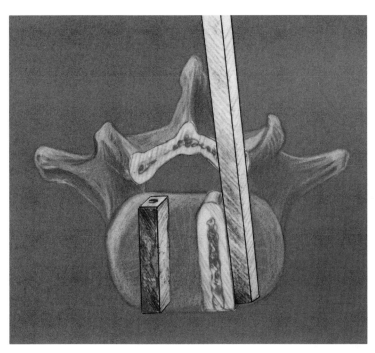

FIG. 13. Puka chisels allow movement of bone block medially.

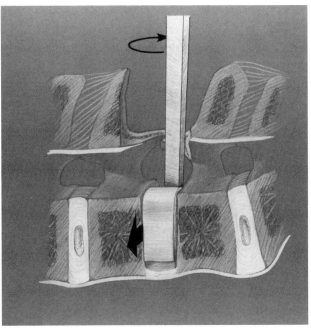

FIG. 14. Manipulation of the Puka chisels for movement of bone block.

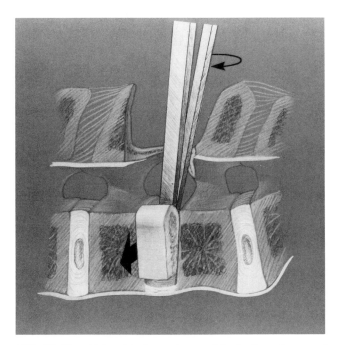

FIG. 15. Two Puka chisels can be used for further placement of bone block beneath the dura.

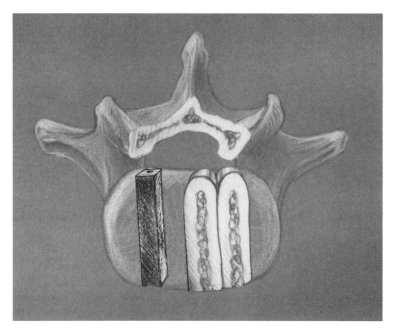

FIG. 16. Placement of the bone blocks should be well between the confines of the vertebral bodies.

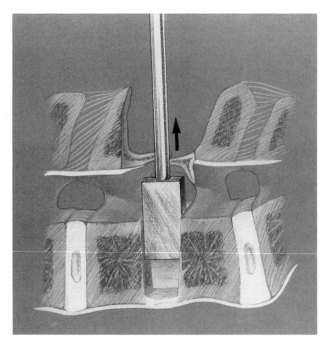

FIG. 17. The spacer is removed following placement of bone blocks on the opposite side.

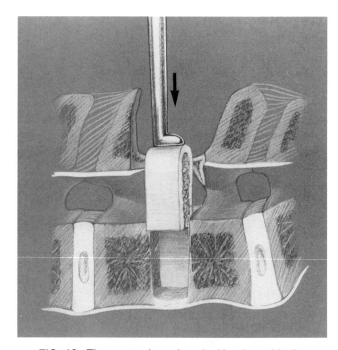

FIG. 18. The spacer is replaced with a bone block.

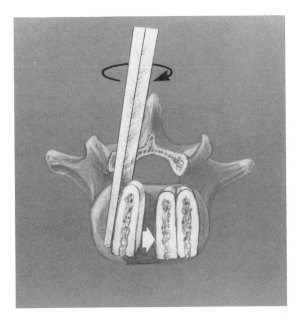

FIG. 19. The pars interarticularis acts as lever for the Puka chisel.

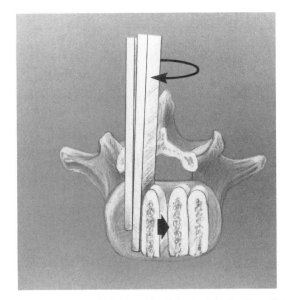

FIG. 20. To obtain tightly packed bone blocks two Puka chisels are used.

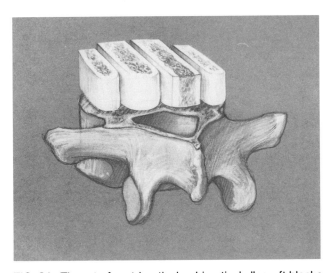

FIG. 21. Three to four tricortical or bicortical allograft blocks tend to fit.

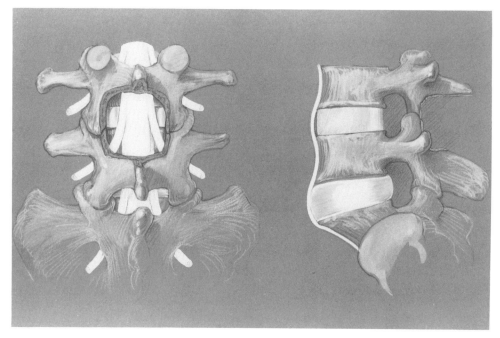

FIG. 22. The graft stabilizes the spine without nerve impingement.

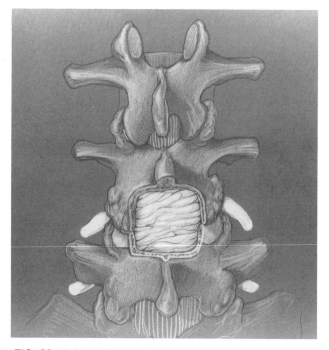

FIG. 23. A fat graft is placed to decrease epidural scarring.

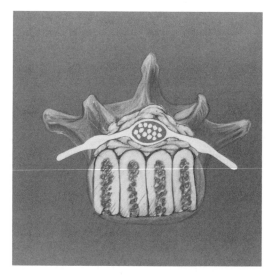

FIG. 24. Axial view of the fat graft.

For spondylolysis or spondylolisthesis, the posterior elements of the involved vertebra are removed (Fig. 25). The ligamentum flavum is removed (Fig. 26) exposing the neural elements (Fig. 27). The decompression is further carried out by removing the superior portion of the S1 apophyseal joints and the posterior elements of the segment involved, out to the pedicle to relieve any bony stenosis (Figs. 28 and 29).

A portion of the posterior superior end plate of S1 or the lower vertebral body of the segment involved is removed (Fig. 30). By using the osteotomes and curettes as previously described, excellent exposure and decompression is obtained (Fig. 31). The deep lamina spreaders can then be placed between the vertebral bodies (Fig. 32). With spreading of the deep laminar spreaders, distracting the vertebral bodies, there is an unfolding effect of the soft tissues as described by Junghanns (29). This unfolding effect or stretching of the anterior longitudinal ligament and annulus appears to decrease the extent of the olisthesis (Fig. 33). The spanners are then used for measurement of the intervertebral width and depth as previously described. The appropriate spacer is inserted in the intervertebral disc space (Fig. 34). An appropriately fashioned bone graft is placed on the opposite side from the spacer (Fig. 35) and the spacer removed (Fig. 36). The intervertebral disc space is filled with bone graft to the extent possible (Figs. 37 and 38).

Text continues on page 1977.

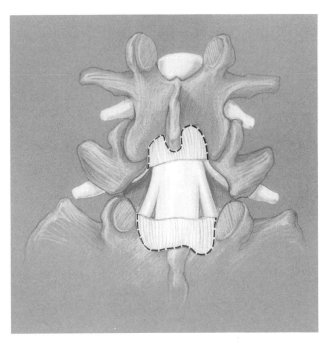

FIG. 26. The ligamentum flavum is removed.

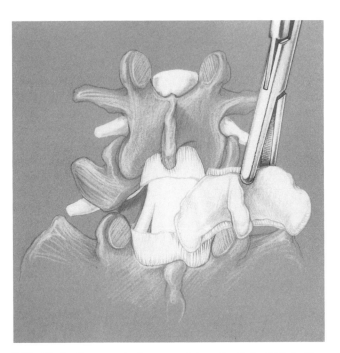

FIG. 25. In the event of a pars interarticularis defect, the loose posterior elements are removed.

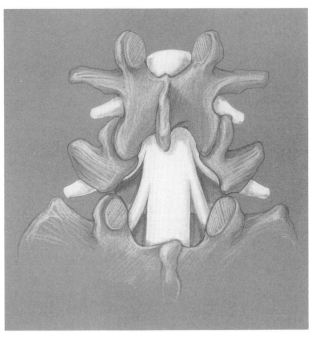

FIG. 27. Excellent exposure of the neural elements is achieved with soft tissue debridement.

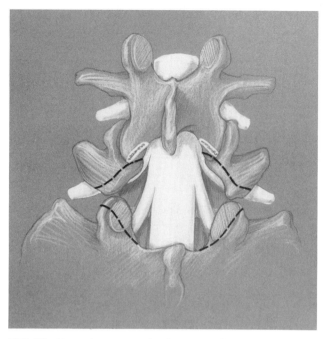

FIG. 28. Bony decompression is accomplished by removing the superior portion of the S1 apophyseal joints and the posterior elements and the L5 pars interarticularis overlying the L5 nerve root.

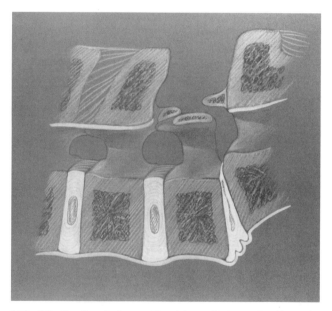

FIG. 29. Sectional view without neural elements. Note the accordion effect of the anterior longitudinal ligament.

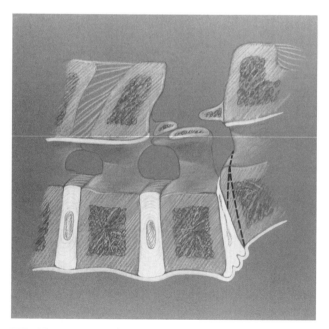

FIG. 30. A portion of the posterior superior end plate may be removed for exposure and fit of the bone block.

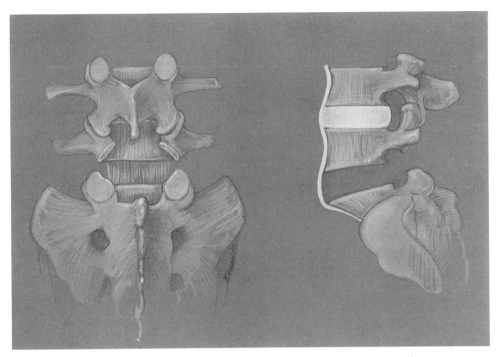

FIG. 31. By using the osteotomes and curettes as previously described, excellent exposure and decompression is obtained.

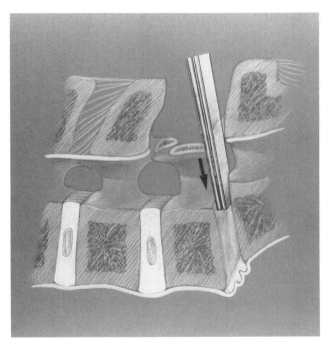

FIG. 32. Deep lamina spreaders are used to distract the vertebral bodies.

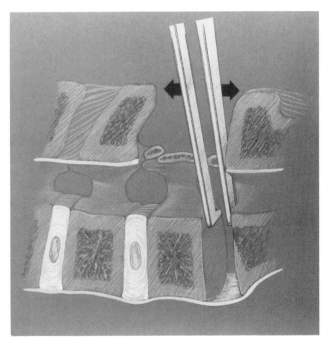

FIG. 33. Stretching the anterior longitudinal ligament allows some reduction of spondylolisthesis.

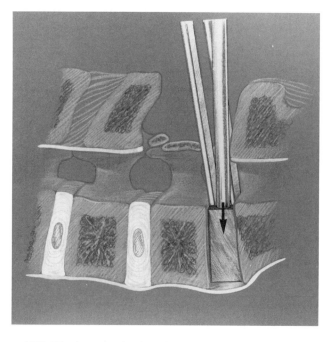

FIG. 34. A spacer is placed to maintain the distraction.

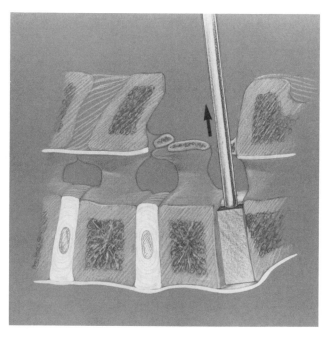

FIG. 36. Spacer is removed.

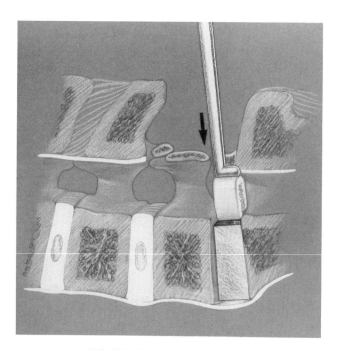

FIG. 35. Bone block is inserted.

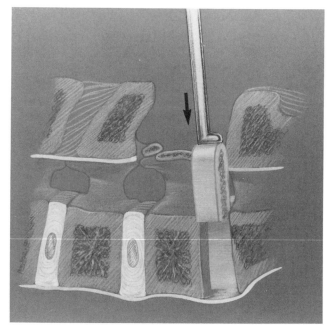

FIG. 37. Bone block is inserted in place of the spacer.

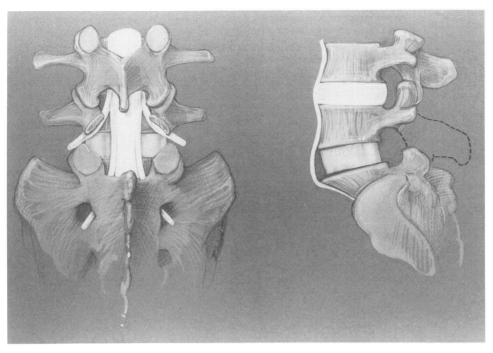

FIG. 38. Disc height is restored and stability accomplished by filling the disc space with bone blocks.

VARIATIONS OF PLIF

Variations of the PLIF have been quite extensive, with apparently excellent results in the hands of those using their own innovations.

Ovens and Williams (42) placed a portion of the spinous process in the intervertebral disc space. Jaslow (27) used a peg of bone in the intervertebral disc space and bone chips from the posterior elements were placed posteriorly (Fig. 39).

The use of the posterior elements cut into corticocancellous chips was described by Briggs (5). When impacted quite briskly into the disc space, after placement of the chips into the disc space with the Ma injection instrument, the fusion rate was found to be quite good (48). The bone chips are packed approximately 5 mm below the posterior border of the vertebral body. Loosening and extrusion of the chips was not found to be a problem. (Figs. 40, 41, 42 and 43).

There is no statistically significant difference in the autogenous blocks and the autogenous chips (48). The decrease in the morbidity certainly would make the utilization of the autogenous chips more feasible if allograft bone is not available (38,48). James and Nisbet (26) describe the use of autogenous fibula for the PLIF. Cloward (9,10) has certainly been the leading proponent for using the PLIF. He originally used autogenous iliac plugs; subsequently, using allograft iliac plugs (Fig. 44).

Text continues on page 1980.

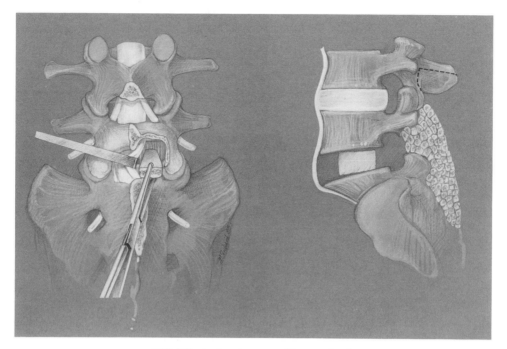

FIG. 39. Jaslow bone grafting method.

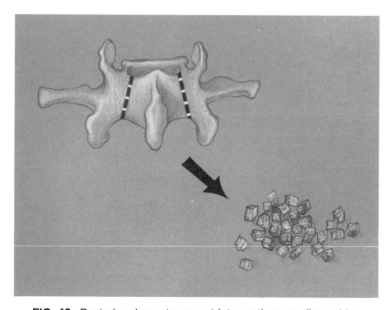

FIG. 40. Posterior elements are cut into corticocancellous chips.

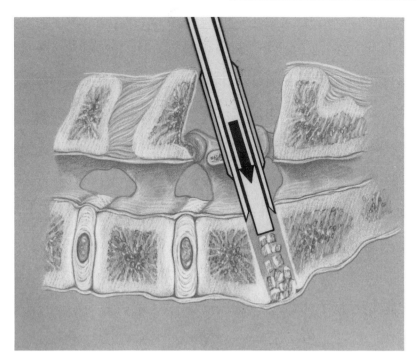

FIG. 41. Chips are inserted using the Ma injection instrument.

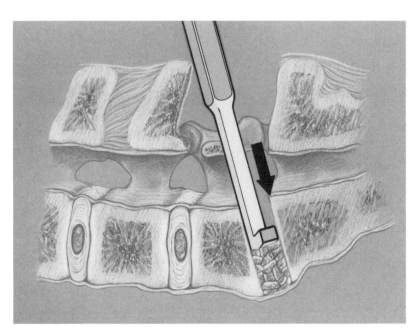

FIG. 42. The bone chips are compressed with an impactor.

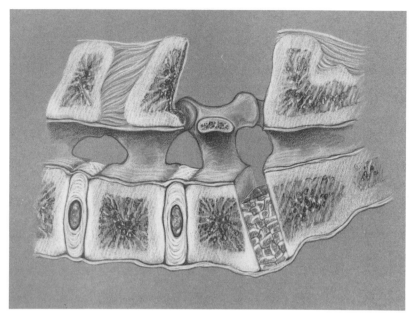

FIG. 43. Impacted autologous bone chips.

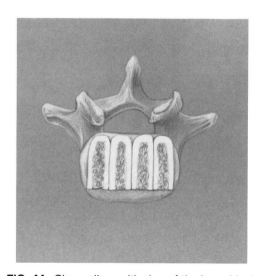

FIG. 44. Cloward's positioning of the bone block.

The PLIF as described by Wiltberger (53) also accomplishes the goals of the PLIF operation. Wiltberger uses iliac dowels (Figs. 45, 46, 47, and 48) but also describes use of the fibula, splitting the fibula plugs and putting cortical bone to cortical bone and making a dowel for insertion in the intervertebral disc space.

Christoferson (8) takes a portion of the lamina and medial facet and fashions it in such a way to fit in the intervertebral disc space as a spacer for stability and fusion.

Hutter (25) uses a slightly different approach creating a "keystone" modeling of the intervertebral disc space to further stabilize the graft and prevent the bone from dislodging out into the spinal canal. He also places some of the autogenous chips taken from the lamina anteriorly to further fill in the disc space (Figs. 49 and 50).

The mortise and chisel method can be used to take autogenous iliac bone and place it in the intervertebral disc space as described by Ma (38) (Figs. 51, 52, 53, and 54).

Blume (1) was quite innovative, sculpturing the end plates to receive layers of wafer-shaped corticocancellous bone taken from the iliac crest placed over anteriorly placed corticocancellous chips (Figs. 55 and 56).

Lin (35) uses a combination of autograft and corticocancellous chips to completely fill the disc space with bone. He also uses a composite of autograft and allograft blocks to fill the intervertebral disc space to whatever extent possible (Fig. 57).

Text continues on page 1985.

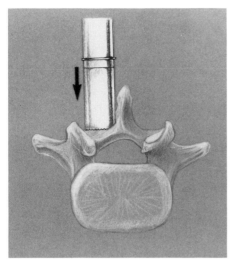

FIG. 45. Dowel cutter is used for laminectomy.

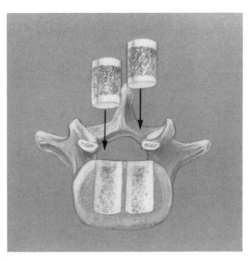

FIG. 47. Insertion of dowels into the prepared intervertebral disc space.

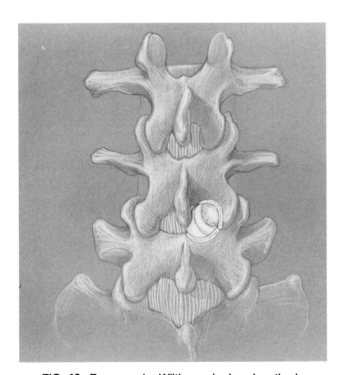

FIG. 46. Exposure by Wiltberger's dowel method.

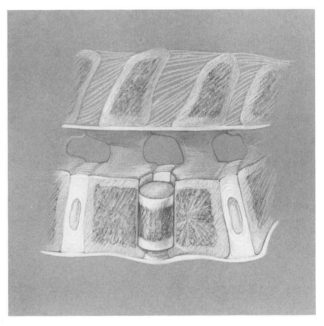

FIG. 48. Dowel placement for a body-to-body fusion.

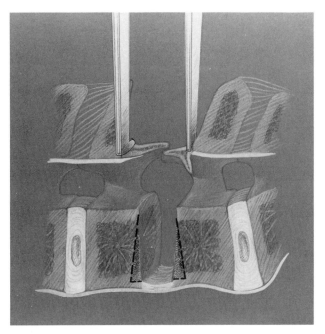

FIG. 49. Preparation of the disc space as described by Hutter.

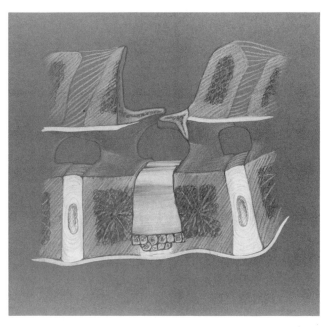

FIG. 50. Autogenous chips from the lamina are placed anteriorly and the Keystone bone blocks are placed posteriorly in the intervertebral disc space.

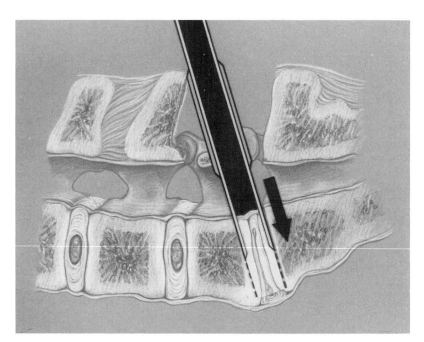

FIG. 51. Removal of the disc and end plates with the Ma chisel.

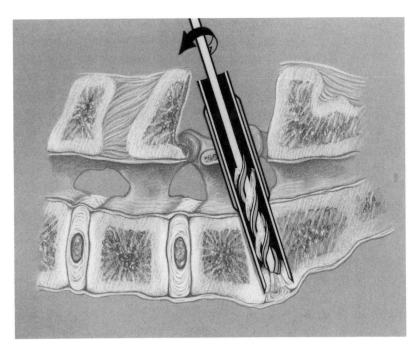

FIG. 52. Ma instrumentation for removal of the disc.

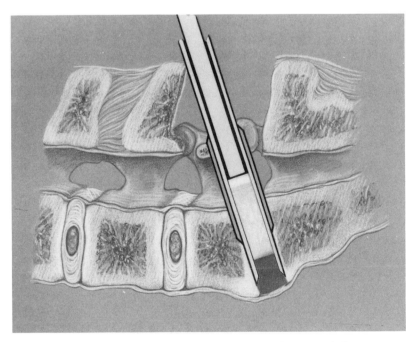

FIG. 53. Insertion of the bone block with Ma instrumentation.

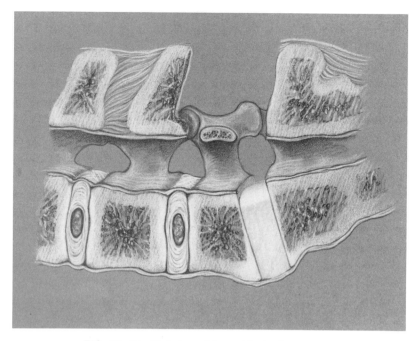

FIG. 54. Sagittal view of bone block placement.

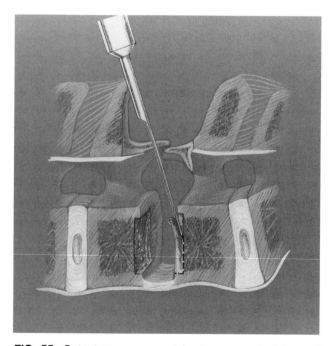

FIG. 55. Osteotomes are used for the removal of the end plates.

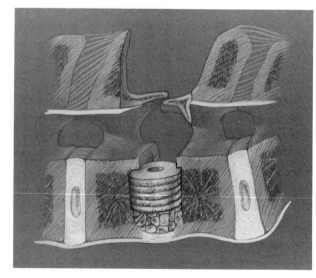

FIG. 56. Wafer-shaped corticocancellous bone and corticocancellous chips are placed to restore height.

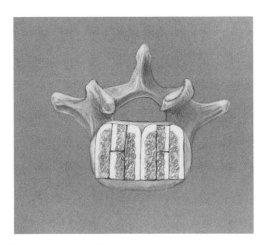

FIG. 57. Bone blocks fill the intervertebral disc space as described by Lin.

RESULTS

The interpretation of PLIF results is very difficult. Most published reports tend to be technique oriented and have relatively short-term clinical follow-up. There is also little uniformity in what constitutes a good result. Certainly residual pain, reliance on medications, or continued interventional care are important clinical factors. However, functional results and return-to-work capacity are just as important, yet probably not directly related. Return-to-work capacity is multifactorial and more dependent on patient population and work type than clinical results. It is possible to have a high clinical success rate but low functional return if revisional work is considered the standard.

Criteria for stability have not been established. Stability is not always radiographically delineated by a bony fusion and may indeed be accomplished without bony union, i.e., fibrous union. Table 1 lists several series in the literature and attempts to quantify the type of PLIF performed, x-ray results, and clinical results.

A posterior lumbar interbody fusion is a technically difficult operation. Potential complications are listed in Table 2 along with a recommended solution. In a skilled surgeon's hands with meticulous attention to detail, a PLIF procedure can be performed safely with an acceptable clinical result.

TABLE 1. *PLIF literature*

Reference	Patients reviewed	Follow-up (years)	Type of PLIF	X-ray results (%)		Clinical results (%)		Return to work (%)	
Cloward (11)	93	*	Iliac: Autograft Allograft	Regular x-rays Bony fusions Fibrous/pseudo	86 14	Excellent Good Poor	89 9 2	*	
Collis (12)	50	>5	Allograft	Regular x-rays Bony fusion Fibrous	94 6	Good Fair Poor	88 4 8	*	
Lin (37)	465	>1	Unicortical autograft	Tomograms Fusion	88	Satisfactory Unsatisfactory	82 18	Full duty Light duty Disabled	61 32 7
Ma (38)	100	>1	Tricortical allograft iliac crest	Regular x-rays Fusion	74	Excellent Good Fair Poor	35 39 17 9	Full duty Light duty Disabled	70 21 9
Blume (1)	216	1–12	"Unilateral" autogenous dowels	*		Excellent Good Fair Poor	72 19 7 2	Same as clinical	
Branch (4)	72	>3	Autogenous keystone and facet fusion	*		Excellent Good Fair Poor	48 33 11 8	*	
Christoferson (8)	418	1–10	Autogenous lamina "wedge"	X-rays: flexion/ extension Tomograms Fusion	10	Excellent/Good Fair/Poor	95 5	Full duty Increased duty Light duty	82 3 15
Wiltberger (53)	46	>2	Cortical tibial dowel Cortical cancellous iliac crest dowel	X-rays: flexion/ extension Fusion Non-fusion	87 13	Good Satisfactory Unsatisfactory	70 17 13	Full duty Return to work	70 89
Hutter (25)	142	>3	Iliac bicortical autograft and chip graft	X-rays: flexion/ extension Fusion	91	Excellent Good Fair Poor	46 32 16 6	*	
Simmons (47, 48)	113	>2	Chip autograft	X-rays: flexion/ extension Stable Unstable	91 9	Good Fair Poor	54 44 2	Full duty Light duty Disabled	54 44 2

* Non-specific.

TABLE 2. *PLIF complications*

Complication	Solution
Blood loss	Layer by layer hemostasis
	Autologous blood
	Cell saver
Epidural bleeding	Positioning of patient
	Bipolar cautery
	Thrombin-gelfoam/packing
End plate bleeding	Good decortication but minimize depth
	Well packed bone graft
Nerve root injury	Careful decompression
	Judicious root retraction
	Lateral disc exposure
	Ample facetectomy/foramenotomy
	Visualization and protection of adjacent nerve root at time of graft impaction
Intra-abdominal vessel injury	Direct visualization of anterior annulus
	Palpable ''feel'' while evacuating disc (instrument on bone)
Graft retropulsion	Appropriate endplate shaping
	Accurate graft sizing
	Place graft 2–4 mm below posterior vertebral margin
	Maintain segmental stability
	Appropriate internal fixation
	Postoperative bracing
Pseudarthrosis	Endplate decortication
	Complete removal of disc and annulus
	Complete packing of disc space
	Maintain stability
	High quality/low antigenicity of either allograft, autograft, or composite bone
	Pulsing electromagnetic fields
Instability	Maintain 2/3 of facet joint
	Maintain supraspinous ligaments
	Graft stability
	Appropriate internal fixation
	Complete filling of disc space
Graft resorption	Low antigenic allograft
	Composite graft
	Avoid overcompression
	Maintain stability
Infection	Pre-operative antibiotics (gram+ and gram−)
	Frequent antibiotic irrigation
	Closed drainage post-operative
	Close dead space
	Debridement of non-viable muscle
Epidural scar	Hemostasis
	Gentle retraction
	Delicate dissection
	Fat graft
	Stabilization
	Appropriate internal fixation
Arachnoiditis	Same as epidural scar
Dural tears	Careful dissection
	Adequate repair

REFERENCES

1. Blume HG, Rojas CH (1981): Unilateral lumbar interbody fusion (posterior approach) utilizing dowel grafts. *J Neurol Orthop Surg* 2(3).
2. Bradford DS (1980): Spinal instability: Orthopedic perspective and prevention. *Clin Neurosurg* 27:591–610.
3. Bradford DS, Gotfried Y (1986): Lumbar spine osteolysis: An entity caused by spinal instability. *Spine* 11:1013–1019.
4. Branch CL, Branch CL Jr (1987): Posterior lumbar interbody fusion with the keystone graft: Technique and results. *Surg Neurol* 27:449–454.
5. Briggs H, Milligan PR (1944): Chip fusion of the low back following exploration of the spinal canal. *J Bone Joint Surg [Am]* 26(1):125–130.
6. Cauthen JC (1983): *Lumbar spine surgery indications, techniques, failures and alternatives.* Baltimore: Williams and Wilkins, p 105.
7. Cautilli RA (1982): Theoretical superiority of PLIF. In: Lin PM, ed., *Posterior lumbar interbody fusion.* Springfield: Charles C Thomas, p 82.
8. Christoferson LA, Selland B (1975): Intervertebral bone implants following excision of protruded lumbar discs. *J Neurosurg* 42:401–405.
9. Cloward RB (1953): The treatment of ruptured lumbar intervertebral discs by vertebral body fusion: Indications, operative technique, after care. *J Neurosurg* 10:154–168.
10. Cloward RB (1963): Lesions of the intervertebral disks and their treatment by interbody fusion methods. *Clin Orthop* 27:51–77.
11. Cloward RB (1981): Spondylolisthesis: Treatment by laminectomy and posterior interbody fusion. Review of 100 cases. *Clin Orthop* 154:74–82.
12. Collis JS (1985): Total disc replacement: A modified posterior lumbar interbody fusion. *Clin Orthop* 193:64–67.
13. Crock HV (1983): *Practice of spinal surgery.* New York: Springer-Verlag.
14. Dupuis PR, Yong-Hing K, Cassidy JD, Kirkaldy-Willis WH (1985): Radiologic diagnosis of degenerative lumbar spinal instability. *Spine* 10:262–276.
15. Evans JH (1985): Biomechanics of lumbar fusion. *Clin Orthop* 193:38–46.
16. Farfan HF (1973): *Mechanical disorders of the low back.* Philadelphia: Lea and Febiger.
17. Farfan HF, Gracovetsky S (1984): The nature of instability. *Spine* 9:714–719.
18. Farfan HF (1985): The use of mechanical etiology to determine the efficacy of active intervention in single joint lumbar intervertebral joint problems. Surgery and chemonucleolysis compared: A prospective study. *Spine* 10:350–358.
19. Finneson BE (1973): *Low back pain.* Philadelphia/Toronto: J.B. Lippincott.
20. Frymoyer JW, Selby DK (1985): Segmental instability. Rationale for treatment. *Spine* 10:280–286.
21. Gertzbein SD, Seligman J, Holtby R, Chan KN, Kapasouri A, Tile M, Cruickshank B (1985): Centrode patterns and segmental instability in degenerative disc disease. *Spine* 10:257–261.
22. Hayes MA, Howard TC, Gruel CR, Kopta JA (1989): Roentgenographic evaluation of lumbar spine flexion-extension in asymptomatic individuals. *Spine* 14:327–331.
23. Hibbs RA, Albee FH (1911): An operation for progressive spinal deformities. *NY State J Med* 93:1013.
24. Hodgson AR, Stock FE (1956): Anterior spinal fusion: A preliminary communication on the radical treatment of Pott's disease and Pott's paraplegia. *Br J Surg* 44:266–275.
25. Hutter CG (1985): Spinal stenosis and posterior lumbar interbody fusion. *Clin Orthop* 193:103–114.
26. James A, Nisbet NW (1953): Posterior intervertebral fusion of lumbar spine. Preliminary report of a new operation. *J Bone Joint Surg [Br]* 35:2:181–187.
27. Jaslow IA (1946): Intercorporal bone graft in spinal fusion after disc removal. *Surg Gyn Obstet* 82:215–218.
28. Junghanns H, Schmorl G (1971): *The human spine in health and disease, 2nd ed.* New York: Grune & Stratton, p 35.
29. Junghanns H (1930): Spondylolisthesen Ohne Spalt im Zwischengelenkstueck (Pseudospondylolisthesen). *Arch Orthop* 29:118–127.
30. Keim HA (1977): Indications for spine fusions and techniques. *Clin Neurosurg* 25:266–275.
31. Kirkaldy-Willis WH, Farfan HF (1982): Instability of the lumbar spine. *Clin Orthop* 165:110–123.
32. Kirkaldy-Willis WH (1983): *Managing low back pain.* New York: Churchill Livingstone.
33. Knutsson F (1944): The instability associated with disc degeneration in the lumbar spine. *Acta Radiologica* 25:593–609.
34. LeVay D (1967): A survey of surgical management of lumbar disc prolapse in the United Kingdom and Eire. *Lancet* 1:1211–1213.
35. Lin PM (1977): A technical modification of Cloward's posterior lumbar interbody fusion. *Neurosurg* 1(2):118–124.
36. Lin PM (1982): *Introduction of PLIF: Biomechanical principals and indications.* Springfield: Charles C Thomas, p. 3.
37. Lin PM, Cautilli RA, Joyce MF (1983): Posterior lumbar interbody fusion. *Clin Orthop* 180:154–168.
38. Ma GW (1985): Posterior lumbar interbody fusion with specialized instruments. *Clin Orthop* 193:57–63.
39. Macnab I (1971): The traction spur: An indicator of segmental instability. *J Bone Joint Surg [Am]* 53:663–670.
40. Mercer W (1936): Spondylolisthesis with a description of a new method of operative treatment and notes of ten cases. *Edinburgh M J* 43:545–572.
41. Mixter WJ, Barr JS (1934): Rupture of the intervertebral disc with involvement of the spinal canal. *N Engl J Med* 211(5):210–215.
42. Ovens JM, Williams HG (1945): Intervertebral spine fusion with removal of herniated intervertebral disk. *Am J Surg* 70(1):24–26.
43. Paris SV (1985): Physical signs of instability. *Spine* 10:277–279.
44. Penning L, Blickman JR (1980): Instability in lumbar spondylolisthesis: A radiologic study of several concepts. *AJR* 134:293–301.
45. Posner I, White AA III, Edwards WT, Hayes WC (1982): A biomechanical analysis of the clinical stability of the lumbar and lumbosacral spine. *Spine* 7:374–389.
46. Putti V (1927): New conceptions in the pathogenesis of sciatic pain. *Lancet* 2:53–60.
47. Simmons JW (1980): Posterior interbody fusions. Abstract presented at the Seventh Annual Meeting of the International Society for the Study of the Lumbar Spine, New Orleans, 1980.
48. Simmons JW (1985): Posterior lumbar interbody fusion with posterior elements as chip grafts. *Clin Orthop* 193:85–89.
49. Simmons JW (1987): Posterior lumbar interbody fusion. In: *Lumbar spine surgery,* White AH, et al, eds. St. Louis: Mosby, p. 286.
50. Stokes IA, Wilder DG, Frymoyer JW, Pope MH (1981): 1980 Volvo Award in Clinical Sciences. Assessment of patients with low-back pain by biplanar radiographic measurement of intervertebral motion. *Spine* 6:233–240.
51. Stokes IA, Frymoyer JW (1987): Segmental motion and instability. *Spine* 12:688–691.
52. White AA, Panjabi MM (1978): *Clinical biomechanics of the spine.* Philadelphia: Lippincott.
53. Wiltberger BR (1957): The dowel intervertebral-body fusion as used in lumbar-disc surgery. *J Bone Joint Surg [Am]* 39(2):284–292.
54. Wiltberger BR (1964): Intervertebral body fusion by the use of posterior bone dowel. *Clin Orthop* 35:69–79.

The Adult Spine: Principles and Practice,
J. W. Frymoyer, Editor-in-Chief.
Raven Press, Ltd., New York © 1991.

CHAPTER 95

Circumferential (360 Degree) Spinal Fusion

David K. Selby and Robert J. Henderson

Circumferential (360 degree) spine fusion can be viewed as an evolving technique whose main purpose is to improve the rate of fusion and the clinical results (Fig. 1). The technique is useful for a small subset of patients with complex spinal disorders such as tumors, difficult deformities, trauma, and failed prior surgery. The greatest controversy is its use in patients with degenerative spinal conditions, particularly when the operation is done as a primary procedure.

As the name implies, circumferential fusion involves both anterior and posterior fusion, with or without instrumentation, performed as a staged procedure or at the same surgical session. The technique is different from the circumduction fusion advocated by Bosworth (3).

In this chapter, we present the history of this procedure, its current indications, the surgical technique, the results, and the complications. A major focus will be on patient selection. The most controversial indication, namely the primary use of 360-degree fusion in patients with degenerative conditions, is analyzed.

D. K. Selby, M.D.: Clinical Professor, Department of Orthopaedic Surgery, University of Texas Southwestern Medical Center; Dallas Spine Group, Dallas, Texas, 74235.

R. J. Henderson, M.D.: Dallas Spine Group, Dallas, Texas, 74235.

HISTORY

Circumferential fusion can be viewed as the evolution of the techniques of anterior and posterior spinal arthrodesis. It is uncertain who first described the procedure. In 1968, Hoover noted a high rate of failure in anterior interbody fusions because of "crumbling" of the graft (17). He reported on six circumferential fusions, three performed as a single-stage procedure and three performed in two separate stages. Four of the six patients achieved excellent results. However, he noted that the operation should be advocated only for cases with "insurmountable difficulties." Later, Goldner advocated staged circumferential fusion in selected cases of previous failed surgery (16). The anterior fusion was performed first. If the anterior bone did not appear to be going on to solid union, a posterior fusion was added. The first formal extensive experience with the combined operation was reported by Dr. John O'Brien (24).

Like many surgeons, our interest in the combined technique resulted from dissatisfaction with fusion rates obtained by the anterior approach, particularly at lumbar motion segments above L5-S1. What has ensued is a rethinking and change of our approach to spinal problems and fusion, which is still evolving and maturing.

A 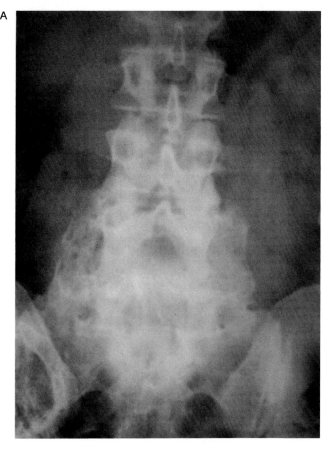 B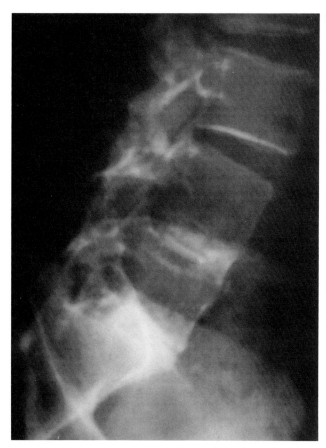

FIG. 1. AP **(A)** and lateral **(B)** radiographs demonstrating 360 degree fusion.

There are three primary criteria for successful spine surgery:

1. Appropriate patient selection, that is, choosing a patient who is able to respond physically and psychosocially to a surgical procedure.
2. Identification of the anatomical source of pain or the "pain generators." These must be understood, and there must be a reasonable likelihood that surgery will relieve the pain.
3. A surgical team with the adaptability, versatility, and expertise to analyze complex patient problems, perform the operation, and manage its potential complications.

SPECIFIC INDICATIONS

In general, indications for circumferential fusions are based on complex instability involving the anterior, middle, and posterior columns. Other chapters summarize the indications for its use in specific pathologic conditions. These include:

1. Complex primary benign osseous tumor, or primary or metastatic malignancy (see Chapter 41).

2. Complex spinal fractures and fracture dislocations (see Chapter 61).
3. Rare spinal infections not amenable to antibiotic therapy involving the posterior and anterior or middle columns.
4. Selected cases with high-grade spondylolisthesis or spondyloptosis at the lumbosacral junction (see Chapter 78).
5. Failure following spinal fusions performed for degenerative conditions (see Chapter 98).

INDICATIONS FOR USE OF 360 DEGREE FUSION IN DEGENERATIVE CONDITIONS

We know from Kirkaldy-Willis's description (19) of the "degenerative cascade" that the spinal motion segment most commonly will undergo concurrent changes in both the anterior and posterior columns (see Chapter 31). It seems logical to deal with both anatomical sites to achieve satisfactory results. Therefore, a thorough evaluation of the patient's sources of pain must be undertaken. If anterior and posterior pathology are confirmed, circumferential fusion is selected.

Our rationale is also based on the biomechanics of

spinal fusion. Rolander (26) analyzed a variety of surgical constructs commonly used in lumbar fusion and determined that there was persistent springy motion. Farfan (10) reported that biomechanical analysis of posterior fusions taken from autopsy specimens revealed less torsional strength than the normal intervertebral joint, but more than the joint with advanced degeneration. Frymoyer (13) radiographically analyzed patients ten or more years after midline lumbar fusion and identified continued motion of a few degrees in many patients, but was uncertain if this finding represented errors in the measurement technique or continued actual motion. However, a more precise analysis, using biplanar radiography, suggested the continued presence of motion following solid spinal arthrodesis (30). Although the addition of rigid internal fixation appears to reduce motion initially, it is uncertain whether this stabilization effect is maintained over the long term, even when a solid arthrodesis is obtained. If the degenerative condition involves the anterior column, and only a posterior fusion is done, continued symptoms are possible even if arthrodesis is solid. This continued pain in psychologically normal individuals who desire to return to work is speculated to be secondary to a discogenic source. Conversely, if an anterior fusion is performed, continued symptoms might result from "micromotion" of diseased facet joints. It is well-known that patients with far-advanced osteoarthritis in peripheral joints often have continued severe pain with only a degree or two of movement.

The specific indication for surgery are, therefore, as follows:

1. Combined anterior and posterior degenerative pathology: Included in this group are patients with anterior column pathology usually revealed by discography, and posterior column involvement usually evident from imaging studies, and sometimes from facet blocks (29).
2. Complex instabilities: The issues surrounding degenerative segmental instability have been reviewed (14,15) (see Chapter 90). Patients with major degenerative instability are considered possible candidates for the procedure, as either a primary or a secondary operation.
3. Disc disruption syndrome at levels other than L5-S1: The classic description of disc disruption has been given by Crock (5) (see Chapter 97). Although he reports excellent results with anterior interbody fusion alone (6,7), others have not had the same experience (25). Review of our early experience with anterior interbody fusion revealed a fusion rate at L5-S1 approaching 90% (2). However, this rate of fusion was not achieved at other levels, particularly at L4-L5, where a non-union rate of 40% to 45% was encoun-

tered. This high non-union rate is probably the result of the torsional forces placed across the interspace as described by Farfan (11).
4. Failed surgery: At our institution, the workup for a patient with failed surgery is no different from that for a primary patient. The basic philosophy is that all potential pain generators must be identified by objective anatomical changes and confirmed by provocative or subjective testing. The major difference between patients with no prior surgery and patients with a failed operation is the psychosocial changes that have occurred in the latter group of patients.

PATIENT EVALUATION

A comprehensive and multidisciplinary evaluation of the patient is mandatory before surgical planning can be done.

History and Physical Evaluation

A careful history is taken. Of particular interest is the mechanism of pain onset. For example, a seated fall that leads to intractable pain suggests a disc disruption syndrome (5). If sclerodermal pain radiation is present in patterns consistent with facet innervation, the facets may be contributing to the patient's pain complaints. However, pain patterns are often non-specific and therefore cannot be relied on in making a surgical judgment. A complete physical examination should rule out the more obvious causes of continuing back and/or leg pain. The initial evaluation should identify a subset of patients with intractable pain who have failed all forms of conservative management and are, therefore, possible candidates for the procedure.

It should be emphasized that circumferential fusion is not a procedure that is done for a simple disc or the relatively recent onset of back pain. Patients who are candidates for this surgery have exhibited symptoms for an average of a year; only on rare occasions is surgery done before a four- to six-month period has elapsed. This reflects the amount of conservative care that is done before considering this major surgery.

Laboratory and Imaging Studies

The possible candidates for the procedure are carefully analyzed by laboratory and imaging techniques.

Electrodiagnostic Studies

In the complicated, difficult patients who are potentially eligible for this type of surgery, an EMG is essential. It may reveal unsuspected peripheral neuropathies, myopathies, or generalized neurologic disease that would contraindicate the surgery. It can also give clues to what further pain provocative tests might be useful, such as a selective nerve root injection.

Imaging Studies

Computerized Axial Tomography. All patients undergo a CT scan particularly focused around exiting nerve roots. It is essential that the CT scan have good sagittal reconstructions that demonstrate each part of the neural foramen. In addition, the CT allows visualization of the uncinate spur and other associated pathology, which is much better delineated by CT scan than by MRI (see Chapter 20).

Magnetic Resonance Imaging. MRI is valuable in demonstrating central and lateral stenosis. We must caution, however, that MRI is exquisitely sensitive and can lead to overdiagnosis of lumbar disc herniation. MRI is invaluable for demonstrating advanced disc degeneration or delineating scars in cases of prior failed decompression.

Discography. The controversies that surround discography have been detailed in Chapter 21. We believe that discography is the only diagnostic test that gives insight into the morphology of the disc itself, while providing an evaluation of the patient's pain response. In our clinic, we routinely perform discograms at every level suspected of causing pain until a non-painful and morphologically normal disc is identified. By this method, an internal control is built into the evaluation. A patient who states that pain is reproduced at more than one morphologically normal level should be suspect, and is unlikely to be a candidate for the procedure.

It is important to confirm, if possible, objective pathology with provocative testing, as discussed by Mooney in Chapter 25. The evaluation often includes selective nerve root injections in those patients who have radicular or claudicatory leg pain. If a selective injection relieves the pain, decompression is warranted as part of the procedure. Similarly, we use the facet injection, although the interpretation of this test is often difficult. Its greatest use is in the patient with obvious facet degeneration, identified by CT, who selectively gets relief of low back and referred pain by the injection. Again, it is useful to inject obviously involved and non-involved joints to get some indication of whether the patient's response is general and non-localized, rather than specific and localized to one or two joints.

Multidisciplinary Evaluation

Any group of patients who might be considered for such an invasive procedure is by definition a complex group to evaluate and treat. Many have failed surgery and have concomitant psychosocial problems and drug dependency. At best, the patient will have experienced a significant period of chronic pain, and only those with the strongest emotional and social support will have escaped without some major psychopathology. Analysis of this complex group of patients must involve a psychiatrist or psychologist, internist, vocational specialist, and physical rehabilitation specialists, including physical therapists, exercise physiologists, or athletic trainers. They must all work together, and input must be made by all members of the team. Cases are presented at a planning conference. All physicians involved in the management must agree with the diagnosis and treatment plan.

To aid in our evaluation and pre-operative planning, we have also developed a Pre-Operative Educational/Evaluation Program (PEP). The evaluation portion includes the following:

1. Medical screening: In addition to the spine evaluation already described, a complete physical examination is conducted by an internist. The goal of the examination is to determine the presence of non-mechanical back symptoms such as ankylosing spondylitis, establish the patient's ability to withstand a three- to five-hour anesthetic and major surgery, and identify unsuspected conditions such as diabetes and coronary artery disease, which require further diagnostic study and treatment. All patients are screened for hepatitis and AIDS as a protection to them and to the operating team.
2. Psychological evaluation: Our staff includes psychologists who are experienced in the general issues of chronic pain and the complex psychosocial issues that relate to chronic spinal disease. Each patient is put through a battery of psychologic tests (21), including the MMPI and the Dallas Pain Questionnaire (23). Other institutions may use different tests (9), but it is critical that all patients be evaluated in a systematic fashion. Those with major behavioral problems may be unable to respond to surgery, no matter how compelling the anatomic cause may appear. However, in our experience, patients with diagnosed psychiatric disorders such as schizophrenia and manic depression appear to do as well as the population with no major psychiatric disease.
3. Patient goals: It is critical that the patient and the surgeon have the same goals, and that they be discussed in an open and forthright manner. The patient must be realistic in his goals and recognize that there is a potential for continuing pain or failure.
4. Vocational evaluation: It is important for all parties to understand the final objective of the surgery. Is the patient going to retire, and the only indication for surgery is an improved quality of life? Is the patient going to enter a retraining program, and if so, how

practical is this objective with respect to his age, education, work background, and forecasted physical status? Is the patient going to return to his old job? Will it be available? We break down these goals into the three "R's": retire, retrain, return to old job. As part of this program, we negotiate a return-to-work date before the operation so that all parties have a definite cutoff date.

5. Legal evaluation: If litigation is involved, the patient's attorney must be contacted, understand the treatment alternatives, and declare whether the patient can "afford to be well." It is desirable, but often not possible, to have the surgery deferred until all legal issues are resolved.

6. Social evaluation: The patient's total psychosocial circumstances need to be understood, including the expectations of the spouse. There are numerous non-organic and environmental circumstances that will promote continued disability and pain behavior (see Chapters 12, 13, and 14).

The educational portion of the program is equally valuable. Its elements are as follows:

1. Education: The patient goes through a formal program to learn about the surgical procedure, recovery process, and potential benefits and risks. The goal of the program is to enable the patient to make a prudent decision regarding surgery. The program includes discussion of the hospital and its routines, the use of analgesia, and the fact that narcotics will be discontinued upon discharge from the hospital and other treatment will be substituted, such as ice, non-steroidal anti-inflammatory medications, and Tylenol. All patients must be totally weaned from narcotics before being considered surgical candidates. Often a pre-operative detoxification program is required to achieve this goal.

2. Physical education: Under the supervision of a physical therapist, the patient is taught body mechanics and is introduced to an exercise program that stresses aerobic fitness and specific muscle strengthening. A simple elastic "sports cord" is used as a substitute for expensive and often unavailable muscle-strengthening equipment. We also emphasize the importance of exercise in promoting recovery from the operation, including the principles of Wolff's law to help the patient understand how exercise promotes bone formation.

At the completion of this extensive evaluation by the multidisciplinary team, only those patients who fulfill the pathologic criteria previously outlined are selected for surgery.

CONTRAINDICATIONS

The evaluation also identifies the patient who is not a candidate for surgery. Contraindications include:

1. A condition, whether primary or secondary to failed surgery, that can be treated with alternative operations such as simple decompression or posterior fusion with or without instrumentation.

2. The clinical history, physical examination, imaging evaluation, or ancillary tests do not provide a definitive explanation for the patient's continued symptoms.

3. The patient has an unresolved drug-abuse problem.

4. The patient's expectations for relief and functional restoration are inconsistent with the probable outcome of the surgery based on a total vocational assessment.

5. Psychological assessment reveals significant dysfunction making a poor surgical result likely. However, a diagnosis of specific psychiatric disorders, under adequate medical treatment, does not preclude the procedure in patients who otherwise fulfill the selection criteria.

6. The patient has an unresolved medical condition that makes a procedure of this magnitude an unacceptable risk for significant pre-operative and post-operative complications.

The rate of pseudarthrosis and complications increases as the number of levels fused increases. The procedure is contraindicated in patients with pathology at three or more levels, with rare exceptions.

Involvement of the L5-S1 disc space in a male is also a relative contraindication. A single-level lesion can be appropriately treated by a posterior interbody fusion at this level, thus reducing the risk of retrograde ejaculation (4). However, in our view, posterior lumbar interbody fusion should not be undertaken in a patient with a prior failed operation with significant scarring even at the L5-S1 level because of the increased possibility of neurologic injury. In these cases, the 360-degree fusion is our procedure of choice.

SURGICAL TECHNIQUE

Anterior Lumbar Fusion

Exposure of the anterior lumbar spine may be by transperitoneal or extraperitoneal approach (28). An extraperitoneal approach reduces post-operative ileus and intraperitoneal adhesions and reduces the potential for complications involving the sympathetic nerve root. A left lower quadrant transverse incision is the incision of choice for one- or two-level interbody fusion (Fig. 2). Its placement is dependent on pelvic geography and the interbody(s) to be fused. An experienced vascular surgeon should make this exposure and be present throughout the anterior portion of the procedure. For fusion of more than two levels, a paramedian incision is best. The extraperitoneal contents and ureter can be retracted across the

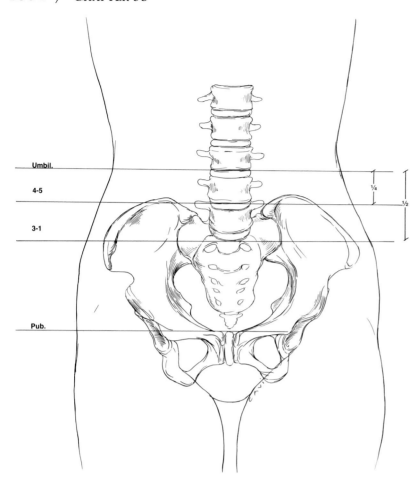

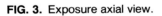

FIG. 2. Location of incision is dependent on level to be approached.

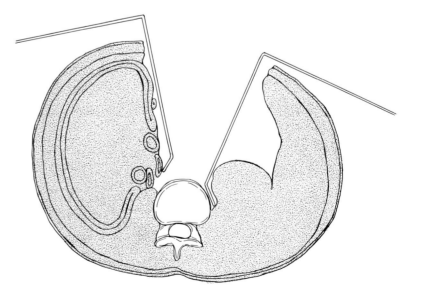

FIG. 3. Exposure axial view.

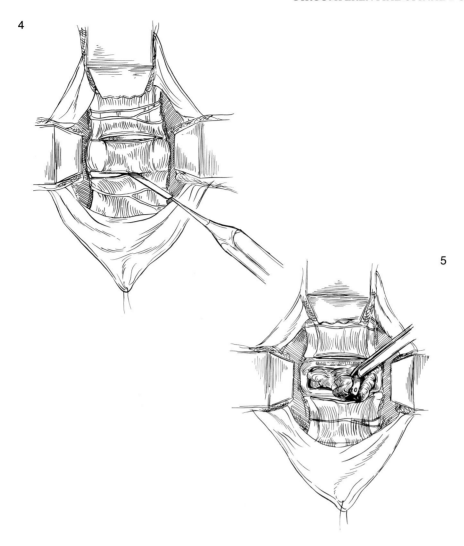

FIG. 4. Exposure axial view with retraction of vessels.

FIG. 5. Disc excision.

spine. Excellent exposure of the anterior portion of the disc space is available, including significant room for technically accomplishing the surgery (Figs. 3 and 4). Location of the level by x-ray is mandatory before starting excision of the disc.

Once the exposure is accomplished, incision with electrocautery into the anterior longitudinal ligament and annulus fibrosus is performed along the line of the end plate (Fig. 5). The periosteal elevator is used to separate the disc from the end plate, which normally separates quite easily in these abnormal discs. Remaining disc material is removed with curettes, being careful to take the end plate down to the bleeding bone throughout the area of the disc space. This accomplishes a very wide and thorough discectomy.

Multiple methods are available for disc replacement with bone. The authors use Crock's dowel technique (7). Using any one of four graduated dowel cutters, two

dowel cuts are made across the interspace (Figs. 6A and 6B). Appropriately sized homografts or allografts are then cut to length and impacted in the previously prepared graft bed. The use of a kidney rest under the patient can be very helpful during this part of the procedure. Raising the kidney rest brings the lumbar spine out of the abdominal cavity, increasing the exposure. This maneuver also opens up the interspace, giving the surgeon increased working room. After the graft is placed, letting the kidney rest down impacts the grafts firmly into the interspace (Figs. 7A and 7B). A closure is then made.

Before the patient is turned for the second half of the operation, pulses in the distal extremities are carefully checked. Older patients are at risk of getting plaque emboli from retraction of the aorta to the right side of the abdominal cavity. Because of this possible complication, we always use a hand retractor and never use fixed re-

A

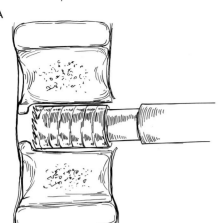

B

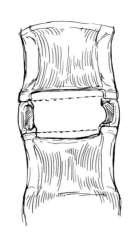

FIG. 6. Cutting dowel holes. **A:** Lateral view. **B:** Anterior view after dowel holes are cut.

A

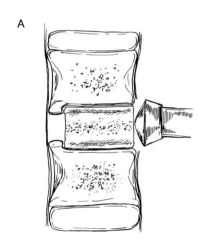

B

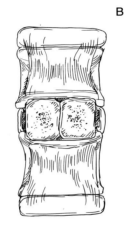

FIG. 7. Graft impacted in place. **A:** Lateral view. **B:** Anterior view.

traction, particularly in patients with significant arteriosclerotic disease of the great vessels. Blood loss should not exceed 100 cc during this portion of the procedure.

Posterior Decompression and Fusion

Exposure and hemostasis are the essential elements for a posterior approach. Hemostasis is obtained by the following:

Patient Position. The patient should be on a frame that allows the abdomen to hang free, thus decreasing the abdominal pressure and the distention of the dural veins. The Wilson frame provides a stable base for surgery and prevents the hyperextension common with most methods that rely on the knee-chest position.

Hypotensive Anesthesia. With some exceptions, it is reasonable for the surgeon to expect hypotensive anesthesia at levels of 80 to 90 mm of mercury systolic. This is a critical factor in a dry field. The dry field allows accurate

delineation of the anatomy and the performance of a procedure that can continue in a methodical and logical fashion.

Vessel Anatomy. The surgeon's knowledge of the anatomy and its arterial supply, which is consistent, allows him to anticipate significant bleeders and prevent blood loss (Fig. 8). There are only four arteries that need to be addressed in this regard:

1. Transverse process artery: This artery appears at the cephalad aspect of the junction of the transverse process and pedicle. Frequently the use of curved forceps facilitates coagulation of this artery.
2. Pars artery: This is lateral to and always closely adjacent to the pars interarticularis. It most commonly comes into play during initial exposure of the spine. Owing to its juxtaposition with the pars, it is easily coagulated with Bayonet forceps over the bleeder by touching the bone at the pars. At the sacrum, this vessel emerges from a recess just below the accumula-

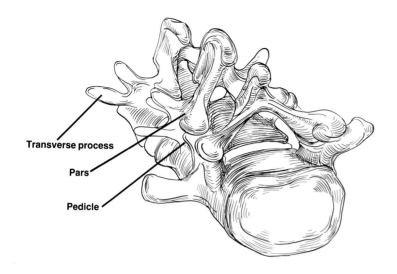

Transverse process

Pars

Pedicle

FIG. 8. Bony anatomy from the dorsal and lateral perspective.

FIG. 9. Outline of incision: midline and graft donor site.

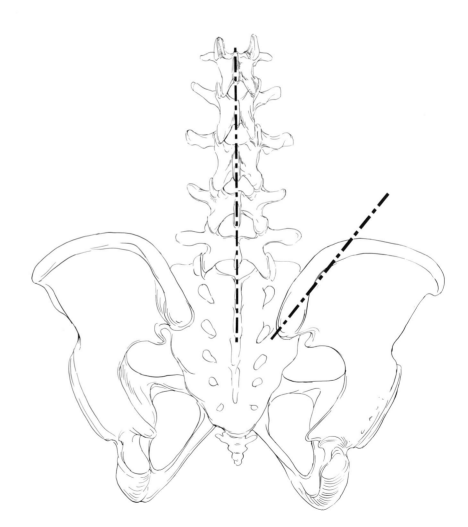

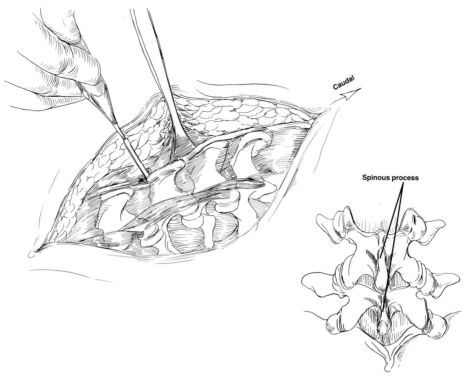

FIG. 10. Exposure down the spinous processes.

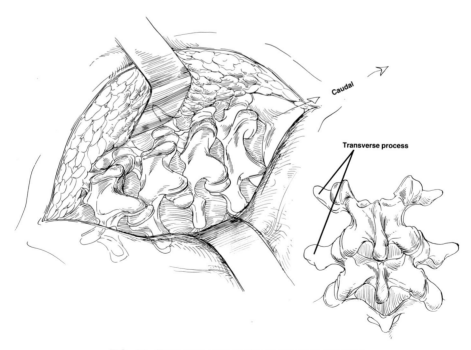

FIG. 11. Exposure across the transverse process.

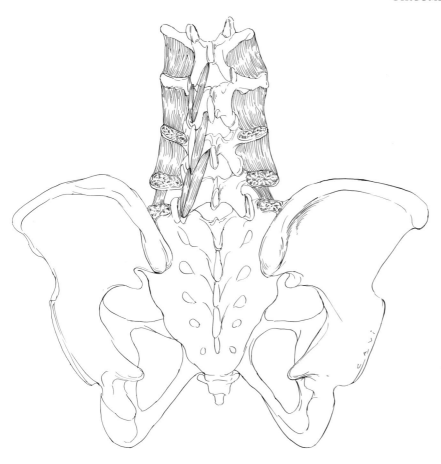

FIG. 12. Posterior view of decorticated transverse processes.

tion of fat, caudal to the inferior articular facet at L5. Coagulation requires the insertion of the forceps into the recess bone.

3. Sacral arteries: These protrude from the sacral foramen and can be difficult to control unless the forceps are inserted into the bony recess for coagulation.

4. Superior gluteal artery: It should be peeled back from the iliac crest and protected during removal of the bone graft. If interrupted, it may be difficult to control, and the use of vascular clips is advised.

The incision is made in the midline over the spinous processes (Fig. 9). It is usually advisable to carry the incision two segments above the proposed fusion level. The lower level should include most of the sacrum. This allows direct visualization of the transverse processes.

The authors avoid a periosteal stripping technique due to the bleeding usually engendered by that process. A more hemostatic technique is to put the tissue on stretch with an elevator and cut with an electrocautery set on the coagulation mode. The dissection should follow the spinous processes down the lamina (Fig. 10) and then clean the lamina laterally. After the lamina has been cleaned, the soft tissue between the lamina can be cut and separated. It is here that one frequently encounters the pars artery. It is advantageous to clear off all bony structures, with particular attention to the pars. The pars

is the anatomical guide to the pedicle and transverse process for the vertebrae. Moving cephalad, the pars runs into the pedicle. By continuing cephalad and laterally, one exposes the mammary process of the transverse process, and just a bit above that, the main body of the

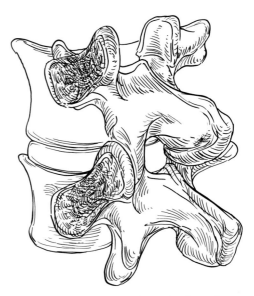

FIG. 13. Lateral view showing decortication of transverse processes and lateral mass.

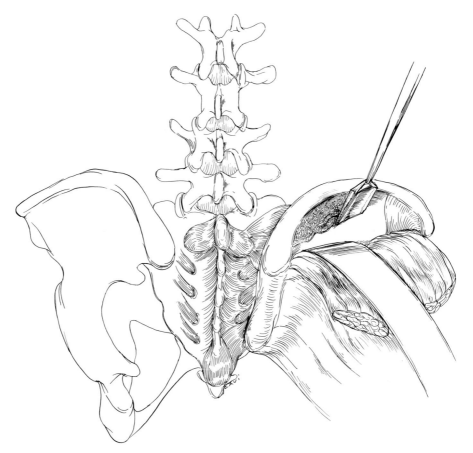

FIG. 14. Bone graft taking the cortical bone.

transverse process. It is relatively easy to become confused about which transverse process (Fig. 11) may be identified at the level of fusion. By careful dissection of the anatomical structures and the use of a pars as a landmark, it becomes easier to identify the specific transverse process of a motion segment.

Decortication of the transverse process must be accomplished under direct vision (Fig. 12). The Hibbs retractor toed in by the assistant will provide excellent exposure. It is important to remove soft tissue from the intertransverse ligaments so that the trough of bone and ligament has no interference by fibrous tissue. The most important part of any grafting procedure is the graft bed, and the most meticulous attention should be paid to its preparation. Thorough decortication should be carried out, not only on the transverse process, but also up the lateral aspect of the pedicle including the facet (Fig. 13). However, the facet at the level above the fusion should be carefully preserved, and no invasion of the capsule should be accomplished during the surgical procedure. Bone graft is taken from the iliac crest (Figs. 14 and 15) and grafts are placed in the previously prepared beds (Fig. 16).

Internal Fixation

A variety of internal fixators are available (see Chapter 92). Mastery of all fixation techniques is not practical, so it is important to gain confidence with several systems that will allow a wide versatility in application.

The advantage of internal fixation is a higher rate of spinal arthrodesis by immobilization of the spinal motion segment (27). Secondary advantages of fixation include the avoidance of external bracing post-operatively and the patient's early participation in a rehabilitation program.

The major disadvantage of instrumentation in the spine is the problem of potential nerve root encroachment from the apparatus. The use of sophisticated fixation devices may greatly increase operative time. The advantages of fixation must be weighed against this concomitant increase in operative time and tissue manipulation, the result of which may be an unacceptable infection rate. Whatever the system employed, care must be taken when inserting hooks, sublaminar wires, or pedicle screws to avoid neurological injury (33). There is minimum room for error when securing the device, and a

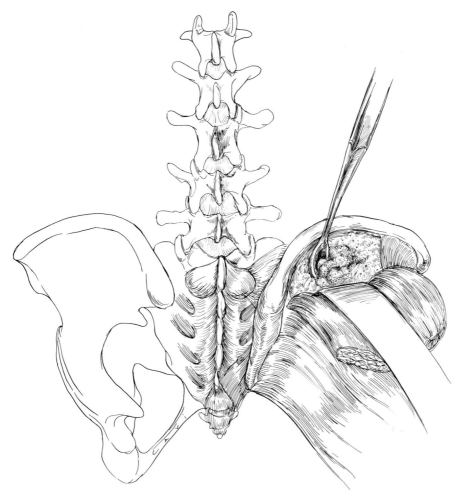

FIG. 15. Bone graft taking the cancellous bone.

high degree of technical proficiency is required. In addition, bone quality should be assessed pre-operatively by plain radiography, duophoton densometry, or quantitative computerized tomography scanning. Since all spinal stabilization systems rely on fixation in the pedicles or lamina, severe osteoporosis represents a surgical problem for many of these devices. A weak lamina might not be able to hold hooks or be available for segmental fixation. Widespread osteoporosis throughout a vertebra may indicate a need for methylmethacrylate insertion in the pedicle to assure good screw purchase. Furthermore, posterior distraction without preservation of lordosis will create a "flat back" syndrome. Finally, all patients should be advised that the hardware may need to be removed at a later date.

A variety of devices have been used (8,20,27). Knodt's rods and the Luque segmental fixation (22) continue to be used whenever possible, and particularly whenever the L5-S1 junction is not spanned. We prefer the simple forms of fixation whenever possible, particularly easily inserted systems that are medially placed, allowing bone to fully cover the transverse process fusion and lateral facets.

Knodt's Rods

Knodt's rods have been an effective way of obtaining fusion over a 20-year period. This fixation is not appropriate when the lamina is removed, and frequently interferes with the sacral nerve roots at its distal insertion, requiring removal in over 30% of cases (8,27). Currently, it is reserved for use in one- or two-level fusion not involving the sacral segment, and in a patient with sufficient lordosis to tolerate the distraction.

The distraction effect of Knodt's rods throws increased weight across the anterior column, therefore giving added compression to the anterior interbody graft. This has a theoretical advantage of increasing the fusion rate in the anterior column.

The Luque Rectangle

The Luque rectangle can be contoured to afford lordosis for a patient. It is a quick, efficacious method of stabilization above the level of the sacrum when the laminae are intact.

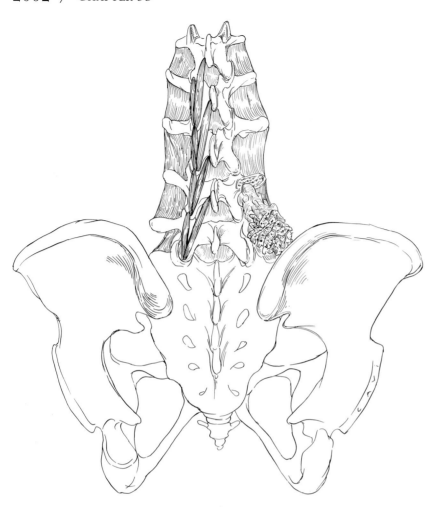

FIG. 16. Posterior view showing grafts in place at transverse processes.

Pedicle Screws

This method of fixation allows stabilization under virtually all circumstances and can be reasonably expected to increase fusion rate. However, accelerated degeneration above the level of fusion is common (32), particularly when a fixation device is used that has greater stiffness than bone. Iatrogenic injury of the facets above the level of fusion may be the most common reason for this problem. Inserting the pedicle screw into the lateral mass is difficult to accomplish without some compromise of the tip of the inferior articular facet and damage to the capsule.

The use of pedicle fixation devices also limits the amount of area available for bony fusion at the transverse processes. More desirable methods of fixation would move the device in a more medial direction, therefore exposing the lateral pedicular cortex and transverse process for bony graft material.

The second problem associated with pedicle screws involves the time and effort required for insertion. An overall complication rate as high as 50% has been reported in the early series of pedicle screws (33), and there is no question that there is a significant learning curve in mastering this technique. Pedicle screw fixation should be avoided whenever possible because of the added operating time, increased infection rate, and potential mechanical neurological problems inherent in the procedure.

Because of these common problems, we prefer distraction systems combined with segmental fixation systems with sacral screws (Figs. 17, 18, 19, and 20), which offer the following advantages:

1. They are medially placed and leave room for the graft.
2. They do not impinge on the facet above the level of the fusion.
3. They can be inserted in a minimal amount of time, usually less than half an hour.

Hardware Removal

We find a high instance of hardware removal, approaching 50%. In a typical case, the patient does well initially, but after four to six months complains of back pain with motion or pressure. Plain x-rays may indicate a loose screw, a "windshield wiper" effect, or even a bro-

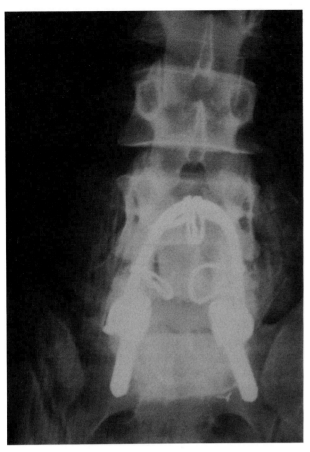

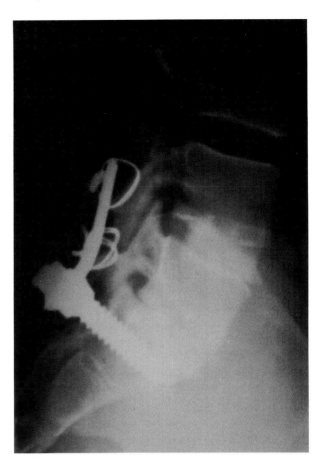

FIG. 17. AP view of segmental fixation with sacral screw.

FIG. 18. Lateral view of segmental fixation with sacral screw.

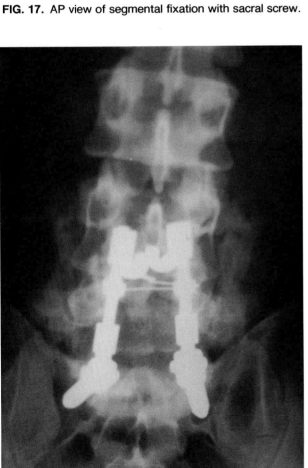

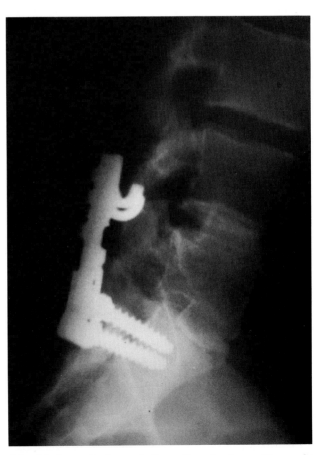

FIG. 19. AP view of distraction fixation with sacral screw.

FIG. 20. Lateral view of distraction fixation with sacral screw.

ken screw. More commonly, a bursitic reaction is present over the screwheads or at the plate ends. An excellent screening test for this latter possibility is an injection of Xylocaine under x-ray control at the screw sites. Relief of pain with injection predicts a high salvage rate from hardware removal. Currently we are considering whether all hardware should be removed on a routine basis.

Bone Grafting

The authors use allograft for the interbody fusion and autograft for the transverse process fusion. In our initial series of 50 patients (unpublished data), the interbody fusion graft was obtained from the anterior iliac crest. The complication rate and morbidity from this grafting technique were unacceptable and led us to use a tricortical graft or cadaver bone. In comparing the next 50 cases (unpublished data), the fusion rate increased slightly in cases using cadaver bone. Conversely, neither allograft nor xenograft has been a satisfactory substitute for the patient's own bone for fusion. In selected cases with a paucity of bone, a unilateral graft technique was employed on the theory that a solid unilateral fusion is better than a bilateral pseudarthrosis. The clinical results seem to be equivalent, and one cannot distinguish between the clinical results of a patient with a solid unilateral versus bilateral fusion. With the use of an autograft technique on transverse processes, early fusion is anticipated and usually occurs within four months, allowing the patient to pursue more vigorous rehabilitation.

Blood Replacement

All patients are given the opportunity to donate two units of autogenous blood forty days before surgery. There is a high acceptance rate among patients; however, the disadvantage is that some patients start surgery with a low hematocrit and hemoglobin.

The routine use of the cell saver during the posterior portion of the procedure reduces the necessity for transfusion. However, with good surgical technique, exposure, and hemostasis, blood loss from a procedure should seldom exceed 500 to 600 cc, and only on a rare occasion exceeds 1,000 cc.

SURGICAL RESULTS

The results will be reported as attainment of the patient's goals and the rate of arthrodesis.

Goals

There is no satisfactory way to absolutely define the benefits of spine surgery of this magnitude. We do think

that a return-to-work criterion in cases of plain herniated nucleus pulposus is a reasonable response, and there should be high correlation with patient satisfaction. This is not true with a circumferential fusion. An end-result criterion of "return to regular job" would place a harsh burden on this type of procedure, with less than 60% of patients achieving this goal. On the other hand, attainment of set goals established by the pre-operative team can result in a success rate well above 95%. Since one criterion produces unfairly low and the other unfairly high results, we have adopted Waddell's criteria (31), which analyze patient satisfaction, i.e., "Was the surgery worth it?" In our series of patients, the results using his criteria are at the 90th percentile. In the working population, particularly those under age 45, we question whether or not the surgery should be done without some expectation of return to at least a modified work status.

One may question the philosophical basis for this surgery without a high return to economic productivity. The surgeon could resolve this problem by offering this procedure to only young, intelligent, vocationally skilled patients.

Fusion Rate

As difficult as it may be to evaluate results in terms of patient function and "goals," it is even more complex to assess simple bony fusion in a patient with an anterior/ posterior graft and internal fixation. The common standard technique has been determination of motion by flexion/extension overlay radiographs. However, with internal fixation and anterior load sharing, it is virtually impossible to determine whether posterior column arthrodesis has occurred using flexion/extension radiographs. By this criterion, our fusion rate is 100%.

The next most commonly used criterion for fusion rate is the CT scan, which is compromised by the metallic fixation. This leaves plain x-rays for evaluation of the anterior and transverse process fusion. An interbody non-union is easy to appraise because of the halo around the graft. A mature, healed interbody fusion with remodeling of the graft and frank trabeculae across the area of the end plate is also easily appraised but usually not apparent for a two- to five-year period. The majority of grafts may or may not be healed, but are at least acting as spacers for the disc. If we accept this middle group as "healed," we can then observe the bony status of the transverse process fusion. Next a decision must be made regarding criteria for each motion segment. Does unilateral posterior bony union constitute a good fusion? A minimal anterior but an excellent bilateral posterior fusion, or vice versa? Independent evaluation of fusion rates from a different study yielded fusion rates of 96% (25). However, we think this is artificially high because of the above-mentioned technical difficulties in determining fusion success.

COMPLICATIONS

Complications of anterior interbody fusion include prolonged operative time, difficult exposures, excessive blood loss, impotence, retrograde ejaculation, and vascular complications in the lower extremities. Three surgical deaths secondary to complications of blood loss from attempted anterior lumbar fusion in three separate regions of the country are known. All of these apparently occurred in the early experience of the surgical teams.

Our surgical experience with anterior fusion has been with 725 patients representing 1,187 anterior intervertebral disc replacements, of which 330 patients had single-level fusions, 320 patients had two-level fusions, 64 patients had three-level fusions, 9 patients had four-level fusions, and 2 patients had six-level fusions. The team experienced virtually all of the known complications of the procedure except patient death (see Table 1), but with a minimal incidence that has decreased with increased experience.

The more significant complications occurred during the early experience, and the demonstration of a learning curve is apparent. This experience reflects the need for proper exposure, proper instrumentation, and a proper team. That team combines a surgeon with vascular expertise and a spine surgeon in attendance throughout the duration of the anterior procedure.

Wound infection is the major complication of the posterior procedure. The occurrence of this complication seems to have a direct correlation to the operative team's experience with pedicle screws. In our experience, during the initial nine-month period the infection rate was 11%. By initiating the following steps, the infection rate for the ensuing nine months decreased to 3.9%:

1. The use of lateral x-rays instead of image intensification to verify position within the pedicle.

2. Decreased use of multilevel pedicle screws and increased use of distraction rods and segmentation fixation, or unilateral fixation with or without sacral pedicle screws.
3. Change of gloves prior to hardware insertion.
4. More meticulous attention to technique of dressing change while on rounds.

In addition, prophylactic antibiotic coverage was changed to include both *Staphylococcus* and gram negative bacteria, because of our suspicion that seeding of gram negative bacteria from the gut was a potential source of hardware infection. We therefore adopted the routine use of cefuroxine sodium given intravenously the night before surgery, at induction of anesthesia, and for three days post-operatively. Over the ensuing four months, there have been no post-operative infections, but a long period of observation will be necessary to validate this early experience.

The other significant complication of posterior fusion is incidental durotomy. This complication rate is directly proportional to the number of patients with previous surgery. Our routine is to repair the rent with an interrupted, horizontal mattress suture and apply a fibrin glue clot made from fresh frozen plasma. A drain is not used. The patient remains at bed rest with slight Trendelenburg for 48 hours before resuming ambulation. We find no long-term complications from incidental durotomy, which agrees with Jones et al. (18). Many patients will have post-operative bone graft pain, which may even imitate sciatica with significant leg pain. To distinguish this from potential nerve injury, we routinely take bone grafts from the side opposite the most significant pain. We do not initiate a workup for leg pain unless there is an associated objective neurological change. Post-operative seromas can occasionally cause significant increase in dural pressure and irritation with concomitant sciatica. This is important only so that the team recognizes this post-operative change and aspirates the seroma.

Because of our immediate (same-day) ambulation program, we have had minimal incidence of thrombophlebitis or pulmonary emboli.

SUMMARY

Circumferential fusion is a logical surgical choice for patients who have pathology involving both the anterior and posterior columns. The procedure should be performed in institutions with teams available, including psychological, vocational, and physical rehabilitation specialists to work with the patient. The procedure should not be undertaken unless the patient has failed considerable conservative care.

In addition, circumferential fusion should not be a common procedure in the average orthopedic institution. Our practice represents a tertiary referral source

TABLE 1. *Complications of spinal fusion*

Complications	Number of cases	%
Permanent retrograde ejaculation	2	0.27
Temporary retrograde ejaculation	5	0.69
Arterial thrombosis	3	0.41
Venous thrombosis	2	0.27
Venous injury	20	2.7
Ileus	24	3.3
Requiring N-G tube	2	0.27
Bladder retention	56	7.7
Requiring indwelling Foley	12	1.6
Temporary sympathetic blockage	61	8.4
Post-sympathectomy syndrome	4	0.55
Incisional hernias	5	0.68
Blood replacement	0	0
Extruded grafts—Anterior	3	0.41
Posterior	2	0.27
Graft infections	0	0
Wound infections	27	3.7

with considerably more complicated patients than would be seen normally. If the procedure is not done by a technically competent team, the chances for catastrophic results are high. It is mandatory that the operative team include a vascular surgeon. The use of internal fixation is highly desirable, and the simplification of posterior fixation devices will lead to a lower complication rate.

Finally, the patient must realize that the operation is but one event in the recovery process. He must understand the importance of rehabilitation and commit to participating. He must be off all narcotics upon leaving the hospital and go through the rehabilitation period without the use of narcotics. Without this strong rehabilitative effort, the chances for success decline considerably.

REFERENCES

1. Beattie FD (1969): Distraction rod fusion. *Clin Orthop* (62):218–222.
2. Blumenthal SL, Baker J, Dossett D, Selby DK (1988): Role of anterior lumbar fusion for internal disc disruption. *Spine* 13:300.
3. Bosworth DM (1956): Circumduction fusion of the spine. *J Bone Joint Surg* [Am] 38:263–269.
4. Cloward RB (1985): Posterior lumbar interbody fusion. Updated. *Clin Orthop* 16–19.
5. Crock HV (1970): A reappraisal of intervertebral disc lesion. *Med J Aust* 1:983–989.
6. Crock HV (1976): Observations on the management of failed spinal operation. *J Bone Joint Surg* [Br] 58:193.
7. Crock HV (1981): Anterior lumbar interbody fusion: Indications for its use and notes on surgical technique. *Clin Orthop* (165):157–163.
8. Dubuc F (1975): Knodt rod grafting. *Orthop Clin North Am* 6:283–287.
9. Fairbank JCT, Cooper J, Davies JB, O'Brien JP (1980): Oswestery disability questionnaire. *Physiotherapy* 66:271.
10. Farfan HF (1975): Comment on paper by Enslin. *Orthop Clin North Am* 6:297.
11. Farfan HF, Cossett JW, Robertson GH (1970): The effects of torsion on the lumbar intervertebral joints: The role of torsion in the production of disc degeneration. *J Bone Joint Surg* [Am] 52:46.
12. Farfan HF, Kirkaldy-Willis WH (1981): The present status of spinal fusion in the treatment of lumbar intervertebral joint disorders. *Clin Orthop* (158):198.
13. Frymoyer JW, Hanley EN, Howe J, Kuhlmann D, Materi R (1979): A comparison of radiographic findings in fusion and non-fusion patients ten or more years following lumbar disc surgery. *Spine* 4:435–440.
14. Frymoyer JW, Krag MH (1986): Spinal stability and instability: Definitions, classification and general principles of management. In: Dunsker SB, Schmidek HA, Frymoyer J, Kahn A, eds. *The unstable spine.* Orlando: Grune and Stratton.
15. Frymoyer JW, Selby DK (1985): Segmental instability rationale for treatment. *Spine* 10:286–288.
16. Goldner JL, Urbaniak JR, McCollum DE (1971): Anterior disc excision and interbody spinal fusion for chronic low back pain. *Orthop Clin North Am* 2:543–568.
17. Hoover NW (1968): Indications for fusion at the time of removal of intervertebral disc. *J Bone Joint Surg* [Am] 50:189–210.
18. Jones AA, Riley S, Torsney B (1989): Assessment of the outcome of lumbar spine surgery. *J Bone Joint Surg* [Br] 70:723–727.
19. Kirkaldy-Willis WH, Wedge JH, Yong-Hing K, Reilly J (1978): Pathology and pathogenesis of lumbar spondylosis and stenosis. *Spine* 3:419.
20. Knodt H, Lavricle R (1964): Distraction fusion of the spine. *Ohio St Med J* 60:1140–1142.
21. Lawlis GF, McCoy CE (1983): Psychological evaluation: Patients with chronic pain. *Orthop Clin North Am* 14:527–530.
22. Luque ER (1982): The anatomic basis and development of segmental spinal instrumentation. *Spine* 7:256.
23. McCoy CE (1989): The development of the Dallas Pain Questionnaire: An assessment of the impact of spinal pain on behavior. *Spine* 14.
24. O'Brien JP (1983): The role of fusion for chronic low back pain. *Orthop Clin North Am* 14:639–647.
25. O'Brien JP (1990): Simultaneous combined anterior and posterior fusion: An independent analysis of a treatment for the disabled low back patient. *Spine* 15.
26. Rolander SD (1966): Motion of the lumbar spine with special reference to the stabilizing effect of posterior fusion. *Acta Orthop Scand* (Suppl) 90:1–144.
27. Selby DK (1986): Internal fixation with Knodt rods. *Clin Orthop* (203):179–184.
28. Selby DK, Henderson RJ, Blumenthal S, Dossett D (1988): Anterior lumbar fusions. In: Cauthen J, ed. *Lumbar spine surgery, 2nd ed.* Baltimore: Williams & Wilkins.
29. Selby DK, Paris SU (1981): Anatomy of facet joints and its clinical correlation with low back pain. *Contemp Orthop* 3:20–23.
30. Stokes IAF, Wilder DG, Frymoyer JW, Pope MH (1981): Assessment of patients with low back pain by biplanar radiographic measurement of intervertebral motion. *Spine* 6:233–239.
31. Waddell G, Stambough JL, Balderston RA, Rothman H (1988): Long-term results of lumbar spine surgery complicated by unintended incidental durotomy. *Spine* 14:443–446.
32. White A (1988): Occult injections of the lumbar spine. Presented at N.A.S.S., Colorado Springs.
33. Whitecloud TW (1988): Complications with the U.S.P. spine system. Presented at N.A.S.S., Colorado Springs.

The Adult Spine: Principles and Practice,
J. W. Frymoyer, Editor-in-Chief.
Raven Press, Ltd., New York © 1991.

CHAPTER 96

Prosthetic Intervertebral Disc

Casey K. Lee, Noshia A. Langrana, John R. Parsons, and Mark C. Zimmerman

The surgical strategies available to manage low back disorders include (a) disc excision; (b) decompression; and (c) spinal fusion with or without supplemental stabilization devices. Although improvements in selection criterion and surgical technique have evolved, the clinical results indicate a significant rate of failure still remains. Improvements in the future must, therefore, be directed towards furthering our knowledge about selection criterion, and then developing the techniques that will have the highest probability for success for a given low back disorder. This chapter will focus on an exciting new prospect for the future: the development of a prosthetic intervertebral disc.

PROBLEMS WITH TECHNIQUES CURRENTLY AVAILABLE

Mixter and Barr's classic report demonstrated that intractable sciatic pain could be satisfactorily relieved by surgical excision of the herniated disc (18). Over the ensuing 50 years, it has been amply demonstrated that as many as 95% of properly selected patients have excellent and lasting relief of their leg pain complaints (10). However, relief of back pain is unpredictable; at least 14% and perhaps as many as 50% of patients have significant and continuing low back pain complaints (10,24). Barr anticipated this problem and advocated spinal fusion to relieve the underlying structural weakness he surmised caused the disc herniation (1). Unfortunately, short- and long-term follow-up analyses showed the expected relief of back symptoms did not occur predictably with spinal fusion (9). Moreover, spinal fusion often created later problems which were worse than the original condition under treatment (9).

As the indications for spinal surgery have broadened, the basic problems reported with lumbar disc excision have been encountered in the surgical treatment of other pathologic conditions. More extensive lumbar decompression has become popular in recent years as the awareness of spinal stenosis has increased. With this procedure the risks of destabilization have also increased, and later disabling low back pain is common. At the same time spinal fusion has become more widely used in the management of less well understood conditions such as disc disruption syndrome and segmental instabilities. The overall success rate achieved is widely variable and ranges from 32% to 99% (5,25,26).

The technical problems encountered have included graft donor site pain, pseudarthrosis, and accelerated degeneration of adjacent motion segments (12,13). In an attempt to overcome these problems attention has been focused on the alternatives such as autogenous bone graft substitutes, and the development of internal fixa-

C. K. Lee, M.D., Professor; J. R. Parsons, Ph.D., Associate Professor; M. C. Zimmerman, Assistant Professor: Orthopaedic Surgery, UMD-New Jersey Medical School, Newark, New Jersey 07103.
N. A. Langrana, Ph.D.: Professor, Mechanical Engineering, Rutgers University, Piscataway, New Jersey 08903.

tion systems. The evolution of these fixation devices has been towards higher rigidity in an attempt to increase stability and the rate of fusion. However, significant problems have been encountered including instrument breakage, neurologic complications, accelerated degeneration of adjacent motion segments (12), and a concern that high-rigidity devices will ultimately cause stress shielding and disuse osteoporosis (17).

From this brief review, it is clear that significant problems remain and there is ample need to improve upon our surgical techniques. The current direction of the treatment for disc herniation is to remove the offending disc herniation with minimum disturbance of normal tissue utilizing techniques of microsurgery and percutaneous nuclectomy, and newer, safer chemonucleolytic agents towards the goal of reducing morbidity and increasing the rate of symptomatic and functional recovery. Further refinements and improvement of surgical instruments and techniques can be expected in the future to make these procedures safer and easier. With these techniques the greater challenge will be to define precisely the indications. In contrast, the challenge in spinal stabilization not only will be to define indications, but to develop the devices that will overcome the inherent limitations of the currently available techniques.

DEVELOPMENT OF A PROSTHETIC INTERVERTEBRAL DISC

Limitations and problems with currently available surgical approaches to low back disorders have led some investigators to explore the radically new concept of a prosthetic intervertebral disc. In recent years, several researchers have attempted to develop prosthetic devices that partially or totally replace symptomatic, dysfunctioning discs. Such devices are designed to relieve symptoms, yet maintain the important functions of the disc: mobility, stability, and weight bearing. If such a device were reliable and safe, and if it could provide equivalent enhanced long-term results relative to the fusion procedure, the choice between such a device and fusion would be clear. Severely degenerated painful joints in other areas of the musculoskeletal system, such as the hip and knee, have been successfully treated with artificial joint replacements, displacing once popular fusion procedures.

GENERAL CONSIDERATIONS FOR A PROSTHETIC INTERVERTEBRAL DISC

Prosthetic intervertebral disc devices are considered "long-term" or permanent implants, unlike many other spinal fixation implants which provide stability and weight bearing functions for a limited time until the repair or fusion is completed. Therefore, these permanent

devices must satisfy important criteria, including but not limited to the following: biocompatibility, mechanical strength, implant material and mechanical stability, acceptable manufacturing process, and safe surgical techniques.

Biocompatibility

Materials used in a permanent or long-term implant must be biocompatible, that is, they should not cause untoward local tissue reaction (inflammatory or foreign body reaction) or untoward systemic effects, such as carcinogenesis or organ toxicity.

Mechanical Strength

The prosthetic disc should have adequate mechanical strength to withstand the continuous but varying degrees of motion and loading. An acceptable prosthetic disc, therefore, will require appropriate maximal failure strength, fatigue strength, as well as optimal axial, torsional, and bending stiffness.

Implant Stability

Various factors affect the temporal stability of prosthetic implants. These include materials degradation characteristics in the in vivo environment, mechanical design, and the host tissue reaction to the implanted device. Some materials, particularly polymers used in prosthetic devices, degrade mechanically in the in vivo environment. Typical problems include embrittlement due to lipid or protein absorption, polymer chain session due to hydrolysis or other factors, or leaching of plasticizers and low molecular weight aligomers on monomers.

The mechanical stability of the implanted device is determined by the mechanical characteristics of the device, the design, and the interface mechanism between the device and the host. Perhaps the greatest concern is the ability to secure the implanted device to the host. Two commonly used methods of securing orthopedic implants are mechanical interlocking (press fitting) and mechanical attachment by either cementing or surface bone ingrowth. Permanent fixation by means of bone ingrowth has been under intense investigation, however it is known to be extremely difficult in the tibial plateau with wide surface areas of cancellous bone. Mechanical interlocking methods have been used in other orthopedic procedures such as in the femoral endoprosthesis. Ultimately, the tissue reaction at the interface governs the stability of the device. The host tissue reaction at the interface is usually determined by the biocompatibility of the materials, and the biomechanical compatibility between the device and the surrounding bone. It is generally accepted that the closer the mechanical properties of the prosthetic disc to the natural disc, the better the tissue tolerance by the host.

Acceptable Manufacturing Process

The manufacturing process of the prosthetic disc should be reliable and reproducible. The final product should not contain any biologically harmful material that may be introduced during the manufacturing process. The implantable device should be able to withstand an acceptable sterilization process without altering the chemical, mechanical, or design characteristics of the materials or device.

Operative Procedure

The safety and ease of the operative procedure for disc replacement is a prerequisite for successful clinical use.

PROSTHETIC INTERVERTEBRAL DISC RESEARCH

Various types of prosthetic intervertebral discs have been described or developed. In general, there are two types: (a) devices that replace only the nucleus pulposus, and (b) devices that replace the total or subtotal of the disc.

Replacement of the Nucleus Pulposus

A spherical metal ball spacer was probably the first implant of this type used in a clinical setting. Fernstrom (7) reported that the majority of his patients showed collapse of the disc space and migration of the metal ball into the vertebral body when evaluated 4 to 7 years later (Fig. 1). Others (4,6) suggested the use of silicone fluid contained in a plastic tube or a silicone rubber nucleus to replace the nucleus pulposus. More recently, a more sophisticated design for nuclear replacement, which consists of two fluid filled semipermeable tubes, has been under investigation (20).

For this type of device, it is hypothesized that painful, dysfunctioning discs may be corrected by restoring the disc height and re-establishing proper weight transmission through the annulus fibrosus and the facet joints. To date, no information is available about the biomechanical behavior of the spinal motion segment before and after such nucleus replacement in normal or degenerated discs.

Total or Subtotal Replacement of the Intervertebral Disc

This type of prosthesis requires removal of the nucleus pulposus and partial or total removal of the annulus fibrosus. Several researchers have tried experimental devices in a limited number of patients. Others have been

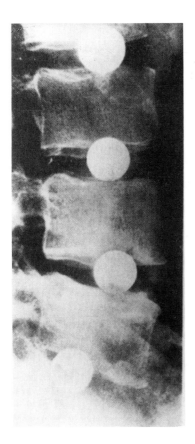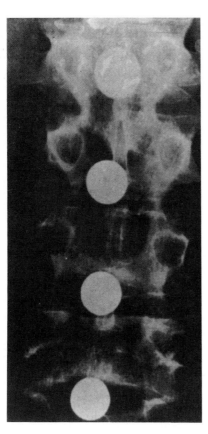

FIG. 1. Spherical metal ball spacer within the disc space at a follow-up evaluation. The metal ball spacer has migrated into the vertebral bodies.

described only in theory while some others have been investigated in the research laboratory.

Low Friction Sliding Surfaces

The device described by Hoogland and Associates (11) and the Link Intervertebral Endoprosthesis/SB Charite (15) are of this type. The device by Hoogland et al. consists of two opposing articulating points made of high density polyethylene. These dome and cup shaped opposing surfaces provide low friction gliding and some mechanical stability for the device. The device is secured in the adjacent vertebral bodies by PMMA bone cement.

The SB Charite lumbar intervertebral disc endoprosthesis is made of three parts: two metal end plates and an interposing polyethylene slide core (Fig. 2). The two metal end plates are secured into the vertebral bodies with mechanical locking spikes. The sliding core is placed between the two metal end plates. Motion from the prosthesis is semi-constrained and is the result of sliding between dome and cup shaped surfaces of the concaved metal end plates and convexed polyethylene core. Weight bearing is transmitted from one end plate through the rigid polyethylene core to the other end plate.

Biomechanical characteristics of the SB Charite endoprosthesis were evaluated under axial compression for hysteresis, dynamic rocking ($\pm 10^{\circ 2} \times 10^{17}$ cycles) and for fatigue strength. The prosthesis (SB II) was found to function adequately under these in vitro testing conditions (3). Because of the prosthetic design with relatively unconstrained movements about all three axes, the prosthesis acts like a ball bearing without providing structural stability and rigidity. The remaining intact structures, especially the posterior facet joints, will probably be required to provide rigidity and stability for the motion segment. The design could allow the polyethylene core to dislocate in vivo, although the probability of this complication is unknown. This device has been implanted in humans with apparently favorable results, but the long-term outcomes are unknown.

Spring System

A system containing springs between metal cups was described by Patil (19), but no detailed information of biomechanical characteristics, in vitro or in vivo is available. Such a system may present various problems such as fatigue failure of the springs and change of mechanical behavior of springs due to tissue interposition. Such a system would be prone to wear and perhaps severe biocompatibility problems due to wear debris.

Contained Fluid Filled Chamber

A fluid filled elastic chamber contained in metal cup-end plates was designed by Froming (8) but no information is available about mechanical characteristics. Ray

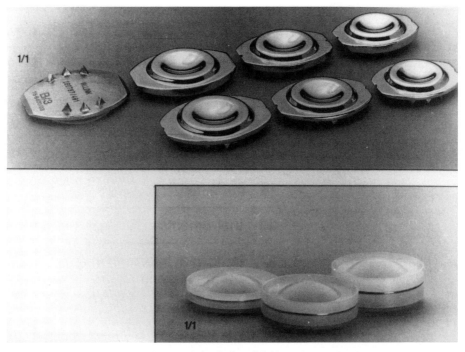

FIG. 2. SB Charite lumbar intervertebral disc (Link) endoprosthesis (with permission from ref. 15).

and Corbin (20) have begun development of fluid filled cylindrical bags with a knit outer covering to encourage soft tissue ingrowth and attachment (Fig. 3). The devices are designed to be implanted in pairs from a posterior approach and theoretically replace the function of the nucleus. This prosthesis design is in the concept/development stage.

Elastic Disc Prosthesis Made of Rubber or Other Elastomers

Stubstad and Associates (23,24) designed a silicon-Dacron reinforced prosthesis, which consists of an intervertebral disc-shaped silicon disc covered with Dacron mesh on the outer surface. Mechanical testing of the device has demonstrated a mechanical behavior similar to the natural disc. The prosthesis was tested in vivo using a chimpanzee model and initially showed promising results. More recently, a similar device made of a rubber material was designed by Steffee (22). The rubber disc is secured to the bone by bone cement with a interposing metal plate. The device has been used clinically in a limited number of patients with early encouraging results.

Elastic "Disc" Incorporated in a Rigid Column

A mechanical device for replacement of the vertebral body has been developed (16). This type of device contains a thin layer of elastic "disc" in a large rigid column of metal to allow some movement. Very few mechanical data are currently available.

Development of Prosthetic Intervertebral Discs at the UMD-New Jersey Medical School

For the past several years, in the authors' orthopedic research laboratories at the New Jersey Medical School, in collaboration with Rutgers University Engineering School and Johnson and Johnson Orthopaedic Research in New Jersey, the authors have been engaged in research, development, and testing a number of disc prostheses (2,14). The overall goal of these research activities has been to produce a prosthetic intervertebral disc design that has biomechanical characteristics similar to the natural disc. Such a prosthetic disc could provide: (a) the best restoration of the function of a spinal motion segment (motion, rigidity, and stability), and (b) the best tolerance by the surrounding structures, especially the interface between the prosthesis and the vertebral bone and the posterior facet joints.

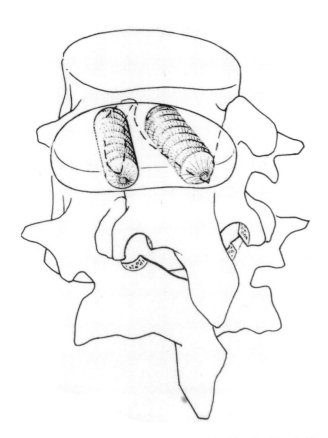

FIG. 3. The prosthetic device designed by Charles Ray (with permission from the designer).

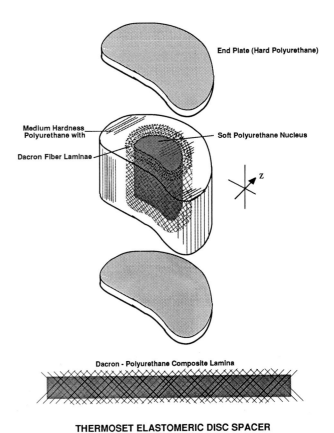

FIG. 4. Fiber reinforced polyurethane disc prosthesis (with permission from UMD-New Jersey Medical School).

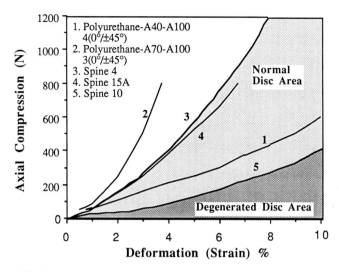

FIG. 5. Compressive response of the fiber reinforced polyurethane disc prosthesis under axial loading in comparison to that of the natural disc.

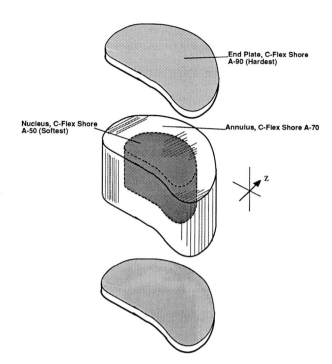

THERMOPLASTIC ELASTOMERIC DISC SPACER
THREE DIFFERENT DUROMETERS:
NUCLEUS, ANNULUS, AND ENDPLATES

FIG. 7. Multi-durometer thermoplastic disc prosthesis design (with permission from UMD-New Jersey Medical School).

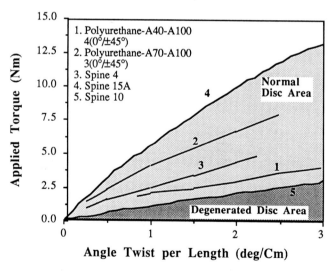

FIG. 6. Torsional response of the fiber reinforced disc prosthesis under combined axial compression and torsion in comparison to the natural disc.

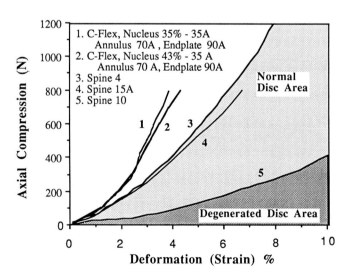

FIG. 8. Biomechanical properties: axial compression test, natural discs versus C-Flex prostheses.

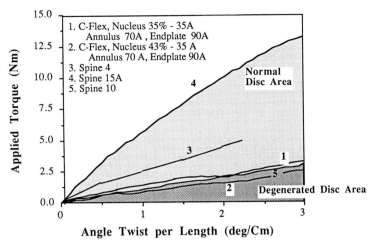

FIG. 9. Biomechanical properties: torsional twist with 800N axial load, natural spine versus C-Flex prostheses.

This research project has included several phases:

1. identification of biocompatible materials that have suitable biomechanical properties;
2. design and fabrication of prosthetic discs;
3. mechanical testing of the various disc prostheses alone and in vitro testing of the prostheses in the cadaveric lumbar spine of human and canine models;
4. finite elements analysis of the prosthetic disc;
5. studies on attachment of the prostheses;
6. in vivo study of prosthetic disc replacement in a canine lumbar spine model for biocompatibility, histopathologic, and biomechanical studies.

During the initial phase, three biomaterials among many examined were identified for potential use: silicone rubber, polyurethane (thermo set), and C-flex (thermoplastic-polysilicone modified styrene-ethylene/butylene block copolymer, Concept Polymer Technologies of Clearwater, Florida). In addition, Dacron fiber among other fiber types was identified as the fiber-reinforcement material in certain disc designs.

Prosthetic intervertebral discs made of homogenous biomaterials of silicone rubber, polyurethane, or C-flex were not suitable, as their mechanical characteristics could not match those of the natural disc. Even by varying polymer durometer (stiffness) it was found that polymers appropriately rigid in axial compression lack sufficient torsional rigidity. Polymers suitably rigid in torsion are far too stiff axially. This inability to match the properties of the natural disc with homogenous polymers arises from the complex anisotropic properties of the natural spine disc. To overcome this fundamental problem, directional fiber reinforcement was used.

Fiber Reinforced Elastomeric Disc Designs

Contrary to the results published by Urbaniak et al. (24), discs fabricated of silicone rubber with or without laminated fiber reinforcement in the annular area demonstrated mechanical strength and rigidity below the lower normal limit of the natural disc.

This finding led to investigation of thermoset urethane elastomers which were stronger, tougher, and of higher stiffness. The design consisted of three components corresponding to the end plates, the annulus, and the nucleus pulposus of the natural disc. Urethanes used for this design were of three different durometers (stiffness): A durometer (Shore A) of A40 was the least stiff and was used for the nucleus pulposus. A70 durometer, an intermediate grade, was used for the annulus, and A100, being the stiffest, was used for the end plates. The annulus was reinforced with laminates of urethane/Dacron fiber, with specific fiber orientations in each layer (0° ± 45°).

The nucleus pulposus analogue was made of homogenous urethane elastomer (A40) and was placed at the center of the prosthetic disc and enclosed within the annulus between two relatively rigid end plates. The end plates were made of homogenous plates of urethane elastomer (A100). When properly manufactured, all three components (nucleus, annulus, and the end plates) were molded under heat and fused into a single unit prosthetic disc.

The results of mechanical testing of this type of fiber reinforced disc prosthesis indicated that the addition of three or four layers of pre-impregnated fiber laminae (0/+45°/−45°) in the annular region resulted in doubling of the axial stiffness, and the torsional stiffness increased by a factor of two to four relative to unreinforced disc prostheses. The results of this study demonstrated that, properly fabricated, this design results in mechanical properties similar to the natural disc (Figs. 4, 5, and 6).

Multi-Component Thermoplastic Design

This design consisted of three C–flex components without fiber reinforcement: a central core (nucleus) of relatively soft polymer, a more rigid annulus containing the central core, and end plates with still more rigid polymer. The relative areas of the annulus and nucleus could be adjusted to provide appropriate mechanical properties in axial compression. The torsional properties of the device were adjustable by varying the amount and durometer of the annular polymer. By using the proper combinations of areas and stiffness of materials, a prosthetic disc which had mechanical properties similar to the natural disc could be manufactured. The results of mechanical testing of such disc prostheses are demonstrated in Figures 7, 8, and 9.

A preliminary study of bone attachment to thermoset urethanes and thermoplast C-flex polymer in the rabbit distal femur demonstrated very satisfactory bone ingrowth into polymer surfaces coated with hydroxyappatite (2). However, the results of a bone ingrowth experiment were less satisfactory when hydroxyappatite was incorporated in the surface of a prosthetic disc implanted in canine lumbar spines. The interface problem between the host bone and the prosthetic disc needs further investigation.

The most current phase of research in this laboratory is a long-term (up to 12 months) animal experiment. Prosthetic discs fabricated using the multi-durometer thermoplastic elastomeric design have been implanted in the canine lumbar disc space to study the biocompatibility and biomechanical response. The preliminary results indicate that prosthetic intervertebral disc replacement in the canine model is well tolerated and provides satisfactory stability and function despite a lack of significant bone ingrowth into the textured hydroxyappatite surface. This experiment is ongoing and design modifications for enhanced fixation are underway.

SUMMARY

An appropriately designed and fabricated prosthetic intervertebral disc may provide an improved alternative to currently available surgical approaches to low back disorders. Such a device may relieve symptoms, yet maintain the important functions of the disc: mobility, stability, and weight bearing.

REFERENCES

1. Barr JS (1947): Ruptured intervertebral disc and sciatic pain. *J Bone Joint Surg* 29:429–437.

2. Boone PS, Zimmerman MC, Guttling E, Lee CK, Parsons JR (1989): Bone attachment to hydroxyappatite coated polymers. *J Biomed Material Research* 23(A2 Suppl):183–199.

3. Buttner-Janz K, Schellnack K, Zippel H (1989): Biomechanics of the SB Charite lumbar intervertebral disc endoprosthesis. *Int Orthop* 13:173–176.

4. Edeland HG (1985): Some additional suggestions for an intervertebral disc prosthesis. *J Biomed Eng* 7:57–62.

5. Evans JH (1981): Paper presented at the annual meeting of the International Society for the Study of the Lumbar Spine, Paris, 1981.

6. Fassio B, Ginestie JF (1978): Prostheses discale en silicone. Etude experimentale et premieres observations cliniques. *Nouv Presse Med* 7:207.

7. Fernstrom U (1966): Arthroplasty with intercorporal endoprosthesis in herniated disc and in painful disc. *Acta Chir Scand* [Suppl] 357:154–159.

8. Froming N (1974): Artificial intervertebral disc. United States Patient File, 1974.

9. Frymoyer JW, Hanley E, Howe J, Kuhlmann D, Matteri R (1978): Disc excision and spine fusion in the management of lumbar disc disease. A minimum ten-year follow-up. *Spine* 3:1–6.

10. Hanley EN Jr, Shapiro DE (1989): The development of low-back pain after excision of a lumbar disc. *J Bone Joint Surg* [Am] 71:719–721.

11. Hoogland T, Steffee AD, Black JD, Greenwald AS (1978): Total lumbar intervertebral disc replacement: Testing of a new articulating spacer in human cadavar spines. Transactions of the 24th annual meeting of the Orthopaedic Research Society, February 21–23, 1978.

12. Hsu KY, Zuckerman J, White AH, Reynolds J, Goldwaite N (1988): Deterioration of motion segments adjacent to lumbar spine fusion. Presented at the annual meeting of the North American Spine Society, Colorado Springs, Colorado, July 24–27, 1988.

13. Lee CK (1988): Accelerated degeneration of the segment adjacent to a lumbar fusion. *Spine* 13:375–377.

14. Lee CK, Langrana NA, Parsons JR, Zimmerman MC, Clemow AJ, Chen EH (1989): Functional disc prosthesis. Transactions of the 35th annual meeting of the Orthopaedic Research Society, Las Vegas, Nevada, February 1989.

15. The Link intervertebral endoprosthesis SB Charite, by Waldemar Link (GMBHK Co.) Barkhausenweg 10, D-2000 Hamburg 63 Germany.

16. Main JA, Wells ME, Strauss AM (1987): Dynamic vertebral body replacement: A proposed prosthetic device. Presented at the winter annual meeting of the American Society of Mechanical Engineers, Boston, Massachusetts, December 13–18, 1987.

17. McAfee PC, Farey ID, Shirado O, Sutterlin C, Gurr K, Woodberry K (1989): A quantitative histologic study of stress shielding with transpedicular instrumentation. A Canine Model. Presented at the annual meeting of the International Society for the Study of the Lumbar Spine, Kyoto, Japan, May, 1989.

18. Mixter WJ, Barr JS (1934): Rupture of the intervertebral disc with involvement of the spinal canal. *New Engl J Med* 211:210–215.

19. Patil AA (1982): Artificial intervertebral disc. United States Patent File, 1982.

20. Ray C (1988): Artificial disc. Presented at the Challenge of the Lumbar Spine '88 meeting, San Antonio, Texas, November 9–13, 1988.

21. Spangfort EV (1972): The lumbar disc herniation. A computer-aided analysis of 2,504 operations. *Acta Orthop Scand* [Suppl] 142:1–95.

22. Steffee A (1988): Artificial disc. Presented at the Challenge of the Lumbar Spine '88 meeting, San Antonio, Texas, November 9–13, 1988.

23. Stubstad JA, Urbaniak JR, Kahn P (1975): Prosthesis for spinal repair. United States Patent File, 1975.

24. Urbaniak JR, Bright DS, Hopkins JE (1973): Replacement of intervertebral discs in chimpanzees by silicone-Dacron implants: A preliminary report. *J Biomed Mater Res* 7:165–186.

25. Watkins RG (1987): Results of anterior interbody fusion. In: *Lumbar spine surgery*. White AH, Rothman RH, Ray CD, eds. St. Louis: C.V. Mosby, p. 408.

26. Zuckerman JF, Selby DK, DeLong WB (1987): Failed posterior lumbar interbody fusion. In: *Lumbar spine surgery*. White AH, Rothman RH, Ray CD, eds. St. Louis; C.V. Mosby, p. 296.

The Adult Spine: Principles and Practice,
J. W. Frymoyer, Editor-in-Chief.
Raven Press, Ltd., New York © 1991.

CHAPTER 97

Internal Disc Disruption

Henry V. Crock

The past ten years have seen a dramatic increase in the number of publications relating to the human spine, as well as extraordinary advances in imaging technology (16,20,24).

The accuracy of diagnosis of disc prolapse has increased with the wider use of computerized tomography and magnetic resonance imaging. The range of surgical methods of its treatment has expanded to include percutaneous discectomy, micro-discectomy, and a variety of intradiscal enzyme therapies (16) although there is little consensus on the indications for the use of these various techniques (3,23). Coupled with these developments has been a wider appreciation of the importance of spinal stenosis.

By contrast, clinical attitudes toward other disc disorders have changed very little. Most practitioners continue to recognize only one entity in addition to disc prolapse, namely disc degeneration.

Disc degeneration used to be defined by changes on plain radiographs of the spine: osteophyte formation on the margins of the vertebral bodies adjacent to the intervertebral discs; variations in the height of the disc space; and narrowing of the facet joints with associated osteophyte formation. The management of patients with disc degeneration is still largely influenced by long-estab-

lished conventions which hold that conservative treatment is usually effective and that surgery may be required in only the few with radiological evidence of spinal instability or spinal stenosis.

Since the application of magnetic resonance imaging (MRI) to the investigation of spinal disorders, a group of patients has been identified in whom plain radiographs are normal but whose MRI shows changes in the discs themselves, especially loss of signal from the nucleus pulposus on T2-weighted sequences. These images are invariably reported in summary as showing "disc degeneration" (Fig. 1).

The classification of disc degeneration has thereby been arbitrarily extended, with the implication that this MRI finding represents an early stage of disc pathology which will inexorably progress to produce the familiar changes of disc degeneration seen on plain radiographs. Disc prolapse fits neatly into this scheme, as it represents the first of the mechanical disorders which may be seen in the natural course of the degenerative process.

It is now becoming apparent that not all patients with "disc degeneration" identified by MRI progress to the traditionally predicted conditions of disc prolapse, vertebral instability, and spinal stenosis. Two other clinically recognizable sub-groups exist among these patients with spinal and limb pains.

The first of these sub-groups is internal disc disruption (IDD), the subject of this chapter. The second is isolated

H. V. Crock, A.O., M.D., M.S., F.R.C.S., F.R.A.C.S.: Cromwell Hospital, London, SW5 0TU, England.

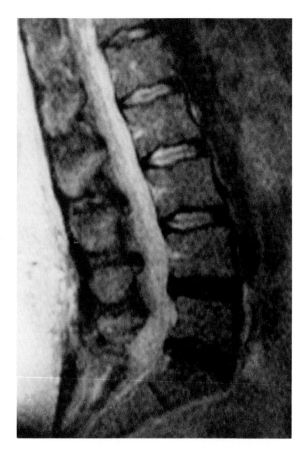

FIG. 1. MRI of the lumbar spine of a female age 36 showing typical changes of IDD at L4-L5 and L5-S1 with loss of the T2-weighted image in both discs, which are not narrowed. The discs visible in the upper lumbar spine appear normal. This patient has remained incapacitated with symptoms typical of post-traumatic IDD following an injury five years ago which occurred when she was working as a nurse and slipped while lifting a heavy hemiplegic patient.

disc resorption (IDR), in which changes both in MRI and plain radiographs proceed to the loss of disc height at a single level, with vertebral sclerosis, minimal osteophyte formation, a vacuum sign in the disc space, and bilateral facet joint subluxation. In IDR, the other discs may remain normal in appearance on plain radiographs even into late middle age. These two disorders produce distinctive syndromes which can be identified on clinical grounds and confirmed with appropriate investigations.

Surgical treatment for disc prolapse, as recommended by Mixter and Barr in 1934 (19), soon became the most common operation performed on the human spine, yet even contemporaries of these two pioneers were dismayed by the failure of their technique to relieve sciatica in many cases, and began to write about elusive "concealed ruptured intervertebral discs" (11). In 1948, Lindblom investigated the possibilities of improving radiological methods of demonstrating intervertebral disc prolapse by injecting radio-opaque dye into the disc, thereby introducing the concept of discography (18).

While discography was taken up and popularized by Cloward (5), its use was soon brought into disrepute by others led by Holt (15). Although this study was later discredited, the impetus for the use of discography had been checked (27). Cloward used discography at first to improve the accuracy of the diagnosis of disc prolapse, previously dependent largely on myelography. He noted later (5a) that in some patients without evidence of disc prolapse, the injection of radio-opaque dye into their discs not only gave a picture of a disordered disc but also reproduced spinal and limb pains; this reaction now serves as an important diagnostic indicator of IDD.

INTERNAL DISC DISRUPTION

The term internal disc disruption (IDD) was first introduced in a paper titled "A Reappraisal of Intervertebral Disc Lesions," published in the *Medical Journal of Australia* in 1970 (6). The information on IDD now presented derives from clinical observations made over a period of more than 20 years. The ideas about this disc disorder originated from the retrospective analysis of hundreds of patients who had continued to complain of disabling symptoms of spinal and limb pains following operations for suspected disc prolapse performed by a number of surgeons in Australia. One group of patients stood out with common features relating to their histories, investigations, and responses to surgery. Nearly all had experienced specific episodes of spinal trauma preceding the onset of pain. These patients had been made worse by the operations designed to remove suspected disc prolapses. Some left hospital complaining of worse pain than they had experienced before surgery, while others relapsed within a short time after operation. A few had undergone more than one similar procedure and had been rendered progressively more disabled.

Their pre-operative investigations had relied heavily on myelography, before CT scanning had become widely used, and long before MRI was available; these myelograms, viewed retrospectively, often provided inconclusive evidence of disc prolapse. The constitutional features of profound loss of energy and of body weight were prominent; psychological disturbances were common.

The value and importance of the use of discography in the further investigation of these disabled patients soon became apparent.

DEFINITION

Internal disc disruption (IDD) is a condition marked by alterations in the internal structure and metabolic functions of one or more discs, usually following significant trauma.

The clinical syndrome includes spinal and limb pains which are made worse by physical activities that increase compressive forces on the affected discs. Profound loss of energy occurs, sometimes associated with significant reduction of body weight, along with a range of psychological disturbances.

It is not associated with the escape of disc fragments from the confines of the disc space. Disc degeneration with loss of disc height and osteophyte formation is not seen, either at the time of the patient's initial presentation or later even after four or five years.

MECHANISMS OF SYMPTOM PRODUCTION

The interpretation of the clinical characteristics of IDD is based on the theory that catabolites pass out of the affected disc, or discs, via the vascular system of the vertebral body (9). These products of protein degradation produce two effects: the first, adverse reactions in the regional nerves in and around the discs and in the spinal canal; the second, constitutional disturbances possibly mediated through the body's immune system.

The intervertebral discs in adults have capillary beds in the vertebral endplate cartilages. These drain into a complex horizontal sub-articular collecting vein system

in the vertebral body (10). This system of veins has tributaries draining both into the main veins of the vertebral body and into the internal vertebral venous plexus in the spinal canal (Fig. 2). Fluids moving into and out of the normal intervertebral disc must flow through the complex vertebral vascular system. Physiological diurnal variations in the height of the intervertebral discs can be understood on this basis (8). Potentially then, the products of protein degradation in IDD produce changes in the intradiscal nerve fibers and in the spinal nerves which are surrounded by the thin-walled veins of the internal vertebral venous plexus, causing spinal and limb pain.

Characteristically, the pain produced by IDD is made worse by activities which force more irritant fluid out of the affected disc or discs. The referred limb pains in these patients are thought to be chemically induced and are not associated with the familiar abnormal neurological signs, ascribed to tension or compression, which are commonly observed in patients with sciatica and brachial neuralgia due to disc prolapse. Recent studies have confirmed that the chemistry of collagen in intervertebral discs is actively influenced by overall compressive loading (2).

The recognition of IDD as an important cause of spinal and referred limb pains calls for a radical reappraisal

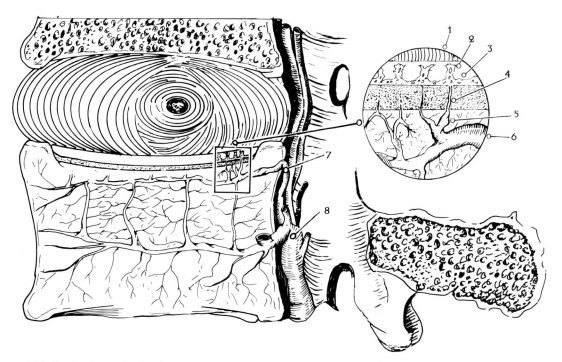

FIG. 2. A schematic drawing to show the spatial relationships of the veins of a typical vertebral body in an adult. 1: intervertebral disc; 2: capillary bed in vertebral endplate cartilage; 3: subchondral post-capillary venous network on the vertebral endplate; 4: vertebral endplate perforated by short vertical venules; 5: vertical tributary from the subchondral post-capillary venous network, draining to the horizontal subarticular collecting vein; 6: horizontal subarticular collecting vein; 7: horizontal subarticular collecting vein joining the anterior internal vertebral venous plexus; 8: system of veins joining the anterior internal vertebral venous plexus (with permission from the editor of *J Bone Joint Surg* [Br], Vol. 55, 1973).

of thinking about disc pathology, with a shift of emphasis from mechanical notions of nerve root compression, traction, and vertebral instability to more complex aspects of biochemical pathology.

EVOLUTION OF THE SYNDROME

The clinical syndrome associated with this disorder usually follows trauma inflicted on the disc, either as the result of sudden and unexpected weight lifting or by forces transmitted through the disc or discs during high speed accidents.

The condition is seen commonly in heavy workers who have been involved in incidents in which weights of up to 200 kilograms have been accidentally or suddenly lifted. For example, a meat worker may slip while carrying a heavy fore-quarter of beef, subjecting his lumbar spine to a massive compression load of short duration. Likewise, nurses not uncommonly develop low back pain having accidentally taken unexpected loads during the lifting of disabled or unconscious heavy patients. The first essential therefore in recognizing IDD is to obtain a detailed history of the likely mechanism of injury. Patients often fail to give accurate accounts of the mechanisms of their injuries, being preoccupied with communicating concern about the severity of their pain.

The spinal pain of which these patients complain has the character of a deep-seated ache. It does not abate rapidly with rest as pain usually does in cases involving mechanical derangements of the spine. Typically, it becomes worse over the course of several months following its onset, aggravated by activity, especially by bending or lifting, and classically by the more vigorous exercises often prescribed by physical therapists. Both the patient's doctor and physical therapist may recognize that these programs are exacerbating the condition and appropriately discontinue therapy. Other clinicians blame the patient for failing to cooperate and may discontinue all treatment for this reason.

Physical exercise may exacerbate spinal pain in patients with symptoms arising from spondylolisthesis or spinal osteoarthritis, but rest usually relieves it rapidly. The use of spinal supports in these patients is often effective in controlling their spinal pain.

In contrast, patients with IDD react quite differently to these conservative measures. The pain resolves only slowly with rest, and is often troublesome, even in bed. Lumbar spinal supports increase abdominal pressure and change the venous blood flow in the spine. This may help to explain why patients with IDD rarely tolerate their use. Paradoxically, this adverse reaction to lumbar bracing should be taken as an indication for recommending spinal fusion in IDD, while in patients with spondylolisthesis or spinal osteoarthritis, it would usually be regarded as a contraindication to spinal fusion.

Whereas limb pain of acute onset may be the initial complaint of patients with disc prolapse, in those with IDD it develops more slowly and they find difficulty in describing its character. Descriptions of the pain as being right inside the limb with an intolerable aching character are common and contrast with the descriptions of intense, fluctuating, sharp pains of sciatica or brachial neuralgia due to disc prolapse, and of the slowly spreading cramp-like pains of spinal stenosis.

IDD patients also commonly complain of feelings of heaviness and impending weakness in the affected limbs. Paresthesia of the type described by those with spinal stenosis is uncommon. Because of the long-term nature of the condition, patients with this syndrome run the high risk of becoming drug dependent, sometimes taking more than 20 different medications daily.

SPINAL MOVEMENT

When attempting to stand up, many patients with IDD have difficulty in rising from the flexed position, often assisting themselves by placing the palms of their hands on the anterior aspects of their thighs, literally climbing up from the stooped position using their hands as props. Similarly, in attempting to sit up from a lying position, they may find it impossible to do so without placing both hands on the bed behind them and exerting pressure on the upper limbs to raise themselves to a sitting position.

At other times they may turn on to one side and get up into a sitting position by rolling their legs over the side of the bed and then levering themselves up slowly and awkwardly, obviously in pain. However, spasm of the paraspinal muscles as seen in cases with disc prolapse and other forms of degenerative spinal disease is uncommon, particularly that associated with pelvic tilt or so-called sciatic scoliosis.

NEUROLOGICAL SIGNS

Abnormal neurological signs in the limbs are uncommon, although complaints of weakness, clumsiness, and of sympathetic nervous system disturbances, such as a feeling of heat in the limb, are often made. It is now more widely accepted that in conditions producing spinal stenosis or nerve root canal stenosis, an absence of objective neurological signs may not contraindicate surgery.

Because patients with IDD also present with normal plain radiographs and normal CT scans, such an absence is often erroneously taken as an absolute contraindication to surgical treatment.

PSYCHOLOGICAL FACTORS IN IDD

Some degree of psychological disturbance is an accepted part of the clinical syndromes seen in a range of spinal disorders. In those with IDD, it often assumes major importance. The diagnosis of the cause of their problems is often long delayed. As they pass through the hands of many different doctors and paramedical practitioners, they soon realize that their symptoms are a mystery not only to themselves but to their doctors and therapists also. On many occasions, the doctors, unaware of the true diagnosis, suggest to the patient and relatives that, despite "thorough investigation," no cause has been found for the pain and that it must therefore be "all in the mind." This leads to antagonism between patient, relatives, and doctor. These patients feel that their problems are being taken too lightly and that even their relatives have turned against them under the influence of the doctor's advice. Psychosexual difficulties may arise, leading to serious marital problems, even to marriage breakdown. Financial worries due to inability to work add to their concerns; eventually the whole fabric of their lives begins to disintegrate, giving rise to an anxiety state or worse.

Mental depression occurs more commonly in patients with IDD than in any of the other chronically painful spinal disorders. Acute psychotic disturbances, with mental confusion and aggressive, violent behavior in the post-operative period following disc excision and anterior interbody fusion have been reported in some cases (25).

The psychological testing of patients with spinal and limb pains is currently regarded as an essential part of the pre-operative studies that should be performed in establishing a diagnosis and in planning surgical treatment. In particular, observations of behavior during the course of physical examinations can be important in determining a patient's likely response to surgery (26).

In patients with IDD, psychological factors must be considered in the context of the syndrome as a whole, with the sure knowledge that even major disturbances in behavior can be reversed after appropriate surgery. Without such an approach, these disabled patients may be denied access to the surgery which, in the present state of knowledge and practice, is most likely to cure them.

CHANGES IN BODY WEIGHT

Patients with lumbar disc prolapse are usually otherwise well, as are those with many of the degenerative forms of spinal disorders which cause chronic back and limb pains, and in whom weight loss is not seen. On the other hand, patients with infective diseases and neoplasms of the spine are often obviously ill and exhibit weight loss.

Because mechanical and degenerative interpretations of disc disorders have so influenced the conventions of history-taking, it is unusual to question patients with spinal pain about their body weight. Consequently, patients

with IDD—despite numerous consultations with different doctors—may never have been asked about changes in their body weight. Vital clinical information will therefore have been overlooked.

In cases of IDD, weight loss ranging from a few to as many as 20 kilograms may occur within the first 3–4 months following the injury and onset of pain. Less often, patients will report a marked increase in their weight, which they usually relate to decreased physical activity.

LOSS OF ENERGY

These patients nearly always complain of profound fatigue after physical activities which aggravate their spinal and limb pain. Parents of young adolescents with this disc disorder often draw attention to this aspect of their child's symptoms.

INVESTIGATIONS

Plain Radiography

Unless clear evidence of vertebral instability can be demonstrated on films taken in flexion and extension, plain radiographs are of no value in establishing this diagnosis (21). However post-operative tomographs provide the best evidence of union in interbody fusion.

Computerized Tomography

CT is likewise of no value in making this diagnosis, unless performed after discography, when the abnormal spread of dye in the disrupted disc can be shown in three planes.

Discography

In the past, this has been the key investigation in the diagnosis of IDD because the other imaging modalities —plain radiography, myelography, computerized tomography, epidurography, venography, and ultrasonography—fail to demonstrate this non-prolapsing disc disorder.

Indications for the use of discography have been clearly defined by the North American Spine Society (22). Discography remains important where more than one lesion is demonstrated by MRI or where there is disagreement in the interpretation of the MRI (Figs. 3, 4, and 5). Discography will then provide a series of images in the radiographs which, with the assistance of CT images in the horizontal, coronal, and sagittal planes, can add to the accuracy of diagnosis. The discogram provides vital information, not only in relation to imaging

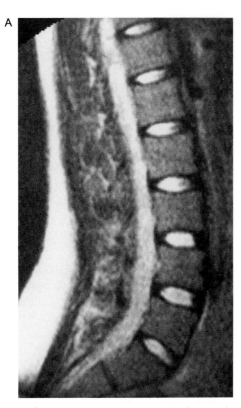

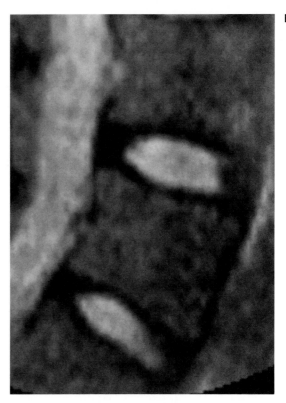

FIG. 3. MRI of the lumbar spine of a female patient age 17. **A:** Lateral mid-sagittal view. On superficial examination all the discs from T11 to the sacrum appear normal. **B:** A detailed view of the discs between L4-L5 and L5-S1. At L5-S1 there is a subtle change in the T2-weighted image of the nucleus with the suggestion of forward extension of nuclear material into the annular fibers of the disc. This patient presented with a classic syndrome of intractable low back pain associated with referred leg pain. Symptoms had been aggravated by physical activities and by physical therapy. The patient had marked loss of energy, and weight loss had occurred early after the onset of symptoms. Plain x-rays and CT scans of the lumbar spine had been reported as normal. Because of these changes at L5-S1, CT discography was undertaken.

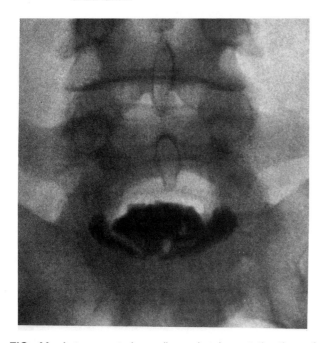

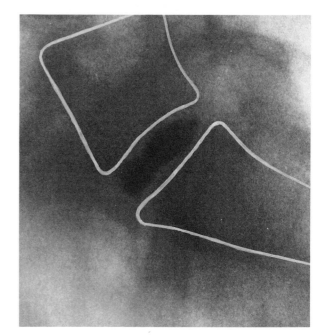

FIG. 4A. Antero-posterior radiograph taken at the time of discography. This discogram was performed using a double-stiletted needle technique with a single transdural midline puncture to position the needle in the midpoint of the disc before injection. In the antero-posterior view, dye can be seen spreading on either side of the nuclear shadow outlined in black.

FIG. 4B. The lateral radiograph showing excessive spread o dye within the disc space. The volume injected was 2.2 ml; the injection of dye with the patient under light narcosis reproduced her back pain.

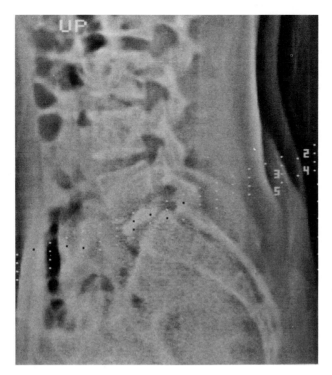

FIG. 5A. Lateral tomogram following discography. The spread of dye in the disc space is abnormal.

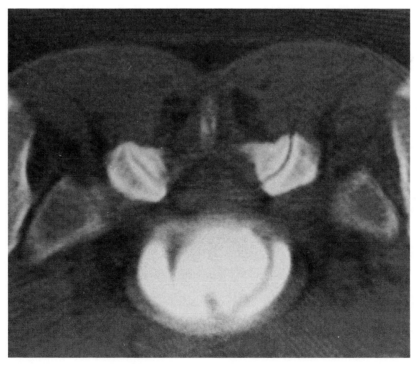

FIG. 5B. CT discogram taken within 15 minutes of the injection of dye into the disc space viewed in the axial plane, showing radial extension of dye on either side of an overfilled nucleus.

in the disc space but also regarding the volume of dye which, usually, should not exceed 1.0–1.5 ml in normal lumbar discs. Any greater volume indicates that the internal structure of the disc is disrupted. Furthermore, the character of the pain reproduced during the injection is similar to that which the patient experiences clinically but is usually of greater severity. In normal discs this pain reaction does not occur; in patients with IDD it is marked and immediate.

Discography has been associated with a significant incidence of discitis, which usually takes the form of localized vertebral endplate erosions on either side of the nucleus, giving rise to excruciating spinal pain and protracted disability in many instances. The research of Fraser (12,13) indicates that the incidence of this complication may be significantly reduced by using stiletted needles—19 gauge to penetrate the skin and 22 gauge passed through the "guide" needle to penetrate the disc —and by mixing the radio-opaque dye with a small volume of a broad-spectrum antibiotic before injecting it into the disc.

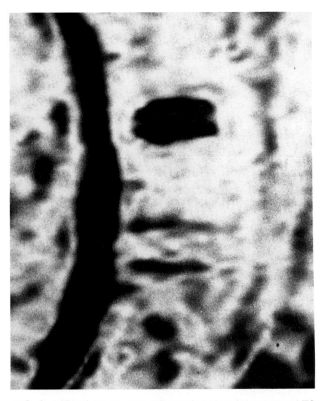

FIG. 6. MRI of the lower lumbar spine showing a normal T2-weighted image of the nucleus of the L4-L5 area. At L5-S1 there has been loss of signal from the nucleus but a high signal is noted in the region of the vertebral endplates on either side of the disc space where the horizontal subarticular collecting veins of the vertebral bodies are found. The images may represent changes in the vertebral marrow surrounding these veins brought about by the movement of irritant catabolites out of the disc (with permission from ref. 8).

Magnetic Resonance Imaging

This has become the most important diagnostic test for IDD, largely replacing discography. Nevertheless, the significance of many of the findings referred to in MRI reports is still not clearly understood.

Patients with IDD show changes in the signals generated from the intervertebral disc and sometimes from signals within the adjacent vertebral bodies (Fig. 6). Surgeons should be confident in diagnosing the condition from the MRI, since recognition of this syndrome is only gradually entering the field of radiology. MRI and CT reports often refer only to space-occupying defects in the spinal canal due to disc pathology or to the pathology of degenerative spinal disease.

It is crucial that an interchange of ideas between spinal surgeon and radiologist be encouraged, for the full value of the use of MRI, and even of CT scanning, will only be realized in future, when radiologists-in-training spend time in spinal clinics and in operating rooms with spinal surgeons. In this way, they would acquire first-hand knowledge of the range of clinical problems and of the pathology seen at operation, and so be able to extend the usefulness of the imaging techniques at their disposal, and to provide more accurate reports for their colleagues.

SITES OF LESIONS

IDD occurs most commonly in the lower lumbar intervertebral discs, often at a single level. Upper lumbar lesions are rare, but should be suspected in patients who complain of high lumbar pain associated with abdominal discomfort.

In the neck, these lesions generally occur at C5-C6 or C6-C7, although discs at higher levels are occasionally affected. IDD in the cervical spine may occur as a result of various mechanisms of injury, including whiplash. The symptom complex usually includes disabling occipito-frontal headache in addition to neck and arm pain and lethargy.

TREATMENT

Surgical treatment is indicated in those patients with IDD who have become seriously disabled and who have failed to respond to routine conservative methods of treatment administered over many months.

Symptoms can be controlled with a small range of drugs: analgesics, non-steroidal anti-inflammatory preparations, narcotics, anticoagulants and antibiotics (at the time of surgery), and psychotropic agents. Steroids have little place in the treatment of this syndrome, even though they have been administered to these patients orally and by injection into discs, facet joints, epidural and intradural spaces.

Disc excision and anterior interbody spinal fusion is the most effective operation for the persistent, disabling symptoms that may occur either in the cervical or lumbar spine. The surgical techniques for this operation are detailed in Chapter 91 and are also described in the books listed in the references (4,7,17).

RESULTS

The overall results of the surgical procedure, as the first operative intervention in patients with IDD, are more than 80% good in cases when one disc is involved and fall to about 70% when there is multi-level involvement (Fig. 7). Two series have carefully analyzed the results, Fujimaki et al. (14) and Blumenthal et al. (1).

Fujimaki (14) analyzed the author's results in 75 male and 75 female patients, who had operations at 188 disc space levels. The age range was from 19 to 62 years, the mean age was 41.6 years. Eighty-four of the cases had this procedure as the first and only spinal operation; a second group of 38 cases had supplementary operations performed following the interbody fusion. In this last group of patients, the second operation was a planned decompression of the spinal or nerve root canal. The majority of the procedures for single-level fusions were at L5-S1, while in double-level fusions, the majority were at L4-L5 and L5-S1.

The overall rate of radiologic union was 96%. Table 1 lists the results as measured by return to work and combines all three patient cohorts.

Blumenthal (1) studied 34 patients who had no prior surgery, and who fulfilled the author's criteria of IDD. Twenty-one (62%) were males, the age range was 15 to

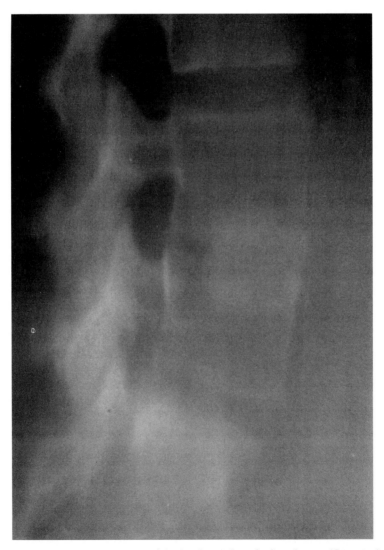

FIG. 7. A lateral tomogram of the lumbar spine of a female age 45 treated for IDD at L4-L5, showing interbody fusion 6 months after operation.

TABLE 1. *Summary of findings*

Group	Occupation		Time off (months)	Resumed same occupation	Other occupation	Did not return to work
1	Nonsedentary	49	11.8	39	7	3
	Home duties	18	3.3	16	1	1
	Sedentary	17	7.4	17	0	0
	Total Group 1	84				
2	Nonsedentary	23	24.0	14	6	3
	Home duties	7	5.6	6	0	1
	Sedentary	8	6.5	7	0	1
	Total Group 2	38				
3	Nonsedentary	19	16.5	10	3	6
	Home duties	5	11.5	3	1	1
	Sedentary	4	12.5	2	0	2
	Total Group 3	28				

With permission from ref. 14.

66, with an average of 36 years. The duration of symptoms ranged from 3 months to 10 years and averaged 29.4 months. The levels fused were 19 (53%) at L5-S1, 11 (32%) at L4-L5, and 5 (15%) at either L3-L4 or L2-L3.

The average duration of follow-up was 29 months and a successful result was defined by return to work or normal activities, no requirements for medications, or a non-steroidal anti-inflammatory agent only. Twenty-five of the 34 patients (74%) achieved a satisfactory clinical outcome, with an average time out of work of 6.1 months. The rate of fusion varied by level and by smoking. The poorest rate of fusion was 55% at L4-L5, while a higher rate of 100% was obtained at the upper lumbar levels, and 80% at L5-S1. It is important to point out that the union rate was overall 82% for non-smokers and 63% for smokers. The clinical success rate did not strictly correlate with the presence or absence of fusion. In patients with a successful result, the union rate was 73%, while for those with non-union, the success was 62.5%.

It is important to point out that allograft was used in all but 7 patients, although the rate of non-union in the small number of patients with autograft was the same as those treated by allograft.

The reported complications in the first series were minimal, attributed to the extraperitoneal approach. Deep vein thrombosis was present in 3%; infections and retrograde ejaculation were rare but not quantified for this series. In Blumenthal's 34 patients two complications were reported, one a graft extrusion, and one retrograde ejaculation.

These two series illustrate that a clinical success rate, as measured by return to work, can be accomplished by proper techniques of anterior interbody fusion in a significant percentage of patients with the diagnosis of IDD.

REHABILITATION

Rehabilitation after anterior spinal fusion commences with mobilization a few days after surgery. The use of a bed which can be tilted to the vertical allows these patients to stand comfortably within 24 hours of surgery and to take a few steps away from the bed within 36 hours. Patients and their relatives should be informed of the likely time schedule of recovery. Even in an uncomplicated case, with fusion at a single level, and performed within a relatively short time (4 to 6 months) of the onset of symptoms, full recovery is likely to take 6 to 9 months, extending to 12 to 18 months for multi-level fusions. Only in exceptional cases can any of these patients return to work in less than 6 months from the time of operation.

In the early months, the importance of maintaining the patient's morale becomes paramount. This is best achieved by team care, the team including the patient's family physician and surgeon, together with a specialist in physical medicine, a physical therapist, and a psychologist or psychiatrist. As the patient struggles to regain mobility, physical fitness, and self-esteem, the slightest set-back from overexertion will lead to mood fluctuations and rising anxiety. During this time, skillful manipulation of drug therapy is often required for the management of problems such as drug dependence, paralytic ileus, gastrointestinal side-effects due to the prolonged use of analgesics, and other reactions to psychotropic drugs.

Many of these patients have been injured at work and have claims for compensation pending. Medical examinations are therefore carried out at the request of insurance companies. These are performed by doctors who do not always contact the patient's treating team. The patient may be forced to perform spinal movements beyond the limits already achieved through carefully supervised physical therapy. Regrettably, the patient may emerge from these encounters in severe pain, thoroughly demoralized and with rehabilitation consequently set back by many months.

CONCLUSION

Internal disc disruption is a form of disc disease usually brought about by trauma. It gives rise to disabling spinal and limb pain, without producing the abnormal neurological signs which are usually found in cases of disc prolapse requiring surgery, namely limitation of straight leg raising, diminution or loss of reflexes in the extremities, and sensory impairment in the dermatomes.

IDD is associated with constitutional disturbances in the patient, reflected in profound loss of energy after activity and often in marked loss of body weight.

Being a non-prolapsing disc disorder, IDD can only be diagnosed with the use of special investigations such as MRI, discography, and CT-discography. Plain radiography, CT scanning, and radiculography—any of which may be useful in identifying disc prolapse—are of no use in the diagnosis of IDD.

Radiological factors such as these, in conjunction with subtle aspects of the patient's presentation, render IDD a condition inherently easy to overlook. Patients with IDD whose symptoms have, in error, been attributed to prolapsed intervertebral disc, will be made worse by the operation of disc fragment excision, an operation which would have produced a good result, had their lesion in fact been a disc prolapse.

The theory presented in this chapter, which has been used to explain IDD, is based on clinical observations supported with the results of special imaging techniques, on the basis of which the operation of disc excision and anterior interbody fusion was performed. The results of these operations have shown that patients with this syndrome can be improved, and many can be cured (1,14).

There is, at present, no proof of the chemical basis of this theory. We hope the challenge of defining the histopathological processes behind this clinical condition will soon be taken up by biochemical scientists. Resolution of this enigma should lead to the future management of disc disorders by pharmaceutical means.

Meanwhile, we should not forget the clinicians and surgeons of the past, who made progress in treating serious diseases long before the identification of their scientific bases. Kocher, for example, was awarded the Nobel Prize for Medicine in 1909 for his work in thyroid surgery. It was not until five years later that Kendall discovered thyroxine.

REFERENCES

1. Blumenthal SL, Baker J, Dossett A, Selby DK (1988): The role of anterior lumbar fusion for internal disc disruption. *Spine* 13:566–569.
2. Brickley-Parsons D, Glimcher MJ (1984): Is the chemistry of collagen in intervertebral discs an expression of Wolff's Law? *Spine* 9:148–163.
3. Brown MD (1983): *Intradiscal therapy.* Chicago: Year Book Medical Publishers, p. 173.
4. Cauthen JC, ed. (1983): *Lumbar spine surgery.* Baltimore: Williams & Wilkins, p. 225.
5. Cloward RB (1952): Lumbar intervertebral disc surgery. *Surgery* 32:852–857.
5a. Cloward RB (1963): Lesions of the intervertebral discs and their treatment by interbody fusion methods. *Clin Orthop* 27:51–77.
6. Crock HV (1970): A reappraisal of intervertebral disc lesions. *Med J Aust* 1:983–989.
7. Crock HV, Bedbrook G (1983): *Practice of spinal surgery.* New York: Springer Verlag, p. 319.
8. Crock HV, Goldwasser M, Yoshizawa H (1988): Vascular anatomy related to the intervertebral disc. In: Ghosh P, ed., *The biology of the intervertebral disc, vol. 1.* Boca Raton: CRC Press, p. 109–133.
9. Crock HV, Yoshizawa H (1977): *The blood supply of the vertebral column and spinal cord in man.* New York: Springer Verlag, p. 129.
10. Crock HV, Yoshizawa H, Kame SK (1973): Observations on the venous drainage of the human vertebral body. *J Bone Joint Surg* [Br] 55:528–533.
11. Dandy WE (1941): Concealed ruptured intervertebral disks: Plea for elimination of contrast mediums in diagnosis. *JAMA* 117:821–823.
12. Fraser RD (1990): Personal communication.
13. Fraser RD, Osti OL, Vernon-Roberts B (1987): Discitis after discography. *J Bone Joint Surg* [Br] 69:26–35.
14. Fujimaki A, Crock HV, Bedbrook GM (1982): The results of 150 anterior lumbar interbody fusion operations performed by two surgeons in Australia. *Clin Orthop and Related Res* (165):164–167.
15. Holt EP Jr (1968): The question of lumbar discography, *J Bone Joint Surg* [Am] 50:720–726.
16. Jason MIV, ed. (1987): *The lumbar spine and back pain.* Edinburgh: Churchill Livingstone, p. 463.
17. Lin P, Gill K, eds. (1989): *Lumbar interbody fusion.* Rockville: Aspen Publishers.
18. Lindblom K (1948): Diagnostic puncture of intervertebral disks in sciatica. *Acta Orthop Scand* 17:231–239.
19. Mixter WJ, Barr JS (1934): Rupture of the intervertebral disc with involvement of the spinal canal. *New Engl J Med* 211:210–215.
20. Modic MT, Masaryk TJ, Ross JS (1989): *Magnetic resonance imaging of the spine.* Chicago: Year Book Medical Publishers, p. 280.
21. Morgan FP, King T (1957): Primary instability of lumbar vertebrae as a common cause of low back pain. *J Bone Joint Surg* [Br] 39:6–22.
22. North American Spine Society (1988): Position statement on discography. *Spine* 13:1343.
23. Onik G, Helms CA, eds. (1988): *Automated lumbar discectomy.* San Francisco: Radiology Research and Education Foundation, p. 144.
24. Rothman SLG, Glenn WV Jr (1985): *Multiplanar CT of the spine.* Baltimore: University Park Press, p. 520.
25. Stevenson HG (1970): Back injury and depression. A medico-legal problem. *Med J Aust* 1:1300–1302.
26. Waddell G, McCulloch JA, Kummel E, Venner RM (1980): Nonorganic physical signs in low-back pain. *Spine* 5:117–125.
27. Weinstein J, Claverie W, Gibson S (1988): The pain of discography. *Spine* 13:1344–1348.

The Adult Spine: Principles and Practice,
J. W. Frymoyer, Editor-in-Chief.
Raven Press, Ltd., New York © 1991.

CHAPTER 98

Failures After Spinal Fusion

Causes and Surgical Treatment Results

John P. Kostuik and John W. Frymoyer

  J. P. Kostuik, M.D., F.R.C.S.(C): Professor of Orthopaedics, University of Toronto, Toronto, Ontario; and Head, Combined Division of Orthopaedic Surgery, Toronto General/Mount Sinai Hospitals; Chief, Dewar Spinal Unit, The Toronto Hospital, Toronto, Ontario, Canada M5G 2C4.
  J. W. Frymoyer, M.D.: Professor of Orthopaedics, Director, McClure Musculoskeletal Research Center, Department of Orthopaedics and Rehabilitation, University of Vermont, Burlington, Vermont, 05405.

The early enthusiasm for lumbar spinal fusion as a treatment for low back pain with or without sciatica had decreased considerably because of the poor results. In the past five years, however, enthusiasm has again increased for a variety of reasons: The causes of failure have become better understood; new operative techniques, such as rigid internal fixation, have allowed fusion to be performed more predictably and more difficult adult deformities to be corrected; and new diagnostic tests such as MRI and discography have led to a better understanding of the causes of lumbar pain, particularly those associated with degenerative conditions. Although some of the diagnoses are still debated, for example "disc disruption," surgeons are treating them aggressively, and are demonstrating good results.

In other instances, surgeons now are dealing with the late consequences of prior fusion, whose treatment may require further stabilization. With these developments, there is an even greater need to understand the sources of failure that accompany spinal fusion and how these problems can be managed when they occur.

In this chapter, we consider an overview of the causes of failure after lumbar fusion and discuss the general approach to the patient with respect to the history, physical, and imaging information that is useful. We then detail the causes of failure in terms of how often they occur, how they are recognized, and how they are treated. Finally, there is an overview of the results that may be obtained. Although spinal fusion is employed for a variety of pathologic conditions, we have focused the chapter on the later failures that follow fusion for degenerative conditions.

Chapters that have dealt with specific pathologies, such as tumor, infection, trauma, and major thoracolumbar deformities, have detailed the failures that follow arthrodesis in those conditions.

OVERVIEW OF FAILURE AFTER LUMBAR FUSION

Failures can be simplistically viewed as being due to three causes, which are known as the three W's: the wrong patient, the wrong diagnosis, and the wrong surgeon. However, this approach does not account for the problems that follow a properly performed fusion in the right patient, for the right diagnosis. Such failures can represent unavoidable complications, or can result from ongoing degenerative disease. Nevertheless, the three W's are a useful starting point.

It is simple to eliminate the wrong surgeon. Jones (36) reviewed 180 residency training programs, of which 88% believed spinal surgery was an important component of clinical practice. However, only 74% provided what was deemed to be adequate training. Today, spinal surgery is about to enter the twenty-first century. The current state of the art in this field is approximately comparable to joint replacement surgery 15 to 20 years ago. Because of the increasing complexity of spinal surgery, and the increasingly sophisticated techniques and instrumentation, we believe the spinal surgeon of tomorrow will need to have completed a fellowship and devote the majority

of his time to spinal problems for these complex techniques to be mastered.

The wrong patient is a more complex problem, and can be divided into two general categories: The patient was chosen for treatment by fusion when the pathology at hand could not be expected to benefit from that operation, or the patient's psychosocial circumstances and expectations simply precluded success. An example of the former is the utilization of spinal fusion for a patient with non-specific, chronic, disabling low back pain, where history, physical examination, and imaging studies indicate no definite pathology. In these circumstances, failure rates as high as 80% are recorded, leading most authorities to conclude that spinal fusion has no role in the management of non-specific spinal pain. Similarly, the psychosocial determinants of success and failure in spinal disease and surgery have been emphasized throughout this text. This issue is again reviewed in Chapter 91 as it relates to arthrodesis and its indications.

The wrong diagnosis is an even more complex issue and ranges in cause from inadequate imaging studies that led to misdiagnosis all the way to a poor choice of surgical technique from the large menu of alternatives that are currently available to the spinal surgeon.

A more specific classification for the failures of spinal fusion is shown in Table 1. Here we have divided these failures by the time of appearance as well as the predominant symptom that occurs. The importance of a temporal division was emphasized by Finnegan (24) in the analysis of failures of both decompression and fusion. When the patient has no immediate relief, the wrong diagnosis or the wrong operation should be suspected. When the patient has immediate relief and then has recurrent symptoms within weeks to months following the operation, new pathology or a complication of the operation should be suspected. When the patient has good relief, and months to years later has recurrent symptoms, new pathology or ongoing degeneration should be suspected. Table 1 shows the relative distribution of failures as a function of time after surgery.

It should be emphasized that in Table 1 we are not referring to leg symptoms that relate to an original decompression performed in conjunction with a fusion, since this topic has been covered extensively in Chapter 89. Rather, we are referring to leg symptoms independent of the original pathology, which in the case of prior fusion are more likely to suggest spinal stenosis rather than a single-level radiculopathy.

In addition to these general sources of failure, there are also specific systemic and local complications that follow spinal fusion. In some instances, these complications may cause symptoms that are at times more devastating to the patient than the condition for which treatment was initially sought. These complications will be detailed later in this chapter.

TABLE 1. *Causes of failure after spinal fusion*

Time	Back pain predominant	Leg symptoms
Early (weeks)	Infection	Nerve impingment by fixation device or cement
Mid-term (months)	Wrong level fused	
	Insufficient levels fused	
	Psychosocial distress	
	Pseudarthrosis	Fixation loose
	Disc disruption	
	Early adjacent disc degeneration	Early adjacent disc degeneration
	Inadequate reconditioning	
	Graft donor site	Graft donor site
Long term (years)	Late pseudarthrosis	Disc with pseudarthrosis
	Adjacent level instability	Adjacent level stenosis
	Acquired spondylolysis	Adjacent level disc
	Abutment syndrome	Stenosis above fusion
	Compression fracture above fusion	

APPROACH TO A PATIENT WITH A FAILURE FOLLOWING FUSION

History and Physical Examination

A complete history and physical examination is essential, and all prior historical records, operative reports, and imaging studies need to be reviewed. A history of never having pain relief strongly suggests that the wrong pre-operative diagnosis was made or wrong operation performed, whereas a long interval of relief and return to function followed by insidious onset of symptoms suggests a late degenerative lesion. Obviously if the patient did not have relief, never returned to function, and had a long pre-operative interval of disability, the possibility of psychosocial dysfunction should be strongly entertained.

The physical examination rarely gives a precise diagnosis, particularly if the original surgery included a decompression. Limitation of spinal motion is a non-specific symptom of failure rather than an identification of its causes (28). Similarly, limitation of motion is frequently associated with psychosocial dysfunction, particularly in patients who appear to have had the right operation and achieved a solid fusion. Leg symptoms should be carefully analyzed. If the patient had no leg symptoms and a normal neurologic examination prior to the first operation, and the current examination shows deficits, this is of major importance and suggests a high probability that there is new pathology or a complication due to a fixation device. If the patient had leg symptoms before the first operation, the neurologic findings are most likely residual, unless an entirely new set of objective deficits is present. If the patient has diffuse leg symptoms as part of the overall pain complaint, it is common for these to be localized to the graft donor site. However, the usual graft donor complaints seem to be highly associated with overall failure of symptomatic relief rather than due to a specific complication at the donor site (29).

Psychological Testing

The psychosocial issues are major in evaluating a patient with failed fusion, particularly in those patients who have not had a pain-free interval and returned to normal function prior to the new onset of symptoms. The numerous techniques available have been detailed by Keefe, and the issues that must be considered in the specific planning for a fusion are presented in Chapter 91.

Plain Radiography

The plain radiographs must be interpreted with care. In post-operative patients it is common to identify disc space narrowing and even excessive motions at the adjacent functional spinal segment. For example, a positive Knuttsen's sign is identified in 20% of patients at the L3-L4 level above an L4 to the sacrum fusion, but few have symptoms (28). However, a number of radiographic signs are particularly useful: (a) the unequivocal presence of a pseudarthrosis; (b) a pars defect above a midline fusion, most commonly at the L3 lamina; or (c) an obvious failure of instrumentation with cutting out of devices attached to the lamina, or breakage of screws; a more subtle sign may be a halo around a pedicle screw, indicating motion in an apparently solid fusion.

The addition of motion radiography is a subject that has been analyzed in Chapter 90. However, this is an important test in the identification of pseudarthrosis, as originally stressed by Bosworth and Cleveland (9). Because some motion is common, particularly in a solid midline fusion, it is important to identify at least four degrees of motion before a pseudarthrosis can be suspected with confidence (28). The major difficulty lies in accurate centering and positioning of the patient for the flexion and extension view. Translation of 3 to 4 mm is also diagnostic of abnormal motion.

Bone scintigraph is rarely indicated, but is helpful on occasion in a patient suspected of having an infection, or occasionally when a pseudarthrosis is suspected but is not confirmed by flexion-extension films and tomography.

Most spinal fusions show increased uptake up to two years following fusion. Significant "hot spots" within the general area of increased uptake or a localized area two years or more following fusion may be indicative of a pseudarthrosis.

CT Scans

The CT scan is invaluable in assessing the bony canal. In one series, it reportedly demonstrated unanticipated failures in 13% of cases, most of which were secondary to improper diagnoses prior to the first operation (62). The test is particularly enhanced by the addition of myelographic dye, which remains the most sensitive mechanism to identify spinal stenosis. In patients with apparent instability and stenotic symptoms, it is important to obtain a flexion and extension view with the dye in place before proceeding to the CT scan. CT scans, especially if enhanced by myelographic dye, are valuable post-surgically for the assessment of canal contents, but may easily miss a transverse pseudarthrosis if the cut is not at the appropriate level. These deficits may be overcome by three-dimensional CT or MRI reconstructions, which may prove to be of great value in the assessment of fusion mass integrity. For example, Laasonen and Soini (47) studied 48 patients with a painful lumbosacral fusion by careful CT scanning. Sixteen had unsuspected fragmented grafts, and 9 had hairline pseudarthrosis, which might have caused their symptoms. Similarly, hypocycoidal frontal plane tomography was investigated by Dawson et al. (16) and revealed unsuspected pseudarthrosis in patients who had previous fusions for scoliosis. The imaging evidence for pseudarthrosis was later confirmed by surgical exploration.

Pseudarthroses occur in two modes: transverse or plate pseudarthroses. The former is the traditional well-known form of pseudarthrosis. The latter is a failure of the graft material to unite with the underlying laminae and/or transverse processes despite the fact that the fusion mass, derived from the graft material, is solid.

Myeloscopy

Myeloscopy was initially felt to provide the answer to many of the problems of continued radicular pain following surgery. This, however, has not met universal enthusiasm and has been abandoned in most centers. Its value may lie in the assessment of arachnoiditis, but not of bone.

Facet Blocks

These are discussed elsewhere (see Chapter 25). The problem with facet blocks in a failed surgical case is that the presence of scarring frequently inhibits an accurate infiltration of the anesthetic agent; hence, in the failed case, this may be of limited value. It is of value in assessing levels proximal in previous fusions, however. As well, the local infiltration of anesthesia into a pseudarthrosis may help delineate whether or not the pseudarthrosis is the cause of the patient's pain. Infiltration may be done into both anterior and posterior pseudarthroses. The infiltration of local anesthesia around internal fixation devices may help to delineate whether these may be a cause of post-operative pain. However, the sensitivity and specificity of these techniques are unknown.

Discography

Discography can be used in two fashions: one to assess disc degeneration and the other as a pain provocative test. As a method of assessing disc degeneration, MRI is at least as valuable and of course is non-invasive.

Discography may be used to diagnose painful levels within an area of obvious disc degeneration as noted on plain radiographs, but it is perhaps more reliably used as an assessment of discs proximal to obvious degenerative levels both to determine minor degrees of degeneration and as part of the pain provocative study.

Macnab (personal communication) has stated that discography is valuable in proving whether posterior pseudarthrosis is a painful source or not. He felt that reproduction of pain on discography at the suspected level of pseudarthrosis proved that the pseudarthrosis was the source of pain. We have not been fully convinced of his belief. It is often technically difficult to perform discography in the presence of a previously performed posterolateral fusion with or without pseudarthrosis. We prefer to do discography from a posterolateral rather than a transdural approach.

The patient with a previous fusion who continues to have pain may have two sources of pain, which can be differentiated with the aid of discography. When the patient has had a previous L4 to the sacrum fusion and presents with pain sometime post-operatively, perhaps many years post-operatively, the use of discography at levels above the fusion may help to see whether these are a source of subsequent pain or continuing pain. Similarly, discography may be of value at interspaces under a previous fusion. In a small number of patients with continuing pain who were normal on plain and dynamic x-rays, and did not have a pseudarthrosis, pain was reproduced on discography (73). Subsequent anterior procedures with disc excision and fusion resulted in relief of pain. We feel that these cases are examples of what Crock

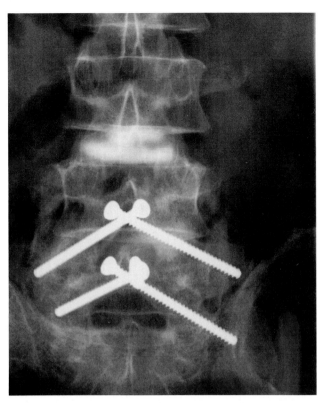

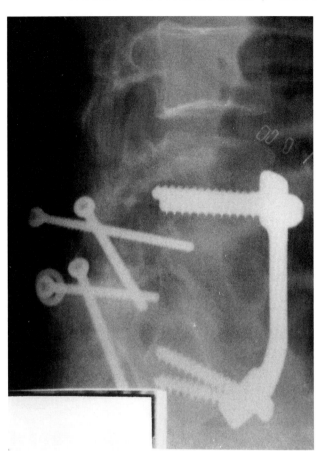

FIG. 1. A 53-year-old male, operated on for segmental instability of L4-S1; AO translaminar screws were used. Pre-operative discography at L4-S1 and L5-S1 reproduced his pain. Post-operatively, pain persisted despite a solid fusion. Repeat discography at L4-L5 reproduced his pain despite the solid fusion. L3-L4 discogram was normal.

FIG. 2. Same patient as in Figure 1. Anterior L4-S1 interbody fusion (I plate was added for fixation) relieved his pain.

(Chapter 97) described as internal disc derangement, which can occur beneath a solid fusion (Figs. 1 and 2).

Nachemson (57) has recently criticized discography. The reason he gave was that the outer part of the annulus has a multilevel nerve supply, as does the dorsal longitudinal ligament. This may result in difficult and false interpretations. The criticism that previously normal pain-free people may have pain from a discogram is not valid, since the point is whether or not the discogram reproduced the patient's typical pain in the same area and of the same quality. As well, in a significantly degenerative disc, pain may not occur with discography, since there are so many annular tears it is impossible to raise the interdiscal pressure to a sufficient degree to reproduce pain. In these instances, the fluid medium used to inject and raise pressure escapes too rapidly.

Discography has, in our hands, helped us to differentiate the painful from non-painful levels and to aid in the assessment of the number of levels requiring fusion. It has been of particular value in the failed back patient.

Use of External Fixator

Esses, Kostuik, and Botsford (23) recently compared pre-operative testing with the AO external fixator (Figs.

3, 4, 5, 6, and 7), plain x-rays, and discography in 30 patients with chronic low back pain. The clinical improvement by use of rigid external fixation proved to be a good predictor of the result of posterior fusion, which was not the case for discography or pain reproduction by discography. However, this series was small and requires repetition with larger numbers. Although Esses et al. (23) have shown that external fixation may be a good predictor of outcome following spinal fusion, a similar unpublished study by Olerud did not come to the same conclusion, after initially reporting (61) success similar to that of Esses et al. Further evaluation of this physical modality as a method of prediction of the outcome of a spinal fusion is necessary.

Let us now look at the specific causes of failure that occur after lumbar spinal arthrodesis.

CAUSES OF EARLY FAILURE

Infection

The rate of infection following lumbar surgery is variable, dependent on the era in which the operation was performed, operative time, history of prior surgery, the approach employed, and the use of antibiotics and in-

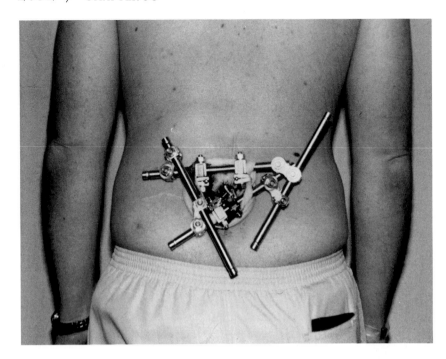

FIG. 3. A 39-year-old male presented with a two-year history of disabling low-back pain. Plain films were unremarkable (except for traction spur). L4-L5 was unstable on flexion-extension radiographs. No discograms were done. See also Figures 4-7.

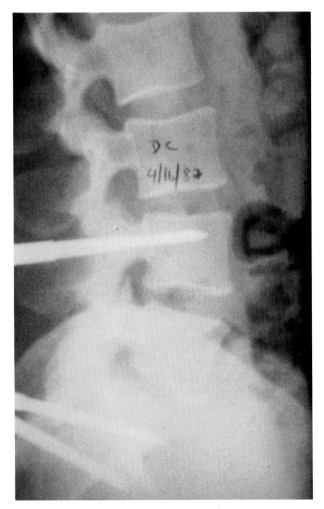

FIG. 4. Same patient as in Figure 3. A temporary internal fixator was placed with relief of symptoms.

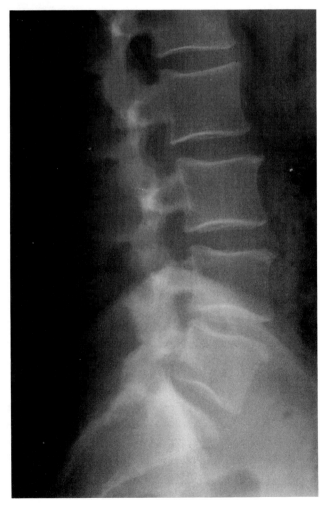

FIG. 5. Same patient. Temporary internal fixator.

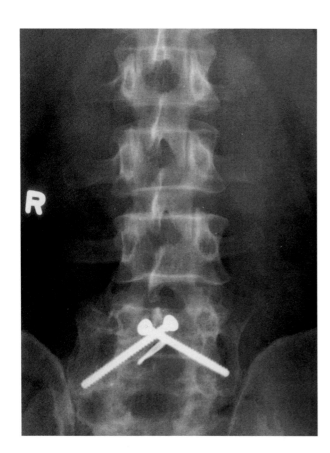

FIG. 6. Same patient then underwent a two-level fusion of L4-L1. Despite a solid fusion, pain persisted.

FIG. 7. Same patient. Discograms done at L3-L4 revealed a degenerative painful disc. L2-L3 was normal. The fusion was extended one level and the pain was relieved.

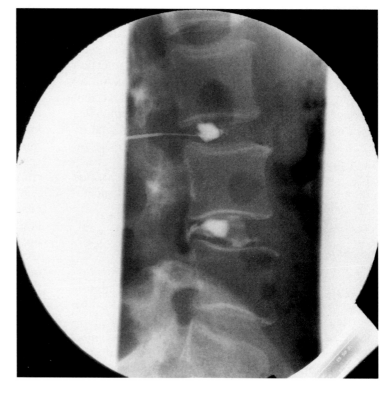

strumentation. Rates less than 1% and greater than 10% have been recorded. In general, the lower figures have been reported in the past decade. In 1966, Prothero (63) reviewed 1,000 cases of midline and intertransverse process fusion and compared patient cohorts treated a decade apart. The operative indications were multiple; the overall infection rate of 3.4% was no different for the two time intervals. At about the same time, Freebody (26) reported an incidence of wound infection of 3.0%. The highest rate of recently reported infection was 13% (77) in patients treated with pedicle fixation, which was attributed to the long operative time that resulted from a steep learning curve, rather than to the use of instrumentation per se. Although there is no certain proof, Kostuik and Hall (45) felt that anterior fusion had a lower rate of infection than the posterior approach. In 100 anterior fusions performed for burst fractures together with decompression and instrumentation, Kostuik noted one deep infection. In 67 cases of anterior fusion and instrumentation performed for degenerative disease or previous failed posterior surgery, no deep infections occurred. One deep infection occurred in 108 cases of anterior instrumentation and fusion for scoliosis. No infections occurred in 205 cases of kyphosis instrumented and fused anteriorly.

Whether this infection rate can be reduced by antibiotics is debatable. A generally accepted but not proven belief is that antibiotics are warranted with fusions, particularly if metallic devices are implanted. In an early retrospective and uncontrolled study, Fogelberg (25) reported lower infection rates in both spine and hip surgery with the use of post-operative penicillin. In a similar, uncontrolled study, Lonstein (52) reported infection rates of 2.8% with antibiotics and 9.3% without antibiotics, in patients treated for scoliosis with and without Harrington instrumentation. If antibiotics are employed for prophylaxis, a general body of basic and clinical research supports the drug being given pre-operatively, intra-operatively, and for as little as 24 hours post-operatively. This teaching is opposed to the historic belief that antibiotics should be administered for longer post-operative intervals.

Presentation

The classic presentation of deep wound infection is five to seven days post-operatively. Rarely, infections can occur in the first twenty-four hours. We have encountered one such patient with *Streptococcal* infection. The clue was a rapidly developing sore throat and a watery hematoma, suggesting bacteriologic fibrinolysis. Dependent on host immunologic competency and the virulence of the organism, the presentation ranges from high-grade fever and severe pain to an indolent course, often accompanied by delay in diagnosis. Superficial

signs may be notably absent in a large, muscular, or obese patient.

Treatment

A superficial wound infection can be appropriately treated by antibiotics and relief of any local wound tension, including drainage to the fascia. In deeper infections, the issue is whether or not to remove instrumentation and/or graft, and whether to debride and leave the wound open, or to debride and close the wound over suction drainage. This decision is dependent on the patient's magnitude of sepsis, the condition for which the operation was performed, and the organism. In general, we have performed debridement, washed the bone graft, left the instrumentation in place, and closed the wound over suction drainage or a suction irrigation system. Exceptions to this general approach may be warranted when a gram negative organism such as *Pseudomonas* is causative. Obviously if the original indication was for severe spinal instability, particularly when associated with neurologic involvement, every effort should be made to retain the fixation device.

Wrong or Insufficient Levels Fused

Patients with wrong or insufficient level fusions usually are identified only when a significant time interval has elapsed after the operation, although their failure for symptomatic relief is noticeable soon after the operation. Usually their post-operative symptoms are attributed to wound healing; later, pseudarthrosis is often suspected. The most apparent source of failure of this type is when a surgeon fails to perform a fusion over the area of obvious pathology, equivalent to failure to decompress a known disc herniation. In the older literature, a common cause of failure was thought to occur when the surgeon overlooked two-level lumbar disc herniations when combined decompression and fusion was performed.

It will be remembered that some clinical reviews recorded that two-level lesions occurred in up to 10% of patients (58). For that reason, many reports stressed the importance of two-level decompressions and fusion in all patients with suspected L5-S1 or L4-L5 disc herniations. Today's sophisticated imaging techniques make these earlier recommendations obsolete. However, this issue is more difficult when subtle pathologic conditions are being treated, such as disc disruption or degenerative scoliosis (see Figs. 6 and 7). Elsewhere in this text (Chapter 22) recommendation is made for performing discography at all lumbar levels until a morphologically normal disc is identified and the patient has no pain reproduction. This is a controversial view. The use of MRI also is controversial in this regard; Zuckerman (77) and Kornberg (41) each report a small group of patients with normal MRIs later shown to have an unequivocally positive discogram.

In the older literature, the extent of the fusion was often based on the plain radiographic findings, such as disc space narrowing and osteophytes. When the primary indication was lumbar disc disease, more than two-level degeneration was used as a contraindication to L4 to the sacrum fusions. For this reason, many authorities believed that a floating fusion at L4-L5 should never be done. Fusion that involved L4-L5 was thought to necessitate an L5-S1 fusion as well. However, Brodsky (5) has shown that satisfactory results can be obtained with the floating fusion, providing the L5-S1 level is carefully analyzed. We have advocated that the extent of a fusion in complex degenerative conditions be determined by pre-operative facet blocks and discography, although the precise sensitivity and specificity of these tests have yet to be established. At this time there is no certain data that tell us how often missed levels cause failures of spinal fusion.

Presentation

As previously noted, fusion at the wrong level is suspected only after a significant time delay in all but the most gross and obvious omissions. Back pain that fails to improve during the first three months would suggest this diagnosis, but frequently it is only when the fusion is solid that this type of failure is suspected. In these instances, the differential diagnosis typically is pseudarthrosis or that the wrong patient was chosen. In the latter instance, the patient may falsely be assumed to have psychosocial or compensation issues that are the cause of symptoms.

Treatment

The treatment is based on establishing that the fusion was inadequate in its extent or the wrong levels were fused. This decision necessitates the use of all of the pre-operative analytic techniques outlined earlier in this chapter (Figs. 5, 6, and 7).

Psychosocial Distress

The issues of psychosocial distress and compensation and their effects on the incidence of later surgical failures have been detailed in prior chapters. The presentation in those chapters was to emphasize that the important time to identify these factors is before the operation, not after it. Finnegan et al. (24) have stressed the importance of this causation.

The analysis of entrants into rehabilitation programs also emphasizes the commonality of psychosocial dis-

tress and compensation in the etiology of fusion failures (1). How commonly this failure occurs is uncertain. In one series in which fusion was performed in conjunction with disc excision, 15% of patients had no obvious causation for their continued pain and disability (28).

Nerve Root Impingement

We are not including here early failures due to pre-operative misdiagnosis, intra-operative errors, or nerve root complications, such as scarring, that follow decompression. These are detailed in Chapter 89. The major cause of nerve root impingement that directly relates to fusion today is usually a result of internal fixation devices, particularly those involving the pedicle. Chapter 97 analyzes these issues, including strategies for its avoidance, in detail. However, the most important insight on this problem is derived from Weinstein's (75) study of screw misplacement, when experienced and inexperienced surgeons performed the operation in cadaver specimens set up to simulate a real procedure, including C-arm radiographic control. Misplacement of the screws occurred in 21% of all pedicles, many of which were in

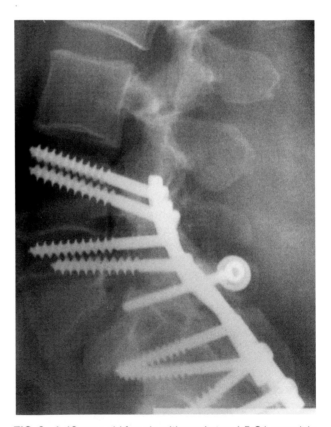

FIG. 8. A 42-year-old female with grade two L5-S1 spondylolisthesis. Discography revealed a typically painful L4-L5 disc. Facet blocks at L4-S1 and L5-S1 relieved her pain. Arthrodesis was done using contoured AO-DCP plates and screws. One screw missed the L5 pedicle resulting in root pain, while two screws appear to be in the disc space of L4-L5.

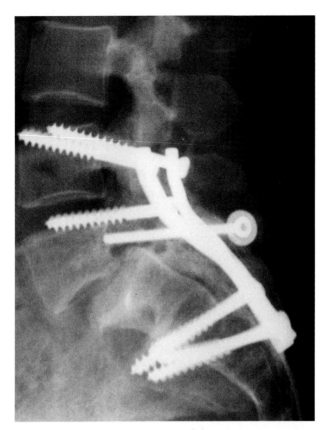

FIG. 9. Same patient as in Figure 8. The screw was removed and symptoms abated. A solid fusion was obtained. The sacral screws are in the ala and thus appear too long in the lateral projection, while one L4-L5 screw remains in the disc space.

close proximity to the nerve (Figs. 8 and 9). The addition of methylmethacrylate to increase holding strength is an additive factor, since thermal and mechanical damage can result (see Chapter 33).

This cause of failure is also observed in devices that depend on laminal fixation, and is usually due to a jumped hook. A particularly high rate of nerve root complications is noted with the Knodt rod.

The problem usually relates to the lumbosacral area, and necessitates rod removal in 20% to 50% of patients (see Chapter 95). In general, nerve root symptoms, when they occur with this device, are a later rather than early complication. Causations of nerve root impingement, specific to one or another fusion technique, include nerve root traction injury or graft extrusion. The incidence of graft extrusion with posterior lumbar interbody fusion varies, and was reported in 1 of Cloward's 321 cases (10), 4 of Lin's 500 cases (50), and 4 of Collis's 750 cases (12). Lin (51) suggests that the overall rate is 0.3% to 2.4%, but for inexperienced operators the rate is a disturbing 9%. The rate of nerve root damage is less certain, although Lin (51) noted a temporary dropped foot in 25 of 500 patients (5%), but all but 3 recovered in 6

months. With posterior fusion techniques, neurologic deficit or pain may occasionally result from graft material becoming dislodged, or from an unrecognized fracture of a facet, producing a fragment that causes nerve impingement. How often this occurs is unknown, but it is probably rare.

Presentation

The diagnosis is most suspect in patients who have had no pre-operative nerve root symptoms and early after their surgery have neurologic deficit or pain. More difficult is a patient who had nerve involvement, had a decompression in combination with the fusion, and whose post-operative symptoms are increased deficit or pain. In these instances, a large differential diagnosis is necessary, as detailed in Chapter 89.

The diagnosis is also complicated because of the presence of metal, which may make imaging techniques such as MRI impossible or CT scans difficult to interpret because of image scatter. In these cases, it may be necessary to resort to polytomal tomography, with or without myelographic enhancement, although when the screw misplacement or fixation displacement is obvious, plain radiographs will suffice (see Figs. 8 and 9).

These same diagnostic issues also come into play when later nerve root symptoms occur. Assuming that the nerve root compression is within the area encompassed by the fusion, fixation device displacement should be considered. Usually when this occurs, there may be obvious clues from plain radiography, e.g., jumped hook, or the diagnosis may be suspected by the presence of a radiolucent "halo" around one or more portions of the device.

Treatment

Dependent on the magnitude of symptoms and neurologic deficits, the options range from doing nothing until the fusion is mature to immediate removal in more severe cases, and replacement of the screw or an alternative fixation device.

CAUSES OF MID-TERM FAILURE

Pseudarthrosis

Pseudarthrosis is the most common cause of failure in spinal fusion. It is also the most difficult to establish as the source of failure, because many patients will have radiographic evidence of fusion failure with no symptoms (17,28).

Conversely, repair of a pseudarthrosis often will not result in symptomatic relief. For example, one long-term follow-up study of patients who had undergone re-fusion demonstrated satisfactory results in only 60% of the patients who had repair of a pseudarthrosis (27). It is, however, anticipated that today with better means of internal fixation this will be improved upon.

The calculation of the rate of pseudarthrosis is highly variable and dependent on the following factors: (a) the number of levels fused; (b) the fusion technique, including the type (e.g., anterior interbody, midline posterior) as well as the presence or absence of internal fixation; (c) the source of bone graft; (d) the underlying pathology for which the fusion was performed; (e) constitutional and other factors, such as age and possibly sex of the patients and their smoking habits; (f) the type of external protection afforded the patient; and (g) the radiographic criteria utilized to assess for the presence or absence of pseudarthrosis. These issues have been discussed in Chapter 91, and again are mentioned here to emphasize that the rate of pseudarthrosis cannot be calculated unless there is full knowledge of the relevant variables that influence its occurrence. In posterior surgery a one-level fusion usually bears an incidence of pseudarthrosis of 5%. For two levels, this may increase to as high as 20%, and for three or more levels, to 40% or greater in fusions performed to the sacrum (54).

In anterior surgery, the incidence of pseudarthrosis for one- or two-level anterior fusions is in the area of 20%. Given the current state of internal fixation devices, no clear statistics are available as to the incidence of pseudarthroses. This is particularly true for failed back surgery. Jacobs et al. (35) have recently shown that with the use of AO translaminar screw fixation (Fig. 10), the incidence of pseudarthrosis is approximately 5%. These were in previously unfused patients. Kostuik (43), in a review of internal fixation devices for various etiologies of low back pain, has shown that in three or more levels of lumbosacral fusion, with the use of Luque sublaminar wires and $\frac{1}{4}$-inch Luque rods, the incidence of pseudarthrosis was reduced to 15% (Fig. 11). This study was done prospectively in a consecutive series and represented a significant decrease from 40% without internal fixation.

The same author studied a series of 56 patients who had previously undergone posterior spinal fusion that had failed because of pseudarthroses (42). Following anterior fusion with the aid of internal fixation devices, including the use of single-cable Dwyer or single-rod or double-rod Zielke systems, the incidence of pseudarthrosis was 18%. When double-rod systems alone are analyzed, the incidence of pseudarthrosis decreased to 9%. Current improved methods of anterior fixation should decrease this even more.

Clinical Presentation

The clinical presentation of pseudarthrosis is highly variable and ranges from no symptoms to significant

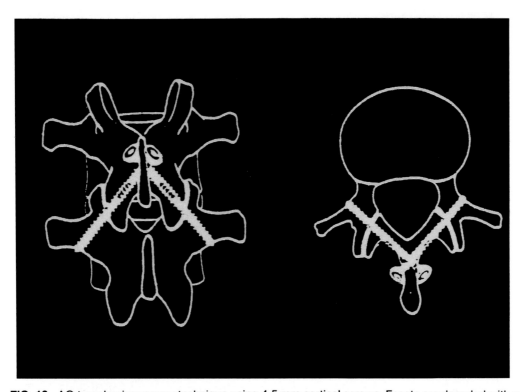

FIG. 10. AO translaminar screw technique using 4.5 mm cortical screws. Facets are denuded with a burr or curette of articular cartilage, and packed with cancellous bone graft. The laminae and transverse processes are decorticated with a burr. The screws aim for the base of the transverse process (with permission from ref. 35). (See also Fig. 1.)

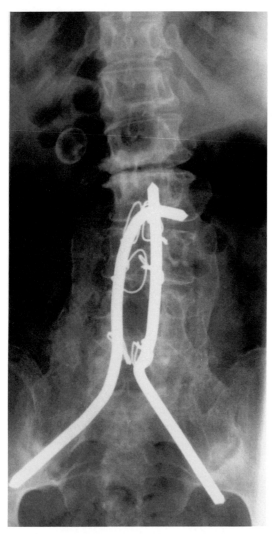

FIG. 11. A 48-year-old female underwent an L3-S1 fusion using Luque rods and sublaminar wires. She did well for ten years but developed mild back pain and degenerative changes above her fusion at L2-L3.

persisting and disabling back pain (17,28). Rarely should pain be ascribed to a pseudarthrosis until a 6-month interval has elapsed, and even then, continued motion may not necessarily indicate that the fusion is a failure. For that reason, we usually do not consider fusion failure to be present until the patient is one year post-operative, unless there are obvious reasons to reach that conclusion, such as graft dislodgement or an obvious failure of fixation. Frequently a pseudarthrosis may remain undetectable for years.

Because pseudarthrosis can be asymptomatic, it is important to evaluate the patients for other sources of continued symptoms or recurrent symptoms. The strategies that have been used to determine a symptomatic pseudarthrosis were presented earlier in this chapter.

Treatment

Because pseudarthrosis frequently accompanies other causes of failure, we will consider surgical treatment of this condition later in this chapter.

Disc Disruption

This issue has been discussed in general during the discussion of wrong diagnosis. However, there is a small subset of patients who achieve a solid arthrodesis yet continue to have symptoms. This usually occurs when the first operation has been a posterior fusion technique, and the continuance or onset of new symptoms occurs in the face of a solid fusion. Biomechanical studies have suggested that an apparently continuous graft may nevertheless allow continued deflections of a magnitude sufficient to cause symptoms (48,65,76). In these instances, discography may be employed to determine the diagnosis, although this technically may be difficult because of obstructing bone between the transverse processes.

Treatment

If a solid posterior fusion is present, the obvious solution is an anterior interbody technique. If disc disruption is part of the presentation of a pseudarthrosis, then anterior fusion or circumferential fusion, with or without instrumentation, may be considered (Figs. 1 and 2).

Early Adjacent Disc Degeneration

Rarely does degeneration cause symptoms in the months after spinal fusion in a segment that was normal prior to the operation. The exceptions may be cases in which rigid internal fixation or possibly circumferential fusion has been performed. Hsu, Zuckerman, and White (34) reported accelerated degeneration with internal fixation, while Dewar (18) reported that this complication occurred with circumferential fusion. This led him to abandon the technique.

Presentation

The typical presentation of degeneration adjacent to a fusion will be detailed later in this chapter, but it is important to stress here that the single most unequivocal indication of accelerated degeneration is a new disc herniation at the level adjacent to the fusion (Fig. 12). More common is the development of disc degeneration, without herniation, resulting in instability (Figs. 13, 14A, and 14B) or spinal stenosis.

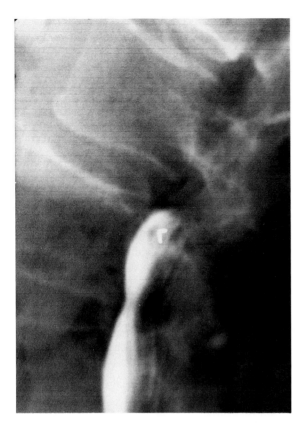

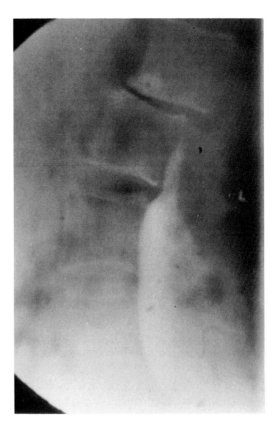

FIG. 12. L5-S1 fusion performed two years previously. The patient developed a degenerative slip 18 months later. An acute disc sequestration was found in addition to the spondylolisthesis at L4-L5. The fusion was extended to L4 with internal fixation following decompression.

FIG. 13. A 58-year-old female had spinal fusion 18 years previously. Myelogram demonstrates flow defects proximal to the fusion (L2-L3) with retrolisthesis at L2-L3 and L1-L2.

A

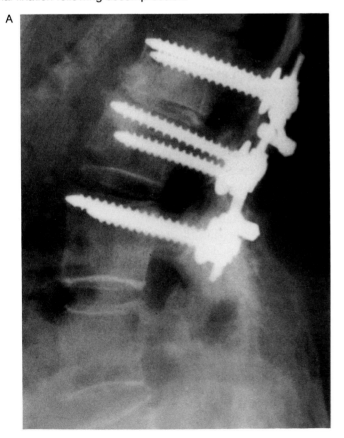

B

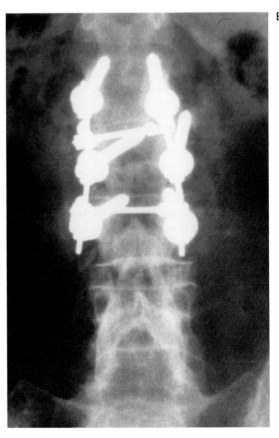

FIG. 14. The fusion was extended to L1 with Zielke instrumentation **(A and B).** Symptoms were relieved.

Treatment

The treatment is identical to that for later degeneration and will be presented there.

Graft Donor Site Problems

This issue is discussed in a separate section later in this chapter.

Inadequate Reconditioning

There is very little data that can establish how often patients are inadequately reconditioned. However, it must be a common problem, based on our clinical experience. Very often patients are referred either because they are thought to have an anatomic failure of fusion or because they are thought to have psychosocial or compensation factors interfering with their recovery. Where those problems leave off and inadequate conditioning enters in is less relevant than the knowledge that the two often go hand in hand. Frequently, these patients have had long periods of disability and deconditioning prior to the first operation, complicated by the fact that posterior fusion techniques denervate the paraspinal muscles.

Clinical Presentation

Continued back pain, particularly that which increases with physical activity (i.e., mechanical pain), must be suspected to be caused by inadequate reconditioning in all patients, unless the causation is obvious and anatomic. Thus, pseudarthrosis cannot be considered the source of symptoms until rehabilitation has occurred.

Treatment

It can be argued that a chronically debilitated patient can be returned to function solely by outpatient physical therapy or a functional restoration program. If these methods are chosen, the operating surgeon must take an active role in monitoring the program and establishing a time limit for achieving the goal. Too often, a patient will continue month after month with a combination of inadequate reconditioning and emphasis on modalities. The general principles and approach outlined by Hazard (Chapter 13) would suggest that more intensive, multidisciplinary rehabilitation is appropriate in those patients who fail to respond to less structured programs. The surgeon constantly finds himself with the problem of when to repeat all studies and consider re-operation versus continuing the rehabilitation program. There is no certain guideline, other than the general principle

that the more certain the anatomic causation for pain, the more reasonable is surgical intervention; the less certain, the greater the reason to continue a non-operative approach.

CAUSES OF LONG-TERM FAILURE

Late Pseudarthrosis

The general issues in pseudarthrosis have already been presented. It is uncommon for a patient who has previously had symptomatic relief to present after one year with pain due to a pseudarthrosis. There are two general exceptions: The first is a disc herniation under a fusion. In a follow-up study of 10 years' minimum duration and an average follow-up of 13.7 years, Frymoyer (29) found that no patient with a solid fusion had a disc herniation. Of 23 patients who required a second operation, 13 required fusion for back pain only, 4 for a recurrent disc herniation at the same level as their previous surgery, and 1 had a new herniation at a new level, under the fusion.

All patients with new or recurrent herniation had a pseudarthrosis. Thus, a patient presenting with a disc herniation under a fusion must be highly suspect of having an accompanying pseudarthrosis. A less certain source of failure is in a patient who had spine fusion and later presents with symptoms and findings indicative of arachnoiditis. In this situation, it is less certain if some of the increasing symptoms can be alleviated by repair of the pseudarthrosis.

Treatment

Treatment of pseudarthrosis will be presented later. Obviously if a disc herniation accompanies the pseudarthrosis, this must be decompressed. The technique is identical for that described in Chapter 89, with the exception that the overlying graft must be removed with either high-speed burrs or osteotomes. The critical part of the procedure is the identification of the old lamina, which may be difficult if the original procedure was a midline fusion. Techniques of repair and approaches to the problem of surgical repair are discussed later in this chapter.

Adjacent Motion Segment Degeneration

Segments adjacent to a previously performed lumbar fusion are at risk for the later development of a variety of degenerative changes, which may be either asymptomatic or symptomatic, and may include the clinical and radiographic features of segmental instability, degenerative spinal stenosis, or lumbar disc herniation (4,49).

These changes are four times more likely to occur at L4-L5 (20%) when the original fusion was performed at L5-S1 for a degenerative condition, than at L3-L4 when the original fusion spanned from L5 to the sacrum, where the rate is 4% to 5% (28). Similarly, when the fusion was performed for thoracolumbar deformities, the magnitude of symptomatic degeneration increases the lower into the lumbar spine the original fusion was extended (11,33,53,56).

The dominant reason for these degenerative changes is mechanical. Fusions cause increased shear stresses, as measured experimentally and in humans with biplanar radiography (48,65,69). Inadvertent damage to facets or denervation may be contributory.

Asymptomatic Degeneration

Asymptomatic degenerative changes may include osteophytes, disc space narrowing, hypermobility with or without translation (i.e., a positive Knuttsen's sign), and spinal stenosis. A comparison of plain radiographic findings 10 or more years after patients were treated with or without fusion is shown in Table 2 (28). This table demonstrates the high rate of degenerative changes, which were unrelated to symptoms. In particular, claw spurs were more common in heavy laboring males above the fusion. Hypermobility was also more common. A subsequent study by Lehmann (49) in 1987 analyzed patients 30 or more years after fusion, and included CT studies as part of the radiologic evaluation. Almost 50% of patients had radiographic evidence of segmental instability and/or spinal stenosis. Again, these radiographic findings in general were unrelated to symptoms. He found, however, that 85% of patients were satisfied with their outcomes 30 or more years after their spinal fusions.

Because there is a high incidence of radiographic changes, the most difficult clinical task is to determine whether the level above the fusion is causing symptoms in a patient who has back pain alone. In these instances, discography is the procedure of choice, in our opinion. If segmental instability is present, the problem is also complex. In these instances, discography, and possibly facet blocks, may again be useful to determine whether the lesion is symptomatic (Figs. 13, 14A, and 14B).

Spinal Stenosis

The diagnostic problem becomes significantly easier if the patient has peripheral symptoms of claudication. Brodsky (4) in particular has stressed that this is the most common cause of recurrent symptoms after a fusion. Although he reported a large number of cases, it was impossible from his study to determine the actual incidence of this late cause of failure (Figs. 15A–15E).

Disc Herniation

This is the easiest problem to diagnose with certainty, because the clinical symptoms, physical findings, and confirmatory images are typical. How often true disc herniation occurs varies widely. In the 10-year study by Frymoyer (29), a 4% rate at L3-L4 was found in fusions that spanned from L4 to the sacrum, which is similar to that reported by DePalma and Rothman (17).

Treatment

The treatment of failures above fusion is largely based on the pathology, but in our opinion should usually include spinal fusion, combined with appropriate decompression based on the pre-operative symptoms, physical findings, and radiologic images. In general, the accompanying fusion should include instrumentation, particularly when the segment is unstable. However, selected cases may be appropriately treated by posterior fusion techniques or anterior interbody fusions with instrumentation (Figs. 16A–16C).

Spinal Stenosis Under a Fusion

This is almost exclusively a problem with posterior midline fusion. Macnab (55) thought it occurred in 20% of all patients treated previously with that technique, but later Brodsky's (4) clinical experience suggested that this was a significant overestimate of the problem. His opinion is supported by Lehmann's (49) finding that a stenotic appearance was common under a midline fusion many years after the operation, but rarely were symp-

TABLE 2. *Comparison of radiographic findings in fusion and non-fusion patients*

Variable	Fusion patients (%)	Non-fusion patients (%)	Significance
Traction spurs L3–L4	14.3	34.3	$0.01 > P < 0.025$
Traction spurs L4–L5	6.1	19.4	$0.01 > P < 0.025$
Claw spurs L3–L4	50.0	22.5	$P = 0.005$
Facet subluxation L1–L2	70.8	45.0	$0.01 > P < 0.025$
Facet subluxation L3–L4	82.8	64.0	$P = 0.025$

With permission from ref. 28.

toms of spinal stenosis present. The presumed etiology is hypertrophy of the graft over time in response to Wolff's law. Interestingly, stenosis has never been reported as occurring beneath a fusion performed in adolescence or adult life for scoliosis. The majority of cases reported by Macnab had had their fusions done prior to the common recognition of the spinal stenosis syndrome. Thus, it is quite possible that they had this condition prior to their first operations (Figs. 17A–17D).

Clinical Presentation

The condition is suspected in a patient with long-standing midline posterior fusion, insidious and progressive symptoms of spinal stenosis, and imaging studies that demonstrate absence of significant stenosis above the fusion and significant stenosis beneath it.

Treatment

The treatment is decompression. This is made difficult by the massive amount of bone that overlies the lamina and the inability to identify the old lamina and scar. In very difficult cases, it may be necessary to go to the next level to identify tissue planes and move back from that level. In that event, the fusion should be extended, unless the level is anatomically normal, and minimal bone sacrifice is necessary.

Acquired Spondylolysis

This is almost exclusively a later cause of failure in posterior midline fusion and is reported in 0% to 2.5% of patients treated by that technique (8,28,32,64,66,72) (Fig. 18). The causation is thought to be secondary to repetitive mechanical forces, and can be produced in the laboratory after simulated posterior midline fusion (65). Weakening of the neural arch by overzealous decortication and possibly interference with the blood supply have also been suggested contributors (55). It has been rarely reported with transverse process fusion (2).

Treatment

The treatment is stabilization and fusion by anterior interbody or posterior intertransverse process fusion, with or without instrumentation.

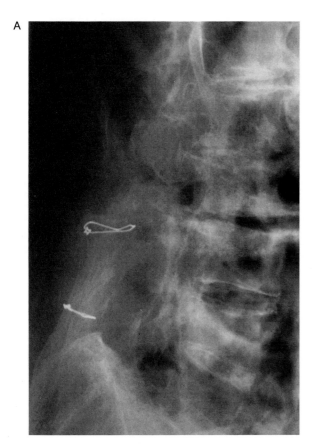
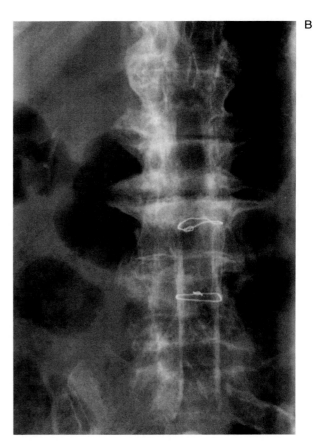

FIG. 15. A 76-year-old female had a three-level midline tibial graft fusion **(A and B)** 35 years previously with an excellent result (she was an orthopedic chairman's secretary). (Figs. 15C–15E follow.)

C
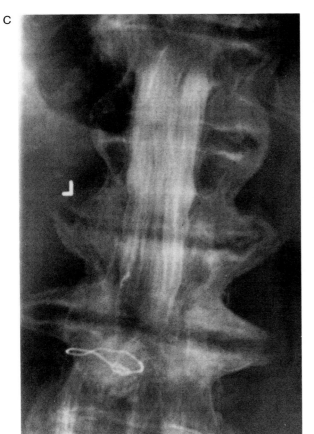

D
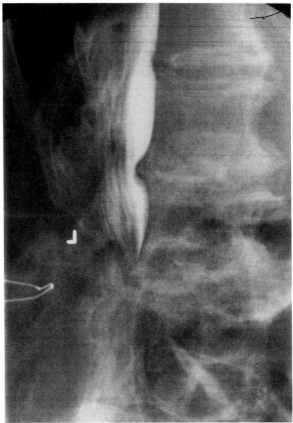

E
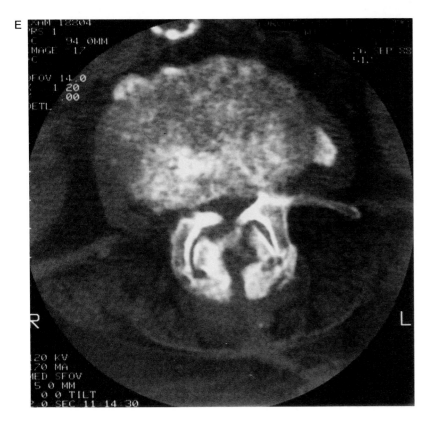

FIG. 15. *Continued.* Pre-operative myelogram **(C and D)** and CT **(E)** demonstrate a complete block with very severe spinal stenosis at the level immediately proximal to the fusion. She became paraparetic with grade 1-2 power and loss of bowel and bladder control. One year following decompression, she walks with one cane and has complete bowel and bladder control.

A

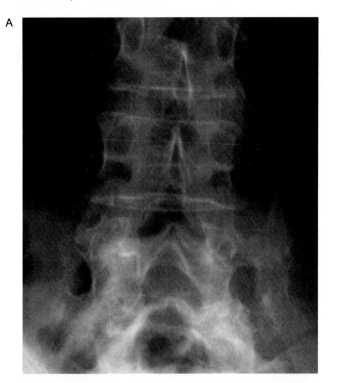

B

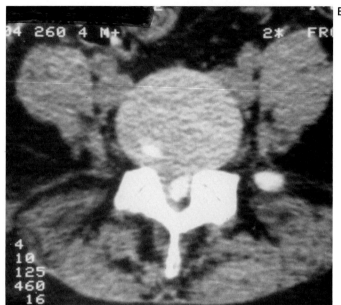

C

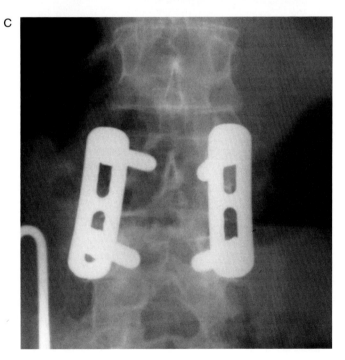

FIG. 16. A 46-year-old female **(A)** had prior disc excisions of L4-L5 and L5-S1. She presented with a solid arthrodesis, but recurrent back and leg pain. Myelographically enhanced CT scan **(B)** demonstrates a disc herniation at L3-L4. Decompression revealed a sequestrated disc **(C).** A fusion supplemented by Steffee plates was performed with symptom relief.

A
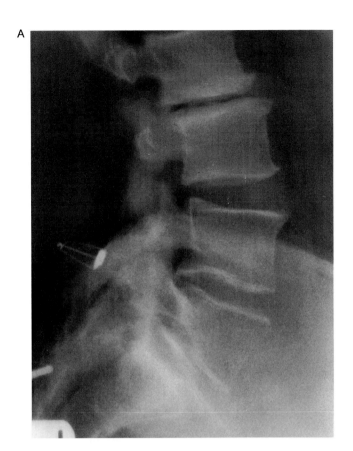

B
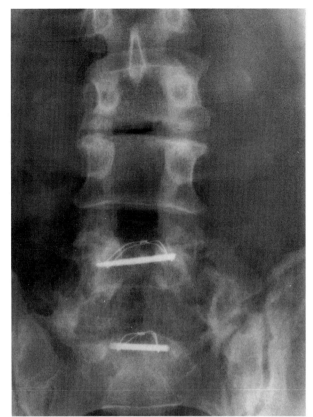

C
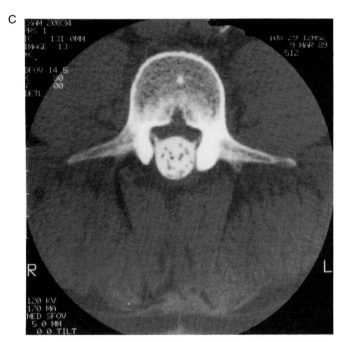

D
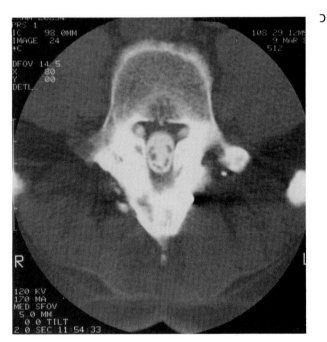

FIG. 17. A 51-year-old male had undergone a two-level fusion 21 years previously **(A and B).** He developed symptoms of spinal stenosis confirmed by myelographically enhanced CT from L2 to L4. He underwent decompression with only partial relief of his symptoms. A repeat myelographically enhanced CT scan **(C)** shows full decompression at L3. At L4-L5, spinal stenosis persists **(D).** A further decompression was done with improvement. It is anticipated that the instability at L2-L3, L3-L4 may increase and require stabilization, which ideally should have been done at the time of the L2-L4 decompression.

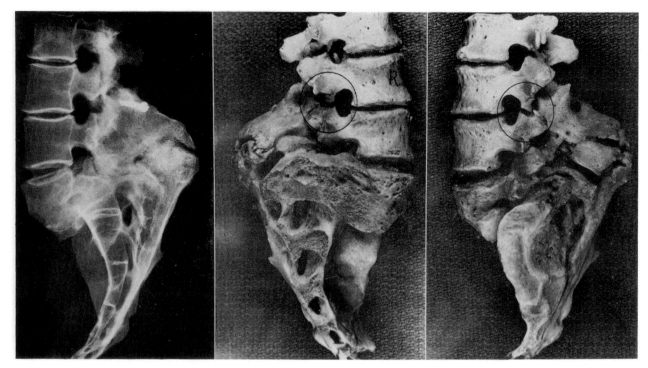

FIG. 18. Acquired spondylolysis above a fusion (from the collection of the late Dr. R. I. Harris). This patient underwent an L4-S1 fusion for a severe spondylolisthesis when she was a young woman. She did well but later in life developed breast cancer and died. At autopsy the spine was harvested. A pseudarthrosis at L4-L5 was found plus an acquired spondylolisthesis at L3-L4, which was not present initially.

Abutment Syndrome

This complication was noted in early literature regarding posterior midline fusions (9) and has been reported in more recent literature to be an overlooked source of failure, particularly when the facets are involved (14,70). The etiology is either overzealous initial graft placement or later hypertrophy. The condition may be considered when motion pain occurs, particularly in extension, and radiographs show a large midline fusion mass, usually at L4, abutting on the spinous process of L3. Diagnostic anesthetic injections can be employed to confirm the diagnosis. Surgical management may include excision of the abutment or extension of the fusion to the next adjacent level.

GRAFT DONOR SITE PROBLEMS

The graft donor site may be a source of problems in general, while specific donor sites are associated with unique complications, particularly nerve entrapments.

Pain

Graft donor site pain is a common complaint of all patients, particularly in the early post-operative phase. How long the pain persists is debatable. Kurz et al. (46) states that it is common in up to 15% in the first three months. However, a long-term study (29) reported that 37% of the patients identified donor site pain 10 or more years after their operations. Statistical analysis made it uncertain whether the pain was actually related to the donor site or was part of a general pain syndrome. When donor site pain was present, it was more common if the graft had been taken from the same side as the original sciatica, and there is a high association among persisting back pain, leg pain, and donor site pain. These complaints occurred independent of any radiographic changes, such as degeneration, that occurred at the donor site. A positive Trendelenburg sign was seen in 18%, but appeared to be independent of patient complaints or sacroiliac disease.

Specific complications can occur, however, which are painful and require later treatment. These include sacroiliac disruption, when the graft is from the posterior iliac crest, herniae in both anterior and posterior grafts, and fracture at the graft donor site, typically from the anterior ilium. Heterotopic bone formation has also been thought to occasionally cause local pain, although in a long-term study, the presence of heterotopic bone bore little relationship to symptoms (27).

Sacroiliac Instability

Sacroiliac instability occurs rarely, and is rarely included in large series as a significant complication. It is discussed in detail in Chapter 104.

Fractures can also occur, usually an avulsion of the anterior wing of the ilium, and may necessitate internal fixation. Fractures extending into the acetabulum have been alluded to in the literature (13).

Similarly, herniae are an infrequent complication and are usually related to full thickness grafts. Bosworth described this complication in posterior iliac graft donor sites, as well as the technique for its repair (3).

Infection

The donor site as a local source of infection is reported by Kurz to be less than 1% (46).

Nerve Pain

Bone graft incisions may cause peripheral nerve injury, or later nerve symptoms may result from entrapments secondary to scar or occasionally heterotopic bone. The classic site is in the anterior ilium, where involvement of the lateral femoral cutaneous nerve produces meralgia paresthetica. This complication is reported in 1% to 14% of patients (74). Even more rarely, other cutaneous nerves such as the ilioinguinal, genitofemoral, or femoral nerve may become involved (13,46,68). In posterior grafting, the cluneal nerves are most commonly involved (Fig. 19). We advocate not using an incision of the crest that extends more than one

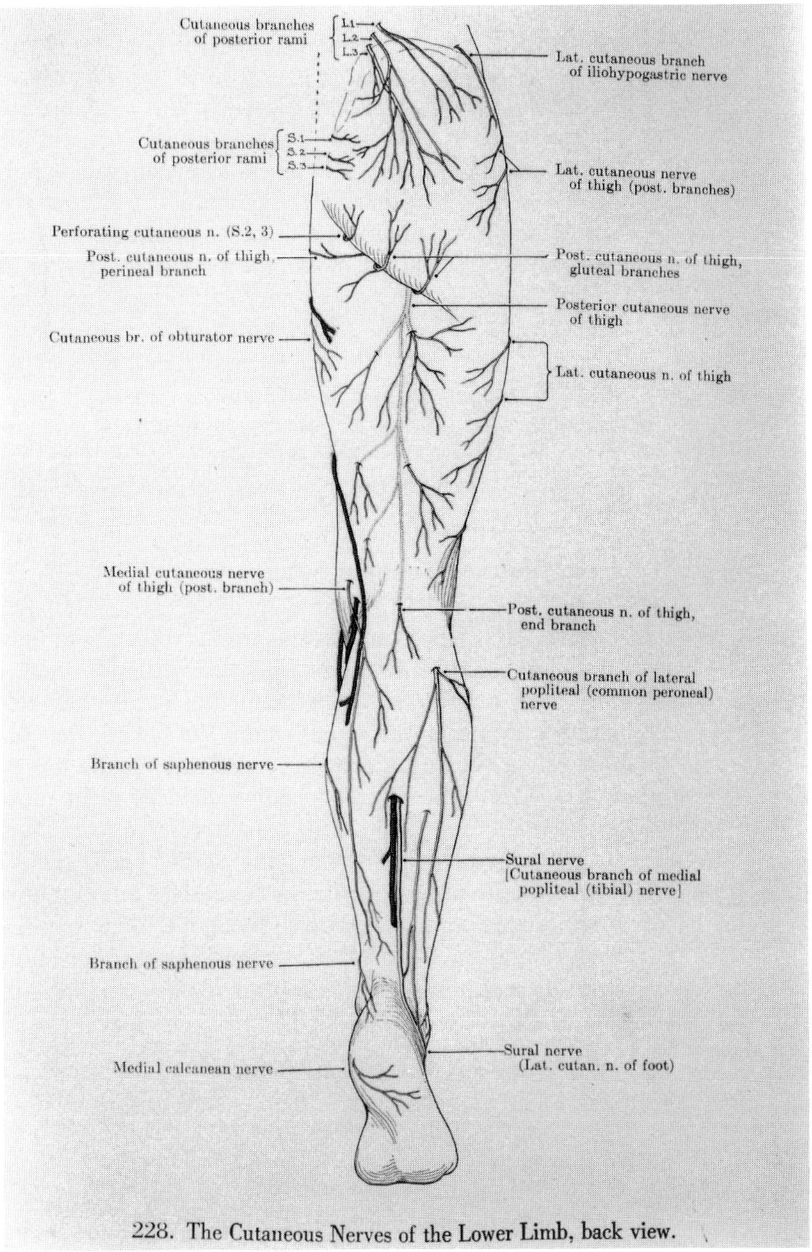

FIG. 19. Cluneal nerves pass over the iliac crest approximately 8 cm from the posterior iliac spine (with permission from *Grant's Atlas of Anatomy, 8th ed.,* Baltimore: Williams & Wilkins, 1983).

228. The Cutaneous Nerves of the Lower Limb, back view.

hand's breadth to help avoid this problem. The use of a hockey stick or tunneling procedure or longitudinal incision will avoid this problem. Drury (19) suggested that the diagnosis of cluneal nerve neuroma could be made by local anesthetic injections, and that resection of the neuroma could relieve that symptom.

In addition, a variety of more dramatic complications may include hemorrhage, particularly from gluteal arteries in posterior iliac grafts, and even visceral injuries.

TABLE 3. *Other complications*

Local	General
Posterior	
Early:	
Hemorrhage	Blood transfusion
Elchymoses	reactions
Wound dehiscence	Hemolysis
Neurological	Anemia
Laminal fracture	Urinary retention
Pedicle fracture	Sepsis
Sepsis	Metabolic disorders
Vascular (anterior)	Psychosis
Iliac crest	Drug overdose
	Hypotension
Anterior	
Early:	
Hemorrhage	Chocycystitis
Vascular (vessel)	Pancreatitis
Ureteric damage	+ All listed from
	Posterior
Renal damage	
Splenic damage	
Bowel damage	
Sympathetic disruption	
Iliac crest hemorrhage	
Iliac crest fracture	
Wound dehiscence	
Sepsis	
Graft extrusion	
Anterior and Posterior	
Intermediate:	
Wound sepsis	
Fracture at fixation points	
Instrumentation failure	
Vascular aneurysm (anterior only)	
Retroperitoneal fractures	
Ureteric obstruction (anterior only)	
Hydronephrosis	
Incisional hernia	
Iliac crest fracture	
Nerve irritation secondary	
to donor site	
Late:	
Late sepsis	
Instrumentation failure	
Donor site problems	
Retroperitoneal fibrosis	
Ureteric obstruction (anterior only)	
Hydronephrosis (anterior only)	
Vascular aneurysm (anterior only)	
Incisional hernia	

GENERAL COMPLICATIONS

Table 3 lists the array of complications that have been associated with lumbar spinal fusions, some of which are specific to a particular technique, and others of which are generic.

SURGICAL TREATMENT

Because there are so many different causes for failure after spinal fusion, the operative choices are numerous and carefully selected. Again, the general principle applies: The more certain the history, physical examination, and imaging studies, the more likely success will occur. In general, the most predictable results will occur in patients with leg symptoms rather than low back pain alone. Alternatively, uncertainty about diagnosis will predictably lead to less assured outcomes, particularly in patients with long-standing disability and psychosocial dysfunction. In this regard, pseudarthrosis is one of the most difficult conditions to assess as a source of symptoms, and not surprisingly the outcome from repair of pseudarthrosis is the most difficult to predict.

It should also be evident that the second, third, or even fourth operation introduces additional risks, including higher rates of infection and lower rates of successful fusion, as well as specific problems related to scarring and devascularization of bone and soft tissues.

A few general principles of surgical treatment are useful as one approaches these complex patients. They are categorized by the type of previous surgery performed.

Failed Previous Posterior Surgery

When adequate bone stock is present, the patient may again be approached posteriorly, particularly when a new level of pathology is present that necessitates decompression and new or re-fusion. We believe that fusion in general should be accompanied by the use of internal fixation, of which pedicle devices seem most useful (Figs. 20 and 21). If the decompression required is wide and involves additional facet sacrifice, serious consideration should be given to a second-stage anterior procedure. This need is particularly evident if there is inadequate bone stock for fusion or rigid posterior fixation cannot be obtained (Figs. 22A and 22B).

Failed Previous Posterior Surgery with Wide Laminectomy

If decompression is not necessary, and stabilization is the major object, this is best obtained with an anterior fusion. The presence of a wide laminectomy usually leaves inadequate bone stock for posterior re-fusion, par-

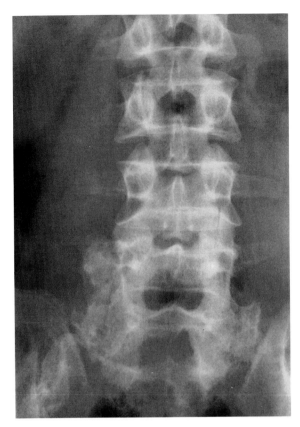

FIG. 20. A 42-year-old male underwent an L4-S1 intertransverse fusion without instrumentation two years previously. A pseudarthrosis at L4-L5 was believed to account for persistent pain.

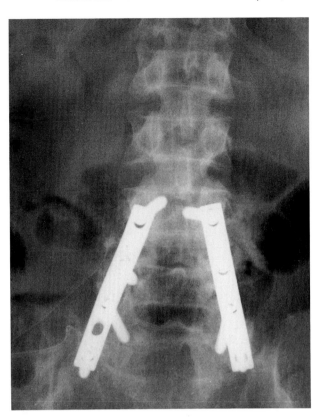

FIG. 21. A fusion at L3-S1 was performed using AO plates. Pre-operatively a discogram also revealed problems at L3-L4. Pseudarthroses were found at L4-L5 and L5-S1. The patient had good posterior bone stock and has gone on to solid fusion.

ticularly when there is extensive scarring and poor blood supply (Figs. 23A, 23B, 24A, 24B, and 25A–25D).

Failure of Two or More Previous Posterior Fusions

Under these circumstances, an anterior fusion is beneficial to achieve stability. Whether this is accompanied by anterior instrumentation will depend on the number of levels, as well as the specific levels, and the assessment of stability that might be achieved without instrumentation (Figs. 26A–26D and 27A–27D).

Failure of Previous Anterior Surgery

If there has been previous anterior surgery and a resultant pseudarthrosis, a posterior approach with internal fixation is the method of choice. However, patients who have had both prior anterior and posterior surgery are again better approached anteriorly. In either event, it is advisable to insert stents up both ureters to prevent inadvertent cutting of these structures, which is a risk because of retroperitoneal scarring. Even though the ureters still may be cut, the complication is easier to recognize and repair.

It is also important to realize that the additional retroperitoneal scarring caused by additional procedures may result in urinary tract obstruction. Fortunately, this complication is rare. However, repeat anterior surgery, in the lumbosacral area in particular, has a definite risk of vascular complication involving both venous and arterial structures. The surgeon must be prepared to deal with the consequences of the injuries. It is also prudent to consider post-operative anticoagulation therapy, because of an increased risk of thromboembolism.

Who Should Have Combined Procedures?

The issue of who should have a combined procedure, i.e., anterior and posterior surgery, is of increasing interest. As already noted, this approach is indicated when a posterior approach is mandated for decompression, but prior decompression and fusion have left inadequate bone stock either for a fusion bed or for the insertion of posterior fixation devices. The stumps of the pedicles, if they remain, are a possible site for the insertion of these devices.

Frequently, the extensive scarring and devascularization make the posterior fusion alone unlikely to succeed,

A

B

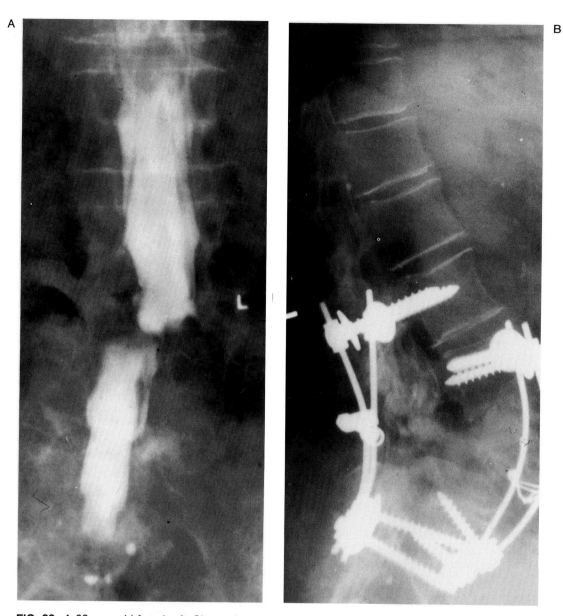

FIG. 22. A 68-year-old female. **A:** Six previous procedures had been performed including attempts at instrumentation using Harrington rods. Severe sepsis had occurred on one occasion. The patient was paraparetic, in a wheelchair. Note the translation of the dye column on myelography. **B:** A two-stage procedure was necessary. First, a posterior approach to decompress and realign the cauda equina. The stubs of the pedicles were used to provide some fixation because of inadequate area for a fusion. As a result of the previous surgery and the laminectomies, there was extensive scarring. The second procedure was done via the anterior approach and consisted of interbody grafts. The internal fixation screws (Zielke) were reinforced with methylmethacrylate bone cement for the severe osteoporosis. The patient walks with canes and has regained bowel and bladder control.

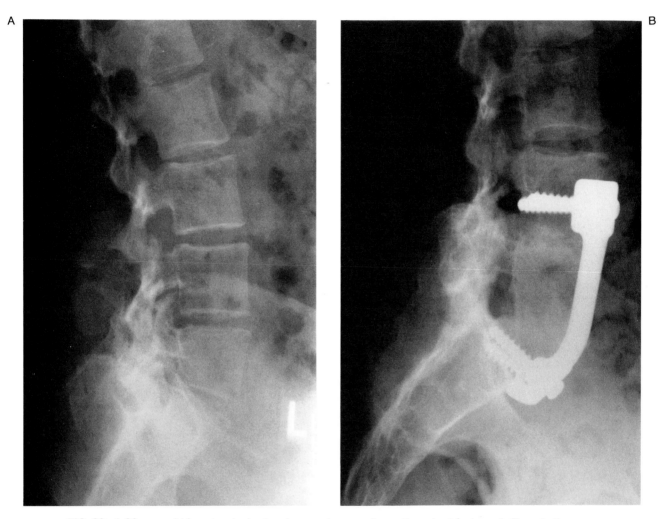

FIG. 23. A 36-year-old female who had undergone two previous attempts at fusions. **A:** Pseudarthroses were located at L4-L5 and L5-S1 on plain radiography and tomography. An anterior interbody fusion of L4-S1 was performed **(B).** An I beam plate was used to enhance fusion. The plate was contoured to the sacral promontory. The patient is pain free and has returned to work.

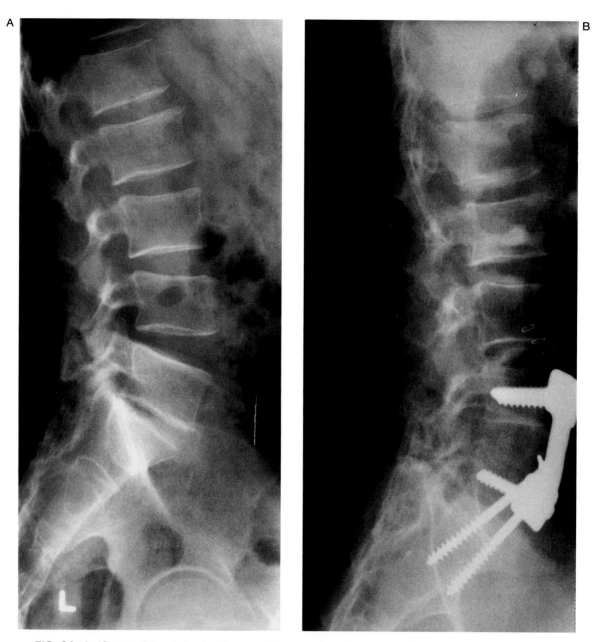

FIG. 24. A 42-year-old male had undergone three previous decompression attempts and fusion plus decompression. **A:** Pseudarthroses were noted at L4-L5 and L5-S1. **B:** An anterior interbody fusion of L4-S1 was successfully done. An I beam plate was used from L4-L5 and two 6.5 mm AO cancellous screws from L5 into the sacrum. If the promontory (L5-S1 angle) is very prominent this screw placement is preferred to contouring the plate.

and the combined anterior-posterior approach is utilized (Figs. 22A, 22B, 27A–27D, and 32A–32G). A second indication is in cases in which there is significant loss of lumbar lordosis from previous surgery. The problems of the iatrogenic flatback deformity have been considered in Chapter 65. Under this circumstance, the anterior procedure is used to mobilize the disc spaces, which are filled with morsellized bone, and anterior internal fixation is contraindicated. A second-stage posterior procedure is used for the correction of the deformity by posterior osteotomy and instrumentation to re-create the lordosis. If a pseudarthrosis is present, this may be used in lieu of the osteotomy, but usually requires widening to achieve the necessary correction.

We do not feel that circumferential fusion is indicated for primary, unoperated upon patients, with the possible exception of some cases of degenerative spondylolisthesis or patients requiring four or more levels of fusion to the sacrum, as noted in the chapter on scoliosis.

Who Should Have a Posterior Lumbar Interbody Fusion?

The use of posterior lumbar interbody fusion in itself is of some controversy because of the high risk of neurologic injury, graft extrusion, and the inability of some to obtain an adequate rate of fusion even in primary cases. The major problem is the wide exposure necessary to obtain placement of the grafts, which the detractors of the procedure feel results in unusual scarring. However, the proponents of the procedure feel that this complication is avoidable (see Chapter 94).

We feel that in cases in which there is a previous failed fusion, the role of posterior lumbar interbody fusion is extremely limited on the basis of technical problems that are encountered as one approaches the dense scar that often is present. If an interbody fusion is felt to be necessary, we feel that the anterior route is preferable, but not everybody agrees.

TECHNICAL DETAILS OF POSTERIOR RE-FUSION

Dependent on the specific condition being treated and the history of prior surgery, certain technical details are useful to keep in mind. First we will look at the general issues in posterior re-fusion.

Fixation

As noted, we prefer pedicle devices whenever possible, if posterior internal fixation is deemed necessary. In failed prior posterior fusion, the anatomic landmarks of the pedicle may be difficult to define, and radiologic control is essential. If there is a large amount of old bone graft present, the screws may be attached into the graft without involving the pedicle. More often this is not the case, or osteoporosis is an additional source of concern. Under these circumstances the pedicle should be defined. Time can be saved by estimating the anatomic point of insertion and making a drill hole. A Kirschner wire is placed in the hole, and fluoroscopic confirmation is obtained. If the devices are not in proper position, slight alterations in level can succeed in achieving the proper entry point, which is then completed with an awl or tap drill.

Once a pedicle fixation system is placed, the linkage must be carefully selected. Plates appear to be more rigid, but are less adaptable. Although they may be contoured for lordosis, it is difficult to adapt them to a rotatory or lateral deviation deformity. Conversely, rods can be easily contoured three-dimensionally, but many of the devices are less rigid than a plate device. Ultimately, the choice of device rests with the surgeon's experience and the pre-operative assessment of which system will best deal with the complexities of the individual patient.

Regardless of the type of device used, it is important to obtain at least two points of fixation, proximal and distal to the pseudarthrosis, such that there are a total of 8 points (Fig. 21). The inclusion of the sacrum also raises a number of technical difficulties. The main problems are screw orientation and the number of screws that can be employed. In our experience, the use of single screws at each side of the sacrum is insufficient, although others have not had that concern (Figs. 28A and 28B). In general, we try to introduce four screws, two on each side. The point for entry is usually at the base of the first sacral pedicle (Figs. 29A and 29B). In the female, access to the sacral promontory from this point of entry is not difficult, but in the narrow male pelvis, the challenge is greater. Thus in males, we have used a similar point of entry but have directed the screw to the thickest part of the ala, aiming distally and laterally at about 30 degrees. A second screw is then introduced into the second sacral pedicle, going directly laterally (Fig. 30). Because of the close proximity of the sacrum to the overlying skin, the use of a bulky fixation device should be avoided if at all possible.

More recently, particularly with the Cotrel-Dubousset form of instrumentation, introduction of two screws, both at the base of the first sacral pedicle, has resulted in more easy alignment and introduction of the device. The first is angled into the promontory and the second is directed laterally into the ala.

Posterior Decortication

In the presence of a pre-existing pseudarthrosis, or when a new laminectomy is required that involves the

Text continues on page 2062.

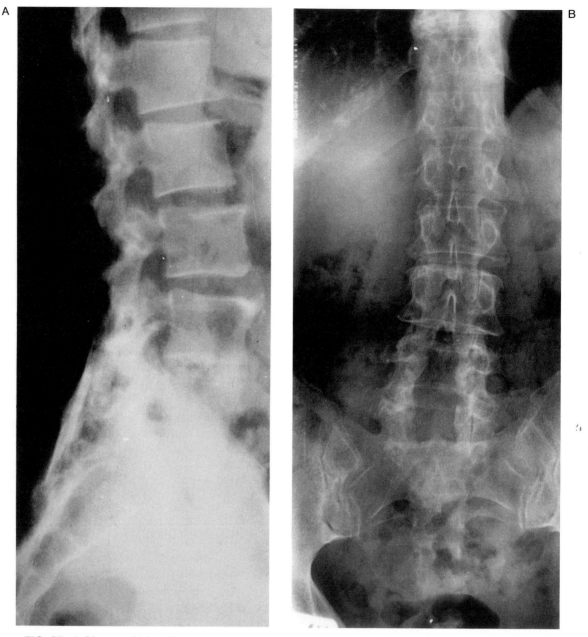

FIG. 25. A 28-year-old female had undergone four previous operations including two decompressions and two posterior attempts at fusion. **A and B:** She had pseudarthroses at L5-S1, L4-L5, L3-L4, and an unstable L2-L3 level with little or no posterior elements. (Figs. 25C–25D follow.)

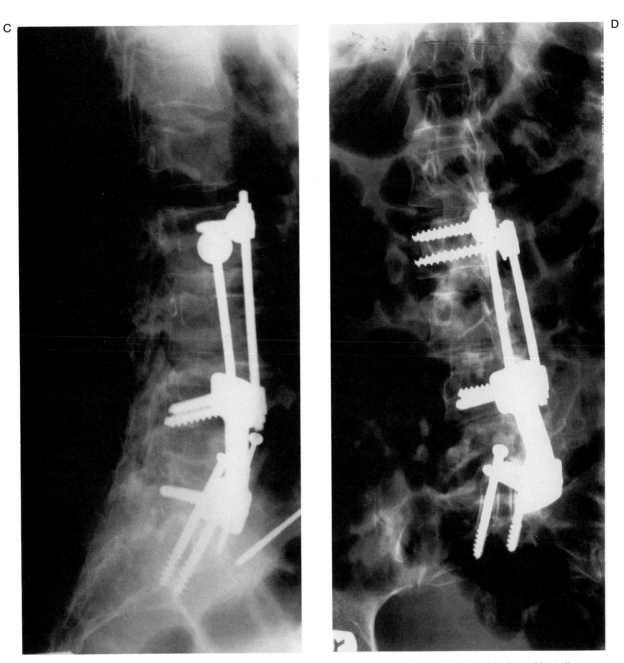

FIG. 25. *Continued.* **C and D:** Interbody grafts were used (iliac crest) for stabilization of L2-L4, Kostuik-Harrington (compression) at L4-L5, and I plate with 6.5 mm AO cancellous screws at L5-S1. Pain has been considerably lessened and the patient is functional.

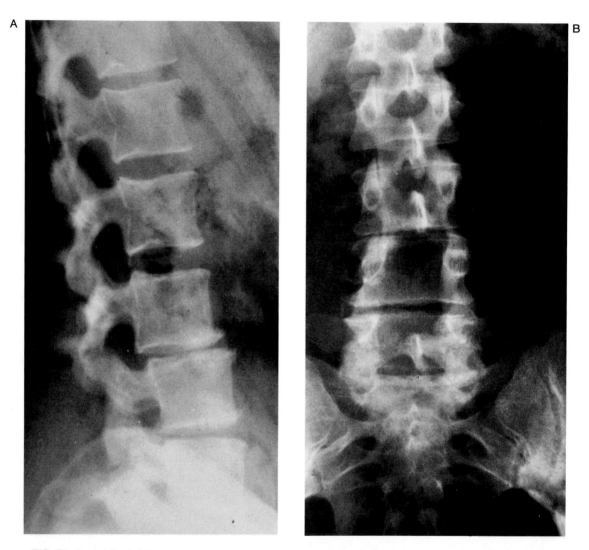

FIG. 26. A and B: A 51-year-old female who had undergone five previous procedures including multiple decompressions and attempts at postero-lateral fusion. L2-L3 was unstable as well. (Figs. 26C–26D follow.)

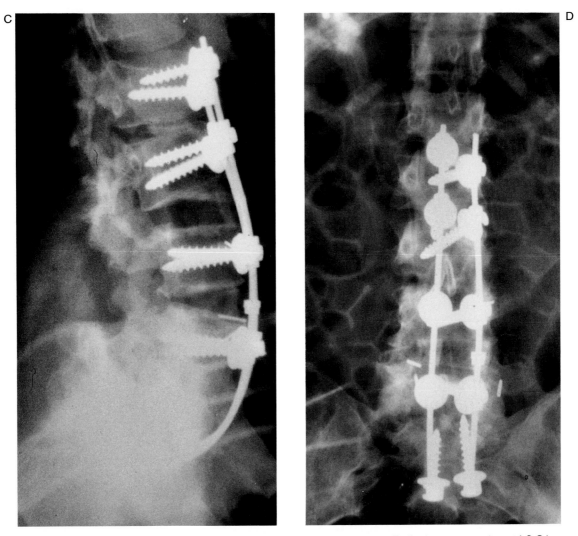

FIG. 26. *Continued.* **C and D:** Interbody fusion (iliac crest) with double Zielke instrumentation at L2-S1. Patient returned to work as a pharmacist assistant after being off work for seven years. Double rods are necessary for rotational control.

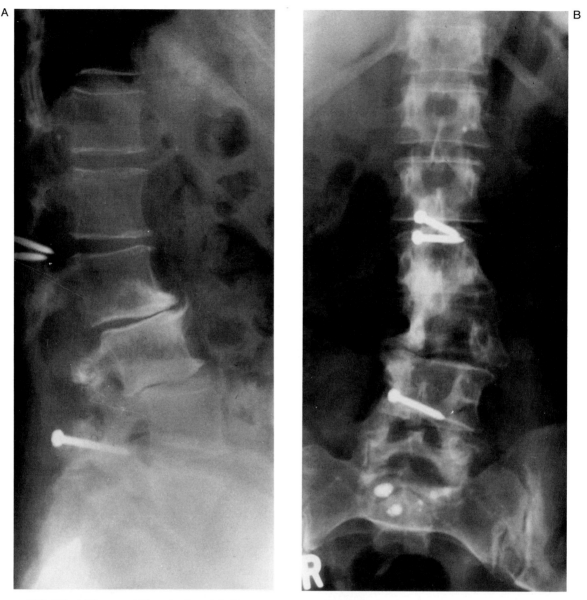

FIG. 27. A 62-year-old female. **A and B:** Six previous procedures had been attempted resulting in severe instability, neurological pain, and back pain. (Figs. 27C–27D follow.)

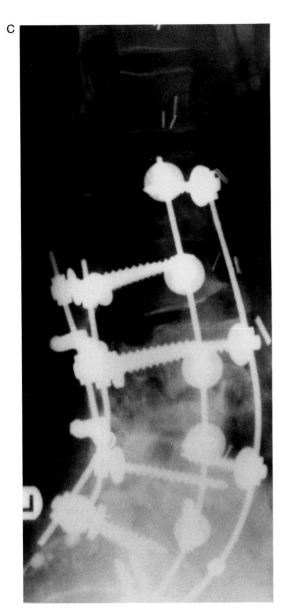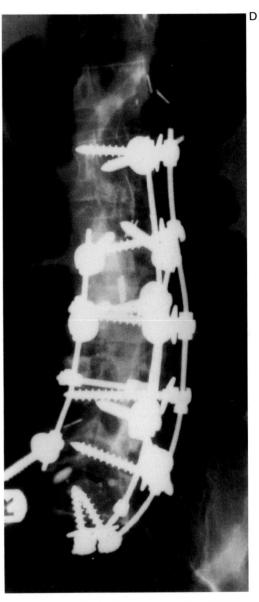

FIG. 27. *Continued.* **C and D:** A two-stage procedure was performed including posterior decompression. The pedicle stumps were used for stabilization posteriorly but because of inadequate bone stock an anterior fusion was done using interbody grafts and double Zielke rods. The patient is remarkably improved five years later and drives from Toronto to Florida annually for holidays.

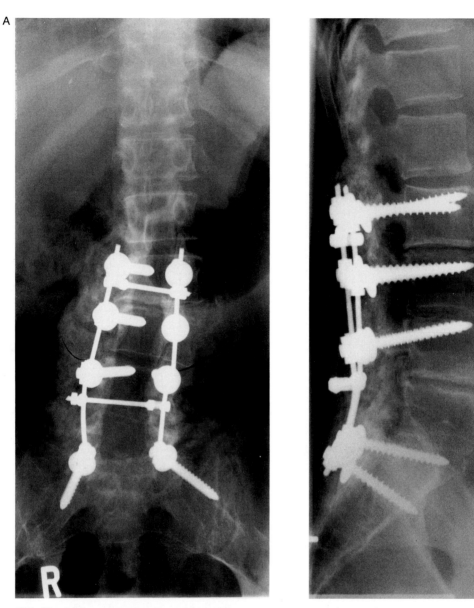

FIG. 28. A 63-year-old female underwent four-level decompression fusion and Zielke instrumentation for severe spinal stenosis 4.5 years previously **(A and B).** Only one screw was used on each side of the sacrum at S1 directed into the arch. She developed pseudarthrosis.

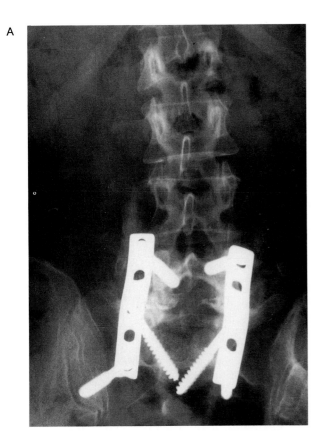
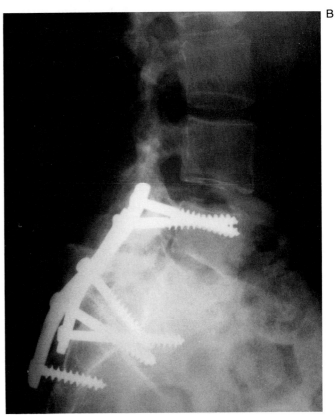

FIG. 29. A 42-year-old female underwent decompression, fusion, and AO plate fixation at L4-S1 for spondylolisthesis **(A and B).** The S1 screws are directed toward the promontory; the S2 screws are directed laterally into the ala. On the lateral view the S2 screws appear to penetrate too far anteriorly but are really in the ala of the sacrum.

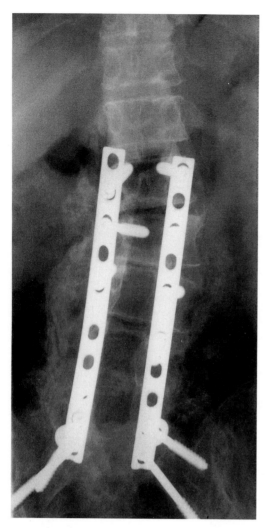

FIG. 30. In the male patient the sacral screws are directed laterally into the thickest part of the ala of the sacrum penetrating both cortexes. In over 300 cases (J.P.K.) we have had no vascular problems.

important to supplement the fusion with autogenous graft. Usually sufficient bone can be harvested from one or the other iliac crest, or both. An alternative is to obtain anterior iliac crest graft before starting the posterior approach.

When the approach is anterior, the decision as to the bone graft source is somewhat more debatable. Although autogenous bone is preferable, allografts may help in this situation.

Management of Osteoporosis

This topic is presented in Chapter 33. This situation presents a number of major challenges. First, the radiographic determination of fusion after a primary intervention is often difficult. Second, fixation devices may be more difficult to apply. As previously noted, we do not advocate the use of methylmethacrylate in the pedicles, with the exception of the first sacral pedicle. However, methylmethacrylate can be injected into the vertebral body to enhance fixation, with minimal risk.

TECHNICAL DETAILS OF ANTERIOR RE-FUSION

Fixation Devices

The role of anterior fixation remains more controversial, particularly because of the increased inherent risks of the procedure and, in general, the less biomechanically favorable devices. The types of devices available are discussed in Chapter 93, together with their indications.

Approaches

The anterior approaches are detailed in Chapter 90. For a single simple approach to L5-S1, a transverse suprapubic incision may be used and is cosmetically more acceptable. A transperitoneal or retroperitoneal approach can then be developed. We prefer the retroperitoneal approach because the bowel contents are well contained, and retraction is easier.

For a two-level approach, a left paramedian incision and retroperitoneal approach are utilized. If fixation devices are affixed to the sacrum and pass beneath the left common iliac system (Fig. 31), we prefer to lay a thin sheet of silicone rubber. This prevents direct adherence of the vessels to the scar, and if later surgery is required, the dissection is facilitated.

For approaches of three levels or more, we prefer a flank approach, but when the fusion is to be extended to the sacrum, the bed of the twelfth rib is used. The incision is carried to the rectus sheath, which is then split, and the incision is then carried down as a paramedian

old fusion, a wide exposure is necessary. Although most pseudarthroses are at right angles to the longitudinal axis of the spine, this is not always the case, and the defect may not be easily identifiable. All too frequently, an exploratory operation fails to identify the pseudarthrosis, even when it was suspected pre-operatively. As already noted, one cause is termed a "plate pseudarthrosis," where the bone graft has consolidated into a solid plate of bone, which has not adhered to the underlying lamina or transverse processes. Failure to recognize this condition is usually due to inadequate pre-operative imaging, including lateral, AP, and axial tomograms and three-dimensional reconstructions.

Sources of Bone Graft

Although it is tempting to use local bone graft obtained from the old fusion, we feel that in most cases it is

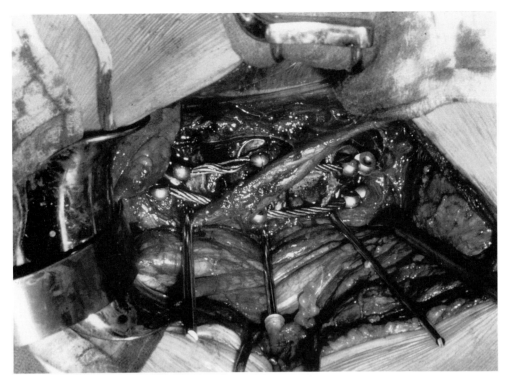

FIG. 31. The left common iliac vessels have been dissected out. In this example, Dwyer cables go from L4-L5 to S1 passing beneath the vessels. The screws pass anterior to posterior. The vessels have been modified by tying off and sectioning the ilio-lumbar vessels.

incision, followed by a retroperitoneal approach (see Chapter 69).

In all patients, rehabilitation of the abdominal musculature is necessary, but in the elderly patient, this may be difficult. Not uncommonly, an incisional hernia is the consequence.

SURGICAL RESULTS OF REPEAT FUSION

As noted previously, the results of a second operation are less predictable. In a simple group of patients treated for pseudarthrosis, where the previous surgery was simple posterior fusion, a success rate of only 60% was obtained, often despite a subsequent solid arthrodesis (28). This analytic problem becomes even more difficult when the published series are a mixed population with respect to original pathology, numerous sources of failures are included, and a variety of surgical techniques have been used. However, a number of studies are instructional and give some broad indication of the results that can be achieved.

The first lesson is that patients properly selected can achieve reasonable, but by no means perfect, results, even when the problems are complex. One of us (Kostuik) has treated 35 patients with fusion and sublaminar wiring. All 35 patients had been off work for an average of 9 years since their last operations. Thirteen were returned to work. Satisfactory results were obtained in an additional 9 patients who had significant decrease in pain, but did not return to work. Pain persisted in 13 patients despite a solid arthrodesis being achieved. A subsequent clinical series was performed between 1984 and 1988 and involved 246 patients treated by a variety of posterior pedicle fixations. At two years, the pseudarthrosis rate was 8%. During the same period, 51 patients underwent anterior salvage surgery with fusion and instrumentation. The most instructive part of this series constituted the 38 patients who were treated by anterior salvage surgery for a posterior pseudarthrosis, while an additional group included 6 patients with degenerative disease above or below the previous fusion. The incidence of pseudarthrosis was 9%. Of those who had developed yet another pseudarthrosis following anterior surgery, 50% had pain relief at more than 2 years following the operation. Almost all of the patients were on long-term disability, yet 43% returned to work despite being off for an average of 4 years. Also of interest is that 57% of the patients had significant psychological problems, yet had satisfactory results. Although these results do not compare to those achieved in primary spine surgery, they do suggest that there is a group of patients who can benefit. The challenge is how to further hone down the selection technique and surgical approach to improve upon these results.

Other series, in general, give somewhat similar results with respect to the later incidence of pseudarthrosis fol-

Text continues on page 2067.

A

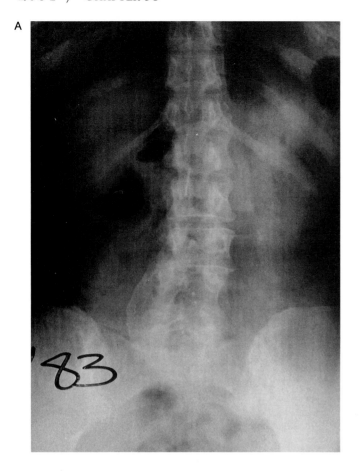

FIG. 32. A 63-year-old female had undergone a two-level L4-S1 fusion 12 years previously. **A:** She developed symptoms of spinal stenosis and segmental instability proximal to L3-L4 and L2-L3. **B:** Her surgeon extended the fusion following posterior decompression at L2-L3 and L3-L4, to T10. One year later, the hooks disengaged. The rods were removed but the pseudarthroses were not repaired. (Figs. 32C–32G follow.)

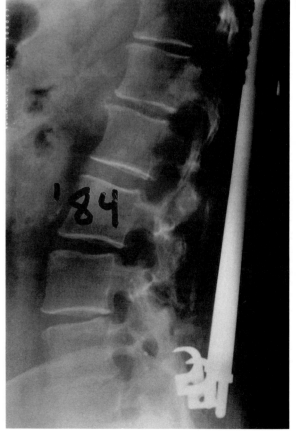

B

C

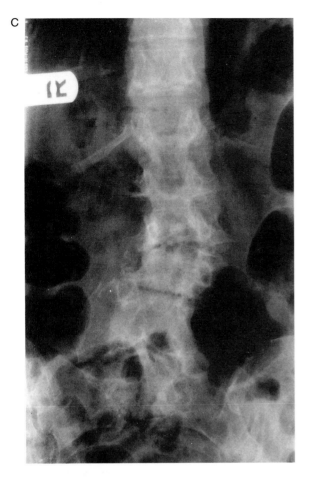

D

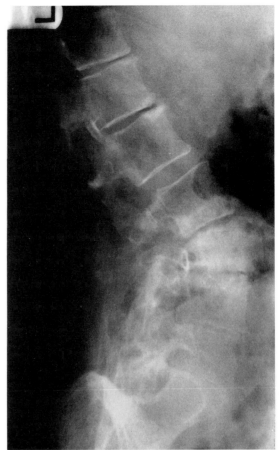

E

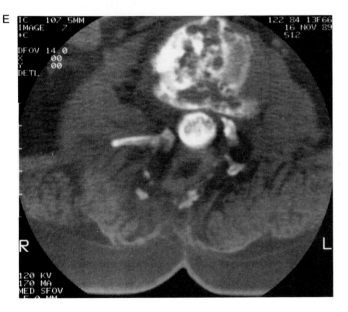

FIG. 32. *Continued.* **C:** Her deformity progressed, together with increased instability and pain. **D:** The L3 vertebral body appears to be avascular. She developed marked lateral quadriceps weakness and could not stand. **E:** A post-myelographic CT shows her residual bone. (Figs. 32F–32G follow.)

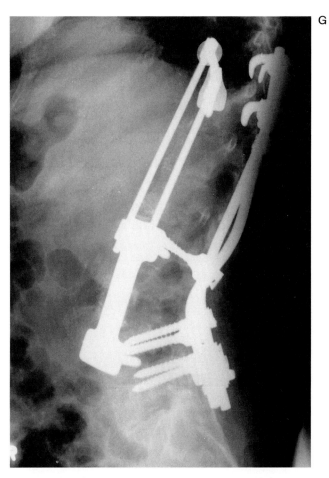

FIG. 32. *Continued.* **F and G:** Posterior decompression was performed together with Cotrel-Dubousset instrumentation and fusion using pedicle screws distally. The L4-S1 fusion was solid, but all other levels had pseudarthroses. Because of the long fusion extending to the fixed sacrum and poor posterior bone stock (small amount with extensive scarring), an anterior fusion was done.

lowing re-fusion. Fujimaki, Crock, and Bedbrook (31) reported on 38 salvage cases treated by anterior interbody fusion without instrumentation. Only one pseudarthrosis occurred.

Thalgott et al. (71) have reported on the use of AO DCP plates for internal fixation in 31 patients with prior failures of fusion. Seventeen of these 31 had failed interbody fusions. Following their surgical intervention, a pseudarthrosis rate of 24% was noted. In 14 patients the fusion failure was for a prior posterior operation, and a lower non-union rate of 14% was obtained.

Zuckerman et al. (77) have used the Steffee system, but their failures included a variety of patients who had not been subjected to previous fusion. Of note was their high rate of screw breakage and infection.

ALTERNATIVE NON-SURGICAL TREATMENT

As noted earlier in this chapter, an alternative for many patients is a vigorous rehabilitation program, particularly in the post-operative course, when the fusion is deemed solid. Additional therapy that may be considered is the use of electrical stimulation in patients with pseudarthrosis. This technique was first proposed by Dwyer (21,22) and has been used by Kane (40) in a controlled study of both primary fusion and repair of pseudarthrosis. A large amount of basic research in the peripheral skeleton, and some experimental work in animals (37,59), has suggested that electrical stimulation enhances bone formation. In primary fusion, Kane (40) has observed a rate of fusion of 91.5%. The comparison group achieved 81% success.

In secondary fusions, less certain data are available, but Kane recommends that the procedure be accompanied by bone grafting. In a randomized prospective study of "difficult patients," 15 of 28 controls achieved fusion (54%) compared with 25 of 31 stimulated controls who gained solid arthrodesis (81%).

As an alternative, the use of pulsating electromagnetic coils, applied externally, has been advocated by Simmons (67). In a preliminary study, 13 patients with failures of posterior interbody fusion were analyzed, 10 of whom showed increased bone formation, and 77% of whom went on to solid arthrodesis. His results have not been replicated by Brodsky (6), who demonstrated only a 36% success rate in patients with posterior fusion and pseudarthrosis.

REFERENCES

1. Beals RK, Hickman NW (1972): Industrial injuries of the back and extremities: Comprehensive evaluation—an aid in prognosis and management; a study of one hundred and eighty patients. *J Bone Joint Surg* [Am] 54:1593–1611.
2. Blasier RD, Munson RC (1987): Acquired spondylolysis after posterolateral spinal fusion. *J Ped Orthop* 7:215–217.
3. Bosworth DM (1955): Repair of herniae through iliac-crest defects. *J Bone Joint Surg* [Am] 37:1069–1073.
4. Brodsky AE (1976): Post-laminectomy and post-fusion stenosis of the lumbar spine. *Clin Orthop* (115):130–139.
5. Brodsky AE, Hendricks RL, Khalil MA, Darden BV, Brotzman TT (1989): Segmental ("floating") lumbar spine fusions. *Spine* 14:447–450.
6. Brodsky AF, Khalil MA (1987): Preliminary report on the use of EBI pulsing electromagnetic field therapy for treatment of pseudoarthrosis of lumbar spine fusion. Presented at North American Spine Society Annual Meeting, Banff Springs, Alberta, Canada, June 27.
7. Brodsky AE, Khalil MA (1988): Efficacy of electrical bone growth stimulation among 97 patients with pseudoarthrosis of the lumbar spine. Presentation North American Spine Society Meeting, Colorado Springs, June.
8. Brunet JA, Wiley JJ (1984): Acquired spondylolysis after spinal fusion. *J Bone Joint Surg* [Br] 66:720–724.
9. Cleveland M, Bosworth DM, Thompson FR (1948): Pseudoarthrosis in the lumbosacral spine. *J Bone Joint Surg* [Am] 30:302–312.
10. Cloward RB (1953): The treatment of ruptured lumbar intervertebral discs by vertebral body fusion: indications. Operative technique, after-care. *J Neurosurg* 10:154–168.
11. Cochran T, Irstam L, Nachemson A (1983): Long-term anatomic and functional changes in patients with adolescent idiopathic scoliosis treated by Harrington rod fusion. *Spine* 8:576–584.
12. Collis JS (1985): Total disc replacement: A modified posterior lumbar interbody fusion. Report of 750 cases. *Clin Orthop* (193):64–67.
13. Cotler JM, Starr AM (1989): Complications of spinal fusions. In: Cotler JM, Cotler HB, eds. *Spinal fusion, science and technique.* New York: Springer Verlag.
14. Crock HV (1976): Observations on the management of failed spinal operations. *J Bone Joint Surg* [Br] 58:193–199.
15. Crock HV (1986): Internal disc disruption: A challenge to disc prolapse fifty years on. *Spine* 11:650–653.
16. Dawson EG, Clader TJ, Bassett LW (1985): A comparison of different methods used to diagnose pseudoarthrosis following posterior spinal fusion for scoliosis. *J Bone Joint Surg* [Am] 67:1153–1159.
17. DePalma AF, Rothman RH (1968): The nature of pseudarthrosis. *Clin Orthop* (59):113–118.
18. Dewar FP (1963): Circumferential fusion for degenerative disc disease, Toronto, unpublished data.
19. Drury BJ (1967): Clinical evaluation of back and leg pain due to irritation of the superior cluneal nerve. *J Bone Joint Surg* [Am] 49:199.
20. Dwyer AF (1973): Experience of anterior correction of scoliosis. *Clin Orthop* (93):191–214.
21. Dwyer AF, Wickham GG (1974): Direct current stimulation in spinal fusion. *Med J Aust* 1:73–75.
22. Dwyer AF, Yau AC, Jeffcoat KW (1974): Use of direct current in spine fusion. *J Bone Joint Surg* [Am] 56:442.
23. Esses SI, Botsford DJ, Kostuik JP (1989): The role of external spinal skeletal fixation in the assessment of low-back disorders. *Spine* 14:594–601.
24. Finnegan WJ, Fenlin JM, Marvel JP, Nardini RJ, Rothman RH (1979): Results of surgical intervention in the symptomatic multiply-operated back patient. Analysis of 67 cases followed for 3–7 years. *J Bone Joint Surg* [Am] 61:1077–1082.
25. Fogelberg EV, Zitzmann EK, Stinchfield FE (1970): Prophylactic penicillin in orthopaedic surgery. *J Bone Joint Surg* [Am] 52:95–98.
26. Freebody D, Bendall R, Taylor RD (1971): Anterior transperitoneal lumbar fusion. *J Bone Joint Surg* [Br] 53:617–627.
27. Frymoyer JW, Hanley E, Howe J, Kuhlmann D, Matteri R (1978): Disc excision and spine fusion in the management of lumbar disc disease; a minimum ten-year follow-up. *Spine* 3:1–6.
28. Frymoyer JW, Hanley EN Jr, Howe J, Kuhlmann D, Matteri RE (1979): A comparison of radiographic findings in fusion and non-fusion patients ten or more years following lumbar disc surgery. *Spine* 4:435–440.
29. Frymoyer JW, Howe J, Kuhlmann D (1978): The long-term effects of spinal fusion on the sacroiliac joints and ilium. *Clin Orthop* (134):196–201.

30. Frymoyer JW, Matteri RE, Hanley EN, Kuhlmann D, Howe J (1978): Failed lumbar disc surgery requiring second operation. A long-term follow-up study. *Spine* 3:7–11.
31. Fujimaki A, Crock HV, Bedbrook GM (1982): The results of 150 anterior lumbar interbody fusion operations performed by two surgeons in Australia. *Clin Orthop* (165):164–167.
32. Harris RI, Wiley JJ (1963): Acquired spondylolysis as a sequel to spine fusion. *J Bone Joint Surg* [Am] 45:1159–1170.
33. Hayes MA, Tompkins SF, Herndon WA, et al (1988): Clinical and radiological evaluation of lumbosacral motion below fusion levels in idiopathic scoliosis. *Spine* 13:1161–1167.
34. Hsu KY, Zuckerman J, White A, Wynne G, Reynolds J, Goldthwaite N, Schofferman J (1988): Deterioration of motion segments adjacent to lumbar fusion. Proceedings of the North American Spine Society Annual Meeting, Colorado Springs.
35. Jacobs RR, Montesano PX, Jackson RP (1989): Enhancement of lumbar spine fusion by use of translaminar facet joint screws. *Spine* 14:12–15.
36. Jones JB (1971): The training of orthopedic surgery residents in lumbar disk surgery. *Clin Orthop* (83):88–92.
37. Kahanovitz N, Arnoczky SP (1987): The efficacy of direct current electrical stimulation to enhance canine posterior spinal fusions. Presented at the North American Spine Society Annual Meeting, Banff Springs, Alberta, Canada, June 27.
38. Kahanovitz N, Arnoczky SP (1990): The efficacy of direct current electrical stimulation to enhance canine spinal fusions. *Clin Orthop Rel Res* (251):295–299.
39. Kahanovitz N, Arnoczky SP, Hulse D, Shires PK (1984): The effect of postoperative electromagnetic pulsing on canine posterior spinal fusions. *Spine* 9:273–279.
40. Kane WJ (1988): Direct current electrical bone growth stimulation for spinal fusion. *Spine* 13:363–365.
41. Kornberg M (1989): Discography and magnetic resonance imaging in the diagnosis of lumbar disc disruption. *Spine* 14:1368–1372.
42. Kostuik JP, Carl A, Ferron S (1986): Anterior interbody fusion and instrumentation for lumbar degenerative disc disease. Unpublished data.
43. Kostuik JP, Carl A, Ferron S, Dowling T, Errico T, Abbitbol JJ (1990): Results of instrumentation and fusion for salvage surgery in degenerative disc disease. Canadian Orthopaedic Association, Vancouver.
44. Kostuik JP, Errico T, Gleason T (1990): Luque instrumentation in degenerative conditions of the lumbar spine. *Spine.* 15:318–321.
45. Kostuik JP, Hall BB (1983): Spinal fusions to the sacrum in adults with scoliosis. *Spine* 8:489–500.
46. Kurz LT, Garfin SR, Booth RE Jr (1989): Harvesting autogenous iliac bone grafts. A review of complications and techniques. *Spine* 14:1324–1331.
47. Laasonen EM, Soini J (1989): Low-back pain after lumbar fusion: Surgical and computed tomographic analysis. *Spine* 14:210–213.
48. Lee CK, Lagranda NA (1984): Lumbosacral spinal fusion: A biomechanical study. *Spine* 9:574–581.
49. Lehmann TR, Spratt KF, Tozzi J (1987): Long-term follow-up of lower lumbar fusion patients. *Spine* 12:97–104.
50. Lin PM (1985): Posterior lumbar interbody fusion complications and pitfalls. *Clin Orthop* (193):90–102.
51. Lin PM (1989): Technique and complications of posterior lumbar interbody fusion. In: Linn PM, Gill K, eds. *Lumbar interbody fusion, principles and techniques in spine surgery.* Rockville, Maryland: Aspen Press.
52. Lonstein J, Winter R, Moe J, Gaines D (1973): Wound infection with Harrington instrumentation and spine fusion for scoliosis. *Clin Orthop* (96):222–233.
53. Luk KD, et al (1987): The effect on the lumbosacral spine of long spinal fusion for idiopathic scoliosis. A minimum 10 year follow-up. *Spine* 12:996–1000.
54. Macdonald G, Pennel G (1966): Lumbar spine fusion. Presented at Workman's Compensation Course, Toronto.
55. Macnab I, Dall D (1971): The blood supply of the lumbar spine and its application to the technique of intertransverse lumbar fusion. *J Bone Joint Surg* [Br] 53:628–638.
56. Michel CR, LaLain JJ (1985): Late result of Harrington's operation. Long-term evolution of the lumbar spine below the fused segments. *Spine* 10:414–420.
57. Nachemson A (1989): Lumbar discography—where are we today? *Spine* 14:555–557.
58. Naylor A (1974): Late results of laminectomy for lumbar disc prolapse: A review after ten to twenty-five years. *J Bone Joint Surg* [Br] 56:17–29.
59. Nerubay J, Marganit B, Bubis JJ, Tadmor A, Katznelson A (1986): Stimulation of bone formation by electrical current on spinal fusion. *Spine* 11:167–169.
60. O'Brien JP, Dawson MH, Heard CW, Momberger B, Speck G (1986): Simultaneous combined anterior and posterior fusion. A solution for failed spinal surgery with a brief review of first 150 patients. *Clin Orthop* (203):191–195.
61. Olerud S, Hamberg M (1986): External fixation as a test for instability after spinal fusion L4-S1. A case report. *Orthopaedics* 9(4):547–549.
62. Phytinen J, Lahde S, Tanska EL, Laitinen J (1983): Computed tomography after lumbar myelography in lower back and extremity pain syndromes. *Diag Imag* 52:1922.
63. Prothero SR, Parkes JC, Stinchfield FE (1966): Complications after low-back fusion in 1,000 patients. *J Bone Joint Surg* [Am] 48:57–65.
64. Quinnell RC, Stockdale HR (1981): Some experimental observations of the influence of a single lumbar floating fusion on the remaining lumbar spine. *Spine* 6:263–267.
65. Rolander SD (1966): Motion of the lumbar spine with special reference to the stabilizing effect of posterior fusion. *Acta Orthop Scand* (Suppl) 90:1–144.
66. Rombold C (1965): Spondylolysis: A complication of spine fusion. *J Bone Joint Surg* [Am] 47:1237–1242.
67. Simmons JW (1985): Treatment of failed posterior lumbar interbody fusion on the spine with pulsing electromagnetic fields. *Clin Orthop* (193):127–132.
68. Smith SE, DeLee JC, Ramamurthy S (1984): Ilioinguinal neuralgia following iliac bone-grafting. Report of two cases and review of the literature. *J Bone Joint Surg* [Am] 66:1306–1308.
69. Stokes IAF, Wilder DG, Frymoyer JW, Pope MH (1981): Assessment of patients with low back pain by biplanar radiographic measurement of intervertebral motion. *Spine* 6:233–239.
70. Terry A, McCall IW, O'Brien JP, Park WM (1981): Graft impingement following posterolateral fusion. Proceedings of the International Society for the Study of the Lumbar Spine.
71. Thalgott JS, LaRocca H, Aebi M, Dwyer AP, Razza BE (1989): Reconstruction of the lumbar spine using AO DCP plate fixation. *Spine* 14:91–95.
72. Uander-Scharin L (1950): Case of spondylolisthesis lumbalis acquisita. *Acta Orthop Scand* 19:536–544.
73. Weatherley CR, et al (1986): Discogenic pain persisting despite solid posterior fusion. *J Bone Joint Surg* [Br] 38:142–143.
74. Weikel AM, Habal MB (1977): Meralgia paresthetica: A complication of iliac bone procurement. *Plast Reconstr Surg* 60:572–574.
75. Weinstein JN, Spratt KF, Spengler D, Brick C (1988): Spinal pedicle fixation: reliability and validity of roentgenogram-based assessment and surgical factors on successful screw placement. *Spine* 13:1012–1018.
76. Yang SW, Langrana NA, Lee CK (1986): Biomechanics of lumbosacral spinal fusion in combined compression-torsion loads. *Spine* 11:937–941.
77. Zuckerman J, Hsu K, White A, Wynne G (1988): Early results of spinal fusion using variable spine plating system. *Spine* 13:570–579.

The Adult Spine: Principles and Practice,
J. W. Frymoyer, Editor-in-Chief.
Raven Press, Ltd., New York © 1991.

CHAPTER 99

Alternative Therapies for the Failed Back Syndrome

Harold A. Wilkinson

"The failed back syndrome" can result from a varied number of specific, but often overlapping, pathoanatomic conditions for which a considerable number of both non-specific and specific therapies are available (24,72,76). Clinically, the syndrome presents as a constellation of pain, dysfunction, and frequently psychosocial disturbances, which follows lumbar discectomies, decompressions, and fusions. In considering the pathoanatomic causation it is useful to divide the symptoms into problems involving predominantly leg pain, problems involving predominantly low back pain, or problems which are sequelae to spinal fusion. Adhesive arachnoiditis may well justify a separate category, since this condition represents one of the major, unsolved dilemmas in the surgery of low back disease and is commonly associated with both lumbago and sciatica.

The focus of this chapter is to consider the non-operative and operative options available to patients with this complex, often discouraging "failed back syndrome." Previous chapters have detailed the causes of failure after surgical decompression or lumbar spinal fusion, and the non-operative and surgical approaches which can be

taken to solve many of the more easily identifiable causes of symptoms. This chapter offers a broad overview of the syndrome, but focuses on the difficult group of patients with nerve root scarring, arachnoiditis, or chronic pain syndromes which may require unconventional therapeutic approaches, many of which attempt to deal with pain, rather than pathoanatomy. I will re-emphasize the importance of determining a specific diagnosis and of aggressive non-surgical management and will consider both proven and unproven remedies to help these patients. The reader is referred to Chapters 12 (psychology of chronic pain), 13 (functional restoration), 14 (pain clinics), and 30 (mechanisms of spinal pain) for additional information about the general pathoanatomy of spinal pain and its rehabilitation and treatment.

OVERVIEW PERSPECTIVES IN DIAGNOSIS AND TREATMENT

Treatment of the failed back syndrome should include surgery for only a small minority of patients, yet a large number of therapeutic options are available. Treatment can be based on general symptoms, using the broad categories previously noted, or can be precisely tailored for a specific pathological entity. Generally, the more invasive

H. A. Wilkinson, M.D., Ph.D.: Professor and Chairman, Division of Neurosurgery, University of Massachusetts Medical School, Worcester, Massachusetts 01655.

TABLE 1. *Potential specific diagnoses in patients with predominantly leg pain*

Retained disc fragment or far lateral disc rupture
Retained foreign body
Arachnoiditis
Nerve root cyst
Lateral recess stenosis
Diabetic mononeuritis
Benign spinal neoplasm
Unresected disc rupture (wrong level)
Nerve root fibrosis or injury
Arachnoidal cyst, post-operative facet synovial cyst
Spinal stenosis
Viral neuritis
Herpetic nerve root involvement

the procedure, the more specific are the indications. Accordingly, the non-invasive treatment for the failed back syndrome may be based on a probable diagnosis or short list of diagnoses within a broad diagnostic category. Conversely, more specific or invasive therapy requires a more precise diagnosis (Tables 1, 2, and 3). As emphasized throughout this text, diagnosis remains founded on the twin pillars of history and physical examination. In this technological age, these basic skills are greatly enhanced, albeit perhaps too profusely and too expensively, by sophisticated imaging techniques (radiographs, isotope scans, myelograms, CT and MRI scans), and by other electrodiagnostic and laboratory examinations. However, even these advanced and often anatomically detailed diagnostic supplements may be insufficient to establish the pathophysiologic causes of pain. Other important information sometimes can be obtained through an analysis of response to therapy (such as medications, bed rest, exercises and orthoses), or from diagnostic injections, including trigger points, facet joints, nerve root or spinal blocks, or contrast or anesthetic discography. Many of the specific therapeutic alternatives referred to in this chapter are discussed in detail in other chapters, but they are included here to present an overview of what is available to deal with the patient with failed back syndrome.

Another vital element to treatment is the attitude of the treating surgeon. The surgeon who operated initially on a patient with a low back disorder should not abandon that patient if his initial therapeutic efforts fail. Faced with an operative failure, new therapy should be structured and rational, keeping in mind the wide range of potential diagnoses and available therapeutic options. In my experience, all too often an early failure of spinal surgery becomes a failed back syndrome because the operating surgeon did not attempt to analyze carefully the cause of the failure and did not offer a rational and structured therapeutic program. Therapy need not be protracted in all patients, particularly if a more involved or more invasive therapy would offer a significantly greater probability of earlier success with an acceptable probability of risk. Indeed, for some patients this complex or more invasive therapy may become the "most conservative" option. Stated another way, "conservative therapy" can be defined as therapy which is maximally effective at minimal risk and cost. Similarly, non-invasive therapy can become "radical" if it is unwisely applied or unduly prolonged. Non-invasive therapy is not without complications, such as muscle or ligamentous weakness, psychological enervation from prolonged inactivity, or gastrointestinal bleeding from anti-inflammatory drugs. Poorly chosen non-invasive therapy also can result in undue prolongation of the illness and inability to perform at work or recreation. The choice, therefore, should be made carefully and appropriately to the patient's condition and expectations.

NON-INVASIVE THERAPY

Non-invasive therapies can often be applied more non-specifically than invasive therapies. This is especially useful if one uses the broad diagnostic categories referred to earlier: problems of predominantly leg pain, problems of predominantly back pain, and problems related to fusion failure. The psychological contributions and reactions to the illness must also be understood and managed effectively.

TABLE 2. *Potential specific diagnoses in patients with predominantly back pain*

Flabby back syndrome	Epidural scar
Meningeal irritation	Pseudomeningocele
Arachnoid cyst	Discitis or aseptic interspace inflammation
Disc space infection	Osteomyelitis
Painful arthropathy of disc (without rupture)	Facet syndrome
Acute or fixed muscle spasm	Trigger point
Ischiogluteal bursitis	Fasciitis, fibromyalgia
Transaponeurotic fat herniation	Spondylolysis with spondylisthesis
Trauma: contusion, sprain, muscle spasm, compression fracture, microfracture	Benign neoplasm
Metastatic neoplasm	Arthritis
Cervical disc disease	Osteoporosis

TABLE 3. *Potential specific diagnoses in patients with fusion problems*

Symptomatic pseudarthrosis
Kissing pseudarthrosis
Trauma: Traumatic avulsion of attachments to fusion, fracture of fusion
Iatrogenic spinal stenosis
Painful bone donor site
Osteomyelitis

Enforced Inactivity and Enforced Activity

Enforced inactivity and enforced activity have long been mainstays of the non-invasive treatment of problems of low back disorders. However, deciding when to advise inactivity, when to advise activity, or when to convert from one to the other may not always be readily apparent. As a generality, patients with predominantly post-operative leg pain are more likely to be suffering an irritative process affecting their nerve roots and are more likely to profit from reduced irritation of the nerve root through enforced inactivity. On the other hand, patients with lumbago are more likely to be suffering from a mechanical disorder of the musculoskeletal structures. While acute pain initially may preclude activity, prolonging inactivity is now generally felt to be inadvisable for the majority of patients. Prolonged inactivity can rapidly lead to further weakening and stiffness, a phenomenon well known to arthritic patients.

Bed rest is the mainstay of inactivity therapy. It is most useful for patients with leg pain, but short periods of bed rest can be quite useful for patients with long-standing back pain (18). I advise my patients to remain recumbent in bed because merely sitting up in or on the side of the bed continues weight bearing on the lumbar area. Bed rest can often be facilitated or made more comfortable by special positioning, such as the use of small supports under the lumbar curve or padding under the calves to elevate the legs and produce slight pelvic rotation. I specify and monitor the duration of bed rest each day, since I believe there may be an important therapeutic difference between 23 hours of bed rest daily and 24 hours. However, even much briefer periods of bed rest, 1 hour at a time, may be helpful during a period of restorative activity or "work hardening."

For some patients I use pelvic traction (Fig. 1). My clinical observations lead me to believe traction may help to overcome painful muscle spasms or to open narrowed disc spaces or neural foramina, and thus may have benefit exceeding the obvious of simply keeping the patient in bed (54). Patients should be cautioned that the first few minutes of pelvic traction may cause increased discomfort. Traction optimally should be used for periods of at least an hour to achieve a therapeutic effect.

Inactivity can be continued while patients are ambulatory through the use of orthoses or crutches. Orthoses

range from lumbosacral belts to spica casts, although it should be recognized that even a spica cast, including one or both hip joints, does not stop all back motion. In general it is advisable to accept a lesser degree of back immobilization and permit greater patient function. Satisfactory immobilization can be achieved through the use of full torso supports such as a Taylor back brace, Orthomold hyperextension brace, or molded orthosis. In addition to the obvious usefulness of this type of immobilization following severe bony trauma, primary fusion, or pseudarthrosis repair, these devices may have diagnostic significance. Relief of lumbago through external immobilization in my view argues strongly for a beneficial result following internal immobilization through spine fusion. However, prolonged bracing promotes pain relief and tissue healing at the expense of progressive weakening of back muscles and ligaments. Less rigid orthoses, such as lumbar corsets, produce relatively little spinal stabilization, but act as helpful reminders to limit activity. Lumbosacral elastic belts provide essentially no stabilization for the back but do provide comforting

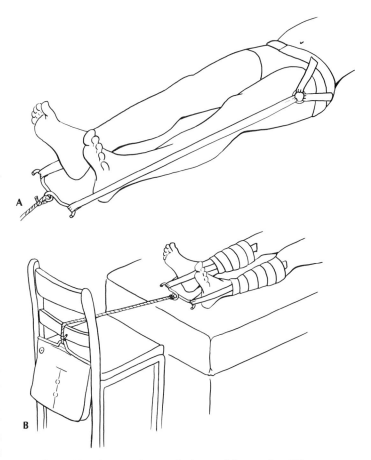

FIG. 1. Traction can be applied as pelvic traction **(A)**, or as leg (Buck's) traction **(B)**. Pelvic traction allows freedom for leg movements and lessens the risk of inducing sciatica through nerve root stretch. When traction is used at home, a chair back can be used as the pulley (with permission from ref. 72).

compression or warmth and do not interfere with full activity.

Enforced activity includes an early return to activities of daily living or work, but generally refers to one of several types of exercise programs that promote increased range of motion, strength, or endurance. Stretch-ing exercises, including the classical "Williams" exer-cises, may be beneficial for patients with painful muscle spasms (Fig. 2). On the other hand, stretching or limber-ing exercises do not improve muscle or ligamentous strength. Simple back strengthening exercises can begin against gravity, such as standing forward, bending at the

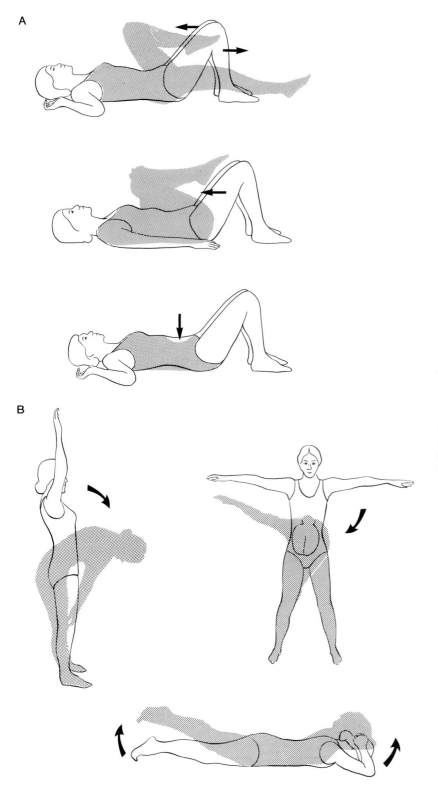

FIG. 2. Exercises can be aimed at improving limberness and stretching out muscle spasms, improving power, or improving endurance. **A:** The classic Williams exercises are stretching exercises but do nothing to strengthen the back. **B:** Strengthening exercises begin by us-ing the upper body as the counterweight. Pro-gressively adding weights increases back mus-cle power and increasing the number of repetitions increases endurance (with permis-sion from ref. 72).

waist, and elevating the thorax or legs while lying prone. More advanced strengthening is essential as a component of the "work hardening" or functional restoration programs described in Chapter 13. The regimen frequently employs resistive exercises such as lifting weights and using exercise equipment, as well as simulated job tasks. The third goal of exercise is endurance. To improve endurance through exercising necessitates increasing the repetitions, often against increasing weight over a prolonged period of time.

Spinal manipulative therapy is a mainstay of chiropractic and osteopathic therapy (8,33,37,53) (see Chapter 73). Several studies have demonstrated that these therapies can bring useful short-term symptomatic relief, but there is no convincing proof that they bring earlier recovery than other forms of enforced activity or inactivity therapy. Instances of further, damaging prolapse of protruding lumbar discs are uncommonly encountered, and instances of lumbar manipulation therapy being applied for incorrect diagnoses seem to be reduced by the more extensive medical training required of osteopaths than of chiropractors (16). How manipulation fits into the treatment of surgical failures is not clear, although patients sometimes self-select these methods.

Topical Therapies

Topical therapies have a hoary tradition ranging from massages given in the Roman baths to oriental moxibustion and remain important today in the therapy of failed back syndrome. Massage, formal myotherapy, liniments, heat or cold applications, and simple topical analgesics have as their goal the reduction of painful muscle contractions and patient relaxation. Despite the debates of therapists regarding the merits of heat and cold, most patients rapidly develop their own personal preference.

Acupuncture and transcutaneous electrical neurostimulation (TENS) may be useful and probably have in common the suppression of pain by induction of intense tactile stimulation, utilizing the physiology of competitive inhibition of sensory transmission in the nervous system (Fig. 3) (60,63,70,71). This mechanism may also be operational with moxibustion, favored by orientals, which involves burning small amounts of materials directly on the skin or on small cups to create intense suction as the cups later cool down. The underlying goal of all these treatments is pain relief, so that tissue healing, restorative activity therapy, and an increase in functional capability can proceed.

Pharmacotherapy

Prescription of medications for patients with the failed back syndrome in clinical practice includes egregious ex-

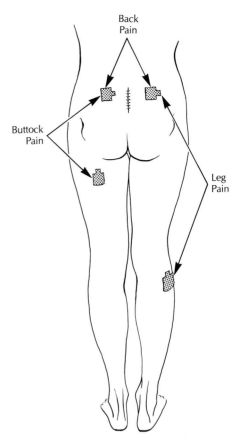

FIG. 3. Transcutaneous electrical nerve stimulation (TENS) is generally most effective when electrodes are applied to bracket the area of pain. Common application sites are illustrated for the relief of back pain, buttock pain, or leg pain (with permission from ref. 72).

amples both of improperly excessive or illogical prescription and of failure to prescribe medications which might be extremely beneficial.

Muscle relaxing medications can be helpful in patients with acute pain, but have minimal usefulness with chronic syndromes and are a poor substitute for strengthening exercises. Furthermore, many of the muscle-relaxing medications have sedating or tranquilizing properties, which can reduce the patient's ability to function. On the other hand, an anxiolytic effect may be helpful in some situations of acutely painful muscle spasm. The practitioner should be familiar with the range of available muscle relaxing medications (see Table 4). An awareness of the varying secondary properties of these medications can help in tailoring the drug(s) selected to the individual patient's needs.

Non-steroidal anti-inflammatory drugs generally have some inherent value as anodynes, in addition to the reduction of local tissue inflammation which results from maintaining sustained therapeutic blood levels. The large number of available anti-inflammatories attests to the complexity of their use and the often idiosyncratic response of the users. Their mechanism of action, side effects, and indications have been given in Chapter 31.

TABLE 4. *Commonly employed muscle relaxing medications*

Generic name	Brand name	Relative muscle relaxing potency[a]	Relative sedating effect[a]
Baclofen	Lioresal	+++	+
Carisoprodol	Soma	+	++
Chlordiazepoxide	Librium	++	+++
Chlorzoxazone	Parafon, Spasgesic	+	++
Cyclobenzaprine	Flexeril	++	++
Dantrolene	Dantrium	+++	+
Diazepam	Valium	++	+++
Meprobamate	Equanil, Miltown	++	++
Metaxalone	Skelaxin	+	++
Methocarbamol	Robaxin	+	++
Quinine sulfate	Quinamm	+	+

[a] Scale of + to +++ based on clinical observations.

These medications can often be extremely beneficial in assisting patients through an exercise or "back hardening" program, and can even be continued through the period of increasing endurance following return to work. Unlike muscle relaxing medications, anti-inflammatory medications may need to be continued for long periods.

Anodynes, or pain relieving medications, seem frequently to be prescribed improperly. It is often easier for a busy clinician to prescribe anodynes to a chronically suffering patient than to spend time listening to and examining the patient in search of means to eliminate the pain source. On the other hand, in the early post-operative period a failure to prescribe anodynes in adequate doses and at appropriately short intervals can prolong pain and distress, teaching patients to fear their pain and to seek overmedication. Anodynes include non-narcotics and narcotics, but muscle relaxers, anti-neuralgic medications, and tranquilizers should not be overlooked as effective pain-relieving therapies.

The opiates are rightly treated with respect because of their potential for addiction and abuse, but respect should not generate unwise fear. For many patients with acute pain, narcotics provide sufficient temporary relief to permit them to begin an earlier restorative or rehabilitation process or even simply to begin early ambulation following spine surgery. Chronic use of narcotics is of course much more dangerous, but mixed agonist-antago-

nist preparations provide excellent analgesia with reduced addictive potential. Occasionally a patient with failed back problems, whose condition is not amenable to cure, can be maintained for many years in a functional state on small and stable doses of narcotics (usually codeine, dihydrocodeinone, or mixed agonist-antagonists) under the careful supervision of the physician. Conversely, detoxifying patients with continued back pain can be followed by a reduction in their symptoms. The underlying physiology of this effect has been discussed in Chapter 14.

Other drugs may be important in controlling pain of neuralgic origin. Included in the list of drugs with proven or possible anti-neuralgic effects are: anticonvulsants, vitamins, one muscle relaxer with central neuronal activity, psychotropics and, if the neuralgic process has an inflammatory component, the non-steroidal anti-inflammatories (see Table 5). Since most anti-neuralgia medications have no direct effect as anodynes, patients should be cautioned that a 2 or 3 week period of steady intake is often necessary before a pain relieving effect is achieved.

Intravenous infusions of lidocaine, or other local anesthetics, offers the possibility of sustained and at times cumulative benefit (20). Outpatient infusions of 1 to 5 mg/kg provide relief of diffuse musculoskeletal, neuralgic, or deafferentation pain for about half of the patients

TABLE 5. *Drugs useful for neuralgic pain*

Generic name	Brand name	Usual dose	Secondary effects
Diphenylhydantoin (phenytoin)	Dilantin	100 mg t.i.d. or q.i.d. or 200 mg b.i.d.	Mildly sedating, frequent allergic rash
Carbamazepine	Tegretol	200 mg b.i.d. to q.i.d.	Rare suppression of white blood count
Clonazepam	Klonopin	0.5 to 2.0 mg b.i.d. to q.i.d. or only q.h.s.	Sedating
Baclofen	Lioresal	10 to 20 mg t.i.d. or q.i.d.	Muscle weakness at higher doses
Thiamine HCL	Vitamin B₁	100 mg b.i.d. to q.i.d.	Uncertain effectiveness
Amitriptyline	Elavil	10 to 50 mg q.h.s.	Sedating or depersonalizing
Trazodone	Desyrel	50 to 100 mg q.h.s.	Sedating or depersonalizing
Haloperidol	Haldol	0.5 to 2 mg q.h.s.	Sedating or depersonalizing

treated, and with relief lasting more than a week in about one-fourth of the responders. The mechanism of the prolonged benefit is unknown, but might be due to desensitization of central or peripheral pain neurons to chemical neurotransmitters.

Lastly, psychotropic drugs may also play an important role in overall pain management. Anxiety and depression are common consequences of pain and disability, especially when these are persistent, and are important potentiators of pain. Tranquilizers or antidepressants can be useful adjuncts to managing the muscle tension and emotional consequences of chronic pain, in addition to having a direct action in reducing central deafferentation, hypersensitivity pain.

Central deafferentation pain, like chronic peripheral pain of nerve root injury, fusion instability, or adhesive arachnoiditis, can be an important factor in chronic pain states. Central deafferentation pain occurs when peripheral sensory input has been interrupted and central pain-transmitting neurons become hypersensitive, so that the patient experiences spontaneous pain in the area of sensory loss (13,47,57,81). It has been demonstrated experimentally that deafferented pain neurons can become so hypersensitive that they fire in response to increased blood levels of circulating biogenic amines, thus explaining in part the increased pain which these patients experience under emotional duress. Central deafferentation pain clinically resembles antalgic sensory loss, but arises from a nearly opposite mechanism. In antalgic sensory loss pain input into the central nervous system is the primary component and sensory loss results from competitive inhibition in a normally functioning central nervous system; relieving the pain by treating its cause restores lost sensation. Thus distinguishing between these two clinical conditions is important, since central deafferentation pain must be treated by therapy aimed at the central nervous system (and is made worse by further peripheral denervation), while antalgic sensory loss is treated by peripheral nervous system or musculoskeletal therapy.

Psychotherapy

The physical aspect of the failed low back syndrome never occurs in isolation from the psychological or human reaction to and contribution to that disease. Diagnostically, it is never easy to separate with certainty those treatable components of an illness which are based on tissue injury from those which are the result of a psychological reaction to that injury. Even more complex is deciphering when and to what degree psychological factors are contributing not only to pain but also to suffering. Those who treat patients with the failed back syndrome must constantly attempt to treat both aspects of each patient's problem at all times (4,26,32,34). It is the operating surgeon's responsibility to play a role in this process and not to rely solely on psychologists and psychiatrists. Not all doctors fully appreciate and exploit the considerable power they can wield in their relationships with patients. Whether inadvertent or intended, casual or calculated actions and words loosed by the physician toward his patient can do great psychological good or harm. The search for "disease," the basic task of establishing a differential diagnosis, is inherently discouraging. It has been suggested that since 80% of all American workers lose some time during their career from back pain, patients with back pain should not be considered to have "a disease," but merely "a symptom" or an unpleasant part of the normal human existence (11). In the management of patients with the failed back syndrome it is important to redefine their problem away from a search for a cure of their "disease" to an emphasis on renewing a more normal life style (26).

Great care must be taken to avoid rejecting the patient. Rejection can dash hope and weaken resolve to recover if the patient is allowed to feel unworthy or untreatable. Rejection can come in a variety of forms, including the doctor who is too busy to spend time with his patient or whose superficial optimism ignores the patient's real concerns and suffering. If referral is made to other health professionals, the patient must not be abandoned, but must receive continuing therapeutic input from the surgeon.

On the other hand, hope and confidence are important allies in the fight against disease and can do much to relieve pain and anxiety. The treating surgeon can offer explanations for anxiety-producing symptoms, treatment for those symptoms when needed and available, or simply the reassurance that specific treatment is not needed. Gaining the patient's confidence and understanding of treatment goals and of the duality of the psychosomatic nature of disease will also permit the later introduction of more formal psychotherapy if deemed necessary.

Psychosexual aspects of disease are also important, but are not always adequately dealt with by doctors. The physician should be aware that disease and suffering frequently cause impotence, dyspareunia, frustration, loss of self-image, and destruction of intimacy between partners. The doctor helps by inquiring about dysfunction in this aspect of life, discussing problems which are uncovered, providing insight on these problems to patients and partners, and by discussing alternative techniques of physical coupling, relaxation techniques, and timing of medications to facilitate love-making.

Suicide is a very real potential complication of the failed back syndrome. Patients who are depressed or discouraged are clearly at risk. Any patient who verbalizes ideas of self-destruction obviously should be considered at higher risk. If suicidal thoughts are expressed, experts have advised asking, "Have you thought how you would do it?" A patient who has contemplated both the act and the method seems to be a particular risk and should be referred for formal psychotherapy.

Several stress reduction techniques couple a psychological with a physical approach. Included are stress reduction clinics or neighborhood classes, support groups or private "lay" instruction in transcendental meditation or yoga. Hypnotherapy is probably best carried out in conjunction with formal psychotherapy. Biofeedback techniques stress physical control but should be coupled with relaxation goals.

Formal psychotherapy usually stresses coping with anxiety or depression more than pain relief, but improvement in anxiety or depression clearly can do much to relieve suffering. Unfortunately the patient suffering from a failed back syndrome often has maladaptive defense mechanisms and a history of overemphasis on work and poor interpersonal relations. For formal psychotherapy to be helpful the patient must first be convinced by the treating surgeon or other physician that pain and suffering which accompany tissue injury can indeed be helped by psychotherapy. The patient must participate in therapy willingly and actively. Since chronic pain treatment centers usually emphasize formal psychotherapy along with other treatment modalities, this need is equally as important when a chronic pain clinic is utilized, as discussed in Chapter 14.

INVASIVE THERAPY: NEEDLE TECHNIQUES

Needle therapy can be either (a) restorative or corrective or (b) destructive or neuroablative. Agents injected for restorative or corrective goals include local anesthetics, corticosteroids, or possibly prolotherapy. The goal of these injections is relaxation of muscle spasm, reduction of local inflammation, or, in the case of prolotherapy, tissue toughening through stimulation of proliferative fibroblastic reaction. Destructive or neuroablative techniques include injection of phenol, alcohol, or hypertonic solutions, or the creation of electrothermal lesions with radiofrequency current. These latter techniques are designed to provide pain relief by interrupting the neural transmission of pain impulses.

Injection techniques commonly provide pain relief of limited duration, but have the attraction that they are generally simpler and carry less risks than open surgery. All invasive procedures, even those employing only a needle, carry some inherent risks, including damage to nerves or other tissues, infection, or hemorrhage. Re-

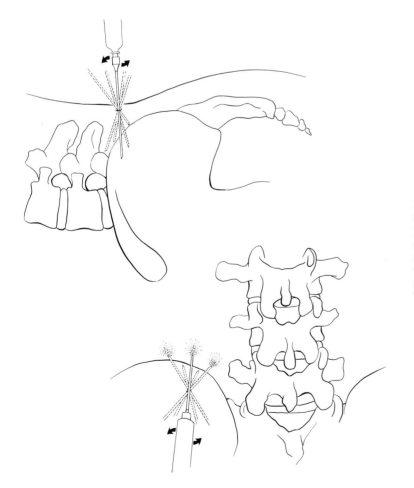

FIG. 4. Painful periosteal trigger points occur most commonly in the vicinity of the posterior/superior iliac spine. Effective relief can best be achieved by systematic injections along the medial and superficial periosteal surface using local anesthetics, often combined with depository corticosteroids or prolotherapy (with permission from ref. 72).

peatability is a major advantage of needle procedures. Long-lasting results are sometimes achieved, and repeated injections may suffice to maintain patients in a functional status.

The needle techniques are aimed at precise tissue targets, so precision of diagnosis is important. Often one goal of these injections is diagnostic: to determine when anatomic abnormalities are indeed physiologically significant and causative of pain.

The combination of pain and local tenderness is encountered in ischiogluteal bursitis, muscular or periosteal trigger points, iliolumbar syndrome, transaponeurotic fat herniation, coccydynia, and fixed muscle spasms (36,50,67,72). More diffuse tenderness and pain is often referred to as "fasciitis," or the "fibromyalgia" or "fibromyositis" syndrome as described by Katz and Liang in Chapter 15 (27).

A study was done by this author on 233 "trigger point" injections given between 1979 and 1984 to 46 of 327 low back patients (Fig. 4) (74). Sixty-nine percent were at the posterior iliac spine and 73% of patients were female. One hundred twenty-five corticosteroid injections brought total or excellent improvement in 57% of injections and poor or no relief in 26%. Improvement lasted an average of 4.5 months for those obtaining relief, and 15% obtained relief for over 6 months. Longer relief was obtained following unilateral injections, in post-operative patients and in males. In a study of prolotherapy 108 injections brought total or excellent relief in 42% of injections given and poor or no relief in 31%. Pain relief lasted an average of 2.4 months in those obtaining relief, with relief lasting 6 months or more in 7% of the patients. Relief was better and more lasting in females and in patients not previously operated upon.

Periosteal trigger points occur most commonly at the posterior superior iliac spine, but may be identified elsewhere over the lumbar spine, sacrum, or pelvic brim (74). Ischiogluteal bursitis and coccydynia both are commonly encountered in failed back syndrome. The local tenderness is aggravated by sitting and in coccydynia may be aggravated as well by bowel movements or sexual intromission. Ischiogluteal bursitis is identified by palpating the tip of the ischium with the hip flexed to rotate off the gluteal muscles, exposing the underlying bursa. Coccydynia is identified by the presence of local tenderness at the sacrococcygeal joint and by manipulating the coccyx bone itself, usually with one gloved finger inserted into the rectum and the thumb outside. Confirmation is obtained by anesthetizing the bursa or within and bilaterally adjacent to the sacrococcygeal joint. Intrabursal or intraarticular corticosteroids can give dramatic and long lasting relief, but sclerosing agents should not be employed.

Whether or not local anesthetics should be combined with corticosteroids for trigger point therapy is not currently scientifically validated. The injection of scleros-

ing solutions, commonly referred to as "prolotherapy," is specifically recommended by its advocates for aponeurotic fat herniations to toughen and strengthen the area of herniation, but this diagnosis is difficult, if not impossible, to confirm. Sclerosing solutions injected into muscle can, of course, be damaging. Prolotherapy is reported to be beneficial for the treatment of periosteal trigger points (26,30,31,36,50,58,72,74). The beneficial effect, if any, might be due to the powerful neurolytic effect of phenol on small unmyelinated pain fibers rather than a fibroblastic proliferant effect. The advocates of prolotherapy also suggest this technique has an advantage over corticosteroid injections because injections are thought to be cumulatively beneficial. One common solution used for prolotherapy is 5% phenol in anhydrous

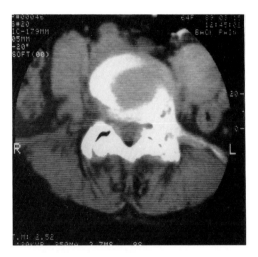

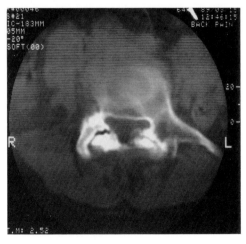

FIG. 5. This CT scan was taken at a motion segment level above a two-level solid lumbosacral fusion and illustrates two syndromes that can result from severe facet degeneration. On the right side, severe degeneration with vacuum phenomenon was associated with a "facet syndrome" of lumbago and pain on hyperextension. On the left side, hypertrophic changes caused lateral recess stenosis with nerve root compression and sciatica but no nerve root entrapment on stretch testing.

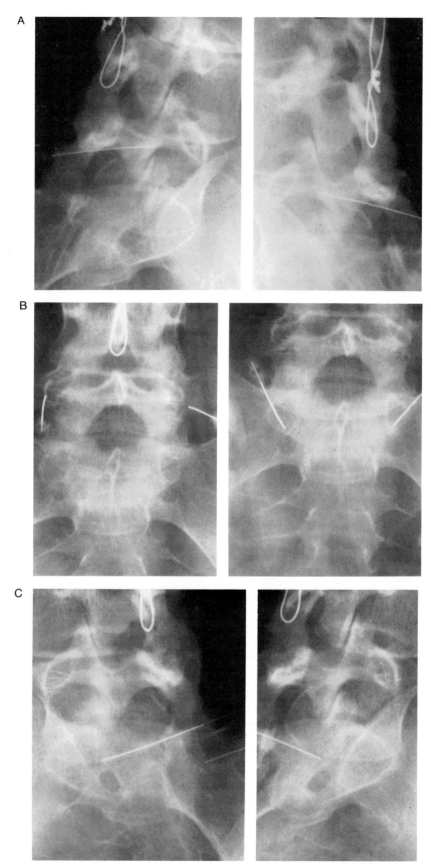

FIG. 6. These radiographs demonstrate needle placements for denervation of superior and inferior facet nerves to provide a "field block" of the lumbosacral facets bilaterally. Needle tips are placed in the vicinity of the superior facet nerves (**A**, right and left; **B**, left), then are shifted to the inferior facet nerves (**B**, right; **C**, right and left).

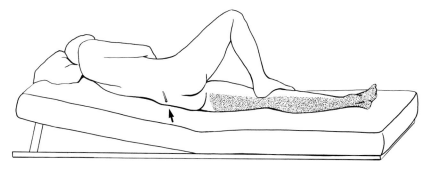

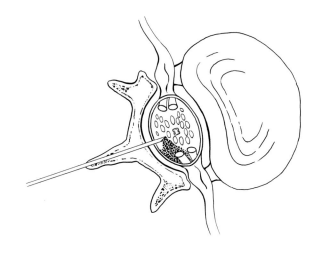

FIG. 7. Intrathecal phenol chemical sensory rhizotomy selectively interrupts pain transmission more than motor outflow. The thecal sac is punctured close to the nerves to be treated, then the hyperbaric solution is positioned gravimetrically in aliquots until sensory loss is achieved in the desired area (stippled). Tilting the patient slightly backwards is intended to increase exposure of dorsal sensory roots to the phenol (with permission from ref. 72).

glycerol mixed 1:4 with 0.5% plain bupivacaine, usually used in volumes of 4 to 10 ml. A few cases of disastrous complications have been reported following prolotherapy injections inadvertently given into the subarachnoid space (40). It must be emphasized that not all believe prolotherapy to be acceptable therapy.

Facets

The rationale, therapeutic effectiveness and techniques of facet anesthetization have been discussed in Chapter 25. As noted in that chapter, the correlation between anatomic changes in the facets and pain production is poor. Placing a needle in an unanesthetized facet joint causes pain in the lumbar paraspinal area with sharp radiation into the buttock and posterior thigh, but rarely below the knee. This same pattern of pain is characteristic of symptomatic facet syndrome and differs from true sciatica in that most of the pain is in the upper leg, whereas most of the pain of true sciatica is in the lower leg (Fig. 5). The pain of disc rupture is usually most severely aggravated by forward bending, while the pain of facet disease is characteristically aggravated principally by hyperextending the back. Anesthetic blocks of the facet joint, especially with radiopacified anesthetics, or of superior and inferior articular nerves, have been quite useful in my experience in determining which facet

is symptomatic, particularly in a failed back syndrome when several facets show degenerative change.

The invasive therapy of symptomatic facets with needle techniques can entail denervation, intraarticular corticosteroids or a combination of both. Even complete interruption of the superior and inferior articular nerves by 5% or 10% phenol or radiofrequency (RF) electrothermal lesioning leaves the joint denervated for only a few months, because the nerves are short and regenerate quickly. Lasting pain relief can at times be obtained by single or repeated facet injections or denervations. These techniques may be used to facilitate a restorative back exercise program. If repeated steroid injections are chosen as an alternative for long-term relief, it is not clear whether this results in hastening degeneration of the joint, or whether the joint simply continues to degenerate while its owner continues a life of increased activity.

Chemical or RF denervation of facets has largely supplanted surgical section of facet nerves. Sectioning also can easily be done at the time of a decompression or posterior fusion to reduce initial operative pain (49). Needle denervation is carried out under fluoroscopy, and permanent radiographs are obtained in case the procedure needs to be repeated (Fig. 6). Phenol is injected through 22 gauge lumbar puncture (LP) needles and RF lesioning is achieved with 12 or 18 gauge electrodes with 10 mm bared tips. The center of the RF electrode or the tip of the LP needle is placed at the anatomically presumed site of the superior and inferior recurrent facet nerves. Since there is no reliable physiologic test, points are selected midway between adjacent facets. This technique permits both facets to be denervated. Care must be taken not to lesion deeper than the intertransverse ligaments to avoid damaging nerve root trunks. Local anesthesia usually suffices for phenol injections (generally 0.5 to 0.75 ml 10% or 20% in glycerol for each site), and has the benefit of alerting the surgeon to inadvertent nerve root injections. Neuroleptanalgesia may be required for RF lesioning (generally 2 minutes at 85° or 90° Celsius).

Another place where local anesthetic injections of facet nerves may be helpful is determining the cause of pain with a pseudarthrosis. This topic has been carefully analyzed in Chapter 98 (Fig. 7). Less commonly, the facet nerves can be clinically significant in patients who have suffered traumatic avulsions of fascial adhesions to their fusion bone. Considerable local tenderness is usually present, often with localized swelling or even ecchymosis, but radiographs usually show no bony abnormality. As is true of pseudarthrotic pain, the regenerated facet nerves often play an important role in transmission of this form of avulsion pain, and diagnostic and therapeutic injections can play a useful role similar to that described for pseudarthrosis.

Discs

Both the injection of chymopapain (or other digestive enzymes) and of corticosteroids into lumbar discs can be therapeutically useful.

Chymopapain chemonucleolysis (discussed in Chapter 81) is not advisable in discs which have once been surgically resected or previously injected and is of relatively little benefit for the failed back syndrome sufferer (15,42). One possible exception, of course, is the patient whose original disc rupture was inadvertently overlooked during the first operation. Nonetheless, the careful study which chymopapain discolysis received is of considerable importance to all patients suffering disorders of the lower back. An international series of double blinded studies compared chymopapain injection to several different types of "placebo" intradiscal injections. It is important and well known that all of these studies showed some beneficial effect from chymopapain, despite its risks and limitations. Equally important, but less often discussed, is the fact that each of these series showed that approximately one-half of those patients injected with "placebo" also obtained relief of their sciatica! In each of these studies patients were selected for chymopapain discolysis only if they fulfilled the "accepted" criteria for the diagnosis of lumbar disc rupture causing sciatica unresponsive to "conventional non-operative therapy" and if their symptoms were severe enough and diagnosed with sufficient certainty to

make them candidates for open surgical resection. The fact that one-half of these patients who were considered to be suitable candidates for either open surgery or chymopapain were relieved by placebo injection raises strong doubts about our understanding of the pathophysiology of lumbar disc rupture and of the adequacy of "accepted non-operative therapy."

Intradiscal injection of both hydrocortisone and depository corticosteroids has been reported in published series to produce successful outcomes in from 60% to 90% of cases (21,29,78). A posterolateral needle technique is employed, similar to that for diagnostic discography or chymopapain chemonucleolysis. Its effects at times can be quite beneficial. Patients most likely to benefit from these intradiscal injections usually present with continuing lumbago greater than sciatica, presumed to be caused by a "painful disc." Imaging studies commonly show degenerative changes in the disc, including the "vacuum phenomenon," but degeneration does not always correlate with pain production. A few patients may have an aseptic inflammatory discitis, possibly on an autoimmune basis, and respond especially well to this therapy. Septic discitis should be first excluded by the absence of fever, imaging changes of bone destruction, or leukocytosis (but with an elevated sedimentation rate), and by barbotage/culture of the disc space contents. Pain on injection of contrast or saline into the disc, followed by a noticeable improvement in pain and range of back motion following disc anesthetization (the so-called "anesthesia discogram"), strongly suggest to me that the disc is a pain source and might respond to intradiscal steroids.

Nerve Roots

Nerve root irritation produces leg pain (sciatica) greater than back pain (lumbago). Nerve root irritation can be secondary to surgical decompression, nerve injury, periradicular scar, adhesive arachnoiditis (especially type I), lateral recess stenosis, synovial cysts, or major or minor trauma (especially when movement of the nerve root is restricted by adhesions). Retained disc fragments or unresected compressive disc ruptures in a patient in whom surgery had been carried out at the wrong level constitute special instances of persistent nerve root irritation and are more likely to require surgery.

Commonly, the pain of nerve root irritation is more or less constant, especially if the irritation is due to direct injury of the nerve, arachnoiditis, or constrictive scar. Activity typically aggravates the sciatica and acutely traumatized but not severely injured nerve roots sometimes can be healed by a period of inactivity.

Nerve root tension or entrapment signs may be absent in patients with lateral recess stenosis, but are usually present in most of the other conditions. Nerve root tension signs are elicited when sciatic radiation of pain is elicited by movements which stretch the nerve root within the neural foramen, such as straight leg raising or added forced ankle dorsiflexion with the leg partly elevated. Pain elicited by these maneuvers which is maximal in the lower back or buttock is more likely to derive from joints, ligaments, or tendons and does not constitute an abnormal nerve root tension response.

Motor, sensory, and reflex loss similarly indicate nerve injury if they occur in a radicular pattern. However, pain which occurs in patients with intact nerve roots not uncommonly produces antalgic anesthesia or antalgic paresis. These conditions are characterized by non-segmental impairment of motor and sensory function, often extending to segments above the level of discopathy, often with a stocking pattern of sensory loss to the knee or hip, accompanied by the preservation of deep tendon reflexes. Antalgic neurologic loss should not be equated with hysterical neurologic loss, since the former is the result of physiologic competitive inhibition within the central nervous system.

Diagnostic Testing

In approaching patients with nerve root symptoms, a variety of imaging techniques may be useful. Myelography remains the definitive way of diagnosing arachnoiditis, especially type I arachnoiditis, but most other conditions can be diagnosed equally well or better with CT scan or MRI. High quality CT scans show bony detail superbly and three dimensional reconstructions give excellent anatomic information about lateral recess stenosis. CT scans usually document the mass effect of extradural scar, disc fragment, or synovial cyst, but cannot image a damaged nerve root not associated with bulky scar. Differentiating extradural scar from disc material is often made possible by the presence of enhancement of scar tissue after intravenous contrast administration. Myelography or CT/myelography may demonstrate swollen nerve roots in the absence of extradural mass and, thus, may raise anatomic suspicion of symptomatic nerve root injury. High quality MRI can often differentiate extradural tissue better than CT scan (especially when coupled with gadolinium enhancement), and has the major advantage of multiplanar imaging. Thermography may detect associated autonomic injury but seems incapable of precisely localizing the pain source. Temperature increases are sometimes observed overlying areas of muscle spasm. The EMG and nerve conduction electrodiagnostic studies may be abnormal if there is associated nerve injury, but abnormalities are frequently noted in the post-operative patient without symptoms.

As noted by Mooney in Chapter 25, diagnostic nerve root anesthetic blocks may be helpful in determining whether pain arises from nerve roots and which nerve roots are involved. However, short-term pain relief from anesthetization of a nerve root does not necessarily predict a long term therapeutic effect because of peripheral overlapping sensory innervation and the later development of central deafferentation hypersensitivity pain (5). In performing these injections, the lateral extraspinal approach probably offers greater specificity of nerve root anesthesia and greater safety in patients with epidural scar, but the medial, epidural approach offers an opportunity for concomitant steroid injection.

Epidural periradicular injection can be especially helpful in patients with persistent sciatica following surgery, especially patients with continued monoradicular pain. The lasting relief which occasionally follows local anesthetic injection presumably occurs by interrupting pain cycles or perhaps by disrupting or stretching local scar. More consistent and at times long lasting relief can be obtained through the use of corticosteroids (5). Periradicular injections are often effective when midline epidural steroid injections fail, perhaps because local scar tissue blocks access of the midline steroid injection to the inflamed nerve root. Periradicular steroid injections must be given cautiously once the nerve root is anesthetized to limit the risk of damage to the root. While there is some suggestion of neurotoxicity of perineural or periradicular depository steroid injection, that risk seems to be slight if the nerve root has not actually been penetrated. The risk of infection can usually be minimized with careful technique and skin preparation. Frequent repetitions seem to increase the risk considerably, apparently because of an increased risk of neurotoxicity and possibly because the steroids reduce the local tissue resistance to infection if organisms are subsequently injected.

Midline Epidural and Intrathecal Injections

A variety of restorative and neuroablative agents and techniques have been used for midline epidural and intrathecal injections. These techniques can be helpful in some patients with either severe back pain or unilateral or bilateral sciatica. Painful inflammation of the dura or its adnexae and painful cicatricial entrapment of nerve roots are conditions which in my experience are most commonly responsive to injections, but relief is sometimes achieved non-specifically in a variety of other causes of the failed back syndrome.

However, the use of epidural and especially intrathecal corticosteroid injections is particularly controversial (2,12,14,19,25,37,62,65,69,74,75,80). The literature documents significant complications following such injections, particularly in patients with complicated medical problems who have received multiple injections (28,51). The literature supporting the efficacy of intrathecal steroids is more limited than that for epidural steroids and is further confused by the large amount of literature regarding the use of frequent injections of intrathecal steroids in the treatment of multiple sclerosis. Except for the septic complications, the neurologic complications often affected the thoracic spinal cord at a distance from the site of injection, even though studies have shown the corticosteroid to concentrate in the lumbar theca. The identification of the corticosteroid as the causative agent for these neurologic complications has been based exclusively on circumstantial evidence. The experimental literature is also confusing, since some investigations emphasize the apparent beneficial effect of intrathecal injections while others emphasize an induced pleocytosis and a possible increased risk of arachnoiditis (22,52,65). This is especially true if corticosteroids are injected with blood or non-water soluble contrast agents. Considerable literature and clinical experience attest to the therapeutic benefit of epidural corticosteroid injections, which may in themselves be curative, or may provide long-term symptomatic relief through judicious repetition, or may facilitate and make possible restorative programs. Several authors have commented that intrathecal steroid injections are at times beneficial when epidural steroid injections have failed. My experience has been that intrathecal steroid injections may at times be the only treatment which can bring intermediate or long-term relief to patients suffering intractably from the pain of lumbar adhesive arachnoiditis (74,75). The practitioner must be aware that the manufacturer of Depo-Medrol (methylprednisolone acetate) has specifically advised against its intrathecal use because of its potential risks, but this potential risk seems smaller than that of repeated surgical intervention, and its use may be justified in the specifically informed patient.

Neuroablative Injections

Neuroablative or destructive intrathecal injections can be considered for longer lasting or semi-permanent sensory fiber interruption in an effort to control pain, especially of radicular origin (5,68,77). Phenol (or carbolic acid) and absolute ethanol are the agents most commonly employed, though iced or hypertonic saline injections enjoyed a brief popularity (1,40). Since these agents cause relatively long-lasting loss of neurologic function, it is important that restorative therapy first be carried out in an attempt to provide relief of sciatic pain before selecting those few patients who may benefit from these denervating and potentially damaging procedures. It is mandatory that the neuroablative injections be preceded by diagnostic blocks in an effort to predict whether or not sensory interruption will bring pain relief rather than aggravating central deafferentation pain. It is also essential to carry out myelography to ensure that the subarachnoid space is open to minimize the risk of loculation of the destructive agent.

The injections are administered via a spinal puncture at or near the level of exit of the painful nerve roots or just at the upper edge of the posterior fusion if the nerve roots exit from beneath a solid fusion mass. The patient is positioned with the painful side down if hyperbaric phenol solutions are to be used or with the painful side up if hypobaric absolute ethanol is to be used (Fig. 8). Angling the patient 10° backward or forward is intended to increase contact between the destructive agent and the sensory portion of the exiting nerve root. A free flow of spinal fluid must be maintained throughout the procedure to ensure subarachnoid injection. Subdural injections give poor or erratic results, including an increased risk of motor loss. It is important that the patient be placed on a hospital bed, table, or x-ray platform that permits Trendelenburg and reverse Trendelenburg posi-

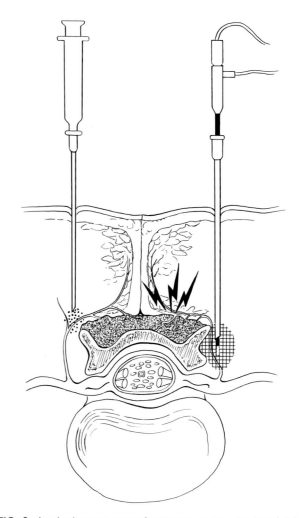

FIG. 8. Lesioning recurrent facet nerves may be helpful for the pain of fusion pseudarthrosis. These nerves regenerate to innervate the fusion bone. If a painful pseudarthrosis develops, the pain is largely transmitted through these nerves. Phenol injection (left, stippled) or radiofrequency lesioning (right, crosshatching) can interrupt nerve transmission and provide months of relief (with permission from ref. 72).

tioning, since the solution is localized gravimetrically by tilting the patient and observing induced sensory loss. Solutions of 5% phenol in anhydrous glycerol give selective sensory interruption greater than motor interruption. Solutions of 7.5% phenol in iophendylate permit radiographic confirmation that the contrast material is in the desired location. However, phenol is more soluble in iophendylate than in spinal fluid and is thus absorbed much more slowly. Consequently the iophendylate must be removed completely to prevent damage to unwanted portions of the nervous system after the patient's position is changed. The induced sensory loss clears in an inversely exponential fashion. Sensory loss is quite rapid over the first 12 hours, then is increasingly slow over many months or even a few years. The volume of phenol in glycerol or of ethanol injected usually should not exceed 1.0 to 1.5 ml. The initial goal of therapy is to create dense sensory loss in the area of pain with only minimal motor weakness, which when present usually clears overnight. Phenol injections have become more popular than ethanol injections since they seem to have a more selective effect on sensory fibers, and spare motor fibers.

Even though neuroablative injections do not involve a formal, operative procedure, they are invasive procedures. The limitations and potential complications of the technique may be long lasting and must be weighed against potential benefit. As mentioned earlier, the production of sensory loss does not always equate with pain relief, even though this usually represents a failure of choice of therapy rather than being a failure of the ablative technique. The duration of induced sensory loss is rarely permanent, and even though the procedure may be repeated, repetitive injections are less likely to be effective due to nerve root scarring. The risk of motor nerve injury also is greater with subsequent injections. Furthermore, even though the neuroablative techniques offer a differential interruption of sensory fibers greater than motor fibers, complete or sufficient sensory interruption may not be possible without producing undesirable motor or autonomic loss. The production of such unwanted deficits represents one of the major complications of the procedure, including the risk of sacral sensory and autonomic loss which is especially great with injections of phenol in iophendylate. Although no precise complication rates are available, perhaps 10% of patients will experience undesirable weakness and 5% impairment of sphincter control, although nearly all recover in 6 to 18 months. Also, neuroablative solutions are inherently irritating. Some meningismus is an expected part of the procedure, and an occasional patient may experience considerable meningismus with secondary painful muscle spasms for several days following the procedure. Planned introduction of the neuroablative agents directly into the high cervical region has been associated with respiratory arrest, which fortunately is usually temporary.

Intraspinal Morphine

Extradural injection of morphine or other agents has been reported as a routine step in lumbar laminectomy, but is usually accomplished via a temporary indwelling epidural or intrathecal catheter (55,64). In chronic pain syndromes percutaneous catheter placement is useful for preliminary testing, but carries an unacceptable risk of sepsis with prolonged use. Fully implantable pump systems are generally expensive and earlier pump versions resulted in numerous reports of pump failure or unreliability. Apparently mechanical device failures accounted for some of the early pessimism regarding habituation to long-term administration of intrathecal or epidural morphine, though this remains a significant potential limitation. Before reliable mechanical pumps were readily available, manually activated systems were more commonly implanted, consisting of a subcutaneous and refillable reservoir with a manual pump (often a CSF shunt/valve). These devices were subject to considerable patient error and the possibility of overdosage through accidental overcompression of the reservoir.

Currently both the Medtronic Corporation and the Infusaid Corporation manufacture fully implantable pump systems. Each version has a reservoir which can be refilled by percutaneous needling, allowing one to two weeks of administration. The catheter is placed epidurally or intrathecally in the lumbar spinal canal through a side-hole Touhey needle after making a small skin incision. Some surgeons prefer a small laminotomy if the catheter is to be placed intrathecally, since this permits placement of a purse-string suture at the dural penetration site. The catheter is tunneled subcutaneously around the trunk to be attached to the pump, which is inserted into a subcutaneous pocket over the lower rib cage anteriorly. Subarachnoid catheter placement permits the administration of smaller narcotic doses than those required for epidural administration, but carries a risk of CSF leakage. Preservation free morphine, now fairly readily available, has been the most widely used agent for pain relief, though a variety of other agents have been studied. Lioresal seems to have a useful role in long term relief of spasticity, and may have a useful role in centrally mediated deafferentation pain (56).

Even with fully implantable pumps, sepsis still remains the major risk in epidural or subarachnoid catheter placement. Careful sterile technique must be followed in percutaneous refilling of pump reservoirs and in drug administration through transcutaneous catheters. Drug concentrations and doses must be carefully selected and the dose to be administered must be carefully formulated. An initial test dose must be given with the patient under close observation to avoid the risk of over sedation or respiratory depression. Subsequently, drug formulation and reservoir refilling must be carried out by professional personnel or by carefully trained family members. This requirement for reservoir refilling, generally at intervals of 1 to 3 weeks, is one of the major limitations of the use of implantable pump systems, since the process is relatively labor intensive. This can pose a particular problem for patients who live at a distance from the implanting facility or who do not have available competent family members.

INVASIVE THERAPY: SURGERY

Surgery is indicated for only a minority of patients suffering from a failed back syndrome. However, this does not imply that appropriate surgery, which has a reasonable likelihood of success, should be avoided or should be unduly delayed. At times the most conservative approach to a problem may in fact be early surgical intervention, if that intervention carries a better risk/benefit ratio than non-surgical alternatives. This is particularly true with retained or new disc fragments.

As emphasized repeatedly in this text, a surgical procedure cannot be successful unless it meets the patient's expectations, and it follows that the patient's expectations can never be met if they are unreasonable because he is ill informed or emotionally incapable of making a clear and tenable decision. No surgery can be uniformly successful and surgical decisions in patients with failed back syndrome are often difficult because the expected success rates are often far from perfect. The decision to undertake surgery in the face of more limited success rates and significant potential for complications must be a carefully considered joint decision between the surgeon, the patient, and preferably the patient's family.

Many of the procedures potentially useful in treating patients with failed back syndrome have been discussed in detail in Chapters 89 and 92–98, such as removal of recurrent or retained disc ruptures, laminectomy for excision or repair of pseudo-meningoceles, bony decompression of individual or multiple nerve roots or for residual stenosis, and the role of fusion for instability. Here I will emphasize other surgical alternatives, such as excision of epidural scar, lysis of intradural arachnoiditis, implantation of dorsal column stimulators, sensory rhizotomy or dorsal root entry zone lesioning, cordotomy, stereotactic placement of brain stimulators or lesions, and cingulotomy. Many of these operations are aimed at pain control and are not specific for spinal disease, so will not be discussed in detail.

Nerve Root Decompression

Deciding which patient becomes a surgical candidate for nerve root decompression for a failed back syndrome is often difficult. Even our most advanced imaging techniques with contrast enhanced CT or MRI cannot infallibly distinguish between extradural scar and disc mate-rial. Furthermore, in the presence of extradural scar even a small amount of additional disc material pressing against a tethered nerve root may cause severe symptoms. Compression and tethering of the nerve root by extradural scar can also be quite symptomatic even without a fragment or disc rupture, and many neurosurgeons still believe decompression may give lasting pain relief, especially if coupled with fat pad grafting to limit the recurrence of scar tissue. However, excision of extradural scar in patients who present principally with lumbago is likely to fail, since nerve root compression causes sciatica, not lumbago, and the extradural scar may be asymptomatic. Even if the extradural scar is deemed to be causing symptoms, surgical intervention often is unnecessary. Many of these patients achieve adequate function and control of symptoms with alternative nonsurgical therapy, such as antineuralgia medications and periradicular epidural steroid injections.

Lysis of Adhesive Arachnoiditis

The surgical lysis of adhesive arachnoiditis plays a limited, but sometimes valuable role in the management of failed back syndrome patients (43,60,73,78). Adhesive arachnoiditis occurs in the context of lumbar disc surgery usually in a form limited to one or two motion segment levels (6,10,44). The arachnoiditis may be classified as type I, which affects a single nerve root exit zone, type II, which causes bilateral or annular constriction with preservation of an open central canal, or type III, where there is total transverse CSF obstruction (Fig. 9) (44). Adhesive arachnoiditis has been variously ascribed to myelographic contrast media, especially non-water soluble media in the presence of blood, and to surgical trauma (6,10,44,51,71,72,74). It clearly can develop spontaneously either as the result of a disc rupture or present de novo, mimicking disc rupture. On rare occasions arachnoiditis is reported as a familial disorder. Implications of myelographic contrast media, especially iophendylate, as a causative agent are confused by the observation that arachnoiditis almost never occurs in patients who have undergone cervical myelography alone and by the observation that arachnoiditis usually occurs at mid to low lumbar levels and almost never in the sacral end of the theca to which retained iophendylate gravitates. Arachnoiditis can be completely asymptomatic, but yet may be of major significance, since its presence can make difficult the diagnosis of alternative or treatable conditions or can divert attention away from a search for those conditions. Arachnoiditis probably becomes symptomatic by mechanical constriction of nerve roots and by interfering with that portion of nerve root nutrition derived from the spinal fluid. The process seems to develop and progress over a course of 6 to 18 months, but rarely further progresses beyond that inter-

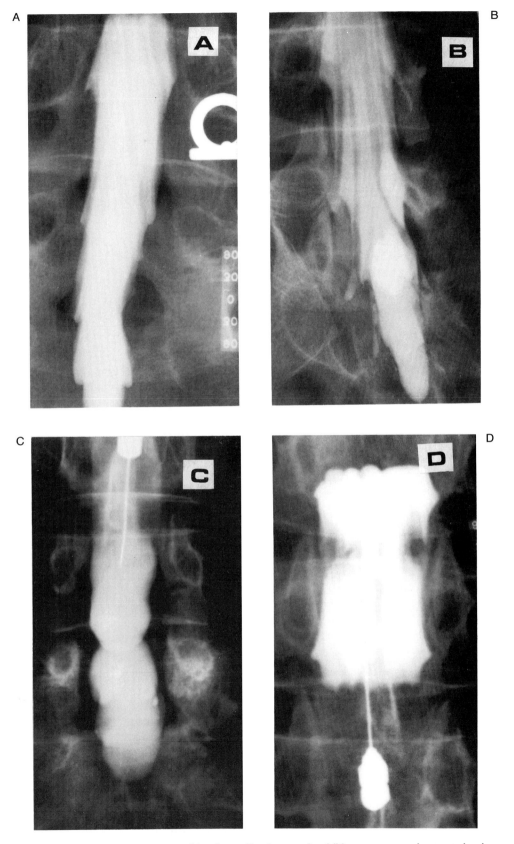

FIG. 9. Three stages or types of lumbar adhesive arachnoiditis are commonly recognized. **A:** Type I entails obliteration of a single nerve root pouch and mimics disc rupture—though the CT scan and surgery in this patient disclosed no disc herniation. **B and C:** Circumferential adhesion of nerve roots constitutes type II and can be localized or extensive. **D:** Despite total transverse obliteration of the subarachnoid space, type III arachnoiditis can be asymptomatic.

val except in the face of continuing trauma from spinal instability or secondary to intercurrent injury which causes stretching of constricted nerves, or localized hemorrhage and edema of nerve roots already compromised by the scarring. Accordingly, patients who develop new symptoms 2 or more years following their initial spinal intervention and who are documented to have adhesive arachnoiditis are quite likely to be symptomatic from a condition other than the arachnoiditis.

As discussed earlier, patients who failed to obtain relief from their arachnoiditis through non-operative therapy can at times be successfully treated with intrathecal methylprednisolone acetate, recognizing the risk and complications of that technique.

Patients with severely symptomatic arachnoiditis may become candidates for microsurgical lysis of the arachnoiditis, especially if their clinical condition is deteriorating progressively within the first year after the surgical intervention. The value of surgical lysis of type I arachnoiditis, confined to a single nerve root exit site and causing monoradiculopathy, has not been quantified. Type I arachnoiditis can occur in association with or following removal of a disc herniation. It also can mimic disc herniation and cause a monoradiculopathy, accompanied by a large myelographic defect, but with little abnormality visualized extradurally on CT or MRI imaging or at the time of surgical exploration. Some of these patients were found to have significant extradural adhesions at the time of primary operative exploration of the disc space. The results of microsurgical lysis of type II or type III arachnoiditis, including ossified arachnoiditis, have been reported in several series. The results have been varied and often less than spectacular (43,60,73,78).

In my series of 17 patients on whom I performed microsurgical lysis, three-fourths of the patients achieved initial improvement in pain or neurologic deficit, but at the end of one year only 50% of these patients maintained a useful degree of improvement (Fig. 10). Furthermore, new neurologic deficits followed surgery in 18% of these patients, most notably bladder and bowel dysfunction. The addition of dural decompressive grafting at the time of microsurgical lysis has resulted in an increased incidence of spinal fluid leaks without apparently improving effectiveness. Other investigators have added intrathecal corticosteroids or digestive enzymes at the conclusion of the lysis, but the data are insufficient to state whether or not these additions have been beneficial. In my series, patients were chosen on the basis of severe and progressive symptomatology and documented severe arachnoiditis. Some of these desperate patients achieved initial and persistent improvement. The severity of the clinical disease was confirmed in those who failed to obtain relief from surgery, since suicide was one alternative chosen by several patients who failed to obtain relief from microsurgical lysis.

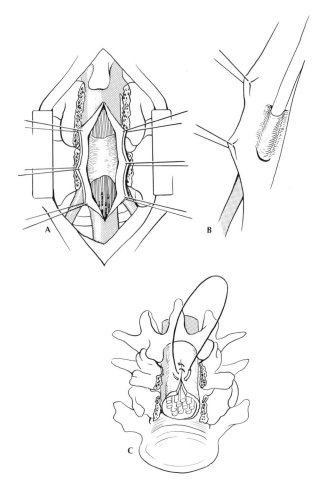

FIG. 10. **A:** Adhesive arachnoiditis can occur as type III or transverse complete obliteration of the subarachnoid space at the level of "disc disease." **B:** Type I arachnoiditis is localized to the nerve root exit site and may be one cause of sciatica. **C:** Dural thickening facilitates water tight closure so excessively vigorous resection of extradural scar is best avoided (with permission from ref. 72).

Excision of Periosteal Trigger Points

Excision of persistently painful and focally tender periosteal trigger points is a therapy of low morbidity but unconfirmed benefit. Focal periosteal trigger points occur with a 70% to 75% frequency at or adjacent to the posterior iliac spine. The combination of localized pain and sharply focalized tenderness, when confirmed by relief of pain and tenderness with local anesthetization, implies a condition which usually responds well to nonsurgical therapy, especially local injection. Recurrent trigger points usually can be obviated by a program of progressive back strengthening exercises. Surgical excision of the trigger point becomes an option to consider for those patients who suffer from typical focal trigger points consistently in the same location, who obtain consistent relief from local injection but who remain severely symptomatic due to persistent recurrences. The area of maximum tenderness can be marked just before surgery by injection of indigo carmine under local anesthesia. The area of periosteal involvement is then excised, underlying bone spurs are removed and an area of bone is partially decorticated in hopes of encouraging more firm tissue reattachment. Ligaments and periosteum are then tightly resutured. The whole procedure can often be accomplished under local anesthesia on a day surgery basis. In a limited number of patients I have been able to achieve lasting improvement (perhaps two-thirds).

Dorsal Column Stimulator Implantation

Dorsal column stimulation (DCS) provides pain relief through competitive sensory stimulation of the dorsal fibers of the spinal cord which transmit tactile and postural information (60,70,71). Dorsal column stimulator implantation offers carefully selected patients with failed back syndrome the possibility of pain relief without destruction of nervous tissue and with relatively limited risk (3,17,45,59,60). The outcome of dorsal column stimulator implantation is generally better in patients who have obtained at least partial pain relief from transcutaneous stimulation (TENS) and seems especially applicable to those patients with widespread back and bilateral leg pain in whom the scope of TENS is not sufficiently wide to relieve all of the painful area. Patients with symptomatic adhesive arachnoiditis or patients who remain severely symptomatic despite extensive surgery and stable fusions most commonly are selected for this technique.

Dorsal column stimulating electrodes can be inserted percutaneously or by open surgical laminotomy, and can be attached to temporary external connections for testing prior to permanent implantation (Fig. 11). The simpler technique of percutaneous electrode placement with temporary externalization for preliminary testing has the obvious attractiveness of permitting preliminary testing of the adequacy of pain relief before committing the patient to more extensive surgery for implantation of a costly internalized device. Unfortunately, two major problems restrict the usefulness of this technique. Despite all precautions, the temporary percutaneous device carries a distinct risk of sepsis. Equally important is that the easily placed percutaneous electrodes do not maintain their position well relative to the spinal cord and tend to shift as the patient resumes a more active lifestyle, thus losing their effectiveness.

The alternative surgical technique, which I prefer, is to proceed directly with permanent implantation once the patient has been determined to be a reasonable candidate, based in large part on the patient's prior response to TENS. Patients who obtain no pain relief whatsoever from TENS have a much reduced chance of obtaining benefit from an implanted system. The epidural stimulating electrode is implanted through a short low thoracic skin incision. One very satisfactory electrode system consists of four small contact plates in a ribbon of silastic rubber. This can be inserted obliquely in the epidural space across the dorsum of the spinal cord in the low thoracic region from a laminotomy on one side to a laminotomy at a higher level on the opposite side. The combination of four contacts allows a variety of stimulation patterns. The wires from the electrode are tunneled subcutaneously around the chest to a subcutaneously created pocket over the lower anterior rib cage. Alternatively, the wires may be tunneled over the shoulder or around the upper thorax above the breast to a pocket in the pectoral area. Either a receiver/transducer or a self-powered stimulating unit is then attached to the electrode wires and implanted in the subcutaneous pocket. Many surgeons prefer to use local anesthesia with light neuroleptanalgesia for DCS implantation, rather than general anesthesia. Having the patient awake during the procedure allows intra-operative stimulation for confirmation of electrode placement, but requires a cooperative patient and may increase the risk of wound infection by increasing the complexity and duration of the operation.

The implanted systems themselves vary widely. The simpler systems involve a single fixed output to one channel so one pair of electrodes must be preselected either through external testing, through manipulation of the electrodes under local anesthesia, or through reliance on anatomical probability. Other systems provide for multiple channels or selection of different channels after implantation. The unit which is implanted may be either a radio receiver/transducer or a battery powered self-contained unit. The receiver/transducer units are powered by externally applied antennae, and stimulus parameters are set easily by the patient using the power transmitter which operates through the antenna. While this can be more inconvenient than the completely implanted battery powered systems, the need for surgical intervention to change batteries is obviated. Under normal usage batteries generally last several years. Stimulus parameters and power output can be changed on the battery powered implanted systems through a transcutaneous control device. If the patient is to control his own stimulus parameters, this entails the purchase of an extra and expensive unit, though alternatively all settings can be made by the surgeon or his designee. The battery powered units can be turned on and off with a simple magnet held in proximity to the device.

Complications from dorsal column stimulator implantation include sepsis, spinal cord compression, device failure, or pain or discomfort. As mentioned earlier, infection is a major consideration in percutaneously tested systems, but any chronically implanted device has the potential for early or later infection, usually necessitating removal of the device, particularly when there is a

A

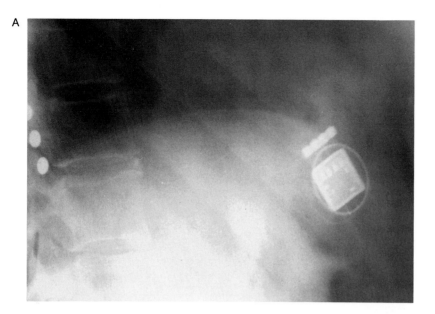

FIG. 11. These radiographs demonstrate an implanted dorsal column stimulator (DCS) receiver placed subcutaneously over the lower rib cage **(A)** and attached by subcutaneously placed wires to a four-contact ribbon electrode placed by two-level laminotomy in the lower thoracic epidural space **(B)**.

B

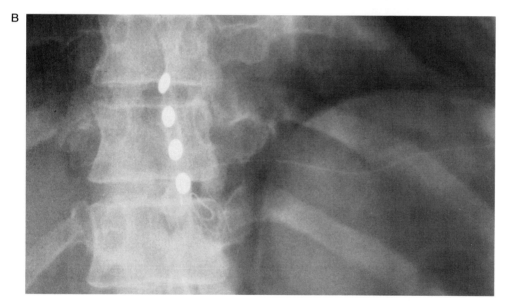

deep infection. Occasionally the electrode has elicited a fibrous reaction, possibly related to tearing of small epidural vessels, which has caused later spinal cord compression. This rare complication requires removal of the electrodes and decompression of the epidural mass. Device failure is most commonly encountered when simple electrodes shift their position. Even well placed and permanently secured electrodes will give varying results depending on patient posture. As the patient bends forward or backward the spinal cord moves within the subarachnoid space, coming either closer to or further from the epidural stimulating electrode. While this is rarely a major problem, it can be annoying to some patients, especially those who have to change positions frequently. A progressive failure to produce pain relief does not necessarily imply device failure, especially if the patient continues to obtain sensory input. On the other hand, a progressive fading of sensory awareness of stimulator input can be due to epidural fibrosis, interruption of implanted wires, corrosion of contacts, or failure of the implanted receiver or battery powered generator. Relatively inexpensive devices are available for percutaneous measurements of the output of the implanted device, but confirmation and correction of the problem often requires surgical intervention. A number of patients will request removal of the device because of discomfort or pain, especially if the original pain for which the device was implanted has not been adequately controlled. Patients commonly experience pain either at the site of electrode penetration into the spine or from the subcutaneous bulk of the implanted receiver or generator. Subcutaneous implantation of the receiver or generator over the upper chest or lower rib cage is preferable to subcutaneous implantation over the abdomen, where the device can be painfully compressed by the rib cage on trunk flexion. At any location, compression by constricting clothing, especially belts or brassieres, can provoke discomfort, and this consideration should also influence device placement.

Rhizotomy and Dorsal Root Entry Zone Lesioning

Monoradicular or biradicular pain which proves refractory to non-operative therapy may be treated by afferent sensory interruption at one or more nerve root levels (72). Nerve root anesthetic blocks, paravertebrally or epidurally, help to define which nerve root(s) are involved and whether or not the pain is more likely to be of peripheral or of central deafferentation origin. Additional information can at times be achieved by segmental spinal subarachnoid or differential spinal anesthetic block techniques. These tests are especially helpful in determining whether or not the radicular pattern of pain is likely to have a central deafferentation origin. Unfortunately, the plasticity of the nervous system limits accurate prediction of long-term pain relief following surgical interruption of sensory nerves, even when short-term pain relief is excellent following diagnostic blocks. Peripheral sensory overlap, peripheral sprouting and central deafferentation hypersensitivity all become more important with time. The published series of sensory rhizotomies report long-term failure rates of pain relief varying widely from as low as 10% to as high as 75% or 80%. Conversely, of course, this data means that from 20% to 90% of patients with refractory sciatica in fact do achieve lasting pain relief.

Sensory ganglionectomy has been advocated by some as an alternative to dorsal sensory rhizotomy, the rationale being that some axonal sensory fibers may reach the cord via ventral roots (81). The technique has not been widely employed and seems to have been used most commonly for thoracic rhizotomy, where there is probably less risk of destabilizing active motion segments by more lateral removal of bone.

Dorsal root entry zone lesioning attempts to provide pain relief to patients suffering from central deafferentation hypersensitivity by destroying cell bodies in the dorsal root entry zone of the spinal cord (17). These cells have been demonstrated pathophysiologically to become hypersensitive following deafferentation to the point that they can fire spontaneously or in response to elevated levels of circulating biogenic amines, which can be promoted by emotional tension or anxiety. This technique has been employed most widely in the cervical region, and as yet extensive data are lacking regarding its efficacy in patients with lumbar radicular pattern pain of central deafferentation origin. In contrast to lesioning in the cervical area, the risk of leg weakness would seem to be reduced by anatomic considerations and hopefully disturbances of bladder or bowel function should not be

severe following unilateral interruption of intermediolateral cell columns and corresponding fiber tracks.

Cordotomy and Stereotaxic Brain Surgery

Anterolateral spinal cordotomy and stereotaxic brain lesioning or electrode implantation are specialized neurosurgical techniques for providing pain relief (9,38). Because of their complexity, potential risk, and imperfect success rates these procedures are usually reserved for failed back syndrome patients with truly desperate and refractory clinical conditions. Cordotomy carries the risk of significant weakness of the leg contralateral to the pain, and at least half of patients seem to lose their pain relief when they are followed for periods exceeding one year. Bilateral brain lesioning in the medial thalamic areas can selectively interrupt the protopathic or suffering component of pain, but carries the risk of ataxia, dysarthria, and impairment of consciousness. Stimulating electrodes placed into periaqueductal gray or lateral thalamic regions produce results similar to, but more powerful than, those achieved with dorsal column electrode implantation and stimulation (38,39,61). Electrode placement must be extremely precise, electrodes may shift with time and habituation of the response to stimulation has been a troublesome development. Cingulotomy seems to provide pain relief by interrupting the selective pathway which maintains conscious awareness of pain through prevention of habituation (34,41,72). It seems to provide relief of persistent pain without blocking awareness of new pain in approximately two-thirds of patients. At times the relief can be spectacularly successful, especially in patients with chronic and steady pain associated with strong emotional reactions in the patient. Cingulotomy has also been used to treat severe depression, but one of my patients, who was dramatically relieved of pain, became profoundly and suicidally depressed when he was no longer distracted by pain but was increasingly aware that he would never be able to return to his former job. The effect of cingulotomy on intellectual performance is generally minimal, though minor blunting of affect is often noted by families. Although there are as yet no published reports, in my longterm follow-up of cingulotomy patients, approximately 20% later developed convulsive seizures.

PAIN CLINIC OR INDIVIDUAL THERAPIST?

Formally organized chronic pain control clinics, especially those with inpatient programs, can provide a valuable asset for the treatment of refractory patients with failed back syndromes, as discussed elsewhere in this book (23,48). These clinics offer a multimodality approach which attempts to address not only the patient's pain but the patient's emotional reaction toward his pain, family interactions, and employment concerns. It is important that patients referred to these clinics be aware of the psychotherapeutic aspect of the treatment they will receive, and that they are educated to accept this aspect of therapy as a valuable part of their rehabilitation process.

Not all aspects of chronic pain clinics are positive however. Success rates measured in terms of pain relief and medication reduction vary considerably from clinic to clinic, and outcomes in terms of return to work status are generally even less favorable. Recidivism and pain recrudescence are commonly encountered with long-term follow-up. Furthermore, only a limited number of such clinics are available in the United States, and referral of a patient to such a center often necessitates the patient traveling to a distant city and to unfamiliar therapists. And, all too often, a referral to a pain clinic is viewed by the patient's operating surgeon as a "one way ticket" for the patient, by which the surgeon is relieved of the necessity of continued involvement in that patient's care. Since the failed back syndrome is usually a non-fatal disorder (barring suicide), and since most patients are relatively young and face a relatively long life expectancy, transferring care to a distant clinic or specialist often deprives the patient of important continuing support and care. While the multimodality aspect of pain clinics is capable of addressing many facets of the patient's problem, the potential inefficiency of "the committee approach" is notorious, and the patient may find himself deprived of a single familiar and reliable source of support and comfort to whom he or she can turn in time of need.

The alternative to formal pain clinics is long-term care by the responsible surgeon who performed the patient's back surgery, with the assistance of local specialists. Good medical practice dictates that a surgeon who undertakes the treatment of a particular medical problem for a patient should continue to be responsible for that patient's care until a successful outcome is achieved. This does not imply that the surgeon must or should work alone, especially in dealing with a disease as complex as a failed back syndrome. The patient's family physician or a rheumatologist or internist might function as the patient's principal contact person, but the operating surgeon should still remain actively involved until a successful outcome has been achieved from his surgery. Additional local specialists and health care therapists can then be called in by the primary medical physician or the surgeon to help assess and treat specific aspects of the patient's problem. Specialists to be considered include not only neurosurgeons, but orthopedists, anesthesiologists, or algologists. A rheumatologist willing to treat patients with non-specific arthralgias can be very helpful in managing anti-inflammatory drugs. Psychiatrists, psychologists, physiatrists, physical therapists, family counselors, social workers, and rehabilitation and job retraining specialists all can be involved at a local and individual level in the patient's care.

REFERENCES

1. Battista AF (1971): Subarachnoid cold saline wash for pain relief. *Arch Surg* 103:672–675.
2. Benzon HT (1986): Epidural steroid injections for low back pain and lumbosacral radiculopathy. *Pain* 24:277–295.
3. Blume H, Richardson R, Rojas C (1982): Epidural nerve stimulation of the lower spinal cord and cauda equina for the relief of intractable pain in failed low back surgery. *Appl Neurophysiol* 45:456–460.
4. Blumer D (1978): Psychiatric and psychological aspects of chronic pain. *Clin Neurosurg* 25:276–283.
5. Brechner VL (1990): Management of pain by conduction anesthesia techniques. In: Youmans JR, ed. *Neurological surgery*, 3rd ed. Philadelphia: WB Saunders, pp. 4007–4025.
6. Brodsky AE (1978): Cauda equina arachnoiditis: a correlative clinical and roentgenologic study. *Spine* 3:51–60.
7. Bronec PR, Nashold BS Jr (1990): Dorsal root entry zone lesions for pain. In: Youmans JR, ed. *Neurological surgery*, 3rd ed. Philadelphia: WB Saunders, pp. 4036–4044.
8. Brunarski DJ (1984): Clinical trials of spinal manipulation: A critical appraisal and review of the literature. *J Manipulative Physiol Ther* 7:243–249.
9. Bullard DE, Nashold BS Jr (1990): Brain stem procedures for pain. In: Youmans JR, ed. *Neurological surgery*, 3rd ed. Philadelphia: WB Saunders, pp. 4070–4085.
10. Burton CV (1978): Lumbosacral arachnoiditis. *Spine* 3:24–30.
11. Carron H, Tanenbaum RL (1987): *Rehabilitation of persons with chronic low back pain*. Washington, D.C.: D:ATA Institute, p. 1.
12. Carron H, Toomey TC (1982): Epidural steroid therapy for low back pain. In: Stanton-Hicks M, Boas R, eds. *Chronic low back pain*. Philadelphia: Grune and Stratton, pp 193–198.
13. Casey KL (1980): Reticular formation and pain: Toward a unifying concept. In: Bonica JJ, ed. *Pain*. New York: Raven Press, pp. 93–105.
14. Cuckler JM, Bernini PA, Wiesel SW, Booth RE Jr, et al. (1985): The use of epidural steroids in the treatment of lumbar radicular pain: a prospective, randomized, double-blind study. *J Bone Joint Surg* [Am] 67:63–66.
15. Dabezies EJ, Langford K, Morris J, Shields CB, Wilkinson HA (1988): Safety and efficacy of chymopapain (Discase) in the treatment of sciatica due to a herniated nucleus pulposus: results of a randomized double-blind study. *Spine* 13:561–565.
16. Dan NG, Saccasan PA (1983): Serious complications of lumbar spinal manipulation. *Med J Aust* 2:672–673.
17. De LaPorte C, Siegfried J (1983): Lumbosacral spinal fibrosis (spinal arachnoiditis): its diagnosis and treatment by spinal cord stimulation. *Spine* 8:593–603.
18. Deyo RA, Diehl AK, Rosenthal M (1986): How many days of bed rest for acute low back pain? A randomized clinical trial. *N Engl J Med* 315:1064–1070.
19. Dilke TF, Burry HC, Grahame R (1973): Extradural corticosteroid injection in management of lumbar nerve root compression. *Br Med J* [Clin Res] 2:635–637.
20. Edwards WT, Habib F, Burney RG, Begin G (1985): Intravenous lidocaine in the management of various pain states: a review of 211 cases. *Reg Anaesth* 10:1–6.
21. Feffer HL (1975): Regional use of steroids in the management of lumbar intervertebral disc disease. *Orthop Clin North Am* 6:249–253.
22. Feldman S, Behar AJ (1961): Effect of intrathecal hydrocortisone on advanced adhesive arachnoiditis and cerebrospinal fluid pleocytosis: an experimental study. *Neurology* 11:251–256.
23. Fordyce WE, Roberts AH, Sternbach RA (1985): The behavioral management of chronic pain: a response to critics. *Pain* 22:113–125.
24. Frymoyer JW (1988): Back pain and sciatica. *N Engl J Med* 318:291–300.
25. Gardner WJ, Goebert HW Jr, Sehgal AD (1961): Intraspinal corticosteroids in the treatment of sciatica. *Transactions of the American Neurological Association* 86:214–215.
26. Gildenberg PL, DeVaul RA (1990): Management of chronic pain refractory to specific therapy. In: Youmans JR, ed. *Neurological surgery*, 3rd ed. Philadelphia: WB Saunders, pp. 4144–4165.

27. Goldenberg DL (1987): Fibromyalgia syndrome: an emerging but controversial condition. *JAMA* 257:2782–2787.

28. Goldstein NP, McKenzie BF, McGuckin WF, Mattox VR (1970): Experimental intrathecal administration of methylprednisolone acetate in multiple sclerosis. *Transactions of the American Neurological Association* 95:243–244.

29. Graham CE (1975): Chemonucleolysis: a preliminary report on a double blind study comparing chemonucleolysis and intradiscal administration of hydrocortisone in the treatment of backache and sciatica. *Orthop Clin North Am* 6:259–263.

30. Hackett GS (1958): *Ligament and tendon relaxation by prolotherapy*, 3rd ed. Springfield, IL: Charles C Thomas.

31. Hackett GS, Huang TC, Raftery A, Dodd TJ (1961): Back pain following trauma and disease—prolotherapy. *Milit Med* 126:517–525.

32. Hackett TP (1972): Pain and prejudice: Why do we doubt that the patient is in pain? *Resident and Staff Physician* 18:101–109.

33. Haldeman S (1983): Spinal manipulative therapy: a status report. *Clin Orthop* 179:62–70.

34. Hebben N (1985): Toward the assessment of clinical pain. In: Aronoff GM, ed. *Evaluation and treatment of chronic pain*. Baltimore: Urban and Schwarzenberg, pp. 451–462.

35. Hendler N (1990): Psychiatric considerations of pain. In: Youmans JR, ed. *Neurological surgery*, 3rd ed. Philadelphia: WB Saunders, pp. 3813–3855.

36. Hirschberg GG, Froetscher L, Naeim F (1979): Iliolumbar syndrome as a common cause of low back pain: diagnosis and prognosis. *Arch Phys Med Rehabil* 60:415–419.

37. Hoehler FK, Tobis JS, Buerger AA (1981): Spinal manipulation for low back pain. *JAMA* 245:1835–1838.

38. Hosobuchi Y (1990): Intracerebral stimulation for the relief of chronic pain. In: Youmans JR, ed. *Neurological surgery*, 3rd ed. Philadelphia: WB Saunders, pp. 4128–4143.

39. Hosobuchi Y, Adams JE, Linchitz R (1977): Pain relief by electrical stimulation of the central gray matter in humans and its reversal by naloxone. *Science* 197:183–186.

40. Hunt WE, Baird WC (1961): Complications following injection of sclerosing agent to precipitate fibro-osseous proliferation. *J Neurosurg* 18:461–465.

41. Hurt RW, Ballantine HT Jr (1974): Stereotactic anterior cingulate lesions for persistent pain: A report on 68 cases. *Clin Neurosurg* 21:334–351.

42. Javid MJ, Nordby EJ, Ford LT, et al. (1983): Safety and efficacy of chymopapain (Chymodiactin) in herniated nucleus pulposus with sciatica: results of a randomized double-blind study. *JAMA* 249:2489–2494.

43. Johnston JD, Matheny JB (1978): Microscopic lysis of lumbar adhesive arachnoiditis. *Spine* 3:36–39.

44. Jorgensen J, Hansen PH, Steenskov V, Ovesen N (1975): A clinical and radiological study of chronic lower spinal arachnoiditis. *Neuroradiology* 9:139–144.

45. Kumar K, Wyant GM, Ekong CEU (1986): Epidural spinal cord stimulation for relief of chronic pain. *The Pain Clinic* 1:91–99.

46. Lloyd JW, Hughes JT, Davies-Jones GA (1972): Relief of severe intractable pain by barbotage of cerebrospinal fluid. *Lancet* 1:354–355.

47. Loeser JD, Ward AA Jr, White LE Jr (1968): Chronic deafferentation of human spinal cord neurons. *J Neurosurg* 29:48–50.

48. Mayer TG, Gatchel RJ, Kishino N, et al. (1986): A prospective short-term study of chronic low back pain patients utilizing novel objective functional measurement. *Pain* 25:53–68.

49. McCulloch JA, Organ LW (1977): Percutaneous radiofrequency lumbar rhizolysis (rhizotomy). *Can Med Assoc J* 116:28–30.

50. Naeim F, Froetscher L, Hirschberg GG (1982): Treatment of the chronic iliolumbar syndrome by infiltration of the iliolumbar ligament. *Western J Med* 136:372–374.

51. Nelson DA (1988): Dangers from methylprednisolone acetate therapy by intraspinal injection. *Arch Neurol* 45:804–806.

52. Oppelt WW, Rall DP (1961): Production of convulsions in the dog with intrathecal corticosteroids. *Neurology* 11:925–927.

53. Ottenbacher K, DiFabio RP (1985): Efficacy of spinal manipulation/mobilization therapy: A meta-analysis. *Spine* 10:833–837.

54. Pal B, Mangion P, Hossain MA, Diffey BL (1986): A controlled trial of continuous lumbar traction in the treatment of back pain and sciatica. *Br J Rheumatol* 25:181–183.

54a.Parry CB (1980): see ref. 81.

55. Penn RD, Paice JA (1987): Chronic intrathecal morphine for intractable pain. *J Neurosurg* 67:182–186.

56. Penn RD, Savoy SM, Corcos D, Latash M, Gottlieb G, et al. (1989): Intrathecal baclofen for severe spinal spasticity. *N Engl J Med* 320:1517–1521.

57. Perlman SL, Kroening RJ (1990): General considerations of pain and its treatment. In: Youmans JR, ed. *Neurological surgery, 3rd ed.* Philadelphia: WB Saunders, pp. 3803–3812.

58. Peterson TH (1963): Injection treatment for back pain. *Am J Orthop* 5:320–325.

59. Ray CD (1981): Electrical and chemical stimulation of the CNS by direct means for pain control: present and future. *Clin Neurosurg* 28:564–588.

60. Ray CD (1990): Percutaneous, peripheral nerve, and spinal cord stimulation for pain. In: Youmans JR, ed. *Neurological surgery, 3rd ed.* Philadelphia: WB Saunders, pp. 3984–4006.

61. Richardson DE, Akil H (1977): Pain reduction by electrical brain stimulation in man. Part 1: Acute administration in periaqueductal and periventricular sites. *J Neurosurg* 47:178–183.

62. Rivera VM (1981): Intraspinal steroid therapy (Letter). *Neurology* 31:1060–1061.

63. Satran R, Goldstein MN (1973): Pain perception: modification of threshold of intolerance and cortical potentials by cutaneous stimulation. *Science* 180:1201–1202.

64. Saunders RL, Coombs DW, Harbaugh RE (1990): Central nervous system infusions for pain. In: Youmans JR, ed. *Neurological surgery, 3rd ed.* Philadelphia: WB Saunders, pp. 4121–4127.

65. Sehgal AD, Gardner WJ (1963): Place of intrathecal methylprednisolone acetate in neurological disorders. *Transactions of the American Neurological Association.* 88:275–276.

66. Shikata J, Yamamuro T, Iida H, Sugimoto M (1989): Surgical treatment for symptomatic spinal adhesive arachnoiditis. *Spine* 14:870–875.

67. Swartout R, Compere EL (1974): Ischiogluteal bursitis: the pain in the arse. *JAMA* 227:551–552.

68. Tank TM, Dohn DF, Gardner WJ (1963): Intrathecal injections of alcohol or phenol for relief of intractable pain. *Cleve Clin J Med* 30:111–117.

69. Tkaczuk H (1976): Intrathecal prednisolone therapy in postoperative arachnoiditis following operation of herniated disc. *Acta Orthop Scand* 47:388–390.

70. Wall PD (1980): The role of substantia gelatinosa as a gate control. In: Bonica JJ, ed. *Pain.* New York: Raven Press, pp. 205–231.

71. Wall PD, and Sweet WH (1967): Temporary abolition of pain in man. *Science* 155:108–109.

72. Wilkinson HA (1983): *The failed back syndrome: Etiology and therapy.* Philadelphia: Lippincott.

73. Wilkinson HA (1985): Lumbar adhesive arachnoiditis. In: Long DM, ed. *Current therapy in neurological surgery.* BC Decker, pp. 198–200.

74. Wilkinson HA (1988): *Aseptic inflammatory complications of spinal surgery. Congress of Neurological Surgeons, Audiotape W128-10.* Info Medix.

75. Wilkinson H (1989): Dangers from methylprednisolone acetate therapy by intraspinal injection (Letter). *Arch Neurol* 46:721.

76. Wilkinson HA (1988): Low back pain with or without sciatica. In: Long D, ed. *Current therapy in neurological surgery.* BC Decker, pp. 269–274.

77. Wilkinson HA, Mark VH, and White JC (1964): Further experiences with intrathecal phenol for the relief of pain. *Journal of Chronic Disabilities* 17:1055–1059.

78. Wilkinson HA, and Schuman N (1979): Results of surgical lysis of lumbar adhesive arachnoiditis. *Neurosurg* 4:401–409.

79. Wilkinson HA, and Schuman N (1980): Intradiscal corticosteroids in the treatment of lumbar and cervical disc problems. *Spine* 5:385–389.

80. Winnie AP, Hartman JT, Meyers HL Jr, Ramamurthy S, Barangan V (1972): Pain Clinic. II. Intrathecal and extradural corticosteroids for sciatica. *Anesth Analg* 51:990–1003.

81. Parry CB (1980): Pain in avulsion lesions of the brachial plexus. *Pain* 9:41–53.

PART VII

Sacrum and Coccyx

The Adult Spine: Principles and Practice,
J. W. Frymoyer, Editor-in-Chief.
Raven Press, Ltd., New York © 1991.

CHAPTER 100

Surgical Anatomy and Operative Approaches to the Sacrum

Stephen I. Esses and D. J. Botsford

The sacrum evolved in lower animals along with the development of hind limbs, as part of the spinal column specialized for connecting the pelvis and the more cranial vertebrae. In primates, this led to a bone consisting of three fused vertebrae to support the intermittently bipedal gait and forward leaning posture of early hominoids. The upright posture of humans required further modifications to the spinal column. These changes included the incorporation of the next two cranial vertebrae into the fused body of the sacrum, the widening of the sacral alae, and a change in the angle that the sacrum forms with the pelvis. These modifications strengthened the sacrum to allow for the greater downward force placed upon it by erect posture.

In addition to bearing the weight of the upper body and connecting the lower limbs with the spine, the sacrum has other functions. It serves as an anchor for the posterior spinal group of muscles which aid in maintaining the curvature of the lumbar spine. It also forms the posterior segment of the pelvic ring, thus protecting the pelvic organs and acting as a part of the obstetrical pelvic canal. Finally, like the other parts of the spine, it protects

the neural elements; in this case, the sacral and coccygeal nerve roots of the cauda equina.

The sacral vertebrae develop from sclerotomes in the same way as other vertebrae, thus maintaining a similar scheme with respect to blood supply (5). The sacrum does, however, have a different pattern of ossification than the other vertebrae. Each sacral vertebra develops from at least three centers of ossification: one for the vertebral body and one for each half of the neural arch. The three or four most cranial sacral vertebrae each have two additional centers on their pelvic surfaces to form the parts of the sacrum which represent the costal elements. Additionally, there are centers for apophyseal plate formation: two on each lateral aspect of the sacrum and one each for the cranial and caudal surface of every vertebral body (10).

At birth, the sacral vertebrae are similar to those of the lumbar spine. The sacral wings do not begin to ossify until late in the first year of life. At this point, the vertebral bodies are separated by intervertebral discs. It is not until approximately the eighteenth year of life that the most caudal two bodies undergo bony fusion. This process of fusion continues cranially for the next decade or so. Thus, between the ages of 25 and 30 years the adult sacrum, consisting of five fused sacral vertebrae, is fully formed. This process of development, however, is dependent on normal weight-bearing. It has been found that patients who are paraplegic from an early age do not go on to fuse the sacral vertebrae (1).

S. I. Esses, M.D., M.Sc., F.R.C.S.: Assistant Professor, Department of Surgery, University of Toronto, Toronto, Ontario; Consultant, Dewar Spine Unit, The Toronto Hospital, Toronto, Ontario, Canada, M5G 2C4.

D. J. Botsford, M.D.: Faculty of Medicine, University of Toronto, Toronto, Ontario, Canada, M5S 1A8.

This chapter reviews the anatomy of the sacrum and its surrounding structures and discusses surgical approaches to the adult sacrum.

BONY ANATOMY

The adult sacrum consists of five sacral vertebrae which are fused in such a way as to make the anterior or pelvic surface concave in two dimensions and the posterior surface convex. The sacrum appears wedge-shaped because of its broad base. It articulates with the lowest lumbar vertebra superiorly, and at its apex, which forms the sacrococcygeal joint, inferiorly. The lateral surface of the upper two or three sacral vertebrae form an ear-shaped surface, which articulates with the ilium on each side, while the lower two or three vertebrae comprise the thin, tapering lower half of the sacrum.

The most prominent features of the anterior surface are the four pairs of pelvic foramina where the ventral rami of the first four sacral nerves pass into the pelvis. Running horizontally between each pair of foramina is a transverse ridge, which represents the area where the intervertebral disc was once located. The first two transverse ridges link the edges of the foramina where they come closest together while the inferior two ridges link the caudal margins of the foramina. The prominent anterior enlargement of the upper portion of the body of the first sacral vertebra is known as the sacral promontory. It is the most anterior part of the sacrum and marks the posterior portion of the pelvic inlet (Fig. 1).

The area lateral to the pelvic foramina is known as the pars lateralis. The pars lateralis is marked by grooves running laterally from the foramina. The groove from the most inferior foramen runs slightly inferiorly. These grooves mark the passage of each of the ventral roots. Between each of the grooves is a ridge of bone which is the origin of the piriformis muscle. The large lateral mass of the first sacral vertebral body is known as the ala. Its most lateral tip is part of the origin of the iliacus muscle.

On the posterior surface, there are dorsal foramina continuous with those on the pelvic surface; however, the dorsal ones are smaller, and the grooves which mark the passage of the dorsal rami are not as prominent. In the midline is the prominent median crest which ends inferiorly in the sacral hiatus. The upper portion of the crest may receive some aponeurotic fibers from the latissimus dorsi muscles. The crest is punctuated by three or four tubercles which represent the spinous processes of

A

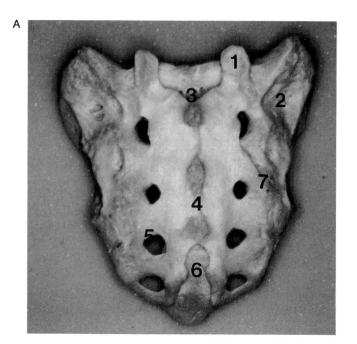

FIG. 1A. Dorsal bony anatomy.

1. superior articular process
2. auricular surface
3. superior sacral notch
4. median crest
5. dorsal foramen
6. sacral hiatus
7. lateral sacral tubercle

B

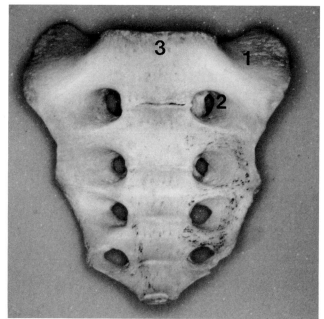

FIG. 1B. Ventral bony anatomy.

1. ala
2. first sacral foramen
3. sacral promontory

the sacral vertebrae. Lateral to the median crest but medial to the foramina lie the indistinct intermediate sacral crests, which give rise to the origin of the multifidus muscle. The origin of the multifidus is surrounded by the origin of the erector spinae, which extends onto the median crest and may partly overlie the fourth dorsal foramina. Lateral to the foramina lies the lateral sacral crest which consists of a series of tubercles. The upper two tubercles comprise the sacral tuberosity. The tuberosity is the attachment site of the posterior sacroiliac ligament, while the lower tubercles are the anchors for the oblique fasciculi of the dorsal sacroiliac ligament and the sacrotuberous ligament. The gluteus maximus has its origin along the inferolateral edge of the dorsal surface of the sacrum. The lamina of the last sacral segment does not close completely over the sacral canal, leaving the gap known as the sacral hiatus. On either side of the hiatus lie the sacral cornua, which are rudimentary inferior facets. These articulate with the cornua of the coccyx (Fig. 1).

At the base of the sacrum is the body of the first sacral vertebra. The anterior surface of the body of S1 is the sacral promontory, while the flattened, triangular-shaped opening for the sacral canal lies posteriorly. Laterally, the body extends into the thicker, wing-shaped alae. Lateral to the opening for the sacral canal, approximately the same distance apart as the width of the body of S1, lie the superior articular facets of the sacrum. These are only slightly C-shaped at this level with the joint surfaces pointing posteriorly and slightly medially and inferiorly. Between the facets and the alae are the superior sacral notches, along which pass the dorsal ramus of the fifth lumbar nerve root. There are a pair of notches at the apex of the sacrum, the sacrococcygeal notches, along which pass the fifth sacral dorsal roots. Between these notches, and slightly caudal, lies a small facet for articulation with the coccyx.

The sacral canal is the continuation of the vertebral canal inferiorly from the lumbar spine. In contrast to the lumbar spine, where the canal in cross-section approximates an equilateral triangle, in the upper portion of the sacrum, it is a flattened triangle with a wide, anterior-facing base. Below the level of the middle of the S1 body, the openings from the canal of the posterior and anterior foramina begin. Here the canal and foramina can be thought of as a Y-shape, with the stem of the Y being the anterior foramen. The dorsal foramen and opening from the sacral canal make up the limbs of the Y. There is marked variation in the orientation of these foramina, but usually the upper pelvic foramina are pointed downward and laterally. The inferior foramina are smaller, and the anterior and posterior roots take a more lateral route out from the canal. The canal continues into the hiatus, which cross-sectionally maintains the flattened triangular shape present at the top of the canal, albeit on a smaller scale (29,46).

JOINTS AND LIGAMENTS

The sacrum articulates with the lumbar spine superiorly via the bilateral facet joints and the lumbosacral intervertebral disc. Inferiorly, it articulates with the coccyx via the cornua and the sacrococcygeal joint. Laterally, there are articulations with the innominate bone and the sacroiliac joints.

For the most part, the lumbosacral joint is similar to the intervertebral joints in the lumbar spine. The inferior facets of the fifth lumbar vertebra articulate with the superior facets of the sacrum; the vertebral bodies are separated by an intervertebral disc; and the ligaments are the same as those higher in the spine. The lumbosacral junction does, however, possess some unique biomechanical features. The facet joints at this level are substantially further apart than the joints one level higher, the joint surface is slightly closer to the frontal plane, and the joint is less C-shaped. These last features allow more lateral rotation to occur.

The anterior longitudinal ligament crosses the anterior surface of the disc space and the sacral promontory to attach to the sacrum between the pelvic foramina, ending at or above the level of the fourth pair of foramina. Likewise, the posterior longitudinal ligament runs across the posterior surface of the lumbosacral disc forming the anterior margin of the sacral canal. The ligamentum flavum connects the last lumbar and sacral laminae, and the interspinous and supraspinous ligaments connect the fifth lumbar spinous process with the rudimentary spines on the median sacral crest.

The lumbosacral angle—the angle between the inferior surface of the last lumbar and the superior surface of the first sacral bodies—is approximately 22°. Ideally, these surfaces should be parallel for the greatest biomechanical stability; since this is not the case, the lumbar spine has a tendency to slip forward on the sacrum. The facet joints are the structures primarily responsible for the resistance of this tendency, aided by the ligamentous and muscular elements. It is for this reason that the facets are oriented close to the frontal plane, as this configuration obviously offers the most resistance to spondylolisthesis. The amount of strain put on the joint by its configuration may help to explain this area's prominence as a source of low back pain (34).

The sacrococcygeal joint possesses a fibrocartilaginous intervertebral disc, which allows the coccyx to move backward on defecation and during parturition. This is not a typical disc, however; it is somewhat thinner and firmer but usually does have a synovial membrane. With increasing age, the joint may undergo bony ankylosis. There are four sets of ligaments which secure this joint. The ventral sacrococcygeal ligament is analogous to the anterior longitudinal ligament. Its sparse fibers link the periosteum of the anterior surfaces of the sacrum and coccyx. The dorsal sacrococcygeal ligament consists of a deep and superficial part; the deep part is analogous to the posterior longitudinal ligament while the superficial part overlays this and is somewhat longer. The combined ligament lies over the sacral hiatus and the inferior end of the sacral canal. The lateral sacrococcygeal ligaments are analogous to the intertransverse ligaments higher in the spine. They connect the inferior surface of the sacrum with the rudimentary transverse processes of the first coccygeal segment. Finally, the intercornual ligaments, which approximate the articular capsules between the facet joints, link the sacral and coccygeal cornua.

The sacroiliac articulation consists of a pair of irregularly shaped joints between the ala and ilium, a small synovial cavity with surrounding ligaments, and three sets of accessory ligaments—the sacrospinous, sacrotuberous, and iliolumbar—which function to strengthen the pelvic girdle. The joint itself consists of hyaline cartilage on the sacral surface and a thin layer of fibrocartilage on the surface of the ilium. The axial cross-sectional shape of the joint is thought to contribute somewhat to its function; that is, support of the sacrum when downward force is applied by the lumbar spine. The center of gravity of the upper body lies anterior to the sacroiliac joints. Consequently, there is a rotatory force applied to the sacrum as well as a downward force. The center of rotation of the sacrum is through the posteroinferior part of the second sacral vertebra. Just superior to this axis, the joint surface is turned slightly anteriorly so that the downward and anterior rotational forces tend to wedge the sacrum more firmly between the ilia. Similarly, inferior to the axis of rotation, the sacral joint surface is turned slightly posteriorly so that the upward and posterior rotation of this part of the sacrum also wedges it into place. It should be noted, however, that significant resistance to rotation is also supplied by the accessory ligaments.

The anterior surface of each sacroiliac joint is strengthened by two ligaments. These are the ventral sacroiliac ligament and the lumbosacral ligament. The latter is also referred to as the inferior band of the iliolumbar ligament. The ventral sacroiliac ligament stretches from the base of the sacrum along the lateral aspect of the body of S1 and the ala to blend with the periosteum of the ilium on its auricular surface and pre-auricular sulcus. The lumbosacral ligament runs from the inferior surface of the transverse process of L5 to merge with the superior portions of the ventral sacroiliac ligament. The ligaments which stabilize the dorsal aspect of the sacroiliac joint, the dorsal and interosseous sacroiliacs, are very strong. The dorsal sacroiliac is divided into deep and superficial parts: the short posterior sacroiliac and long posterior sacroiliac ligaments, respectively. The former passes from the sacral tuberosity to the ileal tuberosity. The long ligament partly overlies the short one and stretches from the posterior superior iliac spine to the

tubercles of the lateral sacral crest. Its lateral portion is continuous with the sacrotuberous ligament. The interosseous ligament is stronger than the dorsal sacroiliac. It underlies and partly blends with the short posterior ligament and also connects the tuberosities of the sacrum and ilium. It fills in the area directly posterior to the joint surface where the sacrum and ilium are in close apposition. Both the dorsal and interosseous ligaments are vital to the integrity of the sacroiliac unit. They both resist the forward and downward rotatory force applied to the top of the sacrum.

There are three sets of important accessory ligaments involved indirectly in stabilizing the sacroiliac joint. The first of these is the iliolumbar ligament, originating on the transverse process of the fifth lumbar vertebra and consisting of a superior band, which passes to the superior surface of the iliac crest, and an inferior band, the lumbosacral ligament, which has already been discussed. The iliolumbar, like the dorsal and interosseous sacroiliac ligaments, prevents forward and downward rotation of the sacrum. The second accessory ligament of the sacroiliac joint is the sacrospinous ligament, a triangularly-shaped ligament with its apex pointing laterally and somewhat inferiorly. Its base connects the lateral and anterolateral surfaces of the sacrum and coccyx with the ischial spine, its apex. The ligament divides the sciatic notch into the greater and lesser sciatic foramina. Inserting on the anterior surface of the ligament as well as a small portion of the sacrum is the coccygeus muscle. The sacrotuberous ligament is an extensive structure. It originates from the posterior superior iliac spine, the fourth and fifth transverse sacral tubercles, the lateral margin of the sacrum, and the lateral edge of the coccyx. It inserts on the posterior surface of the ischial tuberosity. The ligament begins as a broad structure; and as it descends, it narrows to a dense fibrous band. It fans out again at its attachment to the ischium. The origin of the gluteus maximus extends onto the posterior surface of this ligament while the piriformis muscle originates in part from the sacrotuberous ligament's anterior surface. The sacrotuberous and sacrospinous ligaments both serve to resist the posterior and upward rotatory motion of the sacrum below the body of the second sacral vertebra caused by the downward and anterior force applied by the lumbar spine to the top of the sacrum (10).

Despite the extensive ligamentous reinforcement of the sacroiliac joint, it does appear capable of some motion. It is well accepted that during pregnancy, the ligaments relax due to hormonal influences, and the sacrum is capable of a small amount of motion. Older studies seemed to indicate that normally, motion between the sacrum and ilium was limited to a few millimeters (11). This, however, has been disputed by other studies, one of which appears to show movement along the order of one or two centimeters (12,23,25,47). In any case, mobility in this joint may become restricted in later life. The narrow joint space described above very commonly undergoes arthritic changes and may display osteophytes and bony ankylosis, particularly with advancing age. This is more common in males. It appears that perhaps all males over eighty years of age have fusion of their sacroiliac joints (40). While it is clear that this may become symptomatic and cause pain, there is considerable controversy concerning normal and abnormal motion of the joint, and the clinical relevance is uncertain.

VARIATIONS IN THE BONY ANATOMY OF THE SACRUM

The sacrum is the most variable portion of the spine. The most important of these differences are the number of sacral vertebrae present, the development of the posterior aspect of the sacrum, and intersex distinctions.

While it is not very common to find a change in the total number of vertebrae, it is quite common to see one portion of the spine to be lengthened at the expense of an adjacent portion. The most common anomaly is the addition of a coccygeal vertebra to the sacral bone. This has never been demonstrated to be a source of symptoms.

The next most common anomaly is the lengthening or shortening of the lumbar spine; this can be at the expense of or at the addition of the sacrum. Thus, the sacrum can be composed of six segments or, less commonly, of four. While the presence of four sacral vertebrae does not appear to hinder the strength of the sacrum, the presence of a sacralized segment of the lumbar spine may possibly give rise to symptoms. This is an area of great dispute. Bertolotti described the association of back pain with lumbosacral transitional vertebrae (6). Frymoyer et al. reviewed the radiographs of both symptomatic and asymptomatic individuals and found that there was no increase in incidence of transitional vertebrae in patients with low back pain (24). Certainly, there are some instances in which anomalous lumbosacral articulations can give rise to symptoms. In addition, occasionally, the L4 nerve root can become stretched over an enlarged or abnormal L5 transverse process and give rise to radicular complaints (15). It has been suggested that the abnormal joint surfaces from transitional vertebrae are prone to degenerative changes and that these may lead to low back pain (13,26,31). This area remains controversial, and the significance of transitional vertebrae in the production of low back pain warrants further investigation.

In addition to changes in the number of vertebrae, the much rarer deformity of agenesis of the sacrum may occur. This is usually seen in association with other musculoskeletal deformities such as club foot or agenesis of the lower limbs. Most commonly, these patients do not have the function of their lower limbs (3,38).

Another source of variation in sacral anatomy is in the development of the posterior elements. A number of studies have shown that the sacral hiatus, which is normally located at the level of the S4 vertebral body, commonly begins much higher. One study has suggested that 22% of female and 26% of male sacra had a deficiency in the posterior wall of the sacrum while another suggested that approximately 1% of all sacra have sacral canals completely open posteriorly. At the same time, it may be noted that 5% have the opposite abnormality—they have a rudimentary hiatus with an opening smaller than 2.0 mm (32,42,43).

It is often stated that the sacrum differs significantly between the human male and female, and recent anthropometric studies have borne out the fact that there are differences, though these are not as extensive as once believed (4). For instance, the often-mentioned difference in the curvature of the sacrum does not appear to be significant. The body of the first sacral vertebra in the male is cross-sectionally wider and larger in the sagittal plane than the female's while the width of the sacral alae, but not the thickness, is greater in the female. It may well be that any other differences in the shape of the sacrum are more dependent on morphological differences such as weight and race rather than sex. The angle that the sacrum makes with the innominate bone appears to be sex dependent. In the sagittal plane, the female sacrum is tilted forward so that the apex of the sacrum lies further back of the ischium than in the male. Because of this, the sacrospinous ligament is longer and less laterally directed in the female. This arrangement allows for a wider pelvic outlet and allows more room for the fetus's head during delivery (8,16,17).

NEURAL ANATOMY

The sacral canal encompasses the dural sac containing the cauda equina and the sacral and coccygeal nerve roots. The filum terminale continues down the spinal canal from the conus medullaris to emerge from the sacral hiatus, and anchors on the dorsum of the first coccygeal vertebra. The filum is classified into two portions, the filum terminale externum and internum. The former is surrounded by dura, which also contains the cauda at this point, while the latter is merged with the dura distal to the end of the dural sac, usually at the level of the second sacral vertebral body. The end of the dural sac is, like the termination of the cord, cone shaped. The first pair of sacral roots emerges from the sac just where the cone begins to narrow, and the coccygeal nerves and filum terminale emerge from the apex.

The spinal cord itself usually ends high in the lumbar spine, while the sacral spinal nerves emerge from the sacral foramina. Thus, it is necessary for them to travel as far as 26 cm, as in the case of the coccygeal nerve, before exiting the canal. The sacral and coccygeal roots have a loose, wavy appearance as they pass through the lumbar canal; the waves allow straightening of the nerves without excessive tension when the spine is flexed within the normal range of motion. Each root, then, travels in the subarachnoid space of the cistern until it reaches the point at which it leaves the main dural sac which, in the case of the sacral roots, is slightly superior to their respective foramina. At this level, the dorsal and ventral roots are still separate and they each carry out a sleeve of dura and arachnoid matter as they pass out of the sac. This sleeve is continuous with the subarachnoid space in the lumbar cistern and therefore contains cerebrospinal fluid. Just proximal to the dorsal root ganglion, the dural sleeves fuse, and this continuation of the subarachnoid space ends although it may, rarely, extend past the dorsal root ganglia. At this point, the dura becomes continuous with the epineurium, the arachnoid with the perineurium, and the pia with the endoneurium.

In the other segments of the vertebral column, the dorsal root ganglia lie outside of the vertebral canal; however, the sacrum differs from this in that the ganglia lie in the sacral canal; central and superior to the foramina at which the respective rami emerge. In the case of the first sacral roots, this means that the long axis of the oval-shaped ganglia lies at a 45° angle to the vertical; however, the ganglia for the last pair of sacral nerves and the coccygeals are oriented almost vertically. The course of the combined sacral spinal nerves is quite short, only a few millimeters, and lies distal to the dorsal root ganglia entirely within the sacral canal. Distal to this, the nerve divides into dorsal and ventral rami, which exit the canal via the dorsal and pelvic foramina respectively.

The dorsal rami of the sacral nerves are small and become progressively smaller the lower the segment. The first four emerge from the dorsal foramina, the fifth from the lateral aspects of the inferior end of the sacral hiatus, and the coccygeals medial to this. Somewhat lateral and inferior to the foramina from which they emerge, the dorsal rami of the first three sacral roots divide into the medial and lateral branches. These further split into a series of interconnecting arcades.

The ventral rami of the sacral nerves are much larger than the dorsal; the first anterior sacral nerve is often the largest spinal nerve in the body. The first four anterior sacral rami emerge from the pelvic foramina and course along the grooves in the pars lateralis, while the fifth emerges between the sacrum and the coccyx, and the coccygeals enter the pelvis inferior to the first coccygeal segment. Outside the foramina the rami begin to branch, forming together with contributions from the lumbar plexus and the lumbosacral trunk the sacral plexus. The sacral plexus consists of contributions from the fourth and fifth lumbar and the first three sacral spinal nerves. Inferior to this level, the fourth sacral ramus combines with branches from the third and fourth to form the pudendal nerve, while it also sends a branch to join the fifth sacral and first coccygeal segments, thus forming the coccygeal plexus.

The sacral plexus is complex and will be discussed only so far as it relates to the sacrum (Fig. 2). The most superior contribution to it is the lumbosacral trunk, which is comprised in small part of the fourth lumbar nerve. The trunk traverses the anterior aspect of the

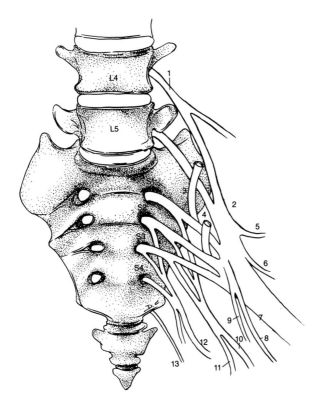

FIG. 2. Sacral plexus.

1. L4 root
2. lumbosacral trunk
3. superior gluteal artery
4. inferior gluteal artery
5. superior gluteal nerve
6. inferior gluteal nerve
7. sciatic nerve
8. nerve to quadratus femoris and inferior gemellus
9. nerve to obturator internus and superior gemellus
10. posterior cutaneous femoral nerve
11. perforating cutaneous nerve
12. pudendal nerve
13. S5 root

transverse process of L5 and curves down to meet the fifth anterior lumbar ramus which completes the trunk. The two merge on the anterior surface of the sacral ala. The superior gluteal artery may lie between them just proximal to their junction or between the trunk and the first sacral nerve. From here, the trunk continues inferolaterally to meet the first sacral anterior ramus on the surface of the piriformis muscle posterior to the internal iliac vessels. This is at about the level of the upper edge of the second pelvic foramen at the furthest lateral edge of the sacrum. Just inferior and slightly lateral to this, the sacral plexus is met by the branches from the second sacral root. The third sacral nerve branches to add to the sacral plexus just inferior to the inferior gluteal artery, which pierces the plexus just lateral to the sacrum. The third nerve root's other branches join with those from the second at about the level of the S4 vertebral body. They continue on to join a branch from the fourth sacral nerve and form the pudendal nerve. The loops of the coccygeal plexus are formed by an inferomedially turning branch of the fourth sacral nerve which meets the fifth sacral and coccygeal nerves as it runs down the anterior surface of the lateral edge of the coccyx. This plexus sends off cutaneous branches to the perianal skin known as the anococcygeal nerves, as mentioned above.

Each of the ventral rami from the fourth lumbar to the second sacral divides into a ventral and a dorsal portion, and while this is not as obvious anatomically as in the brachial plexus, it is useful in describing how the branches of the sacral plexus are formed.

The superior gluteal nerve is formed from the dorsal portions of the fourth and fifth lumbar and first sacral nerves. It runs dorsally and laterally to join the superior gluteal artery and is thus located lateral to the sacrum as it runs through the greater sciatic foramen.

The inferior gluteal nerve is formed from the dorsal portions of the fifth lumbar and first and second sacral ventral rami. It passes through the sciatic notch posterior and lateral to the sciatic nerve itself and thus is also entirely lateral to the sacrum.

The sciatic nerve is formed from the posterior divisions of the fourth and fifth lumbar and the first and second sacral nerves. It is composed of the common peroneal and tibial portions. The tibial nerve is formed from the ventral divisions of the same segments as the common peroneal plus the ventral division of the third sacral anterior ramus. The sciatic nerve is formed in its entirety just lateral to the inferior gluteal artery, which pierces the sacral plexus lateral to the sacrum at about the level of the third pelvic foramen. Arising from the plexus and lying on the anterior surface of the sciatic nerve are the nerve to the quadratus femoris and inferior gemellus and the nerve to obturator internus and the superior gemellus. These nerves are formed from the anterior divisions of the fourth and fifth lumbar and first sacral nerves and the fifth lumbar and first two sacral nerves, respectively.

These nerves pass out of the pelvis with the sciatic nerve (35).

The posterior femoral cutaneous nerve forms from both anterior and posterior divisions of the sacral plexus. It travels posteromedial to the sciatic nerve, and it therefore leaves the pelvis just lateral to the sacrum and the sacrotuberous ligament.

The perforating cutaneous nerve is formed from the posterior division of the second and from part of the third sacral nerve. It travels medial to the posterior femoral cutaneous nerve and pierces the inferior part of the sacrotuberous ligament and curves around the bottom of the gluteus maximus to supply the skin over parts of that muscle.

The area once known as the pudendal plexus, now usually grouped with the rest of the sacral plexus, is formed from the ventral branches of the second, part of the third, and all of the fourth sacral nerves. It lies inferior to the rest of the sacral plexus on the anterior surface of the piriformis muscle lateral to the sacrum. It sends short motor fibers to the levator ani and the coccygeus muscles as well as the perineal branch of the nerve to the external anal sphincter, which it reaches by piercing the coccygeal muscle lateral to the inferior end of the sacrum and the coccyx. This nerve passes out of the pelvis just posterior to where the sacrospinous ligament and the spine of the ischium meet and then continues back into the pelvis through the lesser sciatic foramen, accompanying the internal pudendal artery along the anterior edge of the sacrotuberous ligament.

In addition to the somatic nerve supply discussed above, there is extensive sympathetic and parasympathetic innervation within the pelvis and around the sacrum. The sympathetic trunk continues inferiorly, passing deep to the common iliac artery to run on the anterior surface of the sacrum just medial to the pelvic foramina of the sacrum. It contains four or five ganglia, each of which supplies gray rami communicans to the two adjacent sacral spinal nerves. There are no white rami communicans in this area. The trunks continue inferiorly until they meet on the anterior surface of the coccyx where they form a single ganglion, the ganglion impar. The trunks supply branches to the superior hypogastric plexus, which is the continuation inferiorly of the aortic plexus. This plexus lies on the anterior surface of the upper sacrum, medial to the sympathetic trunks. It crosses the sympathetic trunk just above the level of the first sacral foramina and continues laterally and caudally, until it is joined by branches from the sympathetic trunks and the pelvic splanchnic nerves to form the inferior hypogastric, or pelvic plexus. The pelvic plexus lies embedded in the subperitoneal serosa lateral to the sacrum on the superior surface of the obturator internus muscle. The pelvic splanchnic nerves, which represent the sacral outflow of the parasympathetic nervous system, are formed by small branches from the second,

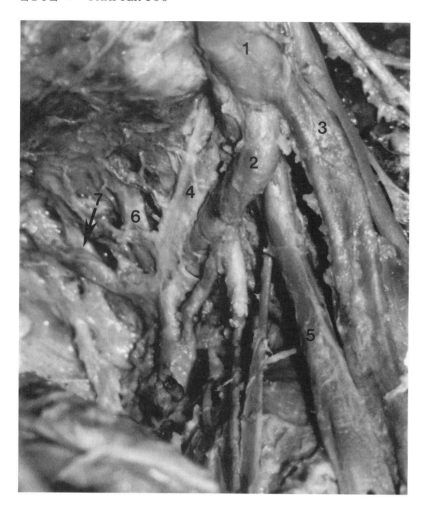

FIG. 3. Anatomic dissection.

1. left common iliac artery
2. left internal iliac artery
3. left external iliac artery
4. left internal iliac vein
5. left external iliac vein
6. first sacral root
7. second sacral root
8. third sacral root
9. fifth sacral root

third, and fourth sacral rami. These pass just anterior to the sacral plexus to supply the pelvic plexus with its parasympathetic innervation. The pelvic plexus sends further parasympathetic innervation to the various secondary plexuses supplying the pelvic organs.

The above brief description of the neural anatomy surrounding the sacrum has referred to the anatomy of the sacrum as if it were always this way. However, the "normal" configuration described above only occurs roughly half of the time. There is an almost endless number of possible variations to the scheme; one attempt to classify these changes has called the two major groups of variations the pre- and post-fixed patterns. The pre-fixed pattern is one in which, among other changes, the sacral plexus is supplied by the third and fourth lumbar nerves, while the post-fixed is one in which the fifth lumbar nerve forks to join both the lumbar and sacral plexuses. While more detail could be provided on these groups of changes, this would be beyond the scope of this text. It would be well, in any case, for the surgeon to be fore-warned that the sacral plexus is highly variable and that the anatomy found in many texts commonly is not the anatomy present in the patient (Fig. 3) (14,28,33,41).

VASCULAR ANATOMY

The vascular anatomy relevant to the sacrum is, like the neural anatomy, quite variable. This is especially so since some of the vessels are often described in relation to nerves of the sacral plexus, the branchings and positions of which are manifold (14). For this reason, the vasculature adjacent to the sacrum will be only briefly discussed with note being made of the most common variations.

The abdominal aorta bifurcates at the level of the fourth lumbar vertebra or at the disc space inferior to it. The small middle sacral artery runs from just proximal to the bifurcation down the midline to the anterior surface of the coccyx. Along the way, it anastomoses with the lateral sacral arteries, and this anastomosis sends branches into the anterior sacral foramina.

The aorta divides into the common iliac arteries which travel inferiorly and laterally to further bifurcate into the external and internal iliac arteries at the level of the lumbosacral disc. The right common iliac artery must cross over the right common iliac vein to lie lateral and anterior to it at the point of the artery's bifurcation, while the left common iliac artery runs parallel, just lateral and anterior to the vein of the same name.

The iliolumbar artery may arise from the common iliac artery, although it more commonly is the first branch of the internal iliac artery. Upon branching from the posterior surface of the internal iliac, it turns superiorly and medially to travel near the lumbosacral trunk. It then turns laterally and upwards to cross behind the common iliac artery. The iliolumbar artery may overlie the superior part of the sacroiliac joint for the medial part of its course.

The lateral sacral artery is usually the second branch of the internal iliac though it may originate from the superior gluteal. The lateral sacral artery crosses the sacroiliac joint at the level of the first or second pelvic sacral foramina and then turns distally to run on the pelvic surface of the piriformis muscle just lateral to the sacral foramina. As discussed above, it anastomoses with the median sacral artery, and this anastomosis sends out branches which enter the sacral canal via the pelvic foramina and exit through the dorsal foramina. There may be two lateral sacral arteries; a superior and an inferior. If this is so, the superior lateral sacral artery runs beside only two or three of the cranial foramina while the inferior lateral sacral artery originates from the internal iliac distal to the origin of the superior one. It then crosses the sacroiliac joint at the level of the inferior two or three foramina, which it runs lateral to.

The superior and inferior gluteal arteries are the next two branches of the internal iliac. The superior gluteal, which is the largest tributary of the internal iliac, passes anteriorly across the lumbosacral trunk as the trunk traverses the ala. It then turns posteriorly and laterally to pierce the sacral plexus above the level of the piriformis and then leaves the pelvis via the greater sciatic foramen. Because of the great variability in the sacral plexus, the constituents of the plexus pierced by the superior gluteal artery are variable. It may pass between the fourth and fifth lumbar rami proximal to where they join to form the lumbosacral trunk, between the trunk and the first sacral nerve, or even more caudally. Similarly, the levels of the plexus pierced by the inferior gluteal artery as it passes anterior to the piriformis and then posterior to the coccygeus are not constant; the artery may run between the branches of the first and second, the second and third, or the third and fourth sacral roots.

The venous anatomy is even more variable than the arterial. Generally speaking, it parallels the arterial anatomy with some important differences and features of note. First, the vena cava lies to the right of the aorta at the branching of the iliac veins, and the right common iliac vein lies to the left of the artery. The right common iliac vein must cross behind the artery and therefore be significantly shorter than its counterpart on the left. The left common iliac is notably variable in its position; indeed, it may lie almost on the midline. Second, the mid-

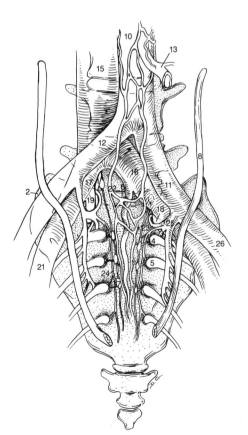

FIG. 4. Composite illustration.

1. L5 nerve root
2. sacroiliac joint
3. superior gluteal artery
4. S1 nerve root
5. S2 nerve root
6. lumbosacsal disc
7. sympathetic trunk
8. ureter
9. L4 vertebral body
10. aorta
11. left common iliac artery
12. right common iliac artery
13. inferior mesenteric artery
14. middle sacral artery
15. vena cava
16. left common iliac vein
17. right common iliac vein
18. left internal iliac vein
19. right internal iliac vein
20. L5 vertebral body
21. right external iliac vein
22. superior hypogastric plexus
23. left iliolumbar artery
24. right lateral sacral artery
25. left internal iliac artery
26. left external iliac artery

dle sacral vein, which may be double, drains into the left common iliac rather than the inferior vena cava. Finally, the iliolumbar veins usually drain into the common iliac veins rather than the internal iliacs. It should also be noted that, in accompanying their arterial counterparts they pass posterior to the common iliac veins (Fig. 4).

POSTERIOR MIDLINE APPROACH

The most common approach to the lumbosacral junction and sacrum is through a posterior midline incision. The patient is placed in the prone position. It is important that the abdomen be free of pressure so that bleeding is minimized. In addition, the chest must be left unconstricted to allow normal ventilation. The Relton-Hall frame was designed with these factors in mind (37). The eyes and elbows should be well padded as they are susceptible to pressure injury. Some consideration should be given to the optimal position of the lumbosacral junction for each individual case. For example, if a lumbosacral fusion is to be undertaken and supplemented with internal fixation, then the lumbosacral junction should be placed in extension. This can easily be achieved by placing pillows or bolsters under the hips.

Once the patient position is satisfactory and after prepping and draping, the midline vertical incision is scratched onto the skin. The subcutaneous tissues are infiltrated with 1/500,000 solution of epinephrine. This minimizes bleeding through vasoconstriction. Spinal needles are used to infiltrate the deeper layers. Great care must be taken to avoid any intra-dural injection of the solution.

The incision is carried down through the subcutaneous tissues until the deep fascia is identified. Using electrocautery, the fascia is dissected off the spinous processes and midline crest of the sacrum. Sharp Cobb elevators are used to carry out a sub-periosteal dissection. This minimizes bleeding and avoids damage to the thoracolumbar fascia, latissimus dorsi, sacrospinalis, and multifidus muscles. The Cobb can be hooked around the facet joints and used to retract these muscle groups laterally. Care must be taken to avoid damaging the capsule of the joints. In the distal part of the dissection, bleeding may be encountered from the sacral foraminal vessels. Gauze is used to pack off the wound and tamponade bleeding.

Accurate assessment of levels is achieved in three ways. The lumbosacral junction is the most caudad level at which motion is detected. Towel clips can be placed through the spinous processes of L5 and S1. By forcibly moving these caudally and cranially, motion can be detected. The sacrum has a distinct sound to palpation. It is hollow and produces a deeper pitch. If there is any doubt as to the location of the lumbosacral junction, then an intra-operative lateral radiograph should be obtained.

POSTERIOR SACROSPINALIS–SPLITTING APPROACH

Wiltse has popularized a paraspinal trans-sacrospinalis approach to the lumbosacral spine (48). The patient is placed in the prone position with consideration given to the factors discussed above. In most instances, two separate incisions are made 5 cm lateral to the midline, medial to the posterior-superior iliac spine. These incisions are carried down through the subcutaneous tissue so that the deep fascia is exposed. The fascia overlying the sacrospinalis muscle is now incised in the same direction as the skin incisions. Caudally, the incisions in the deep fascia can be curved medially to allow for easier retraction. Dissection is carried down through the sacrospinalis muscle to the transverse process of the fifth lumbar vertebra and ala of the sacrum.

This approach is ideal for lumbosacral fusions as exposure of the lateral gutter is excellent. A separate incision in the deep fascia is used for harvesting bone graft from the iliac crest.

This approach may be carried out using a single midline skin incision, providing it is long enough to allow for the two separate incisions in the deep fascia.

OTHER POSTERIOR APPROACHES

Watkins has described a lateral approach to the lumbosacral area which elevates and dissects under the lumbosacral muscle. This approach requires removal of a bicortical section of bone from the posterior-superior iliac crest. This approach, lateral to the sacrospinalis, is associated with a greater blood loss. Although its use is limited, it may be a useful exposure in those cases of lumbosacral pseudarthrosis (44,45).

If the surgery is designed to expose both sacroiliac joints, then it may be preferable to use two longitudinal paramedian incisions over the joints themselves. Horizontal incisions are not recommended unless great care is taken not to divide the paravertebral muscle groups.

ANTERIOR TRANSPERITONEAL APPROACH

Pre-operatively, the patient is given a bowel prep. A urinary catheter is placed so that the bladder is empty throughout the procedure. The patient is positioned supine with a small bolster or rest placed underneath the small of the back. This hyperextends the lumbosacral junction allowing easier access. After appropriate prepping and draping, the skin incision is made. Three different incisions have been described. The most popular is a vertical midline incision (20). Alternatively, a left paramedian incision can be used (39). Rarely, a horizontal smile incision is used. The latter is not routinely recommended as it requires transection of the rectus muscles.

Through the vertical incisions, the linea alba is identified and incised. The peritoneum can now be opened in the midline. The bowel and small intestine are packed off superiorly and laterally. This is made somewhat easier if the patient is tilted into the Trendelenburg position. The posterior peritoneum can now be opened over the sacral promontory. Some authors suggest that the retroperitoneal tissues be first infiltrated with adrenaline and saline (21,22). This may make the dissection of the great vessels and hypogastric plexus easier. Once the posterior peritoneum is opened, blunt dissection is used to identify the lumbosacral disc. It is important not to use diathermy as this can cause damage to the pre-sacral nerves. If there are large middle sacral vessels, then these should be carefully ligated. If the dissection is to be carried on more cranially, then the vessels can be retracted to the right. Usually, this requires ligation of the left iliolumbar vein. Spike retractors are useful in ensuring that the vessels do not drift into the operative field.

At completion of surgery, the posterior peritoneum is closed. The bowel is allowed to fall back into its normal position and should be checked to ensure that there is no inadvertent volvulus. The anterior peritoneum is not usually closed as a separate layer.

ANTERIOR EXTRAPERITONEAL APPROACH

The sacrum may be approached retroperitoneally either through an anterior paramedian incision or through a flank incision with the patient on his side (18). The anterior incision is preferred as it allows greater access to both sides of the sacrum and avoids having to completely mobilize the iliac arteries. In this approach, the patient is positioned supine with a sandbag underneath the lower lumbar spine. A left paramedian incision is made based over the lateral border of the left rectus abdominus muscle. The anterior lamellar rectus sheath is opened, and the rectus muscle can then be retracted to the midline. As this is done, the inferior epigastric vessels are usually identified and cauterized. The posterior rectus sheath is opened carefully so as to avoid perforating the peritoneum. A sponge is used to dissect the peritoneum off of the abdominal wall and to open up the retroperitoneal space. The peritoneum with abdominal contents, along with the ureter, are now retracted to the right. Blunt dissection over the anterior promontory of the sacrum exposes the middle sacral vessels. These can be ligated if necessary. Cautery is not used in this area to avoid unnecessary damage to the hypogastric plexus. Depending on the individual anatomy and extent of exposure necessary, it is occasionally necessary to retract the left iliac vein to the right. If this is to be undertaken, it is important to identify and ligate the left iliolumbar vein as it is easily avulsed.

Alternately, with the patient supine, an oblique incision can be made (27). This is more extensive and is recommended if the more cranial part of the lumbar spine is to be included in the dissection. If this skin incision is used, then the muscle fibers of the external oblique, internal oblique, and transversus abdominus muscles are incised. The retroperitoneal plane is best identified at the point that the transversalis fascia splits to form the lamina of the rectus sheath. Once the retroperitoneal space is identified blunt dissection is used and the peritoneum and ureter are retracted to the right.

Fraser has described an extraperitoneal approach through an oblique incision which is muscle splitting (20). Through an oblique incision, the external oblique muscle is split in line with its fibers, and the fascia is divided downward and medially to the rectus sheath. The fibers of the internal oblique muscle are now split in line with its fibers rather than being incised.

With these approaches, it is important to close the fascia of the muscle layers well in order to avoid a post-operative abdominal hernia.

The anterior retroperitoneal approach can be performed with the patient on his side. A flank incision is made halfway between the iliac crest and 12th rib. The muscle layers of the abdominal wall are incised. The retroperitoneal space and peritoneum are identified in the mid-axillary line. The peritoneum is then bluntly dissected off of the transversalis fascia before its fibers are cut. The remainder of this approach is similar to that described above.

COMPLICATIONS OF ANTERIOR APPROACHES

As described in the section on neural anatomy, the sympathetic autonomic system makes up the superior hypogastric plexus. This plexus is situated in the bifurcation of the aorta. It lies on the fifth lumbar body and lumbosacral disc space just to the left of the midline. This plexus has two major sexually relevant functions (30). It causes the smooth muscle of the seminal vesicles to contract as the bladder neck closes during ejaculation. In addition, it is responsible for spermatozoa transport from the testes to the seminal vesicles via the vas deferens. Thus, damage to the superior hypogastric plexus can theoretically result in sterility through the loss of this normal spermatozoa transport system. Sterility could also occur as the result of retrograde ejaculation due to a failure of the seminal vesicles to contract and the bladder neck to close.

Flynn and Price have reviewed a large clinical experience and the literature with respect to sexual complications of anterior fusion of the lumbar spine (19). They report an incidence of retrograde ejaculation of 0.42%. Although they reported an incidence of impotence, a failure to obtain or maintain an erection, of 0.44%, they note that this was not the result of organic harm to the nerve supply to the penis.

Competency in vascular surgery is important in case inadvertent injury to the great vessels occurs. Raugstad reported two injuries to the right iliac vein in 47 cases (36). Because venous structures are mobilized and retracted, the incidence of post-operative deep vein thrombosis is significant. We routinely use perioperative prophylactic anti-coagulation.

Abdominal incisional hernias will occur unless the muscular layers are approximated and sutured.

REFERENCES

1. Abitbol MM (1987): Evolution of the sacrum in hominoids. *Am J Phys Anthrop* 74:65–81.
2. Anderson JE (1983): *Grant's Atlas of Anatomy, 8th. ed.* Baltimore: Williams and Wilkins.
3. Andrish J, Kalamchi A, MacEwen GD (1979): Sacral agenesis: A clinical evaluation of its management, heredity, and associated anomalies. *Clin Orthop* (139):52–57.
4. Asher MA, Strippgen WE (1986): Anthropometric studies of the human sacrum relating to dorsal transsacral implant designs. *Clin Orthop* (203):58–62.
5. Basmajian JV (1980): *Grant's Method of Anatomy, 10th. ed.* Baltimore: Williams and Wilkins.
6. Bertolotti M (1987): Contributo alla conoscenza dei vici di differenzarione regionale del rachide con speciale riguards all asimilazione sacrale della v. lombare. *Radiologique Medica* 4:113–144.
7. Breathnach AS, ed. (1965): *Frazer's anatomy of the human skeleton, 6th ed.* London: Churchill.
8. Caldwell WE, Moloy HC (1933): Anatomical variations in the female pelvis and their effect in labor with a suggested classification. *Am J Obstet Gynecol* 26:479–505.
9. Clemente CD (1981): *A regional atlas of the human body, 2nd ed.* Baltimore: Urban and Schwartzenberg.
10. Clemente CD, ed. (1985): *Gray's anatomy, 30th American ed.* Philadelphia: Lea and Febiger.
11. Colachis SC Jr, Worden RE, Bechtol CO, Strohm BR (1963): Movement of the sacroiliac joint in the adult male: A preliminary report. *Arch Phys Med Rehab* 44:490–498.
12. Egund N, Olsson TH, Schmid H, Selvik G (1978): Movements in the sacroiliac joints demonstrated with roentgen stereophotogrammetry. *Acta Rad: Diag* 19:833–846.
13. Elster AD (1989): Bertolotti's syndrome revisited: Transitional vertebrae of the lumbar spine. *Spine* 14:1373–1377.
14. Esses SI, Botsford DJ, Huler RJ, Rauschning W (in preparation): Surgical anatomy of the sacrum: A guide for rational screw fixation.
15. Finneson BE (1980): Uncommon causes of low back pain. In: *Low back pain.* Philadelphia: Lippincott. pp. 545–548.
16. Flander LB (1978): Univariate and multivariate methods for sexing the sacrum. *Am J Phys Anthrop* 49:103–110.
17. Flander LB, Corruccini RS (1980): Shape differences in the sacral alae. *Am J Phys Anthrop* 52:399–403.
18. Flynn JC, Hoque MA (1979): Anterior fusion of the lumbar spine. End-result study with long-term follow-up. *J Bone Joint Surg* [Am] 61:1143–1150.
19. Flynn JC, Price CT (1984): Sexual complications of anterior fusion of the lumbar spine. *Spine* 9:489–492.
20. Fraser RD (1982): A wide muscle-splitting approach to the lumbosacral spine. *J Bone Joint Surg* [Br] 64:44–46.
21. Freebody D (1964): Treatment of spondylolisthesis by anterior fusion via the transperitoneal route. *J Bone Joint Surg* [Br] 46:788.
22. Freebody D, Bendall R, Taylor RD (1971): Anterior transperitoneal lumbar fusion. *J Bone Joint Surg* [Br] 53:617–627.
23. Frigerio NA, Stowe RR, Howe JW (1974): Movement of the sacroiliac joint. *Clin Orthop* (100):370–377.
24. Frymoyer JW, Newberg A, Pope MH, Wilder DG, Clements J, MacPherson B (1984): Spine radiographs in patients with low-back pain. *J Bone Joint Surg* [Am] 66:1048–1055.
25. Grieve FM (1982): Mechanical dysfunction of the sacroiliac joint. *Int Rehab Med* 5:46–52.
26. Harmon PH (1966): Congenital and acquired anatomic variations, including degenerative changes of the lower lumbar spine: Role in the production of painful back and lower extremity syndromes. *Clin Orthop* (44):171–186.
27. Hodgson AR, Wong SK (1968): A description of a technic and evaluation of results in anterior spinal fusion for deranged intervertebral disk and spondylolisthesis. *Clin Orthop* (56):133–162.
28. Hollingshead WH (1982): *Anatomy for surgeons, 3rd. ed.* Philadelphia: Harper and Row.
29. Jackson H, Burke JT (1984): The sacral foramina. *Skeletal Radiol* 11:282–288.
30. Johnson RM, McGuire EJ (1981): Urogenital complications of anterior approaches to the lumbar spine. *Clin Orthop* (154):114–118.
31. Jonsson B, Stromqvist B, Egund N (1989): Anomalous lumbosacral articulations and low-back pain: Evaluation and treatment. *Spine* 14:831–834.
32. Letterman GS, Trotter M (1944): Variations of the male sacrum: Their significance in caudal analgesia. *Surg Gynecol Obstet* 78:551–555.
33. McCulloch JA, Waddell G (1980): Variation of the lumbosacral myotomes with bony segmental anomalies. *J Bone Joint Surg* [Br] 62:475–480.
34. Mitchell GAG (1934): The lumbosacral junction. *J Bone Joint Surg* 16:233–254.
35. Peck P, Haughton V (1985): A correlative CT and anatomic study of the sciatic nerve. *AJR* 144:1037–1041.
36. Raugstad TS, Harbo K, Hogberg A, Skeie S (1982): Anterior interbody fusion of the lumbar spine. *Acta Orthop Scand* 53:561–565.
37. Relton JE, Hall JE (1967): An operation frame for spinal fusion. *J Bone Joint Surg* [Br] 49:327–332.
38. Renshaw TS (1978): Sacral agenesis. *J Bone Joint Surg* [Am] 60:373–383.
39. Sacks S (1965): Anterior interbody fusion of the lumbar spine. *J Bone Joint Surg* [Br] 47:211–223.
40. Sashin D (1930): A critical analysis of the anatomy and the pathologic changes in sacroiliac joints. *J Bone Joint Surg* 12:891–910.
41. Sherington CS (1982): Note on the arrangement of some motor fibers in the lumbosacral plexus. *J Physiol* 13:621–772.
42. Trotter M (1947): Variations of the sacral canal: Their significance in administration of caudal analgesia. *Anaesth Analg* 26:192–202.
43. Trotter M, Letterman GS (1944): Variations of the female sacrum: Their significance in continuous caudal anesthesia. *Surg Gynecol Obstet* 78:419–424.
44. Watkins MB (1964): Posterolateral fusion in pseudarthrosis and posterior element defects of the lumbosacral spine. *Clin Orthop* (35):80–85.
45. Watkins MB (1953): Posterolateral fusion of the lumbar and lumbosacral spine. *J Bone Joint Surg* [Am] 35:1014–1018.
46. Whelan MA, Gold RP (1982): Computed tomography of the sacrum: Normal anatomy. *AJR* 139:1183–1190.
47. Wilder DG, Pope MH, Frymoyer JW (1980): The functional topography of the sacroiliac joint. *Spine* 5:575–579.
48. Wiltse LL, Bateman JG, Hutchinson RH, Nelson WE (1968): The paraspinal sacrospinalis-splitting approach to the lumbar spine. *J Bone Joint Surg* [Am] 50:919–926.

The Adult Spine: Principles and Practice,
J. W. Frymoyer, Editor-in-Chief.
Raven Press, Ltd., New York © 1991.

CHAPTER 101

The Sacroiliac Joint Syndrome

Pathophysiology, Diagnosis, and Management

Thomas N. Bernard, Jr., and J. David Cassidy

The sacroiliac joint as a primary source of low back pain is an old hypothesis that is resurgent but still controversial (1,12,25,52,56,59,63,65,97,99,106,114,134, 135). Because of its anatomical location, the sacroiliac joint is difficult to examine; many of the provocative tests also stress the lumbar spine or hip joints. There are other well-recognized pain sensitive structures such as the posterior facet joints, lumbar discs, or nerve roots which may refer pain to the sacroiliac joint region. This has led many to dismiss the sacroiliac joint as a primary source of low back pain.

During the nineteenth century, the sacroiliac joint was known to be susceptible to relaxation after pregnancy,

and for this reason, it was presumed to be a source of pain in post-partum females. In 1905, Goldthwait proposed that the sacroiliac joint could be a source of unexplained low back and leg pain even in patients who were not pregnant (52). Logically, the sacroiliac joint could be a source of pain since it is a synovial joint and is subjected to the same inflammatory, infectious, and dysfunctional conditions affecting other synovial joints.

The objectives of this chapter are to review the pertinent developmental, anatomical, and pathophysiological criteria that support the hypothesis that the sacroiliac joint is a primary source of low back pain. This foundation of knowledge provides the basis for a rational plan of treatment.

T. N. Bernard, Jr., M.D.: Hughston Orthopaedic Clinic, Columbus, Georgia 31995.
J. D. Cassidy, D.C., M.Sc. (Orth.), F.C.C.S.(C): Department of Pathology and Orthopaedics, University Hospital, Saskatoon, Saskatchewan, Canada, S7N 0W0.

DEVELOPMENT AND ANATOMY

Much of the gross bony anatomy of the sacrum has been presented in Chapter 100. Here we will emphasize those anatomic features important to understanding the sacroiliac joint syndrome.

Embryology

The sacroiliac joint first appears between the tenth and twelfth week of intrauterine life and continues to develop until birth (3,131). Initially, this region is occupied by mesenchymal tissue between the cartilage of the sacral anlage and the newly ossified ilium. By the tenth week, the joint space cavitates at the interface between the mesenchyme and the sacrum, thus differing from other peripheral joints, which develop between two cartilage anlages (147).

During the first trimester of intrauterine development, the ilium has ossified while the sacrum is formed in hyaline cartilage. The two sides of the joint develop differently. At cavitation, fetal hyaline cartilage, which is present on the sacral side, undergoes central enchondral ossification leaving a peripheral cap of hyaline cartilage at the joint surface (Fig. 1). On the iliac side a small nest of chondrocytes develops between the surface layer of mesenchyme and the fetal ilium. At birth the iliac side has only a thin layer of stacked chondrocytes covered by a second layer of mesenchymal spindle cells. During infancy, the mesenchymal layer thins and slowly disappears, leaving a thin layer of cartilage that resembles fibrocartilage (11).

At birth, the joint surfaces are smooth and flat, paralleling the long axis of the lumbar spine (135). A gradual change in joint contour and orientation occurs with age (11,149), presumed to be influenced by the mechanical forces of growth and bipedal gait.

Gross Anatomy of the Adult Sacroiliac Joint

The adult sacroiliac joint is auricular or C-shaped, with the convexity facing anteriorly and slightly inferiorly. The longer arm of the joint surface is directed posterolaterally and caudally. The short arm is directed posteriorly and cranially. The sacroiliac joint varies widely from individual to individual and from side to side in the same individual with respect to size, shape, and contour. The average surface area of the sacroiliac joint is 1.5 cm²

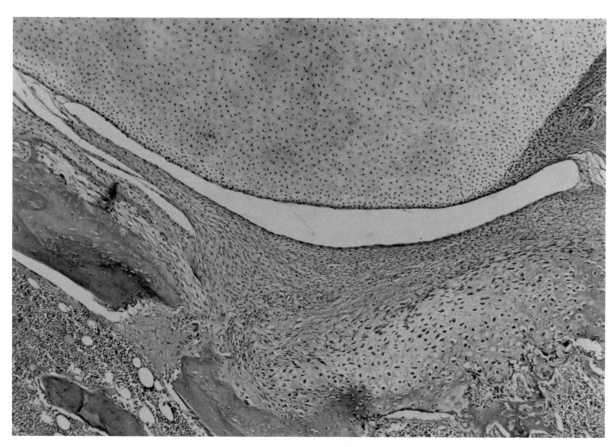

FIG. 1. Histological section through a 25-week gestation female sacroiliac joint. The sacral cartilage anlage (above) has the appearance of fetal hyaline articular cartilage. Below the newly formed joint space, there is a layer of undifferentiated mesenchymal cells overlying a small nest of developing chondrocytes. These chondrocytes are arranged in stacks or rows, parallel to the iliac bone below (×38, Safranin O).

at birth, 7 cm² at puberty, and 17.5 cm² in the adult (16). The articular portion of the sacral side always involves the second sacral segment and rarely includes the L4, L5, or S4 segments. The most common combination is S1, S2, and the mid-portion of S3 (135). In comparative vertebrate anatomy when more weight bearing is required by the hind limbs, the more sacral segments participate in the sacroiliac joint articulation. Amphibians usually have only two segments, whereas mammals commonly have three or four (4). In the adult human there are two elevations on the sacral side with a saddle-shaped depression allowing interdigitation with the ilium (149). These surfaces are not congruent or reciprocally shaped in most individuals.

The Sacroiliac as a Diarthrodial Joint

The sacroiliac joint has been classified as either an amphiarthrosis, meaning two hyaline cartilage articular surfaces joined by fibrocartilage, or a synarthrosis where the articular surfaces are joined by fibrous tissue (88). Much of the confusion results from a lack of appreciation of the unique nature of the sacroiliac cartilage and the age-related changes that occur to this joint. Early

anatomical studies were performed on cadaver or autopsy material. Many of these were older specimens that had advanced degenerative changes with fibrous adhesions that restricted motion. These findings, combined with the appearance of fibrocartilage on the iliac surface, led many to believe that the sacroiliac joint was relatively immobile.

The sacroiliac joint was recognized as a diarthrodial joint by Albinus (1697–1770) and Hunter (1718–1783), but it has taken many years for anatomists to reach a consensus on that point (1,11,16,23,46,50,56,93,118, 120,131,135). It is now agreed that it fulfills the criteria for a synovial joint which include: (a) presence of a joint cavity containing synovial fluid; (b) adjacent bones having ligamentous connections; (c) an outer fibrous joint capsule with an inner synovial lining; and (d) cartilaginous surfaces allowing motion.

The nature of the articular cartilage of the sacroiliac joint is unique. In the adult, the sacral cartilage is usually thicker anteriorly than posteriorly measuring 1 to 3 mm in depth. The sacral cartilage is typically hyaline in appearance with large paired chondrocytes that fill the evenly distributed lacunae (Fig. 2) (11,112). The cartilage matrix appears homogeneous with little fibrous tissue. The sacral cartilage has collagen fibrils arranged par-

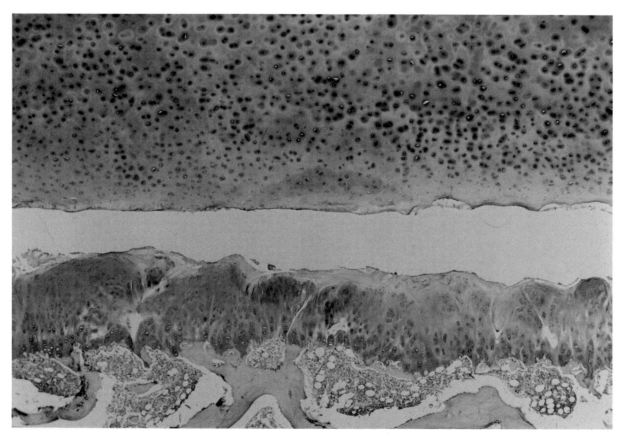

FIG. 2. Histological section through a 20-year-old male sacroiliac joint. The sacral surface (above) has the typical appearance of hyaline cartilage. The iliac surface (below) is much thinner and has the appearance of fibrocartilage (×38, Safranin O).

allel to the joint surface in the superficial zone and randomly in the deeper zones.

The iliac cartilage is thinner, averaging one millimeter in depth. The chondrocytes are arranged in palisades and are clumped together and interspersed between bundles of collagen fibrils (Fig. 2). These fibrils have an orientation parallel to the joint surface, even into the deeper zones. This arrangement gives iliac cartilage a macroscopic and microscopic appearance that resembles fibrocartilage. However, a biochemical study of the iliac collagen revealed Type II collagen, which is found in hyaline cartilage and not Type I collagen, which is found in fibrocartilage (111).

Age-Related Changes

Age-related changes occur that are also unique to the sacroiliac joint (11,16,120,129,131,135,147). Prior to puberty, the sacral side of the joint appears smooth and creamy-white and has the typical appearance of articular cartilage (Fig. 3). The iliac surface is rough and bluish in color reflecting the friable nature of the fibrocartilaginous surface and the bluish color of the underlying trabecular bone. This difference in gross appearance is maintained throughout life.

In the second decade of life, a crescent-shaped ridge develops on the entire length of the iliac surface with a corresponding depression on the sacral side. By the third decade, this interdigitation is well developed and further limits joint motion to x-axis rotation or sacral nutation.

In the joints of males, degenerative changes occur on the iliac side as early as the third decade of life and are manifested by increased joint irregularity, fibrillation, crevice formation, and clumping of the chondrocytes. Similar changes do not affect the sacral side until the fourth or fifth decade.

Age-related changes occur at an accelerated rate, particularly in males over the age of fifty. Fibrous ankylosis is more common at this stage of life, thereby giving the sacroiliac joint the appearance of an amphiarthrosis. Degenerative arthrosis of the sacroiliac joint is histologically similar to that occurring in other joints, but occurs at an earlier stage in life. Whether these changes predispose patients toward developing sacroiliac joint symptoms is not known, since their occurrence may be simply a normal part of aging. Similar age-related changes have been described in the canine and equine sacroiliac joints (21,28,29,42,54).

Accessory sacroiliac articulations are thought to represent acquired fibrocartilaginous joints that result from stresses of weight bearing (3,41,58,131,135,142,143, 149). They develop posterior to the articular surface between a rudimentary transverse process of the second sacral vertebra and the ilium. These articulations have a joint capsule and are saddle-shaped. They may be single, double, unilateral, or bilateral (149). Both fibro- and hyaline cartilage joint surfaces have been reported.

The incidence of accessory sacroiliac joint articulations has been estimated between 8% and 35.8% in the general population, depending on age. In males, the incidence increases with age. Racial difference was noted with accessory sacroiliac joint articulations occurring more frequently in whites than blacks (142). These articulations are rarely seen before the fourth decade of life, and the contribution to sacroiliac pain is unknown.

Anatomy of Sacroiliac Ligaments

The anterior sacroiliac ligament is a thickening of the anterior joint capsule. Posteriorly, the joint capsule is rudimentary or absent, and the interosseous ligament forms the posterior border of the joint (Fig. 4). This liga-

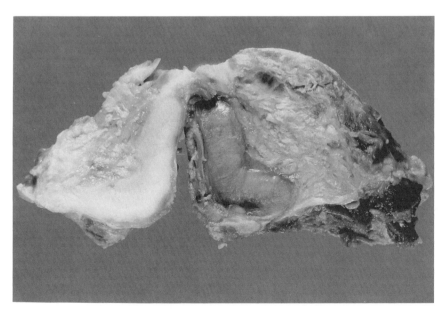

FIG. 3. Gross anatomical appearance of a 6-year-old female sacroiliac joint. The sacral surface (left) has a creamy-white smooth appearance, while the iliac surface has a dark-blue roughened appearance.

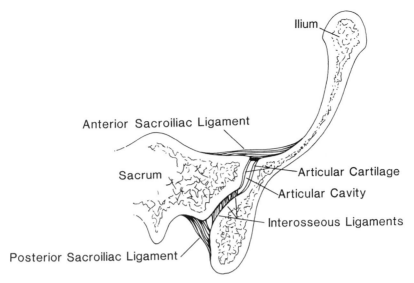

FIG. 4. The sacroiliac joint consists of a ligamentous compartment posteriorly and an articular compartment anteriorly.

ment binds the sacrum and ilium and is the strongest of the sacroiliac ligaments; if the joint is forced apart it usually separates from one bony surface or the other. It rarely fails in midsubstance. The accessory ligaments are the iliolumbar, sacrotuberous, and sacrospinous (Figs. 5 and 6) (148). The adult sacrospinous ligament has a cranially and caudally-directed fascicular orientation which is not seen in the fetus.

The sacroiliac ligament complex immobilizes the sacrum between the two ilia and prevents x-axis rotation secondary to the forces of gravity. After puberty, there is considerable difference between the male and female sacroiliac joint ligaments. In men, the ligaments remain well developed. In women, the ligaments are not as

strong and contribute to the mobility, which is required during pregnancy and delivery.

Blood Supply

The anterior blood supply to the sacroiliac joint occurs by anastomosis between the median sacral artery and the lateral sacral branches from the internal iliac artery. They enter the anterior sacral foramina and anastomose with the posterior sacral iliac blood supply from the gluteal arteries. Venous drainage occurs from tributaries of the median and lateral sacral veins.

Innervation

The innervation of the axial skeleton has been investigated extensively, and this knowledge has given insight into the sacroiliac joint as a pain sensitive structure (8,9,66,75). According to Hilton's law, any nerve crossing a joint gives a branch to that joint (70). Wyke recognizes two types of articular nerves: a specific type reaching the joint capsule as independent branches of peripheral nerves and nonspecific articular branches that are derived from muscles overlying a particular joint (155). These articular nerves are thought to have a unique feedback mechanism on the overlying muscles, which receive the same innervation. This arthrokinetic reflex exists because articular mechanoreceptors regulate muscle tone.

Like the posterior facet joints, the synovial capsule of the sacroiliac joint and overlying ligaments have unmyelinated free nerve endings that transmit pain and thermal sensation. The sacroiliac joint capsule is also inner-

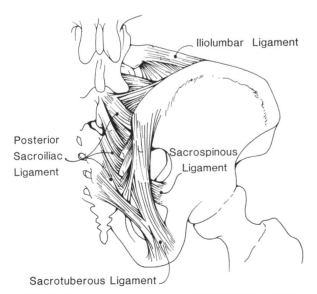

FIG. 5. Posterior accessory sacroiliac joint ligaments.

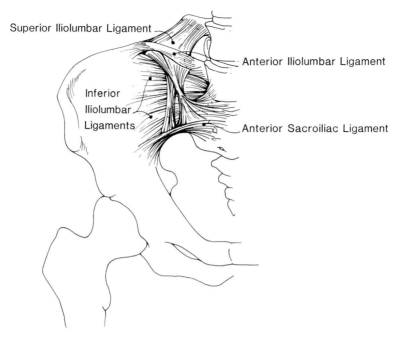

Superior Iliolumbar Ligament

Anterior Iliolumbar Ligament

Inferior Iliolumbar Ligaments

Anterior Sacroiliac Ligament

FIG. 6. Anterior accessory sacroiliac joint ligaments.

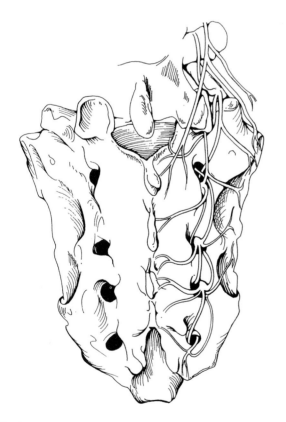

FIG. 7. The lateral branches of the posterior primary rami innervate the posterior sacroiliac joint and overlying ligaments.

vated by encapsulated and complex unencapsulated nerve endings providing pressure and position sense information (12,87,135). Posteriorly, the ligaments and joint capsule are supplied by the lateral branches of the posterior primary rami from L4 to S3 (Fig. 7). The anterior innervation is from L2 to S2 (12,45,135). This is a variable nerve supply which is not constant even in the same individual. This wide range of segmental innervation probably accounts for the variable referred pain patterns seen in sacroiliac joint syndrome. An autonomic nervous system supply to the sacroiliac joint has also been postulated (109,114).

Pain from the sacroiliac joint, like all posterior primary rami innervated structures, may be well localized or referred distally into an extremity (97,114). This referred pain (splanchnic, pseudoradicular, sclerotomal) produces a deep, dull, and often ill-defined sensation that radiates in the sclerotomal distribution (73,74). When saline or local anesthetic is injected into the posterior sacroiliac joint ligaments or joint space, familiar pain may be reproduced which may be referred into an extremity (78,136,137).

Referred pain from the sacroiliac joint is not associated with motor, reflex, or sensory deficits on physical examination. The only possible exception to this could be from an infected sacroiliac joint where swelling of the weaker anterior joint capsule comes in contact with the lumbosacral plexus.

BIOMECHANICS

The postulated functions of the sacroiliac joint are to transmit or to dissipate the loading of the upper trunk to the lower extremities. During pregnancy, the sacroiliac joints have a special role in facilitating parturition by ligamentous relaxation (138).

In the newborn, the joint surfaces are parallel to the lumbar spine axis, but with the stresses of weight bearing, the joint is reoriented in both the coronal and sagittal planes. In the adult, the sacrum is a wedge-shaped structure from anterior to posterior and from cranial to caudal. The ligamentous support (capsular, interosseous, and accessory) and the interdigitating joint surfaces favor stability (36,135). The sacroiliac joint has a higher coefficient of friction than other joints (121).

The sacroiliac joint is surrounded by some of the largest and most powerful muscles of the body, but none of these muscles have direct influence on joint motion. Contraction of the erector spinae, psoas, quadratus lumborum, pyriformis, abdominal obliques, and gluteal muscles places shear and moment loads across the sacroiliac joints in proportion to their contraction forces (105).

The sacroiliac joints resist downward shear loads ranging from 300 to 1,750 N. When a person stands in the relaxed position, the lumbar discs are subjected to a compressive load approximating 1,000 N. Each sacroiliac joint under these circumstances would resist 500 N of downward shear as well as a flexion moment of 20 N-m (105). During the act of lifting, the maximal compressive load at the L3 vertebra has been estimated at 3,500 N. This would translate to a shear load of 1,750 N to each sacroiliac joint. Gunterberg demonstrated a mean downward shear strength of 4,865 N for both sacroiliac joints in cadaver specimens (57).

When compared with a lumbar motion segment, the sacroiliac joint is able to withstand about six times as much medially directed force (lateral shear on a lumbar motion segment) and seven times as much lateral bending force. The lumbar motion segment is able to withstand twenty times as much axial compression and two times as much axial torsion as the sacroiliac joint. This would suggest that the sacroiliac joint is more susceptible to axial compression and torsion that would stress the weaker anterior capsule and ligaments. This type of force would be created by forward bending, lifting, and twisting.

Some motion in the sacroiliac joint is inherent in the transmission of body weight. Both in vivo and in vitro kinematic studies have demonstrated various types of motion in the sacroiliac joints, such as gliding, rotation, tilting, nodding, and translation (3,36,82). The precise nature of this motion in the normal joint is unclear. Sacroiliac motion is affected by motions in the lumbar spine, hip joint, and the symphysis pubis. In the newborn and until the second decade of life, the joint surfaces are flat allowing gliding motion. After puberty, age-related changes in joint topography alter this relationship.

There has been considerable debate concerning sacroiliac joint motion occurring around a fixed axis (2,3). The axes that have been proposed include: (a) the intraosseous ligaments; (b) the second sacral segment; (c) a point anterior to the sacral promontory; and (d) Bonnaire's tubercle, which is located between the caudal and cranial segments of the articular surfaces.

Various plain radiographic and stereoradiographic techniques have also been employed in vivo and in vitro to study sacroiliac joint motion and to determine an axis of rotation (22,24,40,47,150). Although these studies differ in their conclusions, the location of the proposed axes included (a) a point on the second sacral body at the level of the posterior superior iliac spine and (b) the intersection of three axes at the level of the symphysis pubis (88).

Analysis of various studies seems to indicate that sacroiliac joint motion is complex and may not occur around a fixed axis (24,40,47,55,153). In addition, motion around a fixed axis would require significant joint separation. This degree of joint separation is not seen clinically or radiographically.

It is known that whatever motion is present decreases in men between ages forty and fifty and after age fifty in women (94). There is increased motion following pregnancy (93).

Lumbar scoliosis, leg-length inequality, and hip joint disease can affect the physical examination of the sacroiliac joints when motion is being inferred from two bony landmarks (27). Lumbar spinal fusion does not appear to affect sacroiliac joint mobility or hasten degenerative changes in the sacroiliac joints (48), although continued pain at the donor site is a common complaint. Apart from fracture or major trauma, true sacroiliac subluxation or dislocation does not occur.

The precise model of sacroiliac joint motion remains unknown. The predominant motion appears to be x-axis rotation with some degree of z-axis translation (Fig. 8). It is also unclear whether normal motion or its variations are contributing factors in painful conditions in the sacroiliac joint (139).

CONDITIONS AFFECTING THE SACROILIAC JOINT

Table 1 lists the reported pathological conditions affecting the sacroiliac joint. Sacroiliac joint syndrome and inflammatory sacroiliitis are the most common conditions.

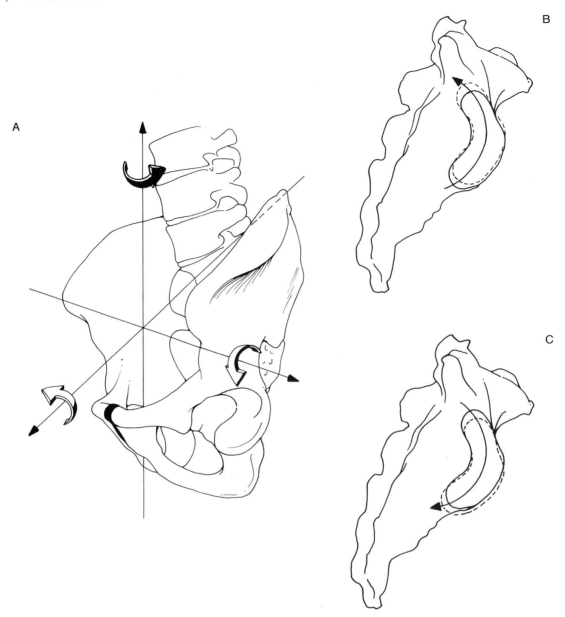

FIG. 8, A. The physiologic motion in the normal sacroiliac joint is a composite of x-axis rotation and z-axis translation. This allows sacral nutation (negative or positive rotation) about the x-axis **(B and C)**.

TABLE 1. *Pathological conditions affecting the sacroiliac joint*

1. Sacroiliac joint syndrome
2. Traumatic
3. Infectious
4. Inflammatory
5. Degenerative
6. Metabolic
7. Tumor, tumor-like conditions
8. Iatrogenic conditions
9. Referred pain from other sources

Sacroiliac Joint Syndrome

Sacroiliac joint syndrome is a common but frequently overlooked source of low back pain. Dysfunction in the sacroiliac joint can cause localized pain in the region of the sacroiliac joint and referred pain into the extremity, thus mimicking other well known causes of low back pain. Sacroiliac joint syndrome may exist alone or in combination with other conditions. The diagnosis of sacroiliac joint syndrome can be established by the appropriate clinical history and confirmed by specific provocative sacroiliac joint stress tests.

The incidence of sacroiliac joint syndrome in the general population is unknown, but it was reported to be the primary source of back pain in 22.5% of 1,293 patients with low back pain (6). In 30% of patients with L5–S1 isthmic spondylolisthesis, Bernard concluded that the radiographic finding was incidental and the sacroiliac joint was the anatomical source of pain (6). The sacroiliac joint is also reported as a common source of low back pain in school children (102).

The following data were derived from a retrospective review of 250 patients we have studied whose symptoms were consistent with sacroiliac joint syndrome. There were 90 men and 160 women whose average ages were 39.5 and 48.9 years, respectively. Onset of symptoms was unknown or attributable to minor trauma in 58% of patients or to a compensable injury in 42% of patients. The symptom duration averaged eleven months, but ten patients were symptomatic for over five years.

The pain was right-sided in 45%, left-sided in 35%, and bilateral in 20%. The pain radiated below the knee in 10%. In 43.6% of patients were associated conditions: posterior facet joint syndrome (38), lateral recess spinal stenosis (31), herniated nucleus pulposus (15), lumbar discogenic syndrome (20), and arachnoiditis (5). Forty-two patients had a history of lumbar spine surgery.

The pain in patients with sacroiliac joint syndrome can be sharp, aching, or dull. It can be referred to the buttocks, groin, posterior thigh, and occasionally below the knee. Symptoms are usually unilateral and have a right-sided predominance. Pain is aggravated by bending, sitting or riding in an automobile and is frequently alleviated by standing or walking. Rarely are there associated neurological symptoms of weakness, paresthesias, or dysesthesias.

The patient's pain drawing may be helpful in the initial evaluation (Figs. 9, 10, and 11). In sacroiliac joint syndrome, the pain is usually unilateral and does not seem to originate in the lumbar area, whereas in posterior facet joint syndrome, the symptoms are often bilateral. In patients with a herniated nucleus pulposus, the pain or sensory aberration often extends into the calf or foot.

The physical findings common to sacroiliac joint syndrome include tenderness over the sacral sulcus and the posterior sacroiliac joint line (Fig. 12). Lumbosacral spine range of motion may elicit pain with flexion and extension, but usually not with lateral bending unless there is a concomitant posterior facet joint lesion. Neurologic findings such as motor, reflex, or sensory deficits, or nerve-root tension signs are absent, but hamstring tightness may be present.

Although there is no direct method for isolating sacroiliac joint pain during physical examination, there are several provocative maneuvers that seem to be selective

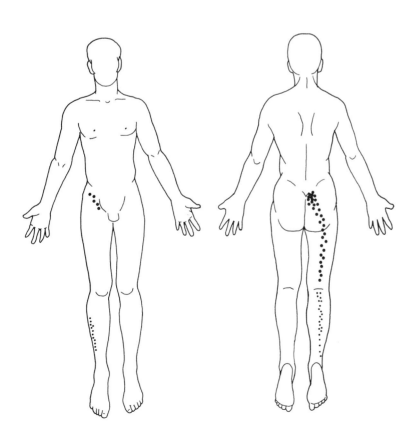

FIG. 9. Pain drawing of a typical sacroiliac joint syndrome.

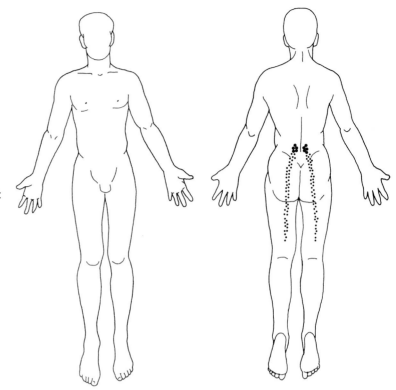

FIG. 10. Pain drawing of a typical posterior facet joint syndrome.

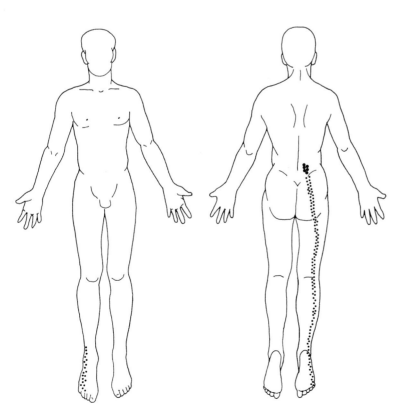

FIG. 11. Pain drawing of a typical herniated nucleus pulposus.

for the sacroiliac joint. A positive test is only significant when the clinical history and remaining physical findings rule out other syndromes.

Numerous tests to detect dysfunction of the sacroiliac joint are described in the chiropractic and manual medicine literature. Although commonly used, many of these tests are difficult to perform or interpret (5,35,37,67,100,115,122,123). The following tests of the sacroiliac joint are easily mastered and have a high degree of interexaminer reliability.

Gillet's test attempts to measure the x-axis rotation of the sacroiliac joint by noting a change in the relationship between the second sacral spinous process and the posterior superior iliac spine with maximal hip flexion. The rotary component of sacroiliac joint motion is amplified at the posterior superior iliac spine which is posterior to the x-axis of rotation (Fig. 13). This test is performed with the patient standing. One of the examiner's thumbs is placed on the second sacral spinous process and the other on the posterior superior iliac spine. Normally, when the patient maximally flexes the hip, the posterior superior iliac spine moves inferiorly in relation to the second sacral spinous process (Fig. 14). In a fixed or dysfunctional sacroiliac joint, the posterior superior iliac spine remains at the level of the second sacral spinous process or, paradoxically, elevates as the patient compensates by tilting the pelvis at terminal hip flexion (Fig. 15). This maneuver is usually painful in symptomatic patients. This test assumes no intrinsic hip abnormality and is compromised by leg length inequality, lumbar scoliosis, and in the obese patient in whom bony landmarks are difficult to palpate.

Patrick's test stresses the hip and sacroiliac joint by flexion, abduction, and external rotation of the hip. A positive test reproduces back, buttocks, or groin pain. Both sacroiliac joints should be tested by this maneuver (Fig. 16).

Gaenslen's test is performed with the patient supine. The hip joint is maximally flexed on one side and the opposite hip joint is extended (Fig. 17). This maneuver stresses both sacroiliac joints simultaneously by counter-rotation at the extreme range of motion. Additionally, this test stresses the hip joints and stretches the femoral nerve on the side of hip extension, and thus, care should be taken to insure normal hip findings or absence of neurologic conditions affecting the femoral nerve.

Yeoman's test stresses the sacroiliac joint by extending the hip and rotating the ilium (Fig. 18). A positive test produces pain over the posterior sacroiliac joint. This test also extends the lumbar spine and stretches the femoral nerve.

The sacroiliac shear test is performed with the patient prone. The palm of the hand is placed over the posterior iliac wing and an inferiorly directed thrust produces a shearing force across the sacroiliac joint (Fig. 19). This maneuver often reproduces familiar pain in a symptomatic sacroiliac joint.

The hip rotation test is an indirect evaluation of sacroiliac joint dysfunction by allowing the examiner to compare the relative lengthening or shortening of the lower extremities with maximal external and internal rotation of the hip joint. This test is performed with the patient supine. Its interpretation assumes no scoliosis, pelvic obliquity, leg length inequality, or intrinsic hip disease. The level of the medial malleoli is noted and a mark is placed on the skin (Fig. 20A). The extremity to be tested is abducted, externally rotated, and then adducted (Figs. 20B and C). Normally, leg lengthening is apparent. Next, the same leg is abducted, internally rotated, and then adducted. Normally, shortening of the extremity is apparent (Figs. 20D and E). These same procedures are then performed with the other extremity. No apparent lengthening or shortening indicates an abnormal test. This maneuver is frequently painful. A positive test is thought to be an indication of an imbalance in the arthrokinetic reflex leading to dysfunction in those muscles whose innervation is similar to that of the sacroiliac joint.

Radiographic Evaluation

Sacroiliac joint syndrome is diagnosed by clinical examination, and radiographic evaluation rarely adds any useful information. A 30 degree cephalad view projects the beam at a right angle to the sacrum allowing good visualization of the anterior and posterior sacroiliac joint lines and can reveal accessory sacroiliac facet joints (Fig. 21). The presence of degenerative changes usually bears no correlation with symptoms because 24.5% of patients over the age of fifty have abnormal appearing sacroiliac joints on plain radiographs (23,77,83,110,124).

There is general agreement that radionuclide scanning of the sacroiliac joints is the procedure of choice for demonstrating infection, inflammation, stress fracture, or neoplasm involving the sacroiliac joint. However, in the presence of structural abnormalities or degenerative lumbar spondylosis, radionuclide scanning can be falsely positive over the sacroiliac joint region (51). There is some debate over the value of quantitative bone scanning of the sacroiliac joints, particularly when the sacrum is used as a reference point (111,144). For all of these reasons, the role of scintigraphy in sacroiliac joint syndrome remains unclear (30,34,72). Some evidence exists that quantitative scintigraphy could be an important objective test for diagnosing sacroiliac joint syndrome. When two or more sacroiliac joint stress tests are positive, there is a statistically significant increased uptake on the symptomatic side (101), suggesting an element of low-grade inflammation in sacroiliac joint syndrome.

Computerized tomography clearly demonstrates bone and soft tissue anatomy of the ligamentous and articular compartments of the sacroiliac joint (Fig. 22). It is of

Text continues on page 2121.

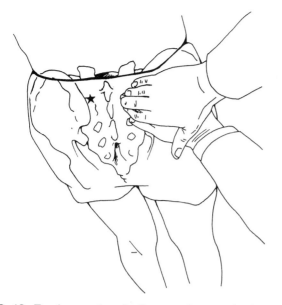

FIG. 12. Tenderness to palpation over the sacral sulcus and posterior sacroiliac joint line is a common physical finding in sacroiliac joint syndrome.

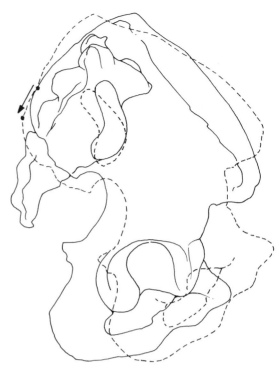

FIG. 13. The physiologic motion in the sacroiliac joint is amplified at the level of the posterior superior iliac spine. This allows this structure to be used as a reference point to detect subtle changes in joint motion.

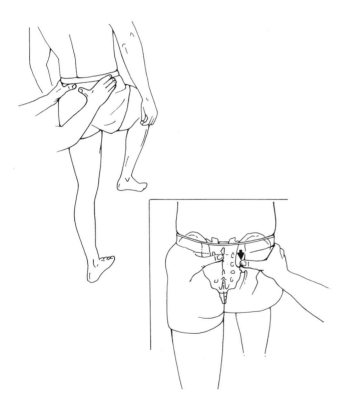

FIG. 14. Gillet's test is designed to detect normal and dysfunctional sacroiliac joint motion. With normal sacroiliac joint function, when raising the right leg the posterior superior iliac spine moves inferior relative to the sacrum.

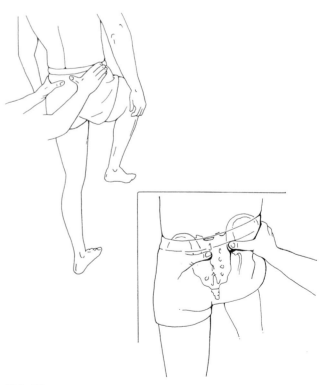

FIG. 15. With dysfunctional motion, patients will tend to compensate by tilting the pelvis. This will cause the posterior superior iliac spine to move superiorly with reference to the sacrum.

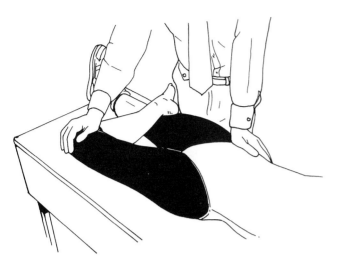

FIG. 16. Patrick's test.

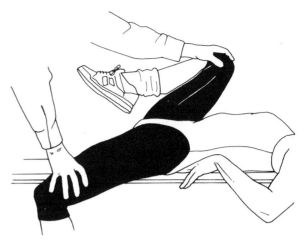

FIG. 17. Gaenslen's test.

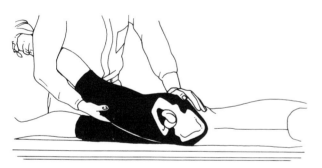

FIG. 18. Yeoman's test.

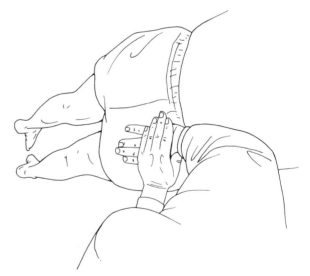

FIG. 19. Sacroiliac joint shear test.

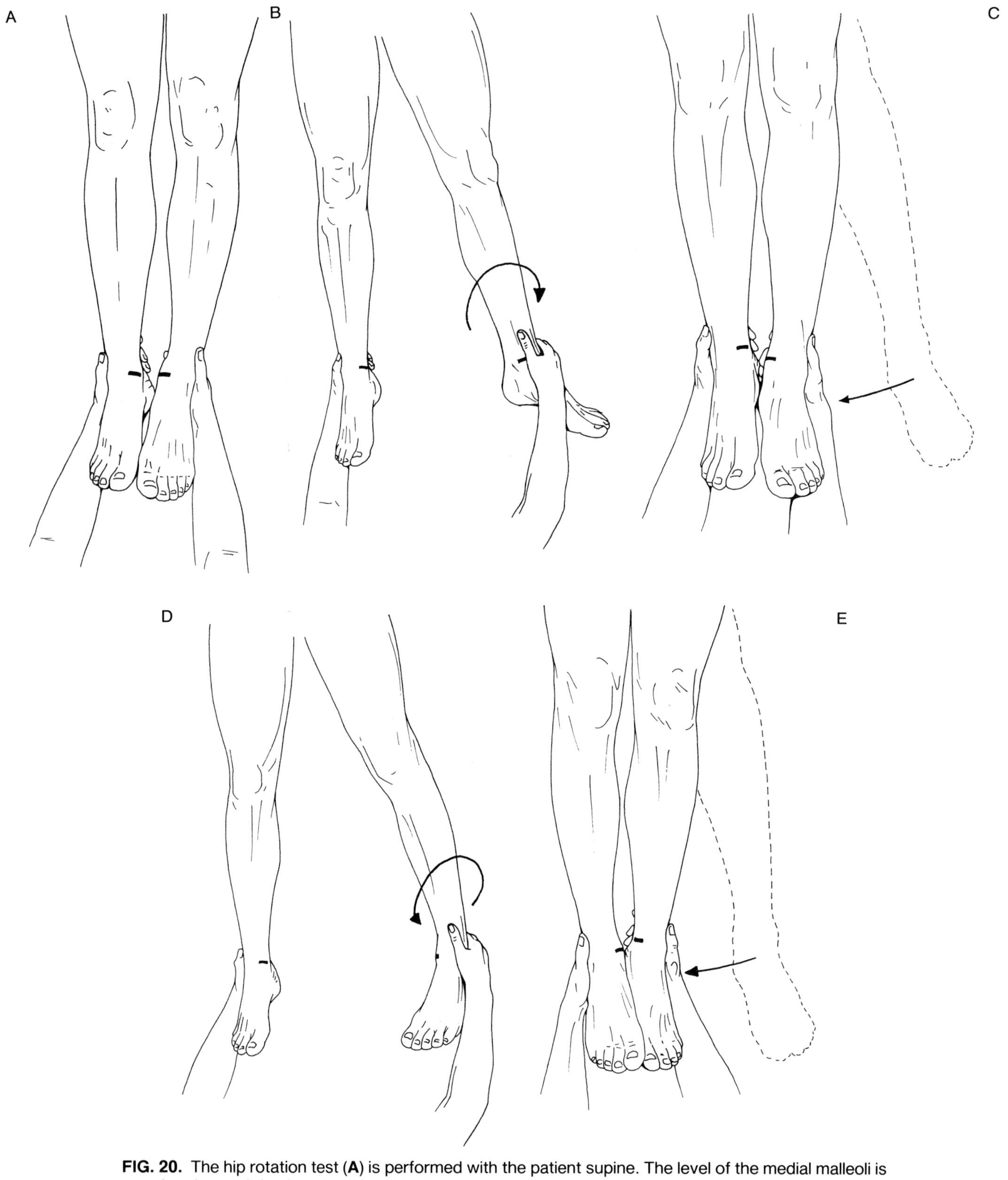

FIG. 20. The hip rotation test (**A**) is performed with the patient supine. The level of the medial malleoli is noted and a mark is placed on the skin. **B:** To test the left sacroiliac joint, the left leg is abducted and externally rotated. **C:** The left leg is then brought back to the neutral position. With normal joint mechanics, the level of the medial malleolus will appear to have moved distally with respect to the right side. **D:** The extremity is next abducted and internally rotated and brought back to the neutral position. **E:** The level of the medial malleolus with normal joint mechanics will appear to have moved proximally with respect to the right side.

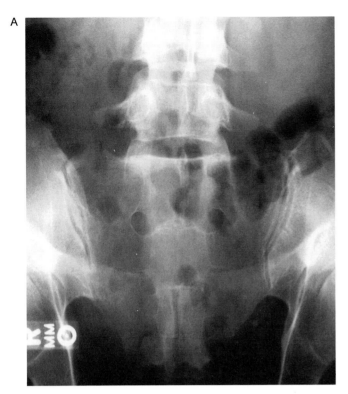

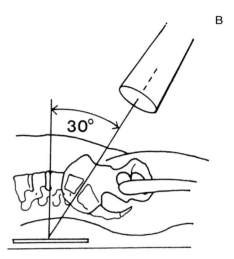

FIG. 21, A and B. Thirty degree cephalad tilt view demonstrating the sacroiliac joint.

greater diagnostic value, however, in areas of infection, inflammation, or trauma (17,124,141). Computerized tomography frequently reveals degenerative changes in patients over the age of thirty years, but these changes often bear no relationship to symptoms (Fig. 23) (89,120,145).

Magnetic resonance imaging reveals details of the soft

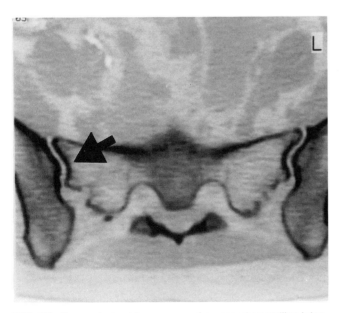

FIG. 22. Computerized tomogram of a normal sacroiliac joint showing the articular compartment (arrow).

tissue anatomy and the articular surfaces of the sacroiliac joint. Its role in the diagnostic evaluation of sacroiliac joint syndrome has not been established but holds considerable promise (Fig. 24).

Thermography, tomography, and arthrography of the sacroiliac joint have been described but have limited application (76,135,154).

From all of these data it can be concluded that the radiographic evaluation of the sacroiliac joint is of most value in ruling out infection, inflammation, metabolic, or traumatic conditions, rather than in providing precise diagnostic information about the sacroiliac joint syndrome.

Trauma

A fracture-dislocation through the sacroiliac joint involves significant trauma and is frequently associated with other injuries, as discussed in Chapter 103. Stress fractures have been reported in military personnel and among joggers or gymnasts (43,61,62,98,104). They occur from extreme physical exertion and are best demonstrated by radionuclide bone scanning.

Infection

Infection to the sacroiliac joint is hematogenously spread from cutaneous sources. Predisposing factors for

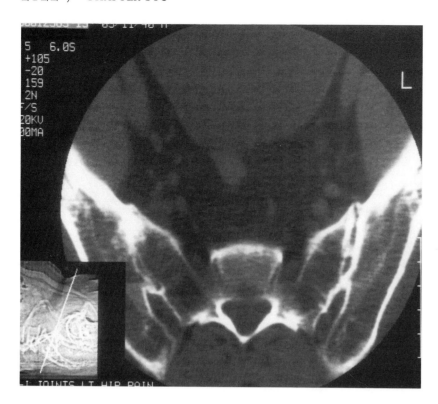

FIG. 23. Computerized tomography is the best radiographic means to demonstrate early degenerative changes in the sacroiliac joint. This patient was symptomatic on the left side. On the right side the joint was ankylosed.

infection include pregnancy, trauma, cutaneous infection, endocarditis, intravenous drug use, and immunosuppression (38,45,140).

Because blood circulation is sluggish in the ilium, infections in this area begin as osteomyelitis and then extend into the sacroiliac joint.

Even though these patients may be febrile and acutely ill, diagnosis is often delayed. A sacroiliac joint infection may distend the anterior joint capsule, and patients will avoid weight bearing and prefer hip flexion. There may be signs of femoral or sciatic nerve root irritation if the distended anterior joint capsule comes in contact with the lumbosacral plexus (53,92).

The white blood cell count and sedimentation rate are usually elevated and blood cultures may be positive. In the early stages of infection, plain radiographs are unremarkable. Radionuclide bone scanning may be abnormal as early as 48 hours and always by two to three weeks

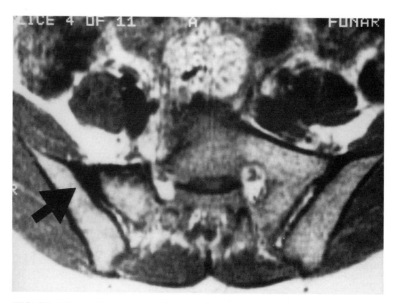

FIG. 24. Magnetic resonance image of a normal sacroiliac joint. The articular cartilage is clearly demonstrated (arrow).

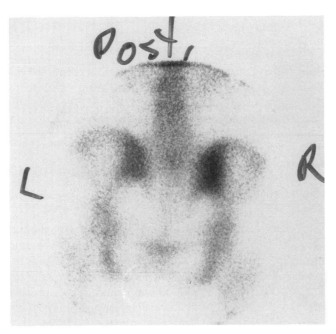

FIG. 25. Radionuclide bone scanning in a patient with a proven sacroiliac joint infection.

(Fig. 25) (79). Obtaining anterior views on bone scans are needed to reduce false negative results (85). Gallium-67 citrate scans may be more sensitive early in the course of an infection than technetium scans when the infection is the result of intravenous drug abuse (7). In an established infection, CT scanning reveals joint space widening with necrotic material in the joint space (Fig. 26). Magnetic resonance imaging has been used to diagnose a sacroiliac joint infection during pregnancy (152).

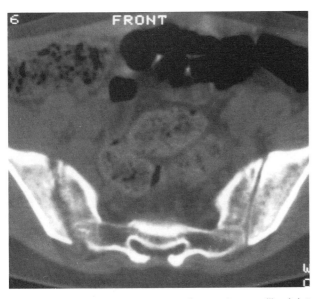

FIG. 26. Computerized tomogram of a septic sacroiliac joint. Note the intra-articular necrotic material and loss of definition of the joint margins.

The diagnostic test of choice is aspiration, but even under computerized tomographic control or general anesthesia, sacroiliac joint aspiration is technically difficult because of irregular joint topography (107). The midportion of the joint can be more easily reached using conventional fluoroscopy with the patient in an oblique position.

The most commonly identified causative organisms are *Staphylococcus aureus, Streptococcus,* and *Pseudomonas* (26,31,79,108,132). *Cryptococcus neoformans* infections of the sacroiliac joint have been reported in immunocompromised patients (13). Microbacterial and treponemal infections of the sacroiliac joint are rare (116,117,125).

Treatment of sacroiliac joint infections consists of two to four weeks of bactericidal intravenous antibiotics followed by oral antibiotics until the sedimentation rate returns to normal. Surgical drainage from a posterior approach is required when the patient has continuing symptoms, radiographic evidence of cortical destruction, or has an abscess.

Inflammatory Diseases

Inflammatory conditions causing sacroiliitis are distinguished from sacroiliac joint syndrome by the associative symptoms and signs particular to the type of inflammatory disease. The most common involvements are in patients with spondyloarthropathies.

Ankylosing spondylitis usually leads to bilateral sacroiliitis and can be confirmed by the typical clinical signs and symptoms and radiographic findings. Symmetrical increased uptake occurs on radionuclide bone scanning early in the course of the disease, frequently before plain radiographs are abnormal (68,69,81,91,112), but the findings are too non-specific to be clinically useful. When plain radiographs become abnormal, there is joint space widening initially, followed by narrowing and complete intra-articular bridging. Other forms of spondyloarthropathies are seen in patients with psoriasis, Reiter's syndrome, and inflammatory bowel disease.

Psoriatic arthritis involvement of the sacroiliac joints is usually bilateral, unlike its manifestation in the peripheral joints (33). Sacroiliitis in Reiter's disease usually has the other stigmata of this disease which include uveitis, urethritis, and a painful heel. Inflammatory bowel disease, such as Crohn's disease or ulcerative colitis, can be associated with sacroiliitis. Rheumatoid arthritis may cause the same type of joint destruction in the sacroiliac joint that it does in the peripheral joints. Juvenile rheumatoid arthritis does not involve the sacroiliac joint without peripheral joint manifestation (18).

Radiographic evidence of sacroiliitis occurs in patients with systemic lupus erythematosus. Quantitative radionuclide bone scanning correlated with the clinical and laboratory evidence of active lupus (32). In Behçet's disease, there is no evidence of an increased frequency of sacroiliitis than in the general population (156).

Sacroiliitis has been reported also in familial Mediterranean fever following a febrile episode in a child of Mediterranean ancestry (15,90). This is an autosomal recessive disease with multisystem involvement including arthritis.

Degenerative Joint Disease

In degenerative joint disease, there is joint space narrowing with anterior-superior and posterior-inferior osteophyte formation. These lead to peri-articular ankylosis with occasional intra-articular gas formation. Radionuclide bone scanning may reveal mild increased uptake in the area of degenerative change. Computerized tomography is a more sensitive test in revealing early joint space narrowing (Fig. 23) (39,44,151). The presence of degenerative changes is common in patients over the age of thirty and do not always correlate with symptoms, and thus it is difficult to assess how commonly symptomatic degeneration occurs.

Osteitis Condensans Ilii

Osteitis condensans ilii occurs in young, multiparous females. This condition is found radiographically following pregnancy. There is increased radiodensity bilaterally on the iliac side of the sacroiliac joint (119). This condition has been proposed to be the aftermath of ligamentous disruption during pregnancy or parturition. It is a self-limiting problem that rarely leads to chronic sacroiliac joint pain.

Metabolic Conditions

Gout and pseudogout are infrequently occurring metabolic conditions affecting the sacroiliac joints (71,80,95). Primary and secondary hyperparathyroidism can widen the joints on x-ray. These conditions usually occur bilaterally and are always associated with peripheral manifestation in other joints. The diagnosis of these conditions is confirmed by their characteristic serologic findings that clearly distinguish them from sacroiliac joint syndrome.

Tumor and Tumorlike Conditions

Metastatic tumors of the sacroiliac joint occur infrequently and are not specific for any particular tissue type. Pigmented villonodular synovitis is a rare tumorlike condition which has been reported in the sacroiliac joint (128).

Iatrogenic Conditions

An unfortunate but frequently occurring problem results when the sacroiliac joint is entered while the physician is obtaining a bone graft. This event can lead to chronic pain from the sacroiliac joint region, and is reported in as many as one-third of the patients with prior bone grafts (48).

Referred Pain to the Sacroiliac Joint from Other Sources

Referred pain to the sacroiliac joint from other sources can occur when the sclerotome or myotome from these syndromes extends to the sacroiliac joint region (6). The syndromes that commonly cause referred pain to the sacroiliac joint region include posterior facet joint syndrome, herniated nucleus pulposus, lateral recess spinal stenosis, contained discogenic disease, hip joint disease, Maigne's syndrome, and some myofascial or muscle syndromes. It is probably this referral pattern that has led critics to doubt primary sacroiliac syndromes.

Posterior facet joint syndrome may be established on physical examination by restricted lumbar motion and the lack of motor, reflex, or sensory deficits and the lack of nerve root tension signs. Dynamic bending lumbar x-rays can reveal dysfunctional motion. Computerized tomographic and magnetic resonance imaging are usually within normal limits or reveal degenerative changes in the posterior facet joints. A favorable response to facet joint mobilization, manipulation, or injection confirms the diagnosis.

Lumbar disc herniation or lateral recess stenosis is usually associated with some signs of nerve root irritation. Computerized tomographic and magnetic resonance imaging are usually abnormal, and confirmatory.

Hip joint disease is most often associated with early loss of internal rotation on physical examination. Plain radiographs, radionuclide bone scanning, or magnetic resonance imaging of the hip joints usually establishes the presence of hip joint disease.

Myofascial, or muscle syndrome, can cause referred pain in the sacroiliac joint region. Common muscle syndromes are gluteus maximus or quadratus lumborum. By careful physical examination and localization of the symptomatic trigger points, this diagnosis can be established particularly when injection of a local anesthetic into the trigger point allows restoration of normal muscle tone and breaks the cycle of pain.

Pain from contained discogenic disease is mediated through the pain sensitive annulus fibrosus and can refer pain to the sacroiliac joint region. Plain radiographs and computerized tomographic scanning are often normal. An abnormal T2-weighted image on magnetic resonance imaging may be indicative of a symptomatic lumbar disc. Reproduction of familiar pain by lumbar discography is a controversial but common means to establish a discogenic cause of the patient's current pain complex.

Adding to the diagnostic dilemma is that patients with sacroiliac joint syndrome can have coexisting sources of pain. This was observed in 33.5% of 1,293 patients with low back pain. The most common combinations are posterior facet joint syndrome and sacroiliac joint syndrome, sacroiliac joint syndrome and lateral recess spinal stenosis, and sacroiliac joint syndrome and herniated nucleus pulposus. Distinguishing the relative contribution of the sacroiliac joint to other causes may be extremely difficult.

TREATMENT

The treatment goals in sacroiliac joint syndrome are directed at restoring the balance between joint kinematics and the overlying muscle function thereby restoring the arthrokinetic reflex to normal. From this perspective, problems in the joint and in the overlying muscles are proposed to lead to an imbalance in the arthrokinetic reflex (Fig. 27). This imbalance opens the gate to nociceptive input, and the patient enters the painful cycle. Exercise, joint mobilization, joint manipulation, or joint injection allow reestablishment of normal muscle tone and joint kinematics. This rebalancing of the arthrokinetic reflex breaks the cycle of pain. This conceptualization is little different from most other approaches to low back disease.

The natural history of untreated sacroiliac joint syndrome is unknown. With the exception of manipulation, there are no controlled prospective trials on the efficacy of any of the commonly used treatment modalities such as bed rest supports, exercise medications, injections, or fusion.

Empirically, the following treatment modalities seem to work. However, prospective controlled trials will be needed to determine whether these treatments, in fact, alter the natural history of sacroiliac joint syndrome.

Exercise

A range-of-motion exercise program for the patient with sacroiliac joint syndrome should promote trunk and hip flexibility and hamstring stretching. It is believed that by restoring normal stretch length in muscles, the Golgi stretch mechanism is reset and the perception of pain is inhibited centrally.

Medications

A one- to two-week regimen of a non-steroidal anti-inflammatory medication may benefit or complement other treatments. This regimen is recommended when the duration of symptoms prior to treatment exceeds three months. Narcotics are to be avoided.

Patient Education

Patient education should include the basic anatomy of the lumbosacral spine and sacroiliac joint. The patient

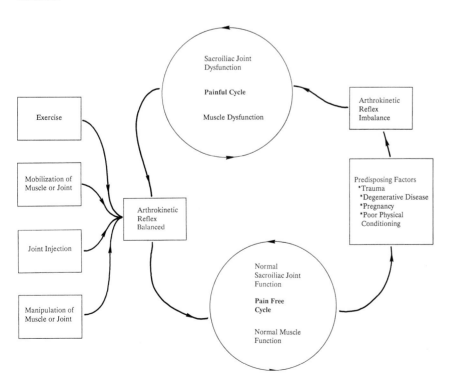

FIG. 27. The arthrokinetic reflex influences normal sacroiliac joint function and dysfunction.

2126 / CHAPTER 101

should be given written materials concerning activities of daily living that affect lower back pain. Ergonomic advice should also be provided.

Mobilization and Manipulation

One unproven theory suggests that the source of sacroiliac joint pain is subluxation or small degrees of displacement of the sacroiliac joint (10,56). This theory has been supported with claims of success from reduction of these displacements by manipulation. Sacroiliac joint subluxation has never been proven in vivo or in vitro, and there is considerable evidence that the physiologic motion in the sacroiliac joint is in fact quite small. It remains to be proven that altering mobility correlates with symptoms (139). The positive response to joint mobilization or manipulation must, therefore, be through a mechanism other than the reduction of a subluxation or a dislocation (14).

Passive motion of small or large amplitude within the physiological range of motion of a joint constitutes mobilization (96). When the motion is carried into the paraphysiological zone, increased joint separation leads to a change in the intra-articular pressure which is followed by liberation of a bubble of nitrogen gas from the synovial tissues (126,127). This bubble rapidly collapses producing an audible crack (Fig. 28). This constitutes a manipulation. A recent randomized controlled study demonstrated an increased passive range of motion after manipulation (103).

One could hypothesize that high velocity, short amplitude manipulation forcefully stretches hypertonic muscles against their muscle spindles leading to a barrage of afferent impulse signals to the central nervous system. Hypothetically, reflex inhibition of gamma and alpha motor neurons therefore may lead to readjustment of muscle tone and relaxation (19). It might, therefore, be possible that manipulation affects joints by stimulating type I and type II articular mechanoreceptors as well as type III mechanoreceptors in the overlying ligaments. These impulses travel along medium and large diameter nerve fibers and inhibit pain impulses traveling through smaller caliber fibers (113).

Joint mobilization followed by an exercise program to maintain mobility and to improve physical fitness is thought to prevent recurrence of sacroiliac joint dysfunction, but this is an unproven hypothesis in the absence of controlled studies or knowledge of the natural history. Side postural manipulation of the posterior-superior iliac spine or ischial tuberosity mobilizes a stiff or dysfunctional sacroiliac joint (Figs. 29 and 30) (20,84). In Cassidy's and Kirkaldy-Willis' studies, a daily, two- to three-week regimen effectively treated 90% of patients with chronic sacroiliac joint syndrome. A maintenance exercise program is also thought to be important to prevent recurrence of symptoms.

Injection

Another effective method of treatment of sacroiliac joint syndrome is an injection of a local anesthetic and cortisone solution into the subligamentous portion of the joint (59,60,64,82,86,130,133,135). This diagnostic and therapeutic procedure is based upon the historic observations of Steindler and Luck. They reported that if familiar pain is reproduced during the initial stage of injection of a structure and is alleviated following the injection, the structure contributes to the patient's current pain complex (137). Because of the joint's topography, it is exceedingly difficult to introduce a needle into the joint space, even under fluoroscopic control. Injection to the posterior capsular region and the overlying ligaments blocks the posterior primary rami to this portion of the joint.

Injection can be performed with conventional overhead fluoroscopy of C-arm image intensification. Patients are examined prior to injection by sacroiliac joint stress maneuvers and then positioned prone. The region over the sacroiliac joint is prepared sterilely, and through anesthetized skin a $3\frac{1}{2}$ inch, 22 gauge spinal needle is positioned under fluoroscopic control to the superior, middle, and inferior portions of the sacroiliac joint (Fig. 31). Next, a solution of 0.25% bupivacaine and a water-soluble steroid is mixed, and 1 cc is injected into the deep ligamentous area or capsular area and 1 cc to the superficial layer.

Frequently, there is precise reproduction of familiar pain and its referral pattern into the buttocks and thigh

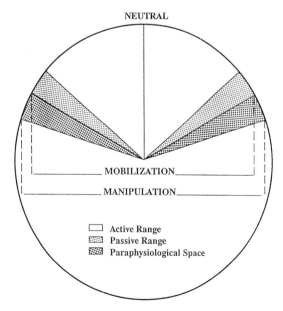

FIG. 28. Exercise, mobilization, and manipulation carry the sacroiliac joint through different limits of motion (ref. 127).

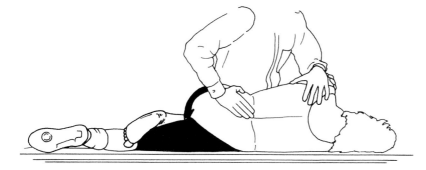

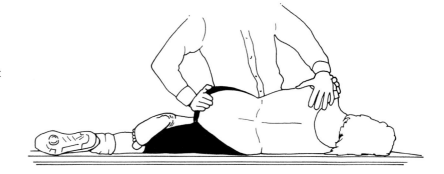

FIG. 29. Side posture superior sacroiliac joint manipulation.

FIG. 30. Side posture inferior sacroiliac joint manipulation.

and occasionally into the calf and foot. After injections, patients continue with exercise or joint mobilization or manipulation. However, it should be emphasized that sacroiliac joint injection is not the primary means of treatment and is reserved for recalcitrant cases which have failed primary exercise, mobilization, or manipulation. The sacroiliac joint injections may be repeated in three months, but not more than three times per year.

These injections only block the posterior primary rami to the sacroiliac joint and not the anterior nerve supply. In spite of this, posterior injections seem to be sufficient. The reported success from injection is 60% to 70.3% (60,110). Among 72 patients who underwent sacroiliac joint injection, 81% experienced satisfactory pain relief at an average follow-up period of nine months. Nine patients with recurring symptoms required repeat injections and had favorable results. In 46 patients there was precise reproduction of familiar pain and its referral pattern.

Arthrodesis

Sacroiliac joint arthrodesis has been suggested as a therapeutic option by some, but the number of patients in these series has been small (49,135,146). It is not recommended for sacroiliac joint syndrome. The only exception may be chronic pain following a major fracture of dislocation, and the rare case of sacroiliac subluxation following overzealous harvesting of bone grafts.

CONCLUSIONS

In this chapter we have proposed that sacroiliac joint syndrome is a frequently occurring cause of low back pain that can cause referred pain in the lower extremities mimicking other well known causes of low back pain. The basis for this focus on the sacroiliac joint is that it shares many anatomical, histological, and biochemical similarities and disease states common to other synovial joints. The debate surrounding the diagnosis is that it shares many of the non-specific complaints typical of

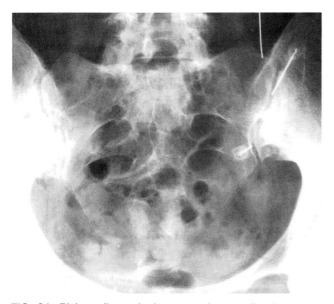

FIG. 31. Plain radiograph demonstrating needle placement for a sacroiliac joint injection.

many low back related complaints. The physical findings are thought by some to be non-specific, and the confirmation by radiographic study is often difficult. These same problems are germane to many commonly diagnosed low back conditions.

We believe the diagnosis of sacroiliac joint syndrome is established by careful clinical history, physical examination, and ruling out other causes of low back pain. Although the radiographic evaluation does not contribute much to the diagnosis, a positive bone scan and at least two positive stress tests are indicative of a sacroiliac joint dysfunction. A favorable response to mobilization, manipulation, or injection also helps confirm the diagnosis and an effective means of treatment. Exercise and improved physical conditioning reduce recurrence of symptoms.

In addition to the general causes of sacroiliac syndrome, this chapter has also included more easily confirmed entities such as spondylitis and infections. Although rarer causes, they are important to consider in patients with sacroiliac pain.

ACKNOWLEDGMENT

We thank the Hughston Sports Medicine Foundation Medical Illustration Department.

REFERENCES

1. Albee FH (1909): A study of the anatomy and the clinical importance of the sacroiliac joint. *JAMA* 53(16):1273–1276.
2. Bakland O, Hansen JH (1984): The "axial sacroiliac joint." *Anat Clin* 6:29–36.
3. Beal MC (1982): The sacroiliac problem: Review of anatomy, mechanics, and diagnosis. *JAOA* 81(10):667–679.
4. Bellamy N, Park W, Rooney PJ (1983): What do we know about the sacroiliac joint? *Semin Arthritis Rheum* 12(3):282–313.
5. Bemis T, Daniel M (1987): Validation of the long sitting test on subjects with iliosacral dysfunction. *J Orthop Sports Phys Ther* 8(7):336–345.
6. Bernard TN Jr, Kirkaldy-Willis WH (1987): Recognizing specific characteristics of nonspecific low back pain. *Clin Orthop* 217:266–280.
7. Bittini A, Dominguez PL, Martinez Pueyo ML, Lopez Longo FJ, Monteagudo I, Carreno L (1985): Comparison of bone and Gallium-67 imaging in heroin users' arthritis. *J Nucl Med* 26:1377–1381.
8. Bogduk N, Wilson AS, Tynan W (1982): The human lumbar dorsal rami. *J Anat* 134:383–397.
9. Bogduk N (1983): The innervation of the lumbar spine. *Spine* 8(3):286–293.
10. Bourdillon JF (1982): Treatment of the joints of the pelvis. In: *Spinal manipulation.* London: William Heinemann Medical Books and New York: Appleton-Century-Crofts, pp. 105–117.
11. Bowen V, Cassidy JD (1981): Macroscopic and microscopic anatomy of the sacroiliac joint from embryonic life until the eighth decade. *Spine* 6(6):620–628.
12. Bradley KC (1974): The anatomy of backache. *Aust NZ J Surg* 44:227–232.
13. Brand C, Warren R, Luxton M, Barraclough D (1985): Crytococcal sacroiliitis. *Ann Rheum Dis* 44:126–127.
14. Bressler HB, Deltoff MN (1984): Sacroiliac syndrome associated with lumbosacral anomalies: A case report. *J Manipulative Physiol Ther* 7:171–173.
15. Brodey PA, Wolff SM (1975): Radiographic changes in the sacroiliac joints in familial Mediterranean fever. *Radiology* 114:331–333.
16. Brooke R (1923–24): The sacro-iliac joint. *J Anat* 58:299–305.
17. Carrera GF (1983): Computed tomography in sacroiliitis. *Clin Rheum* 9(2):403–415.
18. Carter ME, Loewi G (1962): Anatomical changes in normal sacro-iliac joints during childhood and comparison with the changes in Still's disease. *Ann Rheum Dis* 21:121–134.
19. Cassidy JD (1988): Manipulation. In: Kirkaldy-Willis WH, ed. *Managing low back pain, 2nd. ed.* New York: Churchill Livingstone, pp. 287–296.
20. Cassidy JD, Kirkaldy-Willis WH, McGregor M (1985): Spinal manipulation for the treatment of chronic low back and leg pain: An observational study. In: Buerger AA, Greenman PE, eds. *Empirical approaches to the validation of spinal manipulation.* Springfield, IL: Charles C Thomas, pp. 119–148.
21. Cassidy JD, Townsend HGG (1985): Sacroiliac joint strain as a cause of back and leg pain in man—Implications for the horse. *Proceedings of the 31st Annual Convention of the American Association of Equine Practitioners*, p. 317–334.
22. Chamberlain WE (1930): The symphysis pubis in the roentgen examination of the sacroiliac joint. *Am J Roent Radium Ther* 24:621–625.
23. Cohen AS, McNeill JM, Calkins E, Sharp JT, Schubart A (1967): The "normal" sacroiliac joint: Analysis of 88 sacroiliac roentgenograms. *Am J Roent Radium Ther* 100(3):559–563.
24. Colachis SC Jr, Worden RE, Bechtol CO, Strohm BR (1963): Movement of the sacroiliac joint in the adult male: A preliminary report. *Arch Phys Med Rehab* 44:490–498.
25. Cox HH (1927): Sacro-iliac subluxation as a cause of backache. *Surg Gynecol Obstet* 45:637–649.
26. Coy JT 3rd, Wolf CR, Brower TD, Winter WG (1976): Pyogenic arthritis of the sacro-iliac joint. Long-term follow-up. *J Bone Joint Surg* [Am] 58(6): 845–849.
27. Cummings GS, Crowell RD (1988): Source of error in clinical assessment of innominate rotation. A special communication. *Phys Ther* 68(1):77–78.
28. Dalin G, Jeffcott LB (1986): Sacroiliac joint of the horse. 1. Gross morphology. *Anat Histol Embryol* 15:80–94.
29. Dalin G, Jeffcott LB (1986): Sacroiliac joint of the horse. 2. Morphometric features. *Anat Histol Embryol* 15:97–107.
30. Davis P, Lentle BC (1978): Evidence for sacroiliac disease as a common cause of low backache in women. *Lancet* 2(8088):496–497.
31. Delbarre F, Rondier J, Delrieu F, Evrard J, Cayla J, Menkes CJ, Amor B (1975): Pyogenic infection of the sacro-iliac joint. Report of thirteen cases. *J Bone Joint Surg* [Am] 57(6):819–825.
32. De Smet AA, Mahmood T, Robinson RG, Lindsley HB (1984): Elevated sacroiliac joint uptake ratios in systemic lupus erythematosus. *Am J Roent Radium Ther* 143:351–354.
33. Dixon AS, Lience E (1961): Sacro-iliac joint in adult rheumatoid arthritis and psoriatic arthropathy. *Ann Rheum Dis* 20:247–257.
34. Dodig D, Domljan Z, Popovic S, Simonovic I (1988): Effect of imaging time on the values of the sacroiliac index. *Eur J Nucl Med* 14:504–506.
35. DonTigny RL (1979): Dysfunction of the sacroiliac joint and its treatment. *J Orthop Sports Phys Ther* 1(1):23–35.
36. DonTigny RL (1985): Function and pathomechanics of the sacroiliac joint. A Review. *Phys Ther* 65(1):35–44.
37. DonTigny RL (1989): Dialogue on the sacroiliac joint [letter]. *Phys Ther* 69(2):164–165.
38. Dunn EJ, Bryan DM, Nugent JT, Robinson RA (1976): Pyogenic infections of the sacro-iliac joint. *Clin Orthop* 118:113–117.
39. Durback MA, Edelstein G, Schumacher HR Jr (1988): Abnormalities of the sacroiliac joints in diffuse idiopathic skeletal hyperostosis: Demonstration by computed tomography. *J Rheumatol* 15(10):1506–1511.
40. Egund N, Olsson TH, Schmid H, Selvik G (1978): Movements in the sacroiliac joints demonstrated with roentgen stereophotogrammetry. *Acta Rad* [Diag] (Stockh) 19:833–846.
41. Ehara S, El-Khoury GY, Bergman RA (1988): The accessory sa-

croiliac joint: A common anatomic variant. *Am J Roent Radium Ther* 150:857–859.

42. Ekman S, Dalin G, Olsson SE, Jeffcott LB (1986): Sacroiliac joint of the horse. 3. Histological appearance. *Anat Histol Embryol* 15:108–121.

43. Fink-Bennett DM, Benson MT (1984): Unusual exercise-related stress fractures. Two case reports. *Clin Nucl Med* 9:430–434.

44. Firooznia H, Golimbu C, Rafii M, Kricheff II, Marshall C, Beranbaum ER (1984): Computed tomography of the sacroiliac joints: Comparison with complex-motion tomography. *J Comput Assist Tomogr* 8:31–39.

45. Fishbein M, Sundaram M (1988): Radiologic case study. Pyogenic sacroiliitis. *Orthopedics* 11:811–814.

46. Fitch RR (1908–09): Mechanical lesions of the sacroiliac joints. *Am J Orthop Surg* 6:693–698, 731–733.

47. Frigerio NA, Stowe RR, Howe JW (1974): Movement of the sacroiliac joint. *Clin Orthop* 100:370–377.

48. Frymoyer JW, Howe J, Kuhlmann D (1978): The long-term effects of spinal fusion on the sacroiliac joints and ilium. *Clin Orthop* 134:196–201.

49. Gaenslen FJ (1927): Sacro-iliac arthrodesis; indications, author's technic and end-results. *JAMA* 89(24):2031–2035.

50. Gardner E, Gray DJ, O'Rahilly R (1975): *Anatomy: A regional study of human structure. 4th ed.* Philadelphia: W.B. Saunders.

51. Goldberg RP, Genant HK, Shimshak R, Shames D (1978): Applications and limitations of quantitative sacroiliac joint scintigraphy. *Radiology* 128:683–686.

52. Goldthwait JE, Osgood RB (1905): A consideration of the pelvic articulations from an anatomical, pathological and clinical standpoint. *Boston Med Surg J* 152:593–601.

53. Gordon G, Kabins S (1980): Pyogenic sacroiliitis. *Am J Med* 69:50–56.

54. Gregory CR, Cullen JM, Pool R, Vasseur PB (1986): The canine sacroiliac joint. Preliminary study of anatomy, histopathology, and biomechanics. *Spine* 11(10):1044–1048.

55. Grieve EFJ (1983): Mechanical dysfunction of the sacroiliac joint. *Int Rehab Med* 5:46–52.

56. Grieve GP (1988): *Common vertebral joint problems, 2nd. ed.* New York: Churchill Livingstone.

57. Gunterberg B, Romanus B, Stener B (1976): Pelvic strength after major amputation of the sacrum. An experimental study. *Acta Orthop Scand* 47:635–642.

58. Hadley LA (1952): Accessory sacro-iliac articulations. *J Bone Joint Surg* [Am] 34:149–155.

59. Haggart GE (1938): Sciatic pain of unknown origin; effective method of treatment. *J Bone Joint Surg* [Am] 20(4):851–859.

60. Haldeman KO, Soto-Hall R (1938): The diagnosis and treatment of sacro-iliac conditions by the injection of procaine (novocain). *J Bone Joint Surg* [Am] 20(3):675–685.

61. Harris NH (1974): Lesions of the symphysis pubis in women. *Br Med J* [Clin Res] 4(5938):209–211.

62. Harris NH, Murray RO (1974): Lesions of the symphysis in athletes. *Br Med J* [Clin Res] 4(5938):211–214.

63. Hatch ES (1912): Strains and dislocations of the sacroiliac joints. *South Med J* 5:153–157.

64. Hendrix RW, Lin PJ, Kane WJ (1982): Simplified aspiration or injection technique for the sacro-iliac joint. *J Bone Joint Surg* [Am] 64:1249–1252.

65. Hiltz DL (1976): The sacroiliac joint as a source of sciatica. *Phys Ther* 56(12):1373.

66. Hirsch C, Ingelmark B-E, Miller M (1963): The anatomical basis for low back pain. *Acta Orthop Scand* 33:1–17.

67. Hobbs D (1988): Inter- and intra-examiner reliability of palpation for sacroiliac joint dysfunction [Letter]. *J Manipulative Phys Ther* 11(4):336–337.

68. Hollingsworth PN, Owen ET, Dawkins RL (1983): Correlation of HLA B27 with radiographic abnormalities of the sacroiliac joints and with other stigmata of ankylosing spondylitis. *Clin Rheumatol* 9(2):307–322.

69. Hollingsworth PN, Cheah PS, Dawkins RL, Owen ET, Calin A, Wood PHN (1983): Observer variation in grading sacroiliac radiographs in HLA-B27 positive individuals. *J Rheumatol* 10(2):247–254.

70. Hollinshead WH (1982): *The back and limbs. Anatomy for surgeons, 3rd. ed.* Philadelphia: Harper & Row.

71. Hooge WA, Li D (1981): CT of sacroiliac joints in secondary hyperparathyroidism. *Can Assoc Radiol J* 32:42–44.

72. Horgan JG, Walker M, Newman JH, Watt I (1983): Scintigraphy in the diagnosis and management of septic sacroiliitis. *Clin Radiol* 34:337–346.

73. Inman VT, Saunders JBdeC (1944): Referred pain from skeletal structures. *J Nerv Ment Dis* 99:660–667.

74. Inman VT, Saunders JBdeC (1947): Anatomicophysiological aspects of injuries to the intervertebral disc. *J Bone Joint Surg* [Am] 29(2):461–475.

75. Jackson HC 2nd, Winkelmann RK, Bickel WH (1966): Nerve endings in the human lumbar spinal column and related structures. *J Bone Joint Surg* [Am] 48:1272–1281.

76. Jacobsson H, Vesterskold L (1985): The thermographic pattern of the lower back with special reference to the sacro-iliac joints in health and inflammation. *Clin Rheumatol* 4(4):426–432.

77. Jajic I, Jajic Z (1987): The prevalence of osteoarthrosis of the sacroiliac joints in an urban population. *Clin Rheumatol* 6(1):39–41.

78. Kellgren JH (1939): On the distribution of pain arising from deep somatic structures with charts of segmental pain areas. *Clin Sci* 4:35–46.

79. Kerr R (1985): Pyogenic sacroiliitis. *Orthopedics* 8(8):1028–1034.

80. Kerr R (1988): Radiologic case study. Sacroiliac joint involvement by gout and hyperparathyroidism. *Orthopedics* 11(1):185, 185–187, 190.

81. Khan MA, van der Linden SM, Kushner I, Valkenburg HA, Cats A (1985): Spondylitic disease without radiologic evidence of sacroiliitis in relatives of HLA-B27 positive ankylosing spondylitis patients. *Arthritis Rheum* 28(1):40–43.

82. Kim LYS (1984): Pelvic torsion a common cause of low back pain. *Orthop Rev* 13(4):206–211.

83. Kirkaldy-Willis WH (1988): The site and nature of the lesion. In: *Managing low back pain, 2nd. ed.* New York: Churchill Livingstone, pp. 133–154.

84. Kirkaldy-Willis WH, Cassidy JD (1985): Spinal manipulation in the treatment of low back pain. *Canad Fam Physician* 31:535–539.

85. Kumar R, Balachandran S (1983): Unilateral septic sacro-iliitis. Importance of the anterior view of the bone scan. *Clin Nucl Med* 8:413–415.

86. LaBan MM, Meerschaert JR, Taylor RS, Tabor HD (1978): Symphyseal and sacroiliac joint pain associated with pubic symphysis instability. *Arch Phys Med Rehab* 59:470–472.

87. Lamb DW (1979): The neurology of spinal pain. *Phys Ther* 59(8):971–973.

88. Lavignolle B, Vital JM, Senegas J, Destandau J, Toson B, Bouyx P, Morlier P, Delorme G, Calabet A (1983): An approach to the functional anatomy of the sacroiliac joints in vivo. *Anat Clin* 5:169–176.

89. Lawson TL, Foley WD, Carrera GF, Berland LL (1982): The sacroiliac joints: Anatomic, plain roentgenographic, and computed tomographic analysis. *J Comput Assist Tomogr* 6(2):307–314.

90. Lehman TJA, Hanson V, Kornreich H, Peters RS, Schwabe AD (1978): HLA-B27-negative sacroiliitis: A manifestation of familial Mediterranean fever in childhood. *Pediatrics* 61(3):423–426.

91. Lentle BC, Russell AS, Percy JS, Jackson FI (1977): The scintigraphic investigation of sacroiliac disease. *J Nucl Med* 18:529–533.

92. Lourie G, Pruzansky M, Reiner M, Freed J (1986): Pyarthrosis of the sacroiliac joint presenting as lumbar radiculopathy. A case report. *Spine* 11(6):638–640.

93. Lynch FW (1920): The pelvic articulations during pregnancy, labor, and the puerperium, an x-ray study. *Surg Gynec Obstet* 30:575–580.

94. MacDonald GR, Hunt TE (1952): Sacro-iliac joints: Observations on the gross and histological changes in the various age groups. *Canad Med Assoc J* 66:157–163.

95. Malawista SE, Seegmiller JE, Hathaway BE, Sokoloff L (1965): Sacroiliac gout. *JAMA* 194(9):954–956.

96. Maitland GD (1977): *Peripheral manipulation, 2nd. ed.* London: Butterworth.

97. Martin ED (1922): Sacro-iliac sprain. *South Med J* 15(2):135–139.

98. Marymont JV, Lynch MA, Henning CE (1986): Exercise-related stress reaction of the sacroiliac joint. An unusual cause of low back pain in athletes. *Am J Sports Med* 14(4):320–323.

99. McGregor M, Cassidy JD (1983): Post-surgical sacroiliac joint syndrome. *J Manipulative Phys Ther* 6(1):1–11.

100. Macnab I (1977): Lesions of the sacroiliac joints. In: *Backache.* Baltimore: Williams & Wilkins, pp. 64–79.

101. Mierau DR (1989): Radionuclide scanning of sacroiliac joint syndrome. Masters thesis.

102. Mierau DR, Cassidy JD, Hamin T, Milne RA (1984): Sacroiliac joint dysfunction and low back pain in school aged children. *J Manipulative Phys Ther* 7(7):81–84.

103. Mierau D, Cassidy JD, Bowen V, Dupuis P, Noftall F (1988): Manipulation and mobilization of the third metacarpophalangeal joint. A quantitative radiographic and range of motion study. *Manual Medicine* 3:135–140.

104. Milgrom C, Chisin R, Giladi M, Stein M, Kashtan H, Margulies J, Atlan H (1985): Multiple stress fractures. A longitudinal study of a soldier with 13 lesions. *Clin Orthop* 192:174–179.

105. Miller JA, Schultz AB, Andersson GB (1987): Load-displacement behavior of sacroiliac joints. *J Orthop Res* 5:92–101.

106. Miltner LJ, Lowendorf CS (1931): Low back pain; A study of 525 cases of sacro-iliac and sacrolumbar sprain. *J Bone Joint Surg* [Am] 13:16–28.

107. Miskew DB, Block RA, Witt PF (1979): Aspiration of infected sacro-iliac joints. *J Bone Joint Surg* [Am] 61:1071–1072.

108. Ncube BA (1988): Pyogenic sacroiliitis in children. *Br J Clin Pract* 42(4):154–157.

109. Norman GF, May A (1956): Sacroiliac conditions simulating intervertebral disc syndrome. *West J Surg* 64:461–462.

110. Norman GF (1968): Sacroiliac disease and its relationship to lower abdominal pain. *Am J Surg* 116:54–56.

111. Paquin J, Rosenthall L, Esdaile J, Warshawski R, Damtew B (1983): Elevated uptake of ^{99m}technetium methylene diphosphonate in the axial skeleton in ankylosing spondylitis and Reiter's disease: Implications for quantitative sacroiliac scintigraphy. *Arthritis Rheum* 26(2):217–220.

112. Paquin JD, van der Rest M, Marie PJ, Mort JS, Pidoux I, Poole AR, Roughley PJ (1983): Biochemical and morphologic studies of cartilage from the adult human sacroiliac joint. *Arthritis Rheum* 26(7):887–895.

113. Paris SV (1979): Mobilization of the spine. *Phys Ther* 59(8):988–995.

114. Pitkin HC, Pheasant HC (1936): Sacrarthrogenetic telalgia; A study of referred pain. *J Bone Joint Surg* [Am] 18:111–133.

115. Potter NA, Rothstein JM (1985): Intertester reliability for selected clinical tests of the sacroiliac joint. *Phys Ther* 65(11):1671–1675.

116. Pouchot J, Vinceneux P, Barge J, Boussougant Y, Grossin M, Pierre J, Carbon C, Kahn M-F, Esdaile JM (1988): Tuberculosis of the sacroiliac joint: Clinical features, outcome, and evaluation of closed needle biopsy in 11 consecutive cases. *Am J Med* 84:622–628.

117. Reginato AJ, Ferreiro-Seoane JL, Falasca G (1988): Unilateral sacroiliitis in secondary syphilis [letter]. *J Rheumatol* 15(4):717–719.

118. Resnik CS, Resnick D (1985): Radiology of disorders of the sacroiliac joints. *JAMA* 253(19):2863–2866.

119. Resnick D (1977–78): Disorders of the axial skeleton which are lesser known, poorly recognized or misunderstood. *Bull Rheum Dis* 28:932–939.

120. Resnick D, Niwayama G, Goergen TG (1975): Degenerative disease of the sacroiliac joint. *Invest Radiol* 10:608–621.

121. Rothkotter HJ, Berner W (1988): Failure load and displacement of the human sacroiliac joint under in vitro loading. *Arch Orthop Trauma Surg* 107:283–287.

122. Rothman RH, Simeone FA (1982): Arthritis, disorders of the spine. In: *The spine, 2nd. ed.* Philadelphia: W.B. Saunders, pp. 914–916.

123. Russel AS, Maksymowych W, LeClercq S (1981): Clinical examination of the sacroiliac joints: A prospective study. *Arthritis Rheum* 24(12):1575–1577.

124. Ryan LM, Carrera GF, Lightfoot RW Jr, Hoffman RG, Kozin F (1983): The radiographic diagnosis of sacroiliitis. A comparison of different views with computed tomograms of the sacroiliac joint. *Arthritis Rheum* 26(6):760–763.

125. Salomon CG, Ali A, Fordham EW (1986): Bone scintigraphy in tuberculous sacroiliitis. *Clin Nucl Med* 11:407–408.

126. Sandoz R (1976): Some physical mechanisms and effects of spinal adjustments. *Ann Swiss Chir Assn* 6:91–141.

127. Sandoz R (1981): Some reflex phenomena associated with spinal derangements and adjustments. *Ann Swiss Chir Assn* 7:45–65.

128. Sarma NH (1985): Pigmented villonodular synovitis of sacral joint—Report of a case. *Cent Afr J Med* 31(8):156–157.

129. Sashin D (1930): A critical analysis of the anatomy and the pathologic changes in sacro-iliac joints. *J Bone Joint Surg* [Am] 12:891–910.

130. Schuchmann JA, Cannon CL (1986): Sacroiliac strain syndrome: diagnosis and treatment. *Tex Med* 82:33–36.

131. Schunke GB (1938): The anatomy and development of the sacroiliac joint in man. *Anat Rec* 72(3):313–331.

132. Shapiro SK, See CE (1986): Pyogenic sacroiliitis. *Minn Med* 69:201–204.

133. Shealy CN (1976): Facet denervation in the management of back and sciatic pain. *Clin Orthop* (115):157–164.

134. Smith-Petersen MN (1924): Clinical diagnosis of common sacroiliac conditions. *Am J Roent Radium Thera* 12:546–550.

135. Solonen KA (1957): The sacroiliac joint in the light of anatomical, roentgenological and clinical studies. *Acta Orthop Scand Suppl* 27:1–127.

136. Steindler A (1940): The interpretation of sciatic radiation and the syndrome of low-back pain. *J Bone Joint Surg* [Am] 22(1):28–34.

137. Steindler A (1938): Differential diagnosis of pain low in the back; allocation of source of pain by procaine hydrochloride method. *JAMA* 110:106–113.

138. Stewart TD (1984): Pathologic changes in aging sacroiliac joints. A study of dissecting-room skeletons. *Clin Orthop* 183:188–196.

139. Sturesson B, Selvik G, Uden A (1989): Movements of the sacroiliac joints: A roentgen stereophotogrammetric analysis. *Spine* 14:162–165.

140. Sueoka BL, Johnson JF, Enzenauer R, Kolina JS (1985): Infantile infectious sacroiliitis. *Pediatr Radiol* 15:403–405.

141. Taggart AJ, Desai SM, Iveson JM, Verow PW (1984): Computerized tomography of the sacro-iliac joints in the diagnosis of sacroiliitis. *Br J Rheumatol* 23:258–266.

142. Trotter M (1937): Accessory sacro-iliac articulations. *Am J Phys Anthropol* 22(2):247–261.

143. Trotter M (1940): A common anatomical variation in the sacro-iliac region. *J Bone Joint Surg* [Am] 22(2):293–299.

144. Vesterskold L, Axelsson B, Jacobsson H (1985): A method for combined quantitative pertechnetate and bone scintigraphy of the sacro-iliac joints. *Scand J Rheumatol* 14:324–328.

145. Vogler JB 3d, Brown WH, Helms CA, Genant HK (1984): The normal sacroiliac joint: A CT study of asymptomatic patients. *Radiology* 151:433–437.

146. Waisbrod H, Krainick JU, Gerbershagen HU (1987): Sacroiliac joint arthrodesis for chronic lower back pain. *Arch Orthop Trauma Surg* 106:238–240.

147. Walker JM (1986): Age-related differences in the human sacroiliac joint: A histological study; implications for therapy. *J Orthop Sports Phys Ther* 7(6):325–334.

148. Weisl H (1954): The ligaments of the sacro-iliac joint examined with particular reference to their function. *Acta Anat (Basel)* 20(3):201–213.

149. Weisl H (1954): The articular surfaces of the sacro-iliac joint and their relation to the movements of the sacrum. *Acta Anat (Basel)* 22(1):1–14.

150. Weisl H (1955): The movements of the sacro-iliac joint. *Acta Anat (Basel)* 23(1):80–91.

151. Weisz GM, Green L (1986): Progressive sacro-iliac obliteration in Forestier disease. *Int Orthop* 10:47–51.

152. Wilbur AC, Langer BG, Spigos DG (1988): Diagnosis of sacroiliac joint infection in pregnancy by magnetic resonance imaging. *Magn Reson Imaging* 6:341–343.

153. Wilder DG, Pope MH, Frymoyer JW (1980): The functional topography of the sacroiliac joint. *Spine* 5(6):575–579.

154. Wilkinson M, Meikle JAK (1966): Tomography of the sacro-iliac joints. *Ann Rheum Dis* 25:433–440.

155. Wyke B (1967): The neurology of joints. *Ann R Coll Surg Engl* 41:25–50.

156. Yazici H, Tuzlaci M, Yurdakul S (1981): A controlled survey of sacroiliitis in Behcet's disease. *Ann Rheum Dis* 40:558–559.

The Adult Spine: Principles and Practice,
J. W. Frymoyer, Editor-in-Chief.
Raven Press, Ltd., New York © 1991.

CHAPTER 102

Benign and Malignant Tumors of the Sacrum

Eugene R. Mindell and Constantine P. Karakousis

Sacral tumors, both primary and secondary, are rare lesions. The incidence of these tumors among all bone tumors in worldwide studies varies from 1% to 3.5% (1,15). They are unusual even in comparison with the rest of the spine because metastatic carcinoma and marrow cell lesions such as myeloma are seldom seen in the sacrum. They often escape early diagnosis because of their location, requiring rectal examination and a thorough radiographic study.

The sacrum may be the site of any of the tumors, benign as well as malignant, that involve the spine. However, certain lesions such as chordoma do have a predilection for the sacrum. Sacral tumors present special problems in diagnosis and in management because of their unique location.

DIAGNOSIS AND STAGING STUDIES

The history is of utmost importance. Most patients with sacral tumors have the common and non-specific complaint of low back pain, although great variability

E. R. Mindell, M.D.: Professor, Department of Orthopaedic Surgery, State University of New York at Buffalo, Director, Orthopaedic Oncology Division, School of Medicine and Biomedical Sciences, Buffalo, New York; Buffalo General Hospital, Buffalo, New York, 14203.

C. P. Karakousis, M.D.: Associate Chief, Surgical Oncology, Chief, Soft Tissue Melanoma Service, Roswell Park Memorial Institute; Clinical Professor, State University of New York at Buffalo, Buffalo, New York, 14263.

exists in the type and timing of pain. As with tumors in other locations, pain may be present at rest and may not be altered by changes in the patient's physical activities. Radiating pain and paresthesias may be produced by root involvement.

On examination, local tenderness is a common finding. Swelling or a mass is often present which may require careful rectal examination for detection. The patient's gait is usually not altered but may be abnormal if nerve roots are involved or if the sacral tumor has produced marked bony destruction. Delay in accurate diagnosis not infrequently occurs because the patients are sometimes incorrectly considered to have lumbar disc disease. Late in the course of a serious sacral lesion disturbance of urinary and/or bowel control may occur. Soft-tissue extension of a malignant sacral tumor laterally and into the upper thighs may be detected in a late case.

Imaging Studies

The radiographic diagnosis of a sacral tumor is often delayed for long periods of time because of overlying gas and bowel content shadows. The lower bowel must be properly prepared if the sacrum is to be well visualized on routine radiographs. If one suspects a sacral lesion and the routine radiographs appear normal, bone scan, CT scan, and MRI may be revealing. Isotope scans are less helpful in the sacrum than elsewhere, although they are useful in identifying the presence of a lesion. The CT scan is helpful particularly in demonstrating bony abnormalities, while the MRI demonstrates soft-tissue extension quite clearly. Pyelograms, barium enemas, and angiograms also have their place, although they are not used as frequently as they were before the advent of CT and MRI.

A myelogram may be in order if the lesion is located in the upper sacrum and extra-dural extension must be determined.

Biopsy

In most cases an accurate diagnosis requires histologic examination of the lesion. Biopsy is best performed after all of the other necessary staging procedures have been completed. The biopsy must yield an adequate sample and should not contaminate tissue planes unduly. The entry wound either for needle or open biopsy should be in an area which can be easily excised with the definitively resected specimen. A midline vertical posterior approach is usually utilized for biopsying sacral lesions involving posterior elements.

A transrectal needle biopsy for anterior tumor masses risks pelvic contamination if the needle tract is not subsequently excised. Open biopsy of an anterior lesion may be done through a lower midline abdominal incision, or an oblique incision from near the left costal margin to near the pubic symphysis; great care is necessary to avoid dissemination and implantation of the tumor as the biopsy is taken, by walling off the field with multiple laparotomy pads, copious irrigation, and finally closing the pre-sacral fascia over the biopsy incision, when feasible, to prevent later seepage of tumor into the operative field. The necessity for an anterior approach to biopsy should arise rarely, and it is best avoided because it is difficult to eliminate the risk of tumor cell implantation and impossible to perform an en bloc excision of the biopsy tract since the latter involves the posterior half of the lesser pelvis. In most situations, even for lesions protruding anteriorly, it should be possible to obtain a diagnostic biopsy through a posterior incision via the posterior elements of the lower sacral vertebrae (S4 and S5), and from this level the bone biopsy needle may be extended cephalad, as necessary, through the anterior, fused sacral bodies and into the tumor mass; for greater exposure, if necessary, the coccyx may be resected and thus direct visual and palpatory evaluation of the anterior surface of the sacrum obtained for biopsy, but this approach may lead to tumor contamination of the pre-sacral space, although to a far lesser extent than the transabdominal approach.

Not infrequently the proper diagnosis can be suspected before biopsy. Under these circumstances the surgical alternatives can be discussed with the patient before

biopsy. In addition, the pathologist should have the opportunity to review the case with the surgeon prior to the biopsy. If frozen section analysis confirms the surgeon's impression and if planning has been thorough, a definitive surgical procedure should then be carried out. This sequence of events, with resection immediately following biopsy, minimizes local spread of tumor.

Frozen section analysis is useful in confirming the presence of abnormal cells from which the pathologist can make a diagnosis. Unfortunately, the pathologists have usually not been prepared in advance, or the lesion is a rare one and the pathologists want more time to be certain of the exact diagnosis. Certainly it is better to wait than to proceed with improper treatment.

CLASSIFICATION OF SACRAL TUMORS

Sacral tumors can be classified as benign or malignant:

1. Benign tumors
   Aneurysmal bone cyst
   Osteoblastoma
   Giant cell tumor
      Osteochondroma
      Sacral cysts
2. Malignant tumors
   Chordoma
   Chondrosarcoma
   Metastatic carcinoma
   Marrow tumors
      Myeloma
      Ewing's
   Other primary malignant tumors.

BENIGN SACRAL TUMORS

Benign bone lesions in the sacrum should be staged just as they are in other locations: stage 1 (latent), stage 2 (active), and stage 3 (aggressive). Most aneurysmal bone cysts and osteoblastomas of the sacrum are stage 1 or 2, and can be successfully treated by intra-lesional curettage or marginal excision through a posterior approach without difficulty. Adjacent or involved nerve roots are easily seen, unroofed and retracted. If the lesion has expanded anteriorly, perforating the anterior reactive rim, one may find it useful to place an assisting finger (covered with a second glove) in the rectum so that the curettage can be safely completed. However, this maneuver should generally be avoided due to the risk of contamination.

In large, narrowly marginated stage 2 (active) or stage 3 (aggressive) benign bone tumors, especially vascular aneurysmal bone cysts or giant cell tumors, the risk of serious hemorrhage or neurologic loss may make a marginal or wide excision an unattractive choice. Here intralesional curettage and occasionally adjunctive radiotherapy are reasonable.

Aneurysmal Bone Cyst

Aneurysmal bone cyst (ABC) is a cystic, vascular, tumorlike process which expands and destroys bone. Its clinical characteristics cover a broad spectrum ranging from lesions that remain quiescent to aggressive ones that mimic sarcoma (12).

Pathologic Abnormalities

The radiographic hallmark is localized expansion of bone with development of a thin peripheral rim of bone which delineates the edge of the lesion and separates it from adjacent normal soft tissue structures. When located in the spine it may expand into adjacent vertebrae, which can be a helpful diagnostic clue.

Bone scans demonstrate increased uptake, particularly in the peripheral portions, and decreased uptake in its center. This difference is also noted on angiograms where modest vasculature is noted at the rim and relative avascularity in the center.

The peripheral thin rim of bone can be penetrated very easily with an osteotome. The central portion is found to be filled with unclotted blood and contains varying amounts of soft tissue. Although initial bleeding may be quite brisk, it can usually be controlled without difficulty by local pressure, indicating the feeding vessels are small ones. Occasionally, however, brisk bleeding with alarming blood loss may occur, particularly in spine and pelvic locations.

Histologic examination reveals the central tissues to contain blood-filled cavernous sinuses, benign spindle cells, and new bony trabeculae. Multinucleated giant cells are present which are usually smaller than those found in giant cell tumors. Histiocytes and foam cells are also encountered. The peripheral rim of new bone is often quite cellular, with bone formation and resorption often adjacent to large vascular lakes (12).

Clinical Findings

Symptoms and signs vary widely from none at all to markedly disabling. Presenting complaints and signs depend on the location and size of the cyst, and the presence of pathologic fracture or pressure on adjacent vital structures.

The most common locations for aneurysmal bone cysts are in the metaphysis of long tubular bones and the vertebral column. However, they have been detected in virtually every part of the skeleton. Aneurysmal bone cysts are slightly more common in females and are most frequently found between 10 and 20 years of age; they are rare after age thirty. Dahlin found 5 aneurysmal bone cysts in the sacrum out of a total of 134 aneurysmal bone cysts, with an incidence of 3.7% (1).

The diagnosis is usually suspected from radiographs. The staging studies often include isotope scans, which demonstrate the increased uptake at the reactive rim, and CT scans which usually reveal the thin peripheral rim of bone. Biopsy is almost always necessary and usually is an open one although fine needle biopsy can sometimes yield adequate tissue. The practical problem is to obtain tissue representative of the lesion.

In young adults, the usual differential diagnosis is from giant cell tumor. However, the possibility of confusing ABC with telangiectatic osteosarcoma must be emphasized.

Tissue grossly and microscopically identical to ABC can be encountered immediately adjacent to other lesions of bone including many benign abnormalities, and may even be found adjacent to malignant tumors (12).

Pathogenesis

Although the cause of the ABC remains unknown, Lichtenstein (9) and others feel the lesion results from a local change in vascular hemodynamics (12).

Treatment

The treatment offered for ABC depends on the location and size of the lesion, symptoms and signs, and threat to normal function. These lesions are not true neoplasms and will often be cured though incompletely removed. Marginal excision is usually the treatment of choice, often consisting of curettage. However, the behavior of the ABC is unpredictable and recurrences are not uncommon. Marginal excision is also the treatment of choice for recurrences unless vital functions are threatened. Radiation should only be carried out in refractory cases (12).

Results of Treatment

Marginal excision of ABC in general is followed by a recurrence rate of up to 20%. Often these recurrences are noted radiographically, do not progress, and may be of little clinical importance. Of great concern, however, is the occasional ABC which, when treated by marginal excision, recurs massively, destroys the bone graft and leads to marked disability. This aggressive, unpredictable behavior fortunately is quite unusual. Conversely, some lesions will subside spontaneously and become

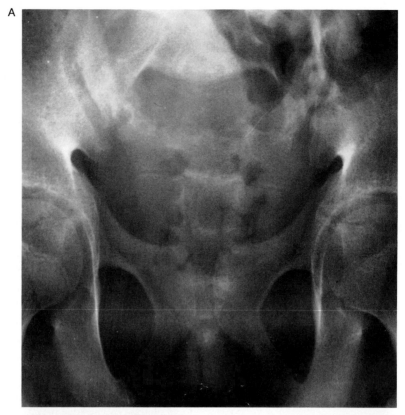

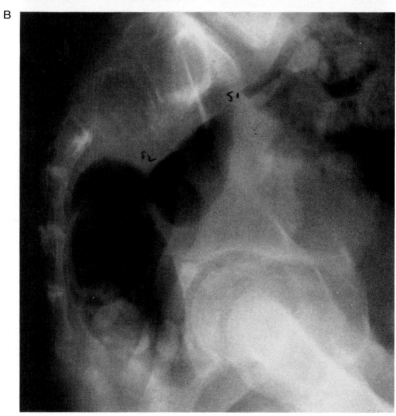

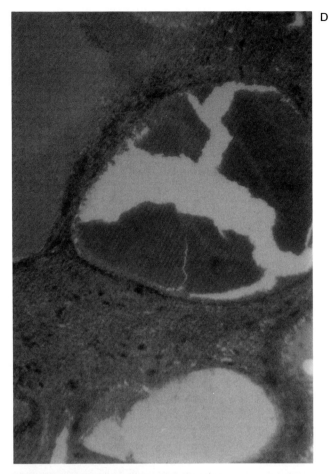

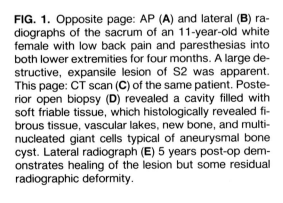

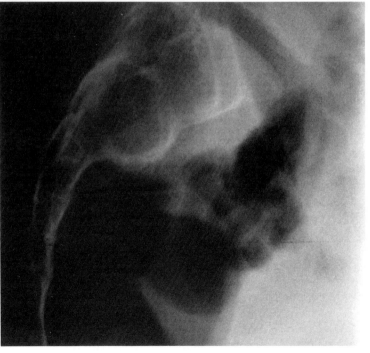

FIG. 1. Opposite page: AP (**A**) and lateral (**B**) radiographs of the sacrum of an 11-year-old white female with low back pain and paresthesias into both lower extremities for four months. A large destructive, expansile lesion of S2 was apparent. This page: CT scan (**C**) of the same patient. Posterior open biopsy (**D**) revealed a cavity filled with soft friable tissue, which histologically revealed fibrous tissue, vascular lakes, new bone, and multinucleated giant cells typical of aneurysmal bone cyst. Lateral radiograph (**E**) 5 years post-op demonstrates healing of the lesion but some residual radiographic deformity.

asymptomatic, although radiographic abnormalities persist (12).

Illustrative Case of Aneurysmal Bone Cyst of the Sacrum

An 11-year-old white female was seen in December 1984 because of increasing low back pain and paresthesias down the back of both thighs that was present for four months. On examination, marked tenderness was present over the sacrum; neurological examination of her lower extremities was normal. Radiographs and CT scan (Figs. 1A–1C) demonstrated a large osteolytic lesion of the sacrum involving S2, with extensive loss of cortex. Biopsy revealed vascular spaces, soft tissue containing benign fibrous tissue, multinucleated giant cells, and trabeculae of immature new bone (Fig. 1D). The lesion was curettaged, accomplishing an intra-lesional excision. Nothing further was done. The patient's symptoms gradually disappeared over a few months. When seen in 1989 for follow-up examination, she was asymptomatic and exhibited normal function. Lateral radiograph of her sacrum (Fig. 1E) five years after surgery demonstrated healing of the lesion with mild residual distention of the sacrum at S2.

Giant Cell Tumor

Giant cell tumors of the spine and sacrum are rare clinical entities that pose a difficult challenge for the surgeon. Complete excision, although the recommended treatment for giant cell tumors, is difficult to achieve. The incidence in spine and sacrum averages between 4% and 12% of all giant cell tumors. Of Dahlin's 264 cases of giant cell tumor, 23 occurred in the sacrum with an incidence of 9% (2). Turcotte, who recently studied 28 sacral giant cell tumors, found that 86% of the sacral lesions had neurologic signs (unpublished data, 1988). They were purely osteolytic on x-ray and eccentrically located. The upper sacrum lesions frequently presented soft-tissue extensions. His recommended treatment was intra-lesional excision for most giant cell tumors. En bloc excision was performed when the lesion was small and in the distal part of the sacrum. When the lesion was large, curettage and bone grafting was the treatment of choice with preservation of sacral roots. Radiation may be a valuable adjunct for lesions that cannot be completely excised or for local recurrences.

Surgery remains the most plausible option for giant cell tumors of the sacrum, although fraught with problems because of the location and the size of tumor. Surgical exposure must be extensive to provide sufficient exposure to remove the tumor completely and to control the bleeding. Wide resection of the tumor has consistently provided better tumor control than intra-lesional curettage, although it often implies a functional deficit and spinal instability if the lesion is located in the upper sacrum.

Other Benign Tumors

Osteochondromas are rarely noted in the sacrum. Hanakita and Suzuki (5) described a sacral osteochondroma that produced sensory disturbances and urinary dysfunction successfully removed via lumbar hemilaminectomy.

Osteoblastomas and neurofibromas are occasionally located in the sacrum, while sacral meningiomas are extremely unusual.

Intra-spinal lipomas are thought to pre-exist from birth, are associated with defects in the laminae, and may be extensions of subcutaneous lipomas. When resection is delayed to adulthood, there is a significant risk of increased neurologic deficit.

MALIGNANT SACRAL TUMORS

Malignant tumors of the sacrum must be staged carefully before treatment (3). The stage will often provide guidelines to treatment. For instance, most of the chordomas are low grade but extra-compartmental, which would be classified as IB and require a wide excision.

Malignant intra-spinal extra-dural tumors are principally metastatic and are extensions of the bony lesion or of a lesion in the pelvis such as extensive rectal adenocarcinoma.

Chordoma

Sacrococcygeal chordoma is a relatively rare, often fatal malignant tumor believed to take its origin from remnants of the notochord. The neoplasm develops most often at either end of the spinal column, grows slowly, but is locally infiltrative and destructive. Symptoms initially may be mild and present months or even years before medical attention is sought. Definitive diagnosis is usually not made until the tumor has attained considerable size. Patients may have back pain or perineal pain and numbness. As the disease progresses, the patient's pain may become intractable and often disabling, despite many forms of treatment. Although metastases occur in some instances, death usually results from complications of extensive local tumor growth.

Constipation is a common complaint; however, rectal bleeding is rare since the neoplasm usually does not penetrate the rectal wall. Fecal incontinence may occur late in the course of the disease. Urinary symptoms such as frequency, urgency, and difficulty starting the stream may eventually progress to incontinence. As the lesion infiltrates pelvic nerves, paresthesias and anesthesias may develop.

A careful rectal examination will almost always reveal the pre-sacral tumor mass which is firm, fixed to the sacrum, and extra-rectal. Although decreased perianal sensation may be found, motor loss is rarely present (8).

Radiographic Features

Radiographic findings reveal the bone destruction and the soft-tissue mass. Irregular areas of osteolysis with expansion of the sacrum due to remodeling about a slowly growing lesion are noted. The soft-tissue mass is usually detected anteriorly. CT scans and MRI are particularly useful in delineating the extent of soft-tissue extension. Increased densities are a frequent finding, due to calcification in the degenerating and necrotic portion of the neoplasm (11).

Gross Pathology

Chordomas are usually soft, vary from firm to semi-liquid, and are grayish in color and semitransparent. Discoloration due to old and recent hemorrhage may be noted. They are lobulated and usually well encapsulated in the soft tissues, although no distinct tumor edge is present where bone is invaded. Soft-tissue extension of the tumor may occur into the sacral canal. Although growth is slow, so much room for expansion is present that the soft-tissue component may become enormous (Fig. 2). The rectum, uterus, bladder, and adnexae may be displaced or even partially surrounded by neoplasm. Eventually the tumor may destroy the sacrum and coccyx, fill the pelvis, extend behind the sacrum, and even exit from the pelvis into the buttock as a huge mass (11).

Histopathology

The histologic hallmark, the physaliferous cell, is vacuolated, containing intra-cytoplasmic mucous droplets. The nucleus is enveloped by a narrow ring of clear cytoplasm, encircled by cytoplasm containing a zone of well-defined vacuoles. Sometimes the nucleus itself is vacuolated. The vacuoles may contain mucin, which when discharged from the vacuoles accumulates between the cells, often as great quantities of acellular mucinous material. The chordoma or physaliferous cells are often arranged in lobules (Fig. 3). Considerable pleomorphism is present, but only rarely are mitotic figures present.

Sometimes few physaliferous cells are present and then the histological diagnosis may be somewhat difficult. Syncytial strands of cells with indistinct cell boundaries lying in an expanse of mucin may be found, which is almost as characteristic as the collections of physalifer-

ous cells. Occasionally, anaplastic spindle cells are present (11).

Diagnosis

The finding of a midline sacral tumor exhibiting radiographic manifestations of bone destruction and with a soft-tissue mass should suggest the diagnosis of chordoma, particularly if a soft-tissue mass is palpated anterior to the sacrum on rectal examination. However, other sacral tumors such as giant cell tumor, metastatic carcinoma, or even ependymoma must be differentiated from chordoma. The diagnosis must be verified histologically. The histological differentiation among chordoma, chondrosarcoma and adenocarcinoma is sometimes difficult (11).

Staging

Staging studies must document the degree of local spread of chordomas as with any malignant bone neoplasm, and the presence of metastases. These studies usually include a technetium bone scan which is useful in providing a rough estimate of the extent of local involvement. CT scan is helpful in demonstrating the soft-tissue extension and the anatomic details of the bone involvement. Barium enema, angiogram, and intravenous pyelogram have been used in the past and occasionally are still useful in providing additional information about extent of tumor. However, in recent years MRI has become most useful for detecting soft-tissue extension. Since metastases occur to the lungs and sometimes bone, chest x-ray and bone scans are of importance. The tumor must be accurately staged before treatment is planned (11).

Biopsy

The biopsy of a sacral lesion suspected of being a chordoma should be carefully planned so as not to interfere with subsequent complete surgical removal by radical resection of the sacrum. For instance, the biopsy should not be done through the rectum, unless removal of the rectum or removal of the needle biopsy site is planned. If the clinical and radiographic findings strongly suggest chordoma, staging studies determining the extent of local spread should be done before biopsy. Not infrequently the history, physical findings, clinical course, and radiographic appearance are so typical of sacral chordoma that definitive surgical treatment may be carried out immediately after open biopsy with frozen section confirmation, provided pre-biopsy planning was carried out. Usually an open biopsy through the direct posterior route is preferred, and definitive surgical resec-

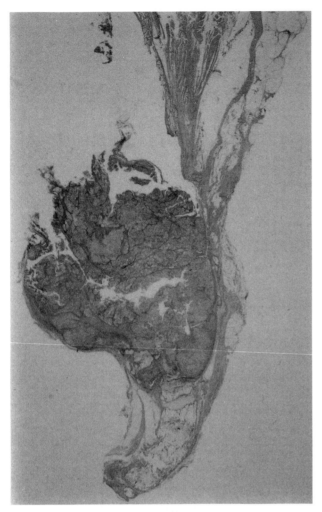

FIG. 2. Large histosection of resected lower sacrum containing a chordoma that has extended anteriorly into soft tissue.

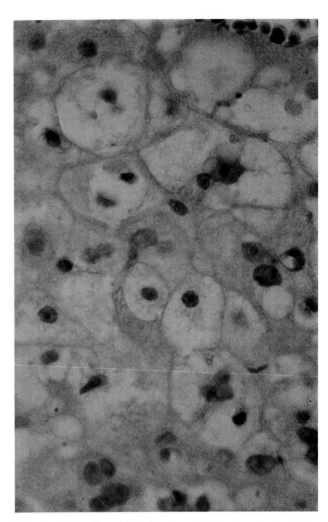

FIG. 3. High power histosection photomicrograph of the chordoma reveals typical physaliferous cells.

tion is usually planned after the diagnosis has been confirmed by examining the final histologic sections (11).

Treatment of Sacrococcygeal Chordoma

In the past most chordomas have been treated by intra-lesional or marginal excisional surgery and/or radiation. Recurrence, local spread, and eventually death has been the rule following such treatment. In recent years, however, it has been established that wide resection of the sacral chordoma can lead to cure and should be attempted whenever possible. This is feasible particularly when the lesion is small, permitting removal of a cuff of normal tissue peripheral to all tumor margins. The surgical plane of excision must pass through normal tissue. Spillage of tumor during surgery must be avoided.

In the past, high sacral amputation was thought to be contraindicated because of the impaired anorectal and urogenital function and loss of pelvic girdle stability that was thought to follow. However, recent studies assessing

the consequences of extensive surgical sacral resections with most of the sacral nerve roots have indicated that such radical procedures are reasonably well tolerated by the patients months and years later.

Gunterberg (4) has found that if only the upper half of the body of S1 remains bilaterally, the pelvic girdle retains sufficient strength to permit standing immediately after resection surgery without the collapse of the bony pelvis.

In 1978, Stener and Gunterberg (13) described a surgical technique for high amputation of the sacrum which, although it results in some disability, offers improved chances for cure. The transection of bone is through the uninvolved vertebra above the tumor and includes a rim of normal soft tissue.

Studies by Stener and Gunterberg (13) indicate that if all the sacral nerve roots are sacrificed on one side and preserved on the other side, practically no functional deficit occurs (11).

Our own experience (7), gained from the hemipelvectomy operation, corroborates these findings and pro-

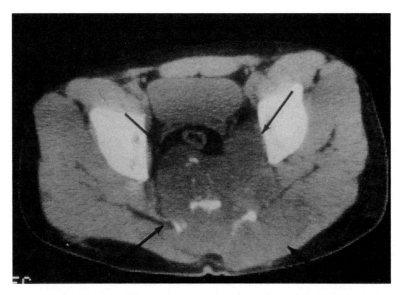

FIG. 4. Pre-operative CT scan in a young male patient with sacral chordoma extending into the surrounding soft tissues.

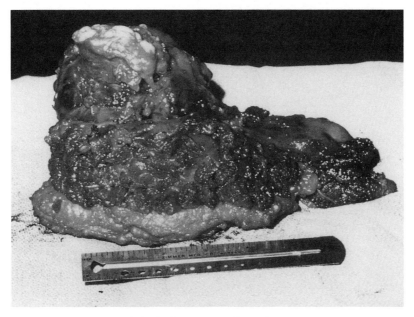

FIG. 5. The resected specimen.

vides a definitive answer to the issue of unilateral interruption of the pudendal nerve or the roots from which it arises. The pudendal nerve, exiting through the greater sciatic notch and around the ischial spine, then reentering the pelvis through the lesser sciatic notch, finally courses in the pudendal canal of the obturator fascia, the latter covering the surface of the obturator internus muscle. It is obvious that this segment of the nerve, which branches to the sphincters, unless specifically dissected, is resected during the procedure of hemipelvectomy. In hemipelvectomy following division of the pubic sym-

physis and the sacroiliac joint (or sacral ala), the dissection is carried out through the loose areolar tissue between the bladder and rectum medially and the wall of the pelvis laterally, definitely interrupting the branches of the pudendal nerve to the sphincters. In our personal experience with 53 hemipelvectomies performed through December 1986 and several since then, none of the patients had any difficulties with sphincteric control of the bladder or rectum or with potency. Bilateral sacrifice of all sacral nerves except S1 results in urinary bladder and urethral sphincter denervation. The

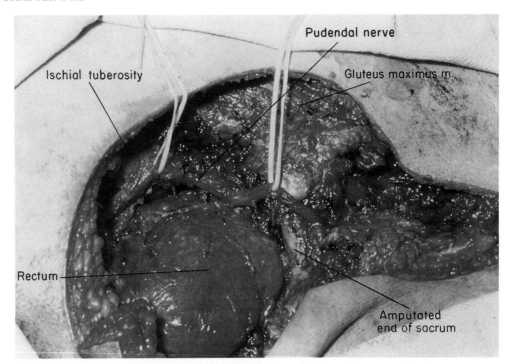

FIG. 6. Operative field of the patient shown in Figures 4 and 5. The left S2 root (and possibly S3) has been preserved along with its continuation to the pudendal nerve. All right-sided roots were divided as they were found to course into tumor. The patient retained sphincteric control and potency and, following adjuvant post-operative radiation, is well 6 years later.

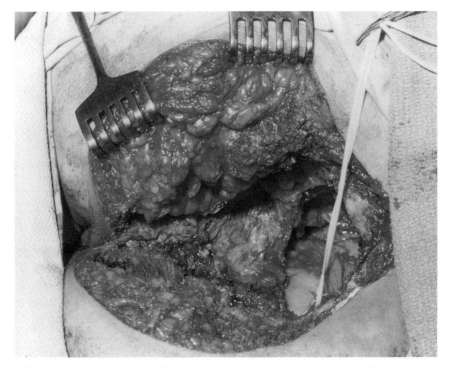

FIG. 7. En-bloc resection of the lower rectum and sacrum for a locally recurrent adenocarcinoma performed in a lateral position through a combined approach. The vessel loop identifies the pudendal nerve on one side. This female patient retained bladder control and is well 2 years later.

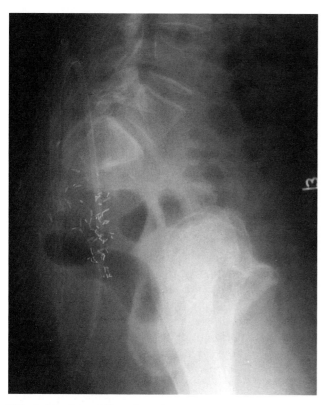

FIG. 8. The lateral film often shows more clearly the level of sacral resection. In this patient the bone was divided just below the S1 vertebra with preservation of continence. Suction drains are still in place post-operatively.

patient is incontinent and will require a urinary collecting device or diapers. Genital function will be impaired, although ejaculation may be preserved. The loss of rectal control is surprisingly well tolerated, since there is usually no constant or frequent leak of feces, but the stool collects in the rectal ampula and every 2 to 3 days needs to be disimpacted. The urine also does not dribble constantly, but tends to collect in the bladder where it is effectively evacuated through self-catheterization with a straight catheter 3 to 4 times daily. Patients usually learn to catheterize themselves fairly quickly. The use of diapers is, of course, essential but overall this marked disability is tolerated surprisingly well by patients.

Fortunately, motor function loss in the lower extremities is minor when both S1 roots are preserved. Gait is normal on level ground, although the resultant partial gluteus maximus muscle functional loss will make climbing somewhat difficult.

Operative Considerations

The technique of resection of chordomas or other malignant tumors of the sacrum may vary somewhat according to the nature of the tumor, its size, and location but some general principles apply. The patient is usually positioned in a right lateral position so that, with appro-

priate prepping and draping of the patient, the abdominal wall is also exposed, should a transabdominal approach be required for proximal anterior exposure and/or control of bleeding. The left side is placed up to facilitate the mobilization of the sigmoid colon, a common antecedent to the mobilization of the rectum. However, for most tumors, with the exception of those with adhesions in the pre-sacral space due to previous surgery or irradiation, it is possible to perform the entire operation through the posterior incision. Any bleeding from branches of the internal iliac artery can usually be controlled through the posterior approach. For tumors without prior surgery or radiation, particularly those extending into the buttocks, a prone position may be preferable. A longitudinal posterior incision over the middle of the sacrum is preferable for biopsy because it provides greater exposure of the posterior sacral surfaces. Localio has described a transverse incision over the lower sacrum for a combined abdominosacral approach in the resection of a low rectal carcinoma and anastomosis under direct vision (10). This transverse incision makes possible the resection of the coccyx and lower sacrum (S4, S5) and provides ample exposure for the resection of low rectal tumors and small, distal sacral tumors but is inadequate for large sacral tumors and those extending proximally.

A longitudinal, usually elliptical incision (in order to circumscribe a previous biopsy tract) is made over the midline, and may be veered off to the left of the midline at the two ends for further improvement in exposure, particularly caudally. Flaps are raised bilaterally, dissecting the surface of the gluteus maximus aponeurosis to beyond the palpable extent of the tumor or the edge of the sacrum. Caudally, the anococcygeal raphe is divided transversely below the tip of the coccyx, and the pre-sacral space entered. With blunt dissection, the potential space between the anterior sacral surface and the rectum is developed. The left index finger in this space provides further guidance as to the exact outline of the bone or tumor, as the fibers of the gluteus maximus are divided. Some dissection with scissors may also be needed in the pre-sacral space, but most of the dissection is blunt, provided that no prior surgery or radiation to this area has been applied. Commonly, the tumor is palpable either from the posterior or more frequently the anterior surface of the sacrum, a situation which provides guidance to the surgeon as to the cephalad extent of the dissection and the level of transection of the sacrum. The level of division of the sacrum is critical in two ways: (a) the provision of an adequately wide surgical margin proximally and (b) the identification of the level with regard to the corresponding sacral vertebra, as this has a direct bearing on the risk of denervation of the pudendal nerve roots.

Determination of an adequate surgical margin is obviously heavily influenced by the anatomical constraints or lack thereof, of the specific region under consideration. Ultimately, an adequate margin is one that is free of microscopic involvement on detailed pathologic examination. A 2 cm margin around the tumor would be satisfactory in the sacral area, although often difficult to attain in the cephalad direction, unless the tumor is located in the distal portion of the sacrum.

Selection of the specific sacral vertebral site for division of the bone is also difficult. One may attempt to count caudad starting from the spinous process of the fifth lumbar vertebra, but the spinous processes of the proximal sacral vertebrae are fused, covered by the posterior intraspinous ligament, and certainly not easily distinguishable. More laterally remaining fibers of the sacrospinalis muscle and ligaments obscure the exposure of the posterior sacral foramina. In most cases the entire posterior surface of the sacrum is not exposed, in order to avoid violating the biopsy track, and therefore there may be difficulty in deciding whether to transect just below the S1 vertebra, through the middle of S2, or just below S2. A useful anatomical landmark in our experience is the line connecting the upper limits of the lateral dissection on both sides of the sacrum. The lateral dissection on either side stops just below the sacroiliac joint or in effect, the inferior aspect of the sacroiliac ligaments. This is the highest point that may be attained with scalpel, scissors, or electrocautery dissection on each side. The line connecting these points is just below the S3 vertebra and therefore division of the sacrum with a Gigli saw (which provides a straight line of division), when the tumor location permits, can be certain in most situations to leave intact the innervation of the sphincters. Division of the bone at a higher level can be carried out with bone instruments (e.g., osteotome), the bone being divided for some distance along the sacroiliac joint on each side and then across the midline. As the subarachnoid space descends to the middle of the second sacral vertebra, resection through this level risks entry into this space. In our experience, if the subarachnoid space should be traversed while dividing with the osteotome through this level, the operative field would be immediately flooded with the leaking cerebrospinal fluid. Should this happen, the dura would need to be carefully closed after completion of the resection. In cases where the S1 vertebra is itself involved and is simply curetted, entry into the subarachnoid space, as it is involved by tumor and reactive changes in this area, may not be appreciated at the time of surgery, although the post-operative drainage and/or the development of meningitis make this plain later. In one of our patients with this complication (meningitis) antibiotics had to be administered for over one month before this condition resolved completely.

Lack of certainty as to the exact level of division of the sacrum and the risks of entry into the subarachnoid space, of injury to the roots of the pudendal nerve, and of cutting into an unexpected cephalad extension of the tumor into the sacral canal limit the usefulness of the osteotome in dividing through the full thickness of the proximal sacrum. As in other areas, but perhaps more importantly here, the surgeon should be as deliberate and conscious of the available choices as possible. With the use of fine rongeurs one may enter the sacral canal at the proposed line of resection posteriorly well above the tumor and through bone (the fused laminae) which grossly at least should look normal, and actually outline the whole line of posterior element division in this fashion (6). It is thus possible to enter the sacral canal first, to identify nerve roots at this level, assess the extent of the tumor, and with the use of pledget dissection displace the dural attachment superiorly. Having exposed and traced the sacral roots at this level to the anterior sacral foramina, and following assessment of the extent of the tumor on the anterior sacral surface, one may then divide the fused sacral bodies at the desired level with the use of an osteotome. The plea for the use of this technique is not for the encouragement of conservative surgery, it is for the encouragement of deliberate surgery.

In large tumors extending into the buttock, the flaps are developed further and the gluteus maximus muscle divided at the appropriate distance from its sacral origin. The ischiorectal fossa is entered just medial to the ischial tuberosity by dividing the sacrotuberous ligament and the pudendal nerve identified on the surface of the obturator internus muscle and then traced proximally. During this process the contributions from the S4 root, and when necessary the S3 root, may be divided next to the nerve trunk, and the pudendal nerve protected in its course over the posterior aspect of the ischial spine, as the short sacrospinous ligament is divided. Even for large chordomas, it may be possible to preserve, unilaterally at least, the pudendal nerve and its continuation with the S2 root (Figs. 4–8).

The removed specimen is sent to the pathologist for frozen section examination of the soft tissues surrounding the bone and for smears from the divided bone surface. An x-ray of the specimen may occasionally be helpful.

Following hemostasis and irrigation, suction drains are placed in the wound and exited as laterally as possible through one of the flaps. Post-operatively, culture of the drainage should be obtained periodically as these wounds, due to the proximity of the anus, are more prone to infection. There is often copious drainage which prevents the removal of the drains for one week or longer. When the drainage rate decreases to below 100 ml per 24 hours, the drains may be removed. Any lymphocele may be aspirated later using sterile technique.

For tumors previously operated on or irradiated, one may start with the posterior incision, but if the dissection of the rectum from the anterior sacral surface is difficult, one may have to resort to a simultaneous, transabdominal approach. The latter becomes necessary when the lower rectum is involved. In this case, for example in locally recurrent adenocarcinoma of the rectum following a low-anterior resection, when the tumor is situated between the rectum and the lower sacrum, an en bloc resection of the rectum and lower sacrum may be performed (i.e., an abdominoperineal resection en bloc with resection of the lower sacrum) in a lateral (Sim's) position (Fig. 7). It is not usually necessary to use the abdominal approach to simply visually expose the anterior upper sacrum or the roots of the sciatic nerve; the latter is best accomplished through the posterior incision by exposing the sciatic nerve immediately lateral to the sacrum.

The abdominal incision is preferably a lower midline incision, because it provides good exposure and leaves the left side of the abdominal wall intact for the construction of an end sigmoid colostomy. If the latter can be precluded in advance with certainty, one may use an oblique incision from below the left costal margin to the pubic symphysis.

Post-operatively, the level of division of the sacrum is determined with anteroposterior and lateral radiographs (Fig. 8).

Post-Operative Management

Wound suction is mandatory post-operatively. Sometimes considerable fluid collects in the dead space. Occasionally, repeated aspiration is necessary.

Patients are treated symptomatically post-operatively with early ambulation recommended. Standing with full weight-bearing within a few days as tolerated and walking assisted by a walker are encouraged.

Patients are evaluated periodically for local recurrence and metastasis.

Several chemotherapeutic agents have been tried but without success.

Irradiation

Irradiation, although not curative offers the possibility of significant palliation in primary and recurrent chordoma, although little objective evidence exists for decrease of tumor size following radiation.

Although chordomas are relatively radioresistant, large doses of radiation may achieve some degree of tumor control. Irradiation to the tumor bed should be considered if residual tumor was left behind. The recommended dosages vary in different centers. A dose of more than 5,000 rads to the tumor may lead to prolonged remission (8).

Recurrent chordoma may be treated with radiation therapy with some improvement expected.

Results and Prognosis

The seriousness of chordoma lies in its critical location adjacent to important structures, its locally aggressive nature, and its extremely high recurrence rate.

According to Sundaresan, patients may live for several years with recurrent disease. Therefore, evaluation of the effects of various modes of treatment is difficult, because of the length of follow-up required. Chordomas metastasize late and by the hematogenous route. The incidence of metastasis is more frequent than was thought in the past. Although the Mayo Clinic estimates that only about 10% of their cases metastasize (2), Sundaresan reported that 39% of his cases eventually exhibited metastases (14). This indicates that chordomas exhibit a wide spectrum of biological behavior.

The outlook is bleak when the diagnosis is made late and surgical treatment is often inadequate, with most such patients succumbing after five to ten years. However, radical surgical procedures in recent years have produced longer survivals and may result in cures when performed early, particularly for small lesions. A plea is made for early diagnosis and early radical surgery, although the usefulness and application of the latter has not yet been thoroughly assessed. However, early reports are encouraging.

REFERENCES

1. Dahlin DC (1981): *Bone tumors, 3rd. ed.* Springfield, Illinois: Charles C Thomas, p. 11.
2. Dahlin DC, MacCarty CS (1952): Chordoma: A study of fifty-nine cases. *Cancer* 5:1170–1178.
3. Enneking WF, Spanier SS, Goodman MA (1980): A system for the surgical staging of musculoskeletal sarcoma. *Clin Orthop* 153:106–120.
4. Gunterberg, B, Romanus B, Stener B (1976): Pelvic strength after major amputations of the sacrum. An experimental study. *Acta Orthop Scand* 47:635–642.
5. Hanakita J, Suzuki T (1988): Solitary sacral osteochondroma compressing the cauda equina. Case report. *Neurol Med Chir (Tokyo)* 28:1010–1013.
6. Karakousis CP (1986): Sacral resection with preservation of continence. *Surg Gynecol Obstet* 162:270–273.
7. Karakousis CP, Emrich LJ, Driscoll DL (1989): Variants of hemipelvectomy and their complications. *Am J Surg* 158:404–408.
8. Karakousis CP, Park JJ, Fleminger R, Friedman M (1981): Chordomas: Diagnosis and management. *Am J Surg* 47:497–501.
9. Lichtenstein L (1950): Aneurysmal bone cyst. *Cancer* 3:279–289.
10. Localio SA, Eng K, Coppa GF (1983): Abdominosacral resection for midrectal cancer. A fifteen-year experience. *Ann Surg* 198:320–324.
11. Mindell ER (1981): Chordoma. *J Bone Joint Surg* [Am] 63:501–505.
12. Mindell ER (1987): Aneurysmal bone cyst. *Iowa Ortho J* 7:39–41.
13. Stener B, Gunterberg B (1978): High amputation of the sacrum for extirpation of tumors. Principles and technique. *Spine* 3:351–366.
14. Sundaresan N, Galicich JH, Chu FC, Huvos AG (1979): Spinal chordomas. *J Neurosurg* 50:312–319.
15. Sung HW, Shu WP, Wang HM, Yuai SY, Tsai YB (1987): Surgical treatment of primary tumors of the sacrum. *Clin Orthop* 215:91–98.
16. Turcotte RE, Sim FH, Unni KK (submitted for publication): Giant cell tumors of the sacrum. *Clin Orthop*

The Adult Spine: Principles and Practice,
J. W. Frymoyer, Editor-in-Chief.
Raven Press, Ltd., New York © 1991.

CHAPTER 103

Fractures of the Sacrum and Coccygodynia

Thomas K. Kristiansen

For good reason, fractures of the sacrum have recently emerged as an area of intense interest (9,11,14,16,21, 22,25,32,43,59,64,65,66,67,78,80,81). Historically, sacral pathology, whether a manifestation of neoplastic disease, developmental abnormality, metabolic bone disease, infection, or trauma, was considered a curiosity. Pertinent literature was sparse, and treatment an enigma. As we have come to better understand the osseous pelvis and spine and, as techniques for treatment of pelvic and spinal pathology have improved, the interposed sacrum has come to present an interesting, important, and difficult challenge. The morphology of the sacrum and its intricate relationship with the sacral plexus complicate matters of treatment considerably, despite available technology.

The increased incidence of motor vehicle and industrial trauma during the twentieth century has led to an increase in fractures of the lower spine, pelvis, and sacrum (4). In the past, many patients with severe pelvic and lower spinal trauma did not survive. Recent advances in the care of polytraumatized patients have, through improved survival rate, increased the incidence of sacral and pelvic fractures requiring treatment (45,54,57,61,72).

In this chapter, I will review the anatomy of the sacrococcygeal region and discuss assessment, classification,

and treatment of sacral and coccygeal fractures and coccygodynia.

ANATOMY OF THE SACROCOCCYGEAL REGION

It is historically relevant that the sacrum was at one time supposed to be the seed from which the body would be resurrected. The anatomy of the sacrococcygeal region (Fig. 1) is well described in Esses's chapter (see Chapter 100).

It is worth emphasizing that the complementary surfaces on the ilium with elevations and depressions on the sacrum allow very little motion but provide anti-rotational and anti-shear features (69). In vivo these joints are extremely stable due to the very thick posterior sacroiliac ligament and the anterior sacroiliac ligament and sacrospinous and sacrotuberous ligaments (Fig. 2).

Also relevant to injuries in this region is re-emphasis of certain features of neuroanatomy. First is the variable size of the foramina. The first sacral foramen is the largest, and the size diminishes at each successive caudal level. These foramina transmit the rami of the first four sacral nerves and their associated vessels. The ratio of nerve root diameter/foramen diameter progressively decreases from $\frac{1}{3}$ to $\frac{1}{6}$ as one proceeds from the S1 to the S4 foramina (11).

Second, there is considerable variation in the anatomy of the sacral canal.

Third, the dural sac usually ends at S2, and the filum terminale penetrates the dural sac and continues to in-

   T. K. Kristiansen, M.D.: Associate Professor, McClure Musculoskeletal Research Center, University of Vermont College of Medicine, Department of Orthopaedics and Rehabilitation, University of Vermont, Burlington, Vermont, 05405.

A

Pelvic surface

Base of sacrum

Superior articular process

Lateral part

Ala

Promontory

Sacral portion of pelvic brim

Transverse lines

Pelvic sacral foramina

Apex of sacrum

Coccyx

Transverse process

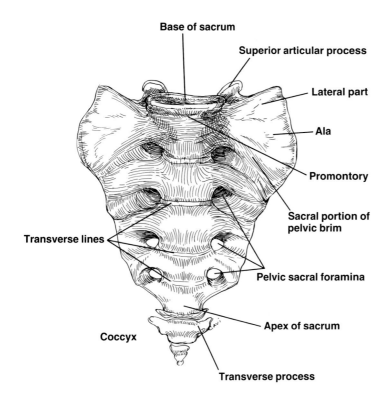

After Netter

FIG. 1. Sacrum and coccyx (**A, B, and C**) (with permission from FH Netter).

C

Dorsal surface

Facets of superior articular processes

Sacral tuberosity

Lateral sacral crest

Median sacral crest

Sacral hiatus

Sacral cornu

Auricular surface

Intermedian sacral crest

Dorsal sacral foramina

Coccygeal cornu

Transverse process

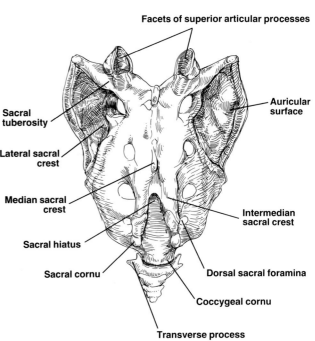

B

Superior articular process

Dorsal surface

Pelvic surface

Sacral canal

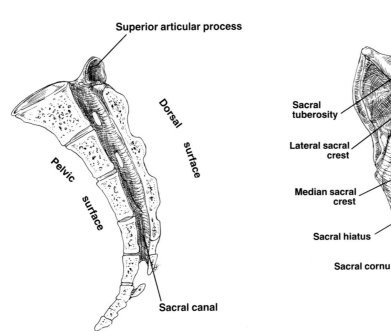

Sacrum and coccyx (median sagittal section)

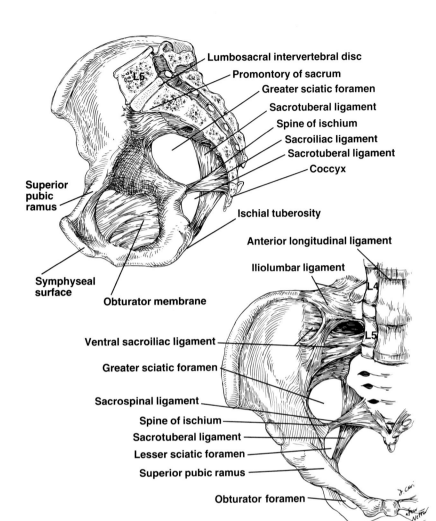

FIG. 2. Vertebral column and pelvis (with permission from FH Netter).

Lumbosacral intervertebral disc
Promontory of sacrum
Greater sciatic foramen
Sacrotuberal ligament
Spine of ischium
Sacroiliac ligament
Sacrotuberal ligament
Coccyx

Ischial tuberosity

Anterior longitudinal ligament
Iliolumbar ligament

Ventral sacroiliac ligament
Greater sciatic foramen
Sacrospinal ligament
Spine of ischium
Sacrotuberal ligament
Lesser sciatic foramen
Superior pubic ramus
Obturator foramen

Superior pubic ramus
Symphyseal surface
Obturator membrane

sert in the coccyx. All of these features influence the risk of neurologic injury. In addition, the sacral plexus anatomy, as reviewed in Chapter 100, is also relevant as it affects both the peripheral neurologic and sexual function (see Figs. 3 and 4).

SACRUM

Visceral Anatomy

The sacral plexus is in close proximity to the ureters and the internal iliac vessels and branches, any of which may be injured in severely displaced sacral fractures. Severe injuries also may be associated with massive bleeding from severed arteries, the bone itself, and the so-called presacral venous plexus. A retroperitoneal hematoma may accumulate in large volume as it extends cephalad into the abdomen, which can lead to hypovole-mic shock and even death if proper resuscitative measures are not promptly undertaken. Regardless of its size, such a hematoma should not be evacuated, as such a course often leads to exsanguination. These factors generally preclude an anterior intra-abdominal approach to the sacrum for the treatment of fresh fractures.

In addition, the anterior pelvis is frequently disrupted in conjunction with a sacral fracture and, if displacement is severe, there is resulting injury to either the bladder or the urethra. This further complicates the evaluation and treatment of a patient with bladder dysfunction following pelvic and sacral disruption.

Radiologic Assessment

As elsewhere in the skeleton, sacral fractures are associated with pain, swelling, ecchymosis, and tenderness to palpation. If there is any clinical suspicion, further radiographic evaluation is necessary. An anteroposterior radiograph of the pelvis is the standard screening test used to evaluate the pelvis in a polytraumatized patient. Because the sacrum is curved (see lateral view of sacrum, Fig. 1B) and because it projects 45° posteriorly from the lumbosacral junction, it is poorly visualized on this view. Although sacral fracture is identified in association with a pelvic fracture in 30% to 74% of cases (15,26,27, 29,42,48,49,75,76), the diagnosis is frequently not made even in the presence of associated neurologic symptoms. A high index of suspicion is therefore warranted. Several findings on the anteroposterior pelvis x-ray suggest the possibility of a pelvic fracture and the need for further evaluation: (a) fracture of a lower lumbar transverse process; (b) significant anterior pelvic fracture without otherwise identifiable posterior pelvic lesions such as sacroiliac joint disruption; (c) discontinuity or asymmetry of the sacral notch; (d) clouding of the radiating trabecular pattern in the lateral sacral mass; or (e) irregularity in the arcuate lines of the upper three sacral foramina (36,52,67).

An anteroposterior view of the sacrum with the beam projected cephalad 30° allows better visualization of the upper half of the sacrum, but no single view on a plain film will allow complete evaluation of the sacrum because of its complex geometry (see Fig. 3). The lateral view must include the lower sacral segments and coccyx and may be very instructive, although a portion of the posterior ilia is superimposed.

If a sacral fracture is suspected on the anteroposterior pelvic view, it is advisable to next obtain anteroposterior and lateral tomograms. If associated neurologic injury is present, computer-assisted tomography may be useful to demonstrate impingement at the foramina or within the sacral spinal canal. The technique should involve tilting of the gantry and thin cuts for good quality images in the reconstructed sagittal plane, or transversely oriented fractures may be missed or poorly visualized (11,23,70,77). In these situations, lateral plane tomography may prove more useful than the CT scan.

Sacral myelography may be useful if the injury is high in the vicinity of S1 but not below, as the dural sac ends at S2 (see Fig. 4). Experience with magnetic resonance imaging (MRI) is lacking, but may prove valuable for evaluating impingement of soft tissue structures in the future (55). Technetium bone scanning may be valuable particularly if osteopenia is present (1,68).

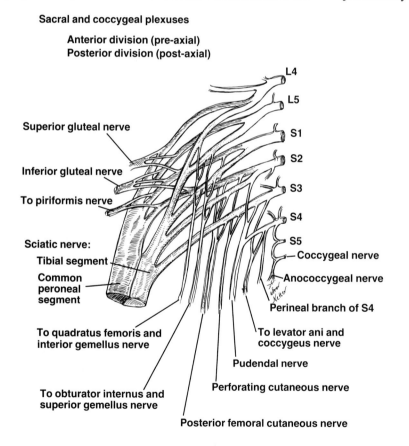

Sacral and coccygeal plexuses

Anterior division (pre-axial)
Posterior division (post-axial)

L4
L5
S1
S2
S3
S4
S5
Coccygeal nerve
Anococcygeal nerve
Perineal branch of S4

Superior gluteal nerve
Inferior gluteal nerve
To piriformis nerve
Sciatic nerve:
Tibial segment
Common peroneal segment
To quadratus femoris and interior gemellus nerve
To obturator internus and superior gemellus nerve
Posterior femoral cutaneous nerve
Pudendal nerve
Perforating cutaneous nerve
To levator ani and coccygeus nerve

FIG. 3. Sacral and coccygeal plexuses (with permission from FH Netter).

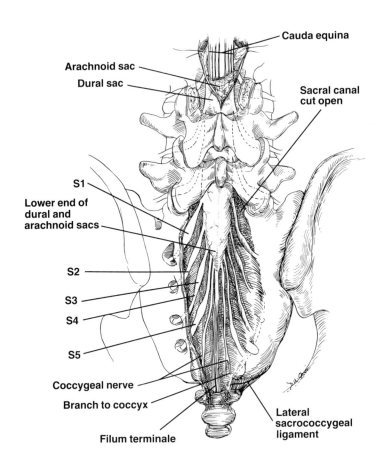

Cauda equina

Arachnoid sac

Dural sac

Sacral canal
cut open

S1

Lower end of
dural and
arachnoid sacs

S2

S3

S4

S5

Coccygeal nerve

Branch to coccyx

Filum terminale

Lateral
sacrococcygeal
ligament

FIG. 4. The sacral canal and its contents (with permission from ref. 73).

Neurologic Assessment

Early careful neurologic evaluation of a patient with a sacral fracture is often not performed, yet may contain the key to accurate diagnosis. Neural injury resulting from sacral fractures, if high in the sacral plexus, i.e., L5, S1, S2, will be manifest in dermatomal sensory loss and lower extremity motor weakness. Injury to the S2–S5 roots results in perineal numbness in a dermatomal distribution often accompanied by bowel, bladder, and sexual dysfunction. Careful evaluation of sensory deficit in the perineum may provide a clue to the precise root injury. Less specific but important information is obtained from evaluation of anal sphincter tone, the anal wink, and bulbocavernosus reflexes. In the multiply traumatized patient these aspects of the physical exam are frequently overlooked, and recognition of the injury occurs days to weeks later when the patient complains of perineal numbness and is unable to void when a urinary catheter is withdrawn.

Injury to the L5 root leads to weakness in the anterior compartment of the leg and sensory changes on the lateral aspect of the lower leg and dorsum of the foot. Injury to the S1 root leads to plantar flexion weakness, diminished ankle jerk, and sensory alteration on the lateral

aspect of the foot. Injury to the superior gluteal nerve is manifested by weakness of hip abduction and internal rotation, which probably is frequently overlooked. The S2 nerve root contributes to the inferior gluteal and sciatic nerves, but is functionally overshadowed in the limb by the S1 root. S1 is the main constituent of the pudendal nerve, and along with the ventral rami of S3 and S4 innervates the striated muscle of the internal and external anal sphincter and provides sensory input from the genitalia and anus.

Coordination of bowel and bladder emptying as well as sexual potency and ejaculation depend on integration of the autonomic nervous system. The inferior hypogastric plexus receives parasympathetic fibers from the ventral rami of S2–S4 and sympathetic input from the sacral splanchnic nerves arising from the S2 and S3 sympathetic ganglia just medial to the ventral foramina.

Conventional electromyography may be useful for evaluation of root injuries affecting L5–S2, but has restricted application during the acute phase of the injury, as abnormality will not appear for several weeks. It may help differentiate between a sacral plexus and nerve root injury or in identifying specific peripheral nerve injuries.

Fountain et al. (24) emphasized the usefulness of cystometography (CMG) in the evaluation of cauda equina damage in sacral fractures (17). Denis et al. (11) echoed this sentiment and found the CMG useful for initial diagnosis and follow-up of neurogenic bladder. They recommend a CMG in all patients with questionable bladder involvement and in all patients with injury to the bony sacral spinal canal.

Classification of Sacral Injuries

Bonnin in 1945 published the first proposed classification scheme for sacral fractures. During the past decade,

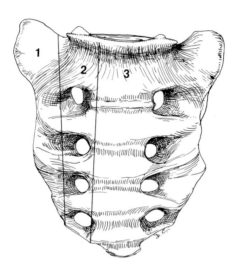

FIG. 5. Classification of sacral fractures (with permission from ref. 11).

at least three classification schemes have followed (11,65,67). Because of its simplicity and its emphasis on neurologic injury, the system of Denis et al. (11) is currently the most useful (see Fig. 5). This scheme expands to incorporate the fracture patterns described in the other schemes and provides guidelines for evaluation, treatment, and prognosis.

Zone I Injuries

Zone I injuries involve a fracture through the ala without damage to the foramina or the central canal. The most common injury in this zone is the result of lateral compression injuries to the pelvis in which the posterior sacral iliac ligaments remain intact and a portion of the ala is compressed anteriorly (Fig. 6). If not displaced vertically, these fractures are stable by virtue of the intact posterior ligaments and the compaction of the cancellous bone. Dissimilar fractures that also occur in Zone I are avulsion fractures of the sacrum at the bulbous enlargement adjacent to the S4 foramen (Fig. 7). This bony site serves as attachment for the sacrospinous and sacrotuberous ligaments. Small juxta-articular fractures of the sacrum may also be caused by ligamentous avulsion by the anterior or posterior sacroiliac ligaments in association with anteroposterior compression injuries or S1 joint dislocation.

Zone II Injuries

The dorsal and ventral foramina appear to act as stress risers as it is relatively common for a fracture line to

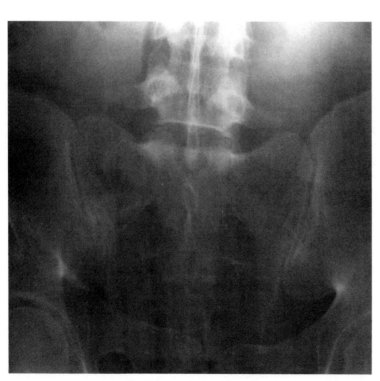

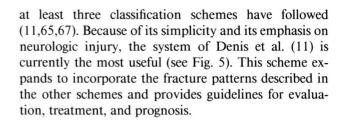

FIG. 6. The upper sacrum is well visualized in this 30° cephalos view and reveals a displaced Zone I fracture involving the sacral ALA on the right.

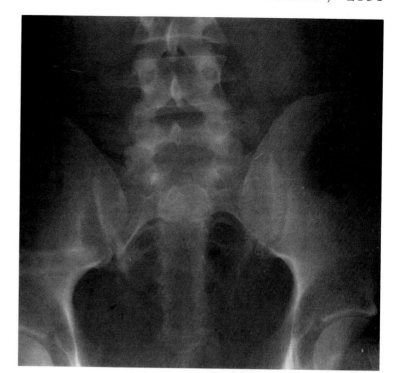

FIG. 7. AP plexus film showing avulsion of the sacrum by the sacrotuberous ligament.

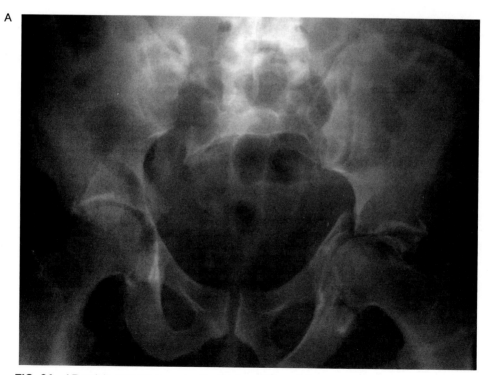

FIG. 8A. AP pelvis reveals a markedly displaced Zone II fracture through the right sacrum and a bilateral acetabular fracture. (Figs. 8B–8C follow.)

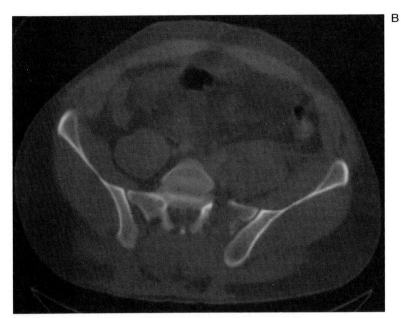

FIG. 8. Continued. B: Computerized tomography reveals no involvement of the central canal at any level. **C:** Same patient following open reduction internal fixation of both acetabulae and sacrum.

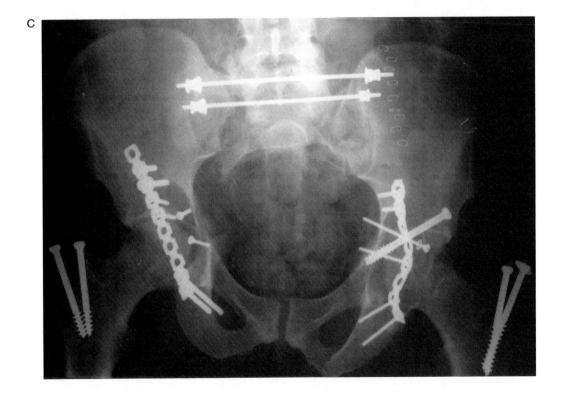

A

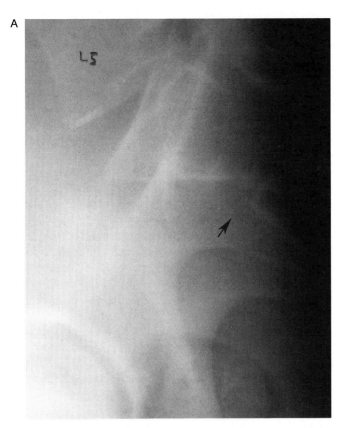

B

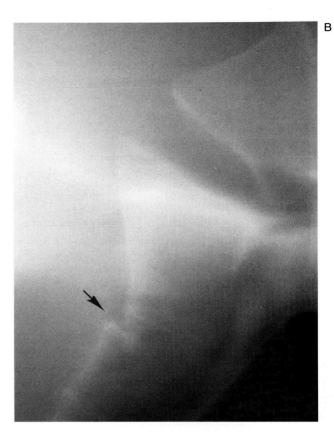

FIG. 9. Plain lateral (**A**) and lateral tomographic (**B**) cut reveals fracture of S2 and the superior fragment projecting posteriorly into the canal.

extend to involve several of the foramina. Zone II fractures involve one or several foramina but not the sacral canal (Fig. 8). These are the Type A fractures according to the classification of Sabiston et al. The fractures are longitudinal (vertical), and the fracture line may exit proximally in various places including the sacral notch or the ala, or distally at virtually any level.

Zone III Injuries

Zone III injuries involve the sacral canal (Fig. 9). These fractures may involve Zones I and II as well. These include high and low transverse fractures (19,20,24), Types B and C of Sabiston et al. (65), and penetrating injuries such as gunshot wounds. Traumatic lumbosacral fracture dislocations should also be included here (6,10,12,18,62).

Neurological Injuries

The cephalad-caudad level of injury influences the neurological injury in each zone (7,30,34,35,44,53,63). That is, high injuries involving L5–S1 will result in limb sensory motor disturbances; S2–S3 injuries are generally accompanied by perineal sensory deficits and bladder

and bowel dysfunction; and low S4–S5 and coccygeal nerve injuries are expected to have minor physiological consequences.

The allure of the classification system proposed by Denis et al. is that it correlates, at least roughly, with neurologic injury. Zone I injuries or fractures are rarely associated with neurologic injuries. A markedly displaced ala fracture associated with vertical shear pelvic fracture conceivably can injure the L5 root or other portion of the sacral plexus. Avulsion fracture and periarticular fracture in and of themselves should not cause injuries. Denis (11) reported that 5.9% of patients with Zone I injury had associated neurologic deficit.

Intuitively, one would expect nerve root injuries in the Zone II injuries group if displacement of the fracture is present. Denis et al. (11) reported that 28% of their Zone II fractures had neurological symptoms attributable to the foraminal fracture. This compared with Sabiston et al., who reported 3 out of 19 patients (16%) who had Type A (Zone II) fractures with a neurologic deficit. The vast majority of these deficits recover with time, but many are missed on examination or poorly documented. Therefore, these figures may represent an underestimation. In general, various unilateral injuries to the upper nerve roots (L5, S1, S2) occur with Zone II injuries, and occasionally cauda equina syndromes are seen. Interestingly, Denis et al. (11) reported that some patients with cauda equina–type symptoms had return of bowel and bladder function, but were left with residual unilateral saddle anesthesia. According to Schmidek et al. (67), unilateral preservation of S2 and S3 will often allow for return of functional urinary and bowel continence.

If the hemipelvis shears off through the sacral foramen and sacral notch and displaces posteriorly and superiorly in association with a pelvic fracture, the L5 nerve root is trapped between the transverse process of L5 and the alar fragment. This is not an uncommon pattern of injury in the Zone II fractures (11,79).

The majority of Zone III fractures are the high and low transverse fractures of Schmidek et al. (67) or the Types B and C of Sabiston et al. (65). Based on 23 cases from the literature, Schmidek et al. reported that transverse fractures were almost invariably associated with neurologic injury in highly variable patterns including roots, multiple roots, or bowel and bladder disorder dysfunctions. In 57% (21 out of 37) of Denis's Zone II patients there was neurologic damage. If one combines the Types B and C fractures of Sabiston et al. (65), 38% of these Zone II patients had neurologic injury. However, their Type C (high transverse or isolated upper segment) fractures had 100% neurologic involvement.

It seems that there is general concurrence that Zone III fractures have a high incidence of neurologic complications, and that it may be important to differentiate between lower and upper transverse sacral fractures within Zone III for purposes of evaluation and treatment.

Treatment of Sacral Injuries

There are two separate issues of treatment: skeletal stabilization, and treatment of neurologic injury and its consequences. The majority of sacral fractures in carefully studied patients are probably Zone I injuries, are stable, and cause no neurological injury. These are dealt with symptomatically and the patient can be mobilized early. Zone I injuries frequently result from lateral compression injuries of the pelvis with intact posterior sacroiliac ligaments and compaction of the anterior lateral mass. Two or more anterior pelvic rami may be fractured in association with the sacral fracture, but the overall situation remains stable. As comfort dictates, the patient can be mobilized, allowing weight bearing early on the uninjured side. However, if there is pelvic instability, the sacral portion of the injury must be handled within the context of the entire injury of the pelvis and/or spine.

If a vertical shear pattern is present with proximal and posterior migration of the hemipelvis and associated with the sacral lateral mass fragment, various options are available. Skeletal traction started early may restore alignment and length to the extremity. In these cases, the pelvic injury is life threatening. Various external fixation resuscitation frames have been proposed for emergent stabilization of the pelvis, with the purpose of reducing hemorrhage and facilitating patient management. In these cases, accurate or acceptable reduction and definitive stabilization may not be possible for several days. Anterior pelvic stabilization is accomplished following reduction by means of an external fixation frame or by open reduction and internal fixation of the pubic symphysis diastasis. No external fixation frame or plate situated anteriorly will adequately stabilize a displaced posterior injury—whether it is a juxta-articular fracture of the ilium, a sacroiliac joint dislocation, or a fracture of the sacrum—making a second operative procedure or continued maintenance of traction necessary in addition to the anterior procedure (47). It is usually difficult to fix the sacrum. The basic strategy is to stabilize indirectly by stabilizing the posterior pelvis. Large "double Cobra plates" are available, as well as threaded metal rod assemblies, both designed to connect the posterior iliac crests posterior to the sacrum and to sandwich the sacrum in between following reduction (so-called posterior tension banding) (13,31,38,47) (Fig. 8C).

The above discussion applies to skeletal stabilization of Zone I and II fractures. The transverse Zone III fractures are usually not associated with massive pelvic disruption. Low transverse fractures most commonly occur through S4 and usually can be handled symptomatically. In markedly displaced fractures, digital reduction through the rectum has been described.

High transverse fractures may require decompression of the contents of the sacral canal only, or if displacement is more severe and associated with intractable pain, these injuries may require reduction. If manual reduction is unsuccessful, threaded pins inserted into the pedicular portion of the sacrum distal to the fracture may provide the purchase necessary.

The majority of neurologic deficits reported in the literature improve without surgical intervention over time (65). Moreover, obtaining and maintaining reduction of the sacral pelvic injury frequently will decompress the acute neural injuries, and no further surgery is needed.

If there is persistent pain (in a sciatic distribution) following reduction, or if there is radiographic evidence of continued nerve root compression, surgical decompression should be contemplated. An anterior approach (transabdominal) is not feasible for reasons already discussed. However, there have been several reports of decompression by means of sacral laminectomy at one or more levels. It is recommended that these procedures be done early, as delayed surgery appears to yield poor results. Information is fragmentary in this regard, but is gradually accumulating. Denis et al. (11) operated on several Zone III injuries by means of sacral laminectomy and foraminotomy to decompress the canal and the foramina. Two patients with high transverse fractures with the sacral vertebral body retropulsed into the canal (sacral burst fracture) were decompressed and recovered completely.

In summary, most sacral fractures can be handled non-operatively. If displacement is associated with neural deficits or if the fractures are markedly displaced, they should be reduced and stabilized. If nerve compression is present, it may improve, but evidence is accumulating that it may be best to perform early for the best clinical result.

COCCYX

Anatomy

The coccyx is formed by fusion of from three to five (usually four) rudimentary vertebrae. In early life they are separate, but are united in the mature adult. The first segment may or may not fuse to the remaining three, and may also fuse to the sacrum with or without the remaining three.

The first coccygeal vertebra has a base for articulation with the apex of the sacrum and vestigial transverse processes as well as paired cornua or vestigial superior anterior processes that are sometimes large enough to articulate with the sacral cornu. The remaining coccygeal vertebrae are only vertebral remnants, the apex being a mere button of bone.

The coccygeal nerves and S5 nerve root exit the sacral hiatus and provide the sensory innervation of the coccyx. The dorsal rami of S4 and S5 join with the coccygeal nerves to innervate the skin in the gluteal cleft over the coccyx. Innervation of the urogenital diaphragm comes in part from the coccygeal plexus, which is derived from the lower sacral nerves and the coccygeal nerve. Apparently, pain fibers pass to these roots via the pelvic splanchnic nerves from the pelvic viscera. This presumably provides a basis to explain referred coccygodynia from non-osseous pelvic pathology. For this reason, we define true coccygodynia as arising from the coccyx while pseudococcygodynia, as arising elsewhere with the pain referred to the coccyx.

The most common cause of the true coccygodynia is trauma, in particular a fall in a partially sitting position or on a narrow object, such that the force strikes the coccyx rather than the ischial tuberosities. This acute variety usually subsides with time, but in some patients may become chronic. Certain anatomic variations of the coccyx have been reported to predispose to this chronicity.

Postacchini et al. (58) reviewed the radiographs of 120 normal individuals and 51 patients with idiopathic coccygodynia. They described four different configurations of the coccyx as follows: In Type I, the coccyx is curved slightly forward, with its apex pointing downward and caudally. In Type II, the curve is more marked and its apex points straight forward. In Type III, the coccyx is sharply angulated forward between the first and second or the second and third coccygeal segments. In Type IV, the coccyx is subluxated anteriorly at the level of the sacrococcygeal joints or the first or second intercoccygeal joint. While they found no correlation between the results following coccygectomy and the pre-operative radiographic pattern of the coccyx, their findings suggest that configuration Types II, III, and IV are more prone to become painful than Type I.

The pain is thought to result from post-traumatic "arthritis" of the sacrococcygeal joint, pseudarthrosis of a fracture of the previously fused coccyx or sacrococcygeal joint, or subluxation or dislocation of the displaced fragments.

Parturition may be considered another form of trauma to the coccyx, and post-partum coccygodynia is a well-recognized entity. Coccygodynia following a history of anal intercourse is also well-recognized and probably should be considered a subset of traumatic coccygodynia. Both these causes may also result in chronic pain recalcitrant to non-operative methods. There are other unusual causes of true coccygodynia that complicate the situation. These include primary and secondary neoplasms involving the coccyx and infections. These present a trap for which the treating physician must be ever vigilant.

Pseudococcygodynia may arise from irritation of lower pelvic structures due to neoplasms (of the rectum or prostate, for example), infection, or other causes of inflammation of the urethra, cervix, bladder, etc. Pseudococcygodynia is sometimes the presenting symptom of a herniated disc. Tumors or other causes of inflammation affecting the sacrum, sacral roots, or portions of the lumbosacral plexus may occasionally produce pseudococcygodynia (51,73,74).

Diagnosis of Coccygodynia

A careful history must be obtained to identify the possible causes of pain. Post-traumatic coccygodynia is usually related to sitting and changing positions, and is relieved by lying down. Pain at night suggests neoplasm. Exacerbation of pain by coughing, sneezing, or defecation suggests more cephalad intraspinal disease. A careful physical exam must be conducted, including dermal sensory examination and rectal examination with careful palpation of the prostate, genitalia, the rectum itself, and the intrapelvic structures in the female. The anterior sacrum and coccyx should be palpated for the presence of masses such as meningoceles, invasive tumors, developmental cysts, and chordomas. The coccyx itself is usually mobile, and in cases of true coccygodynia movement of the coccyx is painful, whereas in the case of referred pain it is not (40,73) (see Table 1).

TABLE 1. *Effect of diagnostic neuroblockade on pain*

Procedure	Coccygodynia	Pseudococcygodynia
Sacrococcygeal joint injection	Decrease	No effect
Sacrococcygeal nerve blocks	Decrease	No effect
Caudal epidural anesthesia*	Decrease	Decrease or no effect
Lumbar epidural anesthesia	No effect	Decrease
Lumbar facet blocks	No effect	Decrease

With permission from ref. 71.
* Blocks pain coming from not only the coccyx but also all structures innervated by the sacral roots and plexus.

Plain anteroposterior radiographs of the sacrum and coccyx may reveal pseudarthrosis, subluxation, dislocation, or destructive processes in the coccyx and sacrum. Bone scan, computer-assisted tomograms with enhancement, and MRI may all reveal causes of pseudococcygodynia. A selective neuroblockade may be used to identify the source of coccygeal pain as described by Traycoff et al. (73) (see Table 1).

Treatment

Coccygodynia is truly a symptom rather than a diagnosis, so a cause must be identified if treatment is to be successful. In cases of pseudococcygodynia, treatment depends on the cause, which is usually not in the orthopedist's or neurosurgeon's domain (41,56,71,73,82).

Post-traumatic coccygodynia that does not spontaneously resolve may respond to seating modifications (e.g., an inflatable doughnut or narrow board that transfers the weight to the ischia) and oral anti-inflammatory agents. If not, infiltration of steroids into the pseudarthrosis or sacrococcygeal junction may provide lasting relief.

For patients with true coccygodynia of non-neoplastic and non-infectious etiology who have intractable incapacitating pain in spite of the conservative measures, coccygectomy may be considered. However, there are skeptics who view the symptom suspect, and the operation rarely, if ever, indicated (3,5,8,33,37,39,40,60).

Coccygectomy

Technique

Coccygectomy is performed with the patient in the prone position and the operating room table flexed at the hips 30°. Pre-operative antibiotics including gram negative coverage are recommended. The buttocks and gluteal crease are carefully prepped and draped, isolating the anus and perianal skin from the field. A two- to three-inch vertical incision is made in the midline and carried down sharply to the bone, exposing it from the sacrococcygeal junction to its distal palpable extent. The

distal portion of the coccyx often extends directly anterior, and in these cases it is difficult to free the tip first as suggested by Gardner (28). Therefore, the portion of the coccyx that is readily accessible proximally is completely exposed posteriorly. The soft tissues between the sacrum and the coccyx should be carefully divided transversely, including the ligaments, keeping close to the bone of the coccyx (see Fig. 10). Paired vessels are encountered here and need to be clamped. Carefully, the proximal coccyx is freed up by pulling up and out of the wound, dissecting close to the bone. As one proceeds distally, it may be necessary to transect the coccyx near its tip and remove it piecemeal with a rongeur and knife. The rectum and attachments of the external sphincter are very close.

The tough fascial tissue that remains should be apposed in the midline to obliterate the dead space and restore as much anatomic integrity as possible. If the distal sacrum is prominent, it should be beveled prior to closure. Post-operatively, careful attention is given to

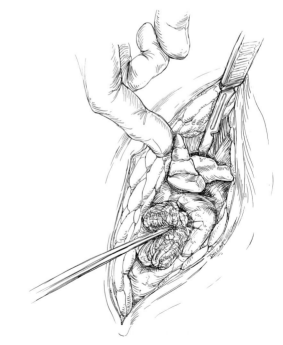

FIG. 10. Artist's interpretation of surgical dissection (with permission from ref. 28).

perineal hygiene and the patients are mobilized as tolerated.

Surgical Results

Bayne et al. (2) evaluated the influence of etiology on results of coccygectomy. They found that patients with post-traumatic recalcitrant coccygodynia did quite well, including those with post-partum coccygodynia, with 75% acceptable results. Patients with "idiopathic" etiology did less well (50% acceptable results), and the patients with prior spine surgery did uniformly poorly (0% acceptable result). They also reported a high gram negative infection rate following coccygectomy of 16.6% and emphasized the importance of not introducing a finger into the rectum during the procedure and the importance of prophylactic antibiotics.

In summary, coccygodynia is a complex problem and demands careful evaluation and accurate diagnosis. It usually responds to conservative measures, with surgical treatment reserved for only recalcitrant, disabling symptoms, particularly patients with post-traumatic etiologies.

REFERENCES

1. Balseiro J, Brower AC, Ziessman HA (1987): Scintigraphic diagnosis of sacral fractures. *AJR* 148:111–113.
2. Bayne O, Bateman JE, Cameron HU (1984): Influence of etiology on the results of coccygectomy. *Clin Orthop* (190):266–272.
3. Beinhaker NA, Ranawat CS, Marchisello P (1977): Coccygodynia: Surgical versus conservative treatment. *Orthop Trans* 1:162.
4. Bonnin JG (1945): Sacral fractures and injuries to the cauda equina. *J Bone Joint Surg* [Br] 27:113–127.
5. Bremer L (1986): The knife for coccygodynia. A failure. *Med Rec* 50:154–155.
6. Bucknill TM, Blackburne JS (1976): Fracture-dislocations of the sacrum: Report of three cases. *J Bone Joint Surg* [Br] 58:467–470.
7. Byrnes DP, Russo GL, Ducker TB, Cowley RA (1977): Sacrum fractures and neurological damage: Report of two cases. *J Neurosurg* 47:459–462.
8. Cameron HU, Fornasier VL, Schatzker J (1975): Coccygodynia. *Can Med Assoc J* 112:557–558.
9. Chiaruttini M (1987): Transverse sacral fracture with transient neurologic complication. *Ann Emerg Med* 16:111–113.
10. Das De S, McCreath SW (1981): Lumbosacral fracture-dislocations: A report of four cases. *J Bone Joint Surg* [Br] 63:58–60.
11. Denis F, Davis S, Comfort T (1988): Sacral fractures: An important problem. Retrospective analysis of 236 cases. *Clin Orthop* (227):67–81.
12. Dewey P, Browne PS (1968): Fracture-dislocation of the lumbosacral spine with cauda equina lesion. *J Bone Joint Surg* [Br] 50:635–638.
13. Dolati B, Beck E (1988): Surgical management of injuries to the dorsal pelvic ring by elastic stabilization. *Unfallchirurgie* 14:199–203.
14. Dowling T, Epstein JA, Epstein NE (1985): S1–S2 sacral fracture involving neural elements of the cauda equina. A case report and review of the literature. *Spine* 10:851–853.
15. Dunn AW, Morris HD (1968): Fractures and dislocations of the pelvis. *J Bone Joint Surg* [Am] 50:1639–1648.
16. Epstein NE, Epstein JA, Carras R (1986): Unilateral S-1 root compression syndrome caused by fracture of the sacrum. *Neurosurgery* 19:1025–1027.
17. Fallon B, Wendt JC, Hawtrey CE (1984): Urological injury and assessment in patients with fractured pelvis. *J Urology* 131:712–714.
18. Fardon DF (1976): Displaced fracture of the lumbosacral spine with delayed cauda equina deficit. *Clin Orthop* (120):155–158.
19. Fardon DF (1979): Displaced transverse fracture of the sacrum with nerve root injury: Report of a case with successful operative management. *J Trauma* 19:119–122.
20. Fardon DF (1980): Intrasacral meningocele complicated by transverse fracture: A case report. *J Bone Joint Surg* [Am] 62:839–841.
21. Ferris B, Hutton P (1983): Anteriorly displaced transverse fracture of the sacrum at the level of the sacroiliac joint: A report of two cases. *J Bone Joint Surg* [Am] 65:407–409.
22. Fisher RG (1988): Sacral fracture with compression of cauda equina: Surgical treatment. *J Trauma* 28:1678–1680.
23. Fishman EK, Magid D, Brooker AF, Siegelman SS (1988): Fractures of the sacrum and sacroiliac joint: Evaluation by computerized tomography with multiplanar reconstruction. *South Med J* 81:171–177.
24. Fountain SS, Hamilton RD, Jameson RM (1977): Transverse fractures of the sacrum: A report of six cases. *J Bone Joint Surg* [Am] 59:486–489.
25. Fredrickson BE, Yuan HA, Miller HE (1982): Treatment of painful long-standing displaced fracture-dislocations of the sacrum: A case report. *Clin Orthop* (166):93–95.
26. Froman C, Stein A (1967): Complicated crushing injuries of the pelvis. *J Bone Joint Surg* [Br] 49:24–32.
27. Furey WW (1942): Fractures of the pelvis with special reference to associated fractures of the sacrum. *AJR* 47:89–96.
28. Gardner RC (1972): An improved technic of coccygectomy. *Clin Orthop and Rel Res* (85):143–145.
29. Gertzbein SD, Chenoweth DR (1977): Occult injuries of the pelvic ring. *Clin Orthop* (128):202–207.
30. Goodell CL (1966): Neurological deficits associated with pelvic fractures. *J Neurosurg* 24:837–842.
31. Gunterberg B (1976): Effects of major resection of the sacrum. *Acta Orthop Scand* [Suppl] (162):1–38.
32. Heckman JD, Keats PK (1978): Fracture of the sacrum in a child. *J Bone Joint Surg* [Am] 60:404–405.
33. Howorth B (1959): The painful coccyx. *Clin Orthop* (14):145–161.
34. Huittinen VM (1972): Lumbosacral nerve injury in fracture of the pelvis. *Acta Chir Scand* [Suppl] 429:3–43.
35. Huittinen VM, Slatis P (1972): Nerve injury in double vertical pelvic fractures. *Acta Chir Scand* 138:571–575.
36. Jackson H, Kam J, Harris JH Jr, Harle TS (1982): The sacral arcuate lines in upper sacral fractures. *Radiology* 145:35–39.
37. Johnson PH (1981): Coccygodynia. *J Ark Med Soc* 77:421–424.
38. Kellam JF, McMurtry RY, Paley D, Tile M (1987): The unstable pelvic fracture. Operative treatment. *Orthop Clin North Am* 18:25–41.
39. Kersey PJ (1980): Non-operative management of coccygodynia. *Lancet* 1:318.
40. Key JA (1937): Operative treatment of coccygodynia. *J Bone Joint Surg* 19:759–764.
41. Kinnett JG, Root L (1979): An obscure cause of coccygodynia. A case report. *J Bone Joint Surg* [Am] 61:299.
42. Laasonen EM (1977): Missed sacral fractures. *Ann Clin Res* 9:84–87.
43. LaFollette BF, Levine MI, McNiesh LM (1986): Bilateral fracture-dislocation of the sacrum. A case report. *J Bone Joint Surg* [Am] 68:1099–1101.
44. Lam CR (1936): Nerve injury in fracture of the pelvis. *Ann Surg* 104:945–951.
45. McMurtry R, Walton D, Dickinson D, Kellam J, Tile M (1980): Pelvic disruption in the polytraumatized patient: A management protocol. *Clin Orthop* (151):22–30.
46. Mears DC, Capito CP, Deleeuw H (1988): Posterior pelvic disruptions managed by the use of the Double Cobra Plate. *Instr Course Lect* 37:143–150.
47. Mears DC, Fu FH (1980): Modern concepts of external skeletal fixation of the pelvis. *Clin Orthop* (151):65–72.
48. Medelman JP (1939): Fractures of the sacrum: Their incidence in fracture of the pelvis. *AJR* 42:100–103.
49. Meyer TL, Wiltberger B (1962): Displaced sacral fractures. *Am J Orthop* 4:187.

50. Moed BR, Morawa LG (1984): Displaced midline longitudinal fracture of the sacrum. *J Trauma* 24:435–437.

51. Nicoll EA (1949): Fractures of the dorsolumbar spine. *J Bone Joint Surg* [Br] 31:376–394.

52. Northrop CH, Eto RT, Loop JW (1975): Vertical fracture of the sacral ala: Significance of non-continuity of the anterior superior sacral foraminal line. *AJR* 124:102–106.

53. Patterson FP, Morton KS (1961): Neurologic complications of fractures and dislocations of the pelvis. *Surg Gynecol Obstet* 112:702–706.

54. Pennal GF, Tile M, Waddell JP, Garside H (1980): Pelvic disruption: Assessment and classification. *Clin Orthop* (151):12–21.

55. Pettersson H, Hudson T, Hamlin D (1985): Magnetic resonance imaging of sacrococcygeal tumors. *Acta Radiol Diagn* (Stockh.) 26:161–165.

56. Peyton FW (1988): Coccygodynia in women. *Indiana Med* 81:697–698.

57. Posner I, White AA 3rd, Edwards WT, Hayes WC (1982): A biomechanical analysis of the clinical stability of the lumbar and lumbosacral spine. *Spine* 7:374–389.

58. Postacchini F, Massobrio M (1983): Idiopathic coccygodynia. Analysis of fifty-one operative cases and a radiographic study of the normal coccyx. *J Bone Joint Surg* [Am] 65:1116–1124.

59. Purser DW (1969): Displaced fracture of the sacrum: Report of a case. *J Bone Joint Surg* [Br] 51:346–347.

60. Pyper JB (1957): Excision of the coccyx for coccydynia. A study of the results in twenty-eight cases. *J Bone Joint Surg* [Br] 39:733–737.

61. Raf L (1966): Double vertical fractures of the pelvis. *Acta Chir Scand* 131:298–305.

62. Resnik CS, Scheer CE, Adelaar RS (1985): Lumbosacral dislocation. *J Can Assoc Radiol* 36:259–261.

63. Rowell CE (1965): Fracture of sacrum with hemisaddle anaesthesia and cerebral spinal fluid leak. *Med J Aust* 1:16–19.

64. Roy-Camille R, Saillant G, Gagna G, Mazel C (1985): Transverse fracture of the upper sacrum. Suicidal jumper's fracture. *Spine* 10:838–845.

65. Sabiston CP, Wing PC (1986): Sacral fractures: Classification and neurologic implications. *J Trauma* 26:1113–1115.

66. Sapkas G, Pantazopoulos T, Efstathiou P (1985): Anteriorly displaced transverse fracture of the sacrum with fracture-dislocation at the L4–L5 lumbar level. *Injury* 16:354–357.

67. Schmidek HH, Smith DA, Kristiansen TK (1984): Sacral fractures. *Neurosurgery* 15:735–746.

68. Schneider R, Yacovone J, Ghelman B (1985): Unsuspected sacral fractures: Detection by radionuclide bone scanning. *AJR* 144:337–341.

69. Solonen KA (1957): The sacroiliac joint in light of anatomical, roentgenological, and clinical studies. *Acta Orthop Scand* [Suppl] 27:1–127.

70. Soye I, Levine E, Batnitzky S, et al. (1982): Computed tomography of sacral and presacral lesions. *Neuroradiology* 24:71–76.

71. Thiele GH (1963): Coccygodynia: Cause and treatment. *Dis Colon Rectum* 6:422–436.

72. Tile M, Pennal GF (1980): Pelvic disruption: Principles of management. *Clin Orthop* (151):56–64.

73. Traycoff RB, Crayton H, Dodson R (1989): Sacrococcygeal pain syndromes: Diagnosis and treatment. *Orthopedics* 12(16):1373–1377.

74. Waddell G, McCulloch JA, Kummel E, et al. (1980): Non-organic physical signs in low back pain. *Spine* 5:117–125.

75. Wakeley CP (1929): Fractures of the pelvis: An analysis of 100 cases. *Br J Surg* 17:22–29.

76. Weaver EN, England GD, Richardson DE (1981): Sacral fracture: Case presentation and review. *Neurosurgery* 9:725–728.

77. Whelan MA, Hilal SK, Gold RP, Luken M, Michelson WJ (1982): Computed tomography of the sacrum: 2. Pathology. *AJNR* 3:555–559.

78. Wiesel SW, Zeide MS, Terry RL (1979): Longitudinal fractures of the sacrum: Case report. *J Trauma* 19:70–71.

79. Wiltse LL, Guyer RD, Spencer CW, Glenn WV, Porter IS (1984): Alar transverse process impingement of the L5 spinal nerve: The far-out syndrome. *Spine* 9:31–41.

80. Woodward AH, Kelly PJ (1974): An unusual fracture of the sacrum. *Minn Med* 57:465–466.

81. Yngve DA (1985): Sacral fractures. *Orthopaedics* 8(4):514, 517–518.

82. Ziegler DK, Batnitzky S (1984): Coccygodynia caused by perineural cyst. *Neurology* 34:829–830.

The Adult Spine: Principles and Practice,
J. W. Frymoyer, Editor-in-Chief.
Raven Press, Ltd., New York © 1991.

CHAPTER 104

Sacral Destabilization and Restabilization

Causes and Treatment

John P. Kostuik and Stephen I. Esses

It is generally recognized that trauma is a major cause of instability of the sacroiliac joint, but other less recognized etiologies may be causative. These include pyogenic and tuberculous infections, primary and metastatic tumors, acquired instability secondary to iliac bone graft harvesting, and idiopathic causes.

Like all spinal conditions, the assessment of sacroiliac joint instability depends on an accurate history, physical examination, and appropriate ancillary radiological investigations.

The classic history of someone with non-traumatic sacroiliac instability is pain originating in the posterior buttock approximate to the sacroiliac joint, often radiating to the greater trochanter and lateral thigh. The pain

J. P. Kostuik, M.D., F.R.C.S.(C): Professor of Orthopaedics, University of Toronto, Toronto, Ontario; and Head, Combined Division of Orthopaedic Surgery, Toronto General/ Mount Sinai Hospitals; Chief, Dewar Spinal Unit, The Toronto Hospital, Toronto, Ontario, Canada M5G 2C4.
S. I. Esses, M.D., M.Sc., F.R.C.S.: Assistant Professor, Department of Surgery, University of Toronto, Toronto, Ontario; and Consultant, Dewar Spinal Unit, The Toronto Hospital, Toronto, Ontario, Canada M5G 2C4.

may also radiate into the anterolateral thigh. Bilateral instability may be present; therefore, bilateral pain should not be regarded simply as referred pain from the low lumbar spine. The patient classically uses his hand to indicate pain in the buttock radiating into the area of the greater trochanter.

Physical examination is not diagnostic but suggestive of sacroiliac problems. Localized tenderness is often noted in people whose pain originates in the lumbar spine rather than from the sacroiliac joint, but specific localized tenderness may be valuable in assessing the sacroiliac joint as a possible source of symptoms.

With instability, forward flexion increases the distance between the posterior superior iliac spine and the sacrum, a differentiating factor from ankylosing spondylitis. However, the diagnostic utility is questionable.

Since the pelvis is a ring, tenderness in the symphysis pubis of an undue nature also may cause the examiner to consider assessing the sacroiliac joint. Physical tests that apply stress to the sacroiliac joint include Patrick's or the so-called cross leg test. The knee is flexed to greater than 90 degrees. The ankle is placed on the opposite thigh, the hip is externally rotated and abducted. Force is applied to the distal femur, which acts as a fulcrum. The hip joint is locked and stress is transferred to the sacroiliac joint. However, as noted in previous chapters, this is an inaccurate test of sacroiliac problems. A more specific test is Gaenslen's test. This consists of the patient lying with the affected side uppermost. The contralateral knee and hip are flexed onto the abdomen in order to lock the pelvis. The uppermost extremity is pulled into extension and stressed. Reproduction of pain is said to be indicative of sacroiliac problems.

Pain from an unstable pelvic ring may be either sacroiliac or symphyseal in origin. If it originates in the sacroiliac joint, it may be indistinguishable from lumbosacral disorders. The pain that originates from the sacroiliac joint usually decreases with recumbency and increases with sitting and walking. The history, per se, does not help to differentiate sacroiliac pain from pain arising from the lumbosacral spine.

RADIOGRAPHIC ANALYSIS OF SACROILIAC JOINT INSTABILITY

The radiographic analysis of the sacroiliac joint may be of considerable value in assessing problems, particularly of stability.

Initial Views

Initial views should consist of an anteroposterior view of the pelvis taken at 90 degrees. Sclerosis or widening of the sacroiliac joint or changes about the symphysis pubis are of limited value. Additional views consist of inlet and outlet views of the pelvis as advocated by Pennal (15,16), which permit an assessment of the proximal migration of the ilium on the sacroiliac joint. Thirty-degree oblique views are also of value in demonstrating the joint.

Aspriation-Injection

Aspiration or injection of the sacroiliac joint is not a commonly performed procedure and is generally recognized as being difficult and time-consuming.

Miskew et al. reported in 1979 (14) a technique of aspirating the most caudal portion of the sacroiliac joint with a needle using a posterior approach under fluoroscopic control (Fig. 1). Hendrix, Lin, and Kane (11) found this technique difficult and time-consuming, and they noted that it was difficult to assess the needle's direction once the tip hit bone. For this reason, they developed a more rapid technique. Under fluoroscopic control, the patient is positioned so that the left hip is raised approximately 10 to 30 degrees from the table. For visualization of the right sacroiliac joint, the right hip is raised similarly. The patient's position is then adjusted until the anterior and posterior orifice of the caudal one third of the joint is seen to be superimposed, which orients the caudal one third of the joint parallel to the x-ray beam (Fig. 2). The prone oblique position of the patient exposes the posterior orifice of the sacroiliac joint and allows direct entry into the joint with a vertically oriented needle. Care must be taken not to advance the needle through the joint into the soft tissues and vessels of the posterior part of the pelvis. Contrast material is then

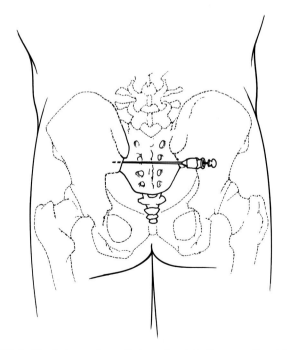

FIG. 1. Technique of needle insertion into the sacroiliac joint.

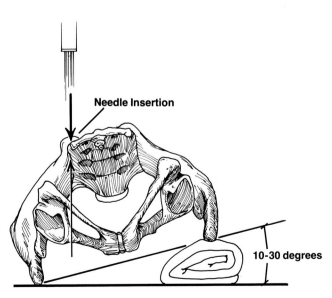

FIG. 2. Portion of the sacroiliac joint in which the anterior and posterior orifices are superimposed, with the walls of the joint parallel to the x-ray beam.

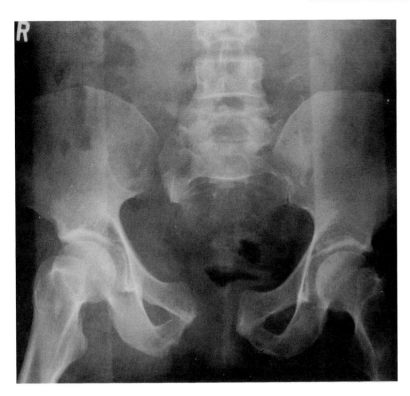

FIG. 5. Radiograph shows Malgaine fracture of the pelvis. There is complete disruption of the symphysis pubis and sacroiliac joint on the ipsilateral side. Note the transverse process fractures on the contralateral side.

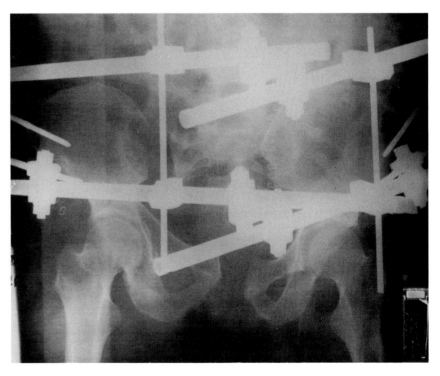

FIG. 6. Radiograph shows anterior external fixation frame on unstable pelvic fracture. The anterior frame is insufficient in stabilizing both the anterior and posterior instability in this injury.

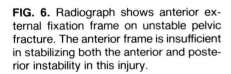

duced, temporary fixation with Kirschner wires can be useful before definitive placement of the stabilization devices.

Plates have been used to secure the sacroiliac joint both posteriorly and anteriorly (Fig. 7). We have had a significant number of wound complications with posteriorly applied plates. Usually, patients being considered for operative stabilization of the sacroiliac joint have a significant amount of soft tissue damage. The dissection required for plate application may further devitalize already compromised tissues. For this reason, applying a plate through an anterior retroperitoneal approach seems attractive, although there are some very significant risks associated with this procedure. In the acute injury, there may be tamponade of bleeding in the retroperitoneal space by hematoma. An anterior exposure of the sacroiliac joint decompresses this hematoma and may lead to hemorrhage with resultant hypotension. This procedure requires the mobilization of the large iliac vessels and occasionally of the lumbosacral plexus or sacral roots. The injury may result in some distortion of the anatomy and, thus, should be undertaken only by somebody experienced in this approach.

An elegant way in which the sacroiliac joint may be stabilized is by the use of screws placed through the ilium posteriorly into the sacral promontory. This technique can be used in those instances in which there is no associated comminution of the sacrum. It can be done with very little soft tissue dissection and thus does not endanger tissue viability. Before inserting these screws it is absolutely essential to examine the CT scan and plan appropriate screw placement (Fig. 8). If this is not done, the screw may inadvertently be placed either into the sacral canal or anterior to the sacrum and cause damage to neurovascular elements. Recently, percutaneous CT-guided stabilization of the sacroiliac joint has been investigated (7). The screws are inserted with the patient lying prone. The lower extremity on the affected side is free draped. In general, we have found that an ideal starting point is two centimeters anterior to the posterior superior iliac spine and two centimeters inferior to the iliac crest. With this starting point, the screw is usually angled 45 degrees anteriorly.

SACROILIAC JOINT DISRUPTION: LATE CASES

If an acute sacroiliac joint disruption is not reduced and stabilized, the incidence of late pain is extremely high. Indeed, sacroiliac joint pain is the major cause of unsatisfactory results following pelvic ring disruption. The pain is caused by either a mal-union or a non-union at the affected sacroiliac joint and is made worse by weight bearing. Some authors have suggested that patients have diminishing pain with time and that in many instances surgical intervention was unnecessary. Those cases that do not have this favorable recovery, and are unresponsive to non-operative modalities of treatment, should be considered candidates for surgical arthrodesis.

Careful assessment should be made of any associated

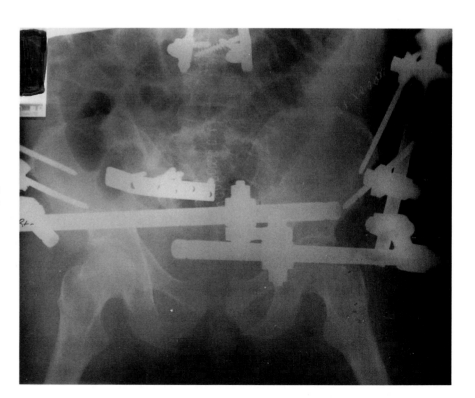

FIG. 7. A posterior sacral plate has been inserted for fixation of the sacroiliac joint injury.

pelvic obliquity. If present, the surgeon should attempt to reduce the sacroiliac joint at the time of fusion in the hope that this will prevent current or later low back pain.

The techniques of sacroiliac joint arthrodesis are discussed elsewhere in this chapter. It is necessary in cases following trauma to meticulously remove all fibrous tissue from the joint in order to be assured of a solid fusion (Fig. 4).

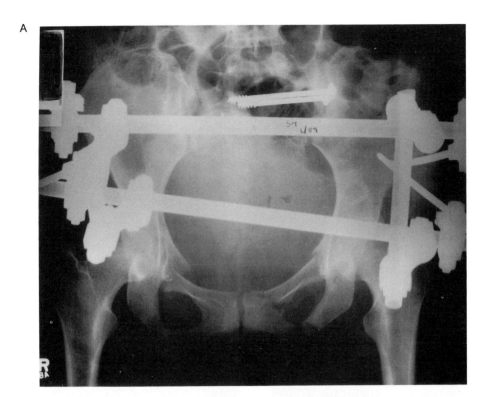

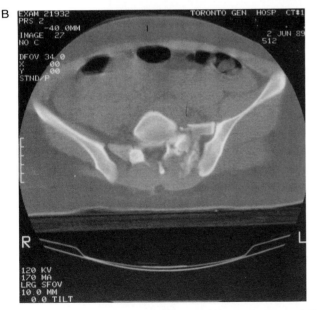

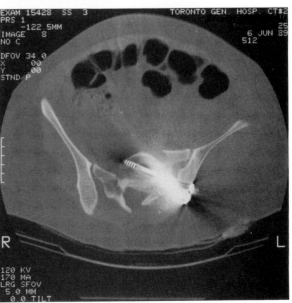

FIG. 8. Radiograph **(A)** shows the position of iliosacral screw used to reduce and fix a dislocated sacroiliac joint. CT scans pre-operatively **(B)** show the instability, and post-operatively **(C)** the location of the screw.

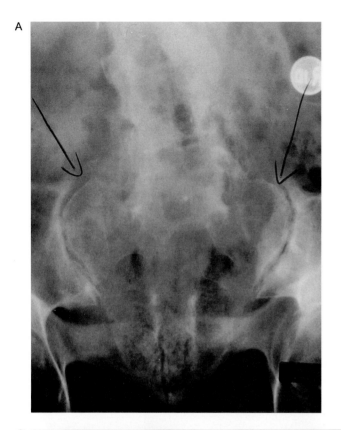

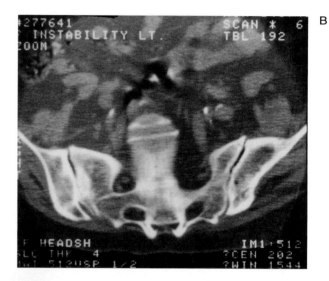

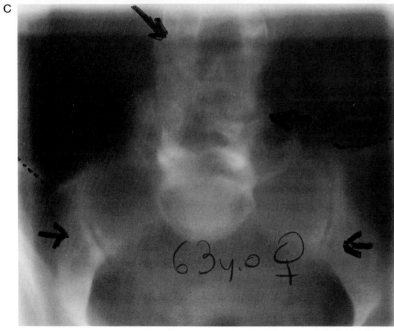

FIG. 9. A 62-year-old female presented with a long history of low back pain. **A, B, and C:** She had had four previous low back procedures including harvesting of bone graft from both iliac crests. She has two persistent lumbar pseudarthroses as well as bilateral sacroiliac instability. Pain was differentiated by the use of local anesthetic blocks. (See also Figs. 10, 11, and 12.)

ACQUIRED PELVIC INSTABILITY

Although it is well known that traumatic interruption of the continuity of the pelvic ring can produce instability, it is generally not recognized that acquired instability may follow the removal of iliac bone for grafting purposes. Lichtblau (13) was the first to report on this complication. He noted that in the course of the procedure of obtaining bone graft, the posterior sacroiliac ligaments were partially destroyed, which could result in later instability. This instability may transfer forces to the pelvic ring, in particular the superior and inferior pubic rami, and result in stress fractures of these bones. In a 1961 report of 45 cases of osteitis pubis, Coventry and Mitchell (3) noted that in one patient the onset seemed to follow removal of iliac bone for a lumbosacral fusion, again suggesting abnormal stress concentration.

In 1972 Coventry and Tapper (4) also reported on six cases in which patients experienced pelvic instability that clearly followed the removal of iliac bone for bone grafting. Pennal has also reported on this syndrome and has fused eight patients who had chronic instability as a result of destruction of the sacroiliac ligaments secondary to the harvesting of iliac bone graft.

Five of the six cases Coventry noted underwent sacroiliac fusion with satisfactory results. One patient had a wedge resection of the symphysis, since the major symptoms seemed to be arriving from the pubis and were symptomatically relieved. A second patient underwent a similar procedure with an unsatisfactory result and was subsequently treated with sacroiliac fusion.

One should suspect such an instability if symptoms persist after the removal of iliac crest bone or if symphyseal pain occurs, especially accompanied by clicking or movement of the pelvis. Continued attention should be given to sacroiliac joints in women who are multiparous and who have radiographic evidence of rather short, straight, flat sacroiliac joints. In these instances, an iliac graft should be taken from an area where the sacroiliac ligaments will not be disturbed.

Recalcitrant or persistent non-union of the sacroiliac joint provides a difficult problem. Solutions to this problem include repeat grafting with internal fixation and immobilization in a bilateral hip spica. Attempts at anterior fusion with internal fixation using either plates or staples may also be done again with post-operative incorporation in a hip spica.

A final option may be the transfer of vascularized bone to the area. Recently, the use of a free vascularized fibular graft has been used to provide transport of viable bone to the sacroiliac joint, and anastomosis was carried out to the superior gluteal vessels (Figs. 9A–9C, 10, 11A, 11B, and 12). This technique may be used for one or both joints if necessary.

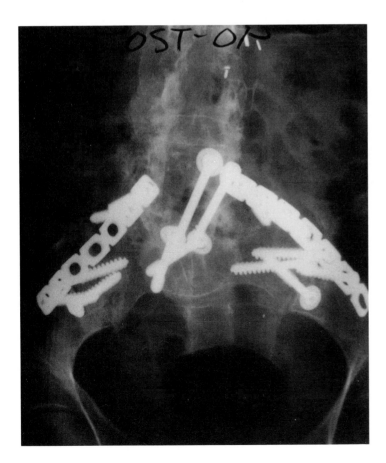

FIG. 10. Same patient as in Figure 9. Following repair of the lumbar pseudarthroses by combined anterior and posterior surgery, both sacroiliac joints were fused using the Smith-Peterson approach. In addition, internal fixation was used together with a bilateral hip spica for three months.

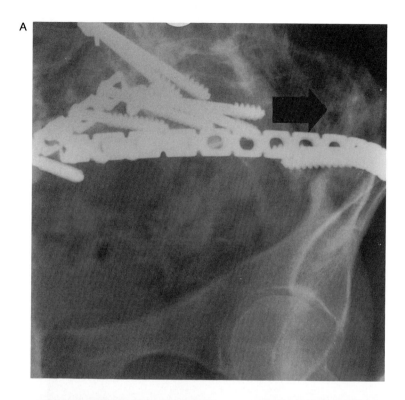

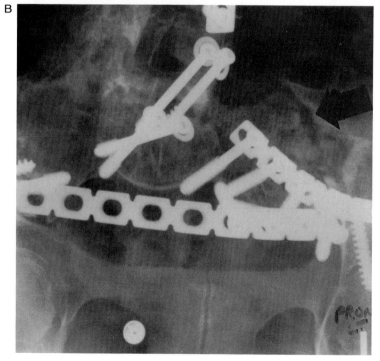

FIG. 11. Same patient as in Figure 9. **A and B:** Non-union persisted (see arrows). An anterior approach (small reconstruction plate) also failed.

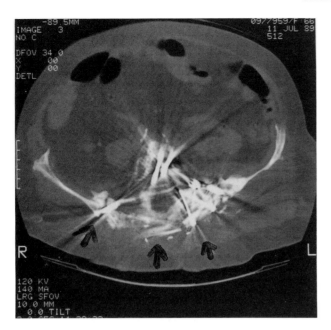

FIG. 12. Same patient. A final procedure using a vascularized fibula (osteotomized for contour) attached to the superior gluteal artery and fixed with screws was done successfully. CT scan (arrows) demonstrates osteotomized fibula. Arrow on the right indicates screw used to hold the fibula.

HOW COMMON IS DONOR SITE INSTABILITY?

Frymoyer (8), in an analysis of the long-term effects of spinal fusion on the sacroiliac joints and ilium, noted in 1978 that there were no differences in patients who had undergone L5-S1 midline fusions between the left and right sacroiliac joints with respect to degenerative changes, although all patients but one had the graft taken from the left ilium. One of the 96 patients exhibited 4 mm of superior subluxation of the ilium at the sacroiliac joint and required codeine for pain. Frymoyer concluded that degenerative changes of the sacroiliac joint were not accelerated by spine fusion. It is certainly this author's (Kostuik) impression that in long fusions done for scoliosis that extend to the sacrum, degenerative changes of the sacroiliac joints are accelerated. This may be bilateral. However, of over 100 patients who have had scoliosis surgery to the sacrum, none has required surgery for disabling sacroiliac pain. Two patients have been referred who had previous long scoliotic fusions to the sacrum and did require surgical intervention related to one sacroiliac joint, with relief following fusion of that joint (Figs. 13A, 13B, and 14).

A
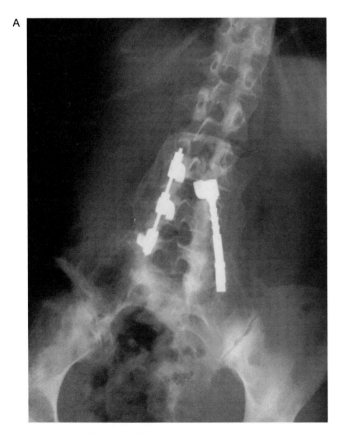

B
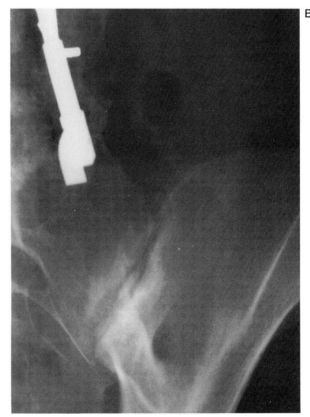

FIG. 13. A 36-year-old female with a history of painful scoliosis was operated on twice. She remained imbalanced with a continuing painful scoliosis and, in addition, a painful left sacroiliac joint. Radiographs **(A and B)** of the left sacroiliac joint reveal widening and sclerosis. Bone scan demonstrated increased uptake. Infiltration with local anesthesia relieved the sacroiliac pain.

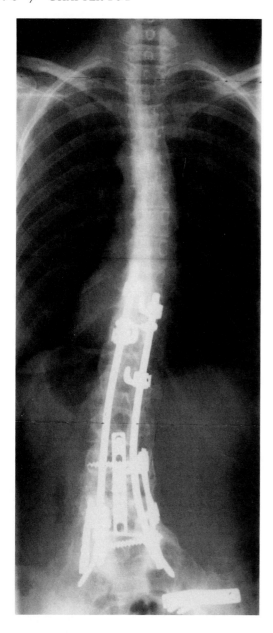

FIG. 14. Same patient as in Figure 13. The scoliosis deformity and pain were corrected by a combined anterior posterior osteotomy to correct her flat back (see Chapter 65) and by extension of her fusion with Cotrel-Dubousset instrumentation. She was then rebalanced in both the frontal and sagittal planes. A left sacroiliac fusion was also done immobilizing the joint with a plate.

INSTABILITY DUE TO INFECTIONS IN THE SACROILIAC JOINT

In the past, most infections of the sacroiliac joint have been tuberculous in nature, but an increased incidence of osteomyelitis is occurring. As with osteomyelitis of the spine, diagnosis is often delayed. Clinical suspicion is substantiated with the use of plain radiography, CT scanning, bone scans, and more recently, MRI.

The differential diagnosis from ankylosing spondylitis may be difficult, since in both infection and inflammatory disease sedimentation rates are elevated and bone scans may be positive. However, the presence of an abscess by CT scan or MRI is diagnostic. However, this finding may not be present. Frequently, infections of the sacroiliac joint may present as a psoas abscess and may not be diagnosed until spontaneous drainage occurs in the groin.

If investigations reveal the presence of a large abscess and there is extensive destruction of the joint, a surgical approach may be necessary.

If the abscess cavity is anterior, as it frequently may be, an anterior approach to the sacroiliac joint may be necessary. Adequate debridement of the joint is essential, including curettage of the infected cartilaginous elements. Subsequent immobilization in a hip spica will frequently result in spontaneous arthrodesis. If this does not occur and late instability is present, a second-stage arthrodesis may be necessary. Shanahan and Ackroyd (17) reported eleven patients who were treated for pyogenic infection of the sacroiliac joint. They noted that this infection accounted for 1.5% of all joint infections in children. Prior to their review, fewer than 120 cases had been reported in the English literature. Before the advent of antibiotics, abscess formation was common, and surgical drainage was frequently needed.

In Shanahan and Ackroyd's (17) review, the average delay in diagnosis was 17 days, but ranged from 2 to 100 days. Differential diagnosis included appendicitis, irritable hip, intervertebral disc disease, and renal abscess. All patients had an elevated sedimentation rate. The most sensitive method to detect early lesions was skeletal scintigraphy with perfusion phase imaging.

The most frequently isolated pyogenic organisms were *Staphylococci* and *Streptococci*. Their treatment in all cases consisted of systemic antibiotics for six weeks with bed rest. No attempt was made to immobilize the patients with casts or traction. Two of the eleven patients went on to spontaneous bony arthrodesis. Two patients had continued pain despite antibiotics for six weeks. One was relieved with further antimicrobial therapy, but the other was treated by aspiration and became asymptomatic. In their series there were no reported cases of late sacroiliac instability, an experience similar to that reported by Dunn (6) and Coy (5).

INSTABILITY DUE TO TUMORS OF THE LUMBOSACRAL ILIAC JUNCTION AND SACRAL TUMORS

The most common tumors in the sacrum are metastatic, followed by multiple myeloma and chordoma. Surgical approaches to these tumors are difficult and warrant detail. Discussion of the diagnosis of tumors in this area is found in Chapter 102 and in the general approach to diagnostic methods for problems related to the sacroiliac and sacrum as noted earlier in this chapter.

Operative Approaches

Tumors of the lumbosacral iliac junction are generally approached by a combined posterior/anterior approach. If the posterior approach is through the spinal canal the anterior approach should be extraperitoneal. Depending on the size of the tumor, the patient is approached from the side, with the patient's affected side uppermost. The patient should be positioned on the table to allow for rotation in order to facilitate the surgical approach. The first step is usually the classic posterior approach of the spine. If the approach is centered over L5 it may be extended proximally or distally as far as necessary. A laminectomy is performed and the dura is exposed. The nerve roots in the intervertebral foramina must be exposed, including L4, L5, and the S1 roots. Following this, an anterolateral approach is created.

The approach extends from the lateral aspect of the rectus muscle halfway, usually between the umbilicus and anterior superior spine, and passes just above the iliac crest to join the posterior midline approach. This

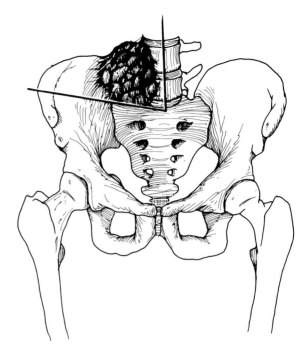

FIG. 15. Resection of the iliac crest allows visualization of the lumbosacral junction.

allows for a retroperitoneal approach and control of the iliac vessels and for an anterior approach to the spine and sacrum.

Through this approach, in order to gain better access to the sacrum, the superior aspect of the ilium may be removed or preferably osteotomized and turned back (Fig. 15).

The ascending lumbar veins and iliolumbar veins must be ligated in order to allow for mobilization of the common iliac vessels (Fig. 16). This is essential in order to allow for good access to the lumbosacral area and sacrum. Healthy tissue must be exposed on all sides of the tumor. Usually, the quadratus lumborum and the erector spinae muscles are divided. The psoas is detached from the transverse processes proximal to the tumor. At the time of laminectomy, the pedicle may be resected posteriorly, thus allowing ease of dissection of the spinal nerves from the intervertebral foramina to the posterolateral aspect of the psoas to the sacrum. The psoas is then separated from the tumor posterior to anterior, with care taken to isolate the lumbar plexus. If, however, the tumor is intimate to the psoas, then this may have to be sacrificed, including as many nerve roots as necessary. The tumor must be visualized at both its upper and lower borders. Distally it may be necessary to free the iliac fascia by excising the upper convex border of the iliac crest to expose the sacroiliac joint and the vessels in this area, including the lumbosacral plexus. An osteotomy, however, of one of the ilium may be preferable (Figs. 15, 16, 17A, and 17B). The tumor, once exposed and isolated, can then be resected en bloc. The

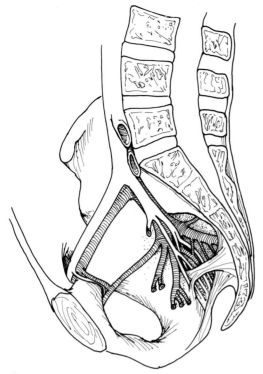

FIG. 16. Ligation of intra-pelvic branches of the internal iliac vessels.

definition of "en bloc" of course depends on the tumor being extradural. If the tumor involves the dura, then this should be excised as well. Conversely, it may be necessary to resect the cauda equina, depending on how far the tumor exists medially. Osteotomes are preferable in dividing healthy bone. Sagittal osteotomies are done. The osteotome is passed from posterior to anterior, protecting the anterior vessels by retractors. Similarly, the upper and lower transverse cuts are done posterior to anterior through healthy bone (Fig. 17). Graft removed from the iliac crest is reshaped to fit the bony defect created following resection, and internal fixation is used (Figs. 18A and 18B). Because of the potential instability in this area, post-operative immobilization in a hip spica is recommended.

If the tumor extends distally to the sacrum, the initial posterior laminectomy must extend to the healthy bone in the sacrum. The iliac crest is divided with an osteotome or saw to the greater sciatic notch in order to resect the superior portion of the iliac crest and remove the iliac side of the sacroiliac joint if the tumor is in this area.

Resection of the ala of the sacrum and the lower sacrum is technically difficult. A midline sagittal osteotomy with an osteotome is directed sagittally from posterior to anterior as well as from cranial to caudad and

A

B

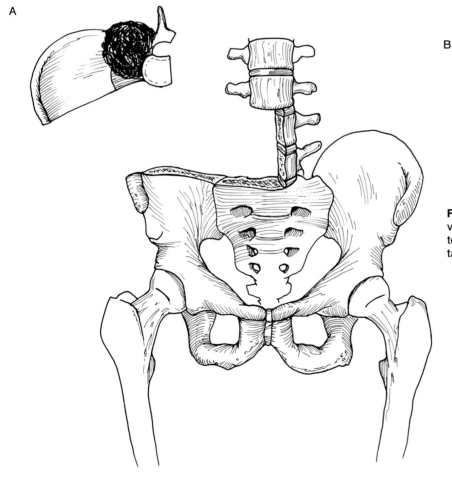

FIG. 17. A: Sagittal osteotomy of involved vertebral bodies from behind using an osteotome. **B:** Anterior-posterior view of sagittal bone section through healthy bone.

parallel to the spinal axis. Care must be taken not to pass the osteotome anterior to the anterior cortex, which should be protected with either retractors or sponges. The ala may be divided using either osteotomes or a saw.

The extent of resection is dependent on the extent of the tumor.

Excision of Sacral Tumors

En bloc resection of sacral tumors was first described by Stener in 1974 (18). Such resection of a tumor, particularly in the upper and middle portion of the sacrum, necessitates an anterior and posterior approach. The anterior approach provides control of neurovascular elements and anterior exposure of the tumor (Figs. 16, 17, 18, and 19). If the rectum must be included in the re-

sected specimen, such as with chordomas, the anterior approach allows for this by dividing the colon at the rectosigmoid junction, freeing the rectum as low as possible. The anus must be sealed. The rectum is removed en bloc with the sacrum through the posterior part of the procedure. The colostomy may be performed prior to turning the patient prone or after. The anterior approach is usually best performed retroperitoneally, although a bilateral approach may be more easily accomplished by a midline transperitoneal approach. In our experience, however, a supra pubic incision will allow for mobilization of either side without the necessity of going transperitoneal (Fig. 19). The lumbosacral trunk is mobilized or retracted. All venous structures from the external and internal iliac veins are ligated and the larger external and internal common iliac vessels retracted.

The anterior osteotomy is done at whatever level is necessary, including through L5 (Fig. 20). In cases of chordoma, it is recommended that the cauda equina at the sacral level be sacrificed; otherwise, the tumor will recur.

Careful pre-operative planning for resection is necessary based on an accurate assessment of magnetic resonance imaging and computerized axial tomography, including reconstruction and three-dimensional views. If a tumor extends into the sacroiliac joints, then these must be sacrificed en bloc. Osteotomy cuts must be done as far lateral as necessary in order to remove the tumor en bloc. After full mobilization of the vessels and, if necessary, the rectum, osteotomy cuts are done proximally in healthy tissue and laterally in healthy tissue. The cuts are made from anterior to posterior.

In our experience, the bone is then best packed with

A

B

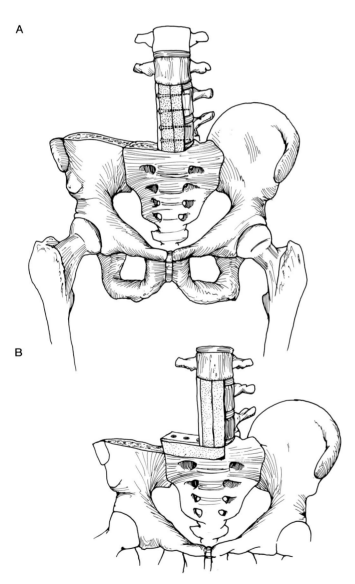

FIG. 18. Reconstruction using interbody grafts and sacroiliac grafts. **A:** Resection to S1. **B:** Resection to S2-S3.

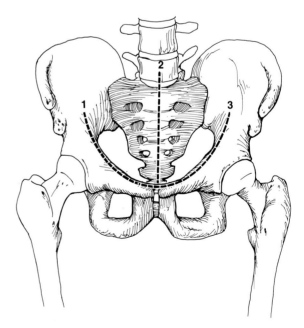

FIG. 19. Anterior approaches. *1:* Suprapubic and subperitoneal. *2:* Vertical. *3:* Transperitoneal or retroperitoneal.

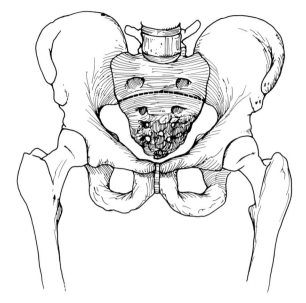

FIG. 20. Anterior horizontal bony section between sacral foraminae.

heavy sponges and the patient turned into the prone position. If there has been a previous biopsy, the posterior incision should include the biopsy scar. The approach posteriorly may be through a straight vertical midline incision or, if a wide lateral approach is made, the vertical limb may be made along the lower lumbar spine and a curvilinear excision made over both ilia. A laminectomy is performed proximal to the level of tumor. Roots are identified and marked. If the roots have been identified anteriorly, they may be more easily located posteriorly. The osteotomy is then carried out, fracturing the remaining cortex and going as far lateral as necessary to be external to the tumor (Fig. 21). The sacral coccygeal area is freed along its lower border and laterally around to its anterior surface. In the area of the sacroiliac joint,

care must be taken of the vascular structures, and the extra pelvic branches of the hypogastric vessels are ligated (Fig. 16).

Reconstruction depends on the extent of the tumor resection. In many chordomas detected early enough, it is possible to preserve the sacroiliac joints and stability is not lost. If, however, stability is lost, stabilization must be achieved with the use of bone grafts between the wings of the ilium together with internal fixation (Figs. 22, 23, and 24).

Gunterberg (10) analyzed pelvic strength after major amputation of the sacrum and found that the pelvic ring was weakened by approximately 30% with the resection of the sacrum between S1 and S2. This increased to 50% when the resection was one centimeter below the sacral promontory. He concluded that it was safe to allow patients with such resections to stand bearing their full weights post-operatively. A resection between S1 and S2 preserves the sacroiliac joints, except for the most inferior part. When resection is carried one centimeter below the sacral promontory, half the sacroiliac joint and ligaments remain on each side in the anterosuperior part. If the resection removes 50% or more of the sacroiliac joints, reconstruction of those joints should be performed (Fig. 25).

SACROILIAC INSTABILITY IN PREGNANCY

The backache of pregnancy and birth is thought to be caused mainly by ligamentous softening as a result of hormonal influence. The onset of this is usually at the sixth or seventh month. Symptoms may become extremely severe and necessitate bed rest. Pain exists over the symphysis pubis and sacroiliac joints. Stressing these joints may reproduce symptoms as reported by Bickel in 1957 (1).

Text continues on page 2178.

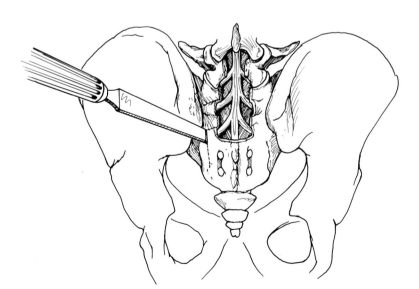

FIG. 21. Posterior osteotomy after laminectomy.

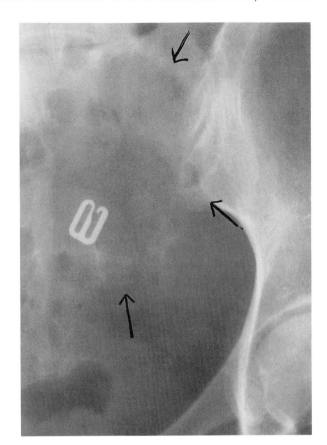

FIG. 22. A 36-year-old female presented with a six month history of low back pain and sciatica. X-rays revealed an eccentric lesion of the sacrum.

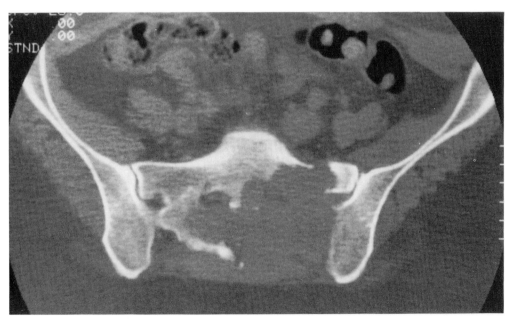

FIG. 23. Same patient as in Figure 22. CT scans revealed extensive destruction of the sacrum involving both sacroiliac joints.

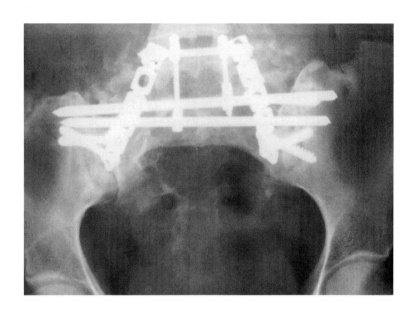

FIG. 24. Same patient. Reconstruction following biopsy, which revealed evidence of a plasmacytoma, consisted of tumor curettage. Pelvic instability was corrected using long sacral bars and pelvic reconstruction plates from the pelvis to L5 with bone graft. The patient was irradiated three months later. She is alive and well three years later.

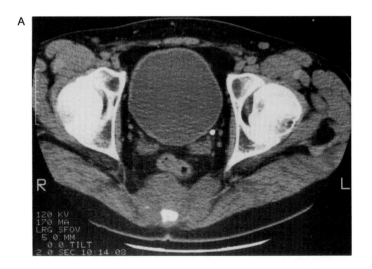

FIG. 25. A 32-year-old male presented with a two year history of low back pain and sciatica. He underwent an L5-S1 fusion and laminectomy. Pain persisted. CT scan after referral **(A)** revealed a large midline mass. (Figs. 25B–25C follow.)

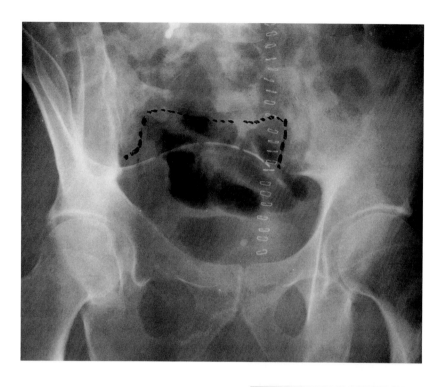

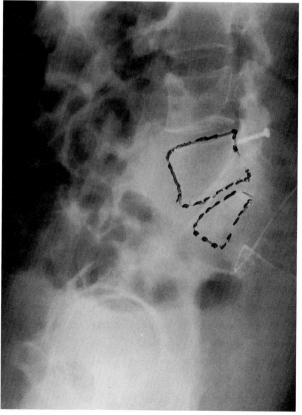

FIG. 25. *Continued.* **B and C:** Resection of the chordoma was through the proximal half of S1 preserving most of the sacroiliac joints. A combined anterior-posterior en bloc resection including colon was done.

Treatment is usually symptomatic, with rest and the use of pelvic support. This may be difficult due to the pregnancy. Residual problems following delivery are unusual.

Should late instability ensue and become troublesome, the approach is as noted in previous sections on iatrogenic instability.

REFERENCES

1. Bickel WH, Romness JO (1957): True diastasis of the sacroiliac joints with hyper mobility. *J Bone Joint Surg* [Am] 39:1381–1384.
2. Bobechko WP, Kostuik JP (1988): Exhibit International Radiological Society of North America, Chicago, November. Canadian Assoc. of Radiologists, Vancouver, June.
3. Coventry MB, Mitchell WC (1961): Osteitis pubis: observations based on a study of 45 patients. *J Am Med Assoc* 17E:898–905.
4. Coventry MB, Tapper EM (1972): Pelvic instability. *J Bone Joint Surg* [Am] 54:83–101.
5. Coy JT 3rd, Wolf CR, Brower TD, Winter WG Jr (1976): Pyogenic arthritis of the sacroiliac joint. Longterm follow-up. *J Bone Joint Surg* [Am] 58:845–849.
6. Dunn EJ, Bryan DM, Nugent JT, Robinson RA (1976): Pyogenic infections of the sacroiliac joint. *Clin Orthop Rel Res* (118):113–117.
7. Ebraheim NA, Rusin JJ, Coombs RJ, Jackson WT, Holiday B (1987): Percutaneous-computed-tomography—stabilization of pelvic fractures: Preliminary report. *J Orthop Trauma* 1:197–204.
8. Frymoyer JW, Howe J, Kuhlmann D (1978): The long-term effects of spinal fusion on the sacroiliac joints and ilium. *Clin Orthop Rel Res* (134):196–201.
9. Gertzbein SD, Chenoweth DR (1977): Occult injuries of the pelvic ring. *Clin Orthop Rel Res* (128):202–207.
10. Gunterberg B, Romanus B, Stener B (1976): Pelvic strength after major amputation of the sacrum. *Acta Orthop Scand* 47:635–642.
11. Hendrix RW, Lin PJ, Kane WJ (1982): Simplified aspiration or injection technique for the sacroiliac joint. *J Bone Joint Surg* [Am] 64:1249–1252.
12. Letournel E (1980): Acetabulum fractures: Classification and management. *Clin Orthop* (151):81–106.
13. Lichtblau S (1962): Dislocation of the sacroiliac joint: A complication of bone grafting. *J Bone Joint Surg* [Am] 44:192–198.
14. Miskew DB, Block RA, Witt PF (1979): Aspiration of infected sacroiliac joints. *J Bone Joint Surg* [Am] 61:1071–1072.
15. Pennal GF, Massiah KA (1980): Nonunion and delayed union of fractures of the pelvis. *Clin Orthop* (151):124–129.
16. Pennal GF, Tile M, Waddell JP, Garside H (1980): Pelvic disruption: Assessment and classification. *Clin Orthop* (151):12–21.
17. Shanahan MD, Ackroyd CE (1985): Pyogenic infection of the sacroiliac joint: A report of 11 cases. *J Bone Joint Surg* [Br] 67:605–608.
18. Stener B (1974): Reseccion de columna en el tralamiento de los tumores vertebrales. *Acta Ortolp Lat Am* 1:189–199.
19. Tile M (1984): *Fractures of the pelvis and acetabulum.* Baltimore: Williams & Wilkins.
20. Wild JJ, Hanson GW, Tullos HS (1982): Unstable fractures of the pelvis treated by external fixation. *J Bone Joint Surg* [Am] 64:1010–1020.

Subject Index

Subject Index

I3